FAMILY NURSE PRACTITIONER
CERTIFICATION REVIEW AND CLINICAL REFERENCE GUIDE

VIRGINIA LAYNG MILLONIG
EDITOR

MARY A. BARONI, SALLY K. MILLER
CONTRIBUTING EDITORS

HEALTH LEADERSHIP ASSOCIATES, INC.

Health Leadership Associates
First in Certification Review

Also offers these publications for your review needs:

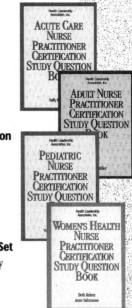

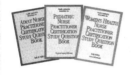
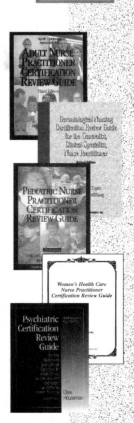

Family Nurse Practitioner Certification Review and Clinical Reference Guide

EDITOR

Virginia Layng Millonig, Ph.D, R.N., C.P.N.P.
President
Health Leadership Associates, Inc.
Potomac, Maryland

CONTRIBUTING EDITORS

Mary A. Baroni, Ph.D., R.N., C.P.N.P.
Director of Practice, Education and Research
Children's Hospital and Regional Medical Center
Seattle, Washington

Sally K. Miller, Ph.D., NP,C., G.N.P., A.N.P., A.C.N.P.
Assistant Professor
College of Nursing
Rutgers
The State University of New Jersey
Newark, New Jersey

Health Leadership Associates
Potomac, Maryland

Health Leadership Associates, Inc.
Managing Editor: Mary A. Riddlemoser
Production Manager: Martha M. Pounsberry
Editorial Assistants: Bridget M. Jones
                        Cheryl C. Patterson
Cover and Design: Merrifield Graphics
Composition: Port City Press, Inc.
Design and Production: Port City Press, Inc.

Printed in the United States of America

Health Leadership Associates, Inc.
P.O. Box 59153
Potomac, Maryland 20859

Library of Congress Cataloging-in-Publication Data

Family nurse practitioner certification review guide / editor,
Virginia Layng Millonig; contributing editors, Mary A. Baroni, Sally K. Miller.
    p.; cm.
    Includes bibliographical references.
    ISBN 1-878028-28-6 (pbk.)
    1. Family nursing—Examinations, questions, etc. 2. Nurse practitioners—Examinations,
questions, etc. I. Millonig, Virginia Layng. II. Baroni, Mary A. III. Miller, Sally K.
    [DNLM: 1. Family Nursing—Examination Questions. 2. Nurse
Practitioners—Examination Questions. WY 18.2 F1983 2001]
RT120.F34 F3532 2001
610.73'076—dc21

        2001026396

10 9 8 7 6 5 4 3

This new addition to Health Leadership Associates' certification review books is dedicated to my daughters Martha, Mary and Bridget and their families. Their contributions and commitment to the success, quality and integrity of Health Leadership Associates has been immeasurable.

Through their dedication and hard work Health Leadership Associates has become the first and foremost provider of certification review in the country and a major player in continuing education.

But most important is the joy and love they have brought to my life and the support they have provided through it all!

And finally to my mother and father, Camilla and Earle Layng who will never know how indebted I am to them for the inspiration, love and faith they instilled in me.

Virginia Layng Millonig

Contributing Authors

Beverly Ruth Bigler, Ed.D., R.N., C.P.N.P.
Professor of Nursing
Department of Nursing
Program Co-Director
Pediatric Nurse Practitioner Program
California State University, Los Angeles
Los Angeles, California
Nurse Practitioner\School Nurse
Alhambra School District
Alhambra, California

Mary A. Baroni, Ph.D., R.N., C.P.N.P.
Director of Practice, Education and Research
Children's Hospital and Regional Medical Center
Seattle, Washington

Leanne C. Busby, D.S.N., R.N.,C.S., F.A.A.N.P.
Chair
Division of Nursing
Cumberland University
Lebanon, Tennessee

Susan E. Chaney, EdD., R.N.,C.S., F.N.P.
Professor
College of Nursing
Family Nurse Practitioner Coordinator
Texas Woman's University
Dallas, Texas

Juanita Conkin Dale, Ph.D., R.N., C.P.N.P.
Pediatric Nurse Practitioner
Center for Cancer and Blood Disorders
Children's Medical Center of Dallas
Dallas, Texas

Jacalyn Peck Dougherty, Ph.D-C., M.A., M.S., R.N., C.P.N.P.
Graduate Student
Prevention Research Center for Family and Child Health
Department of Developmental Psychology
University of Denver
Denver, Colorado

Sandra L. Elvik, M.S., R.N., C.P.N.P.
Associate Professor of Pediatrics
UCLA School of Medicine
Assistant Medical Director
Child Crisis Center
Harbor-UCLA Medical Center
Torrance, California

Sylvia Torres Fletcher, M.S., R.N.,C.S., F.N.P.
Assistant Clinical Professor
College of Nursing
Texas Woman's University
Dallas, Texas

Nancy Dickenson Hazard, M.S.N., R.N., C.P.N.P., F.A.A.N.
Executive Officer
Sigma Theta Tau International
Indianapolis, Indiana

Susan M. Heighway, M.S., R.N.,C.S. P.N.P.
Clinical Professor
School of Nursing
Pediatric Nurse Practitioner
Waisman Center UAP
University of Wisconsin Madison
Madison, Wisconsin

Janet Johnston, M.S.N., R.N., C.P.N.P.
Assistant Professor
Pediatric Pulmonary Center
Department of Pediatrics
Children's Hospital
University of Alabama at Birmingham
Birmingham, Alabama

Nancy E. Kline, Ph.D., R.N., C.P.N.P.
Assistant Professor of Pediatrics
Baylor College of Medicine
Houston, Texas

Mary D. Knudtson, M.S.N., R.N.,C.S., F.N.P., P.N.P
Associate Clinical Professor
Family Medicine
University of California, Irvine
Irvine, California

Debbie G. Kramer, M.S., R.N.,C.S., C.R.N.P.
Clinical Risk Manager\Risk Management Department
Johns Hopkins Bayview Medical Center
Gerontological Nurse Practitioner
VA Maryland Health Care System and EpiHealth Associates
Baltimore, Maryland

Bernadette Mazurek Melnyk, PhD., R.N.,C.S., P.N.P.
Associate Professor of Nursing
Associate Dean for Research
Director, Center for Research and Evidence Based Practice
Director, Pediatric Nurse Practitioner Program
School of Nursing
University of Rochester
Rochester, New York
Pediatric Nurse Practitioner\Consultant
Children and Youth In-Patient Unit
Elmira Psychiatric Center
Elmira, New York

Sally K. Miller, Ph.D., NP,C., G.N.P., A.N.P., A.C.N.P.
Assistant Professor
College of Nursing
Rutgers
The State University of New Jersey
Newark, New Jersey

Susan B. Moskosky, M.S., R.N.C., W.H.N.P.
Woman's Health Nurse Practitioner
Office of Family Planning, Office of Population Affairs
U.S. Department of Health and Human Services
Washington, D.C.

Connie Paczkowski, M.S.N., R.N., C.S., P.N.P.
Pediatric Nurse Practitioner
Hunterdon Pediatric Associates
Flemington, New Jersey

Rosanne Harkey Pruitt, Ph.D., R.N.,C.S., F.N.P.
Professor
Graduate Coordinator
School of Nursing
Clemson University
Clemson, South Carolina

Sister Maria Salerno, O.S.F., D.N.Sc., R.N.,C.S., A.N.P.
Associate Professor
Director Adult and Gerontological Nurse Practitioner Programs
School of Nursing
The Catholic University of America
Nurse Practitioner
Community of Hope Health Services
Washington, D.C.

Alison W. Schultz, Ed.D., R.N., C.P.N.P.
Retired
Waynesboro, Virginia
Formerly
Associate Professor
School of Nursing
University of Rochester
Rochester, New York

Pamela S. Shuler, D.N.Sc., R.N.,C.S., F.N.P.
Family Nurse Practitioner
Consultant
Sylva, North Carolina

Madeline Turkeltaub, Ph.D., R.N.,C.S., A.N.P.
Adult Nurse Practitioner
Private Practice
Greenbelt, Maryland

Karen Uzark, Ph.D., R.N., C.P.N.P.
Director of Process Improvement
and Clinical Outcomes Research
Transplant Nurse Practitioner
Pediatric Cardiology
Children's Hospital Medical Center
Cincinnati, Ohio

Margaret Hadro Venzke, MS., R.N.,C.S., F.N.P.
Instructor
Family Nurse Practitioner Program
College of Nursing and Health Science
George Mason University
Fairfax, Virginia
Family Nurse Practitioner
Student Primary Care Clinic
Georgetown University
Washington, D.C.

Victoria A. Weill, M.S.N., R.N.,C.S., C.P.N.P.
Clinical Coordinator
Pediatric Primary Care Program
School of Nursing
University of Pennsylvania
Pediatric Nurse Practitioner
Emergency Department
Children's Hospital of Philadelphia
Philadelphia, Pennsylvania

Preface

Health Leadership Associates is pleased to introduce one more component to our complement of Nurse Practitioner Certification Review materials. This *Family Nurse Practitioner Certification Review and Clinical Reference Guide* has been developed especially for family nurse practitioners preparing to take certification examinations offered by the American Academy of Nurse Practitioners and the American Nurses Credentialing Center. The purpose of the book is twofold. It will assist individuals engaged in self-study preparation for certification examinations, and may be used as a reference guide in clinical practice. Additional test preparation materials and resources offered by Health Leadership Associates include question books with sample test questions, "live" certification review courses, and independent home study certification review programs.

The book has been organized to provide the reader with critical test-taking strategies and techniques which, when combined with an indepth knowledge base, are key factors in success on the certification examinations. The basis for an integrated knowledge base for the family nurse practitioner is introduced early in the book with comprehensive chapters on growth and development and health maintenance during infancy throughout adolescence. The foundation of nurse practitioner practice continues with discussion of health promotion and evaluation in the adult and elderly population. A special chapter is devoted to the unique aspects of caring for the elderly. A system's approach is used for covering pediatric and adult disorders. Each system includes a separate presentation of pediatric disorders in one section followed by a separate discussion within the same system applicable to the adult population., e.g., endocrine disorders\infancy through adolescence and endocrine disorders in adults. This format allows for a more comprehensive approach to the differences inherent in the presentation, diagnosis, manifestation and management of disorders in different age groups. Common disorders are presented with a succinct summary of definitions, etiology, signs and symptoms, physical findings, differential diagnoses, diagnostic tests\findings and management\treatment plans. Women's health issues are covered in depth both in the pediatric\adolescent populations as well as the adult and elderly including pregnancy, contraception and menopause. The book concludes with the final chapter on advanced practice, trends, issues and health policy.

Following each chapter are test questions, which are intended to serve as an introduction to the testing arena. In addition a bibliography is included for those who need a more indepth discussion of the subject matter in each chapter. These references can serve as additional instructional material for the reader.

Many nurses preparing for certification examinations find that reviewing an extensive body of scientific knowledge requires a very difficult search of many sources that must be synthesized to provide a review base for the examination. This publication provides a succinct, yet comprehensive review of the core material.

The editors and contributing authors are certified nurse practitioners. The have designed this book to assist potential examinees to prepare for success in the certification examination process.

It is assumed that the reader of this certification review and clinical reference guide has completed a course of study in a family nurse practitioner program. It is not intended to be a basic text book.

Certification is a process that has gained recognition both within and outside the profession. For the professional it is a means of gaining special recognition as a certified nurse practitioner which not only demonstrates a level of competency, but may also enhance professional opportunities and advancement. For the consumer, it means that a certified nurse has met certain predetermined standards set by the profession.

CONTENTS

Family Nurse Practitioner

7. **Head, Eye, Ear, Nose, Mouth and Throat Disorders**   *Connie Paczkowski*
Infancy Through Adolescence

8. **Eye, Ear, Nose, and Throat Disorders**   *Margaret Hadro Venzke*
     In Adults

9. **Lower Respiratory Disorders**   *Janet Johnston*
     Infancy through Adolescence

14. Hematological And Oncological Disorders
In Adults

Sister Maria Salerno

15. Gastrointestinal Disorders
Infancy through Adolescence

Victoria A. Weil

16. Gastrointestinal Disorders
In Adults

Sister Maria Salerno

17. **Infectious Diseases**   *Nancy E. Kline*
       Infancy Through Adolescence

18. **Endocrine Disorders**   *Jacalyn Peck Dougherty*
       Infancy Through Adolescence

22. Neurological Disorders
Infancy Through Adolescence

Susan Heighway

23. Neurological Disorders
In Adults

Sally K. Miller

24. Psychosocial Disorders
In Adults

Sister Maria Salerno

25. Dermatologic Conditions
Infancy Through Adolescence

Beverly Bigler

26. Dermatological Disorders In Adults

Sylvia Fletcher
Susan Chaney

27. **Genitourinary And Gynecologic Disorders Adolescent Pregnancy** *Sandra Elvik*
      Infancy Through Adolescence *Mary A. Baroni*

28. **Genitourinary And Gynecologic Disorders** *Pamela A. Shuler*
      In Adults *Mary D. Knudtson*

Test Taking Strategies and Techniques

Nancy A. Dickenson Hazard
Virginia L. Millonig

We all respond to testing situations in different ways. What separates the successful test taker from the unsuccessful one is knowing how to prepare for and take a test. Preparing yourself to be a successful test taker is as important as studying for the test. Each person needs to assess and develop individual test taking strategies and skills. The primary goal of this chapter is to assist potential examinees in knowing how to study for and take a test. Of equal importance to this study preparation is a basic understanding of how certification examinations are developed. They are based upon a universal knowledge foundation. Test items are selected from generally recognized resources available to the examinee, and specific to the type of specialty area.

The purpose of the Family Nurse Practitioner certification examination is to measure one's knowledge of content appropriate to the practice expected of a family nurse practitioner. Examination content areas are those defined as essential to the practice of a family nurse practitioner. Multiple sources are used to prepare these examinations, e.g., national task forces and examination committees composed of expert certified family nurse practitioners who are recognized for their knowledge, expertise and skill in nurse practitioner practice. In addition expert certified nurse practitioners skilled in the area of test question construction are selected as item writers.

Examination committees develop items, coordinate and select appropriate examination content and questions and evaluate the overall certification mechanisms. Certification examinations are either paper and pencil or computer-based. The paper\pencil examinations currently offered are scheduled at prescribed dates throughout the year. The computer-based examination offered by the American Nurse Credentialing Center is offered year round at multiple testing centers throughout the country. Once eligibility has been confirmed, scheduling test site, date and time is at your convenience. Once you have applied to take a certification examination, instructions will be sent to you with information regarding the examination process, sample test questions, where to take the examination and study materials.

Computer knowledge is not required for you to take a computer-based examination. Usually a customized introductory lesson is provided that explains the procedure used to select an answer and movement from question to question. If you are not familiar with using a computer it may be best for you to practice several weeks prior to the examination to acquaint yourself with the keyboard, use of a mouse and the normal mechanics of using a computer.

STRATEGY #1 Know Yourself

When faced with an examination, do you feel threatened, experience butterflies or sweaty palms, have trouble keeping your mind focused on studying or on test questions? These common symptoms of test anxiety plague many of us, but can be used advantageously if understood and handled correctly. Over the years of test taking, each of us has developed certain testing behaviors, some of which are beneficial, while others present obstacles to successful test taking. You can take control of the test taking situation by identifying the undesirable behaviors, maintaining the desirable ones and developing skills to improve test performance.

Technique #1: From the following descriptions of test taking personalities, find yourself (Table 1). Write down those characteristics which describe you even if they are from different personality types. Carefully review the problem list associated with your test taking personality characteristics. Write down the problems which are most troublesome. Then make a list of how you can remedy these problems from the improvement strategies list. Be sure to use these strategies as you prepare for and take examinations.

STRATEGY #2 Develop Your Thinking Skills

Understanding Thought Process: In order to improve your thinking skills and subsequent test performance, it is best to understand the types of thinking as well as the techniques to enhance the thought process.

Everyone has a personal learning style, but we all must proceed through the same process to think.

Thinking occurs on six levels—the lower level of memory and comprehension and the higher levels of application, analysis, synthesis and evaluation (Sides & Korchek, 1994). Memory is the ability to recall facts. Without adequate retrieval of facts, progression through the higher levels of thinking cannot occur easily. Comprehension is the ability to understand memorized facts. To be effective, comprehension skills must allow the person to translate recalled information from one context to another. Application, or the process of using information to know why something occurs, is a higher form of learning. Effective application relies on the use of understood, memorized facts to verify intended action. Analysis is the ability to use abstract or logical forms of thought to show relationships and to distinguish the cause and effect between the variables in a situation.

As related to testing situations, the thought process from memory to analysis occurs quite quickly. Some examination items are designed to test memory and comprehension while others test application and analysis. Examples of memory questions are as follows:

Type 1 diabetes results from dysfunction of the:

a) Liver
b) *Pancreas*
c) Adrenal glands
d) Pituitary gland

A normal child is expected to walk by:

a) 6 months
b) 10 months
c) *14 months*
d) 18 months

To answer these questions correctly, the individual has to retrieve a memorized fact. Understanding

Table 1

Test Taker Profile

Type	Characteristics	Pitfalls	Improvement Strategies
The Rusher	• Rushes to complete the test before the studied facts are forgotten	• Unable to read question and situation completely	• Practice progressive relaxation techniques
	• Arrives at test site early and waits anxiously	• At high risk for misreading, misinterpreting and mistakes	• Develop a study plan with sufficient time to review important content
	• Mumbles studied facts	• Difficult items heighten anxiety	• Avoid cramming and last minute studying
	• Tense body posture	• Likely to make quick, not well-thought-out guesses	• Take practice tests focusing on slowing down and reading and answering each option carefully
	• Accelerated pulse, respiration and neuromuscular excitement		• Read instructions and questions slowly
	• Answers questions rapidly and is generally one of the first to complete		
	• Experiences exhaustion once test is over		
The Turtle	• Moves slowly, methodically, deliberately through each question	• Last to finish; often does not complete the exam	• Take practice tests focusing on time spent per item
	• Repeated rereading, underlining and checking	• Has to quickly complete questions in last part of exam, increasing errors	• Place watch in convenient place to keep track of time
	• Takes 60 to 90 seconds per question versus an average of 45 to 60 seconds	• Has difficulty completing timed examinations	• Mark answer sheet in paper/pencil examination indicating where one should be halfway through exam based on total number of questions and total amount of time for exam
			• Study concepts not details
			• Attempt to answer each question as you progress through the exam
The Personalizer	• Mature person who has personal knowledge and insight from life experiences	• Risk in relying on what has been learned through observation and experience since one may develop false understandings and stereotypes	• Focus on principles and standards that support nursing practice
		• Personal beliefs and experiences are frequently not the norm or standard tested	• Avoid making connections between patients in exam clinical situations and personal clinical experience
		• Has difficulty identifying expected standards measured by standardized examination	• Focus on generalities not experiences
The Squisher	• View exams as threat, rather than an expected event in education	• Procrastinates studying for exams	• Establish a plan of progressive, disciplined study
	• Preoccupied with grades and personal accomplishment	• Unable to study effectively since waits until last minute	• Use defined time frames for studying content and taking practice exams
	• Attempts to avoid responsibility and accountability associated with testing in order to reduce anxiety	• Increased anxiety over test since procrastinating study impairs ability to learn and perform	• Use relaxation techniques • Return to difficult items • Read carefully

(Table continued on next page)

Type	Characteristics	Pitfalls	Improvement Strategies
The Philosopher	• Academically successful person who is well disciplined and structured in study habits • Displays great intensity and concentration during exam • Searches questions for hidden or unintended meaning • Experiences anxiety over not knowing everything	• Over analysis causes loss of sight of actual intent of question • Reads information into questions answering with own added information rather than answering the actual intent of question	• Focus on questions as they are written • Work on self confidence and not on question. Initial response is usually correct • Avoid multiple rereadings of questions • Avoid adding own information and unintended meanings • Practice, practice, practice with sample tests
The Second Guesser	• Answers questions twice, first as an examinee, second as an examiner • Believes second look will allow one to find and correct errors • Frequently changes initial responses (i.e., grades own test)	• Altering an initial response frequently results in an incorrect answer • Frequently changes answers because the pattern of response appears incorrect (i.e., too many "true" or too many correct responses)	• Reread only the few items of which one is unsure. Avoid changing initial responses • Take exam carefully and progressively first time, allowing little or no time for rereading • Study facts • Avoid reading into questions
The Lawyer	• Attempts to place words or ideas into the question (leads the witness) • Occurs most frequently with psychosocial or communication questions which ask for the most appropriate response	• Veers from the obvious answer and provides response from own point of view • Reads a question, jumps to a conclusion then finds a response that leads to predetermined conclusion	• Focus on distinguishing what is said in question and not on what is read into question • Avoid formulating responses aimed at obtaining certain information • Choose responses that allow expression of feelings which encourage hope, not catastrophe, those which are intended to clarify, which identify feeling tones or which avoid negating or confronting feelings • Carefully read entire question before selecting a response

From: "Making the grades as a test-taker," by N. Dickenson-Hazard, (1989) *Pediatric Nursing, 15,* p. 303. Adapted from: *Nurse's guide to successful test-taking* by M. B. Sides and N. B. Cailles, 1989. Philadelphia: J. B. Lippincott, Co., pp 59–70, 199–203. Copyright 1989 by A. J. Jannetti, Inc. Reprinted by permission.

the fact, knowing why it is important or analyzing what should be done in this situation is not needed. Examples of questions which test comprehension are as follows:

You are taking a history on a 47 year-old white female during a routine health assessment visit. She reports that in the past month she has experienced increased thirst and needs to urinate frequently. She reports recurrent episodes of vaginitis and is concerned about an abrasion on her leg which will not heal. You note that her blood pressure is recorded at 150/90 and that she is overweight. You would most likely suspect which of the following?

a)　Hyperthyroidism
b)　Type 1 diabetes mellitus

c) Essential hypertension
d) *Type 2 diabetes mellitus*

To answer this question correctly, an individual must retrieve facts about the physiology of diabetes mellitus in order to understand and differentiate the presenting symptoms.

The mother of an otherwise healthy 11-month-old boy voices concern that her son is not yet walking but her daughter walked at this age. You should know that:

a) Girls generally walk before boys
b) *Her son should be walking by 14 months of age*
c) The mother is demonstrating overanxious behavior
d) Her son is delayed developmentally

To answer this question correctly, an individual must receive the fact that walking well is not always achieved until 14 months of age, and understand that in this situation, a child of 11 months would not necessarily be expected to have achieved this developmental milestone.

In answering an examination question that requires a higher level of thought, an individual must be able to recall a fact, understand that fact in the context of the question, and apply this understanding to determine why one answer is correct, after analyzing possible answer choices as they relate to the situation (Sides & Korchek, 1994). Examples of application analysis questions are as follows:

A 48 year-old diabetic woman wants to enroll in a low-impact aerobics class. Her diabetes is well managed with twice daily insulin injections. Your best advice is to:

a) Increase daily doses of insulin
b) *Have an extra snack before exercise class*
c) Administer a dose of regular insulin after exercise is completed
d) Tell her participating in the class is not advisable

To answer this question correctly, the individual must recall physiologic facts of insulin dependent diabetes, understand what is happening in this situation, consider each option and how it applies to the patient's condition and analyze why each advice option works or doesn't work for this patient.

After administrating the Denver Developmental Screening Test (Denver II), you note that an 18-month-old boy is not walking. The child's mother is voicing concern about this. Your most appropriate action is to:

a) Repeat the Denver II in 6 months
b) *Consult with pediatrician*
c) Reassure the mother that the child's not walking is normal at this age
d) Recommend exercises to strenghthen the lower extremities

To answer this question correctly, the individual must recall the fact at which age walking should be achieved; understand if it is normal or abnormal for an 18-month-old child not to walk as depicted in this situation; apply this knowledge to each option, understanding why it may or may not be correct; and analyze each option for what action is most appropriate for this situation.

Application/analysis questions require the examinee to use logical rationale, based on a well defined principle or fact. Problem solving ability becomes important as the examinee must think through each question option, determining its relevance and importance to the situation in the question.

Building your thinking skills: Effective memorization is the cornerstone to learning and building thinking skills (Olney, 1989). We have all experienced "memory power outages" at some time, due in part to trying to memorize too much, too fast, too ineffectively. Developing skills to improve memorization is important to increasing the effectiveness of your thinking and subsequent test performance.

Technique #1:   Quantity is NOT quality, so concentrate on learning important content. For example, it is important to know the various pharmacologic agents appropriate for the management of chronic obstructive pulmanary disease (COPD), not the specific dosages for each medication.

Technique #2:   Memory from repetition, or saying something over and over again to remember it, usually fades. Developing memory skills which trigger retrieval of needed facts is more useful. Such skills are as follows:

Acronyms: These are mental crutches which facilitate recall. Some are already established such as PERRLA (pupils equal, round, react to light, and accommodation), C.H.F. for (congestive heart failure), or T.I.A. for (transient ischemic attack). Developing your own acronyms can be particularly useful since they are your own word association arrangements in a singular word. Nonsense words or funny, unusual ones are often more useful since they attract your attention.

Acrostics: This mental tool arranges words into catchy phrases. The first letter of each word stands for something which is recalled as the phrase is said. Your own acrostics are most valuable in triggering recall of learned information since they are your individual situation associations. An example of an acrostic is as follows:

Sam **E**xercises **B**y **W**eight-lifting and **R**unning stands for the aspects of non-drug therapy/management for hypertension: **S**alt restriction, **E**xercise, **B**iofeedback, **W**eight reduction, and **R**elaxation techniques.

Mom **C**arried **N**ell **E**very **P**lace **S**he **W**ent stands for the areas of assessment for a cast check: movement, color, numbness, edema, pulse, sensation and warmth.

ABCs: This technique facilitates information retrieval by using the alphabet as a crutch. Each letter stands for a symptom, which when put together creates a picture of the clinical presentation of the disease. For example, the characteristics of peptic ulcer disease using the ABC technique is as follows:

   a) Antacids relieve pain
   b) Burning epigastric pain
   c) Cycle of pain two hours after eating
   d) Discomfort awakens at night

e) Experiences weight loss

f) Food sometimes aggravates pain

Imaging: This technique can be used in two ways. The first is to develop a nickname for a clinical problem which when said produces a mental picture. For example, "thin, barrel-chested, pink puffer" might be used to visualize a patient with emphysema who has a muscle-wasted body appearance, absent central cyanosis, hypertrophy of respiratory accessory muscles and an AP chest diameter greater than the transverse chest. A second form of imaging is to visualize a specific patient while you are trying to understand or solve a clinical problem when studying or answering a question. For example, imagine a young woman who is experiencing an acute asthma attack. You are trying to analyze the situation and place her in a position which maximizes respiratory effort. In your mind you visualize her in various positions of sidelying, angular and forward, imaging what will happen to the woman and her respiratory effort in each position.

Rhymes, music & links: The absurd is easier to remember than the most common. Rhymes, music or links can add absurdity and humor to learning and remembering (Olney, 1989). These retrieval tools are developed by the individual for specific content. For example, making up a rhyme about diabetes may be helpful in remembering the predominant female incidence, origin of disease, primary symptoms and management as illustrated by:

There once was a girl
  whose beta cells failed
She grew quite thirsty
  and her glucose levels sailed
Her lack of insulin caused her to
  increase her intake
And her increased urinary output
  was certainly not fake
So she learned to watch her diet
  and administer injections
That kept her healthy, growing
  and free of complications.

Setting content to music is sometimes useful to remembering. Melodies which are repetitious jog the memory by the ups and downs of the notes and the rhythm of the music.

Links connect key words from the content by using them in a story. An example given by Olney (1989) for remembering the parts of an eye is IRIS watched a PUPIL through the LENS of a RED TIN telescope while eating CORN-EA on the cob.

Additional memory aids may also include the use of color or drawing for improving recall. Use different colored pens or paper to accentuate the material being learned. For example, highlight or make notes in blue for content about respiratory problems and in red for cardiovascular content. Drawing assists with visualizing content as well. This is particularly helpful for remembering the pathophysiology of the specific health problem.

The important thing to remember about remembering is to use good recall techniques.

Technique #3: Improving higher level thinking skills involves exercising the application and analysis of memorized facts. Small group review is particularly useful for enhancing these high level skills. Small group interaction allows verbalization of thought processes and receipt of input about content and thought process from others (Sides & Korchek, 1994). Individuals not only hear how they think, but how others think as well. This interaction allows individuals to identify flaws in their thought process as well as to strengthen their positive points.

Taking practice tests are also helpful in developing application/analysis thinking skills. Practice tests permit the individual to analyze thinking patterns as well as the cause and effect relationships between the question and its options. The problem solving skills needed to answer application/ analysis questions are tested, giving the individual more experience through practice (Dickenson-Hazard, 1990).

Health leadership Associates publishes study question books which enable individuals to conduct this process. Furthermore their certification review books contribute additional questions as well as specific related content which reinforces the practice-test process.

Practice tests alone are not the best way to prepare for certification examinations. A sound knowledge base and expertise in test-taking skills is the foundation for successful performance on the certification examinations and application of this knowledge in the practice setting.

STRATEGY #3 Know The Content

Your ability to study is directly influenced by organization and concentration (Dickenson-Hazard, 1990). If effort is spent on both of these aspects of exam preparation, examination success can be increased.

Preparation for studying: Getting organized. Study habits are developed early in our education experiences. Some of our habits enhance learning while others do not. To increase study effectiveness, organization of study materials and time is essential. Organization decreases frustration, allows for easy resumption of study and increases concentrated study time.

Technique #1: Create your own study space. Select a study area that is yours alone, free from distractions, comfortable and well lighted. The ventilation and room temperature should be comfortable since a cold room makes it difficult to concentrate and a warm room may make you sleepy (Burkle & Marshak, 1989). All study materials should be left in a specific study space. The basic premise of a study space is that it facilitates a mind set that you are there to study. When study is interrupted, it is best to leave study materials just as they are. Don't close books or put away notes as they will have to be relocated, wasting valuable time, when study is resumed.

Technique #2: Define and organize the content. Secure an outline or the content parameters which are to be examined from the examining body. If outline is sketchy, develop a more detailed one for yourself using the recommended texts as a guideline. Next, identify available study resources: class notes, old exams, handouts, textbooks, review courses and books, home study programs, or study groups. For national standardized exams, such as initial licensing or certification, it is best to identify a few resources which cover the content being tested and stick to them. Attempting to review all available resources is not only mind boggling, but increases anxiety and frustration as well. Make your selections and stay with them.

Again, Health Leadership Associates, pioneer in certification review, offers many of these resources, which have resulted in successful performance on national certification examinations.

Technique #3:   Conduct a content assessment. Using a simple rating scale of:

    1 = requires no review
    2 = requires minimal review
    3 = requires intensive review
    4 = start from the beginning

Read through the content outline and rate each content area (Dickenson-Hazard, 1990). Table 2 provides a sample exam content assessment. Be honest with your assessment. It is far better to recognize your content weaknesses when you can study and remedy them, rather than wishing during the exam that you had studied more. Likewise with content strengths: If you know the material, don't waste time studying it.

Technique #4:   Develop a study plan. Coordinate the content which needs to be studied with the time available (Sides & Korchek, 1994). Prioritize your study needs, starting with weak areas first. Allow for a general review at the end of the study plan. Finally, establish an overall goal for yourself; something that will motivate you when brought to mind.

Table 3 illustrates a study plan developed on the basis of the exam content assessment in Table 2. Conducting an assessment and developing a study plan should require no more than 50 minutes. It is a wise investment of time with potential payoffs of reduced study stress and exam success.

Technique #5:   Begin now and use your time wisely. The smart test taker begins the study process early (Olney, 1989). Sit down, conduct the content assessment and develop a study plan as soon as you know about the exam. DON'T PROCRASTINATE!

Getting Down To Business—The Actual Studying: There is no better way to prepare for an examination than individual study (Dickenson-Hazard, 1989). The responsibility to achieve the goal you set for this exam lies with you alone. The means you employ to achieve this goal do vary and should begin with identifying your peak study times and using techniques to maximize them.

Technique #1:   Study in short bursts. Each of us have our own biologic clock which dictates when we are at our peak during the day. If you are a morning person, you are generally active and alert early in the day, slowing down and becoming drowsy by evening. If you are an evening person, you don't completely wake up until late morning and hit your peak in the afternoon and evening. Each person generally has several peaks during the day. It is best to study during those times when your alertness is at its peak (Dickenson-Hazard, 1990).

Table 2

Sample Content Assessment

Exam Content: Gastrointestinal Health Problems of the Adult	
Category: Provided by Examining Body	*Rating: Provided by Examinee*

I. Peptic Ulcer Disease
    A. Etiology 4
    B. Pathophysiology 3
    C. Symptomatology 3
    D. Differential Diagnosis 4
    E. Diagnostic Tests 3
    F. Management/Treatment 4

II. Esophagitis
    A. Etiology 3
    B. Pathophysiology 3
    C. Symptomatology 2
    D. Differential Diagnosis 3
    E. Diagnostic Tests 2
    F. Management/Treatment 4

III. Cholecystitis
    A. Etiology 2
    B. Pathophysiology 2
    C. Symptomatology 1
    D. Differential Diagnosis 2
    E. Diagnostic Tests 4
    F. Management/Treatment 4

IV. Appendicitis
    A. Etiology 3
    B. Pathophysiology 4
    C. Symptomatology 3
    D. Differential Diagnosis 2
    E. Diagnostic Tests 3
    F. Management/Treatment 4

V. Diverticulitis
    A. Etiology 3
    B. Pathophysiology 4
    C. Symptomatology 3
    D. Differential Diagnosis 3
    E. Diagnostic Tests 2
    F. Management/Treatment 4

VI. Hepatitis
    A. Etiology 3
    B. Pathophysiology 4
    C. Symptomatology 4
    D. Differential Diagnosis 4
    E. Diagnostic Tests 2
    F. Management/Treatment 4

VII. Acute Gastroenteritis
    A. Etiology 2
    B. Pathophysiology 3
    C. Symptomatology 2
    D. Differential Diagnosis 3
    E. Diagnostic Tests 4
    F. Management/Treatment 3

VIII. Irritable Bowel Syndrome
    A. Etiology 3
    B. Pathophysiology 3
    C. Symptomatology 3
    D. Differential Diagnosis 4
    E. Diagnostic Tests 4
    F. Management/Treatment 3

Table 3

Sample Study Plan

Goal: Master Content on the Gastrointestinal Problems of the Adult Patient. Test Time Available: 2 Weeks

Objective	Activity	Date Accomplished
Master content on diverticulitis	Read Chapter 26. Take notes on chapter content according to outline	Feb. 5 & 6, 1 hour
	Review class notes combined with chapter notes	Feb. 6, 1 hour
	Review sample test questions	Feb. 6, 1 hour
Understand content on peptic ulcer disease	Read Chapter 25. Take notes on chapter content according to content outline	Feb. 7, 2 hours
	Review class notes combined with chapter notes.	Feb. 8, $1\frac{1}{2}$ hours
Master content on cholecystitis	Read Chapter 24. Take notes on chapter content according to content outline	Feb. 10, 2 hours
	Review class notes combined with chapter notes	Feb. 11, $\frac{1}{2}$ hours
	Review sample test questions	Feb. 12, $1\frac{1}{2}$ hours
Know material on irritable bowel syndrome	Scan Chapter 27. Review class notes supplementing with text notes	Feb. 14, 2 hours
Know material on esophagitis	Scan Chapter 23. Review class notes supplementing with text notes	Feb. 15, 2 hours
Know material on hepatitis	Scan Chapter 28. Review highlights and important concepts	Feb. 16, 2 hours
Know material on appendicitis and acute gastroenteritis	Scan Chapter 29. Review highlights and important concepts	Feb. 17, 2 hours
Demonstrate understanding of all material	Review with another person	Feb. 18, 2 hours
	Review all notes	Feb. 19, $1\frac{1}{2}$ hours
	Take sample test questions	Feb. 19, $1\frac{1}{2}$ hours
Think positively	SMILE	ON GOING
	Take frequent breaks	
	Reward myself after each study session	
	Keep my goal in mind	

During our concentration peaks, there are mini peaks, or bursts of alertness (Olney, 1989). These alertness (''mini'') peaks occur during a concentration peak because levels of concentration are at their highest during the first part and last part of a study period. These bursts can vary from ten minutes to one hour depending on the extent of concentration. If studying is sustained for one hour there are only two mini peaks; one at the beginning and one at the end. There are eight mini peaks if that same hour is divided into four, 10-minute intervals. Hence it is more helpful to study in short bursts (Olney, 1989). More can be learned in less time.

Technique #2:   Cramming can be useful. Since concentration ability is highly variable, some individuals can sustain their mini peaks for 15, 20 or even 30 minutes at a time. Pushing your concentration beyond its peak is fruitless and verges on cramming, which in general is a poor study technique. There are, however, times when cramming, a short term memory tool, is useful. Short term memory generally is at its best in the morning. A quick review or cram of content in the morning can be useful the day of the exam (Olney, 1989). Most studying, however, is best accomplished in the afternoon or evening when long term memory functions at its peak.

Technique #3: Give your brain breaks. Regular times during study to rest and absorb the content is needed by the brain. The best approach to breaks is to plan them and give yourself a conscious break (Dickenson-Hazard, 1990). This approach eliminates the ''day dreaming'' or ''wandering thought'' approach to breaks that many of us use. It is better to get up, leave the study area and do something non-study related for longer breaks. For shorter breaks of five minutes or so, leave your desk, gaze out the window or do some stretching exercises. When your brain says to give it a rest, accommodate it! You'll learn more in less stress free time.

Technique #4: Study the correct content. It is easy for all of us to become bogged down in the detail of the content we are studying. However, it is best to focus on the major concepts or the ''state of the art'' content. Leave the details, the suppositions and the experience at the door of your study area. Concentrate on the major textbook facts and concepts which revolve around the subject matter being tested.

Technique #5: Fit your studying to the test type. The best way to prepare for an objective test is to study facts, particularly anything printed in italics. Memory enhancing techniques are particularly useful when preparing for an objective test. If preparing for an essay test, study generalities, examples and concepts. Application techniques are helpful when studying for this type of an exam (Burkle & Marshak, 1989).

Technique #6: Use your study plan wisely. Your study plan is meant to be a guide, not a rigid schedule. You should take your time with studying. Don't rush through the content just to remain on schedule. Occasionally study plans need revision. If you take more or less time than planned, readjust the plan for the time gained or lost. The plan can guide you, but you must go at your own pace.

Technique #7: Actively study. Being an active participant in study rather than trying to absorb the printed word is also helpful. Ways to be active include taking notes on the content as you study; constructing questions and answering them; taking practice tests and discussing the content with yourself. Also, using your individual study quirks is encouraged. Some people stand, others walk around and some play background music. Whatever helps you to concentrate and study better, you should use.

Technique #8: Use study aids. While there is no substitute for individual studying, several resources, if available, are useful in facilitating learning. Review courses, such as those offered by Health Leadership Associates, are an excellent means for organizing or summarizing your individual study. They generally provide the content parameters and the major concepts of the content which you need to know. Review courses also provide an opportunity to clarify not-well-understood content, as well as to review known material (Dickenson-Hazard, 1990). Study guides/certification review books and home study programs are useful for organizing study. They provide detail on the content which is important to the exam. Study groups are an excellent resource for summarizing and refining content. They provide an opportunity for thinking through your knowledge base, with the advantage of hearing another person's point of view. Each of these study aids increases understanding of content and when used correctly, increases effectiveness of knowledge application.

Technique #9: Know when to quit. It is best to stop studying when your concentration ebbs. It is unproductive and frustrating to force yourself to study. It is far better to rest or unwind, then resume at a later point in the day. Avoid studying outside your A.M. or P.M. concentration peaks and focus your study energy on your right time of day or evening.

STRATEGY #4 Become Test-wise

Most nursing examinations are composed of multiple choice questions (MCQ). This type of question requires the examinee to select the best response(s) for a specific circumstance or condition. Successful test taking is dependent not only on content knowledge but on test taking skill as well. If you are unable to impart your knowledge through the vehicle used for its conveyance, i.e., the MCQ, your test taking success is in jeopardy.

Computer based examinations are a new method of testing for some certification examinations. Eventually all of the certification paper and pencil examinations will be replaced with the computer method. Computer based testing has several advantages such as flexibility in taking the examinations at your convenience and earlier notification of test results. If the certification examination you are planning to take is computerized, the instructions will be provided both prior to the examination as well as at the time of the examination. No computer experience is required, and tutorials or introductory lessons precede the computer-based testing to familiarize you with the process.

It is important to understand that outstanding computer proficiency alone will not lead to success on the certification examination if your knowledge base is deficient or weak. Thus computer-based practice tests exclusively, will not prepare you for the certification examinations.

Moreover, the strategies used to develop effective test-taking skills are applicable to both the traditional paper/pencil and computerized forms of the certification examinations (Sides & Korchek, 1994).

Technique #1: Recognize the purpose of a test question. Most test questions are developed to examine knowledge at two separate levels: memory and comprehension or application and analysis. A memory question requires the examinee to recall facts from their knowledge base while an application question requires the examinee to use and apply the knowledge. Memory questions test recall while application questions test synthesis and problem-solving skills. When taking a test, you need to be aware when you are being asked to recall a fact, and when you are being asked to use that fact.

Technique #2: Recognize the components of a test question. Multiple choice questions may include the basic components of a background statement, a stem and a list of options. The background statement presents information which facilitates the examinee in answering the question. The stem asks or states the intent of the question. The options are 3 to 5 possible responses to the question. The correct option is called the keyed response and all other options are called distractors (ABP, 1989). Knowing the components of a test question helps you sift through the information presented and focus on the question's intent (see Table 4).

Technique #3: Identify the key word(s) in a test question. Don't jump to conclusions when you read the stem. Key words are generally included in the stem of a test question, whereas key concepts or conditions appear in the background statement. You should pay particular attention to the key words in the stem and their impact on the intent of the question (See Table 5). Never "read" into a question or make assumptions beyond the information given.

Technique #4:   Recognize the item types. Basically two styles of MCQs are used for examinations. One requires the examinee to select the one best answer; the other requires selection of multiple correct answers. Among the one best answer styles there are three types. The A type requires the selection of the best response among those offered. The B type requires the examinee to match the options with the appropriate statement. C type items require the examinee to compare or contrast two related conditions. The X type asks the examinee to respond either true or false to each option (ABP, 1989). Table 6 illustrates these item types. Many standardized tests such as those used for certification are composed of three to five option-A type questions.

Table 4

Anatomy Of A Test Question

Background Statement:	A 32 year-old African-American female is being seen for a complaint of sores in the vaginal area. She has been experiencing a low-grade fever, headache and malaise over the past five days. Physical examination reveals inguinal lymphadenopathy, vaginal erythema and multiple labial and vaginal vesicular lesions.
Stem:	Which of the following causative organisms would you most likely suspect?
Options:	(A) *Herpes simplex virus 2* (B) Condylomata lata (C) Herpes simplex virus 1 (D) Treponema pallidum

Table 5

Test Question Key Words And Phrases

First	Priority	True Statements
Best	Advice	Correct Statements
Most	Approach	Contributing to
Initial	Consideration	Of the following
Important	Management	Which of the following
Major	Expectation	Each of the following
Common	Intervention	
Least	Assessment	
Except	Contraindication	
Not	Evaluation	
Greatest	Counseling	
Earliest	Facilitative	
Useful	Indicative	
Leading	Suggestive	
Significant	Appropriate	
Immediate	Accurately	
Helpful	Likely	
Closely	Characteristics	

From "Anatomy of a test question" by N. Dickenson-Hazard, 1989, *Pediatric Nursing 15*, p. 395. Copyright 1989 by A. J. Jannetti, Inc. Reprinted by permission.

Technique #5:   Read the directions to the questions carefully. Since an examination may have several types of questions, it is imperative to read the directions carefully. If different item types are used on an exam, they are generally grouped together by type and marked clearly with directions. Be on the lookout for changing item types and be sure you understand how you are to answer before you begin reading the question.

Technique #6:   Apply the basic rules of test taking. Examination candidates can avert many problems associated with test taking if they give thought to the mechanics of sitting down, reading the question and noting their answers. Timing yourself to avoid spending too much time on a question, returning to difficult questions, and not changing your answers are all techniques that can improve performance. Table 7 provides helpful hints for the basic rules of test-taking. Review these and apply them to the testing situation.

Technique #7   Make educated guesses. This type of guessing is the selection of an option (answer) when certainty of the correct answer is questionable. Elimination of all options except for two of them, followed by a reevaluation of these options based upon your correct knowledge base then allows you to make an educated guess.

There are some examinations that will give credit when correct answers are selected and give no credit for incorrect answers. Directions for this type of examination may state that credit will be given for correct answers, therefore all questions should be answered and you will not be penalized for guessing.

Other kinds of examinations will only give credit for correct answers, and subtract credit for incorrect answers. Directions for this type of examination will instruct you not to guess, or that there is a penalty for guessing. However, even with this kind of an examination, it is still to your advantage to make an educated guess if you can reduce your possibilities to two options and then select the best of the two. **WILD GUESSING** should be avoided since it may not be to your advantage (Nugent & Vitale, 1997).

Technique #8:   Practice, practice, practice. Taking practice tests, such as those published by Health Leadership Associates, can improve performance. While they can assist in evaluation of your knowledge, *their primary benefit is to assist you with test taking skills.* You should use them to evaluate your thinking process, your ability to read, understand and interpret questions, and your skills in completing the mechanics of the test.

Technique #9:   Be prepared for exam day. It is important to familiarize yourself with the test site, the building, the parking and travel route prior to the exam day. If you must travel, arrive early to allow time for this familiarization. It is helpful to make a list of things you need on the exam day: pencils, admission card, watch and a few pieces of hard candy as a quick energy source. On exam day allow yourself plenty of time to arrive at the site. Wear comfortable clothes and have a good breakfast that morning. The night before the exam, go to bed at a reasonable hour, and avoid excessive drinking or eating (Sides & Korchek, 1994). The idea is to arrive on time at the test site, prepared and as rested as possible.

TABLE 6

Item Type Examples

A TYPE

Directions for One Best Choice Items: This item-type requires that you indicate the one best answer from the lettered alternatives offered for each item. After you have decided on the one BEST answer, completely blacken the corresponding lettered circle on the answer sheet.

#1 A 46 year-old white female is being seen in follow-up for the treatment of migraine headaches. Your management plan would most appropriately include counseling on which of the following preventive techniques?
   a. Limiting intake of high calcium foods
   b. Encouraging additional sleep hours
   c. *Learning biofeedback techniques*
   d. Massaging posterior head and neck areas regularly
   e. Developing a rigorous exercise routine

B TYPE

Directions: Each group of questions below consists of five lettered headings followed by a list of numbered words or statements. For each numbered word or statement, select the one lettered heading that is most closely associated with it and fill in the circle beneath the corresponding letter on the answer sheet. Each lettered heading may be selected once, more than once, or not at all.

#2-#4
Medication Types::
   a. Anti-fungal
   b. Anti-protozoan
   c. Antiseptic
   d. Anti-viral
Most useful for treatment of:
   2. Trichomoniasis (B)
   3. Candidiasis (A)
   4. Bacterial vaginosis (B)

C TYPE

Directions: Each set of lettered headings below is followed by a list of numbered words or phrases. For each numbered word or phrase fill in the circle on the answer sheet under A if the item is associated with (A) only, B if the item is associated with (B) only, C if the item is associated with both (A) and (B), D if the item is associated with neither (A) nor (B).
   (A) Diabetic acidosis
   (B) Insulin shock
   (C) Both
   (D) Neither
#5 — Elevated bicarbonate level in serum (D)
#6 — The duration of the condition before proper treatment is begun may influence the prognosis (C)
#7 — Deep breathing (A)
#8 — Coma (C)
#9 — Moist skin (B)

X TYPE

Directions: Each of the questions or incomplete statements below is followed by five suggested answers or completions. For EACH lettered alternative completely blacken one lettered circle in either column T or F on the answer sheet.
   True statements about fractures in school aged children include:
   (A) Assessment of fractures is less difficult in school aged children than adults
   (B) *The initial treatment for sprains and fractures is elevation and application of an ice pack*
   (C) After a plaster cast is applied, little care is necessary
   (D) *Fractures in children heal faster than fractures in adults*
   (E) Clavicular fractures are generally benign

Adapted from ''Anatomy of a test question.'' by N. Dickenson-Hazard, 1989, *Pediatric Nursing 15*, p. 396. Copyright 1989 by A. J. Jannetti, Inc. Adapted by permission.

TABLE 7

Basic Rules For Test Taking

Basic Rule	Helpful Hints
Use time wisely and effectively	Allow no more than 1 minute per question—if you can't answer question, make an intelligent guess

Know the parts of a question
    Background statement: Informational
    scenario
    Stem: Specific question or intent statement
	Select the option that best completes question or solves the problem
	Relate options to question and balance against each other
	Consider all options

Read question carefully	Understand stem first, then look for answer Note key words in background information and stem (i.e., first, best, initial, early, most, appropriate, except, least, not)
Identify intent of item based on information given	Don't assume any information not given Don't read in or add any information not given Actively reason through question
Answer difficult questions by eliminating obviously incorrect options first	Select the best of the viable, available options using logical thought Reread stem; select strongest option Skip difficult questions and return to them later or make an educated guess
Select responses guided by principles of communication	Choose therapeutic, respectful, communication enhancing options Avoid inappropriate, punitive responses
Know the principles of nursing practice	Select options that relate to common need or the population in general Select options that are correct without exception Select options which reflect nursing judgement
Know and use test-taking principles	Avoid changing answers without good reason Attempt every question Don't rely on flaws in test construction Be systematic and use problem-solving techniques in answering questions

From "Making the grade as a test-taker" by N. Dickenson-Hazard, 1989. *Pediatric Nursing 15,* p. 304. Adapted from *How to take tests.* (pp 15-57) by J. Millman and W. Paul, 1969, New York: McGraw-Hill Co. and from *Nurses's guide to successful test taking.* (pp 43-53) by M. B. Sides and N. B. Cailles, 1989, Philadelphia: J. B. Lippincott Co. Copyright 1989 A. J. Jannetti, Inc. Reprinted and adapted by permission.

STRATEGY #5 Psych Yourself Up: Taking tests is stressful

While a little stress can be productive, too much can incapacitate you in your studying and test taking (Divine & Kylen, 1979). Your attitude and approach to test taking and studying can influence your outcomes. Psyching yourself up can have a positive effect and make examinations a non-anxiety laden experience (Dickenson-Hazard, 1990). The following techniques are based on the principles of successful test taking as presented by Sides & Cailles (1989). Incorporation of these techniques can improve response and performance in examination situations.

Technique #1: Adopt an "I can" attitude. Believing you can succeed is the key to success. Self belief inspires and gives you the power to achieve your goals. Without a success attitude, the road to your goal is much harder. We all stand an equal chance of success in this world. It is those who believe they can who achieve it. This "I can" attitude must permeate all your efforts in test taking from studying to improving your skills, to actually writing the test.

Technique #2: Take control. By identifying your goal, deciding how to accomplish it and developing a plan for achieving it, you take control. Do not leave your success or failure to chance; control it through action and attitude.

Technique #3: Think positively. Examinations are generally based on a standard which is the same for all individuals. Everyone can potentially pass. Performance is influenced not only by knowledge and skill but attitude as well. Those individuals who regard an exam as an opportunity or challenge will be more successful.

Technique #4: Project a positive self-fulfilling prophecy. While preparing for an examination, project thoughts of the positive outcomes you will experience when you succeed. Self-talk is self-fulfilling. Expect success, not failure, of yourself.

Technique #5: Feel good about yourself. Without feeling a sense of positive self worth, passing an examination is difficult. Recognize your professional contributions and give yourself credit for your accomplishments. Think ''I will pass,'' not ''I suppose I can.''

Technique #6: Know yourself. Focus exam preparation and test taking on your strengths. Try to alter your weaknesses instead of becoming hung up on them. If you tend to overanalyze, study and read test questions at face value. If you're a speed demon when taking a test, slow down and read more carefully.

Technique #7: Failure is a possibility. We all have failed at something at some point in our lives. Rather than dwelling on the failure, making excuses and believing you'll fail again, recognize your mistakes and remedy them. Failure is a time to begin again; use it as a motivator to do better. It is not the end of the world unless you allow it to be. It is best to deal with the failure and move on, otherwise it interferes with your success.

Technique #8: Persevere, persevere, persevere! Endurance must underlie all your efforts. Call forth those reserve energies when you've had all you think you can take. Rely upon yourself and your support systems to help you maintain a sense of direction and keep your goal in the forefront.

Technique #9: Motivation is muscle. Most individuals are motivated by fear or desire. The fear in an exam situation may be one of failure, the unknown or discovery of imperfection. Put your fear into perspective; realize you are not the only one with fear and that all have an equal opportunity for success. Develop strategies to reduce fear and use fear to your advantage by improving the imperfections. Desire is a powerful motivator and you should keep the rewards of your desire foremost in your mind. Whatever motivates you, use it to make you successful. Reward yourself during your exam preparation and once the exam has been completed. You alone hold the key to success; use what you have wisely.

Technique #10: Overprepare. One of the best ways to reduce test anxiety is to overprepare. The more prepared you are the more confident you will be. Overpreparation requires you to study the same information over again even when you know the information. This activity will reinforce your learning and will build confidence and reduce anxiety when it comes time to take the examination.

Overpreparation can not occur unless adequate time is allowed for this process. A last minute cramming approach will not lead to an overprepared test taker. Being over prepared definitely places an individual in control and in a position of power and confidence (Nugent & Vitale, 1997).

This chapter has provided concepts, strategies and techniques for improving study and test taking skills. Your first task in improvement is to know yourself, how you study and how you take a test. You should use your strengths and remedy the weaknesses. Next you need to develop your thinking skills. Work on techniques to improve memory and reasoning. Now you need to organize your study and concentrate on using these new and used skills to be successful. Create a study space, develop a plan of action, then implement that plan during your periods of peak concentration. Before taking the exam be sure you understand the components of a test question, can identify key words and phrases and have practiced. Apply the test taking rules during the exam process. Finally, believe in yourself, your knowledge and your talent. Believing you can accomplish your goal facilitates the fact that you will.

BIBLIOGRAPHY

American Board of Pediatrics. (1989). *Developing questions and critiques.* Unpublished material.

Burke, M. M., & Walsh, M. B. (1992). *Gerontologic nursing.* St. Louis: Mosby Year Book.

Burkle, C. A., & Marshak, D. (1989). *Study program: Level 1.* Reston, VA: National Association of Secondary School Principals.

Dickenson-Hazard, N. (1989). Making the grade as a test taker. *Pediatric Nursing, 15,* 302–304.

Dickenson-Hazard, N. (1989). Anatomy of a test question. *Pediatric Nursing, 15,* 395–399.

Dickenson-Hazard, N. (1990). The psychology of successful test taking. *Pediatric Nursing, 16,* 66–67.

Dickenson-Hazard, N. (1990). Study smart. *Pediatric Nursing, 16,* 314–316.

Dickenson-Hazard, N. (1990). Study effectiveness: Are you 10 a.m. or p.m. scholar? *Pediatric Nursing, 16,* 419–420.

Dickenson-Hazard, N. (1990). Develop your thinking skills for improved test taking. *Pediatric Nursing, 16,* 480–481.

Divine, J. H., & Kylen, D. W. (1979). *How to beat test anxiety.* New York: Barrons Educational Series, Inc.

Goroll, A., May, L., & Mulley, A. (Eds.). (1988). *Primary care medicine* (2nd ed.). Philadelphia: J. B. Lippincott.

Health Leadership Associates website—www.healthleadership.com

Kelsey, B., & Salomone, A. (Eds.). (1999). *Women's Health nurse practitioner certification study question book.* Potomac, MD: Health Leadership Associates.

Miller, S. K. (Ed.). (1999). *Adult nurse practitioner certification study question book.* Potomac, MD: Health Leadership Associates.

Millman, J., & Pauk, W. (1969). *How to take tests.* New York: McGraw-Hill Book Co.

Millonig, V. L. (Ed.). (1999). *Pediatric nurse practitioner certification study question book.* Potomac, MD: Health Leadership Associates.

Nugent, P. M., & Vitale, B. A. (1997). *Test success.* (2nd ed.). Philadelphia: F. A. Davis.

Olney, C. W. (1989). *Where there's a will, there's an A.* New Jersey: Chesterbrook Educational Publishers.

Sides, M., & Cailles, N. B. (1989). *Nurse's guide to successful test taking.* Philadelphia: J. B. Lippincott Co.

Sides, M., & Korchek, N. (1994). *Nurse's guide to successful test taking* (2nd ed.). Philadelphia: J. B. Lippincott.

Human Growth and Development Infancy Through Adolescence

Mary A. Baroni

Human Growth and Development: Underlying Theory and Science of Child Health

- Definition: How and why a person changes and/or stays the same over time (Berger, 2000)
    1. Nature (heredity and genetic predisposition) vs. nurture (environmental influence)
    2. Continuity (continual process) vs. discontinuity (distinct stages)
- Three Fundamental Domains: Conceptual distinctions but overlapping processes in reality
    1. Physical domain
        a. Genetic factors
        b. Physical stature and appearance
        c. Nutritional status
        d. Physical health and well-being
        e. Fine and gross motor abilities
    2. Cognitive domain
        a. Perception, thinking, information processing and memory
        b. Communication—receptive and expressive language
    3. Psychological and social domain
        a. Temperament and personality
        b. Interpersonal relationships
        c. Home environment and other social contexts

Classic Developmental Theories and Theorists

- Nature Positions: Emphasis on heredity and maturational process
    1. Jacque Rousseau (1712–1778)
        a. *Emile—Treatise on Education*
        b. Child as an "untamed savage"
    2. Charles Darwin (1809–1882)
        a. *Origin of the Species*—human evolution (phylogeny)
        b. First use of "baby journal" as systematic method to document observed behavioral development
    3. Alfred Binet (1857–1911) and Theophile Simon (1873–1961)
        a. First standardized measurement of intelligence
        b. Intention was to identify "mentally defective" children needing specialized education
    4. G. Stanley Hall (1844–1924)

  a. *Adolescence* (1904)—classic work that first described adolescence as a critical developmental period of "Sturm und Drang" or "Storm and Stress."

  b. Development of questionnaires as method for the study of child development via adult retrospective recall

5. Arnold Gesell (1880–1961)

  a. Maturational-organismic theory—biological basis of development

  b. *The Atlas of Infant Behavior* (1934)—developmental milestones

  c. Developed one of the earliest infant tests

6. Sigmund Freud (1856–1939)

  a. *Three Contributions to the Sexual Theory* (1905)

  b. Stage theory of psychosexual development

    (1) Infancy: Oral stage

    (2) Toddler: Anal stage

    (3) Preschool: Phallic stage

    (4) School age: Latency stage

    (5) Adolescence: Genital stage

  c. Key principles

    (1) Id: Principle of pleasure

    (2) Ego: Principle of reality and/or self-interest

    (3) Superego: Principle of morality or conscience

7. Neo-Freudian: Erik Erikson (1902–)—stage theory of life span psychosocial development

  a. Infancy: Trust vs. Mistrust

  b. Toddler: Autonomy vs. shame and doubt

  c. Preschool: Initiative vs. guilt

  d. School age: Industry vs. inferiority

  e. Adolescence: Identity vs. role confusion

  f. Young Adult: Intimacy vs. isolation

  g. Middle-age: Generativity vs. stagnation

  h. Older Adulthood: Integrity vs. despair

8. Neo-Freudian: Margaret Mahler—psychological birth of the infant

  a. Psychological birth of the child with emerging sense of self as separate from mother

    b.   Inadequate early mothering and "psychological birth" results in mental illness

    c.   Phases of "psychological birth"

        (1)   Autism from 0 to 2 months—no real social awareness or concept of self

        (2)   Symbiosis from 2 to 5 months—mother-infant dependency

        (3)   Separation-individuation from 6 to 36 months

            (a)   Differentiation and practicing (6 to 12 months)— beginning awareness of self as separate from mother

            (b)   Rapprochment (12 to 24 months)—exploration, emotional refueling, and ability to sustain brief separations

            (c)   Consolidation (24 to 36 months)—increased ability to cope with separations through symbolic play

9.   Jean Piaget (1896–1980)

    a.   Interactionist—structuralist stage theory of cognitive development

    b.   Sensori-motor stage: Birth to 2 years

    c.   Preoperational thinking: 2 to 7 years

    d.   Concrete operational thinking (7 to 12 years)

    e.   Formal operational thinking (12 years +)

- Nurture Positions: Emphasis on learning and environment

1.   John Locke (1632–1704)

    a.   *Essay Concerning Human Understanding and Some Thoughts Concerning Education*

    b.   Child as "tabula rasa" or "blank slate"

2.   John B. Watson (1878–1958)—behaviorism

    a.   *Classical conditioning*—neutral stimulus associated with meaningful one over time leading "conditioned" response that can be elicited by neutral stimulus alone as though it were the meaningful one

    b.   *Psychological Care of the Infant and Child* (1928)

3.   B. F. Skinner—student of Watson

    a.   Mechanistic-learning theory

    b.   *Operant or instrumental conditioning*—behavior is reinforced or extinguished by positive or negatively experienced consequences such as use of "time-out" for misbehavior

4.   Albert Bandura and Walter Mischel—social learning theory

    a.   Influenced by both behaviorism and psychodynamic theories

   b. Behavior results from interaction of individual characteristics, the environment and the behavior itself

   c. Modeling—learning from direct observation and subsequent imitation of what is seen and done by significant others in the proximal environment

- Ethologic Theories

   1. Konrad Lorenz—*sensitive periods* as biologically-programmed periods predisposed for particular learning, e.g., *imprinting*

   2. Harry Harlow—Wisconsin primate laboratory's classic rhesus monkey experiments on separation, isolation and "terry cloth vs. wire surrogate mothers"

      a. Maternal separation and social isolation resulted in dramatic impairment of social-emotional development

      b. Physical contact and comfort as necessary for normal social and emotional development

   3. John Bowlby: *Attachment and Loss* (1969)

      a. Attachment defined as "an affectional tie the infant forms to another specific person that binds the two together in space and endures over time"

      b. Importance of early mothering and consequences of "maternal deprivation" as observed in orphanages and asylums

   4. Marshall Klaus and John Kennel—*Maternal-Infant Bonding* (1976)

      a. Seminal studies on the impact of early contact vs. separation on maternal-infant bonding

      b. Influential in advocating change in hospital policies regarding rooming-in and father participation in the delivery room

   5. Mary Ainsworth: *Patterns of Attachment: A Study of the Strange Situation* (1978)—developed laboratory paradigm "Strange Situation" to assess security or insecurity of the attachment relationship

      a. Early maternal responsiveness to infant needs promotes secure attachment

      b. Secure maternal-infant attachment provides "safe base" from which the child can begin to actively explore the environment and a source of comfort when distressed

      c. Securely attached infants show more optimal cognitive gains and later school performance, illustrating the interconnectedness of psychosocial and cognitive domains

- Humanistic Theories

   1. Abraham Maslow (1908–1970)

      a. Theory of basic needs and human potential derived from study of healthy, creative individuals; few people achieve self-actualization

      b.   Hierarchy of needs

         (1) Physiologic

         (2) Safety, security and stability

         (3) Affiliation, acceptance and love

         (4) Ego, self-worth, confidence, competence and success

         (5) Self-actualization

2. Carl Rogers

      a.   Client-centered approach from a phenomenologic perspective

      b.   Key strategies for intervention

         (1) Unconditional positive regard, empathy and genuineness

         (2) Empathy

         (3) Congruence or the ability to be genuine

- Moral Development

  1. Lawrence Kohlberg's stages of moral development

      a.   Based on his original cross-sectional study of 84 school-aged boys (10 to 16 years) recruited from two suburban Chicago schools who were later followed longitudinally

      b.   Responses to hypothetic moral dilemmas

      c.   Preconventional or pre-moral level

         (1) Stage 1: Punishment-obedience—child behaves to avoid punishment.

         (2) Stage 2: Instrumental-exchange—child behaves well for some gain or reward

      d.   Conventional level

         (1) Stage 3: Good-boy/good-girl orientation—child behaves for approval

         (2) Stage 4: Law and order perspective—child behaves to avoid getting caught

      e.   Postconventional level

         (1) Stage 5: Social contract—child/adolescent behaves in accordance with generally accepted social norms

         (2) Stage 6: Universal ethical principles—child/adolescent decides on moral standards of behavior through individual reflection and reasoning

  2. Carol Gilligan: Gender differences in moral development

      a.   Male social development orients to ethic of *principles* with moral issues decided on the basis of fairness and justice

b. Female social development orients to ethic of *interpersonal relationships* with moral issues decided on the basis of compassion and caring

- Language Development: L. S. Vygotsky (1896–1934)

    1. Language as biologically-programmed but children learn language actively through direct experience and culture

    2. Zone of proximal development (ZPD): Zone between child's opportunity to observe/participate and ability to internalize the learned behavior

Transactional and Contextual Theories of Development

- Heredity-Environment Interactions

    1. Growth and developmental outcomes result from "main effects" and "interaction effects" of and between both heredity (nature) and environment (nurture)

    2. *Reaction Range*—range of phenotypes that may emerge from similar genotypes developing under varied environmental contexts

- Transactional and Resiliency as Models of Development

    1. Transaction model first described in 1975 as a "continuum of reproductive risk and caretaking casualties" by Arnold Sameroff and Michael Chandler

    2. Research based on transactional model emerged in 1980s describes risk and protective factors associated with vulnerability and resilience in the face of adversity

        a. Emmy Werner (1982)—Kauai longitudinal study from birth to adulthood to explore perinatal risk and environmental factors on subsequent developmental outcomes

        b. Michael Rutter (1979; 1987)—epidemiological studies of children of mentally ill parents to examine risk and protective factors influencing subsequent psychopathology

        c. Alan Sroufe's longitudinal study of competence as a developmental construct

    3. Examples of clinical problems with multifactorial etiology better understood through a transactional perspective include failure-to-thrive, child abuse, attention deficit hyperactivity, conduct, and eating disorders

- Ecological Model or "Development in Context"

    1. Developed and described by Urie Bronfenbrenner in 1979 publication—*Ecology of Human Development: Experiments by Nature and Design.*

    2. Person-place-process model

        a. Microsystems—immediate settings within which a child spends time during development (e.g., home, school, hospital)

        b. Mesosystem—relationship or linkages between microsystems (e.g., service coordination)

    c.   Exosystem—settings that may indirectly influence development (e.g., parent's work place, school boards)

    d.   Macrosystem—broad-based historical, cultural, demographic and institutional context, (e.g., managed care and welfare reform initiatives)

3. Understanding how and why a child changes or stays the same over time requires examination not only of the child's emerging capabilities but the quality of the settings (places and processes) where children spend time, communication/linkages between these settings, influence of policy decisions, and overall social, cultural, and political context

4. Examples of clinical interventions better understood through an ecological perspective include early intervention services, home visiting services, and care coordination/case management strategies

Infant Growth and Development (Birth to 2 years)

- Physical Domain: Major tasks—physiologic regulation/motor control

  1. Definitions

    a.   Preterm—newborn with gestational age estimated as less than 37 weeks

    b.   Low birth weight (LBW)— < 2500 g

        (1) Very low birth weight (VLBW)— < 1500 g

        (2) Extremely low birth weight (ELBW)— < 1000 g

    c.   Assessment of weight for gestational age

        (1) AGA—appropriate for gestational age

        (2) LGA—large for gestational age; weight > 90th percentile; often associated with diabetic pregnancies

        (3) SGA—small for gestational age

            (a) Symmetric intrauterine growth retardation (IUGR)—weight, length and head circumference are SGA; reflects long-standing compromise and/ or intrinsic to infant

            (b) Asymmetric intrauterine growth retardation (IUGR)—underweight for length and head circumference; reflects acute compromise extrinsic to fetus such as placental insufficiency

  2. Average U.S. newborn is 20 to 21 inches (51 cm), weighs approximately 7 pounds (3.1 kg), with head circumference of 13 to 14 inches (33.0 to 35.6 cm) and with chest circumference measuring approximately 2 cm less than head circumference

  3. Initial 10% weight loss in average newborn in first 3 to 4 days of life is usually regained by 14 days

  4. Weight doubles by 4 months, triples by one year and quadruples by 2 years

    a.   6 to 8 oz weight gain per week during first 6 months

b. 3 to 4 oz weight gain per week during 6 to 12 months

c. Average weight gain in second year is 8 to 9 oz (.25 kg) per month

5. Length usually increases by 50% by one year, doubles by 4 years and triples by 13 years—increases by 1 inch per month during first 6 months then $\frac{1}{2}$ inch per month through first year

6. Head circumference increases $\frac{1}{2}$ inch per month during first 6 months then $\frac{1}{4}$ inch per month through first year

7. Serial measurements and observation over time with use of standardized growth charts—National Center for Health Statistics (NCHS)

8. Dental development

a. Formation of teeth begins during the third fetal month and continues through adolescence

b. Primary or deciduous teeth are first set of teeth that are later replaced by permanent teeth

c. Eruption timing can vary greatly but eruption sequence of deciduous teeth is generally consistent—see Table 1

Table 1
Timetable: Primary Teeth Eruption

Primary Teeth	Maxillary Eruption	Mandibular Eruption
(1) Central incisors	6–8 months	5–7 months
(2) Lateral incisors	8–11 months	7–10 months
(3) Cuspids (Canines)	16–20 months	16–20 months
(4) First molars	10–16 months	10–16 months
(5) Second molars	20–30 months	20–30 months

9. Motor development

a. Early reflexive responses—involuntary responses to stimuli that may be viewed as precursors to late motor skills

(1) Survival reflexes

(a) Breathing, hiccups, sneezes, spitting up as infant tries to regulate breathing, sucking and swallowing

(b) Temperature control reflexes—cry, shivering, tucking legs close to body

(c) Feeding reflexes—sucking, rooting, crying, and swallowing

(2) Nonsurvival reflexes—Babinski, stepping, swimming, grasping, moro or startle

b. Gross and fine motor milestones—age of attainment varies but sequence is generally consistent (see Tables 2 and 3)

Table 2
Gross Motor Milestones

Milestone	Age
Good head control	2–3 months
Rolls—front to back	4–5 months
Rolls—back to front	5–6 months
Sits alone	5–6 months
Creeps or crawls	7–8 months
Pulls to standing, cruises	9–10 months
Stands alone	11–12 months
Walks—forward	12–14 months
Walks—backwards	14–16 months
Walks—up steps with assistance	16–18 months
Walks—up and down steps alone	22–24 months
Jumps with both feet	24–28 months

Table 3
Fine Motor Milestones

Milestone	Age
Grasp and shakes rattle	2–3 months
Reaches for object or person	3–4 months
Brings hands to mid-line	4–5 months
Hand-to-hand object transfer	5–6 months
Unilateral reaching	6–7 months
Raking grasp	6–7 months
Finger feeding	7–9 months
Pincer grasp	8–10 months
Simple games—pat-a-cake	9–10 months
Makes marks on paper with pencil/crayon	10–12 months
Opens book, turns pages	12–13 months
Stacks 2 blocks	12–15 months
Uses eating utensils	15–17 months
Stacks 3 blocks	17–18 months
Simple puzzles—circles shapes first	18–20 months
Stacks 6–7 blocks	22–24 months

- Cognitive Development: Major tasks—sensorimotor and early language development
    1. Vision
        a. Presence of blink reflex and pupil constriction to light are indications of new-born vision
        b. Newborns can focus on objects between 4 to 30 inches including mother's face during feeding
        c. Binocular vision develops between 4 to 6 months
        d. Visual acuity is difficult to measure during infancy; distance acuity has been estimated between 20/150 to 20/400 in newborns; improves to 20/70 by 2 years and 20/30 by 5 years

2. Hearing

    a. Infants have greater auditory acuity for high rather than low frequency sounds

    b. Responsiveness to "motherese" as high-pitched "baby talk"

3. Sensori-motor development (Piaget)

    a. Reflexes (birth to 1 month)

    b. Primary circular reactions (1 to 4 months)—adaptation of reflexes to the environment through coordination of 2 actions such as seeing and grasping

    c. Secondary circular reactions (4 to 8 months)—increased awareness of objects, persons and expected responses

    d. Coordination of means and ends (8-12 months)—object permanence introduces this substage with awareness that people and objects continue to exist when out of sight

    e. Tertiary circular reactions—active exploration and trial-and-error learning (12 to 18 months)

    f. Mental combinations—ability to problem-solve simple situations without trial-and-error (18 to 24 months)

4. Language development—receptive language precedes expressive abilities (see Table 4)

Table 4
Language Milestones

Milestone	Age
Responds to sounds	Birth
Smiles and coos	2–3 months
Laughs, expresses delight	4–5 months
Babbles	5–6 months
"Dada" & "mama"	8–9 months
Waves "bye-bye"	8–9 months
Understands "no"	9–10 months
2 words other than "mama/dada"	11–12 months
Jabbering	12–13 months
Begins to point to body parts	15–18 months
2-word phrases & sentences	18–22 months
30-50 word vocabulary	22–24 months

- Psychosocial Development: Major tasks—goodness of fit between temperament and environment; development of secure attachment relationship

    1. Temperament—the "how" of behavior rather than "what" or "why"

        a. New York Longitudinal Study (NYLS) defined 9 dimensions of temperament—activity, rhythmicity, approachability, adaptability, intensity, threshold of arousal, mood, distractibility, and attention

        b. Categories of temperamental profiles

(1) Easy—rhythmic, approachable, adaptable, positive moods, and low intensity (40%)

(2) Slow-to-warm-up—less active, more avoidant, less adaptable, more negative moods and low intensity (15%)

(3) Difficult—arrhythmic, more avoidant, less adaptable, more negative moods and high intensity (10%)

(4) Intermediate high and intermediate low (35%)

2. Parent-infant interaction and the attachment relationship

a. Synchrony—sensitive, coordinated, mutually regulated and reciprocal style of social interactions that evolve between parent and infant during the first year of life leading to a secure attachment by one year

b. Emotional development begins with physiologic experience and expression of "comfort/discomfort" which later differentiates into more fine-tuned emotions

(1) Social smile in response to persons begins around 6 weeks

(2) Emergence of fears and anxiety accompanies the cognitive milestone of object permanency as the infant distinguishes "mother" from "stranger;" fear of strangers (stranger anxiety) begins around 6 months and peaks about 12 months; separation anxiety begins between 8 to 9 months and peaks around 14 months

c. Attachment (definition)—the enduring and specific, affective bond that develops over the first year of life

(1) Secure attachment—underlying emotion is love

(2) Insecure-avoidant—underlying emotion is anger

(3) Insecure-anxious—underlying emotion is anxiety/ambivalence

(4) Insecure-disorganized—underlying process is confusion/ dysfunction

Toddler and Preschooler Growth and Development

- Physical Domain: Major tasks—locomotion and continued motor development

1. Physical growth

a. Reduced rate of growth between 2 to 6 years resulting in fewer caloric needs and decreased appetite

b. Growth in length is approximately 3 inches (7 cm) per year and weight gain approximately 4 $\frac{1}{2}$ pounds (2 kg) per year

c. Average U.S. 6 year old weighs about 46 pounds (21 kg) and is 46 inches (117 cm) tall

2. Motor development

Table 5
Gross and Fine Motor Milestones

Gross Motor Milestones	Mean Age
(1) Balance on each foot 2 seconds	2 $\frac{1}{2}$ years
(2) Hops	3 $\frac{1}{2}$ years
(3) Walks upstairs alternating feet	3 $\frac{1}{2}$ years
(4) Walks on tip toes	3 $\frac{1}{2}$ years
(5) Heel-to-toe walking	4 $\frac{1}{2}$ years

Fine Motor Milestones	Mean Age
(1) Tower of 8 cubes	2 $\frac{1}{2}$ years
(2) Thumb wiggle	2 $\frac{1}{2}$ year
(3) Copies circle	3 to 3 $\frac{1}{2}$ years
(4) Draws a person with 6 parts	4 $\frac{1}{2}$ years
(5) Copies square	5 years

    a. CNS maturation during toddler and preschool years allows for better control and coordination of both gross motor and fine motor skills

    b. Motor developmental milestones—see Table 5

3. Cognitive development—symbolic thinking and increased language development

    a. Pre-operational thinking (Piaget)

        (1) Preconceptual (2 to 4 years)

        (2) Intuitive (2 to 7 years)

    b. Centration—preschoolers' tendency to focus on one idea or characteristic feature of an object or situation at one time

        (1) Egocentrism—tendency to focus thinking and understanding about the world from their own perspective only

        (2) Animism—everything animate or inanimate thinks and feels the way the preschooler does

    c. Difficulty distinguishing fact from fantasy—normative "lying," nightmares, imaginary friends, and potential to feel responsible for bad or good things happening based on their own thoughts, feelings, or behaviors

    d. Language development

        (1) Expressive language

            (a) Up to 425 word vocabulary with 75% speech understandable—2 $\frac{1}{2}$ years

            (b) Increased complexity of sentences including 4 to 5 words—3 $\frac{1}{2}$ years

        (2) Receptive language

            (a) Carries out 2 to 3 item commands—3 years

        (b)   Understands opposite analogies—4 years

        (c)   Understands "if," "because" and "when"—5 years

4.   Psychosocial development: Major tasks—autonomy, impulse control/discipline and gender identity

   a.   Parenting styles and discipline

      (1)   Authoritarian parent—strict parenting with firm or harsh discipline and without questioning; high expectations, low support, low parent-child communication

      (2)   Permissive parenting—few demands and low expectations

         (a)   Democratic-indulgent—low expectations with high support and high parent-child communication

         (b)   Permissive-neglectful—low expectations with low support and low parent-child communication

      (3)   Authoritative parenting—firm limits but opportunity for dialogue; high expectations, high support and high parent-child communication; associated with best-child outcomes

   b.   Aggression and impulse control

      (1)   Instrumental aggression—common form of aggression among preschoolers focused on retrieving an object, space or special privilege; frequency decreases with increased understanding of sharing and impulse control

      (2)   Hostile aggression—person-oriented aggression that is not common among preschoolers but may emerge with school entry if impulse control remains problematic

   c.   Play as the major medium for early mastery of a variety of physical, cognitive and social skills has been appropriately described as the "work of children"

      (1)   Infancy—solitary play as the earliest level of sensorimotor or skill mastery play; associated with little awareness of other children

      (2)   Toddlers

         (a)   Onlooker play is common at this age with curious watching of other children playing

         (b)   Parallel play—becomes predominant style of play with toddlers engaged in similar play activity but with minimal interaction

      (3)   Preschoolers play—more social in character including:

         (a)   Associative play—some interaction and sharing of toys may occur but not organized and consistent enough to be called a game

         (b)   Cooperative play—children are taking turns and actively playing together

(c) Dramatic or pretend play—make believe play during which the children create and act out a scene such as "playing house"

(d) Rough-and-tumble play—physical play involving gross motor activities like running, jumping, chasing and wrestling that appears aggressive but is actually playful

d. Fears

(1) Nightmares

(2) Night terrors—partial arousal for deep non-REM sleep with minimal recollection of screaming/thrashing

e. Gender identity—emerging sense of self as a male or female person

(1) 2-year-olds can distinguish gender and will identify themselves as boy or girl

(2) 3- to 4-year-olds tend to show sex-typed preferences; gender identity is usually firmly established and unlikely to change

(3) 5- to 6-year-olds begin to express notions about how males and females should dress, behave and feel

School-Aged Development

- Physical Domain: Motor coordination and skill development

1. Physical growth—relatively stable, smooth and uneventful

a. Average school-aged child gains about 5 pounds and $2\frac{1}{2}$ inches per year

b. By age 10, the average school-aged child weighs about 70 pounds and is 54 inches tall

2. Motor development—few gender differences except for stronger forearm strength in males and increased flexibility in females

3. Permanent teeth timing and eruption sequence—see Table 6

Table 6
Timetable: Permanent Teeth Eruption

Permanent Teeth	Maxillary Eruption	Mandibular Eruption
a. Central incisors	7–8 years	6–7 years
b. Lateral incisors	8–9 years	7–8 years
c. Cuspids (Canines)	11–12 years	9–11 years
d. First premolar (Bicuspids)	10–11 years	10–12 years
e. Second premolar (Bicuspids)	10–12 years	11–13 years
f. First molars	6–7 years	6–7 years
g. Second molars	12–13 years	12–13 years
h. Third molars	17–22 years	17–22 years

- Cognitive Development: Major task—concrete thinking and adaptation to school
  1. Concrete operational thought (Piaget)
     a. "5 to 7 shift"—transition period between preoperational and concrete operational thinking
     b. Logical operations include:
        (1) Reversibility—ability to reverse a process or action such as understanding that if $2 + 3 = 5$ then $5 - 3 = 2$
        (2) Conservation (number, mass and volume)—understanding that certain aspect or quality of an object can change in appearance without changing the object itself
        (3) Classification—ability to group objects on the basis of similar characteristics such as color or shape
        (4) Seriation—arrangement of items in a series such as by increasing size
  2. School readiness
     a. School entry is a major transition for children
     b. School refusal may reflect separation anxiety masked as vague somatic complaints
- Psychosocial Development: Major tasks—self-esteem, peers, and after school activites
  1. Self-esteem—competence to think, learn, and make decisions as well as believe that one is worthy of love and respectful treatment from others
  2. Peers and development of prosocial behavior through cooperative games, sports, and activities
  3. The need for organized after school activities has become critical with the increasing numbers of children who are regularly left unsupervised after school because of parental work schedules and variations in family structure in the U.S.

Adolescent Development

- Physical Domain: Major tasks—puberty, sexual maturation
  1. Physical growth
     a. Average U.S. female gains about 38 pounds (17 kg) and $9\frac{1}{2}$ inches (24 cm) between 10 to 14 years.
     b. Average U.S. male gains about 42 pound (19 kg) and $9\frac{1}{2}$ inches (24 cm) between 12 to 16 years.
  2. Puberty—period of rapid physical growth and sexual maturation resulting in adult size, shape and reproductive potential
     a. Sequence of puberty—individual variation in onset but sequence of somatic and physiologic changes is relatively set

    (1)   Females

        (a)   Puberty onset 9 to 10 years

        (b)   Precocious puberty < 8 years

        (c)   Delayed puberty > 13 years

        (d)   First physical sign—breast buds

        (e)   Peak height velocity—12.4 years

        (f)   Menarche—12.5 years

        (g)   Fertility—15 years

    (2)   Males

        (a)   Puberty onset 11 to 12 years

        (b)   Precocious puberty < 9 years

        (c)   Delayed puberty > 14 years

        (d)   First physical sign—testicular growth

        (e)   Peak height velocity—14.4 years

        (f)   Spermarche—13 to 14 years

        (g)   Fertility—15 years

b. Anovulatory cycles are common during the first two years after menarche (50% of cycles vs. 20% after 5 years)

c. Stages of genital maturity in males—takes approximately 4 years to move from stage 2 to 5 (Tanner staging)

    (1)   Stage 1: Pre-adolescent testes, scrotum and penis

    (2)   Stage 2: Enlargement of scrotum and testes; scrotum reddens and roughens

    (3)   Stage 3: Penis enlarges primarily in length

    (4)   Stage 4: Penis enlarges in breadth and development of glans

    (5)   Stage 5: Adult size and shape

d. Stages of breast development in females (Tanner staging)

    (1)   Stage 1: Pre-adolescent breast with nipple elevation

    (2)   Stage 2: Breast buds with areolar enlargement

    (3)   Stage 3: Breast enlargement without separate contour with nipple

    (4)   Stage 4: Projection of areola and nipple as secondary mound to breast

    (5)   Stage 5: Adult breast with areola receding and nipple projecting from breast

e. Stages of pubic hair development in males and females (Tanner staging)

(1) Stage 1: Pre-adolescent without pubic hair

(2) Stage 2: Sparse, pale, fine pubic hair

(3) Stage 3: Darker, more curled, increased amount of pubic hair

(4) Stage 4: Hair is adult in character but doesn't cover entire pubic area

(5) Stage 5: Adult distribution in quantity, quality and pattern

- Cognitive Development: Major tasks—ability to abstract and decision-making

    1. Formal operational thought—ability to abstract (Piaget)

    2. Characteristic ways of thinking

        a. Egocentrism—difficulty an adolescent may have in thinking rationally about their own personal experiences as completely unique

        b. Invincibility fable—sense of invincibility that can lead to risk-taking behaviors

        c. Personal fable—variation of adolescent egocentrism whereby adolescent feels personally gifted in some way

        d. Imaginary audience—exaggerated sense that everyone is watching and focused on the adolescent resulting in feeling self-conscious

- Psychosocial Development: Major tasks—independence, intimacy, vocation or career goals

    1. Majority of adolescents cope well with their transition to adulthood and do not experience "storm and stress" as once assumed

    2. A second phase of "separation-individuation" occurs during adolescence that requires new approaches to parenting, communication, decision-making and independence

    3. Three psychosocial periods of adolescence

        a. Early adolescence—middle school (11 to 14 years)

            (1) Importance of peers and feeling "normal"

            (2) Moodiness

        b. Middle adolescence—high school (15 to 17 years)

            (1) Body image, sexuality, dating

            (2) Asserting independence

        c. Late adolescence—vocation and career choices (18 to 21 years)

            (1) Identity formation—achievement, moratorium, foreclosure, diffusion

            (2) Vocation and career choices including college, military, and employment opportunities

            (3) Intimacy in relationships

The Changing American Family as Context for Growth and Development

- Demographic Changes

    1. Increasing rates of divorce and remarriage

    2. Delays and declines in child-bearing

    3. Rise in female participation in work force—voluntary, dual earner families, female head of household, and welfare reform work requirements

    4. Increasing incidence of single parent families, childhood poverty, and homelessness

- Variations in Family Structure

    1. Decrease in "traditional" two-parent family

    2. Increase in single-parent households—divorce, births to unmarried mothers, death of spouse, adoption

    3. Remarriage, blended families, and step-parenting

    4. Extended and/or "skip generation" families with grandparents as primary caregivers and/or with several generations living together

    5. Foster families—estimated 300,000 children in foster care at any given time

    6. Group living including homeless shelters—estimated 43% of the homeless population include families with children

    7. Gay and lesbian families—estimated 5 million lesbian mothers and 3 million gay fathers caring for between 6 to 14 million children

- Family Functioning: Critical concepts

    1. Family functioning is more directly related to healthy growth and development than is family structure

    2. Components of family functioning include provision of a stable and safe physical environment as well as financial and emotional resources necessary to provide supportive and nurturing care with appropriate supervision and guidance

    3. Screening and assessment tools

        a. Family Inventory of Life Events (FILE)

        b. Family Coping Strategies (F-COPES)

        c. Adolescent-Family Inventory of Life Events and Changes (A-FILE)

        d. Parenting Stress Index (PSI)

    4. Family-centered care—Institute for Family-Centered Care

        a. Recognition that the family is the constant in a child's life

        b. Family-professional collaboration at all levels

        c. Respect for family diversity in structure, race, ethnicity, culture and socioeconomic status

    d.   Recognition of family strengths, uniqueness and diversity in coping strategies

    e.   Communication and sharing of information on an ongoing basis with families in a supportive and non-judgmental manner

    f.   Support and facilitation of family-to-family support

    g.   Understand and incorporate strategies supportive of growth and developmental needs of children and their families into health care settings/systems

    h.   Implementation of policies and programs to support emotional and financial well-being of families

    i.   Accessible health care that is flexible, culturally competent and responsive to family-centered need

  5. Resources: Institute for Family-Centered Care
                  http://www.familycenteredcare.org

Deviations in Physical Growth and Behavioral Development

Failure-to-Thrive (FTT)

- Definition

  1. No consensus on definition

  2. Descriptive rather than diagnostic term

  3. Generally refers to infants and young children whose weight is below the 3rd percentile on National Center for Health Statistics (NCHS) growth standards and/or whose weight trajectory has decreased by two major growth percentiles

  4. Traditional categories include organic FTT, non-organic FTT, and mixed etiology FTT

  5. Newer categories include neurodevelopmental FTT and socioemotional FTT

- Etiology/Incidence

  1. Multifactorial etiology including underlying organic disease or predisposing medical condition, maladaptive parent-infant interaction, maternal depression, poverty, deficits in parenting information and skills, child abuse and neglect

  2. Accounts for between 3% to 5% of all pediatric admissions of infants less than one year with as many as 50% without underlying medical condition

  3. Males and females are equally affected

- Clinical Findings

  1. Inadequate intake—inadequate milk production, mechanical problems with suck/swallow coordination, systemic disease, errors in formula preparation, misunderstanding about infant needs and feeding practices

  2. Increased losses or decreased utilization—vomiting and/or malabsorption

3. Increased caloric requirements--underlying disease process including cardiac, respiratory, hyperthyroid, cancer, recurrent infection

4. Altered growth potential—prenatal insult, genetic disorder or endocrine dysfunction

- Differential Diagnosis

   1. Organic causes

      a. Gastrointestinal—gastroesophageal reflux (GER), pyloric stenosis, cleft palate, lactose intolerance, Hirschprung disease, milk-protein intolerance, hepatitis, malabsorption

      b. Cardiopulmonary—cardiac defects, bronchopulmonary dysplasia (BPD), asthma, cystic fibrosis (CF), tracheobronchial malformations

      c. Endocrine—hypothyroid, diabetes, adrenal insufficiency, pituitary disorders, growth hormone deficiency

      d. Infection—parasitic or bacterial, TB, HIV

      e. Neurologic—mental retardation, fetal alcohol syndrome, lead poisoning, prematurity, neuroregulatory difficulties

      f. Genetic—mitochondrial diseases

   2. Social-emotional and environmental causes

      a. Maternal depression, isolation, marital difficulties

      b. Poverty/inadequate resources

      c. Inadequate parenting knowledge and skills

      d. Difficult temperament

      e. Child abuse and neglect

- Diagnostic Methods/Findings

   1. History—prenatal, perinatal, neonatal; complete diet history and feeding practices; environmental, social, and family history

   2. Identification of risk factors—premature, LBW, difficult temperament, regulation problems, social stresses

   3. Height, weight, head circumference; review longitudinal growth data, corrected for gestational age as appropriate; vital signs including blood pressure if child is over 3 years

   4. Physical examination—signs of underlying organic disease; severity of malnutrition, evidence of abuse or neglect

   5. Developmental assessment and caregiver concerns

   6. Feeding observation to assess behavioral or interactional contributing factors

   7. Home visit or public health nurse referral to assess environmental factors.

   8. Laboratory assessment should be judicious based on history and clinical findings;

CBC, UA if applicable; serum creatinine, total protein/albumin; electrolyte screen; other labs as indicated by history, blood lead levels, TB test; thyroid function; test for reflux/malabsorption; sweat test, stool specimen for parasites; bone age if height is poor

- Management/Treatment
    1. Importance of developing therapeutic alliance with caregiver
    2. Usually managed on an outpatient basis if possible with hospitalization indicated when there is evidence of abuse or severe neglect, severe malnutrition, medical instability or when outpatient management has failed
    3. Interdisciplinary approach is optimal utilizing health care, nutritional, mental health and social services
    4. Provide caregivers with necessary information regarding nutritional needs of child and appropriate feeding skills to promote optimal growth
    5. Close monitoring and follow-up on growth and development, social environment and interdisciplinary/interagency communication

Stuttering

- Definition: Speech dysfluency with initial onset during the preschool years that is characterized by repetitions of sounds, syllables, and/or short words as well as pauses in timing of speech.
    1. Mild or developmental stuttering—speech dysfluency most notable when a preschool-aged child is tired or excited that usually resolves spontaneously if not given excessive attention
    2. Moderate or severe stuttering (sometimes referred to as acquired stuttering)—persistent speech dysfluency that is inappropriate for age and usually has a neurologic and/or psychogenic etiology
- Etiology/Incidence
    1. Multifactorial etiology with a 3:1 male to female ratio of occurrence
    2. Prevalence estimated at 1% among pre-pubertal children with decrease to 0.8% estimate post-puberty
    3. Mild developmental stuttering occurs in 4% to 5% of children between 2 to 5 years that spontaneously resolves; approximately 20% of early stuttering does not resolve without intervention
- Clinical Findings
    1. Repetition and/or prolongation of sounds, syllables or short words
    2. Pauses within words or sentences
    3. Signs of physical tension and struggling with speech such as eye blinking and trembling lips

4. Avoidance of words that cause particular problems

5. Child and/or parents are frustrated and/or embarrassed by stuttering posing difficulty at home, in school, or with peers

- Differential Diagnosis

    1. Normal developmental dysfluency

    2. Hearing impairment

    3. Speech-motor deficit

- Management/Treatment

    1. Assess frequency, type and duration of dysfluency

    2. Encourage parents to avoid excessive attention to dysfluency and be patient in listening to child's speech

    3. Refer to speech and language pathologist for assessment if child is showing signs of embarrassment, speech dysfluency interferes with communication and/or parent expresses significant concern regardless of severity

    4. Stuttering Foundation of America
       PO Box 11749
       Memphis, TN 38111-0749
       (800) 992-9392

Autism and Pervasive Developmental Disorder (PDD)

- Definition: Type of pervasive developmental disability characterized by a spectrum of symptoms and characteristics that may range in severity but usually manifest themselves within the first three years of life; symptoms include altered responses to sensory stimuli, impairments in communication, language, play and other social interactions; DSM-IV-TR and International Categories of Disease-10 (ICD-10) categorize PDD similarly to include:

    1. Autistic disorder or autism

    2. Pervasive developmental disorder, not otherwise specified (PDD-NOS) or atypical autism

    3. Asperger's syndrome

    4. Rett's disorder

    5. Childhood disintegrative disorder

- Etiology/Incidence

    1. Underlying neurological disorder caused by brain insult/injury during fetal development and not by psychosocial circumstances as previously believed

    2. Associated etiological factors include genetic link (10%) as well as history of perinatal infection; no clear etiological determination for majority of children with autism

3. Rates are 4 times higher among males than females; occurrence in females tends to be severe; no racial, ethnic, or socioeconomic differences; epidemiological data indicate overall incidence rates of 2 to 5 per 10,000

- Clinical Findings

    1. Normal growth and development usually reported until 2 to 2 $\frac{1}{2}$ years when parents notice delays in language, symbolic or imaginative play, and/or other social interactions; onset of such delay or abnormal behavioral pattern before 3 years of age is considered part of diagnostic criteria.

    2. DSM-IV-TR (2000) diagnostic criteria require a total of six behavioral manifestations from three categories including:

        a. Qualitative impairment in social interaction—poor eye contact; lack of shared enjoyment in activities with peers or family

        b. Qualitative impairment in communication—delayed or deviant language development; lack of interest in toys, activities for symbolic or imaginative play appropriate for age

        c. Restrictive repetitive and stereotypic patterns of behavior, interests and/or activities—repetitive rituals or motor movements such as spinning or hand flapping

    3. Associated problems may include other cognitive delays, problems learning, unusual responses to sensory stimuli, difficulties with sleeping and eating, differences in emotional responsiveness, and seizure activity

    4. Significant variation in clusters of symptoms and characteristics ranging from mild to severely affected

- Diagnostic Tests/Findings

    1. No specific medical diagnostic test for autism

    2. EEG indicated for associated problems including seizures and language delay

    3. Laboratory studies to assess etiological factors

        a. Urine amino acids and organic acids; metabolic screen for metabolic disorders such as PKU

        b. DNA probe for fragile X on blood plasma

    4. MRI or CT scan may show structural abnormalities in cerebellum but otherwise not particularly helpful in absence of clinical signs such as asymmetries, focal tremors or paralyses

- Differential Diagnosis

    1. Mental retardation

    2. Sensory impairment (hearing or vision)

    3. Severe abuse or neglect

4. Subtypes of pervasive developmental disorders

5. Childhood psychosis

6. Gifted child

7. Tourette's syndrome

8. Fragile X

- Management/Treatment

    1. No specific medical interventions currently available

    2. Early screening, diagnosis and referral to early intervention is critical

    3. Treatment is primarily psychoeducation requiring individualized plan

    4. Interdisciplinary team to coordinate care including parents, teachers, primary care provider, psychologist, physical therapy, speech and language and other early intervention staff as appropriate

    5. Address associated problems through specific therapies (sensory integration) counseling (family adjustment, behavioral management), medications (seizures and behavioral problems)

    6. Community education, resource identification and parent-to-parent support

        a. Autism Society of America
        7910 Woodmont Avenue, Suite 650
        Bethesda, MD 20814-3015

        b. CHAT—checklist for autism in toddlers (Baron-Cohen, Cox, Baird, Swettenham, Nightengale, Morgan, Drew, & Chaman, 1996)

Obesity

- Definition

    1. Excess accumulation of body fat relative to lean body mass that results from excessive caloric intake relative to energy expenditure

    2. Operational definitions (cut-off values) vary in the literature

- Etiology/Incidence

    1. Multifactorial etiology with interaction of genetic, environmental, developmental and behavioral factors

        a. Genetic predisposition and parental obesity

        b. Dietary patterns

        c. Inactivity (television, video games)

        d. Cultural and familial food preferences

        e. Use of food as emotional buffer

f. Physical disorders with decreased energy expenditure (spina bifida, Down syndrome, Prader-Willi syndrome)

2. Most prevalent nutritional problem in U.S.

3. Childhood obesity prevalence is rising with current estimates ranging from 15% to 30% depending on definition and cut-off values

- Clinical Findings

  1. Parent and/or child concern regarding body weight

  2. Clinical observation of large size and/or excess fat on child

- Differential Diagnosis

  1. Endocrine dysfunction

  2. Congenital disorders/short stature

  3. Large frame

  4. Muscular hypertrophy

  5. Medication induced obesity (corticosteroids, psychotropic drugs)

- Diagnostic Tests/Findings

  1. History includes detailed dietary and activity level history (past and present), family history of obesity and related morbidities including hypertension, cardiovascular disease, hyperlipidemia, diabetes, depression; review of systems for associated morbidity (glucose intolerance, orthopedic difficulties); developmental milestones, psychosocial concerns about weight

  2. Physical examination, vital signs, blood pressure

  3. Anthropometric measurements

     a. Weight for height ratio greater than 95th percentile on NCHS growth charts is commonly used but doesn't account for large frame or increased muscle mass

     b. Percent of ideal body weight greater or equal to 120%; calculated by dividing child's actual weight by ideal body weight (50th percentile for age and sex) and multiplied by 100

     c. Skin-fold thickness per calibrated caliper measurements at or above 85th percentile for age, sex, and race; tricep measurements are most common and reference charts are available

     d. Body Mass Index (BMI) considered most useful index

        (1) Weight in kilograms/height in meters^2

        (2) Screening classifications using BMI in adolescents

           (a) Obesity—BMI equal or greater than 95th percentile for age and gender

      (b)   At risk for obesity—between 85th and 95th percentile or with rapid weight gain of > 2 BMI units in one year

    (3)   No current consensus on BMI classification of obesity among younger children

    (4)   More recent reference percentiles provide age, gender and ethnic-specific distributions (Rosner, Prineas, Loggie & Daniels, 1998)

  e.   New NHANES III growth chart reference standards will include BMI distributions

  4.   CBC, UA, thyroid function, lipid profile

- Management/Treatment

  1.   Prevention in infancy through parent education regarding nutritional needs and feeding strategies

  2.   Discuss moderate modification of diet and caloric content while increasing exercise program

  3.   Goal for younger child is weight maintenance rather than weight reduction while linear growth catches up; goal for adolescent may include weight reduction if treated after growth spurt

  4.   Behavior modification strategies directed at alternative coping measures to deal with stress, maintain motivation, and reinforce regimen

  5.   Involvement of family in therapeutic program increases likelihood of success

  6.   Refer to and collaborate with available community resources as appropriate

Child Abuse and Neglect

- Definition: Abuse usually refers to actual "acts of commission" and neglect refers to "acts of omission" although there remains no consensus on specific definitions

  1.   First described as "Battered Child Syndrome" by Dr. Henry Kempe in 1962

  2.   Legal definitions and reporting requirements vary from State to State but all 50 States have mandated reporting of suspected abuse or neglect by health care providers

  3.   Categories include physical, sexual and emotional abuse, negligent care, and Munchausen syndrome by proxy (MSP)

    a.   Soft tissue injuries most common—bruises, abrasions and lacerations

    b.   Head injuries less frequent but cause majority of deaths— "Shaken Baby Syndrome" (altered consciousness with or without signs of head injuries)

    c.   Burns account for 10% of abuse injuries

    d.   Abdominal injuries—usually blunt injuries from hitting or kicking; liver lacerations; kidney/pancreas contusions

     e.   Fractures—rib, spiral and multiple fractures at same or various ages should trigger suspicion

     f.   Sexual abuse—probably least reported and underdiagnosed

     g.   Munchausen syndrome by proxy (MSP)—disturbed parent-child relationship with fabrication or actual harm to produce symptoms of illness requiring medical attention

- Etiology/Incidence:

1. Etiological factors associated with abuse and neglect

     a.   Perpetrator—history of being maltreated as a child; cognitive or psychiatric impairment; socially isolated; inadequate parenting knowledge and skills including unrealistic expectations of child

     b.   Victim—unwanted pregnancy; difficult temperament; premature and/or disabled; no significant gender differences

     c.   Social context—violence (family/community); poverty; unemployment; substance abuse

2. An estimated one million children were victims of substantiated reports to Child Protective Services (CPS) from 47 states in 1996 (U.S. Department of Health and Human Services, 1998)

     a.   Neglect (52%) is most common form of maltreatment followed by physical abuse (24%), sexual abuse (12%), emotional abuse (6%), medical neglect (3%) and other forms (16%)

     b.   Approximately equal numbers of males (48%) and females (52%) experienced documented child maltreatment in 1996

     c.   African-American and Native American children had rates twice as high as national average

     d.   Most (80%) perpetrators are parents

3. Child abuse/neglect is a significant cause of pediatric mortality in infants (second to SIDS) and young children (second to accidents)

     a.   1,077 deaths resulting from abuse or neglect were reported in 1996

     b.   Most deaths (75%) were of children 3 years or younger

- Clinical Findings

1. History is vague, inconsistent and/or incompatible with child's developmental stage and severity of injury

2. History may change during course of interview

3. Delay in seeking medical attention for injury

4. History of recurrent injuries

5. Soft tissue injuries with markings characteristic of source of abuse such as hand marks, curved mark of a belt, burn mark in shape of electric iron

6. Bruises in various stages of healing

7. Burn markings characteristic of immersion

8. Undernutrition, poor hygiene

9. Developmental delays

10. Inappropriate parent-child interaction

- Differential Diagnosis

    1. Unintentional injury

    2. Inadequate parenting skills

    3. Underlying disease process, e.g., hemophilia, leukemia, osteogenesis imperfecta

    4. Birth marks, Mongolian spots, and/or other variations in skin pigmentation

    5. Folk-medicine and cultural practices, e.g., coin rubbing

    6. Sudden Infant Death Syndrome (SIDS)

- Diagnostic Tests/Findings

    1. History to determine and precisely document type of injury, alleged circumstances and action taken by caregiver

    2. Observation of parent and child for behavioral extremes or exaggerated responses

    3. Physical examination to assess location, type, and characteristic of any lesions or burns for characteristic pattern, shape or outline; bruises should be noted for coloring

    4. Coagulation studies for severe bruising; radiographs of long bones, ribs and/or skull series as indicated by history and physical examination; ultrasound for suspected visceral injury

- Management/Treatment

    1. Appropriate medical care for child including immediate hospitalization if indicated by severity of injuries

    2. Ensure safety of child utilizing foster care or relatives if necessary

    3. Communicate identified concerns (moderate or severe injuries or threats to child's well-being) and legal imperative to notify child protective services as a mandated reporter of suspected child maltreatment

    4. Assessment of siblings for maltreatment and assurance of safety

    5. Identify and make appropriate referrals to available community resources to facilitate interdisciplinary and interagency collaboration—child protective services, public health, parenting classes, child care/school programs

    6. Education and prevention

    a. Identify families with risk factors associated with child maltreatment and make referrals to appropriate community-based preventive resources before serious abuse occurs

    b. Close primary care supervision and acute care follow-up for at-risk families and children

    c. Early reporting of suspected abuse or neglect

    d. Support community-based child abuse prevention efforts

Attention Deficit Hyperactivity Disorder (ADHD)

- Definition

    1. A behavioral syndrome characterized by a persistent pattern of inattention, poor concentration, impulsivity and overactivity that exceeds normal developmental variation

    2. DSM-IV-TR (2000) defined sub-types

       a. Attention deficit/hyperactivity disorder—predominantly inattention type

       b. Attention deficit/hyperactivity disorder—predominantly hyperactive-impulsive type

       c. Attention deficit disorder—combined type

- Etiology/Incidence

    1. Multifactorial etiology that remains poorly understood but may be associated with:

       a. Delayed CNS maturation

       b. Genetic factors

       c. Prenatal, perinatal, or postnatal trauma or illness

       d. Dysfunction of catecholamine neurotransmitters

       e. Male-to-female ratio ranges from 4:1 (general population) to 9:1 (clinic populations)

    2. Controlled studies have not demonstrated evidence of additives, sugar or salicylates as associated factors

    3. Approximately 3% to 5% of school-aged children meet DSM-IV criteria

- Clinical Findings: DSM-IV-TR (2000) diagnostic criteria for ADHD include:

    1. Six (or more) symptoms of inattention

       a. Poor attention to detail/careless mistakes

       b. Difficulty maintaining attention during activities

       c. Failure to listen even when directly spoken to

       d. Problems following directions and/or with completion of assignments or tasks

       e. Disorganized in activities and tasks

   f.   Avoids activities that require focused mental attention

   g.   Frequently loses items necessary for successful completion of task, activity or assignment

   h.   Easily distracted by external stimuli

   i.   Forgetful
         or

2.   Six (or more) symptoms of hyperactivity/impulsivity

   a.   Fidgets and squirms

   b.   Difficulty staying seated when expected or appropriate

   c.   Excessive running and climbing

   d.   Difficulty with quiet play activities

   e.   Very high energy and activity level

   f.   Excessively verbal and talkative

   g.   Answers questions abruptly before question is completed

   h.   Difficulty waiting for turn

   i.   Frequently interrupts others and acts intrusively
         and

3.   Symptom onset prior to 7 years of age

4.   Symptoms identified as problemsome in at least two settings, e.g., home and school

5.   Negative impact of symptoms on social, academic and/or work performance

6.   Symptoms not attributed to more significant underlying psychiatric or medical disorder

- Differential Diagnosis

   1.   Age appropriate for highly active child

   2.   Inadequate environments (understimulating or chaotic)

   3.   Learning disabilities/sensory impairment

   4.   Seizures or mental retardation

   5.   Situational anxiety and/or depressive reaction

   6.   Oppositional behavior and/or conduct disorder

- Diagnostic Tests/Findings

   1.   History—Perinatal (maternal substance abuse); past (early health problems including ear infections, lead poisoning, iron deficiency anemia, frequent injuries due to activity), present (frequency, severity and context of symptoms at home and school); social and developmental; parenting style; review of systems

2. Physical examination, screen for "neurological soft signs;" affective behavior; laboratory data of limited value; CBC, lead screen

3. Height, weight, blood pressure, vital signs

4. Vision and hearing screen

5. Sample behavioral assessment from multiple settings—(home, babysitter/child care, relatives, school) using rating scale of direct observation

   a. Connor's Abbreviated Parent-Teacher Questionnaire

   b. ADHD Comprehensive Teacher rating scale

   c. Achenbach and Edelbrach's Child Behavior Checklist

   d. Edelbrach Child Attention Problem Scale

   e. DuPaul ADHD Rating Scale for Teachers

6. Psychological evaluation and cognitive testing

- Management/Treatment

  1. Provide structured environment—regular routine, clear and simple rules, firm limits, minimize distraction, overstimulation and fatigue

  2. Behavioral management—formal operant conditioning techniques to reward/reinforce good behaviors; punishment strategies (time-out) or extinction techniques (systematic ignoring) to decrease unacceptable behaviors

  3. Evaluate need for mental health referral

     a. Child-based therapy for depression, anxiety, low self-esteem; cognitive-behavioral training to increase self-control

     b. Parenting classes or family therapy for relationship difficulties

  4. CNS stimulant medication—(children > 5 years)

     a. Methylphenidate—effective in 75% to 80% with trial of at least 2 to 3 weeks; give 20 to 30 minutes before meals to maximize activity; avoid p.m. doses to minimize insomnia

     b. Dextroamphetamine—effectiveness in 70% to 75% with rapid response

     c. Amphetamine mixture—newer drug being utilized that is a combination of dextroamphetamine and amphetamine; onset of action is slower and smoother than methylphenidate or dextroamphetamine; adequate clinical trials are still pending

     d. Magnesium pemoline—effective in 65% to 70% with trial of 2 to 3 weeks; can cause liver toxicity

     e. Desipramine and imipramine (tricyclic antidepressants)—effectiveness with 60% to 70% when other medications are ineffective or have unacceptable side-effects; may work better with children having underlying depression

5. Close follow-up assessment and monitoring of growth and response to medication and behavioral management plan every 3 to 4 months

6. Ongoing coordination and communication with family, school personnel, primary care provider and mental health resources is critical to successful management

7. Medication may be discontinued after 2 to 3 month trial if no change in behavior

8. Non-conventional treatments (no documented evidence of effectiveness in controlled studies)

    a. Megavitamins/mineral therapy

    b. Elimination of sugar, additives, coloring

    c. Neurophysiologic interventions (patterning, sensory integration, optometric training)

9. Community resources

    a. Children and Adults with Attention Deficit Disorder (CHADD)
       International non-profit parent support organization
       499 N.W. 70th Ave., Suite 109
       Plantation, Florida 33317
       (305) 587-3700

    b. National Attention Deficit Disorder Association
       (800) 487-2282
       http://www.add.org

Aggression, Defiance and Disruptive Behavioral Disorders

- Normal behavior vs. dysfunctional patterns and clinical disorders

    1. Most children manifest some degree of developmentally normative aggressive, defiant and disruptive behavior during infancy and early childhood, e.g., breath-holding, temper tantrums, lying, fighting, breaking things

    2. Almost half of all parents consult with primary care providers regarding difficulty managing disruptive and defiant behaviors of their preschoolers

    3. Repetitive and persistent patterns of aggressive, defiant, and disruptive behaviors lasting over 6 months warrant detailed assessment and possible mental health referral

- Conduct Disorder: A repetitive and persistent dysfunctional pattern of aggressive behavior and/or violation of the law, social norms, and basic human rights

    1. Etiology/Incidence

        a. Multifactorial etiology—biological-genetic component suggested from twin/adoption studies

        b. Child onset (less than 10 years) has graver prognosis with increased risk of later substance abuse and anti-social personality disorder than adolescent-onset

c. Incidence greater among males with estimates of 6% to 16%; female estimates of 2% to 9%

2. Clinical Findings—DSM-IV-TR (2000) criteria include:

   a. Aggressive/threatening behavior to people or animals

   b. Deliberate, intentional destruction of property

   c. Lying, stealing

   d. Serious rule violations such as staying out all night, running away, truancy

3. Differential Diagnosis:

   a. Adjustment disorder

   b. ADHD

   c. Oppositional-defiant disorder

   d. Manic episode

4. Diagnostic Tests/Findings

   a. Separate interview with parent and child

   b. Assessment of parental anxiety regarding dependency/control issues; impact on family functioning

   c. Severity of behaviors with respect to intensity, frequency, duration, context, and developmental stage

   d. Identify contributing psychosocial risk factors—poverty, abuse, neglect, exposure to violence, parental mental illness and/or substance abuse

5. Management/Treatment

   a. Identify and communicate concern for child and family well-being

   b. Refer for psychological/psychiatric evaluation and intervention

   c. Refer to social service and/or other community resources for parenting education, support, and to reduce family stress and potential for violence

- Oppositional-Defiant Disorder: A repetitive and persistent dysfunctional pattern characterized by negative, disobedient, defiant and hostile behavior directed at authority figures

  1. Etiology/Incidence

     a. Multifactorial etiology associated with difficult temperament, disruption in early caregiving environment, harsh, inconsistent and/or neglectful parenting; history of psychiatric disorder in at least one parent including maternal depression

     b. Incidence among males is greater than females until puberty after which rates become more equal; overall estimates range from 2% to 16% depending on population

  2. Clinical Findings

    a. Loses temper easily

    b. Argumentative with adult authority figures

    c. Actively defiant of rules and adult requests

    d. Deliberately annoys other people

    e. Blames others for mistakes and misbehavior

    f. Edgy and easily annoyed

    g. Frequently resentful or angry

    h. Spiteful and vindictive behavior

3. Differential Diagnosis

    a. Within normal range of oppositional behavior for age and developmental level

    b. Conduct disorder

    c. ADHD

    d. Mental retardation

4. Management/Treatment

    a. Early identification and monitoring of defiant, aggressive, and oppositional behaviors

    b. Parenting education, support, and effective discipline

    c. Refer for family therapy/intervention if child manifests four or more of clinical behavioral features that have persisted for longer than 6 months

Learning Disabilities (LD)

- Definition

    1. Generic term referring to a heterogeneous cluster of disorders manifested by significant difficulties in the acquisition and use of language, listening, reading (dyslexia), writing (dysgraphia), reasoning, or mathematical abilities (dyscalculia)

    2. School performance in deficit areas significantly below that expected for age, grade, and level of intelligence

- Etiology/Incidence

    1. Multifactorial etiology of genetic and environmental factors

    2. Possible abnormal function in parietal and/or occipital lobes of brain

    3. Conditions associated with LD

        a. Developmental delay

        b. Lead poisoning

        c. Fetal alcohol syndrome

       d.   Fragile-X syndrome

   4.   General prevalence estimated at 6% to 11% of school-age children

   5.   Dyslexia—most common LD, affects 2% to 10% of general population

- Clinical Findings

   1.   Specific academic skill deficits

       a.   Basic reading skills, reading comprehension, spelling

       b.   Mathematical calculations and reasoning

       c.   Disorders of written expression and writing skills

   2.   Perceptual-motor impairments

       a.   Distinguishing shapes and sizes

       b.   Fine motor skills, e.g., writing, coloring, cutting

       c.   May make letter and number reversals

   3.   Memory and thinking impairment (integrative processing)

       a.   Haphazard, ineffective study habits and strategies for memorization

       b.   Sequencing of data

       c.   Understanding abstract concepts, e.g., time, space, parts, whole

       d.   Lacking skills for effective problem-solving and task completion

   4.   Speech and language deficits

       a.   Language delay

       b.   Difficulty with grammar (syntax), meaning (semantics) and/or social use of words (pragmatics)

   5.   Attention deficits—difficulty concentrating and staying on task

   6.   Hyperactivity—difficulty sitting still, constantly in motion

   7.   Impulsiveness

       a.   Often acting without thinking

       b.   Poor planning skills

       c.   Lack of self-regulation skills

   8.   General deficits in coordination—clumsiness

   9.   Emotional problems

       a.   Lability and moodiness

       b.   Often isolated or rejected by peers

       c.   May exhibit inappropriate attention-getting behaviors

       d.   Difficulty reading nonverbal social cues

e. May be passive learners

- Differential Diagnosis

  1. Undiagnosed sensory impairment—vision or hearing deficits

  2. Attention deficit hyperactivity disorder (ADHD)

  3. Seizure disorder

  4. Mental retardation

  5. Maladaptation to chronic disease

  6. Social and environmental factors

     a. Child abuse and neglect

     b. Situational anxiety or depressive reaction

     c. Ethnic or cultural minority

- Physical Findings

  1. Neurological soft signs commonly present

     a. Poor fine motor coordination and tactile discrimination

     b. Strabismus

     c. Poor hand-eye coordination

     d. Balance problems

  2. Phenotypic features of associated conditions—FAS, Fragile-X

  3. Other abnormal physical findings likely to be related to LD

- Diagnostic Studies/Findings: Diagnosis requires multidimensional assessment

  1. Complete medical and social history

  2. Developmental and behavioral history

  3. Educational history and school functioning

  4. Physical examination—soft neurological signs

  5. Laboratory studies—associated conditions

     a. Lead screening

     b. EEG if seizures suspected

  6. Psychoeducational testing

  7. Analysis of history, test results, and academic achievement leads to diagnosis

- Managment/Treatment

  1. Developmental surveillance, early identification and referral is critical

  2. Early intervention to optimize learning and minimize emotional sequelae

3. Thorough psychoeducational evaluation to determine skills and deficits

4. Interdisciplinary conference to evaluate findings (M-team)

5. Individualized education plan (IEP) developed based on multidimentional assessment

6. Yearly re-evaluation of IEP with revisions as needed

7. Address other associated behavioral, social and family issues through counseling and direct instruction

8. Inform parents of legal rights under Individuals with Disabilities Education Act (IDEA) and availability of appropriate special services

Eating Disorders: Anorexia Nervosa and Bulimia Nervosa

- Definition: Chronic and often severe disturbances in eating behavior accompanied by distorted perception of body weight, size and shape

    1. Anorexia nervosa—eating disturbance associated with weight loss and refusal to maintain body weight at minimally normal level (85% of expected body weight for age and sex) with subsequent amenorrhea

    2. Bulimia nervosa—eating disturbance associated with episodic binge eating followed by compensatory efforts to prevent weight gain (self-induced vomiting, dieting, fasting, excessive exercise or misuse of laxatives, enemas and/or diuretics)

    3. Anorexia may occur with or without associated binging/purging (restricting vs. binge-eating/purging types); bulimia may occur with or without purging (purging vs. non-purging types)

- Etiology/Incidence

    1. Family enmeshment hypothesis—rigid, overprotective families with difficulty with conflict resolution; separation-individuation

    2. Fear of sexual maturation; history of sexual abuse

    3. Social pressure to be thin

    4. Ballet dancers and gymnasts at particular risk

    5. Associated with psychological profile of low self-esteem in spite of outward successfulness.

    6. Both disorders are more common among females.

    7. Anorexia affects approximately 1% of white middle/upper class females; 5% to 10% of cases are male often associated with gender identity conflict

    8. Bimodal distribution with one peak at 14 years and second at 18 years

    9. Bulimia is more common than anorexia with later age onset

    10. Suicide rates of 2% to 5% of those with chronic anorexia with overall mortality rate as high as 10%

11. Normal to high intelligence, overachievers, perfectionists

- Clinical Findings

    1. Self-imposed weight loss

    2. Anemia, jaundice, and secondary amenorrhea

    3. Vigorous exercise regimen to increase weight loss

    4. Constipation (chronic laxatives) and reflux esophagitis (self-induced vomiting)

    5. Dry skin, brittle nails

    6. Lower body temperature, blood pressure and heart rate

    7. Lanugo

    8. Sore throat, calluses on dorsum of fingers, loss of tooth enamel (from induced vomiting)

- Differential Diagnosis

    1. General medical condition—gastrointestinal disease, diabetes, thyroid disorder, AIDS, systemic lupus erythematosus

    2. Pregnancy

    3. Depressive disorder or substance abuse

- Diagnostic Tests/Findings

    1. History—include nutritional patterns as well as effort to lose weight (dieting, exercise, vomiting); preoccupation with food and/or feeling "fat"; past medical, family and social; review of systems (amenorrhea)

    2. Weight and height percentiles—degree of malnutrition determined as percentage below ideal weight (IBW)

        a. Mild malnutrition— < 20% below IBW

        b. Moderate malnutrition—20% to 30% below IBW

        c. Severe malnutrition— > 30% below IBW

    3. Physical examination—signs of malnutrition; dry skin, brittle nails, muscle weakness, flat affect, decreased blood pressure, pulse and body temperature; Tanner staging delays

    4. CBC, serum albumin, glucose, electrolytes, thyroid function, ECG; others as appropriate based on history and clinical findings

- Management/Treatment

    1. Interdisciplinary treatment plan including nutritional intervention, behavior modification techniques, psychotherapy (individual, family and/or group therapy), pharmacologic management with antidepressants if appropriate

    2. Hospitalization for rehydration and refeeding if condition warrants

3. Approximately one half of patients show varying degrees of improvement; 25% show long-term improvement; 25% do poorly regardless of intervention

4. Refer to appropriate community resources for assessment tool, support and education:

Eating Disorder Inventory-2
Psychological Assessment Resources, Inc.
PO Box 998
Odessa, Florida 33556

Foundation for Education about Eating Disorders
PO Box 1637
Baltimore, MD 21210
(410) 467-0603

The American Anorexia and Bulimia Association
293 Central Park West, Suite 1R
NY, NY 10024
(212) 501-8351
http://members.aol.com/amambu

National Association of Anorexia Nervosa and Associated Disorders
PO Box 7
Highland Park, IL 60035
(847) 831-3438
http://www.anad.org

Childhood Depression

- Definition: Behavioral pattern lasting at least two weeks that is characterized by affective and behavioral symptoms including sad or tearful moods, irritability and/or social withdrawal with associated decreased interest and pleasure in developmentally appropriate activities

- Etiology/Incidence: Multifactorial etiology with associated risk factors including:

1. History of traumatic event(s) involving significant separation(s) or loss(s) of parent, caregiver or significant other

2. Family history of depression especially in mother; evidence of genetic component from twin and adoption studies

3. Chronic neglect and lack of nurturance due to family disruptions or dysfunction including long-term effects of poverty and/or homelessness

4. Substance abuse, physical or sexual abuse in household

5. Chronic illness and/or disability may increase risk especially with familial predisposition

6. Estimated incidence of 3% for overall pediatric population and as high as 9% for adolescents; no gender differences in early childhood depression but increases among females in adolescence with ratio of 5:1

- Clinical Findings

  1. Major depressive episode—significant distress and/or interference with normal daily functioning lasting at least 2 weeks associated with:

     a. Depressed or irritable mood and/or decreased interest and pleasure in developmentally appropriate activities and a minimum of 4 additional symptoms

     b. Appetite changes with associated weight gain or loss

     c. Insomnia or hypersomnia

     d. Difficulty concentrating; decline in school performance

     e. Feelings of worthlessness, guilt, fearfulness, isolation

     f. Social withdrawal from friends, family, school refusal and/or truancy

     g. General somatic complaints of aches and pains with non-specific etiology, e.g., fatigue, headaches, stomachaches

     h. Agitation, irritability and/or disruptive behavior

     i. Recurrent thoughts of death and/or suicidal ideation

  2. Dysthymic disorder—long-standing depressed or irritable mood lasting one year or more but symptoms of distress and interference with normal daily functioning not as pronounced as a major depressive episode

  3. Adjustment disorder with depressed mood—depressed or irritable mood, sadness, tearfulness and/or feelings of hopelessness causing some degree of impairment of daily functioning that occurs within 3 months of a significant and identifiable stressful life event

- Differential Diagnosis

  1. Normal periods of sadness and/or mood swings

  2. Acute depressive reactions/adjustment disorder with depressed mood in response to identifiable life stress

  3. Masked depressive disorder—somatization and denial of feelings

  4. Underlying physical disorder

  5. Substance abuse

  6. Psychiatric depressive disorder with suicidal risk

- Diagnostic Tests/Findings

  1. Behavioral symptoms according to DSM-IV-TR diagnostic criteria

  2. History—developmental, family, social and school; current medications; chronic disease/disability

  3. Separate interview with child or adolescent is essential

  4. Physical examination—neurological screening

5. Height, weight, vital signs, assess for recent weight loss or gain

6. Laboratory tests—as indicated by history (drug screen; pregnancy test)

- Management/Treatment

   1. Early screening and identification of children and adolescents at risk for depression

      a. Center for Epidemiologic Studies Depression Scale for Children

      b. Children's Depression Rating Scale

      c. Children's Depression Inventory

      d. Child Behavior Checklist

      e. Rose Institute Adolescent Depression Scale

      f. Mood Questionnaire for Adolescents

   2. Evaluate severity of depression including suicidal risk and make appropriate referrals

   3. Psychiatric intervention is necessary for major depressive episode or dysthymic disorder

      a. Family and/or individual psychotherapy

      b. Pharmacotherapy—may be included as part of multimodal treatment plan

         (1) Selective serotonin reuptake inhibitors (SSRI)—most effective medication for major depressive episodes (fluoxetine or sertraline)

         (2) Tricyclic antidepressants have limited clinical use with equivocal effectiveness demonstrated in controlled studies (monitor blood levels)

   4. Supportive counseling for adjustment disorder with depressed mood

   5. Resources

      Depression/Awareness, Recognition, and Treatment (D/ART)
      National Institutes of Mental Health
      Room 10-85
      5600 Fishers Lane
      Rockville, Maryland 20857

Suicidal Behavior

- Definition: Passive or active thoughts/wishes about death and dying (suicidal ideation); talking and/or threatening to take one's life, or self-injury without intent to die (suicidal gesture); deliberate self-injury with the intent to die but not resulting in death (suicide attempt) and self-inflicted death (completed suicide)

- Etiology/Incidence

   1. Accounts for 10% of teenage deaths representing second leading cause of adolescent mortality

2. 15% to 40% of completed suicides were preceded by one or more suicide gestures/attempts

3. Females have higher rates of suicide attempts; males have higher rates of completed suicides

4. Higher rates among Native American, Asian, and chronically ill adolescents

5. Ingestion of medication is most common method; violent methods (hanging and shooting) are more frequently used by males than females and are more often fatal

- Clinical Findings

   1. Severe and/or chronic depression

   2. Hopelessness

   3. Previous suicidal gestures

   4. History of suicide in family

   5. Existence of specific plan

- Differential Diagnosis

   1. Unintentional injuries due to carelessness and/or adolescent sense of "invincibility"

   2. Suicidal gesture as desperate call for help

   3. Imminent risk/acute suicidal intent

   4. Psychotic episode

- Diagnostic Tests/Findings

   1. History—past and present health, chronic depression, chronic illness or disability; school performance; family history of depression and/ or suicide; current medications; substance abuse

   2. Suicidal risk—suicidal ideation, extent of premeditation and existence of plan; likelihood of rescue; suicide notes, previous suicidal gestures

   3. Observation and/or reports of suicidal behavior by family, teachers, or peers

- Management/Treatment

   1. Refer immediately for crisis intervention resources, e.g., 24 hour hot-line

   2. Suicidal ideation and/or gestures with existence of plan requires immediate psychological evaluation

   3. Assure safe environment for child/adolescent including hospitalization if necessary

   4. Short-term hospitalization is recommended for all suicide attempts; attending to emergency treatment and/or surgical management is necessary but insufficient without additional follow-up intervention

   5. Treat underlying depression

6. Inform child/adolescent of seriousness of concern and need to notify family and mobilize necessary community resources

    a. The Youth Suicide National Center
1825 I Street NW
Washington, DC 20006
(202) 429-0190

    b. National Adolescent Suicide Hotline
(800) 621-4000

    c. American Association of Suicidology
2459 South Ash
Denver, Colorado 80222
(303) 692-0985
http://www.cyberpsych.org/aas.htm.

Substance Abuse (Tobacco, Alcohol, and Other Drugs)

- Definition: Use of any drug or chemical for purposes of stimulation, pleasure or in a way that interferes with normal functioning and/or threatens health; includes misuse of legal 'recreational' drugs, prescribed or non-prescribed medications, as well as illegal substances; DSM-IV-TR distinguishes substance abuse from dependence (APA, 1994):

  1. Substance abuse—a maladaptive pattern of substance use associated with significant impairment or distress including inability to meet expected daily obligations, use of substance in situations/context that may be hazardous to self or others, and/or resulting in legal and/or other interpersonal conflicts

  2. Substance dependence—a pattern of repeated substance abuse that results in tolerance, withdrawal, and/or compulsive use that can be psychological and/or physiologic-based

  3. Categories of substances include—alcohol; marijuana (cannabis); nicotine; amphetamines; caffeine; cocaine; hallucinogens; inhalants; opioids; phencyclidine (PCP); sedatives and hypnotics; anabolic steroids

- Etiology/Incidence

  1. Multifactorial etiology including some evidence of biological predisposition along with psychosocial and environmental risks such as impulsivity, non-conformity/rebellion, peer pressure, ineffective coping with stress, undiagnosed depression, family dysfunction, history of child abuse or neglect, parental substance abuse

  2. Majority of adolescents will engage in some form of drug use at some point

  3. More frequent use of all substances among males vs. females

  4. Highest overall incidence of substance abuse among Caucasian teen-agers followed by Hispanic youth, lowest incidence among African-American teen-agers (O'Malley, Johnston, & Bachman, 1995)

5. Most recent national drug use survey reported increasing prevalence of current illicit drug use—11.4% teen-agers from 12 to 17 years of age (SAMSA, 1998)

- Clinical Findings:

   1. Nicotine—decreased exercise tolerance, fatigue, muscle weakness; pallor; tachycardia; staining of teeth; tobacco odor on breath and clothes

   2. Alcohol—initial euphoria and talkativeness; grogginess; impaired short-term memory; decreased reaction time; hypoglycemia

   3. Marijuana (THC, pot, cannabis, joint, reefer, weed, hash, grass)—euphoria; drowsiness; slowed reaction time and motor coordination; time distortions; tachycardia and transient hypertension; blood shot eyes

   4. Amphetamines—dilated pupils, tachycardia, anorexia, insomnia, weight loss, anxiety and suicidal behavior

   5. Cocaine (coke, free-base, crack, nose, flake)—agitation, hyperactivity, euphoria followed by depression, confused thinking, occasional paranoid ideation; tachycardia; habitual ''snorting'' induced nasal septum scabbing or necrosis

   6. Hallucinogens

      a. LSD—dilated pupils; visual and auditory hallucinations and flashbacks; disorganized and confused thinking; increased attention to stimuli; chronic use can lead to psychosis and major personality changes

      b. PCP—euphoria, motor incoordination, hallucinations; paranoia with aggressive/violent behavior

   7. Inhalants/volatile substances (glue, hydrocarbons)—relaxation, hallucinations, light headedness, giddiness; seizures, coma, cardiac arrhythmias and sudden death

   8. Anabolic steroids—used to increase muscle mass and strength (non-substantiated effect); fluid retention, mood swings, menstrual abnormalities; male gynecomastia, female hirsutism, breast atrophy

   9. Opiates include naturally occurring (e.g., morphine, codeine); semisynthetic (e.g., heroine, dilaudid) and synthetic (e.g., fentanyl, meperidine, methadone); constricted pupils; respiratory depression; euphoria, analgesia; dermatologic lesions ''tracks''; tattoos in unusual places to conceal track marks; chronic infections (skin, HIV, scarring and cellulitis); constipation, decrease in libido; urinary retention

- Differential Diagnosis

   1. Social recreational use of legal substances

   2. Experimentation vs. abuse

   3. Chronic depression

   4. Neurological disorder

   5. Learning disabilities

- Diagnostic Tests/Findings

  1. History—past and present, environmental, family, social, and academic history; review of systems; current medications; specific drug history including specific drugs, frequency of use, settings of use, impairment of daily functioning including suspensions or legal difficulties

  2. Interviews with and observations from child/adolescent, parents, school personnel, peers

  3. Physical examination with close assessment of skin integrity (nasal septum, skin lesions/track marks); neurological assessment; vital signs, weight, height, blood pressure

  4. Serum and urine toxicology; HIV testing; others as appropriate to specific history

- Management/Treatment

  1. Assure appropriate privacy, confidentiality and non-judgmental atmosphere

  2. Referral to appropriate substance abuse treatment resources

  3. Identify and provide appropriate referrals for management of underlying psychosocial difficulties contributing to substance abuse

  4. Educate and counsel regarding legal and physical risks of substance abuse

  5. Support community-based prevention programs

  6. Additional National Resources

     National Institute on Drug Abuse (NIDA)
     Hotline: (800) 662-HELP
     National Institute on Drug Abuse Prevention
     (800) 638-2045
     National Federation of Parents for Drug-Free Youth
     (800) 544-KIDS
     National Clearinghouse for Alcohol and Drug Abuse Information
     (800) 729-6686

Health Supervision as Ongoing Surveillance, Screening and Assessment of Physical Growth and Behavioral Development

- Definitions:

  1. Surveillance: A continuous process of periodic assessment and monitoring of growth and development overtime through a variety of methods including direct observation, health history, parent/child interviews, and physical examination

  2. Screening: Use of standardized or generally accepted methods with essentially well populations in order to identify individuals who may be at risk for physical, cognitive or psychosocial abnormality and warrant further assessment; good screening tools are simple, inexpensive, acceptable, valid and reliable

3. Assessment: A more systematic evaluation using a standardized or generally accepted method leading to recommendations for intervention

4. Sensitivity: Proportion of those with the abnormality who are correctly identified through screening (true positives)

5. Specificity: Proportion of those without the abnormality who are correctly identified as negative through screening (true negatives)

6. Positive predictive value (PPV): Proportion of those individuals correctly screened as positive of all those who actually have the abnormality

- Examples of Screening and Assessment Tests Used in Child Health Supervision

    1. Physical assessment and laboratory screening

        a. Newborn genetic screening (blood spot on filter paper)

            (1) Newborn screening for hypothyroidism and phenylketonuria (PKU) required in all States; galactosemia and hemoglobinopathies required in the majority of States

            (2) Newborn screening for additional conditions include—biotinidase deficiency, maple syrup urine disease (MSUD), congenital adrenal hyperplasia, cystic fibrosis, homocystinuria, congenital toxoplasmosis, tyrosinemia

            (3) Requirements for voluntary vs. mandatory screening vary by State

        b. Anthropometric body measurements—weight (wt), length or height (ht), head circumference (hc), skin-fold thickness

            (1) American Academy of Pediatrics (AAP) recommendations:

                (a) Birth to 2 years (wt, length, and hc) at each visit

                (b) 3 to 5 years (wt, ht) annually

                (c) 6 to 20 years (wt, ht) every other year

            (2) NCHS age and gender specific growth charts for serial measurements

            (3) Body mass index (BMI)—adolescents

            (4) Risks—growth retardation, malnutrition, obesity, eating disorders

        c. Blood pressure screening

            (1) AAP recommendations:

                (a) Annually from 3 to 6 years

                (b) Every other year thereafter

            (2) Risks—hypertension

        d. Cholesterol screening (serum levels)

            (1) AAP recommendations:

(a) Universal screening not recommended

(b) Children > 2 years with family history of hypercholesterolemia and/or premature cardiovascular disease

(2) Risks—coronary artery disease in adulthood

e. Anemia screening (hemoglobin/hematocrit)

(1) AAP recommendations—measure once during

(a) Infancy (6 to 9 months)

(b) Early childhood (1 to 5 years)

(c) School-age (5 to 12 years)

(d) Adolescents (14 to 20 years)

(2) Risks—iron deficiency anemia

f. Lead screening—AAP recommends targeted screening based on well-child surveillance of risk

g. Tuberculosis (TB) screening

(1) Methods include Mantoux (PPD) and multiple puncture (tine)

(2) Mantoux is preferred method with better sensitivity and specificity

(3) AAP recommends targeted screening based on degree of risk

(a) Annual testing for high-risk children

(b) Periodic testing for low-risk children living in high prevalence environments—between 4 to 6 years and again between 11 to 16 years

h. Urine screening (urine analysis)—AAP recommendations 6 months, 2, 8, and 18 years

i. Vision screening (visual acuity)

(1) AAP recommendations—ages 3, 4, 5, 6, 8, 12, and 18 years

(2) Methods—visual acuity

(a) Preschool children—Illiterate (tumbling) E; Allen picture cards, HOTV

(b) School-age children and adolescents—Snellen letters

j. Hearing screening

(1) NIH Consensus Statement on Early Identification of Hearing Impairment in Infants and Young Children (1993)

(a) Evoked otoacoustic emissions (EOAE) to screen all newborns

(b) Auditory Brainstem Response Audiometry (ABR) for all newborns who fail EOAE

(2) AAP recommendations

    (a) Low-risk children—pure-tone audiometry at 4, 5, 12, and 18 years

    (b) High-risk neonates and young children— audiology screening preferably before discharge (neonates), and no later than 3 months after being identified at risk

k. Dental screening—AAP recommends first dental screening by 3 years of age

2. Developmental screening and assessment

  a. Global development

    (1) Newborn Behavioral Assessment Scale (NBAS)—assessment of newborn's behavioral capacities including state control, autonomic reactivity, reflexes, habituation, and responsiveness to visual and auditory stimuli

    (2) Bayley Infant Neurodevelopmental Screener (BINS)— screens for basic neurological, receptive, expressive, and cognitive functions in infants between 3 to 24 months

    (3) Bayley Scales of Infant Development (second edition (BSID-II)—current ''gold-standard'' for diagnosing developmental delays and recommending intervention for children birth through 42 months with separate mental, motor, and behavioral rating scales

    (4) Ages and Stages Questionnaires (ASQ)—parent-completed child monitoring system for children 4 to 48 months

    (5) Denver II—screens in personal-social, fine motor-adaptive, language and gross motor domains in children birth to 6 years

    (6) First Step—screening test for evaluating preschoolers

  b. Cognitive development-intelligence

    (1) McCarthy Scales of Children's Abilities

    (2) Weschler Preschool and Primary Scale of Intelligence Revised (WPPSIR)

    (3) Weschler Intelligence Scale for Children-WISC III

  c. Language

    (1) Early Language Milestones Scale (ELM)—(0 to 42 months)

    (2) Receptive and Expressive Emergent Language Scale (REEL)—(0 to 36 months)

    (3) Clinical Linguistic and Auditory Milestone Test (CLAMS)—(0 to 36 months)

   (4)   Language Development Survey—screening tool for toddlers using vocabulary checklist for enumeration of words

   (5)   The MacArthur Communicative Development Inventory—words and gestures

   (6)   The MacArthur Communicative Development Inventory—words and sentences

d.   Behaviors

   (1)   Achenbach's Child Behavior Checklist (ACBCL)

   (2)   Connor's Abbreviated Parent-Teacher Questionnaire

e.   Temperament

   (1)   Infant Temperament Questionnaire—4 to 8 months

   (2)   Toddler Temperament Scale—1 to 3 years

   (3)   Behavioral Style Questionnaire—3 to 7 years

   (4)   Middle Childhood Temperament Questionnaire—8 to 12 years

3.   Parent-child relationship and home environment

   a.   Parenting Stress Index (PSI)

   b.   Home Observation for Measurement of the Environment (HOME scale)—infant, preschool and elementary school versions

   c.   Pediatric Review and Observation of Children's Environmental Support and Stimulation Inventory (PROCESS)

   d.   Nursing Child Assessment Feeding (NCAF) and Teaching (NCAT) scales

4.   Mental health screening and diagnostic classifications

   a.   0–3 Diagnostic classification of mental health and developmental disorders of infancy and early childhood (1995)

   b.   DSM-PC Classification of child and adolescent mental diagnoses in primary care (1996)

   c.   DSM-IV-TR Diagnostic and statistical manual of mental disorders (2000)

Questions
Select the best answer

1. Most stage-based theories of development focus primarily on:

   a. The continuity of development
   b. The discontinuity of development
   c. Persistence of inherent personality characteristics
   d. The influence of context on development

2. The common practice of using ''time-outs'' with young children is a direct application of:

   a. Operant conditioning
   b. Classical conditioning
   c. Separation-individuation
   d. Maturational reinforcement

3. Good communication between families, schools and primary care providers is an example of which ecological concept?

   a. Microsytem
   b. Mesosystem
   c. Exosystem
   d. Macrosystem

4. Which of the following findings would be most likely associated with asymmetric intrauterine growth retardation:

   a. Weight, length and head circumference ranging from 3rd to 5th percentile
   b. Heavy maternal smoking throughout pregnancy
   c. Weight at 3rd percentile and length at 25th
   d. Gestational diabetes

5. Early reflexive responses that are not related to survival include all but:

   a. Babinski
   b. Moro
   c. Swimming
   d. Rooting

6. The most likely weight of a one-year-old child whose weight at birth was $6\frac{1}{2}$ pounds would be:

   a. 19-20 pounds
   b. 13-14 pounds
   c. 25-26 pounds
   d. Impossible to estimate

7. One of the major psychosocial tasks of infancy is:

a. Development of secure attachment
b. Separation-individuation
c. Symbiosis
d. Regulation

8. Which developmental theory best explains the multifactorial etiology of failure-to-thrive?

a. Organismic-maturational theory
b. Social learning theory
c. Transactional theory
d. Psychoanalytic theory

9. Most healthy infants are able to reach, grasp and hold onto a rattle or other small toy by about:

a. 2 months
b. 6 months
c. 8 months
d. 10 months

10. The pincer grasp is a fine motor skill that involves the ability to pick up a small object such as a raisin or piece of cereal with the thumb and forefinger that usually is mastered around:

a. 4 months
b. 6 months
c. 9 months
d. 16 months

11. The majority of American infants are able to walk by about:

a. 11 months
b. 12 months
c. 13 months
d. 14 months

12. A young child should have had a first dental screening by:

a. 2 years
b. 3 years
c. 4 years
d. School entry

13. You would be concerned about the language development of a child who:

a. Repeats simple phrases at 32 months
b. Stutters when excited or tired at 42 months
c. Has a vocabulary of 10 words at 12 months
d. Pronounces words that are not understandable at 36 months

14. The most common temperamental profile is:

a. Easy
b. Difficult
c. Slow-to-warm-up
d. Intermediate

15. The underlying emotion of an insecurely attached (avoidant) relationship is:

    a. Ambivalence
    b. Deprivation
    c. Anger
    d. Conditional love

16. The stage of cognitive development that Piaget decribed as characteristic of the way preschool-ers think is the:

    a. Preoperational stage
    b. Mental combinations stage
    c. Tertiary circular function stage
    d. Sensorimotor stage

17. A preschool boy whose parents have separated and are beginning divorce procedures:

    a. May think that he caused the divorce by misbehaving
    b. Should not be told of the impending divorce until the parents are sure of their decision
    c. Is likely to experience gender identity confusion
    d. Should be able to make a decision about which parent he prefers living with

18. Which behavior would you expect to decrease during the preschool years?

    a. Rough-and-tumble play
    b. Instrumental aggression
    c. Hostile aggression
    d. Cooperative play

19. A preschool child who says that the sky is blue because it is his favorite color is illustrating the concept of:

    a. Symbolic thinking
    b. Egocentrism
    c. Centration
    d. Imaginary audience

20. Which of the following strategies would not be appropriate to include as part of your manage-ment of a 9 year old boy who is obese?

    a. Referral to nutritionist for weight reduction plan
    b. Increase physical exercise
    c. Behavior modification strategies to deal with stress and/or reinforce treatment plan
    d. Involve family in management program

21. Which of the following issues or concepts is relevant to the school-aged child?

    a. Operational thinking
    b. Initiative
    c. Concrete operations
    d. Separation-individuation

22. The first physical sign indicating the onset of female puberty is:

    a. Sparsely distributed fine, pale pubic hairs.
    b. Breast buds
    c. Menarche
    d. Peak height velocity

23. Which of the following findings would be helpful in distinguishing obesity vs. large body frame in an adolescent who is concerned with her weight?

    a. Tricep skinfold measurement
    b. Weight-for-height ratio
    c. Body mass index
    d. Percent of ideal body weight

24. The most common form of child abuse seen in pediatric primary care is:

    a. Burns
    b. Fractures
    c. Soft tissue injuries
    d. Shaken baby syndrome

25. A differential diagnosis for child abuse would include all of the following except:

    a. Birth marks
    b. Unintentional injury
    c. Inadequate parenting
    d. Prader-Willi syndrome

26. Which of the following symptoms are not typical of a child with ADHD?

    a. Easily distracted
    b. Difficulty playing quietly
    c. Doesn't follow directions
    d. Frequently angry and resentful

27. Which of the following clinical findings would not suggest an eating disorder with a purging component?

    a. Sore throat
    b. Brittle nails
    c. Constipation
    d. Finger calluses

28. Which of the following situations does not necessarily warrent immediate mental health assessment and/or referral?

    a. 13 year old girl who has been "down" for the last month with varied somatic complaints
    b. 9 year old boy whose parents recently separated and filed for a divorce and seems to be doing well
    c. 16 year old girl who has a history of long-standing depression but seems to be doing well in school
    d. 15 year old boy who expresses suicidal thoughts

29. Which of the following is not a test for visual acuity?

    a. HOTV
    b. Allen figures
    c. Snellen chart
    d. ELM

30. The preferred method for tuberculosis screening is:

    a. Mantoux
    b. MPT
    c. HOTV
    d. DASE

31. Which adolescent would be at greatest risk for developing anorexia nervosa?

    a. 12 year old female who just had her first period
    b. 14 year old gymnist
    c. 16 year old male runner
    d. 18 year old female college student

32. Which of the following substances is associated with pupillary constriction?

    a. Amphetamines
    b. LSD
    c. Heroin
    d. Nicotine

33. A newborn infant who was recently tested and failed the evoked otoacoustic emissions audiometry (EOAE) prior to discharge should be referred for:

    a. Pure tone audiometry
    b. Complete diagnostic evaluation
    c. Auditory brainstem response
    d. Repeat EOAE within 3 months

34. A risk factor that is common to many psychosocial pediatric problems including failure to thrive, conduct or oppositional disorders, and childhood depression is:

    a. Maternal depression or other psychiatric disorder

     b. Substance abuse

     c. Prematurity

     d. History of sexual abuse

35. Which of the following diagnoses is not more common among males?

     a. ADHD

     b. Conduct Disorders

     c. Suicide

     d. FTT

36. Newborn genetic screening is required in all or most states for all of the following disorders except:

     a. Hypothyroidism

     b. PKU

     c. Galactosemia

     d. Cystic Fibrosis

37. The diagnostic criteria for Autistic disorders includes which of the following?

     a. Speech delay, ataxia, mental retardation

     b. Impairments in social interactions, interpersonal communication and staring spells

     c. Mental retardation, impairments in social interactions and stereotypical restricted pattern of interests and activities

     d. Impairments in social interactions, in interpersonal communication and stereotypical restricted pattern of interests and activities

38. In addition to specific academic skill deficits, learning disabilities are commonly associated with which of the following characteristics?

     a. Perceptual-motor impairments, normal motor function

     b. Perceptual motor impairment, impulsiveness

     c. Perceptual motor impairments, Down syndrome

     d. Lack of impulsiveness, perceptual motor impairment

Answers

1. b	14. a	27. b
2. a	15. c	28. b
3. b	16. a	29. d
4. c	17. a	30. a
5. d	18. b	31. b
6. a	19. b	32. c
7. a	20. a	33. c
8. c	21. c	34. a
9. b	22. b	35. d
10. c	23. c	36. d
11. d	24. c	37. d
12. b	25. d	38. b
13. d	26. d	

Bibliography

American Academy of Pediatrics (1996). *The classification of child and adolescent mental diagnoses in primary care.* Elk Grove, IL: Author

American Academy of Pediatrics (2000). Clinical practice guidelines: Diagnosis and evaluation of the child with attention-deficit/hyperactivity disorder. *Pediatrics, 105*(5), 1158-1170.

American Psychiatric Association. (2000). *Diagnostic and statistical manual of mental disorders—text revision* (4th ed.). Washington, DC: American Psychiatric Association.

Avery, M. E., & First, L. R. (1994). *Pediatric medicine* (2nd ed.). Baltimore: Williams & Wilkins.

Baron-Cohen, S., Cox, A., Swettenham, J., Nightengale, N., Morgan, K., Drew, A., & Charman, T. (1996). Psychological markers in the detection of autism in infancy. *British Journal of Psychiatry, 168*(2), 158-163.

Behrman, R. E., Kliegman, R. M., & Jenson, H. B. (2000). *Nelson textbook of pediatrics* (16th ed.). Philadelphia: W.B. Saunders Company.

Berger, K. S., & Straub, R. (2000). *The developing person through the life span.* NY: Worth Publishers.

Burns, C. E., Brady, M. A., Dunn, A. M., & Starr, N. (2000). *Pediatric primary care: A handbook for nurse practitioners* (2nd ed.). Philadelphia: W. B. Saunders Company.

Dixon, S. D., & Stein, M. T. (2000). *Encounters with children: Pediatric behavior and development* (3rd ed.). St. Louis: Mosby Year Book, Inc.

Green, M. (2000). *Bright futures: Guidelines for health supervision of infants, children and adolescents* (2nd ed.) Arlington, VA: National Center for Education in Maternal and Child Health.

Hanson, S. M. H., & Boyde, S. T. (1996). *Family health care nursing: Theory, practice and research.* Philadelphia: R. A. Davis.

Hoekelman, R. A., Adam, H. M., Nelson, N. M., Weitzman, M. L., & Wilson, M. H. (2001). *Primary pediatric care* (4th ed.). St. Louis: Mosby Year Book, Inc.

Hofmann, A., & Greydanus, D. (1997). *Adolescent Medicine.* (3rd ed.) Stamford, Conn.: Appletone & Lange.

Johnson, B. H., Jeppson, E. S., & Redburn, L. (1992). *Caring for children and families: Guidelines for hospitals.* Bethesda, MD: Association for the Care of Children's Health.

Lemley, K. B., O'Grady, E. T., Rauckhorst, L., Russell, D. D., & Small, N. (1994). Baseline data on the delivery of clinical preventive services provided by nurse practitioners. *The Nurse Practitioner: The American Journal of Primary Health Care, 19*(5), 57-63.

Levine, M., Carey, W., & Crocker, A. (1999). *Developmental-behavioral pediatrics* (3rd ed.). Philadelphia: W. B. Saunders.

McMillan, J. (1999). *Oski's pediatrics. Principles and practice.* Philadelphia: Lippincott, Williams & Wilkins.

Mercugliano, M., Powers, T., & Blum, N. (1999). *The clinician's practical guide to attention-deficit/hyperactivity disorder.* Baltimore: Paul H. Brooks Publishing.

Meisels, S. J., & Fenichel, E. (1996). *New visions for the developmental assessment of infants and young children.* Washington, DC: Zero to Three.

O'Malley, P. M., Johnston, L. D., & Bachman, J. G. (1995). Adolescent substance use: Epidemiology and implications for public policy. *The Pediatric Clinics of North America, 42*(2), 241-260.

Rosner, B., Prineas, R., Loggie, J., & Daniels, S. R. (1998). Percentiles for body mass index in U.S. children 5 to 17 years of age. *J. Pediatrics, 132*(2), 211-222.

Rudolph, A. M., Hoffman, J. I., & Rudolph, C. D. (1996). *Rudolph's pediatrics* (20th ed.). Stanford, CT: Appleton & Lange.

Substance abuse and mental health services administration (S.A.M.S.A.) (1998). Preliminary results from the 1997 National Household Survey on Drug Abuse, Substance Abuse and Mental Health Services Administration. http://wwwsamsa.gov/press/98082/ohtm

Tanner, J. M. (1978). *Fetus into man: Physical growth from conception to maturity.* Cambridge, MA: Harvard University Press.

U.S. Department of Health and Human Services. (1998). *Clinician's handbook of preventive services* (2nd ed.). Washington, DC: U.S. Government Printing Office.

U.S. Department of Health and Human Services. (1996). *Healthy people 2000: Midcourse review and 1995 revisions.* Washington, DC: U.S. Government Printing Office.

U.S. Department of Health and Human Services. (1998). *Child maltreatment 1996: Reports from the states to the national child abuse and neglect data system.* Washington, DC: U.S. Government Printing Office.

Valadian, I., & Porter, D. (1977). *Physical growth and development.* Boston: Little, Brown & Co.

Zero to Three. (1995). *Diagnostic classification: 0-3: Diagnostic classification of mental health and developmental disorders of infancy and early childhood.* Washington, DC: Zero to Three.

Health Maintenance
and
Health Promotion
Infancy Through Adolescence

Bernadette Mazurek Melnyk

Overview: Health Maintenance and Health Promotion

For years, family nurse practitioners have been maintaining and promoting optimal health in children and their families. Because of their understanding of the multiple factors that may influence health and development of children, family nurse practitioners are able to implement individualized and group interventions and appropriately involve all family members to enhance children's outcomes.

One strategy for enhancing health and developmental outcomes in children and their families is the implementation of routine child health supervision. Health supervision is comprised of those measures which promote health, prevent morbidity and mortality, and facilitate development and maturation within the context of the family and community. It involves health visits which include health promotion strategies, anticipatory guidance, as well as specific screening procedures at regular, timed intervals throughout childhood and adolescence.

Child Health Supervision

- Components
    1. The parent/child interview
    2. Developmental and educational surveillance
    3. Observation of parent/child interaction
    4. Physical examination
    5. Screening
    6. Assessment of strengths and vulnerabilities (concerns, problems and stressors affecting the child and family)
    7. Individualized interventions, including health promotion strategies and anticipatory guidance

- General Interviewing Approaches
    1. Determine who will be present for interview
    2. Provide privacy and empathetic environment
    3. Maintain good eye contact and relaxed facial expressions
    4. State you will be taking notes during interview to enhance accuracy of recorded data
    5. Obtain history with child clothed
    6. Begin with open ended questions, e.g., "Tell me what concerns you today."
    7. Use direct questions to obtain specific information, e.g., "How old is Bobby?"
    8. Avoid leading questions, e.g., "Your child doesn't have behavioral problems, does he?"

9. Use language parents and child understand

10. Provide undivided attention; listen carefully

11. Build self-esteem and confidence throughout interview

12. Conduct interview with cultural sensitivity

- Communication with Parents (same as general approaches, plus)

    1. Obtain parent's perception of any concerns or problems; if both parents present, obtain each parent's view of concerns or problems

    2. Restate parental concerns to ensure accuracy and understanding

    3. Be supportive, not judgmental, e.g., ''Why didn't you bring your child in earlier?''

- Communication with Young Children (less than six years of age)

    1. Talk to child at his/her eye level

    2. Use play to enhance comfort

    3. Use projective techniques to elicit information about how child is feeling, e.g., ''Tell me how your bear is feeling today.''

    4. Use nonthreatening words, e.g., tube instead of needle; opening instead of cut, since young children engage in magical thinking

    5. Allow adequate time for responses

    6. Remember that young children have difficulty giving detailed information

- Communication with Younger School-age Children

    1. Communicate with parent first if child is initially shy

    2. Ask questions and give explanations using concrete terminology

    3. Use simple diagrams when asking child to describe location of symptoms

    4. Allow time for responses

    5. Give permission to express fears and concerns

- Communication with Older School-age Children and Adolescents

    1. If parent is present, conduct part of interview (questions dealing with personal or sensitive information) when alone with the older child or adolescent

    2. Interview while fully clothed

    3. Start interview with nonthreatening questions

    4. Inform older child/adolescent that all questions you are asking have to do with his/her health; that you ask all older children/adolescents these questions

    5. Acknowledge that, although all of your questions are necessary, some may feel uncomfortable to answer

6. Inform older child/adolescent that information shared is confidential unless he/she tells you about wanting to hurt him/herself or someone else has hurt him/her

7. Encourage expression of feelings and concerns

8. Enhance self-esteem and provide positive feedback during interview

- Confidentiality Issues and Informed Consent

    1. Health care providers are required by law to keep the information gathered in the course of a child's care confidential

    2. Privileged information may only be shared among health care professionals involved in the care of a child or in medical emergencies when release of information is in the best interest of the child and necessary for the provision of care

    3. Many States mandate reporting by health care professionals of special circumstances (reasonable cause to suspect child physical or sexual abuse or neglect; suicidal intent; gunshot and stab wounds)

    4. Some States require reporting of births, deaths, certain diseases, and other vital statistics.

    5. Consents should be signed by child's parent or legal guardian before information concerning child is released; emancipated minor (under the age of 18 years and married; parent of his or her own child; or self-sufficiently living away from home with parental consent) also may sign consents

    6. Minor's informed consent laws vary across States by status (emancipated) and conditions

        a. Most states have statutes allowing access to contraceptives, pregnancy testing/prenatal care as well as the diagnosis, treatment and prevention of sexually transmitted diseases per consent of minor

        b. Approximately half of the States have statutes allowing HIV testing and treatment per consent of minor

The Pediatric History

During the examination of a pediatric patient, the history is critical in the early detection of problems and prevention of long-term negative outcomes. Approximately 80% of the information used to arrive at a diagnosis is derived from the history.

- New Patient History

    1. Identifying data—demographic data; name and reliability of person providing the history as well as his/her relationship to child

    2. Chief complaint (C.C.)—purpose of visit

    3. Interim health—health since child was last seen by their primary care provider

    4. Current health

        a. Nutrition

b.   Elimination

c.   Sleep

d.   Development—including school performance; daily activities; recreation and hobbies; social adjustment; behavior; and temperament

e.   Discipline

f.   Safety

g.   Immunizations and screening

h.   Allergies—including type of response

i.   Medications

j.   Substance use—alcohol, drug, cigarette, tobacco, caffeine use

5.   Past medical history

a.   Birth—obtain if child is less than 3 years of age or if child is older than 3 years and having developmental or neurological problems

(1)   Prenatal

(a)   Planned or unplanned pregnancy

(b)   Onset of prenatal care

(c)   Medications, drugs, alcohol use during pregnancy

(d)   Medical problems during pregnancy—e.g., bleeding; infections; toxemia

(2)   Perinatal

(a)   Length of labor and delivery

(b)   Type of delivery

(c)   Medications or anesthesia

(d)   Complications

(e)   Birth weight

(f)   Gestation at birth; Apgar scores

(g)   If multiple births, birth order

(3)   Postnatal

(a)   Maternal and infant problems

(b)   Age and weight at discharge

b.   Illnesses and injuries

c.   Hospitalizations and surgeries

d.   Growth and development

      (1) Physical growth

      (2) Developmental milestones

      (3) Social-emotional development—e.g., temperament, relationships

      (4) School—e.g., performance; attendance; problems; early intervention or Head Start

6. Family history

   a. Family profile and medical history (use pedigree chart)—include serious chronic, inherited and congenital problems in immediate family (blood relatives); drug and alcohol abuse; mental health problems; and age of first myocardial infarction if applicable

   b. Family social history—members of household and their relationship to the child; physical environment; employment/financial situation of parents or legal guardian; health care coverage; child care; family stressors (e.g., marital separation; illness); exposure to conflict or violence; presence of social support

7. Review of systems—does this child now or has this child ever had problems with any of the following systems?

   a. General

   b. Head/eyes/ears/nose/throat (HEENT)

   c. Lymph

   d. Respiratory

   e. Cardiac

   f. Gastrointestinal

   g. Genitourinary

   h. Musculoskeletal

   i. Skin

   j. Hematological

   k. Neurological

   l. Psychological

   m. Sexual/reproductive

- Interval History

  1. Chief complaint (C.C.)

  2. Interim health—since last visit

  3. Current health—e.g., nutrition; elimination; sleep; development; allergies; immunizations

  4. Update any changes in history since last visit

5. Review of systems since last history

- History of Present Illness (H.P.I.) or Problem

  1. Description of present illness or problem

     a. Onset

     b. Location; character

     c. Temporal aspects

     d. Precipitating/aggravating factors; relieving factors

     e. Past treatment

     f. Associated symptoms

     g. Course

     h. Effect on daily activities

     i. Similar symptoms in family members or friends

     j. Pertinent negatives

     k. Other current illnesses/health problems

     l. Allergies

- Telephone History (telephone triage)

  1. Requires triage decision

     a. Telephone management

     b. Office visit

     c. Refer to emergency department or other health care provider

  2. Telephone protocol books are helpful in assessment and management of common illnesses and problems encountered by phone

  3. Critical elements

     a. Identify yourself

     b. Identify caller, his or her relationship to child, and caller's telephone number

     c. Obtain child's name, age and approximate weight

     d. Ascertain thorough history of present illness or problem

     e. If not medically necessary to see child, explain rationale and evaluate comfort of caller in home management

     f. Tell caller when to call back which includes advising on signs of worsening status

     g. Ask caller to telephone again to give progress report if there are any concerns about the child; if caller does not telephone as requested, IT IS CRITICAL TO MAKE THE FOLLOW-UP CALL

    h. Ask caller to write down information that has been given or at least to repeat the information

    i. Offer simple, understandable explanations

    j. Advise caller to contact you again with any questions

    k. Convey warmth, empathy and support

    l. Document all telephone conversations, including history, diagnosis, and management plan

- Sexual/Reproductive History

  1. Inform child that these questions are asked of all older school-age children and adolescents

  2. Reenforce that, although these questions are very personal or sensitive, they are necessary to gain a complete picture of that child or adolescent's health

  3. Reassure child or adolescent that the information he or she shares is confidential unless information about harm to self or others is revealed

  4. Progress from least to most sensitive questions

  5. It is best to phrase questions—"When was the first time you had intercourse?" instead of "Have you ever had intercourse?"

  6. Make sure older child or adolescent understands meaning of terms used

  7. Essential elements of sexual/reproductive history

     a. Date of menarche (first menses)

     b. Frequency, length and quantity of menses with associated symptoms, e.g., cramping, headache or backache

     c. Date of last menses

     d. Use of tampons or pads

     e. Age of first intercourse; date of last intercourse

     f. Sexual preference, e.g., males, females, or both; same sex exploration is common in teenagers; number of sexual partners

     g. Types of sexual practices, e.g., male, female; oral sex, intercourse

     h. Reasons for sexual activity, e.g., increases self-esteem; enjoyment; peer pressure

     i. Pregnancies and outcomes

     j. Current contraception

     k. History of any sexually transmitted diseases (STD), naming each disease, e.g., gonorrhea, chlamydia, etc.

     l. Vaginal or penile discharge

    m.   Date of last pelvic examination

    n.   Contraceptive history; current contraception; use of condoms

    o.   Knowledge of STDs, AIDS, pregnancy, and prevention measures

    p.   Date of prior test or desire for HIV testing

    q.   Performance of self-breast or testicular exam

    r.   History of sexual abuse

The Pediatric Physical Examination

- General Information

  1. Examination should be comprehensive and systematic

  2. Observation is first critical component of the examination beginning as soon as the child is seen

  3. Use examination to teach child about his or her body

- Age-related Issues (Infants)

  1. Developmental considerations

     a. Stage of trust versus mistrust

     b. Stranger anxiety develops at 6 to 7 months

     c. Separation anxiety develops at 8 to 9 months

     d. Major fears—separation from parents and pain

  2. Approaches to physical examination

     a. Approach slowly

     b. Conduct as much of examination with infant on parent's lap

     c. Provide infant with security objects, e.g., special blanket or toy

     d. Use distraction and engaging facial expressions during the examination

     e. Conduct examination using noninvasive to invasive sequence, e.g., auscultate heart and lung sounds first; examine ears and throat last

     f. Allow for brief break if infant is hungry or stressed

- Age-related Issues (Toddlers)

  1. Developmental considerations

     a. Stage of autonomy versus shame/doubt

     b. Striving for independence

     c. Negativism and temper tantrums (common)

     d. Beginning of magical thinking

    e. Major fears—separation from parents; intrusion of body orifices; loss of control; pain

  2. Approaches to physical examination

    a. Use of distraction is helpful

    b. Allow child to touch and hold equipment before examination

    c. Demonstrate examination on doll, toy, or parent before conducting examination on child

    d. Give child choices when possible

    e. When necessary, tell child what you are going to do instead of gaining permission, e.g., ''I am going to check your tummy'' versus ''Is it OK with you if I check your tummy?''

    f. Conduct as much of examination as possible on parent's lap

    g. Conduct examination using noninvasive to an invasive sequence

- Age-Related Issues (Preschool Children)

  1. Developmental considerations

    a. Stage of initiative versus guilt

    b. Magical thinking

    c. Egocentrism

    d. Major fears—separation from parents; loss of control; body mutilation; pain

  2. Approaches to physical examination

    a. Inform child what you are going to do and what he/she can do to help

    b. Role play with equipment, e.g., let child examine ears of doll first

    c. Head to toe examination sequence can usually be implemented

    d. Choose words carefully due to magical thinking

    e. Allow choices whenever possible

    f. Teach child about his/her body during course of examination

    g. Praise child for helping and attempting to cooperate

- Age-Related Issues (School-age Children)

  1. Developmental considerations

    a. Industry versus inferiority

    b. Concrete thinking

    c. Desires to act brave

    d. Enjoys gathering scientific information

e. Modesty emerges with older school-age child

f. Major fears—separation from peers; loss of control; pain; death, beginning at age 9 years

2. Approaches to physical examination

   a. Head to toe sequence

   b. Scientific terminology with concrete explanations

   c. Answer questions factually with age-appropriate vocabulary

   d. Explain use of equipment, e.g., otoscope

- Age-Related Issues (Adolescents)

1. Developmental considerations

   a. Stage of identity versus role diffusion

   b. Striving for independence and control

   c. Formal operational thinking

   d. Bodily concerns

   e. Concerns about being different

   f. Major fears—change in body image; separation from peers; loss of control; death

2. Approaches to physical examination

   a. Assure privacy

   b. Examine without parent unless adolescent prefers parent remain in room

   c. Inform adolescent of each step of examination

   d. Give choices whenever possible

   e. Cover parts of body not currently being examined

   f. Assure privacy

   g. Teach adolescent about his/her body during course of examination

   h. Provide reassurance of ''normalcy'' during course of examination

   i. Recognize and discuss apprehension about breast, pelvic and testicular examinations

- Measurement of Vital Signs

1. Temperature

   a. Rectal temperature—most accurate method, but proper technique must be used to avoid injury

   b. Tympanic membrane temperature—quick and noninvasive measurement, reliability is a problem

    c. Temperature of 100.4° F (38° C) and above is considered a fever

2. Pulse

    a. Norms   Beats/minute

		Beats/minute
(1)	Newborn	120–170
(2)	1 year	80–160
(3)	3 years	80–120
(4)	6 years	75–115
(5)	10 years	70–110
(6)	17 years	60–100

    b. Conditions that commonly elevate pulse

        (1) Temperature—for every 1 degree of temperature elevation in fahrenheit, pulse increases by 10 beats per minute

        (2) Anxiety/stress; excitement

        (3) Exercise

        (4) Severe anemia

        (5) Hyperthyroidism

        (6) Hypoxia

        (7) Heart disease

3. Respirations

    a. Norms   Breaths per minute

		Breaths per minute
(1)	Newborn	30–80
(2)	1 year	20–40
(3)	3 years	20–30
(4)	6 years	16–20
(5)	10 years	16–20
(6)	17 years	12–20

    b. Conditions that commonly elevate respirations

        (1) Temperature—for every 1 degree of temperature elevation in fahrenheit, respirations increase by 4 breaths per minute

        (2) Anxiety/stress; excitement

        (3) Pain

        (4) Respiratory conditions, e.g., pneumonia

(5) Heart disease

4. Blood Pressure

    a. Appropriate cuff size required for accurate reading

       (1) Bladder width should not be more than $\frac{2}{3}$ the length of upper arm

       (2) Bladder length should cover $\frac{3}{4}$ of the arm circumference

    b. Use Korotkoff sound IV (muffling sound) as diastolic blood pressure in children under 13 years of age; use Korotkoff sound V (disappearance of sound) as the diastolic blood pressure in children 13 years of age and older

    c. Plot blood pressure on standard blood pressure graphs for boys or girls

    d. Begin to measure blood pressure at well-child visits, starting at 3 years of age

    e. A single elevated blood pressure measurement in an apparently healthy child does not necessarily reflect disease

    f. Hypertension—average systolic and/or diastolic blood pressure $\geq$ 95th percentile for age and sex on at least 3 separate occasions using the same arm, same cuff, and same position

Age	Systolic (mm Hg)	Diastolic (mm Hg)
Infant	$\geq$ 112	$\geq$ 74
3–5 years	$\geq$ 116	$\geq$ 76
6–9 years	$\geq$ 122	$\geq$ 78
10–12 years	$\geq$ 126	$\geq$ 82
13–15 years	$\geq$ 136	$\geq$ 86
16–18 years	$\geq$ 142	$\geq$ 92

    g. Taller, heavier children have higher blood pressure than smaller children of same age

    h. Pulse pressure—difference between systolic and diastolic blood pressures (normal is 20 to 50 mm Hg)

       (1) Wide pulse pressure from high systolic pressure is usually due to fever, exercise, or excitement

       (2) Wide pulse pressure from low diastolic pressure is usually due to patent ductus arteriosus, aortic regurgitation, or other serious heart disease

Specific Normal Findings and Common Variations

- Head and Neck

    1. History indicating possible abnormalities

       a. Difficult birth; use of forceps

b. Unusual head shape or preferred position at rest

c. Poor head control for age

d. Lack of neonatal screening for hypothyroidism

2. Selected physical examination findings

a. Head circumference is approximately 2 cm larger than chest during first year of life; head and chest circumferences should be equal at 1 year of age; during childhood, chest is usually 5 to 7 cm larger than head

b. Fontanels—best to assess while infant is sitting up and not crying

(1) Posterior fontanel rarely palpable at birth; closes by 2 months of age

(2) Size of anterior fontanel should be no larger than 4 to 5 cm in diameter

(3) Anterior fontanel closes between 9 to 18 months of age

(a) Early closure usually leads to synostosis

(b) Late closure is commonly seen with increased intracranial pressure, hypothyroidism, rickets; syphilis, Down syndrome, osteogenesis imperfecta

(4) Large anterior fontanel may indicate:

(a) Chronically increased intracranial pressure

(b) Subdural hematoma

(c) Rickets

(d) Hypothyroidism

(e) Osteogenesis imperfecta

(5) Bulging anterior fontanel is usually seen with conditions that cause increased intracranial pressure, e.g., meningitis/encephalitis, fluid overload

(6) Sunken anterior fontanel is usually seen with severe dehydration (more than 10%)

c. Unusual head size or shape

(1) Hydrocephalus—excessively large head at birth or head that grows abnormally rapid; usually associated with distended scalp veins, widely separated cranial sutures, large and tense anterior fontanel, and "sunset eyes"

(2) Microcephaly—head circumference > 2 standard deviations below the mean for age, sex and gestation; reflects an abnormally small brain; common causes are intrauterine infections (e.g., herpes, rubella, syphilis); genetic defects; drug usage during pregnancy (especially alcohol)

(3) Macrocephaly—head circumference > 2 standard deviations above the mean for age, sex and gestation; common causes are hydrocephalus,

masses, increased intracranial pressure; skeletal dysplasias (osteogenesis imperfecta)

(4) Head tilt—common causes include strabismus, CNS lesions, or short sternocleidomastoid muscle

(5) Caput succedaneum—diffuse edema of the soft tissue of the scalp which usually crosses suture lines; may be seen with bruising due to traumatic vaginal birth; seen at birth; no specific treatment necessary; usually resolves in 2 to 3 days

(6) Cephalohematoma—subperiosteal collection of blood which does not cross suture lines; often does not appear until several hours after birth and may increase over 24 hours; no specific treatment indicated; resolves over a few weeks to months; observe for hyperbilirubinemia

(7) Premature or irregular closure of suture lines can cause unusual head shape (craniosynostosis)

(8) Bossing (bulging) of frontal area is associated with rickets and prematurity

d. Head Control

(1) By 4 months of age, head should be held erect and in midline

(2) By 6 months of age, there should be no head lag when infant is pulled from supine to sitting position—if present, may indicate neuromuscular disorder; may be the *first sign* of cerebral palsy

e. Neck

(1) Pain and resistance to flexion may indicate meningeal irritation

(2) Torticollis (restriction of motion)—can result from birth trauma (e.g., injury to the sternocleidomastoid muscle with bleeding into the muscle); muscle spasm, viral infection, or drug ingestion

(3) Webbed neck—common in Turner's syndrome, a chromosomal abnormality, occurring 99% of the time in females, which results in webbed neck, widespread nipples, abnormal ears, micrognathia and lymphedema of hands and feet

(4) Unusual position of trachea could indicate serious lung problem

(5) Mass in the neck

(a) Thyroglossal duct cyst—usually seen near midline of neck; cyst moves up and down with protrusion of tongue; may become infected and present as an abscess; surgical excision recommended

(b) Brachial cleft cyst—can appear as swelling anterior to sternocleidomastoid (SCM) muscle or as opening along anterior border of SCM, may drain and become infected

(c) Hematoma (of sternocleidomastoid muscle)—more common in breech deliveries

(d) Enlarged thyroid—due to hyperthyroidism or hypothyroidism; visible thyroid gland is almost always enlarged

(e) Enlarged lymph node—most frequent cause of lateral neck mass

- Face

    1. History indicating possible abnormalities

        a. Difficult delivery; use of forceps

        b. Asymmetry of face when crying or speaking

        c. Facial features which are unusual or do not match family characteristics

        d. Drug or alcohol use during pregnancy

    2. Selected physical examination findings

        a. Asymmetry of nasolabial folds or drooping mouth indicates facial nerve impairment or Bell's palsy

        b. Child who demonstrates open mouth breathing and facial contortions may have allergic rhinitis

        c. Dysmorphic facial features are hallmark of numerous syndromes (e.g. fetal alcohol syndrome) and diagnosis should be pursued

- Eyes

    1. History indicating possible abnormalities

        a. Premature infant who required resuscitation; needed ventilator or oxygen support; had retinopathy of prematurity

        b. Infant who does not track faces or objects; absent blink in response to bright lights or sudden movements

        c. Children less than 6 years of age who:

            (1) Rub eyes excessively, squint, have photophobia

            (2) Have difficulty reaching for or picking up small objects

            (3) Engage in head tilting

            (4) Hold objects close to face

        d. School-age children (same as young children, plus) who:

            (1) Sit close to blackboard or TV in order to see

            (2) Are making poor progress in school not explained by intellectual deficit or learning disability

        e. Any age child who:

    (1)   Demonstrates white area in pupil visible in photographs (retino-blastoma)

    (2)   Complains of headaches not present upon awakening, but progress during the day (accommodative errors)

    (3)   Has problems with excessive tearing—allergies, (accommodative errors)

    (4)   Has an eye which turns in or out (strabismus)

2.   Selected physical examination findings

   a.   Position and placement—inner canthal distance averages 2.5 cm; epicanthal folds present in Asian children; palpebral fissures lie horizontally

    (1)   Hypertelorism (wide set eyes)—present in Down syndrome

    (2)   Epicanthal folds can be frequently seen in Down syndrome, renal agenesis, or glycogen storage disease

    (3)   Ptosis could be normal or may indicate paralysis of oculomotor nerve

    (4)   Exophthalmos (protruding eyeballs)—can be seen with hyperthyroidism

   b.   Eyelids normally same color as surrounding skin

    (1)   "Stork Bite" mark—telangiectatic nevi disappear by 12 months

    (2)   Blocked tear duct (dacryostenosis)—may lead to infection of lacrimal sac evidenced by swelling, redness, and purulent discharge (dacryocystitis)

    (3)   Periorbital edema—soft swelling that may be associated with renal or cardiac problems or sinusitis; acute onset of unilateral eyelid edema with erythema, induration and tenderness indicates periorbital cellulitis

   c.   "Allergic shiners"—bluish discoloration and soft edema below eyes usually indicates allergies

   d.   Sclera and conjunctiva

    (1)   Sclera is shiny, clear and white

    (2)   Bulbar conjunctiva (covers sclera) is moist and transparent and palpebral conjunctiva (lines the eyelids) is pink and moist

    (3)   Spots of brown melanin may be seen in dark skinned races

    (4)   Yellow sclera indicates jaundice

    (5)   Redness may indicate bacterial or viral infection, allergy or irritation, e.g., chemicals

    (6)   Excessive pallor of the palpebral conjunctiva indicates anemia

    (7)   Cobblestone appearance of palpebral conjunctiva (lining the eyelids) can indicate severe allergy or contact lens irritation

   e.   Pupils and iris

(1) Unequal pupils (anisocoria)—usually congenital and normal, but can indicate increased intracranial pressure from head trauma or other intracranial disease processes, e.g., meningitis

(2) Dilated, fixed pupils—usually indicate severe brain damage

(3) Dilated pupils—may result from use of anticholinergic drugs (e.g., atropine) and substance abuse (e.g., amphetamines)

(4) Abnormally small pupils—may result from brain damage, use of morphine, or substance abuse (e.g., cocaine)

f. By 3 to 4 months, infants should have binocular vision (ability to fixate on one visual field with both eyes simultaneously)

(1) Assessment techniques to elicit phoria (movement of eye when covered) or tropia (obvious turning in or out of eye without coverage) (e.g., strabismus)

(a) Cover-uncover test (when eye is covered, it may deviate in (esophoria) or out (exophoria) and return to midline when uncovered

(b) Corneal light reflex (Hirschberg's test)—with light held 12 to 14 inches from eyes, reflection of light should be the same on both corneas; if unequal, it is suggestive of phoria or tropia

(2) Intermittent alternating convergent strabismus—normal from 0 to 6 months of age

3. Ophthalmoscopic examination—red reflex should be elicited in every newborn and at each well-child visit

a. Absence of red reflex or an opacity of the lens may indicate cataracts in the newborn

b. Presence of white instead of red reflex may indicate retinoblastoma

- Ears

1. History indicating possible abnormalities

a. Prenatal exposure to maternal infection, irradiation, or drug abuse

b. Birth weight less than 1500 g

c. Anoxia in neonatal period

d. Ototoxic antibiotic usage (e.g., gentamycin)

e. Cleft palate

f. Infections

g. Meningitis

h. Encephalitis

i. Recurrent or chronic otitis media

2. Behaviors suggestive of hearing loss

    a. No reaction to loud or strange noises

    b. No babbling in infant after 6 months

    c. No communicative speech; reliance on gestures after 15 months of age

    d. Language delays

3. Selected physical examination findings

    a. Position and placement—low or obliquely set ears may indicate genitourinary or chromosomal abnormality or a multisystem syndrome

    b. Pain

        (1) Pain produced by manipulation of auricle or pressure on tragus may indicate otitis externa

        (2) Pain and tenderness over mastoid process may indicate mastoiditis

    c. Examination of tympanic membrane (TM)

        (1) For best visualization of TM—pull auricle down and back in children under 3 years of age; pull auricle up and back for children over 3 years of age

        (2) Crying produces erythema of TM bilaterally; landmarks are still visible with succinct light reflexes and +4 TM mobility

        (3) Pneumatic otoscopy is critical for assessment of fluid in middle ear

            (a) Decreased TM mobility—indicates fluid in middle ear

            (b) In child with pressure equalization (PE) tubes, decreased mobility of TM indicates obstruction or dysfunction of tubes

- Nose and Sinuses

  1. History indicating possible abnormalities

    a. Inability to move air through both nares

    b. Discharge

    c. Nasal flaring or narrowing on inspection

    d. Hypernasal voice—snoring, hypertrophied adenoids

  2. Selected physical examination findings

    a. Flattened nasal bridge (in other than Asian or African-American children) may indicate congenital anomalies

    b. Boggy nasal mucous membranes (bluish, pale, edematous) with serous drainage indicates allergic rhinitis

    c. Persistent copious or purulent discharge is indicative of sinusitis

    d. Unilateral purulent discharge suggests foreign body

- Throat/Mouth
  1. History indicating possible abnormalities
     a. Lack of, or excessive fluoride supplementation or fluoridated water
     b. Infant or toddler who goes to sleep with bottle of milk or juice
     c. Thumbsucking or pacifier use beyond 2 years of age
     d. Unusual sequence of tooth eruption
  2. Selected physical examination findings
     a. Lips
        (1) Cherry red color indicates acidosis
        (2) Drooping of one side of lips indicates facial nerve impairment
        (3) Fissures at corners of mouth may indicate riboflavin or niacin deficiency
     b. Teeth
        (1) Mottling may indicate excessive fluoride intake
        (2) Green or black staining can result from oral iron intake
     c. Palate—decay of maxillary incisors may result from baby bottle caries syndrome
        (1) Palpation of palate is important in newborns to detect submucosal cleft
        (2) Uvula rises and remains in midline when saying "ah"; deviation or absence of movement indicates involvement of glossopharyngeal or vagus nerves
        (3) Bifed uvula is suggestive of a submucosal cleft palate
     d. Tonsils
        (1) During childhood, tonsillar hypertrophy is a normal immunological response; largest in size between 8 and 9 years of age and decreases in size after puberty
        (2) Asymmetrically enlarged tonsil without infection may suggest tonsillar lymphoma
     e. Voice
        (1) Nasal quality indicates enlarged adenoids
        (2) Hoarse cry may indicate croup, cretinism or tetany
        (3) Chronic hoarseness may indicate vocal cord polyps
        (4) Shrill, high-pitched cry may indicate increased intracranial pressure
     f. Temporomandibular joint (TMJ)

(1) Findings indicative of TMJ dysfunction—pain upon palpation of TMJ; decrease in mandibular movement; TMJ sounds (popping and clicking); malocclusion; and abnormal morphology of mandible (micrognathia)

(2) Inability to open jaw (trismus) associated with fever and sore throat is suggestive of peritonsillar abscess

- Heart

  1. History indicating possible abnormalities

     a. Infant

        (1) Increased respirations, especially during sleep

        (2) Prolonged feeding time; tires during feedings

        (3) Cyanosis of mucous membranes of mouth

        (4) Eyelid edema

     b. Child

        (1) Increased respirations, especially during sleep

        (2) Squatting or sleeping in knee chest position

        (3) Eyelid edema

        (4) Cyanosis of mucous membranes of mouth

        (5) Exercise intolerance

  2. Selected physical examination findings

     a. Heart sounds and area of clearest auscultation

        (1) S_1 (closure of mitral and tricuspid valves)—heard best at apex

        (2) S_2 (closure of aortic and pulmonic valves)—heard best at aortic and pulmonic areas

        (3) Physiological splitting of S_2 during inspiration is normal; if fixed (heard upon inspiration and expiration), may indicate atrial septal defect or pulmonic stenosis

        (4) S_3—heard best at apex (sounds like Kentucky); due to blood rushing through mitral valve and hitting an empty ventricle; normal in almost all children; if loud in character, may indicate high diastolic pressure in involved ventricle as found in acute ventricular failure

        (5) S_4—heard best at apex (sounds like Tennessee); almost never normal; indicates high pressure in either ventricle as found in pulmonic and aortic stenosis and systemic hypertension

     b. Normal variations in heart rhythm—in sinus arrythmia, heart rate increases with inspiration and decreases with expiration; disappears with exercise or holding breath

    c. Innocent (functional) murmurs—present in approximately 50% of children

      (1) Characteristics

         (a) Usually systolic in timing

         (b) Usually soft; never more than Grade III

         (c) Rarely transmitted

         (d) Low pitched, vibratory, musical, or twangy

         (e) Short duration

         (f) Usually loudest at left lower sternal border or at the second or third intercostal space

         (g) Varies in loudness and presence from time to time

         (h) Heard loudest in the recumbent position, during expiration, and after exercise

         (i) Diminishes with change in positioning from recumbent to sitting

         (j) No cyanosis

         (k) Normal pulses, respiratory rate and BP

         (l) Normal growth and development

         (m) Absence of a thrill (vibratory sensation felt over murmur with palm of hand)

      (2) Types of innocent heart murmurs in children

         (a) *Pulmonary ejection murmur* (heard at the pulmonic area)—early to mid systole; distinct gap between first heart sound and murmur and end of murmur and second heart sound

         (b) *Vibratory or Still's murmur*—musical or vibratory murmur; heard best at the lower left sternal border

         (c) *Venous hum*—heard best above or below clavicles, second or third interspaces; more coarse quality; very dependent upon position; disappears when child lies down or turns neck which decreases blood velocity through internal jugular veins

      (3) Conditions that increase intensity of innocent heart murmurs—exercise, fever, and anemia due to increased cardiac output

      (4) Innocent murmurs in the newborn

         (a) Transition from fetal to adult circulation may take up to 48 hours

         (b) Usually grade I or II

         (c) Systolic

         (d) Not associated with other signs and symptoms

(5) Point of Maximal Impulse (PMI)

    (a) Children less than 8 years of age—4th intercostal space, mid-clavicular line

    (b) Children more than 8 years of age—5th intercostal space, slightly right of mid-clavicular line

    (c) Displacement of PMI with cardiac enlargement

    (d) Increased pulsation of PMI indicates conditions which increase cardiac output, e.g., anemia, anxiety, fever, fluid overload

(6) Peripheral pulses—normally palpable, equal in intensity and rhythm; weak or absent femoral pulses may indicate coarctation of the aorta

- Lungs

1. History indicating possible abnormalities

    a. Family history of tuberculosis, cystic fibrosis, allergy, asthma, atopic dermatitis

    b. Infants and young children

        (1) Premature infant with any respiratory complications

        (2) Sudden onset of coughing or difficulty breathing

        (3) Difficulty feeding

        (4) Apnea episodes

    c. Older children and adolescents

        (1) Smoking

        (2) Cocaine use

        (3) Recurrent or chronic cough

        (4) Exercise intolerance

2. Selected physical examination findings

    a. Normal breath sounds—breath sounds are best heard by having child breath through mouth

        (1) Vesicular—low pitch, soft intensity; inspiration is more than expiration with a ratio of 5:2; heard over peripheral lung fields

        (2) Bronchovesicular—medium pitch, moderate intensity; inspiration equals expiration with a ratio of 1:1; heard over main bronchus

        (3) Bronchial/tracheal—high pitch, loud intensity; inspiration less than expiration with a ratio of 1:2

    b. Abnormal breath sounds

(1) Rhonchi—course sounds heard on expiration that are indicative of secretions in the large airways; usually present in bronchitis; clear with coughing; associated with rhonchal fremitus (course vibrations felt with hand on chest as air passes through exudate in bronchi)

(2) Transmitted rhonchi—course sounds that result from the transmission of sound from congested nasal passages to the chest; can be avoided by having child breathe through mouth

(3) Wheezing—high pitched musical or whistling sounds produced as air passes through narrowed airways; heard in bronchiolitis, asthma; cystic fibrosis; foreign body aspiration (unilateral wheezing)

(4) Crackles—fine crackling sounds heard upon inspiration indicative of air passing through moisture in alveoli; usually suggests pneumonia or congestive heart failure

(5) Pleural friction rub—creaking or grating sound caused by inflamed parietal and visceral pleural linings rubbing together; usually inspiratory and expiratory; subsides when child holds breath

c. Chest movement

(1) Children under 7 years of age are diaphragmatic (abdominal) breathers

(2) Girls over 7 years of age become thoracic breathers; boys continue as abdominal breathers

(3) Chest structural abnormalities may compromise lung function

(a) Pectus carinatum—protuberant sternum

(b) Pectus excavatum—depressed sternum

- Breasts (see Endocrine Disorders chapter)

1. History indicating possible abnormalities

a. Prepubertal breast enlargement in girls

b. Gynecomastia in boys at any age

c. Breast mass

d. Galactorrhea not associated with childbearing

2. Selected physical examination findings

a. Neonate may have gynecomastia and milky discharge which disappears within 2 weeks (or, at least, 3 months)

b. Gynecomastia can be normal variant in males due to temporary estrogen/testosterone imbalance (usually begins at Tanner Stage II to III and can last for 1 to 2 years); most commonly felt as small, tender, oval subareolar mass measuring up to 2 to 3 cm in diameter

c. Gynecomastia also may be indicative of

(1) Obesity or increased muscle (pseudo-gynecomastia)

(2) Testicular tumor (testes must be palpated in any male with gynecomastia)

(3) Medication usage—estrogen, steroids, tricyclic antidepressants (e.g., imipramine), respiridol, mellaril, amphetamines, digoxin, cimetidine

(4) Klinefelter's syndrome (47XXY)—associated with small penis and testes, scoliosis, aspermia, decreased testosterone levels, and height greater than 6 feet

d. Asymmetric breast development is normal in the adolescent female

e. Galactorrhea may be indicative of:

(1) Pregnancy

(2) Recent abortion

(3) Pituitary tumor—associated with increased prolactin level; increased headaches; amenorrhea; peripheral vision loss

(4) Drug use—marijuana; opiates (codeine, heroin, morphine); amphetamines; hormones (oral contraceptives); digoxin; valium; cimetidine; phenothiazines (thorazine, mellaril); haloperidol; tricyclic antidepressants; respiridol

(5) Hypothyroidism

d. Breast masses in adolescents

(1) Benign breast masses (obtain ultrasound versus mammogram due to dense breast tissue in adolescents)

(a) Fibroadenoma—most common breast mass in adolescents; increased incidence in African-Americans

(i) Characteristics—single, unilateral mass; round or discoid in shape; firm and smooth in consistency; no retraction; mobile; nontender

(ii) No variation with menstrual cycle

(b) Fibrocystic breasts—usually result of hormonal imbalance

(i) Characteristics—breast pain with or without lumps; symptoms worsen a few days before menses and resolve with completion of menses

(ii) Mobile cysts or areas are more dense and fibrous; usually resolve in 1 to 3 months

(2) Neoplastic breast masses (very rare)—firm; nonmobile; painless; overlying skin changes; nipple discharge

- Abdomen

  1. History indicating possible abnormalities

     a. Birth weight under 1500 g places infant at high risk for necrotizing enterocolitis

     b. Failure to pass first meconium stool within 24 hours

     c. Jaundice

     d. Failure to grow or unexplained weight loss

     e. Projectile vomiting or blood in emesis

     f. Chronic diarrhea or constipation

     g. Enlargement of the abdomen with or without pain

     h. Abdominal or pelvic pain

  2. Selected physical examination findings—flexion of knees and hips facilitates examination

     a. Prominent abdomen (pot-belly)—normal in early childhood in sitting and supine positions due to poorly developed musculature; children up to 13 years of age may have prominent abdomen in standing position

     b. Liver edge—may be palpable 1 to 2 cm below right costal margin, especially with deep inspiration

     c. Spleen tip—may be palpable 1 to 2 cm below left costal margin, especially with deep inspiration

     d. Diastasis recti—separation of rectus abdominis muscles several cm wide from xiphoid bone to umbilicus; may extend to symphysis pubis; normal as long as not associated with hernia

     e. Bowel sounds

        (1) Active bowel sounds—heard every 5 to 15 seconds; range of 4 to 12 sounds per minute

        (2) Hypoactive bowel sounds—heard at more than 15 second intervals or less than 4 sounds per minute

        (3) Hyperactive bowel sounds—heard less than every 5 seconds or more than 12 sounds per minute

     f. Palpation of fecal mass in LLQ common with constipation

- Reproductive System

  1. History indicating possible abnormalities

     a. Discharge or bleeding from vagina or penis

     b. History or suspicion of sexual abuse

     c. Sexual intercourse without use of contraceptives

  d. Scrotal swelling with crying or bowel movement

  e. "Empty" scrotum versus retractable testes

  f. Unusual voiding pattern

 2. Selected physical examination findings (see Human Growth and Development Infancy through Adolescence chapter for Tanner stages and sequence of pubertal development)

  a. Signs and symptoms of possible sexual abuse

   (1) Evidence of general physical abuse or neglect

   (2) Evidence of trauma or scarring in genital, anal or perianal areas

   (3) Changes in skin color or pigmentation in genital or anal area

   (4) Any sexually transmitted disease

   (5) Anorectal itching, bleeding, pain or poor sphincter tone

   (6) Rashes, sores or discharge in genital area

   (7) Dysuria, frequency of urination, enuresis

   (8) Behavioral or emotional changes

   (9) Deterioration in school performance

   (10) Inappropriate sexual behavior for developmental level

  b. Labial adhesions

   (1) Rule out ambiguous genitalia

   (2) Adhesions of labia minora most common in young infants

  c. Male genitalia

   (1) Phimosis—foreskin that cannot be easily retracted over the glans penis before 5 years of age

   (2) Undescended testes (cryptorchidism)—if testicle can be "milked" down into scrotum, consider it descended; refer undescended testicle after 1 year of age

   (3) Hypospadias or epispadias should be referred

   (4) Large scrotum—hydrocele; spermatocele; varicocele

    (a) Testicular tumor (common in adolescents and young men)

    (b) Indirect inguinal hernia

- Musculoskeletal System (see Musculoskeletal Disorders: Infancy through Adolescence chapter)

 1. History indicating possible abnormalities

    a. Birth history—large for gestational age; abnormal presentation; anoxia in perinatal period

    b. Delay in motor developmental milestones

    c. Unusual style of movement—dragging of legs while crawling

    d. Hand dominance in an infant—may indicate weakness of other hand

    e. Leg pain/limp

2. Selected physical examination findings

    a. Barlow and Ortolani tests to detect hip dislocation or subluxation in infants—more common in females and breech deliveries

        (1) Barlow's test—hip is flexed and thigh is adducted which causes displacement of femoral head from acetabulum with a palpable "clunk"

        (2) Ortolani's test—hip is flexed at 90 degree angle and abducted with examiner's finger over the greater trochanter which reduces dislocated hip; a "clunk" is heard and felt

    b. Allis sign to detect hip dislocation or shortened femur—unequal leg length is abnormal

    c. Trendelenburg test to detect hip dislocation—child stands and raises one leg off the ground; lowering of iliac crest on side opposite weight-bearing leg indicates defect in weight bearing hip

    d. Gower's sign shows generalized muscle weakness; often indicative of muscular dystrophy—use of hands on legs to push self to standing position is abnormal

    e. Scoliosis (lateral curvature of the spine)

        (1) Functional—child can voluntarily straighten spine; disappears when child is recumbent

        (2) Structural—persistent curvature; unequal height of shoulders and iliac crests when standing erect; presence of rib hump when leaning forward

    f. Developmental differences

        (1) Longitudinal arch of foot can be obscured by fat pad until 3 years of age; child appears "flat footed"

        (2) Bowlegs (genu varum) and wide-based gait—common in toddlers

        (3) Knock knees (genu valgum)—common in preschool children

    g. "Turned-in" foot may have different causes

        (1) Femoral anteversion—most common between 3 and 8 years; 99% resolve by 8 years of age

        (2) Tibial torsion—most common between 1 and 3 years of age; growth alone will correct 99% of cases

Table 1
Infant Reflexes

Reflex	Appearance	Disappearance
Palmar grasp	birth	2–3 months
Plantar grasp	birth	10–12 months
Moro	birth	4–6 months
Stepping	birth	3–4 months
Tonic neck	birth to 6 weeks	4–6 months
Rooting	birth	3–4 months, except during sleep up to 12 months

　　　　　(3)　Metatarsus adductus

　　　h.　Hip should always be examined in child complaining of knee pain

- Neurologic System

　　1.　History indicating possible abnormalities

　　　a.　Delay or regression in developmental milestones; unusual behavior for age; learning or school difficulties

　　　b.　Headaches/seizures

　　　c.　Clumsiness or progressive weakness; irritability or lethargy

　　2.　Selected physical examination findings

　　　a.　Infant reflexes (automatisms)—see Table 1

　　　b.　Absence of infantile automatisms or persistence beyond expected time of disappearance may indicate severe CNS dysfunction

　　　c.　Spasticity—may be early sign of cerebral palsy

　　　d.　Use of Denver II or other general developmental screening tool yields much data regarding age appropriate skills

　　　e.　Babinski sign—normal up to 2 years of age

　　　f.　Age of disappearance of individual "soft signs" is typically 8 years

- Dermatologic System (see Dermatologic Conditions: Infancy through Adolescence chapter)

　　1.　History indicating possible abnormalities

　　　a.　Family history of atopic dermatitis, allergic skin disorders, familial hair loss, or unusual pigmentation patterns

　　　b.　Chronic or repeated acute episodes of skin lesions

　　　c.　Frequent scratching or rubbing of body area

　　2.　Selected physical examination findings

　　　a.　Birthmarks (nevi)

      (1)   Salmon patch (stork-bite)—common on eyelids, nasolabial region or nape of neck; disappears by 12 months

      (2)   Nevus flammeus (port-wine stain)—enlarges as child grows

      (3)   Strawberry nevus (raised hemangioma)

          (a)   Begins as circumscribed grayish white area; later becomes red and raised; not always present at birth

          (b)   Majority resolve spontaneously by 10 years of age

      (4)   Mongolian spot (hyperpigmented nevi)

          (a)   Usually in sacral or gluteal areas

          (b)   Generally seen in newborns of African-American, Asian or Latin descent

      (5)   Café-au-lait spots (light brown, flat patches)—6 or more may be associated with neurofibromatosis

  b.   Common color changes in newborns

      (1)   Acrocyanosis—cyanosis of hands and feet due to vascular instability

      (2)   Cutis marmorata—transient mottling when infant is exposed to decreased temperature

      (3)   Erythema toxicum—transient, benign, pink papular rash with vesicles on thorax, back, buttocks and abdomen

      (4)   Harlequin color change—as infant lies on side, dependent portion of body becomes pink and upper portion is pale

      (5)   Jaundice (see Hematological/Oncological/Immunologic Disorders: Infancy through Adolescence chapter)—skin blanches yellow with pressure instead of white as with carotinemia

          (a)   Jaundice appears first on head and then progresses down body

          (b)   Approximate level of hyperbilirubinemia by cephalocaudal distribution—nose (3 mg/dL); face (5 mg/dL); chest (7 mg/dL); abdomen (10 mg/dL); legs (12 mg/dL); palms (20 mg/dL)

          (c)   Physiological jaundice—appears 2 to 3 days after birth

          (d)   Appearance of jaundice in first 24 hours indicates hemolytic disease or infection

          (e)   Breast feeding infants who develop jaundice in the second to third week may have breast milk jaundice

          (f)   First appearance of jaundice at 2 to 3 weeks of age—must suspect biliary atresia (indirect bilirubin is elevated and AST and ALT also may be elevated)

      (g) Factors contributing to development of hyperbilirubinemia—metabolic acidosis, lowered albumin levels, free fatty acids, drugs (maternal or fetal), other conditions (e.g., fetal distress, hypoxia, hypothermia, hypoglycemia, infant bruising, maternal or fetal infection

  c. Degree of dehydration can be estimated by length of time skin retains "tenting" after it is pinched

     (1) < 2 seconds = < 5% loss of body weight

     (2) 2 to 3 seconds = 5% to 8% loss of body weight

     (3) 3 to 4 seconds = 9% to 10% loss of body weight

     (4) > 4 seconds = > 10% loss of body weight

- Lymph Nodes

  1. History indicating possible abnormalities

     a. Recurrent infections—tonsillitis, adenoiditis, bacterial infections, oral candidiasis, chronic diarrhea

     b. Poor growth; failure to thrive

     c. Maternal HIV infection

     d. IV drug use

     e. Multiple and indiscriminate sexual contacts

  2. Selected physical examination findings

     a. Normal size is up to 1 cm in inguinal area; 2 cm in cervical area; in other areas, up to 3 mm is normal

     b. Nodes enlarged due to infection are firm, or fluctuant, warm, tender, mobile, and may be accompanied by redness of overlying skin

     c. "Shotty" nodes (e.g., under 0.5 cm in diameter, firm, mobile and non-tender) can be present at any time in childhood and usually indicate past infection

     d. Suspect malignancy or tuberculosis if supraclavicular nodes are palpated

Selected Laboratory Tests and Values

- General Considerations

  1. Cost, pain, and invasiveness versus need for data to make accurate diagnosis

  2. Anesthetic cream used topically can ease venipuncture, especially in highly anxious children

  3. Laboratory values should be referenced against specified norms of laboratory conducting the testing since normal values may vary from laboratory to laboratory

- Hematology—CBC with differential

Table 2
Normal Range of Values
CBC

	Newborn	1 month	1 year	2–6 yrs	6–12 yrs	12–18 yrs
Hgb (g/dL)	14–24	11–17	11–15	11–15	11.5–15	12–16 (Males) 11.5–16 (Females)
Hct (%)	42–60	33–55	33–41	34–42	34–43	37–50 (Males) 36–44 (Females)
RBC (mill/mm^3)	4.1–7.5	4.2–5.2	4.1–5.1	3.9–5.3	4. 0–5.2	4.5–5.3 (Males) 4.1–5.1 (Females)
WBC × 1000/mm^3	9–30	5–19.5	6–17	5–15.5	4.5–13.5	4.5–13.5
Neutrophils (Segs%)	33–60	32–60	31–60	33–60	33–60	33–60
Bands (%) (Immature neutrophils)	0–5	0–5	0–5	0–5	0–5	0–5
Lymphocytes (%)	25–33	31–57	31–61	31–59	31–57	20–45
Monocytes (%)	3–7	3–7	3–7	3–7	3–7	3–10
Eosinophils (%)	1–4	1–4	1–4	1–4	1–4	1– 7
Basophils (%)	0–.75	0–.75	0–.75	0–.75	0–.75	0–.75
Platelets (10^3/mm^3)	84–478	150–400	150–400	150–400	150–400	150–400
Reticulocyte count (%)	3–7	.2–2	.2–2.8	.5–4	.5–4	.5–1.5
MCV (Mean Cell Volume$^+$; μm^3)	95–120	70–95	70–95	70–95	70–95	78–100
MCHC (Mean Cell Hemoglobin Concentration*)	31–37	31–37	31–37	31–37	31–37	31–37

+ Mean cell volume—average size of red cells
* Mean cell hemoglobin concentration—ratio of hemoglobin weight to hematocrit; helps to distinguish between normal colored cells (normochromic cells) and paler (hypochromic) cells

1. Normal range of values for complete blood count (CBC) with differential (see Table 2)

2. Common causes of variation in CBC with differential

    a. Hemoglobin variations

        (1) Increased—may indicate polycythemia (an overproduction of RBCs as a result of hypoxia); dehydration, or intravascular hemolysis

        (2) Decreased—may indicate anemia, hemodilution, sickle cell anemia, thalassemia; hemorrhage, or hyperthyroidism

    b. Hematocrit variations

        (1) Increased—may indicate polycythemia, dehydration or erythrocytosis

        (2) Decreased—may indicate anemia, hemorrhage; hyperthyroidism; leukemia, or cirrhosis

    c. Red blood cell variations

        (1) Increased—may indicate dehydration; hemorrhage; severe diarrhea; acute poisoning

        (2) Decreased—may indicate blood loss, low iron intake, lead poisoning, leukemia, rheumatic fever; systemic lupus erythematosis, or subacute bacterial endocarditis

d. White blood cell variations

   (1) Increased—first week of life; may signal bacterial infection (e.g., tonsillitis, sepsis, meningitis, appendicitis), or indicate acute hemorrhage, serum sickness, steroid use; hemolysis or leukemia

   (2) Decreased—indicates bone marrow depression which may result from viral infection; rickettsial infection; hypersplenia; leukemia; certain drugs (e.g., antiseizure medications, antibiotics, antihistamines, diuretics, analgesics, tricyclic antidepressants)

e. Neutrophils variations

   (1) Increased—may indicate bacterial infection; ischemic necrosis from burn injuries; metabolic disorders (e.g., diabetic ketoacidosis); stress response, emotional distress; inflammatory diseases (e.g. rheumatic arthritis), or hemolysis

   (2) Decreased (neutropenia)—viral infections (e.g., hepatitis, mononucleosis); chemotherapy or radiation; immune deficiencies; malignancies

f. Band cell or stab (immature neutrophil) variations—increased (known as a shift to the left); usually indicates severe bacterial infection (e.g., sepsis, pneumonia)

g. Lymphocytes variations

   (1) Increased—may indicate a viral infection; lymphocytic leukemia; ulcerative colitis; immune diseases

   (2) Decreased—indicates severe debilitating illnesses (e.g., congestive heart or renal failure, advanced TB); immunosuppressive therapy; Hodgkin's disease; after burns or trauma; Cushing syndrome; corticosteroid usage; HIV infection

   (3) Atypical lymphocytes—common in premature and healthy newborn infants; may indicate viral infection (e.g., mononucleosis, hepatitis); lymphocytic leukemia; ulcerative colitis; immune diseases

h. Monocyte variations

   (1) Increased—may indicate recovery from acute infection; SBE; leukemia; Hodgkin's disease; rickettsial infection; SLE; rheumatoid arthritis; hepatitis

   (2) Decreased—may indicate rheumatoid arthritis; HIV infection; prednisone usage

i. Eosinophil variations

   (1) Increased—may indicate allergic disorders (e.g., asthma, allergic rhinitis, atopic dermatitis) or parasite infection

   (2) Decreased—stress responses due to trauma, shock, burns, and emotional stress; Cushing syndrome

j. Basophil variations

  (1) Increased—may indicate certain leukemias, Hodgkin's disease, inflammatory conditions (e.g. ulcerative colitis); polycythemia, chronic hemolytic anemia; infections such as TB, varicella, influenza

  (2) Decreased—may indicate hyperthyroidism, pregnancy, stress, prolonged use of steroids, allergic reaction

k. Platelet variations

  (1) Increased—may indicate acute infection; malignancy; post-splenectomy; trauma; rheumatoid arthritis; Kawasaki disease

  (2) Decreased (thrombocytopenia)—may indicate leukemia; idiopathic thrombocytopenic purpura (ITP); autoimmune disorders; drugs (e.g., penicillin, ampicillin, cephalothin); hemolytic uremic syndrome; DIC; viral infection; HIV infection

l. Reticulocyte count variations

  (1) Increased—may indicate hemorrhage/blood loss; increased destruction of RBCs; response to initiation of iron therapy

  (2) Decreased—may indicate iron deficiency anemia; chronic infection; radiation; aplastic anemia

m. MCV variations

  (1) Increased—may indicate macrocytic anemia due to folic acid or vitamin B_{12} deficiency

  (2) Decreased—may indicate microcytic anemias caused by iron deficiency and thalassemia; anemia of chronic disease or lead poisoning

n. MCHC variations

  (1) Increased—may indicate spherocytosis

  (2) Decreased—suggests hypochromic anemia caused by iron deficiency; chronic blood loss or thalassemia

- Chemistry

1. Sodium chloride (mEq/L)

  a. Newborn—134 to 144

  b. Child—135 to 145

  c. Increased—dehydration; vomiting or diarrhea; diabetes insipidus; Cushing syndrome

  d. Decreased—vomiting; diarrhea; burns; diabetic ketoacidosis; Addison's disease; acute or chronic renal failure; syndrome of inappropriate antidiuretic hormone (SIADH)

2. Potassium (mEq/L)

    a.   Newborn—3.7 to 5.9

    b.   Child—3.5 to 5.0

    c.   Increased—may indicate acidosis or renal failure

    d.   Decreased—may indicate diarrhea, vomiting, dehydration, malabsorption, use of diuretics or anti-inflammatory drugs

3. Blood urea nitrogen (BUN)

    a.   Normal range—5 to 20 mg/dL

    b.   Increased—may indicate a high protein diet; renal or urinary obstruction or disease; GI hemorrhage; malignancies; dehydration; shock

    c.   Decreased—hemodilution; pregnancy; nephrotic syndrome; liver failure

4. Creatinine (more sensitive indicator of renal function than BUN)

    a.   Normal value—0.3 to 1 mg/dL

    b.   Increased—may indicate renal dysfunction; urinary tract obstruction, dehydration, muscle disease

5. Bilirubin (mg/dL)

    a.   Birth—1.5

    b.   Three to four days postnatal

        (1)   Breastfed—7.3

        (2)   Bottlefed—5.7

    c.   Older infant and child

        (1)   Total—less than 1.5

        (2)   Direct (conjugated)—0.2 to 0.4 (higher levels require investigation for pathology)

        (3)   Indirect (unconjugated) bilirubin—0.4 to 0.8 (levels greater than 20 mg/dL may be neurotoxic to brain)

6. Cholesterol (mg/100 mL)

    a.   Full-term newborn—45 to 167

    b.   Infant—70 to 190

    c.   Child and adolescent—less than 170

7. Lead—normal value (less than 10 μg/dL)

- Urine

1. pH

    a.   Newborn—5.0 to 7.0

    b.   Older infant and child—4.8 to 7.8

c. Increased (alkaline)—may indicate urinary tract infection; salicylate intoxication

d. Decreased (acidic)—may indicate acidosis; renal failure; diarrhea or dehydration

2. Specific gravity

a. Newborn—1.001 to 1.020

b. Older infant and child—1.001 to 1.030

c. Increased—may indicate dehydration, nephrosis, glomerulonephritis

d. Decreased—may indicate diabetes insipidus; severe renal damage

3. Glucose (should be negative)—presence of sugar may indicate diabetes mellitus or other metabolic disorders; liver disease or renal tubular disorders

4. Protein (should be negative)—presence of protein may indicate renal disease (e.g., nephritis, nephrosis); exercise; SLE; orthostatic proteinuria; asymptomatic proteinuria

5. Ketones (should be negative)—presence of ketones may indicate fever, dehydration, anorexia, diarrhea, fasting, prolonged vomiting or anorexia

6. Nitrites (should be negative)—presence of nitrites strongly suggests urinary tract infection

7. WBC

a. Normal range—0 to 4 WBC/HPF

b. Increased—may indicate urinary tract infection; fever; pyelonephritis; TB; nephrosis

8. RBC

a. Normal range 1 to 2 RBCs/HPF

b. Increased—may indicate urinary tract infection; pyelonephritis; SLE; renal stones; trauma; TB; hemophilia; ployarteritis nodosa; malignant hypertension

9. Bacteria (should be negative)—100,000 colonies/mL or more of a single pathogen on urine culture by clean catch method confirms a urinary tract infection; repeat urine culture should be obtained for a result of 10,000 to 100,000 colonies/mL

- Cerebrospinal fluid (CSF)

1. Pressure—70 to 180 mm H_2O; higher indicates increased intracranial pressure which may be the result of a tumor; cerebral hemorrhage; meningitis; obstructed shunt

2. Appearance—Clear

a. Bloody—may indicate traumatic tap; cerebral hemorrhage

b. Yellow—may indicate hyperbilirubinemia or metastatic melanoma

c. Cloudy—suggests increased WBC as found in bacterial meningitis

3. Glucose—60 to 80 mg/dL

    a. Increased—diabetes

    b. Decreased—may indicate bacterial meningitis, TB meningitis; hypoglycemia; leukemia with metastasis

4. Protein—15 to 45 mg/dL; increased in encephalitis; bacterial meningitis; TB meningitis; acoustic neuroma

5. Cell count

    a. Infant—0 to 20 WBC/mm^3

    b. Child and adolescent—0 to 10 WBC/mm^3

    c. Increased—bacterial meningitis; early viral meningitis; cerebral abscess

Selected Screening Tests

- Newborn Screening

  1. Screening should be conducted according to State law

  2. Most States require testing for:

     a. Hypothyroidism

     b. Phenylketonuria (PKU)

     c. Galactosemia

     d. Hemoglobinopathies (e.g., sickle cell disease)

  3. Other tests may include screening for:

     a. Maple syrup urine disease

     b. Homocystinuria

     c. Biotinidase deficiency

     d. Tyrosinemia

     e. Congenital adrenal hyperplasia

     f. Cystic fibrosis

     g. Toxoplasmosis

  4. Initial specimens should be obtained at least 24 hours after birth, but not more than 7 days of age

  5. Most States recommend a second metabolic screening in the first week of life for those infants tested before the first 36 to 48 hours of life

- Vision Screening

  1. Identify risk factors

     a. Prenatal infections

    b. Congenital cyanotic heart disease

    c. Structural malformation

    d. Family history of eye or vision problems

    e. Excessive oxygenation in neonatal period

    f. Hearing problems

    g. Parent concern about the child's visual functioning

    h. Deterioration in school performance

2. Conduct age appropriate screening measures

    a. Young infant

        (1) Assess pupillary response to light

        (2) Illicit blink reflex

        (3) Determine ability to fix on and follow an object

        (4) Assess red reflex

    b. Older infant and toddler

        (1) Determine ability to fix on and follow an object

        (2) Perform corneal light reflex test (Hirschberg)

        (3) Perform cover/uncover test

        (4) Assess red reflex

    c. Preschool child (same as toddler, plus)

        (1) Conduct visual acuity tests (Allen figures, HOTV, Sjogren hand, illiterate E)—refer for further evaluation with visual acuity of 20/50 or worse or a two-line difference or more in scores between eyes

        (2) Use Ishihara for color perception

    d. School-age child and adolescent (preschool child, plus)

        (1) Far vision—Snellen chart

        (2) Near vision—Rosenbaum or Jaeger card

        (3) Refer children for further evaluation with:

            (a) Abnormal or asymmetric red reflex

            (b) Asymmetric corneal light reflex

            (c) Abnormal cover/uncover test

            (d) Structural abnormality

            (e) Failure to follow object equally when covering each eye

            (f) Visual acuity of 20/30 or worse at 7 years of age

(g) Two line difference or more in scores between eyes

- Hearing Screening
    1. Identify infants and children at risk for hearing problems
        a. Neonatal risk criteria
            (1) Affected family member
            (2) Bilirubin > 20 mg/dL
            (3) Congenital CMV, herpes, rubella
            (4) Defects in ENT structure
            (5) Birth weight < 1500 g
            (6) Bacterial meningitis
            (7) Use of ototoxic medications for more than 5 days
            (8) Mechanical ventilation for cardiopulmonary disease for more than 48 hours
            (9) Intracranial hemorrhage
        b. Risk criteria for children less than 2 years of age (neonatal risk factors, plus)
            (1) Parental concerns regarding hearing or language development
            (2) Head trauma with temporal bone fracture
            (3) Infections known to cause sensorineural hearing loss (e.g., measles, mumps)
            (4) Recurrent otitis media or middle ear effusion
    2. Conduct age-appropriate screening measures
        a. Newborn
            (1) Healthy infants—observe responses to voices, loud noises
            (2) High-risk infants—auditory brainstem response (ABR) or evoked otoacoustic emissions (EOAE)
            (3) AAP goal of early identification of infants with hearing loss before 3 months with intervention implemented prior to 6 months of age (AAP, 1995)
        b. Four to 24 months (same as newborn, plus)
            (1) Observe orientation to sound
            (2) Assess language development
        c. Two to 3 years (same as above, plus)—play audiometry
        d. Older than 3 years

(1) Examine ears using an otoscope with pneumatic otoscopy before conducting audiometry

(2) Conduct pure tone audiometry—test each ear at 500, 1000, 2000 and 4000 Hz (hand-held audiometers have not proven effective in screening children)

(3) Use tympanometry to further assess middle ear air pressure and tympanic membrane compliance if pneumatic otoscopy was abnormal

3. Refer children to an audiologist for further evaluation if hearing threshold levels are greater than 20 dB at any of the above frequencies; if the reliability of a test with an individual child is uncertain, repeat screening before referral

- Tuberculosis screening

1. Mantoux test should be used for testing; uses .1 cc of purified protein derivative (PPD) which contains 5 tuberculin units; administer via intradermal injection to produce a 6 to 10 mm wheal; multiple-puncture tests do not have adequate specificity and sensitivity

2. Test should be read 48 to 72 hours following injection by a measurement of the area of *INDURATION,* not redness

3. Positive skin tests include children who have reaction of:

a. At least 15 mm *INDURATION* with no risk factors

b. At least 10 mm *INDURATION* who are less than 4 years of age or those with medical risk factors (e.g., born in, or whose parents were born, in areas of prevalent TB or exposed to adults who are HIV positive; homeless)

c. At least 5 mm *INDURATION* who are household contacts of active or previously active TB cases

4. Current recommendations for TB testing currently based on degree of risk rather than routine, universal screening

5. Annual TB testing for children at high risk

a. Exposure to confirmed or suspected TB

b. Recent immigration from country with endemic TB

c. Institutionalized and/or incarcerated children and youth

d. HIV positive or living with HIV infected person

6. Periodic TB testing between 4 to 6 years and again between 11 and 16 years for children living in high prevalence areas or with uncertain history of risk factors

7. See most recent AAP *Red Book* for specific updated guidelines

- Lead Screening

1. CDC revised guidelines (1997) no longer recommend universal screening; targeted

screening should be based on surveillance of risk (see Hematological/Oncological/
Immunologic Disorders: Infancy through Adolescence chapter)

2. Structured questionnaires such as the one developed by the Center for Disease Control and Prevention (CDC) should be used to assess risk for lead poisoning (refer to *The Clinician's Handbook of Preventive Services, 1994,* p. 27)

3. The blood lead level is more specific and sensitive than the erythrocyte protoporphyrin (EP) level (only 50% of children with a blood lead level of 32 μg/dL have elevated EP leads)

4. Venous blood samples are more reliable than capillary samples

5. The CDC defines lead poisoning as a blood level of ≥ 10 μg/dL; all children with blood lead levels equal to or more than 20 μg/dL should be screened for iron deficiency and receive treatment as recommended by CDC

6. Children who have blood lead levels of 10 to 14 μg/dL need periodic testing, but no treatment

7. Children who have blood lead levels between 15 to 19 μg/dL need education and dietary advice

- Cholesterol Screening

  1. Universal screening for all children not recommended

  2. Children more than 2 years of age who have a parent with a total cholesterol level of 240 mg/dL or greater should receive a total cholesterol screen

  3. Children more than 2 years of age with a family history of premature cardiovascular disease (e.g., a parent or grandparent with a myocardial infarction, sudden cardiac death, angina pectoris, coronary arteriography for diagnostic purposes, or cardiac bypass surgery at the age of 55 years or younger) should be screened with a serum lipid profile

  4. Children receiving total cholesterol screening may eat a normal diet before the test

  5. Children receiving a serum lipid profile should fast for 12 hours (except for water) before their blood is drawn

- Urine Screening

  1. Routine screening should be performed at 6 months and again at 2, 8, and 18 years of age

  2. Positive results of bacteriuria from a bagged urine specimen on an infant should be confirmed by catheterization or suprapubic aspiration

  3. "Clean catch" mid-stream urine specimens in children and adolescents are best for reliable results

- Sexually Transmitted Diseases/HIV

  1. All sexually active adolescents should be screened for gonorrhea and chlamydia as

well as have a Pap smear performed as a screening for Human Papillomavirus (HPV)

2. High-risk adolescents should be screened for syphilis and offered HIV testing (e.g., those with multiple sexual partners, who reside in areas with a high prevalence of STD/HIV infection, who have been sexually abused by or have had sexual contact with individuals with documented STD/HIV infection or parenteral drug use)

Special Examinations

- The Newborn Examination

    1. Immediately after birth, obtain APGAR scores at 1 and 5 minutes; composite scores range from 0 to 10 based on 5 criteria

Criteria	0	1	2
Heart rate	Absent	Slow (< 100)	> 100
Respiratory rate	Absent	Slow, irregular	Good strong cry
Muscle tone	Limp	Some flexion of extremities	Active motion
Reflex irritability	No response	Grimace	Cough or sneeze
Color	Blue, pale	Body pink, extremities blue	Completely pink

2. Obtain length, weight, head circumference percentiles, and vital signs

3. Assess vision and hearing

4. Assess gestational age (Ballard, Dubowitz)

5. HEENT

    a. Palpate anterior and posterior fontanels—note presence of molding, craniosynostosis, cephalohematomas, asymmetry

    b. Assess presence of red reflex

    c. Note size, shape and position of ears and characteristics of TM

    d. Assess for patency of nares, intact palate, and any unusual findings in the mouth

6. Assess neck for webbing; palpate for masses

7. Auscultate lungs and assess thorax for shape, symmetry, and character of respirations

8. Perform cardiac evaluation, including auscultation for murmurs and assessment of brachial and femoral pulses

9. Conduct abdominal examination, including the number of blood vessels in cord

(two umbilical arteries and one umbilical vein), cord appearance, and condition of stump

10. Assess genitourinary system, including prominence of labia; number of testicles and position; position of urethra; circumcision prior to discharge

11. Conduct musculoskeletal examination, including hips; feet; range of motion; presence of crepitus; Ortolani and Barlow maneuvers

12. Perform neurological examination, including assessment of head lag and muscle tone; illicit the following reflexes

    a. Root/suck

    b. Gag reflex

    c. Moro

    d. Plantar/palmar

    e. Stepping

    f. Tonic neck

13. Assess skin for cyanosis, jaundice, meconium staining, rashes, lesions and birthmarks

- The Sports Evaluation

  1. Purpose

     a. Identify risk factors associated with morbidity and mortality

     b. Identify conditions that place the child at risk for injury

     c. Identify conditions which could worsen with sports participation

     d. Determine appropriate sports activities for child's abilities

  2. Most important history-taking question—has the child ever fainted or lost consciousness during exercise?

  3. The physical examination should be comprehensive with emphasis on:

     a. Cardiac examination, including blood pressure

        (1) Presence of a systolic murmur that increases on sitting or with valsalva maneuver requires an echocardiogram

        (2) An arrythmia that does not subside with exercise requires referral to a cardiologist

     b. Musculoskeletal examination

        (1) Perform scoliosis screen

        (2) Have child perform the "duck walk" (squat on heels, walk 4 steps, and stand up)

        (3) Assess shoulder flexion and rotation

     c. Genitalia exam

       (1) Tanner stage

       (2) Presence of hernias

       (3) Presence of both testicles in males

4. Excluding conditions for contact collision sports include:

    a. Atlantoaxial instability (as found in Down syndrome)

    b. Carditis

    c. Absence of a paired organ (e.g., kidneys)

    d. Hepatosplenomegaly

    e. Poorly controlled seizure disorder

    f. Ventriculoperitoneal (VP) shunt

- Breast and Pelvic Examinations

1. Breast

    a. Although breast disease is rare in adolescent females, assessment of the breasts should be performed routinely as part of the well child physical examination from the start of puberty (as soon as breast budding occurs)

    b. In addition to detection of disease, the breast examination is a wonderful opportunity to teach adolescents about breast development and self-breast examination as well as provide reassurance about the "normalcy" of their breasts

2. Pelvic

    a. Recognize the pelvic examination produces much fear and anxiety for adolescents, especially those who are experiencing it for the first time, have had a prior difficult experience, and have been sexually abused

    b. Prepare the adolescent for the examination by showing her illustrations of the reproductive system and explaining the procedure

    c. Provide concrete objective information about sensations the adolescent will feel during course of the examination which will help her cope better with the experience

    d. Suggest ways to maintain control and decrease anxiety during examination (e.g., relaxation techniques)

    e. Use largest speculum that will fit comfortably within vagina (usually small plastic or Pederson speculum work best for this age group)

    f. Warm speculum before insertion

    g. Inform adolescent of what you are doing throughout the examination

    h. Encourage the adolescent to become involved with the examination if she desires (e.g., a mirror can be positioned to see the area being examined)

i. Verbal or visual modes of distraction are helpful (e.g., interesting posters on the ceiling or wall)

j. Use examination to teach adolescent about her body and to reassure her of "normalcy"

k. Provide as much privacy as possible, e.g., while dressing

l. Give positive feedback to the adolescent for her cooperation or assistance

m. Recognize that cervical ectopy is a normal finding during the examination, especially in adolescents taking hormonal contraceptives

Problem-Oriented Health Record

- Organized system for recording health visits to allow for thorough, concise data, easy retrieval of data, enhanced communication between health professionals; documentation of problem assessment/management, and decreased risk of liability

- Components of the problem-oriented health record

  1. Data base—medical history, physical examination, growth charts, developmental flow sheets, screening and laboratory tests, and problem-specific progress notes

  2. Problem list—conditions that require diagnostic work-up or ongoing management

  3. Management plan—includes information related to the diagnosis, management, education and follow-up for specific health problem

  4. Progress notes—includes documentation of each patient visit and is usually recorded in SOAP format

     a. **S**—subjective information provided by child and parent or caregiver

     b. **O**—objective information which consists of observations, physical examination, and laboratory findings

     c. **A**—assessment (diagnosis)

     d. **P**—plan

        (1) Medications

        (2) Treatments (e.g., warm compresses)

        (3) Further laboratory studies

        (4) Consultations or referrals

        (5) Diet or activity modifications

        (6) Teaching

        (7) Follow-up schedule (visit or telephone contact)

Child Health Supervision Schedule of Visits with Key Issues (Nutrition, Development, Screening, Immunizations, Anticipatory Guidance and Health Education)

- Prenatal Visit

  1. General Considerations

     a. Major purposes—ensure the health of the fetus, child, family; establish relationship with family; answer questions; provide anticipatory guidance and plan of care

     b. Timing—between 30 to 35 weeks gestation

     c. Include both parents and/or grandparents if single parent

  2. Family history—parents and siblings' ages; health of parents, siblings, and blood relatives, including chronic illnesses such as asthma, cystic fibrosis, and heart disease as well as mental disorders

  3. Obstetrical history—current gestational age; beginning of prenatal care; ultrasound or amniocentesis results; name of obstetrician; medications, drugs, cigarettes or alcohol usage during this pregnancy; prior pregnancies and outcomes

  4. Preparation for childbirth and infant

     a. Readiness for parenthood

     b. Planned or unplanned pregnancy

     c. Prenatal classes, childbirth preparation

     d. Sibling preparation, if applicable

     e. Choice of infant feeding (breast/bottle)—this visit is an excellent time to encourage breastfeeding, clarify misperceptions, and answer questions

     f. Circumcision, if applicable

     g. Genetic testing, if applicable

     h. Arrangements for child care

     i. Special concerns of prospective parents

     j. Current life stressors

  5. Social history

     a. Family type—single parent, nuclear

     b. Number and types of pets

     c. Perceived social support

     d. Health care practices/religion

     e. Financial information, including insurance

     f. Cultural issues

  6. Plan of care and anticipatory guidance

    a. Timing of health supervision visits

    b. Immunizations

    c. Organization of practice, e.g., team approach with nurse practitioners and physicians

    d. How and where to access care when needed; available hours

    e. Fees/medical coverage

    f. Need for transportation

    g. General infant care and supplies needed

    h. Safety information, e.g., car seats; pets

    i. Psychological adjustment of parents and siblings

- Newborn Visit

  1. Purposes—obtain complete history; physical examination; anticipatory guidance and plan of care

  2. Initial history—from chart review and parent/s

    a. General health of mother

      (1) Mother's age and gestation at first prenatal visit; regularity of visits

      (2) History of maternal infection and prenatal complications

      (3) Substance abuse, tobacco use

      (4) History of chronic disease

      (5) Medications during pregnancy

      (6) Weight gain; nutritional status

      (7) Number of weeks of gestation

      (8) Number of living children

    b. Labor and delivery

      (1) Length of labor

      (2) Medications used—anesthesia

      (3) Type of facility—birthing center, hospital, other

      (4) Type of delivery—spontaneous, C-section (explanation needed if yes)

      (5) Blood type, including Rh factor

    c. Infant's status at delivery

      (1) Identification verified

      (2) Term, preterm (number of weeks)

      (3) Determination of gestational age (Ballard/Dubowitz)

       (4)   Apgar scores

       (5)   Complications

       (6)   Oxygen or any other treatment(s) required

       (7)   Blood, type, Rh Factor; other values

       (8)   Length, weight, head and chest circumference (including percentiles)

       (9)   Physical examination results—note any abnormal findings

     (10)   Correct date of birth

  d. Nursery course—presence of jaundice; type of treatments; medications, immunizations; length of stay; circumcision/cord condition

  e. Family history—maternal/paternal

       (1)   Review of systems (ROS)—includes physical and mental health problems

       (2)   Home environment—members of household; pets; smokers; infant supplies and sleeping arrangements

  f. Common parental concerns

       (1)   Initial weight loss, appearance of infant (cephalohematoma, molding); normalcy of infant

       (2)   Rashes, skin markings—telangiectasis, cafe-au-lait, hemangiomas

       (3)   Infant's habits—feeding, stooling, sleeping, development, normal crying

       (4)   Female infant—breast engorgement, vaginal discharge

  g. Objective data

       (1)   Verify identification of mother, infant

       (2)   Parent/infant interaction—eye contact; holding; response to crying, vocalization

       (3)   Behavioral—consolability, self-quieting

       (4)   Physical examination (see Newborn Examination under Special Examinations in this chapter)

  h. Plan of care

       (1)   Reinforce infant care; cord care; circumcision care; instructions on when to seek medical advice

       (2)   Emphasize individual variability of infant temperament noting positive aspects and challenges

       (3)   Breast-feeding mothers

          (a)   Quiet alert state optimal time for nursing

(b) Initial feedings 3 to 5 minutes/each breast every $1\frac{1}{2}$ to 2 hours; increase time as tolerated

(c) Supplemental formula unnecessary

(d) Colostrum present first 2 to 4 days

(e) Increase maternal fluid intake especially at 6 weeks and 3 months during infant growth spurts

(f) Adequate infant intake indicated by 6 or more voids/day

(g) Vitamins unnecessary unless at risk for nutritional deficiencies, e.g. inadequate sunlight as vitamin D source

(4) Bottle-feeding mothers

(a) Alleviate guilt if it exists for not breast-feeding

(b) Amount and frequency varies

(1) 0 to 1 month—2 to 4 oz. every 3 to 4 hours

(2) 2 to 4 months—5 to 7 oz. every 4 to 5 hours

(c) Inform them that iron-fortified formulas are best

(d) Suggest partial hydrolysate formula if infant at risk for atopic disease, e.g., strong family history of atopic disease

(5) Crying—infant's first way of communicating needs

(a) Less than 2 hours/day during first month; peaks at 6 weeks

(b) Decreases as infant learns other ways to communicate

(6) Colic—excessive crying in otherwise healthy infants beginning at 2 to 3 weeks; may last 3 to 4 months

(a) Rule out physical problems

(b) Assess for over/under feeding

(c) Acknowledge stressful situation; encourage breaks from infant if possible; reassure that it usually subsides by 3 to 4 months

(d) Avoid sudden and overstimulation of infant

(e) If nursing, eliminate possible offending sources from maternal diet, e.g., coffee, spices, chocolate, milk, gas-forming foods

(f) Soothing techniques—rocking, walking, background "white noise," car rides

(g) Antiflatulent if indicated by history and examination

(7) Sleep patterns

(a) Usually sleeps 8 hours by 3 months

(b) Early introduction of solids—doesn't cause infants to sleep through the night

(c) Position on side or supine as SIDS preventive measure unless medically contraindicated

(8) Bowel movements

(a) Usually after feeding (especially if breast fed); normal variation may be up to one/week

(b) Avoid laxatives; use stool softener if constipated

(9) Reminder to schedule office visit for 2 weeks-of-age

- Interim Visits—2 Weeks to 1 Year (2 weeks; 2, 4, 6, 9 & 12 months)

1. Subjective information

    a. Feeding—type, amounts, time at breast, name of formula

    b. Elimination—frequency, color, consistency of stools; number of saturated diapers per day

    c. Sleep

    d. Development, including behavior and temperament

    e. Concerns of parent, caregiver

    f. Interval history—health since last visit; emergency care; illnesses, medications used

2. Objective data

    a. Age, height, weight, head circumference percentiles; vital signs

    b. Caregiver/infant interaction

    c. Vision and hearing screening

    d. Physical examination

    e. Developmental screening—Denver II or equivalent and results

    f. Laboratory

        (1) Bilirubin, if indicated

        (2) Urinalysis at 6 months unless indicated otherwise

        (3) Hematocrit between 6 and 9 months or if indicated otherwise

        (4) Blood lead level between 9 to 12 months or sooner if indicated

3. Plan of care, including health promotion strategies and anticipatory guidance

    a. Administer immunizations as indicated after obtaining consent and assessing response to previous immunizations—see Tables 3 to 9

        (1) Inform parents of common side effects of immunizations

(2) The National Childhood Vaccine Injury Act of 1986 requires all health providers who administer vaccines to report occurrences of certain adverse events stipulated in the Act—see Table 9 "Reportable Events Following Immunization"

b. Inform parents of any medications prescribed, including name, rationale, dosage, frequency, course and potential side effects

c. Implement health promotion strategies and anticipatory guidance appropriate for age and developmental level (ideally should be done before or at the very beginning of a developmental stage or problem); best to focus on one or two per visit with input from the parent or caregiver

4. Anticipatory guidance—nutrition and feeding

a. Nutritional requirements are 110 to 120 calories/kg/day

b. Consumption of more than 32 oz of formula per day usually indicative of need for solids once an infant is at least 4 months of age

c. Formula recommended up to 1 year of age; whole milk until two years of age

d. Judicious use of juices—some fortified with vitamin C; best to place in cup versus bottle

e. Best to avoid giving infants a bottle in bed, especially containing formula or juice (leads to dental caries)

f. Introduction of solids

(1) Usually best to delay introduction of solids until 6 months of age—earlier introduction may lead to overfeeding and allergies

(2) Cereal usually first food added to diet followed by vegetables, fruits and meats

(3) Add only 1 new food every 3 to 5 days

(4) Do not give common allergenic foods until one year of age, e.g. cow's milk, egg whites, wheat, citrus fruits

(5) Avoid the following until 3 years of age to prevent choking—nuts, potato chips, popcorn, raw celery and carrots; hotdogs; fish with bones; tough meat; small, hard candies

g. Introduction of cup—when infant loses interest in bottle (7 to 10 months); spout cup may be used initially

h. Weaning (breast or bottle)—gradually decrease number of feedings over several weeks; night feeding usually last to be eliminated

5. Anticipatory guidance—sleep

a. 2 to 4 month old infant—8 to 12 hours at night; 2 to 3 naps

b. 6 to 12 month old infant—11 to 12 hours at night; 2 to 3 naps

    c. Side-lying or supine sleep position through 6 months

    d. Strategies for parents

        (1) Put infant in crib when drowsy rather than asleep

        (2) Quiet, non-stimulating night feedings

        (3) Night waking once night feedings stop—briefly stroke infant lightly; don't pick infant up

        (4) Avoid pattern of placing infant in parent's bed

6. Anticipatory guidance—infant stimulation

    a. Provide variety of age-appropriate stimulation

    b. Formal infant stimulation programs for infants at risk for developmental delays

7. Anticipatory guidance—teeth

    a. Eruption typically begins at approximately 6 months of age

    b. Signs and symptoms—local sensitivity and inflammation; increased drooling, biting, irritability

    c. No evidence that teething causes fever, diarrhea, or other systemic illnesses

    d. Comfort measures—hard rubber teething toy, chilled teething ring; wet wash cloth; avoid liquid filled teething rings

8. Stranger/anxiety—emerging awareness and preference for mother/ primary caregiver; early indicator of healthy attachment process emerging around 6 months

9. Separation anxiety—emerging awareness that infant is an individual distinct from primary attachment figure/caregiver

    a. Develops around 9 months; peaks at around 18 months

    b. Suggestions for parents

        (1) Recognize that bedtime, going to daycare, having a babysitter at home are all separations

        (2) Gradually introduce child to new situations and caretakers

        (3) The child learns to accept separation through multiple, brief separations and reunions

        (4) Games such as ''peek-a-boo'' and ''hide-and-seek'' may be helpful

10. Safety—prevention of ingestion/aspiration of foreign objects

    a. Keep pins, buttons, and other small objects off the floor and out of reach

    b. Do not feed infants hard foods (e.g., nuts, hard candies)

    c. Discard broken or cracked rattles with beads

    d. Do not give infant balloons

e. Do not prop infant's bottle

f. Select pacifier with shield too large to enter infant's mouth

g. Learn emergency procedure for dealing effectively with choking

11. Injury prevention

a. Keep electrical wires out of reach; outlets covered; cabinet safety locks; medicines, poisons out of reach

b. Install smoke detectors in household

c. Keep syrup of ipecac readily available in case of accidental poisoning; Poison Control telephone number available, other emergency phone numbers

d. Use car seat appropriate for infant's weight and age

e. Avoid walkers and stairs; use gate to barricade doorways and unsafe areas, e.g., kitchen and bathroom

f. Do not place necklaces or pacifier cords around infant's neck

g. Discourage infant jewelry

h. Position crib or playpen away from window blind or curtain cords

i. Use a crib with side rails spaced no more than $2 \frac{3}{8}$ inches apart

j. Secure infant with belt on changing table

k. Lower crib mattress when infant begins to stand

12. Water safety—prevention of drowning and burns

a. Set hot water heater temperature at 120° F or less

b. Do not leave infant unattended in bathtub

c. Do not allow child to play in water unattended, e.g., toilet bowls, sinks, buckets of water

d. Use of safety devices around swimming pools, lakes and in boats, e.g., life jackets

e. Lock fences around swimming pools

f. Continuous supervision around water

g. Do not leave other children in charge of infants around any body of water

13. Sun safety and sunburn protection—use lotion with sun protective factor (SPF) of at least 15; avoid use around eyes; use caps with sun visors or bonnets to protect eyes; keep infants in shaded areas, even with sunscreen; sun avoidance for infants < 6 months

14. Alternative child care arrangements—babysitters and day care; appropriate supervision and stimulation/activities (language, visual and motor)

15. Emphasize positive qualities of the infant and the parent-child relationship and

mutually agree upon a plan with the parent to strengthen needed areas

16. Make referrals to other nurse practitioners, physicians, clinics and community resources as needed

17. Schedule for next visit

- Interim Visits—Toddler (1 to 3 years) (12, 15, 18, & 24 months)

    1. Subjective data—nutrition/appetite; elimination; sleep; development; parental concerns; health since last visit

    2. Objective Data

        a. Assess parent-child interaction and parenting style

        b. Height, weight; head circumference (up to 2 years)

        c. Vision and hearing screening

        d. Physical examination

        e. Developmental screening—Denver II or equivalent and results

        f. Laboratory

            (1) Hematocrit at 2 years or if otherwise indicated

            (2) Urinalysis at 2 years of age or if otherwise indicated

            (3) Lead screening by 2 years of age as appropriate based on well-child surveillance of risk (CDC) (See Hematological/Oncological/Immunologic Disorders: Infancy through Adolescence chapter)

- Management

    a. Update immunizations (see Tables 3 to 9 for immunizations); inform parents of common side-effects of immunizations

    b. Advise parents of any medications prescribed, including vitamins and fluoride, e.g., name, rationale, dosage, frequency, course and potential side effects

    c. Nutrition appropriate for age

        (1) Nutritional requirements are 102 cal/kg

        (2) Provide foods from the five major food groups in realistic amounts; $\frac{1}{4}$ to $\frac{1}{3}$ of adult portion or one measuring tablespoon for each year of the child's age

        (3) Physiological anorexia is common between 15 and 18 months of age

        (4) Parental concerns regarding nutrition—decreased appetite; food jags; rituals; variable intake; definite likes and dislikes

        (5) Potential nutritional problems—iron deficiency anemia (especially if toddler is drinking more than 32 oz of milk per day); low intake of calcium, vitamin A, zinc, ascorbic acid; obesity

Table 3
Recommended Childhood Immunization Schedule
United States, January — December 2001

Vaccines[1] are listed under routinely recommended ages. Bars indicate range of recommended ages for immunization. Any dose not given at the recommended age should be given as a "catch-up" immunization at any subsequent visit when indicated and feasible. The circled, bold italic type indicate vaccines to be given if previously recommended doses were missed or given earlier than the recommended minimum age.

Age → / Vaccine ↓	Birth	1 mo	2 mos	4 mos	6 mos	12 mos	15 mos	18 mos	24 mos	4-6 yrs	11-12 yrs	14-18 yrs
Hepatitis B[2]	HepB#1	HepB#1	HepB#2		HepB#3	HepB#3	HepB#3				HepB[2]	
Diptheria, Tetnus, Pertussis[3]			DTaP	DTaP	DTaP		DTaP[3]	DTaP[3]		DTaP	Td	
Type b H. Influenza[4]			Hib	Hib	Hib	Hib						
Polio[5]			IPV	IPV	IPV[5]	IPV[5]	IPV[5]			IPV[5]		
MMR[6]						MMR	MMR			MMR 6	MMR[6]	
**Pneumo-coccal conjugate[7]			PCV	PCV	PCV	PCV						
Varicella[8]						Var	Var				Var[8]	
Hepatitis A[9]									HepA-In selected areas[9]	HepA-In selected areas[9]		

Approved by the Advisory Committee on Immunization Practices (ACIP), the American Academy of Pediatrics (AAP), and the American Academy of Family Physicians (AAFP)

1.This schedule indicates the recommended ages for routine administration of currently licensed childhood vaccines, as of 11/1/00, for children through 18 years of age. Additional vaccines may be licensed and recommended during the year. Licensed combination vaccines may be used whenever any components of the combination are indicated and its other components are not contraindicated. Providers should consult the manufacturers' package inserts for detailed recommendations.

2. **Infants born to HBsAg-negative mothers** should receive the 1st dose of hepatitis B (HepB) vaccine by age 2 months. The 2nd dose should be at least one month after the 1st dose. The 3rd dose should be administered at least 4 months after the 1st dose and at least 2 months after the 2nd dose, but not before 6 months of age for infants.

Infants born to HBsAg-positive mothers should receive hepatitis B vaccine and 0. 5 mL hepatitis B immune globulin (HBIG) within 12 hours of birth at separate sites. The 2nd dose is recommended at 1-2 months of age and the 3rd dose at 6 months of age.

Infants born to mothers whose HBsAg status is unknown should receive hepatitis B vaccine within 12 hours of birth. Maternal blood should be drawn at the time of delivery to determine the mother's HBsAg status; if the HBsAg test is positive, the infant should receive HBIG as soon as possible (no later than 1 week of age).

All children and adolescents who have not been immunized against hepatitis B should begin the series during any visit. Special efforts should be made to immunize children who were born in or whose parents were born in areas of

(Notes continued on next page)

the world with moderate or high endemicity of hepatitis B virus infection.

3. The 4th dose of DTaP (diphtheria and tetanus toxoids and acellular pertussis vaccine) may be administered as early as 12 months of age, provided 6 months have elapsed since the 3rd dose and the child is unlikely to return at age 15-18 months. Td (tetanus and diphtheria toxoids) is recommended at 11-12 years of age if at least 5 years have elapsed since the last dose of DTP, DTaP or DT. Subsequent routine Td boosters are recommended every 10 years.

4. Three Haemophilus influenzae type b (Hib) conjugate vaccines are licensed for infant use. If PRP-OMP (PedvaxHIB ® or ComVax ®[Merck]) is administered at 2 and 4 months of age, a dose at 6 months is not required. Because clinical studies in infants have demonstrated that using some combination products may induce a lower immune response to the Hib vaccine component, DTaP/Hib combination products should not be used for primary immunization in infants at 2, 4, or 6 months of age, unless FDA-approved for these ages.

5. An all-IPV schedule is recommended for routine childhood polio vaccination in the United States. All children should receive four doses of IPV at 2 months, 4 months, 6-18 months, and 4 to 6 years. Oral Polio Vaccine (OPV) should be used only in selected circumstances. (See MMWR *Morb Mortal Wkly Rep* May 19, 2000/49(RR-5);1-22).

6. The 2nd dose of measles, mumps, and rubella (MMR) vaccine is recommended routinely at 4-6 years of age but may be administered during any visit, provided at least 4 weeks have elapsed since receipt of the 1st dose and that both doses are administered beginning at or after 12 months of age. Those who have not previously received the second dose should complete the schedule by the 11-12 year old visit.

7. The heptavalent conjugate pneumococcal vaccine (PCV) is recommended for all children 2-23 months of age. It is also recommended for certain children 24-59 months of age. (See MMWR *Morb Mortal Wkly Rep* Oct. 6, 2000/49(RR-9);1-35). Table 5 provides PCV immunization information for children less than 23 months who have not been previously immunized (**Academy of Pediatrics Policy Statement, 2000 vol.106, no.02).

8. Varicella (Var) vaccine is recommended at any visit on or after the first birthday for susceptible children, i.e. those who lack a reliable history of chickenpox (as judged by a health care provider) and who have not been immunized. Susceptible persons 13 years of age or older should receive 2 doses, given at least 4 weeks apart.

9. Hepatitis A (HepA) is shaded to indicate its recommended use in selected states and/or regions, and for certain high risk groups; consult your local public health authority. (See *MMWR Morb Mortal Wkly Rep* Oct. 1, 1999/ 48(RR-12);1-37).

10. The Meningococcal vaccine has recently been encouraged for the following individuals:
    1. college bound adolescents 15-24 years of age residing in dormitories or residence halls
    2. anyone in close contact with a known case
    3. anyone with an upper respiratory infection and a compromised immune system
    4. any one travelling to endemic areas.

This vaccine provides protection for 3-5 years (CDC, October 20, 1999 press release).

For additional information about the vaccines listed above, please visit the National Immunization Program Home Page at www.cdc.gov/nip *or all the National Immunization Hotline at 800-232-2522 (English) or 800-232-0233 (Spanish)*

From: American Academy of Pediatrics. In: L.K.Pickering (Ed). *Red Book 2000: Report of the committee on infectious diseases.* 25th ed. Elk Grove Village, IL: American Academy of Pediatrics; 2000: pp. 22-23. Reprinted with permission. Updated from Academy of Pediatrics press release January 8, 2001 (http://www.aap.org/advocacy/releases/janimmun.htm).

Table 4

Recommended Immunization Schedules for Children Not Immunized in the First Year of Life*

Recommended Time/Age	*Immunization(s)†*	*Comments*
Younger Than 7 Years		
First visit	DTaP, Hib‡, HBV, MMR	If indicated, tuberculin testing may be done at same visit. If child is 5 y of age or older, Hib is not indicated in most circumstances.
Interval after first visit 1mo (4 wk)	DTaP, IPV, HBV, Var§	The second dose of IPV may be given if accelerated poliomyelitis immunization is necessary, such as for travelers to areas where polio is endemic.
2 mo	DTaP, Hib,‡ IPV	Second dose of Hib is indicated only if the first dose was received when younger than 15 mo.
≥8mo	DTaP, HBV, IPV	IPV and HBV are not given if the third doses were given earlier.
Age 4-6 y (at or before school entry)	DTaP, IPV, MMRΠ	DTaP is not necessary if the fourth dose was given after the fourth birthday; IPV is not necessary if the third dose was given after the fourth birthday.
Age 11-12 y	see Table 3	
7-12 Years		
First visit	HBV, MMR, dT, IPV	
Interval after first visit 2 mo (8 wk)	HBV, MMRΠ, Var§, dT, IPV	IPV also may be given 1 mo after the first visit if accelerated poliomyelitis immunization is necessary.
8-14mo	HBV ± dT, IPV	IPV is not given if the third dose was given earlier.
Age ll-l2y	See Table 3	

* Table is not completely consistent with all package inserts. For products used, also consult manufacturer's package insert for instructions on storage, handling, dosage, and administration. Biologics prepared by different manufacturers may vary; and package inserts of the same manufacturer may change. Therefore, the physician should be aware of the contents of the current package insert. Vaccine abbreviations: HBV indicates hepatitis B virus; Var, varicella; DTaP, diphtheria and tetanus toxoids and acellular pertussis; Hib, Haemophilus influenzae type b conjugate; IPV, inactivated poliovirus; MMR, live measles-mumps-rubella; dT, adult tetanus toxoid (full dose) and diphtheria toxoid (reduced dose), for children 7 years of age or older and adults.

† If all needed vaccines cannot be administered simultaneously, priority should be given to protecting the child against the diseases that pose the greatest immediate risk. In the United States, these diseases for children younger than 2 years usually are measles and *Haemophilus influenzae* type b infection; for children older than 7 years, they are measles, mumps, and rubella. Before 13 years of age, immunity against hepatitis B and varicella should be ensured. DTaP, HBV, Hib, MMR, and Var can be given simultaneously at separate sites if failure of the patient to return for future immunizations is a concern.

‡ See *Haemophilus influenzae* Infections, Pickering, L.K, (Ed.) *Red Book 2000: Report of the committee on infectious diseases. 25th ed.* Elk Grove Village, IL: American Academy of Pediatrics p 262, and Table 3.11 (p 268).

§ Varicella vaccine can be administered to susceptible children any time after 12 months of age. Unimmunized children who lack a reliable history of varicella should be immunized before their 13th birthday.

Π Minimal interval between doses of MMR is 1 month (4 wk).

± HBV may be given earlier in a 0-, 2-, and 4-month schedule.

From: American Academy of Pediatrics. In: Pickering, L.K. (Ed.). *Red Book 2000: Report of the committee on infectious diseases.* 25th ed. Elk Grove Village, IL: American Academy of Pediatrics; 2000: pp. 24-25. Reprinted with permission.

Table 5

Recommended Primary Series and Catch-up Immunization Schedule for the Pneumococcal Conjugate Vaccine (PCV7) in Previously Unvaccinated Children

Age at first dose	Primary series	Booster dose*
2-6 Months (8-24 weeks)	3 Doses, 6-8 weeks apart	1 Dose at 12-15 months of age
7-11 Months (28-44 weeks)	2 Doses, 6-8 weeks apart	1 Dose at 12-15 months of age
12-23 Months	2 Doses, 6-8 weeks apart	
24 Months and older	1 Dose	

* Booster doses should be given at least 6-8 weeks after the final dose of the primary series

From: American Academy of Pediatrics Committee on Infectious Diseases. *Policy statement: Recommendations for the prevention of pneumococcal infections, including the use of pneumococcal conjugate vaccine (Prevnar), pneumococcal polysaccharide vaccine, and antibiotic prophylaxis.* June 6, 2000. pp. 1-3.

Table 6

Currently Recommended Regimens for Routine *Haemophilus influenzae* Type b Conjugate Immunization for Children Immunized Beginning at 2 to 6 Months of Age*

Vaccine Product at Initiation	Total No. of Doses To Be Administered	Recommended Regimen
HbOC or PRP-T	4	3 doses at 2 mo intervals initially; fourth dose at 12 to 15 mo of age; any conjugate vaccine for dose 4†
PRP-OMP	3	2 doses at 2-mo interval initially; when feasible, same vaccine for doses 1 and 2; third dose at 12-15 mo of age; any conjugate vaccine for dose 3†

* See text and Table 3.10 in The Red Book, 2000 for further information about specific vaccines and for explanation of the abbreviations. These vaccines may be given in combination products or as reconstituted products with DTaP or DTP, provided the combination or reconstituted vaccine is approved by the US Food and Drug Administration for the child's age and administration of the other vaccine component(s) also is justified.

† The safety and efficacy of PRP-OMP, PRP-T, HbOC, and, PRP-D are likely to be equivalent for children 12 months of age and older. If a different product is given for dose 2, then the recommendations for that product (eg, HbOC or PRP-T) apply.

From: American Academy of Pediatrics. In: Pickering, L.K. (Ed.) Red Book 2000: Report of the committee on infectious diseases. 25th ed. Elk Grove Village, IL: American Academy of Pediatrics; 2000: p. 268. Reprinted with permission.

      (6)   Provide regular meals and snacks

      (7)   Avoid food battles

  d.   Toilet Training

      (1)   Most children are psychologically and physiologically ready between 18 to 30 months

      (2)   Majority of children achieve daytime bowel and bladder training simultaneously; average age is 28 months

      (3)   Nighttime control generally occurs about 1 year after daytime control is achieved

      (4)   Toilet training should not be started when family is unduly stressed (e.g., new baby, moving, holidays, divorce)

Table 7

Recommendations for *Haemophilus influenzae* Type b Conjugate Immunization for Children in Whom Initial Immunization Is Delayed Until 7 Months of Age or Older*

Age at Initiation of Immunization, mo	Vaccine Product at Initiation	Total No. of Doses To Be Administered	Recommended Vaccine Regimens
7-11	HbOC, PRP-T, or PRP-OMP	3	2 doses at 2-mo intervals; third dose at 12-15 mo of age, given at 2 mo after dose 2; any conjugate vaccine for dose 3[†]
12-14	HbOC, PRP-T, PRP-OMP, or PRP-D	2	2-mo interval between doses
15-59	HbOC, PRP-T, PRP-OMP, or PRP-D	1[‡]	Any conjugate vaccine
60 and older[§]	HbOC, PRP-T, PRP-OMP, or PRP-D	1 or 2[‡]	Any conjugate vaccine

* See text and Table 3.10 in Red Book, 2000 for further information about specific vaccines and for explanation of the abbreviations. These vaccines may be given in combination products or as reconstituted products with DTaP or DPT provided the combination or reconstituted vaccine is approved by the US Food and Drug Administration for the child's age and administration of the other vaccine component(s) also is justified.

† The safety and efficacy of PRP-OMP, PRP-T, HbOC or PRP-D are likely to be equivalent for use as a booster dose for children 12 months or older.

‡ Two doses separated by 2 months are recommended by some experts for children with certain underlying diseases associated with increased risk of disease and impaired antibody responses to H influenzae type b conjugate vaccination (see text).

§ Only for children with chronic illness known to be associated with an increased risk for H influenzae type b disease (see text).

From: American Academy of Pediatrics. In: Pickering, L.K. (Ed.) *Red Book 2000: Report of the committee on infectious diseases.* 25th ed. Elk Grove Village, IL: American Academy of Pediatrics; 2000: pp. 269. Reprinted with permission.

Table 8

Recommendations for *Haemophilus influenzae* Type b Conjugate Immunization in Children With a Lapse in Administration*

Age at Presentation, mo	Previous Vaccination History	Recommended Regimen
7-11	1 dose of HbOC or PRP-T	1 dose of conjugate vaccine at 7-11 mo of age (depending on age), with a booster dose given at least 2 mo later, at 12-15 mo
	2 doses of HbOC or PRP-T or 1 dose of PRP-OMP	1 dose of conjugate vaccine at 7-11 mo of age with a booster dose given at least 2 mo later at 12-15 mo
12-14	2 doses before 12 mo of age[†]	A single dose of any licensed conjugate vaccine[‡]
12-14	1 dose before 12 mo of age[†]	2 additional doses of any licensed conjugate vaccine, separated by 2 mo[‡]
15-59	Any incomplete schedule	A single dose of any licensed conjugate vaccine[‡]

* See text and Table 3.10 in Red Book, 2000 for further information about specific vaccines and for explanation of abbreviations. These vaccines may be given in combination products or as reconstituted products with DtaP or DTP; provided the combination or reconstituted vaccine is approved by the US Food and Drug Administration for the child's age and the administration of the other vaccine component(s) also is justified.

† PRP-OMP, PRP-T, or HbOC.

‡ The safety and efficacy of PRP-OMP, PRP-T, or HbOC or PRP-D are likely to be equivalent when used for children 12 months of age or older.

From: American Academy of Pediatrics. In: Pickering, L.K. (Ed.) *Red Book 2000: Report of the committee on infectious diseases.* 25th ed. Elk Grove Village, IL: American Academy of Pediatrics; 2000: pp. 271. Reprinted with permission.

Table 9
National Childhood Vaccine Injury Act Reporting and Compensation Table*

	Vaccine	Adverse Event	Interval from Vaccination to Onset of Event For Reporting[†]	For Compensation[‡]
I.	Tetanus toxoid—containing vaccines (eg, DTaP, DTP, DTP-Hib; DT; dT, or TT)	A. Anaphylaxis or anaphylactic shock B. Brachial neuritis C. Any acute complication or sequela (including death) of above events D. Events described in manufacturer's package insert as contraindications to additional doses of vaccine	0-7d 0-28d No limit No limit	0-4h 2-28d No limit Not applicable
II.	Pertussis antigen—containing vaccines (eg, DTaP, DTP, P, DTP-Hib)	A. Anaphylaxis or anaphylactic shock B. Encephalopathy (or encephalitis) C. Any acute complication or sequela (including death) of above events D. Events described in manufacturer's package insert as contraindications to additional doses of vaccine	0-7d 0-7d No limit No limit	0-4h 0-72h No limit Not applicable
III.	Measles, mumps, and rubella virus—containing vaccines in any combination (eg, MMR, MR, M,R)	A. Anaphylaxis or anaphylactic shock B. Encephalopathy (or encephalitis) C. Any acute complication or sequela (including death) of above events D. Events described in manufacturer's package insert as contraindications to additional doses of vaccine	0-7d 0-15d No limit No limit	0-4h 5-15d No limit Not applicable
IV.	Rubella virus—containing vaccines (eg, MMR, MR, R)	A. Chronic arthritis B. Any acute complication or sequela (including death) of above event C. Events described in manufacturer's package insert as contraindications to additional doses of vaccine	0-42d No limit No limit	7-42d No limit Not applicable
V.	Measles virus—containing vaccines (eg, MMR, MR, M)	A. Thrombocytopenic purpura B. Vaccine-strain measles viral infection in an immunodeficient recipient C. Any acute complication or sequela (including death) of above events D. Events described in manufacturer's package insert as contraindications to additional doses of vaccine	0-30d 0-6 mo No limit No limit	7-30d 0-6 mo No limit Not applicable

VI.	Live poliovirus—containing vaccines (OPV)	A. Paralytic polio
		  • in a nonimmunodeficient recipient
		  • in an immunodeficient recipient
		  • in a vaccine-associated community case
		B. Vaccine-strain polio viral infection
		  • in a nonimmunodeficient recipient
		  • in an immunodeficient recipient
		  • in a vaccine-associated community case
		C. Any acute complication or sequela (including death) of above events
		D. Events described in manufacturer's package insert as contraindications to additional doses of vaccine
			
			0-30 d
			0-6mo
			No limit
			
			0-30 d
			0-6mo
			No limit
			No limit
			No limit
				
				0-30 d
				0-6mo
				No limit
				
				0-30 d
				0-6mo
				No limit
				No limit
				Not applicable

VII.	Polio inactivated	A. Anaphylaxis or anaphylactic shock B. Any acute complication or sequela (including death) of above event C. Events described in manufacturer's package insert as contraindications to additional doses of vaccine	0-7d No limit No limit	0-4h No limit Not applicable
VIII.	Hepatitis B antigen—containing vaccines	A. Anaphylaxis or anaphylactic shock B. Any acute complication or sequela (including death) of above event C. Events described in manufacturer's package insert as contraindications to additional doses of vaccine	0-7d No limit No limit	0-4h No limit Not applicable
IX.	*Haemophilus influenzae* type b polysaccharide vaccines (unconjugated, PRP vaccines)	A. Early-onset Hib disease B. Any acute complication or sequela (including death) of above event C. Events described in manufacmrer's package insert as contraindications to additional doses of vaccine	0-7d No limit No limit	0-7d No limit Not applicable
X.	*Haemophilus influenzae* type b polysaccharide conjugate vaccines	A. No condition specified for compensation B. Events described in manufacturer's package insert as contra-indications to additional doses of vaccine	Not applicable No limit	Not applicable Not applicable
XI.	Varicella virus—containing vaccine	A. No condition specified for compensation B. Events described in manufacturer's package insert as contraindications to additional doses of vaccine	Not applicable No limit	Not applicable Not applicable
XII.	Any new vaccine recommended by the CDC for routine administration to children, after publication by Secretary HHS of a notice of coverage	A. No condition specified for compensation B. Events described in manufacturer's package insert as contraindications to additional doses of vaccine		

See next page for notes

* *Effective date: October 22, 1998. DTaP, diphtheria and tetanus toxoids and acellular pertussis; DTP, diphtheria and tetanus toxoids and pertussis; Hib, Haemophilus influenzae type b; DT, diphtheria and tetanus toxoids; dT, adult-type diphtheria and tetanus toxoids; TT, tetanus toxoid vaccine; OPV, oral poliovirus; PRP, polyribosyl ribitol phosphate polysaccharide; CDC, Centers for Disease Control and Prevention; and HHS, US Department of Health and Human Services.*

† Taken from the Reportable Events Table (RET), which lists conditions reportable by law (42 USC §300aa-25) to the Vaccine Adverse Event Reporting System (VAERS), including conditions found in the manufacturer's package insert. In addition, physicians are encouraged to report ANY clinically significant or unexpected events (even if you are not certain the vaccine caused the event) for ANY vaccine, whether or not it is listed on the RET. Manufacturers also are required by regulation (21 CFR §600.80) to report to the VAERS program all adverse events made known to them for any vaccine. VAERS reporting forms and information can be obtained by calling 1-800-822-7967 or from the Web site (http://www.fda.gov/cber/vaers/report.htm).

‡ Taken from the Vaccine Injury Table (VIT) used in adjudication of claims filed with the National Vaccine Injury Compensation Program. Claims also may be filed for a condition with onset outside the designated time intervals or a condition not included in the VIT. The Qualifications and Aids to Interpretation below define conditions or injuries listed on the VIT. Information on filing a claim can be obtained by calling 1-800-338-2382 or through the Vaccine Injury Compensation Program Web site (http://www.hrsa.gov/bhpr/vicp/).

Qualifications and Aids to Interpretation

(1) *Anaphylaxis and anaphylactic shock* mean an acute, severe, and potentially lethal systemic allergic reaction. Most cases resolve without sequelae. Signs and symptoms begin minutes to a few hours after exposure. Death, if it occurs, usually results from airway obstruction caused by laryngeal edema or bronchospasm and may be associated with cardiovascular collapse. Other significant clinical signs and symptoms include the following: cyanosis, hypotension, bradycardia, tachycardia, arrhythmia, edema of the pharynx and/or trachea and/or larynx with stridor and dyspnea. Autopsy findings may include acute emphysema, which results from lower respiratory tract obstruction, edema of the hypopharynx, epiglottis, larynx, or trachea, and minimal findings of eosinophilia in the liver, spleen, and lungs. When death occurs within minutes of exposure and without signs of respiratory distress, there may not be significant pathologic findings.

(2) *Encephalopathy* For purposes of the Vaccine Injury Table (VIT), a vaccine recipient shall be considered to have suffered an encephalopathy only if such recipient manifests, within the applicable period, an injury meeting the following description of an acute encephalopathy, and then a chronic encephalopathy persists in such person for more than 6 months beyond the date of vaccination.

  (i) *An acute encephalopathy* is one that is sufficiently severe so as to require hospitalization (whether or not hospitalization occurred).

    (A) *For children younger than 18 months of age* who present without an associated seizure event, an acute encephalopathy is indicated by a 'significantly decreased level of consciousness' (see 'D' below) lasting for at least 24 hours. Children younger than 18 months of age who present following a seizure shall be viewed as having an acute encephalopathy if their significantly decreased level of consciousness persists beyond 24 hours and cannot be attributed to a postictal state (seizure) or medication.

    (B) *For adults and children 18 months of age or older,* an acute encephalopathy is one that persists for at least 24 hours and is characterized by at least 2 of the following:

      (1) A significant change in mental status that is not medication-related, specifically a confusional state, a delirium, or a psychosis;

      (2) A significantly decreased level of consciousness, which is independent of a seizure and cannot be attributed to the effects of medication; and

      (3) A seizure associated with loss of consciousness

    (C) Increased intracranial pressure may be a clinical feature of acute encephalopathy in any age group.

    (D) A "significantly decreased level of consciousness" is indicated by the presence of at least one of the following clinical signs for at least 24 hours or greater (see paragraphs (2)(i)(A) and (2)(i)(B) of this section for applicable time frames):

      (1) Decreased or absent response to environment (responds, if at all, only to loud voice or painful stimuli);

      (2) Decreased or absent eye contact (does not fix gaze on family members or other persons); or

      (3) Inconsistent or absent responses to external stimuli (does not recognize familiar people or things).

    (E) The following clinical features alone or in combination do not demonstrate an acute encephalopathy or a significant change in either mental status or level of consciousness as described above: sleepiness, irritability (fussiness), high-pitched and unusual screaming and persistent inconsolable crying and bulging fontanelle. Seizures in themselves are not sufficient ro constitute a diagnosis of encephalopathy. In the absence of other evidence of an acute encephalopathy, seizures shall nor be viewed as the first symptom or manifestation of the onset of an acute encephalopathy.

  (ii) *Chronic encephalopathy* occurs when a change in mental or neurologic status, first manifested during the applicable time period, persists for a period of at least 6 months from the date of vaccination. Persons who return to a normal neurologic state after the acute encephalopathy shall nor be presumed to have suffered residual neurologic damage from that event; any subsequent chronic encephalopathy shall not be presumed to be a sequela of the acute encephalopathy. If a preponderance of the evidence indicates that a child's chronic encephalopathy is secondary to genetic, prenatal, or perinatal factors, that chronic encephalopathy shall not be considered to be a condition set forth in the VIT.

  (iii) An encephalopathy shall not be considered to be a condition set forth in the VIT if, in a proceeding on a petition, it is shown by a preponderance of the evidence that the encephalopathy was caused by an infection, a toxin, a metabolic disturbance, a structural lesion, a genetic disorder, or trauma (without regard to whether the cause of the infection, toxin, trauma, metabolic disturbance, structural lesion, or genetic disorder is known). If at the time a decision is made on a petition filed under section 2111(b) of the Act for a vaccine-related injury or death it is not possible to determine the cause by a preponderance of the evidence of an encephalopathy, the encephalopathy shall be considered to be a condition set forth in the VIT.

  (iv) In determining whether or not an encephalopathy is a condition set forth in the VIT, the Court shall consider the entire medical record.

(3) *Residual seizure disorder.* A petitioner may be considered to have suffered a residual seizure disorder for purposes of the VIT, if the first seizure or convulsion occurred 5 to 15 days (not < 5 days and not > 15 days) after administration of the vaccine and 2 or more additional distinct seizure or convulsion episodes occurred within 1 year after the administration of the vaccine that were unaccompanied by fever (defined as a rectal temperature equal to or greater than 34.4°C (≥ 101.0°F) or an oral temperature equal to or greater than 37.8°C (≥ 100.0°F). A distinct seizure or convulsion episode ordinarily is defined as including all seizure or convulsivc activity occurring within a 24-hour period, unless competent and qualified expert neurological testimony is presented to the contrary in a particular case.

  For purposes of the VIT, a petitioner shall not be considered to have suffered a residual seizure disorder if the petitioner suffered a seizure or convulsion unaccompanied by fever (as defined above) before the fifth day after the administration of the vaccine involved.

(4) *Seizure and convulsion.* For purposes of paragraphs (2) and (3) of this section, the terms, "seizure" and "convulsion" include myoclonic, generalized tonic-clonic (grand mal), and simple and complex partial seizures. Absence (petit mal) seizures shall not be considered to be a condition set forth in the VIT. Jerking movements or staring episodes alone are not necessarily an indication of seizure activity.

(5) *Sequela.* The term sequela means a condition or event that actually was caused by a condition listed in the VIT.

(6) *Chronic arthritis.* For purposes of the VIT, chronic arthritis may be found in a person with no history in the 3 years before vaccination of arthropathy (joint disease) on the basis of:

    (A) Medical documentation, recorded within 30 days after the onset, of objective signs of acute arthritis (joint swelling) that occurred between 7 and 42 days after a rubella vaccination;

(B) Medical documentation (recorded within 3 years after the onset of acute arthritis) of the persistence of objective signs of intermittent or continuous arthritis for more than 6 months after vaccination;

(C) Medical documentation of an antibody response to the rubella virus

For purposes of the VIT, the following shall not be considered as chronic arthritis: Musculoskeletal disorders such as diffuse connective tissue diseases (including but not limited to rheumatoid arthritis, juvenile rheumatoid arthritis, systemic lupus erythematosus, systemic sclerosis, mixed connective tissue disease, polymyositis/dermatomyositis, fibromyalgia, necrorizing vasculitis and vasculopathies and Sjögren syndrome), degenerative joint disease, infectious agents other than rubella (whether by direct invasion or as an immune reaction), metabolic and endocrine diseases, trauma, neoplasms, neuropathic disorders, bone and cartilage disorders, and arthritis associated with ankylosing spondylitis, psoriasis, inflammatory bowel disease, Reiter syndrome, or blood disorders. Arthralgia (joint pain) or stiffness without joint swelling shall not be viewed as chronic arthritis for purposes of the VIT

(7) *Brachial neuritis* is defined as dysfunction limited to the upper extremity nerve plexus (ie, its trunks, divisions, or cords) without involvement of other peripheral (eg, nerve roots or a single peripheral nerve) or central (eg, spinal cord) nervous system structures. A deep, steady, often severe aching pain in the shoulder and upper arm usually heralds onset of the condition. The pain is followed in days or weeks by weakness and atrophy in upper extremity muscle groups. Sensory loss may accompany the motor deficits but is generally a less notable clinical feature. The neuritis, or plexopathy, may be present on the same side as or the opposite side of the injection; it is sometimes bilateral, affecting both upper extremities. Weakness is required before the diagnosis can he made. Motor, sensory, and reflex findings on physical examination and the results of nerve conduction and electromyographic studies must be consistent in confirming that dysfunction is attributable to the brachial plexus. The condition should thereby be distinguishable from conditions that may give rise to dysfunction of nerve roots (ie, radiculopathies) and peripheral nerves (ie, including multiple mononeuropathies), as well as other peripheral and central nervous system structures (eg, cranial neuropathies and myelopathies).

(8) *Thrombocytopenic purpura* is defined by a serum platelet count less than $50 \times 10^3/\mu L$ ($50 \times 10^9/L$). Thrombocytopenic purpura does not include cases of thrombocytopenia associated with other causes such as hypersplenism, autoimmune disorders (including alloantibodies from previous transfusions) myelodysplasias, lymphoproliferative disorders, congenital thrombocytopenia, or hemolytic uremic syndrome. This does not include cases of immune (formerly called idiopathic) thrombocytopenic purpura that are mediated, for example, by viral or fungal infections, toxins, or drugs. Thrombocytopenic purpura does not include cases of thrombocytopenia associated with disseminated intravascular coagulation, as observed with bacterial and viral infections. Viral infections include, for example, those infections secondary to Epstein-Barr virus, cytomegalovirus, hepatitis A and B, rhinovirus, human immunodeficiency virus, adenovirus, and dengue virus. An antecedent viral infection may be demonstrated by clinical signs and symptoms and need not be confirmed by culture or serologic testing. Bone marrow examination, if performed, must reveal a normal or an increased number of megakaryocytes in an otherwise normal marrow.

(9) *Vaccine-strain measles viral infection* is defined as a disease caused by the vaccine-strain that should be determined by vaccine-specific monoclonal antibody or polymerase chain reaction tests.

(10) *Vaccine-strain polio viral infection* is defined as a disease caused by poliovirus that is isolated from the affected tissue and should be determined to be the vaccine-strain by oligonucleotide or polymerase chain reaction. Isolation of poliovirus from the stool is not sufficient to establish a tissue specific infection or disease caused by vaccine-strain poliovirus.

(11) *Early-onset Hib disease* is defined as invasive bacterial illness associated with the presence of Hib organism on culture of normally sterile body fluids or tissue or clinical findings consistent with the diagnosis of epiglottitis. Hib pneumonia qualifies as invasive Hib disease when radiographic findings consistent with the diagnosis of pneumonitis are accompanied by a blood culture positive for the Hib organism. Otitis media, in the absence of the above findings, does not qualify as invasive bacterial disease. A child is considered to have suffered this injury only if the vaccine was the first Hib immunization received by the child.

From: American Academy of Pediatrics. In: Pickering, L.K. (Ed.) *Red Book 2000: Report of the committee on infectious diseases.* 25th ed. Elk Grove Village, IL: American Academy of Pediatrics; 2000: pp. 760-765. Reprinted with permission.

(5) Suggestions for parents—praise all efforts; expect accidents to happen; don't punish; if child is resistant, try again in a few weeks; follow usual pattern of elimination; limit time on potty to 5 to 10 minutes

e. Sleep

(1) One to 3 year olds usually sleep 10 to 12 hours at night and take 1 to 2 naps

(2) Toddlers need rituals and consistency at bedtime as well as security objects, e.g., blanket, special toy

(3) Nightmares start at approximately 3 years; child generally wakens and remembers dream

(4) Night terrors generally occur between 2 to 4 years; child does not waken

(5) Tips for parents—quietly reassure child; let child fall asleep in own bed

f. Negativism

(1) Normal behaviors in toddlers as they strive to develop sense of autonomy

(2) Expressed as "no," temper tantrums, breathholding

(3) Tips for parents

    (a) Give child as much control as possible (e.g, offer choice of two acceptable objects or actions); allow independence when possible

    (b) Ignore temper tantrums, however expect a "response burst" initially when ignored

g. Sibling rivalry

  (1) Can occur throughout childhood; is often most troublesome just after birth of new baby if older sibling is under 2 years

  (2) Tips for parents

    (a) Involve children in preparation for new baby

    (b) Praise "big-kid" behaviors; ignore regression

    (c) Provide special time for each child every day

    (d) Stay out of minor sibling conflicts, but discipline if aggression occurs

    (e) Foster individual interests of each child and avoid comparing children

h. Thumb Sucking—peaks between 18 to 21 months; ignore before age 4 unless child is not thriving

i. Safety—apply recommendations given earlier that are appropriate for toddlers, plus

  (1) Emphasize street safety—begin teaching the basic rules of pedestrian and traffic safety

  (2) Avoid strangers; teach child methods to avoid encounters with strangers which can be harmful

  (3) Continued use of car seats according to weight—all toddlers should ride forward-facing and upright (studies show safest place for the child is middle of back seat)

  (4) Keep medicine and poisons out of reach in locked cabinets—highest incidence of poisoning occurs in 2-year-olds

  (5) Use of helmets with any type of bicycle use, either as a passenger or alone

  (6) Enroll child in swimming lessons and always supervise when in or around water

j. Dental care—use of toothbrush; first dental visit recommended at approximately 3 years of age

k. Parenting and Discipline

      (1)   Use limit setting and time-out for inappropriate behavior—1 minute of time-out for each year of age

      (2)   Praise good behavior

      (3)   Emphasize consistency especially between parents

      (4)   Spend time with child; read to child on a daily basis

      (5)   Parents set example as role models

      (6)   Assign chores appropriate for age, e.g., put toys away

      (7)   Begin socialization with other children

  l. Television

      (1)   Limit television viewing to appropriate children's programs

      (2)   Limit time spent watching TV

      (3)   Strong correlation between viewing aggression-type programs and child's level of aggressive play

      (4)   TV fosters negative outcomes—rapid paced, superficial problem-solving; obesity

      (5)   Watch TV with child and provide reality base; opportunity to discuss values, and stereotypes

      (6)   Set good example through parenteral TV habits

  m. Child care arrangements—day care; head start programs; nursery school; pre-school programs; babysitters

  n. Emphasize positive qualities of the child and the parent-child relationship and mutually agree upon a plan with the parent to strengthen needed areas

  o. Make referrals to other nurse practitioners, physicians, clinics and community resources as needed

  p. Schedule for next visit

- Interim Visits For Preschool Child (Ages 3, 4 & 5 years)

  1. Subjective information—nutrition/appetite; elimination; sleep; development, including behavior and temperament; caregiver concerns; interim health since last visit including stressful life changes, e.g., move, divorce

  2. Objective Data

    a. Assess parent-child interaction and parenting style

    b. Height, weight and blood pressure (starting at age 3 years)

    c. Vision and hearing screening

    d. Physical examination

    e. Developmental screening—Denver II or equivalent and results

    f. Laboratory

        (1) Mantoux test for TB screening between 4 and 6 years of age if at risk

        (2) Cholesterol screening if indicated

3. Management

    a. Immunizations—review status and update as indicated; inform parents of common side-effects of immunizations

    b. Advise parents of any medications prescribed, including vitamins and fluoride, e.g., name, rationale, dosage frequency and potential side effects

    c. Nutrition appropriate for age

        (1) Nutritional requirements are 90 cal/kg

        (2) Provide foods from the five major food groups in realistic amounts

        (3) Provide nutritious snacks during television viewing (e.g., fruits, vegetables) instead of high-fat foods (e.g., potato chips, cookies)

        (4) Potential nutritional problems (same as in the toddler years)

    d. Elimination—expect occasional night-time accidents until 4 years of age; do not punish or embarrass child

    e. Sleep

        (1) The 3 to 5-year-old child usually sleeps 8 to 12 hours per night and gradually eliminates naps

        (2) Prepare parents for an increase in nightmares

    f. Development

        (1) Discuss the change from the pleasing 3-year-old to the sometimes aggressive, frustrating behavior of the 4-year-old; provide reassurance that "calmness" usually begins at age 5 years

        (2) Emphasize the "magical thinking" of the preschool child and how it places the child at risk for accidental injury and an increase in fears

        (3) Discuss the child's rigid superego and how children this age feel guilty for negative events

        (4) Inform parents that they can expect "tall tales," the use of "toilet talk" and the construction of imaginary playmates

        (5) Discuss need for peer companionship and school readiness

    g. Sex education—begins in infancy and toddlerhood when parents label the genitals and accept genital exploration and masturbation as normal activities

(1) Preschool children are curious about gender differences and "how babies are made," their questions should be answered briefly and accurately

(2) Explore parents' feelings about masturbation and prepare for a possible increase in this behavior

(3) Talk with child about "good touch" and "bad touch"; encourage parents to re-enforce prevention

h. Dental care

(1) Brush teeth after each meal if possible and at bedtime

(2) Recommend first dental visit if not previously done

(3) If thumbsucking is persistent at age 4, have dental evaluation to rule out malocclusion; speech evaluation if tongue thrust is suspected

i. Safety—apply recommendations given earlier that are appropriate for preschool children, plus

(1) Reinforce pedestrian safety—children ages 3 to 7 years are more frequently involved in pedestrian-related motor vehicle accidents

(2) Teach guidelines for bicycle safety; avoid busy streets

(3) Devise fire escape plan and teach the child; conduct routine fire drills

(4) Teach child to roll and to smother clothing if it catches on fire

(5) Teach safety—the danger of matches, open flames

(6) Always supervise child when swimming or near any water

(7) Frequently check playground equipment for stability, loose nuts and bolts, and suitable landing surface

(8) Keep child away from power equipment, including lawn mowers

(9) Never clean or handle a gun in the presence of the child

(10) Discard old refrigerators and other large appliances or remove all doors during storage to avoid entrapment during play or exploration

(11) Do not allow chewing gum or eating while running or jumping

j. Exercise—encourage frequent periods of outdoor activities and limit television viewing

k. Emphasize positive qualities of the child and the parent-child relationship and mutually agree upon a plan with the parent to strengthen needed areas

l. Make referrals to other nurse practitioners, physicians, clinics and community resources as needed

m. Schedule for next visit

• Interim Visits: School-age Children—annual visit (6 to 12 years)

1. Subjective Data

    a. Nutrition/appetite

    b. Elimination—especially constipation and enuresis

    c. Sleep

    d. Development—include school, activities, exercise, friends, behavior and family relationships

    e. Allergies and reactions

    f. Medications

    g. Drug, alcohol, cigarette and caffeine usage (for older school-age child)

    h. Concerns of child and caregiver; current/recent stressors, e.g., move, divorce

    i. Interim health since last visit (include review of systems); for older school-age children, obtain sexual/reproductive history as indicated

2. Objective

    a. Assess parent-child interaction and child behavior

    b. Height and weight, including percentiles

    c. Vital signs, including blood pressure

    d. Vision and hearing screening

    e. Physical examination, including assessment for scoliosis and Tanner staging

    f. Laboratory

        (1) Mantoux test for TB screening of high-risk child if not performed in the pre-school period

        (2) Hematocrit at 8 years of age

        (3) Urinalysis at 8 years of age; cholesterol, if indicated

        (4) Cholesterol if indicated

3. Management

    a. Immunization—review status and update as indicated (see tables 3 through 9); inform parents of common side-effects

    b. Advise parents of any medications prescribed, including vitamins and fluoride, e.g., on name, rationale, dosage, frequency and potential side effects

    c. Nutrition

        (1) Nutritional requirements are approximately 70 cal/kg

        (2) Most behavioral problems with food resolved

        (3) Potential nutritional problems—obesity, iron deficiency

        (4)   Encourage good nutritional practices (e.g., balanced meals, nutritious snacks, no meal skipping)

    d.   Development characteristics and behaviors

        (1)   Ages 6 to 7—nervous mannerisms; restless activity; egocentric thinking; rigid superego

        (2)   Ages 8 to 10—takes on idols and heros; friends serve as allies against adults; less rigid superego

        (3)   Ages 10 to 12—increased self-awareness and self-consciousness; body image concerns; mood swings, stormy behavior; need for independence

        (4)   Inform parents that use of dirty words may occur

        (5)   Prepare for pubertal changes and menstruation in girls

        (6)   Discuss with parents the importance of and strategies for bolstering the child's self-esteem

    e.   Good health habits—assist child and parents to establish early patterns of behavior, e.g., regular exercise, sufficient sleep, regular dental care, avoidance of drugs, alcohol, tobacco

    f.   Communication—encourage parents to assist child in developing good communication skills, problem-solving strategies and stress management

    g.   Drugs, smoking and alcohol—encourage parent/child discussions

    h.   Sex education—anatomy and physiology; sexual activity; values clarification; decision making; contraception; prevention of STDs and AIDS

    i   Parenting strategies

        (1)   Although the child is maturing, quality time, attention and affection from parents is important (evidence exists supporting ''connectedness'' to parents and/or another adult decreases risk-taking behaviors)

        (2)   Encourage independence and decision-making

        (3)   Promote responsibility and accountability by assigning appropriate chores

        (4)   Maintain adequate supervision

        (5)   Discuss methods of discipline; use positive re-enforcement and appropriate consequences for inappropriate behavior

        (6)   Establish fair rules

        (7)   Respect the child's need for privacy

        (8)   Set example by being a good role model

        (9)   Provide child with an allowance

        (10)   Select movies and TV programming and video games that are appropriate for child's developmental level

        (11)   Praise child for achievements

        (12)   Encourage school attendance

        (13)   Refer parents to resources that can assist them in building assets and preventing psychosocial morbidities (Melnyk et al., in press)

    j.   Safety

        (1)   Bicycle, skateboarding, rollerblading; use of helmets and protection padding

        (2)   Seat belt use

        (3)   Prevention of sexual abuse, e.g., inappropriate touching; what to do if it occurs

        (4)   Water safety; swimming

        (5)   Fire prevention safety; home fire drill; proper use of appliances

        (6)   Sunburn prevention

        (7)   Prevention of violence in home; lock up guns, ammunition; teach child gun safety

        (8)   Pedestrian safety

    k.   Lying and cheating (common in school-age children)

        (1)   School-age children lie to avoid trouble or gain an advantage

        (2)   Appropriate response—confront child in a positive way; try to understand reason for lie; follow through with age-appropriate discipline when needed

        (3)   Adults should model honesty

    l.   Sports

        (1)   For 6 to 8-year-olds, sports participation should be noncompetitive and focused on learning rules, teamwork and having fun

        (2)   Older school-aged children and teenagers should have a pre-participation physical examination

    m.   Emphasize positive qualities of the child and the parent-child relationship and mutually agree upon a plan with the parent to strengthen needed areas

    n.   Make referrals as needed

    o.   Schedule for next visit

- Interim Visits: Adolescent—annual visit (13 to 18 Years)

    1.   Subjective information—gather "sensitive" information when alone with the adolescent

        a.   Nutrition—especially appetite; meal-skipping

b. Elimination—especially use of aids such as laxatives, diuretics

c. Sleep practices

d. Development—special emphasis on assessment of mental and emotional health (including school performance and attendance; self-esteem, friends and relationships; family functioning and "connectedness"; hobbies; activities; work; stress and anger management; coping skills; risk-taking behaviors, such as driving while drinking and use of weapons; violent or aggressive behavior; ideations about hurting self or others)

e. Allergies

f. Medications

g. Drug, alcohol, cigarette, and caffeine consumption

h. Sexual activities, reproductive issues

i. Concerns/worries; current and recent stressors

j. Interim health since last visit—include review of systems, with special emphasis on gathering psychological and sexual/reproductive data

k. Specific questions when alone with parent

    (1) Family communication patterns and relationship with the adolescent

    (2) Parent's description of the adolescent's strong and weak points, attitudes, and behaviors

    (3) Discipline practices and response

    (4) Specific concerns and worries about the adolescent

2. Objective data

a. Observation of parent-adolescent interaction (e.g., parental support of adolescent; does the parent allow the adolescent to answer questions)

b. Height and weight; percentiles

c. Vital signs, including blood pressure

d. Vision and hearing screening

e. Physical examination—including scoliosis screen, Tanner stage, and breast examination; pelvic examination if adolescent female is sexually active, having irregular menses, or is more than 16 years of age

f. Laboratory

    (1) Urinalysis

    (2) Hematocrit

    (3) VDRL, GC, Chlamydia and HIV if sexually active or history of sexual abuse

    (4) Pap smear if pelvic examination performed

(5) Liver function tests (if history of drug usage); cholesterol, if indicated

3. Management

   a. Update immunizations—offer hepatitis B vaccine series, especially for sexually active adolescents or those who are using IV drugs; provide information on common side effects

   b. Advise regarding any medications prescribed, e.g., include name, rationale, dosage, frequency, course and potential side effects

   c. Nutrition appropriate for age

      (1) The adolescent diet should be similar to an active adult with extra calories during rapid growth periods; prudent consumption of high fat foods, e.g., red meats, butter, and eggs

      (2) Nutritional issues—irregular meals, chaotic lifestyle; increase in meals eaten away from home; increase in snacks; skipping of meals; fad diets; vegetarianism

      (3) Potential nutritional problems—increased need for calcium, iron, zinc; eating disorders; obesity

      (4) Encourage well-balanced meals and nutritious snacks

      (5) Discuss adolescent's perception of his/her weight

      (6) Encourage healthy weight loss strategies if indicated, e.g., decreasing fat intake; increasing exercise

   d. Safety—same as school age child, plus

      (1) Emphasize the possible consequences of drinking and use of drugs while driving

      (2) Discourage being a passenger when the driver has been drinking or using drugs

      (3) Discuss typical high-risk situations and how to avoid them; role play healthy behaviors to use in high-risk situations

      (4) Encourage safe swimming and diving practices

      (5) Discuss proper use of safe sports equipment and maintenance

      (6) Instruct adolescent in proper training and warm-up exercises for sports and physical activities

      (7) Educate regarding safe and proper use of firearms and other potentially dangerous objects such as firecrackers

      (8) Discuss use and misuse of over-the-counter medications

   e. Developmental Issues

      (1) Discuss dating and peer pressure

(2) Encourage open communication with parents, peers, and school personnel

(3) Teach stress reduction techniques and coping skills

(4) Educate regarding healthy outlets for anger

(5) Discuss plans for the future—further education; work; recreation; hobbies; marriage; parenthood

(6) Educate regarding acne—e.g., cause, myths and proper skin care

f. Discuss issues related to sexuality—decision making; mature relationships; assertiveness; safe sex/prevention of STDs, including HIV; pregnancy and contraception; implications of potential parenthood; ''normalcy'' of occasional masturbation

g. Encourage good health habits—e.g., regular exercise; sufficient sleep, regular dental care

h. Continue education regarding use of drugs, alcohol, cigarettes, and caffeine

i. Inform parents of major developmental characteristics of adolescents

(1) Increased self-awareness, self-consciousness and self-appraisal

(2) Body image concerns

(3) Mood swings and stormy behavior

(4) Need for independence

(5) Using peer values as criteria with which to judge own values, but still needing family to provide acceptance and feeling of self-worth

(6) Interest in opposite sex

j. Parenting strategies with adolescents

(1) Fairness in rules and reasonable limit setting

(2) Allow decision making

(3) Respect adolescent's privacy

(4) Expect periods of estrangement (be available; adolescent needs supportive family)

(5) Praise achievements at home, school, extracurricular activities

(6) Bolster self-esteem

(7) Supervision as needed

(8) Encourage independence, new experiences, after-school activities, including part-time job

(9) Promote family communication

 (10) Serve as role model—practice good health habits, e.g., parents should not smoke if they do not want child to imitate their behavior

 (11) Recognize signs of probable substance abuse—drop in school performance; personality change; mood swings; sleepiness or fatigue; depression

 k. Emphasize positive qualities of the adolescent and the parent-adolescent relationship and mutually agree upon a plan to strengthen needed areas

 l. Make referrals as needed

 m. Refer parents to resources that can assist them in building their teen's assets as well as with their parenting skills (Melnyk et al., in press)

 n. Schedule for next visit

Note: The author would like to thank Leigh Small, MS, RNCS, PNP, doctoral student, University of Rochester School of Nursing and Pediatric Nurse Practitioner, Genesee Health Services, Rochester, New York for her contributions and review of this chapter.

Questions
Select the best answer

1. Sixteen-year-old Sarah makes the following statements to you during a health visit. Which of the following pieces of information should not be kept confidential?

   a. "I have been sexually active with three of my boyfriends."
   b. "I sometimes smoke marijuana."
   c. "I want to get pregnant."
   d. "Sometimes I feel like ending my life."

2. In performing a physical examination on a nine-month-old infant, which of the following developmental fears would not be appropriate for you to consider?

   a. Stranger anxiety
   b. Pain
   c. Separation from parents
   d. Bodily harm

3. When performing a physical examination on a toddler, which of the following body parts would you examine last?

   a. Heart and lungs
   b. Abdomen and genitals
   c. Ears and throat
   d. Hips and extremities

4. Role play with equipment during the course of a physical examination would be most beneficial with which of the following age groups?

   a. Toddlers
   b. Preschoolers
   c. Young school-age children
   d. Older school-age children

5. Providing reassurance of "normalcy" during the course of an examination would be most important for:

   a. Preschool children
   b. Young school-age children
   c. Older school-age children
   d. Adolescents

6. Which of the following would not elevate the pulse of a child?

   a. Fever
   b. Anemia
   c. Hypothyroidism
   d. Exercise

7. Which of the following sounds should be considered the diastolic blood pressure in children under 13 years of age?

    a. The muffling sound (Korotkoff IV)
    b. The disappearance of sound (Korotkoff V)
    c. Korotkoff sound I
    d. Korotkoff sound II

8. Blood pressure should be measured at well child visits, beginning at age:

    a. 2 years
    b. 3 years
    c. 4 years
    d. 5 years

9. A wide pulse pressure that results from a high systolic blood pressure is usually not due to which of the following?

    a. Fever
    b. Exercise
    c. Excitement
    d. A patent ductus arteriosus

10. Head and chest circumferences should be equal at:

    a. 6 months of age
    b. 1 year of age
    c. 2 years of age
    d. 3 years of age

11. The anterior fontanel usually closes by:

    a. 2 months of age
    b. 6 months of age
    c. 18 months of age
    d. 24 months of age

12. Diffuse edema of the soft tissue of the scalp which usually crosses suture lines in the newborn is:

    a. Bossing
    b. Caput succedaneum
    c. Cephalohematoma
    d. Macrocephaly

13. An infant should no longer have a head lag when pulled from the supine to sitting position at what age?

    a. 2 months
    b. 4 months

    c. 6 months

    d. 9 months

14. "Boggy" nasal mucous membranes with serous drainage upon examination usually suggests:

    a. Sinusitis

    b. Polyps

    c. URI

    d. Allergic rhinitis

15. A white instead of red reflex upon eye examination of a 1-year-old child would suggest:

    a. An accommodative error

    b. Retinoblastoma

    c. Papilledema

    d. Retinal detachment

16. A cobblestone appearance of the palpebral conjunctiva usually indicates:

    a. Bacterial infection

    b. Chemical irritation

    c. Viral infection

    d. Severe allergy

17. An eye that deviates in when covered but returns to midline when uncovered is an:

    a. Esophoria

    b. Exophoria

    c. Esotropia

    d. Exotropia

18. Pain produced by manipulation of the auricle or pressure on the tragus suggests:

    a. Acute otitis media

    b. Otitis externa

    c. Otitis media with effusion

    d. Mastoiditis

19. A hypernasal voice and snoring in a child is suggestive of:

    a. Polyps of the larynx

    b. Nasopharyngeal tumor

    c. Hypertrophied adenoids

    d. Cleft palate

20. Physiological splitting of the second heart sound during inspiration in a child:

    a. Is normal

    b. Should be evaluated with an EKG

    c. Suggests an ASD

    d. Should be referred to a cardiologist

21. Which of the following is not characteristics of innocent heart murmurs in children?

    a. Systolic in timing
    b. Varies in loudness with positioning
    c. Usually transmitted to the neck
    d. Usually loudest at lower left sternal border or at second or third intercostal space

22. A Grade II musical or vibratory murmur heard best at the lower left sternal border that changes with positioning is suggestive of a:

    a. Pulmonary ejection murmur
    b. Ventricular septal defect
    c. Venous hum
    d. Vibratory or Still's murmur

23. Wheezing in a child may not be found in which of the following conditions?

    a. Asthma
    b. Bronchiolitis
    c. Pleural friction rub
    d. Cystic fibrosis

24. Gynecomastia in a male may not be a finding in which of the following?

    a. Normal pubertal development
    b. Steroid usage
    c. Hyperthyroidism
    d. Testicular tumor

25. Which of the following would usually not be considered a sign of a pituitary tumor in an adolescent female?

    a. Dysfunctional uterine bleeding
    b. Galactorrhea
    c. Loss of peripheral vision
    d. Increase in headaches

26. Which of the following is not a specific examination test for a dislocated hip?

    a. Barlow's test
    b. Ortolani's test
    c. Trendelenburg test
    d. Gower's test

27. In addition to the knee, which of the following should be examined in a child complaining of knee pain?

    a. Foot

  b. Ankle
  c. Hip
  d. Spine

28. Which of the following infant reflexes should not disappear by 6 months of age?

  a. Moro
  b. Rooting
  c. Tonic neck
  d. Plantar grasp

29. Spasticity in an infant may be an early sign of:

  a. Neurofibromatosis
  b. Hydrocephalus
  c. Cerebral palsy
  d. Muscular dystrophy

30. A shift to the left is present when which of the following are elevated?

  a. Neutrophils
  b. Bands or stabs
  c. Lymphocytes
  d. Eosinophils

31. Which of the following is usually elevated with viral infections?

  a. Neutrophils
  b. Eosinophils
  c. Lymphocytes
  d. Basophils

32. Decreased platelets may not be found in which of the following?

  a. Leukemia
  b. Anemia
  c. ITP
  d. Medication usage (e.g., ampicillin, cephalothin)

33. Which of the following does not suggest a urinary tract infection?

  a. Increased protein
  b. Increased WBCs
  c. Increased RBCs
  d. Increased nitrites

34. A Mantoux test in a child with no risk factors is considered positive with a reaction of:

  a. At least 5 mm induration
  b. At least 8 mm induration

    c. At least 10 mm induration

    d. At least 15 mm induration

35. Children should receive TB testing at which of the following ages if low risk but is living in a high prevalence neighborhood?

    a. 4 and 14 years of age

    b. 1, 2, 4, and 10 years of age

    c. 1, 4, 10 and 18 years of age

    d. 4, 10 and 14 years of age

36. Cholesterol screening should be done:

    a. Once for all children at 3 years of age

    b. Once for all children at 6 years of age

    c. Once for children whose parents have a total cholesterol level of 200mg/ dL or greater

    d. Only for children with a family history of premature cardiovascular disease

37. For which of the following screening tests should children fast for 12 hours before the test is done?

    a. Total cholesterol

    b. Serum chemistry profile

    c. Serum lipid profile

    d. Hematocrit

38. Which of the following is the most important history-taking question for a sports evaluation?

    a. Has the child ever had a head injury?

    b. Has the child ever fainted or lost consciousness during exercise?

    c. Does the child ever get short of breath with exercise?

    d. Has the child ever had prior surgeries?

39. Which of the following conditions would not exclude a child from participating in contact collision sports?

    a. Hepatosplenomegaly

    b. Absence of a paired organ

    c. Atlantoaxial instability

    d. Prior head injury

40. Which of the following topics would not be appropriate to include when providing anticipatory guidance to the parent of a 4-month-old infant?

    a. Introduction of solid foods

    b. Teething

    c. Negativism

    d. Introduction of a cup

41. Which is the correct order for introduction of solid foods to an infant?

    a. Fruits, cereal, vegetables, and meats
    b. Cereal, meats, vegetables, and fruits
    c. Fruits, cereal, meats, and vegetables
    d. Cereal, vegetables, fruits, and meats

42. Which of the following topics is not appropriate to include when providing anticipatory guidance to the parent of an 18-month-old?

    a. Temper tantrums
    b. Toilet training
    c. Dental care
    d. Stranger anxiety

43. Appropriate anticipatory guidance for the parents of an 8-year-old girl should not include:

    a. Preparation for an increase in nervous mannerisms and restless activity
    b. Preparation for pubertal changes
    c. Information that friends begin to serve as allies against adults
    d. Information that their daughter will take on idols and heroes

44. Which of the following children could routinely receive the MMR vaccine?

    a. A child who has had an anaphylactic reaction to the ingestion of eggs
    b. A child whose mother is pregnant
    c. A child who is receiving chemotherapy
    d. A pregnant adolescent

45. A pelvic examination should not be performed on which of the following adolescents?

    a. A 14-year-old who is sexually active
    b. A 15-year-old who has just started menarche
    c. A 17-year-old who is having irregular menses
    d. An 18-year-old healthy female

Answers

1. d	16. d	31. c
2. d	17. a	32. b
3. c	18. b	33. a
4. b	19. c	34. d
5. d	20. a	35. a
6. c	21. c	36. d
7. a	22. d	37. c
8. b	23. c	38. b
9. d	24. c	39. d
10. b	25. a	40. c
11. c	26. d	41. d
12. b	27. c	42. d
13. c	28. d	43. a
14. d	29. c	44. b
15. b	30. b	45. b

Bibliography

American Academy of Pediatrics. (1995). Joint committee on infant hearing 1994 position statement. *Pediatrics*, 95(1), 152–156.

American Academy of Pediatrics. (2000). In L. K. Pickering (Ed.). *Red Book 2000: Report of the committee on infectious diseases* (25th ed.). Elk Grove Village, IL: Author.

American Nurses Association. (1997). *Clinician's handbook of preventive services.* Waldorf, Maryland: American Nurses Publishing.

Boynton, R. W., Dunn, E. S., & Stephens G. R. (1998). *Manual of ambulatory pediatrics* (4th ed.). Philadelphia: J. B. Lippincott.

Burns, C. E., Barber, N., Brady, M. A., Dunn, A. M. (2000). *Pediatric primary care: A handbook for nurse practitioners* (2nd ed.). Philadelphia: W. B. Saunders.

Fox, J. A. (Ed.). (1997). *Primary health care of children.* St. Louis: Mosby.

Green, M. (Ed.). (1994). *Bright futures: Guidelines for health supervision of infants, children and adolescents.* Arlington, VA: National Center for Education in Maternal and Child Health.

Hoekelman, R. A., Adam, H. M., Nelson, N. M., Weitzman, M. L. & Wilson, M. H. (Eds). (2001). *Primary pediatric care* (4th ed.). St. Louis: Mosby Yearbook.

Melnyk, B. M., Moldenhauer, Z., Veenema, T., Gullo, S., Small, L., & Tuttle, J. (in press). The KySS (keep your children/yourself Safe and Secure Campaign: NAPNAP's national effort to prevent and decrease psychosocial morbidities in children and adolescents. *Journal of Pediatric Health Care, 15*(2).

National Association of Pediatric Nurse Associates and Practitioner (NAPNAP). (2000). *Childhood immunization: A continuing education workbook for pediatric nurse practitioners.* Cherry Hill, NJ: Author.

Neinstein, L. S. (1996). *Adolescent health care: A practical guide* (3rd ed.) Baltimore: Williams & Wilkins.

Health Promotion and Evaluation In Adults

Rosanne H. Pruitt

Theoretical Aspects: Health Promotion Theories and Models

- High Level Wellness—a *continuum* that demonstrates dynamic interaction of health and environment as one moves toward high level wellness; health is dynamic with a continuous need for health promoting activity to maintain and improve one's health

- Maslow's Hierarchy of Needs (Maslow, 1954)

  1. Survival needs—food, water, sleep

  2. Safety and security—protection from physical hazards

  3. Love and belonging—affection, companionship

  4. Self-esteem—sense of self worth, recognition

  5. Self-actualization—achievement of personal potential

- Health Belief Model (Becker, 1972)—health is influenced by age, sex, race, ethnicity, and income

  1. Threats to health

     a. Perceived susceptibility

     b. Perceived seriousness of condition

  2. Outcome expectation of health action

     a. Perceived benefits of action

     b. Perceived barriers to taking action

     c. Efficacy expectations

- Self-Efficacy Theory (Bandura, 1977) explains human behavior in terms of a dynamic, reciprocal interaction between behavior, personal factors, and environmental influences—key concepts include:

  1. Personal factors which include the ability to symbolize behavior meaning, to foresee outcomes of given behavior, to learn by observing others, to self-determine and self regulate, and to reflect and analyze experience

  2. Reciprocal determinism refers to behavior as dynamic and dependent on environmental and personal constructs that influence each other simultaneously

- Health Promotion Model (Pender, 1996)—health promoting behaviors are motivated by multiple cognitive-perceptual factors such as the importance of health and perceived benefits, perceived control of health and self-efficacy, and modified by factors such as demographics and interpersonal influences

- Erikson's Stages of Psychosocial Development (Erikson, 1963)—degree of success in accomplishing developmental tasks influences the accomplishment of tasks of older adults

  1. Trust versus mistrust—trust of self and others

  2. Autonomy versus shame and doubt—self expression and cooperation with others

  3. Initiative versus guilt—focus on purposeful behavior

4. Industry versus inferiority—belief in one's ability

5. Identity versus role confusion—clear sense of self

6. Intimacy versus role confusion—capacity for reciprocal love relationships

7. Generativity versus stagnation—creativity and productivity

8. Ego identity versus despair—acceptance of one's life as worthwhile and unique

- Health Behavior Change Models

   1. PRECEDE Model (Green & Kreuter, 1991)—involves identifying, assessing the learner=s quality of life; identifying health problems and risk factors; The acronym PRECEDE stands for Predisposing, Reinforcing and Enabling Causes in Educational Diagnosis and Evaluation: Predisposing factors (perception, knowledge, and attitudes), Reinforcing factors (significant others), and Enabling factors (environmental factors of accessibility and costs) are used to develop educational interventions for change and policies to support change

   2. Change Theory (Lewin)—advanced practice environments are dynamic; planned change involves unfreezing of current approach, implementing change, refreezing or creating, and acceptance and regular use of new approach (Cohen, 1996)

   3. Transtheoretical Model (Prochaskov & Velicir, 1997)—temporal model of behavioral change, model emerged from comparative analysis of over 300 theories

      a. Precontemplation—no intention to take action within next six months; not ready and often resistant to health promotion change efforts; appropriate to use consciousness raising education

      b. Contemplation—intention to take action within next six months; not ready and ambivalent toward change; appropriate to use consciousness raising education

      c. Preparation—intends to take action within 30 days and has taken some behavioral steps in this direction; individuals at this stage should be recruited for action toward behavior change

      d. Action—individual has changed behavior for less than six months

      e. Maintenance—individual has changed overt behavior for more than six months; support and encouragement pf continued behavior change

- System Theories

   1. General Systems Theory (von Bertalanffy, 1968) views world in terms of sets of integrated reactions in an effort to see parts in relation to the whole—key concepts include:

      a. System—goal directed unit with interdependent, interacting parts that also interact with environment

      b. Boundaries regulate exchange of energy, information, and matter between systems; may be open or closed depending on interaction with surrounding environment

      c.   Input, output, and feedback loop provide for an exchange of energy, information, and matter

    2.   Neuman's Systems Model (Neuman, 1995)—uses a systems format and includes levels of prevention as well as multiple dimensions of health promotion (physical, psychological, spiritual, and social); health promotion efforts are used to strengthen line barriers of defense

Related Concepts

- Levels of prevention from public health science are used by most authorities when differentiating health promotion activities from other interventions. *Healthy People 2010* and other federal documents use a broader interpretation including health protection, with specific screenings and safety factors which are also included in this chapter

    1.   Primary prevention includes measures to promote optimum health prior to the onset of any problems—health promotion, care intended to minimize risk factors and subsequent disease e.g., promoting a healthy diet, exercise, stress management, safety, avoiding harmful substances

    2.   Secondary prevention focuses on early identification and treatment of existing health problems, e.g., screening for disease, pap smear, mamogram

    3.   Tertiary Prevention is care intended to improve the course of a disease; the rehabilitation and restoration to health, e.g., cardiac rehabilitation

- Cultural influence must be considered with any health encounter. Cultural beliefs of disease causation influence health practices e.g., magic or evil spirits (Latino); violation of a natural law (American Indian); imbalance between "hot" or "cold" forces (Asian, Latino). Varied beliefs affect the acceptance of practices such as handwashing and immunizations. There are differences between and among cultural groups. Certain beliefs are common among cultural groups (Clark, 1999)

    1.   Native Americans—harmony with nature and supernatural forces are important factors in health beliefs; social networking is also important; note taking is often considered taboo; silence is a sign of respect

    2.   Hispanic American—extended family is important in decision making; illness may be related to imbalance of hot and cold; sustaining eye contact is considered rude (mal ojo); higher risk of vitamin A, iron and calcium deficiency due to dietary habits

    3.   Asian Americans—naturalistic beliefs are common; saying no is considered rude and is avoided; eye contact may be avoided out of respect; a need to balance hot and cold through food and medication is prevalent; use of acupuncture therapy is widespread

    4.   African-Americans—diverse group with beliefs that include "health is harmony with nature" and "life is a process, not a state;" maternal grandmother is often important in decision making

Lifestyle/Health Behaviors

- Stress Management: Stress is an imbalance between environmental demands and one's individual and social resources required to cope with those demands

  1. Types of stressors

     a. Major life events—discrete events that disrupt normal functioning (e.g., marriage, divorce, death of family member)

     b. Daily hassles—minor daily events perceived as frustrating

     c. Chronic strains—challenges, hardships, and problems

     d. Cataclysmic events—sudden disasters that require major adaptive responses (e.g., natural disasters)

     e. Ambient stressors—continuous and often unchanging conditions in physical environment, such as chronic pollution or noise

  2. Theoretical basis of stress

     a. General Adaptation Syndrome—Selye's (1974) continuum demonstrates how small amounts of stress are motivating and improve the quality of life (eustress or good stress), however beyond a certain point the stress becomes psychologically and physically debilitating (distress)

     b. Physical indicators of stress

        (1) Gastrointestinal symptoms—upset stomach, change of appetite

        (2) Headache, muscle tension, elevated blood pressure (BP)

        (3) Restlessness

        (4) Cold, sweaty palms

     c. Emotional indicators of stress

        (1) Irritability, emotional outbursts, crying

        (2) Depression, withdrawal

        (3) Hostility, tendency to blame others

        (4) Anxiety, suspiciousness

     d. Behavioral indicators of stress

        (1) Lethargy, loss of interest

        (2) Poor concentration, forgetfulness

        (3) Decreased productivity, absenteeism

        (4) Sleep disturbance

     e. Related terminology—Karoshi (Japanese) death by overwork; associated with long hours and stressful working conditions

  3. Stress management intervention techniques

    a. Stress reduction techniques

        (1) Time management—determine goals and priorities, set time priorities, and learn to say no to nongoal related activities

        (2) Time blocking—set aside time to adapt to change and incorporate it into daily routine

        (3) Change avoidance—during periods of high life change, avoid unnecessary change to prevent need to make multiple adjustments simultaneously

        (4) Habituation—incorporate routine into daily activities during stressful situation (e.g., park in same place to avoid having to look for car upon return)

        (5) Environmental modification—identify experiences and/ or personalities that are abrasive or stress producing and minimize contact as much as possible

        (6) Involvement with activities of interest—doing something for others and helping with activities of interest to decrease focus on self

    b. Behavioral aspects to build stress resistance

        (1) Increase self esteem—focus on own strengths and attributes

        (2) Increase assertiveness—substitute positive assertive behavior for negative passive actions

        (3) Meditation/prayer (includes Zen and yoga)

    c. Counter-conditioning to lower stress response

        (1) Autogenic training repetition of autogenic suggestions such as ''my arms and legs are heavy''

        (2) Imagery—image visualization used to relax, or assist with past frightening experiences

        (3) Tension-relaxation exercises—tense muscles for 8 to 10 seconds, then relax; longer training sessions are usually required initially to enhance benefits (may be contraindicated in severe heart disease or hypertension)

        (4) Biofeedback—awareness and control to influence response that is not ordinarily under voluntary control

            (a) Electromyography—measures the amount of electrical discharge in muscle fibers (usually forearm and forehead)

            (b) Skin temperature feedback—peripheral temperature measurement by vasomotor control found in bio-dots, mood rings, etc.

        (5) Exercise—produces physiological changes that counteract effects of stress

    d.   Contraindications for stress management

       (1)   Severe depression

       (2)   Hallucinations or delusions

       (3)   Temporary hypotensive or hypoglycemic states

       (4)   Severe pain

- Social Support: Supportive relationships (Friedman, 1998)

   1.   Four types of supporting behaviors

    a.   Emotional support—provision of empathy, love, trust and caring (strongest, most consistent relationship to positive health status)

    b.   Instrumental support, such as direct assistance or services

    c.   Informational support such as advice, suggestions and information for problem solving

    d.   Appraisal support or provision of information useful for self-evaluation purposes (feedback, affirmation)

   2.   Related research

    a.   Research evidence suggests that quality of supportive relationships rather than quantity is a better predictor of health—relationships are thought to provide buffering effects to protect people from the negative consequences of stressful situations

    b.   The importance of social support has been demonstrated in multiple studies related to recovery from illness, disaster, success with weight loss and other positive life changes; support groups can provide encouragement for those without a strong positive social network (Pender, 1996)

- Nutrition

   1.   Healthy diet guidelines

    a.   Eat a variety of foods, more fruit, vegetables, whole grains, poultry and fish (herbs/spices can enhance diminished taste associated with normal aging)

    b.   Calorie breakdown—55 to 60% carbohydrates, < 30% fat with remainder protein (.8 to 1.0 g/kg)

    c.   Limit total fat to less than 30% of total calories and saturated fat to less than 10% of total calories

    d.   Limit cholesterol intake to 300 mg/day

    e.   Use sugar, salt and sodium in moderation

    f.   The food guide pyramid (U.S. Department of Agriculture) includes the following daily recommendations

       (1)   Bread, cereal, rice—6 to 11 servings

Table 1

Recommended Calcium Intakes

	Amount mg/day
Young Adults (11–24 years) Pregnant/Lactating Women	1,300–1,500
Women, 25–29 years (premenopausal) Women, 50–64 years (postmenopausal, taking estrogen) Men, 25–64 years	1,000
Men and women, 65+ years Women, 50-64 years (postmenopausal, not taking estrogen)	1,500

Food sources of calcium: Yogurt, milk, cheese, calcium fortified juices and cereal, turnip and mustard greens, collards, kale, broccoli, sardines and salmon with bones

        (2)   Vegetable and fruit groups—3 to 5 servings

        (3)   Milk, yogurt, and cheese—2 to 3 servings

        (4)   Meat, poultry, fish, dry beans, eggs, and nuts—2 to 3 servings

        (5)   Oils, sweets, and fats used sparingly

    g.   Multivitamins with folic acid (0.4mg/day) are recommended for all women of childbearing age

    h.   Vitamin D is needed for proper calcium absorption—200 to 800 IU/day

    i.   Calcium (NIH Consensus Panel, 1994), See Table 1

2.   Assessment for weight loss

    a.   Symptoms indicative of underlying pathology (associated with and/or aggravated by excessive weight)

        (1)   Polyuria/polyphagia/polydipsia (diabetes)

        (2)   Joint pain or marked swelling (osteoarthritis or gout)

        (3)   Angina/palpitations/dyspnea (cardiovascular disease)

        (4)   Edema/cold intolerance (hypothyroidism)

        (5)   Recent weight gain with edema, pruritus (renal disease)

    b.   Contraindications for weight loss

        (1)   Pregnancy

        (2)   Chemotherapy due to already compromised nutritional status and potential impact on therapy

3.   Body mass determinations—useful in determining both under-and-over nutrition or

Table 2

Body Mass Formula

1. To convert weight to kilograms, divide pounds (without clothes) by 2.2
2. To convert to meters, divide height in inches (without shoes) by 39.4, then square it
3. Divide weight in kilograms (#1) by meters squared (#2)

Table 3

Body Mass Index Chart

Weight	Height(feet/inches)							
(lbs)	5′0	5′2″	5′4″	5′6″	5′8″	5′10″	6′0″	6′2″
125	24	23	22	20	19	18	17	16
130	25	24	22	21	20	19	18	17
135	26	25	23	22	21	19	18	17
140	27	26	24	23	21	20	19	18
145	28	27	25	23	22	21	20	19
150	29	27	26	24	23	22	20	19
155	30	28	27	25	24	22	21	20
160	31	29	28	26	24	23	22	21
165	32	30	28	27	25	24	22	21
170	33	31	29	28	26	24	23	22
175	34	32	30	28	27	25	24	23
180	35	33	31	29	27	26	25	23
185	36	34	32	30	28	27	25	24
190	37	35	33	31	29	27	26	24
195	38	36	34	32	30	28	27	25
200	39	37	34	32	30	29	27	26
205	40	38	35	33	31	29	28	26
210	41	38	36	34	32	30	29	27
215	42	39	37	35	33	31	29	28
220	43	40	38	36	34	32	30	28
225	44	41	39	36	34	32	31	29
230	45	42	40	37	35	33	31	30

	BMI
Overweight	25-29.9
Obese	30 and above

NHLBI June 17, 1998

weight-for-frame-size; calculate the body mass using the body mass formula in Table 2 or the body mass index chart in Table 3; body mass index is weight (in kilograms) divided by the squared height (in meters)

4. Guidelines for healthy weight loss should include:

   a. A diet deficient in calories, not nutrients, with a focus on diet composition/preparation methods

   b. A balanced diet (food guide pyramid); should not depend on vitamins, weight loss pills, prepared liquids, "fad diets"

   c. A diet that supplies all essential vitamins and minerals

   d. Adequate fiber for proper GI functioning

   e. Adequate fluid for renal functioning

   f. Enough fat to supply essential fatty acid linoleic acid

g. Consumption of a variety of highly nutritious foods

h. A goal of up to 3 lbs/wk (gradual) weight loss

i. A focus on regular meals, avoiding snacks and modifying bad eating habits

5. Weight control strategies

   a. Regular physical activity increases caloric use, aids and sustains weight loss, preserves lean body mass and metabolism

   b. Social support by family, friends, colleagues, and support groups

   c. Focus on internal motivation for loss (e.g., control, personal goals, self-monitoring) and positive health benefits

   d. Smaller, more frequent meals to maintain blood sugar levels and avoid feelings of hunger

   e. Control home environment (e.g., limit eating to one room, sit down at table without watching television)

   f. Control eating environment (e.g., avoid serving bowls at the table, use smaller plates and glasses, and eat slowly)

   g. Limit snacks (e.g., keep low calorie snacks available, ready to eat)

   h. Control work environment (e.g., eat away from your desk, store food away from work area, and take exercise breaks)

   i. Use a shopping list, do not shop when hungry

   j. Food diary (thoughts and feelings regarding eating patterns for two weeks) to guide intervention strategies

6. Health effects of severe dieting (metabolic response to starvation)

   a. Lower metabolic rate

   b. Hypertension as a result of norepinephrine release

   c. Overcompensation, gain beyond pre-diet weight

   d. Loss of fat and protein, regain fat

   e. Fat cells multiply as protective response against starvation

7. Weight loss prognostic factors

   a. Stability of present weight—number of years at present weight

   b. Motivation to change, conditions making weight loss a high priority

   c. Realistic expectations

8. Nutritional risk factors for older adults—three or more factors indicate a moderate nutritional risk (U.S. Dept. of Health and Human Services, 1994)

   a. Presence of illness or condition affecting amount and kind of food eaten or dental/mouth problems which make eating difficult

b. Eats < 2 meals/day, few fruits, vegetables or dairy products

c. Inadequate finances for food

d. Physically unable to shop, cook or feed self

e. Three or more drinks of beer, wine or liquor daily

f. Unintentional loss or gain of 10 pounds in past 6 months

g. Three or more different medications taken daily

- Exercise: Any exercise performed regularly for a total of 30 minutes a day is beneficial, if sedentary, a gradual increase is recommended; added benefit may be derived from further increases (NIH Consensus panel, 1995)

   1. Physical fitness

      a. Psychological benefits

         (1) Increased alertness

         (2) Improved self esteem, feeling better

         (3) Decreased depression

         (4) Lower stress

      b. Physical benefits

         (1) Heart—increases efficiency, lowers heart rate, lowers BP, increases oxygen capacity

         (2) Decreases LDL, increases HDL

         (3) Muscles—improves strength and endurance

         (4) Improves flexibility

         (5) Increases BMR during and after exercise

         (6) Weight loss of fat, not muscle

         (7) Body composition—lowers fat percentage

         (8) Anti-aging effect

      c. Components of effective exercise

         (1) Performed most, but preferably all days of the week

         (2) Enjoyable for participant

         (3) Rhythmic movement with alternating relaxation and contraction of large muscle groups

         (4) Moderate intensity for at least 30 minutes; talk test— one should be able to talk with some labored breathing during exercise

      d. Components of an exercise plan

(1) Warm up (increases blood flow, loosens and strengthens muscles), e.g., brisk walk and deep breathing

(2) Stretch (maintains and increases flexibility), e.g., stretch slowly and hold position several seconds to point of tightness, not pain; do not bounce

(3) Endurance—select a variety of activities to work different muscle groups; start slow and build up gradually

(4) Cool down period allows body temperature and heart rate to decrease slowly, prevents pooling of blood in extremities and decreases muscle soreness, e.g., walk, deep breathe and loosely shake extremities

e. Exercise counseling

(1) Exercises to avoid

(a) Bouncing with stretch (strains involved joints)

(b) Sit-ups with legs straight or double leg lifts (strains lower back)

(c) Duck walk (bent knee walk) (stresses knees)

(d) Toe touching (stresses hamstrings)

(e) Leg splits and leg thrusts in kneeling position (stresses legs and groin area and also creates potential hip strain)

(2) Exercise self-care

(a) Appropriate clothing with layers in winter

(b) Caps for cold weather and summer heat

(c) Appropriate footwear, snug socks

(d) Plenty of fluids before, during and after exercise

(e) Alternate exercise program during weather extremes, e.g., stationary bike, treadmills, steppers etc

(3) Tolerance barometer—refers to potentially dangerous physical symptoms or early signs of injury

(a) Breathlessness (inability to talk while exercising)

(b) Excessive fatigue—fatigue for more than one hour after exercise

(c) Chest discomfort, dizziness, faintness, exertional dyspnea, nausea or vomiting

(d) Stiffness in joints with slight loss of motion

(e) Swelling and localized pain

f. Exercise prescription components:

(1) Specify duration, intensity, and frequency

(2) Progression of physical activity—gradual onset, increasing in intensity/duration, e.g., begin walking, then gradually replace with jogging

(3) Individualized to client capabilities

(4) Client motivation, goals, and interest (motivators)—adolescent females—weight control, improved appearance; adolescent males—increased skills, strength, competition; women—weight control, appearance, stress reduction; men—pleasure, fun, and challenge abilities (Jones, 1997)

(5) Based on available time, equipment, and facilities

(6) Refer individuals with abnormal exercise stress tests (bicycle ergometer or treadmill), chronic/recent heart or lung pathology, or any positive cardiac risk factors to the appropriate health care provider

g. Physical fitness evaluation

(1) Cardiorespiratory endurance or aerobic fitness is usually measured by performance on 1.5 mile run, step test (5 minute pulse-recovery step test), bicycle ergometer test or swimming test

(2) Skinfold test or other determination of body fat composition

(3) Back flexibility of back—hyperextension, sit/reach test

(4) Muscle strength—tested by determining maximum amount of weight that can be lifted comfortably, a single time, by four different muscle groups; test is usually conducted following completion of approximately six weeks of training

(5) Muscle endurance—determined by push-ups (shoulder, arm and chest muscle endurance) and bent knee sit-ups (abdominals)

(6) Leg power—tested by height of vertical jump from squat position

h. Nutrition for athletic performance

(1) Drink 17 ounces of fluid approximately 2 hours prior to exercise to promote hydration; allow time for excretion of excess ingested fluid; drink approximately two cups of fluid for every pound of weight loss during extended athletic activities

(2) Maintain well balanced diet—adequate carbohydrates to optimize respiratory metabolism, adequate protein to preserve lean body mass, adequate minerals to maximize oxygen delivery, and calcium to develop high density bones (Kenney, 1996)

- Safety and Environment
  1. General
     a. Fire safety (smoke alarms, fire extinguishers)
     b. Home safety (secure locks on doors and windows)

  c. Automobile (use of safety belts, harnesses, defensive driving)

  d. Helmets (bikes, motorcycles, roller blades)

  e. Personal safety (avoid risk-taking behaviors; always be on the defensive, especially women)

 2. Safety for aging adult

  a. Home safety

   (1) Adequate lighting especially around stairs; light switches near doorways and accessible from bed

   (2) Home should be surveyed for risk factors that may create walking hazards (loose rugs, furniture placement, electrical cords); traffic lanes in each room free of hazards

   (3) Nightlight or flashlight by bed is recommended to avoid falls or disorientation in the dark

   (4) Avoid housekeeping hazards by cleaning up spills as they occur and avoiding clutter on floors/stairways

   (5) Bathroom—non-slip mat in tub/shower, secure "grab bar"

   (6) Stairwell—secure handrail, steps in good repair

  b. Personal safety

   (1) Avoid dangers of hypothermia with adequate heat and caloric intake

   (2) Set up daily surveillance system with others

   (3) Assess ability to take medications correctly

  c. Physical deficit concerns

   (1) Gait and balance problems

    (a) Slippery or irregular surfaces

    (b) Clutter or obstructions

    (c) Stairs, steep or without rails

    (d) Lack of space to maneuver assistive device (e.g., walker)

    (e) Bathtub without rail or slip guards

   (2) Decreased vision

    (a) Inadequate lighting

    (b) Poorly marked stairs

   (3) Decreased sensitivity to pain/heat

    (a) Hot water bottle/heating pad

    (b) Hot bath water

      (4)   Potential driving/traffic hazards

          (a)   Decreased visual acuity and hearing

          (b)   Decreased reaction time

          (c)   Difficulty moving head (arthritis)

          (d)   Ambulation too slow for traffic signals

3. Four categories of environmental hazards

   a. Biological (e.g., viruses, microorganisms)

   b. Chemical (e.g., lead, asbestos)

   c. Physical (e.g., natural disasters)

   d. Sociological and psychological hazards (e.g., overcrowding, lack of resources)

4. Components of an environmental assessment

   a. Home hazards—fire safety, pest control, inadequate heat or toilet facilities

   b. Work-site hazards and protection—noise, inhalants, lifting, hazardous materials; related exposures

   c. Neighborhood hazards—noise, air/water pollution, inadequate police protection, overcrowding or isolation from neighbors

   d. Community hazards—lack of availability of grocery stores, drugstores, public transportation

Health Evaluation Across the Lifespan

- Health History: Important in identifying risk behaviors and need for health education

   1. Demographics and biographical data

   2. History of present illness

      a. Symptom analysis

         (1) Location and radiation

         (2) Quality or character

         (3) Quantity, frequency, intensity, duration, effect on daily activities

         (4) Gradual, abrupt onset, course, length of time, pattern

         (5) Setting

         (6) Aggravating and alleviating factors

         (7) Associated symptom/manifestations

      b. Reason for seeking health care or chief complaint—signs/symptoms and duration; preferably in client's own words

   3. Past medical history (Swartz, 1994)

a. General state of health (client's perception)

b. Past illnesses (hospitalizations)

c. Past injuries, surgery (dates, treatment, and follow-up)

d. Emotional health (past problems including assistance, history of domestic violence)

e. Sexual health (obstetric and contraceptive history, number of partners, sexual preference, sexual problems, disease prevention efforts)

f. Food or drug allergies (specify reaction and treatment, if any)

g. Medications (prescription and over the counter)

h. Immunizations (type and date)

i. Sleep patterns (approximate hours, difficulties)

j. Last examinations (physical, dental, vision, hearing, radiography, electrocardiogram (ECG), cancer screenings)

4. Personal habits

a. Tobacco use—cigarettes, pipe, cigars, smokeless; record number of cigarettes per day, number of use years, if stopped, how long ago; approach adolescents with declarative statements related to drugs at school, drugs in common use at school, drugs used by friends, and by individuals; inquire about tobacco use in terms of number of packs smoked daily

b. Alcohol and drug use (type, amount)

c. Use of caffeine (coffee, colas, etc.)

d. Diet (24 hour intake, including nutritional supplements)

e. Exercise (type, frequency)

f. Leisure activities (type, frequency)

g. Sports (type, frequency)

h. Additional questions may be required regarding sports participation, especially contact sports that may include:

(1) Have you ever been dizzy or passed out during or after exercise?

(2) Have you had a seizure, concussion or been unconscious?

(3) Are you able to run ½ mile or more?

(4) Are you missing a kidney?

(5) Have you ever had a heart murmur, high blood pressure or heart abnormality?

5. Psychosocial history

a. Living situation at present

b. Education—for adolescents ask, if in school, grades, positive or negative attitudes toward school

c. Religious beliefs in relation to health and treatment

d. Positive or negative perspective of the future

e. Perception of ''typical day''

f. Stress, stress management

g. Depression or anxiety, suicide ideation (adolescents and young adults require direct questioning, e.g., have you ever thought of killing yourself)

h. Support systems

6. Family history: Include age, health status or cause of death of parents, siblings, children in a genogram, (diabetes, heart disease, cancer, hypertension, lung disease, alcoholism, blood disorders, birth defects and any other illnesses that seem to run in the family)

7. Occupational and environmental history

a. Type of work, former occupation(s)

b. Hazardous exposures at home or work

c. Military service, wartime employment, if any

d. Location of home, length of time

e. Home location adjacent to factories, shipyards, or other potentially hazardous facilities

f. Hobbies, potential exposures

8. Adolescent interviewing guidelines

a. Adolescent is primary historian, interviewed alone

b. Explain ground rules—unless serious problem emerges threatening life or health, interview is confidential

c. Home, Education, Activities, Drugs, Sex, Suicide (HEADSS) interview format is widely suggested—see age related anticipatory guidance

- Risk Factor Identification: Virtually every disease, condition has risk factors; select conditions are presented related to prevalence, in addition to protective factors.

1. Research over the past 20 years has identified factors associated with physical health and longer healthier life. (Pender, 1996)

a. Exercise—regular, (see exercise, this chapter)

b. Non-smoker, recently extended to smoke-free environment

c. Seven to eight hours of sleep

d. Moderate or no alcohol

e. Regular and moderate eating (including breakfast)

f. Weight control

g. Ample exercise, good nutrition and healthy lifestyle to slow aging process

2. Cardiac risk factors:

a. Age—male 45+, female 55+ or premature menopause without estrogen replacement therapy

b. Family history of premature heart disease, myocardial infarction or death of father/first degree male relative < 55, mother/female relative < 65

c. Cigarette smoking

d. Hypertension ≥ 140/90 mm Hg, or on anti-hypertensive medication

e. Low HDL cholesterol < 35mg/dL, (> 60 mg/dL negative risk)

f. LDL > 160mg/dL (< 130 mL negative risk)

g. Diabetes mellitus

3. Obesity (20% above desirable weight)—mortality rates increase with weights 10% above desirable weights; obesity is associated with multiple attendant health risks (Clinical Preventive Services, 1997)

a. Three times more prevalent in hypertensives and type 2 diabetes

b. Increased risk of high cholesterol and coronary artery disease

c. Increased risk of cancer (colon, rectal, prostate, gallbladder, biliary tract, breast, cervical, endometrial, and ovarian)

d. Abdominal adiposity associated with increased risk of stroke and death from all causes

4. Suicide risk factors

a. Family history of psychiatric disorders (especially depression or suicide)

b. Previous suicide attempts

c. Family violence (verbal, physical or sexual abuse)

d. Family instability (frequent separation from, or loss of loved one)

e. Alcohol or substance abuse

f. Availability and accessibility of firearms in the home

- Age Related Health Monitoring (if asymptomatic)—Specific health screenings are part of secondary prevention, see Table 4

1. Screening guidelines

a. Generalized screening indicated for diseases of high prevalence in the population and diseases with profound morbidity/ mortality if not diagnosed

Table 4
Adult Screening Guidelines (U.S. Preventive Services Task Force, 1996, American Cancer Society, 1994)

Service	Who Needs	Frequency*	Risk Factors
Blood Pressure	All Adults	Every 2 years	male, blk, fam hx
Cholesterol	All Adults	Every 5 years	Male, tob, htn, fam hx
Dental	All Adults	Annual	
ECG	Adults 40+	Annual (only with cardiac risk factors)	
Pap Smear	Women 18+	Annual recommended every 3 years after two normal exams for women without risk factors**	
Self-Breast Exam	All Women 20+	Monthly	
Breast exam	Women 40+	Annual (age 20–39 every 3 yrs)	
Mammogram (ACS)	Women 40+	Annual	
Colorectal screen (fecal occult + flexible sigmoidoscopy every 5 yrs or colonoscopy every 10 yrs)	Adults 50+	Annual	
Prostate specific antigen (PSA)	Men 50+	Annual (ACS)	blk, fam hx
Glaucoma screen	Adults 40+	Annual	***
Hearing	Only w/excessive noise exposure		
Chest x-ray	Not recommended		
Thyroid palpation	Adults 20 to 39	Every 3 years	
	Adults 40+	Annual	
Urinalysis	Controversy		Yes, w/sx, preg., dm.
Hgb/Hct	Controversy		Yes, w/sx, pregnancy
Health ed/prom. (nutrition, exercise, stress management, substance abuse, safety, safe sex and cancer prevention)	All Adults	Every encounter	

*Increased frequency in the presence of risk factors
**Risk factors for cervical cancer—history of STD, multiple partners, tobacco use(tob), first intercourse before age 18
***Risk factors for glaucoma—myopia, diabetes mellitus(dm), family history (fam hx), African-American(blk) > 40
The term controversy indicates that the U.S. Task Force recommends against routine screening.
Adopted from the U.S. Preventative Task Force *Guide to Clinical Preventive Services,* 1996 and American Cancer Society. Consult full reports for details

     b.   Screening tests must be reliable with acceptable technical process; must include appropriate follow-up

     c.   Test should be sensitive (true positive, those with disease screen positive) and specific (true negative, those without disease screen negative)

  2.   Adolescence (12 to 19 years of age)—American Medical Association (AMA) recommends three visit intervals 11 to 14 years, 15 to 17 years, and 18 to 21 years unless more frequent examinations are indicated (AMA, 1999)

     a.   Complete physical examination including:

      (1)   Height/weight (use anthropometric chart)

          (a)   Screen for eating disorders if indicated

          (b)   Assess perception of food, weight

      (2)   Complete skin examination

      (3)   Assessment for gingivitis, caries, and malalignment

      (4)   Assessment for signs of abuse or neglect

      (5)   Hearing assessment (if exposed to excessive noise), and vision

b. Blood pressure (BP) every two years, normal systolic 110 to 135 mm Hg, diastolic 60 to 85; refer BP > 140/90

c. Tuberculin skin test (PPD) every two years with any exposure or if at risk

d. Female

      (1)   Teach self-breast examination (SBE)

      (2)   Determine Tanner stage (Hay, Groothuis, Hayward, Levin (1995)

          (a)   Tanner Stages usual sequence of pubertal events —**T**elarche (breast development), **P**ubarche (growth of axillary and pubic hair), **A**drenarche (increased secretion of adrenal androgens), **G**rowth spurt and **M**enarche (first menstrual period) (TPAGM)

          (b)   Stage I—growth spurt (height and weight) average age for girls 10 years

          (c)   Stage II—breast bud, sparse pubic hair

          (d)   Stage III–IV—breast development

          (e)   Stage V—mature stage

      (3)   If sexually active or 18 years old—Papanicolaou (pap) smear

e. Male

      (1)   Teach self-testicular examination (STE)

      (2)   Determine Tanner stage

          (a)   Stage I—growth spurt (height and weight) average age for boys 12.5 years

          (b)   Stage II—sparse pubic hair

          (c)   Stage III–IV—male organ enlargement

          (d)   Stage V—mature stage

f. If high risk, counseling and test for human immunodeficiency virus (HIV) and VDRL; assess knowledge of contraceptives and protective barriers

g. Immunization

      (1)   Tetanus-diptheria booster (Td)

      (2)   Others if needed; see Immunization Guidelines this chapter

  h. Remain alert for depressive symptoms, any suicide risk factors

  i. Dental checkup with cleaning annually

3. Young adult (20 to 39 years of age) (see Table 4)

  a. Complete physical examination (age 20, then every 5 to 6 years

  b. BP every 2 years; normal systolic 110 to 135 mm Hg, diastolic 60 to 85 mm Hg

  c. Total cholesterol every 5 years with additional tests if total cholesterol exceeds 200 mg/dL

  d. Female

      (1)   SBE monthly

      (2)   Pap and pelvic examination every 3 years , GC and chlamydia tests

      (3)   Clinical breast examination (by health professional) every 3 years

  e. Male—STE monthly

  f. PPD if exposed to tuberculosis

  g. Immunizations—Td every ten years

  h. Self-skin examination

  i. Dental checkup with cleaning annually

4. Middle-aged adult (40 to 59 years of age) (see Table 4)

  a. Complete physical examination (every 5 to 6 years)

  b. B.P. every 2 years; normal systolic 110 to 135 mm Hg, diastolic 60 to 85 mm Hg

  c. Total cholesterol every 5 years with additional tests if total cholesterol exceeds 200 mg/dL

  d. ECG, age 40+ with cardiac risk factors

  e. Female

      (1)   SBE monthly

      (2)   Clinical breast exam yearly (performed by a health professional)

      (3)   Mammogram annually age 50 years

      (4)   Pap and pelvic examination every 3 years

  f. Male—STE monthly

  g. Colorectal screen (fecal occult or sigmoidoscopy)—age 50 annually

    h. Glaucoma screen, annually

    i. Dental examination with cleaning every 6 to 12 months

    j. Cancer screening yearly

    k. Immunizations—tetanus every 10 years

5. Elderly adult (60 + years of age) (see Table 4)

    a. Complete physical examination every 2 years with laboratory assessments

    b. BP every 2 years, normal systolic 110 to 135mm Hg, diastolic 60 to 85mm Hg

    c. Total cholesterol every 5 years with additional tests if total cholesterol exceeds 200 mg/dL

    d. ECG annually with cardiac risk factors

    e. Female

        (1) SBE monthly

        (2) Annual mammogram

        (3) Pap and pelvic examination every 3 years

    f. Male—STE monthly

    g. Colorectal screen (fecal occult or sigmoidoscopy) age 50—annually

    h. Glaucoma screen—annually

    i. Dental examination with cleaning every 6 to 12 months

    j. Immunizations—tetanus every 10 years, pneumococcal vaccine once, and annual influenza vaccine

- Age Related Anticipatory Guidance (Allender, 1998)

1. Adolescence (12 to 19 years of age)

    a. Leading causes of death—motor vehicle accidents (MVA), suicide, other accidents, homicide, malignancy, cardiovascular disease, congenital disease

    b. Normal growth and development

        (1) Physical changes with puberty

        (2) Need for increased self responsibilities for own health— nutrition, exercise, adequate sleep and safety habits

    c. Nutrition

        (1) Variety of foods, including breakfast

        (2) Nutritious snacks, limit sweets and fast food

    d. Skin care/skin protection

    e. Dental care (brushing and flossing)

        (1)   Fluoride supplementation

        (2)   Dental visits with cleaning every 6 to 12 months

  f. Injury prevention

        (1)   Athletics, safety helmets, pads, mouthguards

        (2)   Safety belts

        (3)   Firearm safety

        (4)   Defensive driving, driver education

        (5)   Violent behavior/gangs

  g. Physical activity

        (1)   Need for regular physical activity

        (2)   Encourage team activities, peer interaction

        (3)   Encourage participation in after school and/or church activities

  h. Substance abuse

        (1)   Tobacco use avoidance or cessation emphasizing unattractive cosmetic effects (stained teeth and fingernails, foul smelling breath and clothes) and athletic consequences (decreased endurance, shortness of breath)

        (2)   Smokeless tobacco is not safer, can be addicting/life-threatening

        (3)   Alcohol and other drugs

  i. Sexuality

        (1)   Dating

        (2)   Responsible sexual behaviors, abstinence, contraception

        (3)   Risks, sexually transmitted diseases, unwanted pregnancy

2. Young adult (20 to 39 years of age)

  a. Leading causes of death—motor vehicle accidents, homicide, suicide, injuries, heart disease, AIDS

  b. Nutrition and exercise

        (1)   Weight management with changing basal metabolic rate

        (2)   Selection of exercise program

  c. Dental care

  d. Sexuality

        (1)   Family planning, contraception

        (2)   Sexually transmitted diseases

    e. Cancer warning signs/skin protection

    f. Substance use/abuse

        (1) Tobacco cessation/primary prevention

        (2) Alcohol and other drugs

    g. Injury prevention

        (1) Athletics

        (2) Safety belts/safety helmets

        (3) Firearm safety

        (4) Defensive driving

        (5) Violent behavior

    h. Lifestyle choices

        (1) Family and parenting skills

        (2) Stress management

    i. Safety and environmental health

3. Middle aged adult (40 to 59 years of age)

    a. Leading causes of death—heart disease, accidents, lung cancer, cerebrovascular disease, breast and colorectal cancer, obstructive lung disease

    b. Nutrition and exercise

        (1) Weight management with changing basal metabolic rate

        (2) Selection of exercise program

    c. Dental care

    d. Sexuality

        (1) Menopause

        (2) Sexual changes due to aging

        (3) Sexually transmitted diseases

    e. Cancer warning signs/skin protection

    f. Substance use/abuse

        (1) Tobacco cessation/primary prevention

        (2) Alcohol and other drugs

    g. Injury prevention

        (1) Athletics

        (2) Safety belts/safety helmets

        (3) Firearm safety

  (4) Defensive driving

  (5) Violent behavior

 h. Midlife changes

  (1) Empty nest syndrome, grandparenting

  (2) Planning for retirement

  (3) Stress management

 i. Safety and environmental health

4. Elderly adult (age 60+ years of age)

 a. Leading causes of death—heart disease, cerebrovascular disease, obstructive lung disease, pneumonia and/or influenza, lung and colorectal cancer

 b. Nutrition and exercise

  (1) Weight management with changing basal metabolic rate

  (2) Selection of exercise program

 c. Dental care

 d. Sexuality

  (1) Sexual changes due to aging

  (2) Sexually transmitted diseases

 e. Cancer warning signs/skin protection

 f. Substance use/abuse

  (1) Tobacco cessation/primary prevention

  (2) Alcohol and other drugs

 g. Injury prevention

  (1) Athletics

  (2) Safety belts/safety helmets

  (3) Firearm safety

  (4) Defensive driving

  (5) Violent behavior

 h. Life changes

  (1) Retirement

  (2) Loss of spouse, friends

  (3) Physical changes (vision, hearing, reaction time, alterations of bowel and bladder habits)

 i. Safety and environmental health

        (a)   Home safety

        (b)   Personal safety

- Immunization Guidelines (Centers for Disease Control and Prevention (CDC) (1998)

  1. Tetanus-diptheria vaccine (Td)—primary series is recommended if not completed during childhood with two doses at least four weeks apart and a third dose 6 to 12 months after the second; Td booster is recommended every 10 years; adolescents 14–16 years of age should receive booster if no dose in past 5 years

  2. Measles-Mumps-Rubella vaccine (MMR)—recommended for adolescents who have not received two doses at or after 12 months of age; second dose is now given routinely as part of preschool immunizations or at age 12 to 14, or prior to post secondary education or military service; adults without documentation of disease or immunization need only one dose; adults born prior to 1956 are considered immune due to prevalence of diseases before that time

  3. Varicella vaccine—recommended for individuals who have never had chicken pox; adolescents and adults need two doses 4 to 8 weeks apart

  4. Influenza vaccine—recommended annually for adults and children with chronic disorders of the pulmonary and cardiovascular systems including asthma, diabetes and renal disease, persons 50 years of age or older and persons with any chronic health condition

     a. Groups that can transmit influenza to high risk persons should be immunized (e.g., health care workers and household members)

     b. Optimal time for immunization (mid-October through mid-November)

     c. Contraindications—history of anaphylactic hypersensitivity to eggs or other components; refer to physician for appropriate therapy and possible allergy evaluation

  5. Pneumococcal vaccine—recommended for any person over two years of age who is at increased risk of complications due to chronic illness (e.g., heart or lung disease and diabetes, alcoholism, Hodgkin's disease, cirrhosis, sickle cell disease) and individuals who work or live with high risk individuals); anyone over age 65 and persons without a spleen; revaccination after five or more years is recommended for those at highest risk of antibody decline, e.g., renal disease or organ transplant and persons vaccinated before age 65

  6. Hepatitis B vaccine (HBV)—three dose regimen recommended for all individuals who are or will be at increased risk of infection; the second dose is given one month after the first with a third dose six months later; categories include health care workers, individuals at high risk of exposure to blood and blood products, and individuals at increased risk of exposure due to sexual practices; the timing and need for periodic boosters is determined by serologic testing; recommended for all adolescents who were not previously immunized

  7. Hepatitis A vaccine (HAV)—two to three doses recommended for individuals working in or traveling to countries with high levels of HAV infection; men who have

sex with men, parenteral drug use, persons exposed to non-human primates, persons with chronic liver disease; adolescents up to eighteen require three doses, the first two doses one month apart and the third dose 6 to 12 months later; adults (>18) require two doses 6 to 12 months apart

8. Polio—inactivated poliovirus vaccine-enhanced potency (IVP-e) is indicated for unimmunized adults who are traveling outside the U.S. and healthcare workers; partially immunized or unimmunized adults with close contact with children receiving OPV; the second dose is given one month after the first with a third dose six months later

9. Catch up schedule, contraindications and precautions

   a. For individuals with uncertain immunization histories (lacking documentation):

      (1) First visit—Td, IPV, MMR, HBV; HAV, varicella, influenza, pneumococccal are optional depending upon risk factors

      (2) Second visit (4 to 6 weeks after first visit)—Td, IPV, HBV, with second dose of HAV, varicella, if given initially

      (3) Third visit (6 months after second visit)—Td, IPV, HBV, with third dose of HAV for adolescents

   b. Contraindications

      (1) Anaphylactic reaction to known component:

         (a) MMR and influenza (eggs)

         (b) Hepatitis (Bakers yeast)

         (c) IPV (streptomycin, polymixin B or neomycin)

         (d) Varicella (gelatin or neomycin)

      (2) Moderate to severe illness (fever > 100.4°F)

      (3) Immunocompromised individuals (no live virus)

   c. Precaution with MMR—delay pregnancy for 3 months following immunization

10. Immunization schedule synopsis for adolescents and adults with documentation of immunizations during childhood

    a. Adolescents and adults

       (1) Hepatitis B Series

       (2) Td Booster, repeat every 10 years

       (3) Varicella, if needed, two doses 4 to 8 weeks apart

       (4) MMR if born after 1956

    b. Adults over 65, chronic disease (heart, lung or diabetes; those who work or live with high risk individuals)

       (1)   Influenza vaccine each fall

       (2)   Pneumococcal vaccine

Resources

Agency for Health Care Policy and Research (AHCPR)
(800) 358-9295
FAX (301) 594-2800
http://www.ahcpr.gov/
AHCPR Publications Clearinghouse
P.O. Box 8547,
Silver Spring, MD 20907
Automated instructions available 24 hours/day
(Pocket guide on smoking cessation, etc.)

American Association for Retired Persons
(202) 872-4700
1909 K Street N.W. Fifth Floor
Washington, D. C. 20049
http://www.aarp.org
Services for age 50 and older include lobby for senior citizens, mail-order pharmacy, bi-monthly magazine, support group for widowed persons.

National Cancer Institute Cancer Information Service
(800) 4-CANCER (800) 422-6237
http://www.nci.nih.gov/
Johns Hopkins Oncology Center
550 N. Broadway, Ste 301
Baltimore, MD 20824-0105
(Pamphlets on breast examination, pap smear, colorectal screening)

National Heart, Lung and Blood Information Center, (NHLBI)
(800) 575-WELL (800) 575-9355
or (301) 251-1222
Fax (301) 251-1223
http://www.nhlbi.nih.gov/
P.O. Box 30105,
Bethesda, MD 20824-0105

National Institute on Aging Information Officer
(800) 622-2225
http://www.nih.gov/nia/health
Building 31, Room 5C-35
9000 Rockville Pike
Bethesda, MD 20205
Self-care and Self-help groups for the elderly (Directory)

National Institutes of Health Consensus Conference.
(800) NIH-OMAR
Fax (301) 480-5144
http://text.nlm.nih.gov
NIH Consensus Development Program

Office of Disease Prevention and Health Promotion
(800) 336-4797
http://www.health.gov
Dietary Guidelines for Americans, 2000

Additional internet resources for Health Promotion

American College of Nurse Practitioners http://www.nurse.org/acnp
American Dietetic Asociation http://www.eatright.com
American Health Line http://www.apn.com/info/am   health/
American Red Cross http://www.redcross.org
American Nurses Association http://www.nursingworld.org
American Journal of Nursing http://www.ajn.org

Centers for Disease Control and Prevention
(888) 232-3299
http://www.cdc.gov
Provides health information and information for international travel

Food and Drug Administration http://www.fda.gov/
Food Insight
Current topics in food safety and nutrition
http://ificinfo.health.org

Health Canada http://www.hwc.ca/
Health Care Financing Administration U.S. Dept. of Health and Human Services (Medicare/ Medicaid) http://www.os.dhhs.gov/

Healthgate http://www3.healthgate.com
Healthy People http://www.health.gov/healthypeople
Health Information for Consumers http://www.healthfinder.gov

International Food Information Council http://www.ificinfo.health.org

Modern Healthcare http://modernhealthcare.com
National Health Information Center http://nhic-nt.health.org
New England Medical Journal On-line http://www.nejm.org
NOAH http://www.noah.health.org

National Institutes of Safety and Health http://www.cdc.gov/niosh/homepage.htm
National Library of Medicine http://www.nlm.nih.gov/
Safety Checklist for the Elderly http://www.usc.edu/dept/gero/hmap/library/safety.html
US Department of Health and Human Services http://www.os.dhhs.gov/
World Health Organization http://www.who.int/

Check the telephone directory for local chapters of:

American Cancer Society Cancer Response System
(800) 227-2345
http://www.cancer.org
2525 Ridge Point Dr. Ste 100
Austin, TX 78754

American Heart Association
(800) AHA-USA1 (800) 242-8721
http://www.americanheart.org
7320 Greenville Avenue
Dallas TX 75231

American Lung Association
(800) LUNG-USA
http://www.lungusa.org/
1740 Broadway
P.O. Box 596
New York, NY 10019

Questions
Select the best answer

1. Using the Health Belief Model, determine which of the following individuals would be most motivated for behavior change?

   a. 42-year-old married female with excess weight for over 20 years
   b. 16-year-old female with poorly controlled sugar levels and poor dietary habits consistent with her friends
   c. 50-year-old male with recent myocardial infarction, whose prognosis is good with positive changes in diet and weight loss
   d. 40-year-old who reports spouse wants him to lose weight

2. Which of the following activities would prepare an individual planning retirement to successfully resolve the final developmental tasks proposed by Erickson?

   a. Plan to simultaneously complete any community obligations
   b. Become involved with community activities
   c. Plan several extended trips early in retirement while able
   d. Avoid any commitments initially, wait for opportunities to present themselves

3. Screening for breast cancer is which level of prevention?

   a. Primary
   b. Secondary
   c. Tertiary
   d. Preliminary

4. Client (age 70) comes into your clinic the first week of November for health screening. Her last immunization, a Td (tetanus) was ten years ago. Which immunization will you recommend?

   a. Td, influenza and pneumococcal vaccine
   b. Influenza and pneumococcal vaccine and schedule Td within three months.
   c. Td and influenza
   d. Td only

5. A temporary certificate for school attendance is given following initial immunizations for a 14-year-old boy. When should the adolescent return for more immunizations?

   a. Six months
   b. Four to six weeks
   c. One year
   d. Four months

6. Female, age 19 will be entering college in January. She is not pregnant. Without evidence of recent immunization, she should receive which of the following today?

   a. Second MMR, Td and polio boosters
   b. Hemophilus influenzae (HIB) and a tetanus booster

    c. Second MMR and Td

    d. Immunization for rubella, tetanus, and influenza

7. Joe, age 15, has just moved to your community and is staying in a temporary foster home. He has no record of any immunizations. Which of the following does Joe need today?

    a. MMR, Td, and varicella

    b. IPV, MMR, HBV and Td

    c. Td only

    d. MMR and Td

8. According to research, which type of social support has the strongest relationship with health status?

    a. Emotional

    b. Instrumental

    c. Informational

    d. Appraisal

9. According to research, how much sleep is associated with a longer healthier life?

    a. 5–6 hours

    b. 6–7 hours

    c. 7–8 hours

    d. 8–9 hours

10. Josh, age 32, is ready to start exercising and wants to jog. Guidelines should include which of the following?

    a. Jog one mile initially, then add distance daily until goal is reached.

    b. Jog at least once a week for 30 minutes to condition your heart and lungs.

    c. Begin with brisk walking and gradually replace with jogging.

    d. Warm up exercises before or after jogging.

11. Several cups of coffee immediately prior to the clinic visit would likely elevate which of the following?

    a. Heart rate

    b. Respiratory rate

    c. Cholesterol

    d. Blood sugar

12. Jim asks why cooling down is necessary for an exercise plan?

    a. Allows body temperature and heart rate to decrease slowly

    b. Loosens and strengthens muscles

    c. Maintains and increases flexibility

    d. Sustains heart rate for longer period of time

13. According to the Transtheoretical Model, intervention at which level is most likely to result in behavior change?

    a. Maintenance
    b. Contemplation
    c. Precontemplation
    d. Preparation

14. Which stress management technique would be most appropriate for a newly diagnosed diabetic?

    a. Change avoidance
    b. Habituation
    c. Time blocking
    d. Imagery

15. According to the U.S. Preventive Services Task Force Recommendations, a woman age 21 needs which of the following annually?

    a. Blood pressure and cholesterol
    b. Clinical breast exam
    c. Pap and pelvic
    d. Dental screen

16. Your female client age 49, has had a normal baseline mammogram. She asks when she should get her next mammogram:

    a. Annually beginning next year at age 50
    b. Every other year from age 50 to 59, then yearly
    c. Every three years until you are age 60
    d. Every 5 years for the rest of your life

17. Which of the following individuals has a body mass index at the desirable level?

    a. Male, 6 feet 2 inches, 200 pounds (BMI 26)
    b. Female, 5 feet 6 inches, 125 pounds (BMI 20)
    c. Female, 5 feet 10 inches, 160 pounds (BMI 23)
    d. Male, 5 feet 10 inches, 145 pounds (BMI 21)

Answers

1. c
2. b
3. b
4. a
5. b
6. c
7. b
8. a
9. c
10. c
11. a
12. a
13. d
14. c
15. d
16. a
17. c

Bibliography

Allender, M. (1998). Adolescent. In C. Edelman & C. Mandle (Eds.). *Health promotion throughout the lifespan* (4th ed.). Baltimore: Mosby.

American Cancer Society. (2000). *Summary of the American Cancer Society recommendations for the early detection of cancer in asymptomatic people.* Atlanta, Georgia, GA: American Cancer Society.

American Nurses Association. (1997). *Clinician's handbook of preventive services: Put prevention into practice.* Waldorf, MD: American Nurses Publishing.

American Medical Association. (1999). *Guidelines for adolescent preventative services.* http://www.ama-assn.org/adolhlth/

Bandura, A. (1986). *Social foundations of thought and action.* Englewood Cliffs, NJ: Prentice-Hall.

Becker, M. (1972). The health belief model and personal health behavior. *Health Education Monographs 2, 326–7.*

Centers for Disease Control and Prevention. (1998). Summary of adolescent/adult immunizations: Recommendations of the Advisory Committee on Immunization Practices, American Academy of Pediatrics, the American Academy of Family Physicians, and the American Medical Association. http://www.cdc.gov/hip/

Cohen, E. (1996). *Nurse case management in the 21st Century.* St. Louis: Mosby.

Clark, M. (1999). *Nursing in the community* (3rd ed.). Norwalk, CT: Appleton & Lange.

Erikson, E. (1963). *Childhood and society* (2nd ed.). NY: Norton.

Friedman, M. (1998). *Family nursing: Research, theory, and practice* (4th ed.). Stanford, CT: Appleton & Lange.

Green, L., & Kreuer, M. (1991). *Health promotion planning: An educational and environmental approach* (2nd ed.). Mountain View, CA: Mayfield.

Jones, K., & Jones, J. (1997). Physical activity & exercise. *Clinician Reviews, 7*(3) 81–102.

Keller,C., Oveland, D., & Hudson, S. (1997). Strategies for weight control success in adults. *Nurse Practitioner, 22*(3), 33–54.

Kenney, W. (1996). *American college of sports medicine fitness book.* Champaign, IL: Human Kinetics.

Maslow, A. (1954). *Motivation and personality.* New York: Harper & Row.

Neuman, B. (1995). *The Neuman systems model.* Norwalk, CT: Appleton & Lange.

NIH Consensus Statement. (1994). *Optimal Calcium intake.* 12(4), 1–31.

NIH Consensus Statement. (1995). *Physical activity and cardiovascular health.* December 18–20, 13(3), 1–33.

Pender, N. (1996). *Health promotion in nursing practice* (3rd ed.). Norwalk, CT: Appleton & Lange.

Prochaska, J., & Velicir, W. (1997). The transtheoretical model of health behavior change. *American Journal of Health Promotion,* 12(1).

Public Health Service. (2000). *Healthy people 2010.* Washington, DC: Department of Health and Human Services.

U.S. Department of Health and Human Services. (1997). *Clinical handbook of preventive services: Put prevention into practice* (2nd ed.). http://www.ahcpr.gov/ppip/

Selye, H. (1974). *Stress without distress.* NY: J. B. Lippincott.

Swartz, M. (1998). *Textbook of physical diagnosis* (3rd ed.). Philadelphia: W. B. Saunders.

von Bertalanffy (1968). *General systems theory.* New York: George Braziller.

Care of the Aging Adult

Debbie G. Kramer

Demographics of Older Adults

The elderly population in America is increasing rapidly. The rates are significantly higher than for other segments of the population. A greater number of aged persons are living longer and healthier due to improved health care and a healthier lifestyle. The average U.S. life span has increased appreciably since the beginning of the century. The average life expectancy at birth increased by almost two years during the past decade. The term "elderly" is generally accepted as referring to persons 65 years and older.

- Definitions of Late Adulthood:

    1. Age 65 to 74 years—the young-old

    2. Age 75 to 84 years—the middle-old

    3. Age 85 and over—the oldest-old

- Population Statistics (U.S. Census Bureau, 1995)

    1. In 1900, individuals aged 65 and over numbered 3.1 million persons—one in every 25 Americans

    2. By 1994, the elderly comprised one in eight (33.2 million); an 11-fold increase

    3. The Census Bureau projects the elderly population will more than double to 80 million, one in five persons, between now and 2050

    4. Fastest growing subgroup is the oldest-old, also referred to as the frail elderly—3 million persons and 10% of the elderly

    5. The elderly population is estimated at 13% utilizing 25% of total health care expenditures and prescription drugs

    6. Greatest growth spurt will be seen when the "baby-boomers" enter the 65 and over group, between the years of 2010 and 2030

    7. The "baby-boomers" will number 19 million in 2050 when they become the oldest-old, making them 24% of elderly Americans and 5% of all Americans

    8. The leading causes of death age 65 and over are heart disease, cancer, stroke, chronic obstructive pulmonary disease and pneumonia/influenza

- Gender Statistics

    1. Elderly women outnumber elderly men by three to two—20 million to 14 million (1994 data)

    2. In 1993, the life expectancy for women was 79 years and 72 years for men

    3. Men have higher death rates at each age

- Marital Status and Living Arrangements

    1. In 1993, 75% of non-institutionalized elderly men were married and living with their spouses

    2. 41% of their female counterparts were married and living with their spouses

3. Older women were three times more likely than men to be widowed—48% versus 14%; eight out of ten elderly persons living alone are women

4. The likelihood of living alone or in a residential care facility increases with age

5. Only 9% of non-institutionalized persons aged 65 to 69 years needed assistance with their activities of daily living (ADL), whereas 50% of the 85 and over age group required such assistance

- Income and Poverty

  1. Living below the government defined poverty level increases with age

  2. Older women (16%) have higher poverty rate than older men (9%)

  3. Elderly African-Americans (33%) and Hispanics (22%) outnumber Whites (11%) with low income levels

  4. Within each race/ethnic group, poverty is more prevalent for women than men; income varies with differences in age, gender, race, ethnicity, marital status, living arrangements, educational level, former occupation, and work history

- Educational Status

  1. Better education is correlated with a healthier, longer life

  2. In 1993, 60% of non-institutionalized elderly as compared to 85% of those under age 65 completed high school

  3. The oldest-old were more likely to have only an eighth grade education or less (24% versus 6%); the level of education decreases with age

  4. 12% of the elderly have college degrees versus 20% of those aged 55 to 59 and 27% of persons aged 45 to 49

- Racial/Ethnic Diversity

  1. In 1995, 85 out of 100 elderly were White

  2. By 2050, 67 out of 100 persons will be non-White

  3. Hispanics will rise from 4% to 16% of the older population

Theories of Aging (Spirduso, 1995)

Aging is a process that occurs to an organism with the passage of time, eventually resulting in death. Understanding by scientists of the mechanisms of the theories of aging may show an interaction and inter-relatedness among the theories in the future.

- Genetic Theories

  1. Gene—process of aging is dictated by preprogrammed genetic components influenced by biological markers such as puberty and menopause; one or more genes control cellular aging process and specific genes may influence longevity

  2. Error - catastrophe—an early theory suggesting errors occur through somatic mutations, chromosomal rearrangements or genetic material transcriptions

3. DNA—mutations occur in the mitochondria of DNA and continually mount upwards throughout an individual's lifetime, causing aging

4. Hayflick limit or cell aging—cells will multiply and divide only a finite number of times; genetically preprogrammed

- Damage Theories
  1. Chemical—chemical reactions occur naturally and result in irreversible molecular defects; may occur from air, food, smoking and the like; if insults and injuries outweigh the repairing process, the system fails

  2. Cross-linkage—atoms or molecules have chemical sites that may link to DNA in the cell; damaged DNA is repaired by body's defense mechanism; if cross-linkage impedes transport of nutrients and information, the damage cannot be repaired

  3. Free-radical—free radicals are oxygen metabolites produced by one-electron reduction of oxygen that can produce damage and lead to cell death

- Gradual Imbalance Theories
  1. Autoimmune—immune system loses its ability to distinguish normal material from foreign antigens and begins to destroy its host

  2. Gradual imbalance—brain, endocrine or immune system begins to fail, possibly at different rates, causing an imbalance and decreased effectiveness

  3. Neuroendocrine regulatory system—enables body to adapt to real or perceived challenges such as changes in workload, temperature, or psychological threats

- Wear and Tear—mechanical and biological features of aging; irreversible damage occurs over time

- Social Theories
  1. Disengagement theory (not currently supported)—individuals inevitably become withdrawn from society as a function of aging; acceptable to both the individual and society

  2. Activity theory—maintenance of activity, social roles and social supports directly related to satisfaction with life and self-concept; quality of activities more important than quantity

- Developmental Theories
  1. Erik Erickson's resolution of psychological conflict—ego integrity vs. despair

  2. Robert Peck expanded upon Erickson's conflict of aging
     a. Ego differentiation vs. work role preoccupation
     b. Body transcendence vs. body preoccupation
     c. Ego transcendence vs. ego preoccupation

  3. Daniel Levinson's Seasons of Life—individual must ultimately come to terms with

the inevitability of death; focus is on the relationship of physical changes to personality

4. Developmental tasks theory

    a. Adjust to decreasing physical strength and health

    b. Adjust to retirement and reduced income

    c. Adjust to death of partner

    d. Establish affiliation with peers

    e. Adapt to social rules

    f. Establish satisfactory physical living arrangements

Interview and Health History

Geriatric intervention goals are care vs cure, and improvement or maintenance of function and quality of life. The goal of the interview is to obtain a complete and accurate health history. It is a subjective account of the individual's status. Much of the information obtained will be utilized to formulate diagnoses and a plan of care.

- Develop a Relationship

  1. Develop a climate of trust

  2. Establish a caring relationship

  3. Identify the chief complaint

  4. Maintain a goal-directed interview, as older adults may have long and complex histories

    a. Direct flow of conversation—avoid a "positive" review of systems-answering "yes" to all questions

    b. Ask specific questions, but allow individual to elaborate

    c. Design questions to address one issue at a time

  5. Be aware that gender and age can influence the patient-provider relationship

  6. Family may be present to assist in the evaluation. The patient may rely on the family for answers to interview questions

  7. Sensitive issues such as incontinence, abuse, failing cognition and sexual dysfunction need to be addressed. It is critical that the patient not feel trust or confidence is betrayed

- Communication

  1. Speak slowly; do not shout; lower octaves are generally heard more clearly

  2. Help interpret patient's feelings; ask for clarification

  3. Convey warmth and concern through listening, appropriate touch

    4. Observe for signs of anxiety, exhaustion, nervousness

    5. Understand social mores, cultural differences, language barriers, personal biases

- Environment

    1. Provide a quiet, private setting

    2. Set time limit, as the elderly may tire

    3. Sit face-to-face to ensure eye contact; exhibit a relaxed, but concerned atmosphere

    4. Provide good lighting and ventilation; avoid light source shining from behind you as it creates shadows and glares

- Health History: Format (assess reliability of historian)

    1. Biographical data—important to obtain name and phone number of closest relative

    2. Family history

        a. Parents' health history; cause of death (if applicable)

        b. History of diabetes, heart and kidney disease, cancer, alcoholism, drug abuse, mental illness and other major medical problems in family

        c. Special attention should be given to neurodegenerative or mood disorders

    3. Occupation—any environmental or occupational exposure to pulmonary toxins; adjustment to retirement; source of income

    4. Medications—prescriptions, over-the counter, nontraditional modalities, home remedies

    5. Smoking history, illegal drug use history

    6. Allergies, drug sensitivities, foods

    7. Mental health problems

    8. Nutrition evaluation

        a. General

            (1) Attitude towards eating—alone, with family or caregiver

            (2) Appetite

            (3) Consumption, special dietary restrictions

            (4) Meal preparation

            (5) Shopping

            (6) Alcohol use/abuse

        b. Significant weight loss (at least 5% of usual body weight)— sudden (days to weeks) vs. gradual weight loss

        c. Common causes of weight loss

            (1) Cancer (lung, GI, lymphoma, GU)—up to 36% of cases

(2)   Diabetes and hyperthyroidism

(3)   Depression, anxiety and dementia

(4)   AIDS—do not rule out high-risk behaviors in elderly such as homosexuality, IV drug abuse, history of blood transfusion or infected spouse

9. Sleep

a. Note patterns—hour of bedtime/sleep, daytime fatigue/naps, insomnia

b. Sleep aids—pharmacological and non-pharmacological

c. Normal changes of sleep patterns with aging

(1)   Longer stage 1, light sleep

(2)   Shorter stages 3 and 4, decreased 20%—deep sleep shorter, therefore less restful nights

(3)   Increased sleep apnea of 10 seconds or more without awakening

(4)   Increased time awake during night

10. Exercise patterns, recreational profile

11. Review of systems

a. Systematic review of elderly individual

b. Subjective data collected

c. Diseases may present atypically

12. Preventive health practices—check frequency of screening tests such as Papanicolaou smear, testicular and prostate exams, stool guaiac test, sigmoidoscopy, cholesterol level, mammograms

● Past Medical History

1. Hospitalization and operations

2. Vaccinations—influenza, pneumonia, hepatitis, tetanus

3. Accidents, injuries, falls

4. Childhood and adult illnesses

5. Communicable disease history

a. Tuberculosis

b. Influenza

c. HIV status

d. Sexually transmitted diseases

e. Streptococcal infections

f. Hepatitis

- Health Practices, Religious Implications

    1. Blood transfusion acceptance/denial

    2. Dietary restrictions

    3. Fasting on certain holidays

    4. Sabbath restrictions for procedures, activities

- Safety Assessment

    1. Environment

        a. Home—stairs, scatter rugs, electrical wires, telephone cords, locks on doors and windows

        b. Neighborhood—sidewalks, location of stores, banks, post office, pharmacy

        c. Community services

        d. Crime

    2. Driving—loss of independence if taken away (difficult decision); must weigh the risks versus benefits of action

    3. Elder abuse—recent and increasingly common form of domestic violence

        a. Estimated to be approximately 1 million persons

        b. Abuser frequently is caregiver or family

        c. Physical or psychological abuse, neglect

- Patient Self-Determination Act (1990)—encourage patient to discuss this with family and health care provider and act upon wishes

    1. Advance directives—indicates intent of patient based on his/her wishes with right to refuse any or all interventions of medical care

    2. Living will—a contract specifying the patient's wishes concerning the end of his/her life; varies according to state in which he/she resides; a copy should be given to the health care provider and family member

    3. Durable power of attorney for health care—authorizes an agent to make medical decisions on behalf of the patient when the patient is unable

    4. Physician-assisted suicide may become an issue

Living Situations and Income Status

    1. Socialization

    2. Support systems in place such as family and friends

    3. Available resources in the community

4. Effect of change in financial resources upon retirement or disability

5. Assess role and status of caregiver; care of the caregiver

Functional Assessment

- Definition—method used to measure an individual's impairment and/or disability through physical, emotional, cognitive and social parameters

    1. Physical function identifies sensorimotor ability

    2. Emotional function focuses on coping mechanisms

    3. Cognitive function identifies intellectual and reasoning capabilities

    4. Social function evaluates ability to maintain social roles

- Certain deficits affect functional status

    1. Visual and auditory deficits may precipitate or worsen confusion

    2. Unfamiliar surroundings may cause confusion, sleep disturbances

    3. Musculoskeletal injury resulting in mobility impairment, dependence, loss of control and sleep disturbances

- Determine ability to perform activities of daily living (ADL) and self-care activities independently using the Index of Independence in Activities of Daily Living Scale (Katz, 1983)

    1. Elderly tend to overrate abilities; underrate disabilities

    2. Family members tend to underrate abilities

    3. Index ranks ability to perform basic functions such as bathing, dressing, feeding and continence

- Determine ability to perform Instrumental Activities of Daily Living (IADL) (Katz, 1983)

    1. More complex personal tasks such as cooking and shopping

    2. More complex independent functions such as taking care of finances, banking and managing medications

- Cognitive status assessments are used to detect causes of cognitive impairment

    1. Short Portable Mental Status Questionnaire (SPMSQ) is used to identify the presence and degree of intellectual impairment by testing orientation, memory concerning self-care, remote memory and math (Pfeiffer, 1975)

    2. The Mini-Mental State Exam (MMSE) is used to identify cognitive aspects of mental functions such as orientation, attention, recall and language (Folstein, Folstein & McHugh, 1975)

- Other functional issues may be assessed such as medical conditions, communication, senses, resources and behavior problems

Physical Assessment

An essential component of the evaluation from which valuable information can be obtained; an organized, systematic approach such as head-to-toe or major organ system should be utilized

- General Inspection
    1. Provide initial assessment of health status
    2. Identify specific characteristics—posture, gait, appearance
    3. Determine if exhibiting altered concentration due to pain, memory loss, agitation, and other signs of focusing deficits
    4. Identify strengths, disabilities and limitations
- Normal Aging Changes in the Elderly: General Appearance
    1. Fat increases by 30% and water decreases by 53% by age 70; fat distribution shifts from extremities to trunk
    2. Weight increases until about age 50 and then begins to fall; longevity favors individuals who are "ideal" weight or slightly above
    3. Anatomic size and height—elderly lose one to two inches due to thinning of cartilage between vertebrae and poor posture; kyphosis; males and females lose approximately one-sixteenth of an inch each year beginning around age 30
- Integumentary System
    1. Anatomical and physiological changes
        a. Decreased elasticity—increased wrinkles, folds, sagging, dry skin resulting in poor turgor
        b. Decreased perspiration—increased heat tolerance, poor temperature regulation; tendency towards hypo/hyperthermia
        c. Body and facial hair grays, thins; increased facial hair on women
        d. Nail growth slows, thickens; hypertrophy common
        e. Eyebrows coarse, bristle-like
        f. Cell regeneration slower
        g. Thinning of epithelial cells and subcutaneous fat layers
    2. Clinical implications
        a. Increased risk of infection
        b. Decreased wound healing
        c. Pruritus
        d. Poorly supported blood vessels rupture easily causing purpura
        e. Common benign skin lesions

(1) Seborrheic/senile keratosis—macular-papular, dark, warty areas seen on face, neck and trunk

(2) Cherry angioma—small, round, red, domed papules seen on trunk and proximal extremities

(3) Cutaneous skin tags—pedunculated papillomas seen on neck, chest and intertriginous sites

(4) Common blue nevus—benign, firm, dark-blue/gray/ black, well-defined papule, usually seen on hands and feet

f. Sun exposure changes

(1) Solar lentigo—flat, brown, pigmented macule on exposed areas only

(2) Solar keratosis—single or multiple discreet, dry, rough, scaly lesions on face, neck and hands

3. Abnormal changes and disease

a. Infections—viral, bacterial, fungal

b. Skin ulcerations

c. Ingrown toenails

d. Bunions, corns, calluses

e. Onychomycosis—fungal infection of nails

f. Abnormal skin lesions

(1) Actinic keratosis—pre-cancerous macular, irregular, scaly lesions seen on hands, arms, neck and face

(2) Squamous cell carcinoma—malignant soft, red-brown lesion of skin and mucous membrane arises as result of exogenous carcinogens such as sunlight or x-rays; seen on exposed areas, especially face, ears, scalp and arms

(3) Basal cell carcinoma—most common type of skin cancer; hard pearly-gray or pink, round, oval lesion with depressed center; usually on forehead, eyelids, nose and lips

(4) Malignant melanoma—round, oval, brown or tan irregular macular lesions seen mostly on trunk, arms, legs; familial tendency, not as common in older population

• Cardiovascular System

1. Anatomical and physiological changes

a. Slight decrease in heart size

b. Decreased cardiac output and cardiac reserve; heart fills and expels blood less efficiently

c. Increased peripheral vascular resistance

    d. Increased ectopic activity

    e. Decreased resting heart rate; increased with exercise/stress, takes longer to return to baseline; decreased exercise tolerance

    f. Increased rigidity and thickness of valves

2. Clinical implications

    a. Orthostatic hypotension

    b. Increased narrow or wide pulse pressure

    c. Unilateral or bilateral pain or swelling in lower extremities

    d. Varicosities—tortuous peripheral vessels

    e. Functional systolic murmurs increase with age; systolic heart murmurs are reported in 1/3 of 80 years olds; assess to determine etiology

    f. S_4 commonly heard

    g. Heart rate < 60 or > 90 beats per minute may be diagnostically significant

    h. BP of 90/60 to 140/90 acceptable

3. Abnormal changes and disease

    a. Hypertension or isolated systolic hypertension

    b. Coronary artery disease—may present with fatigue, confusion, dizziness, dyspnea, palpitations; may *not* present with pain

    c. Cerebrovascular disease—may present as confusion, headache

    d. Congestive heart failure—may present as confusion/delirium, anxiety, shortness of breath, cough and/or palpitations

    e. Arrhythmias—may present with restlessness, diaphoresis, syncope

    f. Peripheral vascular disease

        (1) Arterial—claudication

        (2) Venous—stasis

        (3) Trophic changes with decreased peripheral hair distribution

    g. Valvular pathology and cardiac dysfunction are most common causes of murmurs

- Respiratory System

1. Anatomical and physiological changes

    a. Decreased vital capacity, decreased tissue elasticity

    b. Increased residual volume, decrease in functional alveoli

    c. Increased diameter of the chest

    d. Decreased ability to clear lungs, less efficient cough

    e. Decreased diffusion of gases

    f. Decreased strength of expiratory muscles, more rigid intercostal muscles

    g. Decreased clearance of congestion

    h. Kyphosis may be present

2. Clinical implications

    a. Increased antero-posterior diameter

    b. Barrel chest, retraction

    c. Decreased ventilation at lung bases

    d. Pallor, cyanosis

    e. Nail clubbing

    f. Vesicular breath sounds, bilateral basilar crackles

    g. Decreased reserve

    h. Decreased response to exercise, stress and disease

3. Abnormal changes and disease

    a. Asthma, bronchitis, emphysema

    b. Tumor, lung cancer

    c. Pleural effusion

    d. Pneumonia—atypical presentation of tachypnea, confusion, chest pain, dyspnea and often no fever or low grade fever

    e. Tuberculosis

    f. Atelectasis

    g. Infection

    h. Adventitious sounds—rhonchi, crackles, wheezing, pleural friction rub

    i. Tachypnea, irregular breathing, labored breathing

    j. No breath sounds

- Breasts

    1. Anatomical and physiological changes

        a. Atrophy of fatty tissue and glands, pendulous breasts

        b. May appear nodular

        c. Increased sagging

        d. Nipples are lower

        e. Elderly men may have increased breast size

    2. Clinical implications

a. Wide variation of size, symmetry, contour, texture, pigmentation

b. Gynecomastia for men

3. Abnormal changes and disease

a. Unilateral mass, pain, tenderness, cancer

b. Grossly unequal

c. Redness, bloody discharge

d. Dimpling

e. Fixed inversion or retraction of nipple

- Gastrointestinal System

1. Anatomical and physiological changes

a. Decreased saliva

b. Decreased mastication

c. Decreased peristalsis

d. Weakening of lower esophageal sphincter

e. Lower esophageal sphincter often fails to relax

f. Decreased gastric acid secretion

g. Decreased hepatic metabolism

h. Decreased pancreatic secretion

i. Decreased insulin release

2. Clinical implications

a. Constipation, fecal impaction

b. Indigestion

c. Increased sensitivity to medication in GI tract

d. Increased response to alcohol, nicotine, chocolate, peppermint and caffeine

e. Periodontal disease

f. Malnutrition

3. Abnormal changes and disease

a. Diabetes

b. Nutritional deficiencies

c. Gastroesophageal reflux disease

d. Hiatal hernia

e. Intestinal obstruction, jaundice

    f.   Stool changes—black, tarry; blood; mucus; light tan or gray color

- Genitourinary and Reproductive Systems

   1. Anatomical and physiological changes

      a.   Renal changes

         (1) Decreased kidney function, number of nephrons and glomerular filtration rate (GFR)

         (2) Decreased bladder capacity and muscle tone

         (3) Decreased sphincter control

         (4) Increased frequency, urgency, nocturia

      b.   Hormonal changes

         (1) Decreased estrogen in females

         (2) Decreased testosterone in males

         (3) Atrophy of ovaries, uterus and vagina

         (4) Development of firmer testes, may be smaller

         (5) Sclerosis of penile arteries and veins

         (6) Decreased seminal fluid, sperm number, motility

         (7) Pubic hair thins and grays

         (8) Prostate gland enlargement

         (9) Decreased vaginal secretions

   2. Clinical implications

      a.   Asymptomatic urinary tract infections

      b.   Urinary incontinence

      c.   Atrophic vaginitis, foul-smelling vaginal discharge

      d.   Pelvic prolapse

      e.   Benign prostatic hypertrophy

      f.   Drug toxicity

      g.   Urinary retention

      h.   Impotency

      i.   Testicular enlargement, nodules

   3. Abnormal changes and disease

      a.   Cervical, ovarian cancer/disease/nodules

      b.   Testicular, penile cancer/lesions/nodules

      c.   Bladder, kidney cancer/disease/lesions

- Endocrine System
    1. Anatomical and physiological changes
        a. Decreased size, number and activity of sweat glands
        b. Decline in body's cooling mechanism
        c. Decreased ability to perspire
        d. Decreased ability to metabolize glucose
        e. Reduced insulin secretion
        f. Delayed insulin response
    2. Clinical implications
        a. Dehydration
        b. Hyperthermia
        c. Hypoglycemia
    3. Abnormal changes and disease
        a. Diabetes mellitus
        b. Tumors
        c. Thyroid disease
- Musculoskeletal System
    1. Anatomical and physiological changes
        a. Bone demineralization
        b. Decreased strength and endurance, range of motion
        c. Joint and cartilage erosion
        d. Loss of flexibility in the joints
        e. Bony growths at joints
        f. Decreased muscle mass
        g. Bony prominences develop
    2. Clinical implications
        a. Gait disturbances
        b. Falls
        c. Loss of height
        d. Hallus valgus—bunions
        e. Hammer toes
        f. Valgus, varus deformities

g. Lordosis, scoliosis, kyphosis

h. Stiffness and decreased range of motion of joints

3. Abnormal changes and disease

a. Osteoporosis

b. Degenerative joint disease

c. Fractures—vertebrae, hip, colles' (fracture of lower end of radius)

d. Extra-articular pathologic changes—bursitis, fibrositis

e. Swelling, tenderness pain in joints

f. Neuropathy and ischemia

- Sensory System

1. Vision

a. Anatomical and physiological changes

(1) Lens yellows and clouds

(2) Pupils smaller, but remain equal

(3) Decreased tear production

(4) Lens stiffen

(5) Decreased peripheral vision

(6) Difficulty in color discrimination

(7) Eyelids thinning, increased stretching, poor fit; entropion and ectropion

(8) Conjunctiva pale and less white

(9) Arcus senilis

b. Clinical implications

(1) Decreased visual acuity

(2) Decreased adaptation to darkness

(3) Corneal irritation

(4) Decreased peripheral vision

(5) Dry appearance

(6) Progressive eyelid relaxation

c. Abnormal changes and disease

(1) Macular degeneration

(2) Blindness

(3) Retinal detachment

          (4)   Glaucoma

          (5)   Cataracts

  2.   Hearing

     a.   Anatomical and physiological changes

          (1)   Decreased discrimination of pitch and acuity

          (2)   Decreased sensitivity to higher frequency sounds

          (3)   Excessive cerumen, hair growth in canal

          (4)   Tympanic membranes may lose mobility

     b.   Clinical implications

          (1)   Vertigo, tinnitus

          (2)   Diminished hearing

          (3)   Auricle loses elasticity, lobe elongates

     c.   Abnormal changes and disease

          (1)   Tumors

          (2)   Deafness

          (3)   Presbycusis

          (4)   Otosclerosis

          (5)   Impacted cerumen

          (6)   Tophi, pain

  3.   Head/throat/neck/nose

     a.   Anatomical and physiological changes

          (1)   Decreased sense of smell; difficulty distinguishing specific odors

          (2)   Decreased size of thyroid gland

          (3)   Atrophy of pharynx, larynx

          (4)   Nose sags, appears longer

          (5)   Lymph nodes may be noted—less than 1 cm in size, soft discrete and mobile considered normal variation

     b.   Clinical implications

          (1)   Marked asymmetry of face

          (2)   Increased size of lymph nodes

          (3)   Soft voice

          (4)   Difficulty swallowing

          (5)   Postnasal drip

    c. Abnormal changes and disease

       (1) Loss of smell

       (2) Allergic rhinitis

       (3) Cracks, fissures of lips

       (4) Head, neck, throat nodules/cancer

4. Taste

    a. Anatomical and physiological changes

       (1) Decreased number of taste buds, papillary atrophy

       (2) Difficulty distinguishing specific tastes

       (3) Teeth yellow, increased space between teeth

       (4) Decreased ability to chew

    b. Clinical implications

       (1) Loss of interest in eating

       (2) Poor fitting dentures, loose or broken teeth

       (3) Dehydration

    c. Abnormal changes and disease

       (1) Oral cancer

       (2) Ulcerations

5. Touch

    a. Anatomical and physiological changes

       (1) Decreased receptors

       (2) Lower ability to distinguish temperature and pain

    b. Clinical implications

       (1) Decreased sensation

       (2) Numbness, tingling

       (3) Potential for burns, injury

    c. Abnormal changes and disease

       (1) Loss of feeling

       (2) Scalding, frostbite

- Neurological system

1. Anatomical and physiological changes

    a. General decrease in cerebral blood flow

    b. Global brain atrophy

    c. Slowed response to heat and cold

    d. General slowing of reaction time

    e. Sluggish deep tendon reflexes

    f. Loss of vibratory sensation

2. Clinical implications

    a. Benign senile tremors

    b. Decreased coordination and balance

    c. Wide-based gait

    d. Nystagmus

    e. Decreased response to pain

3. Abnormal changes and disease

    a. Ataxia

    b. Dysphasia, aphasia

    c. Dysarthria

    d. Parkinson's disease

    e. Senile dementia/Alzheimer's disease

    f. Delirium

    g. Cerebrovascular accident (CVA)

    h. Vertigo

Common Selected Problems of the Older Adlut

For review of other common health problems that affect the elderly see "Gerontological Nursing Certification Review Guide," published by Health Leadership Associates

Common Neurological Disorders and Mental Health Issues

- Delirium—acute change of mental status with disturbance of attention and cognition due to an organic cause; common problem of hospitalized elderly

    1. Definitive diagnostic features

        a. Acute onset; may be worse at night; "sundowning"

        b. Varying course

        c. Psychotic symptoms

            (1) Often iatrogenic—related to medications or fluid and electrolyte imbalance

    (2)   Initial presentation of many serious and treatable medical disorders

    (3)   Initial presentation in many common disorders, for example:

       (a)   Urinary tract infection

       (b)   Long history of alcohol abuse combined with an anticholinergic or narcotic

  d. Visual and auditory hallucinations

  e. Frequent disorientation

2. Common medications causing delirium

  a. Narcotics

  b. Benzodiazepines

  c. Anticholinergics

  d. Antidepressants

  e. Barbiturates

  f. Antihypertensives

  g. Digoxin

  h. Antibiotics such as cephalosporins, aminoglycosides and metronidazole

  i. H_2 blockers such as cimetidine

3. Conditions predisposing the elderly to development of delirium

  a. Head injury

  b. Dementia

  c. History of significant substance abuse

  d. Advanced medical illness or organ failure

4. Effective treatment

  a. May be difficult; interventions that help orientation

  b. Keep out of bed during waking hours

  c. Presence of family members

  d. Bedroom lights kept on at night; use of clock and calendar

  e. Regular schedule

  f. Trial of low-dose neuroleptic medication or high-potency antipsychotic

- Dementia—gradual regression and loss of intellectual functioning, such as thinking, remembering, and reasoning, of sufficient severity to interfere with daily functioning

  1. Definitive diagnostic features

    a. Impaired judgement

      b. Change in personality

      c. Mood swings

      d. Erratic behavior

      e. Significant short term memory impairment

      f. Impairment in abstract thinking

      g. Aphasia, apraxia, agnosia

2. Major causes of dementia

      a. Alzheimer's disease (AD)

          (1) Affects 2.5 million Americans, increasing from 0.6% from age 65 to 70 to 8.4% over age 85

          (2) Most common type of dementia; 16% of women and 6% of men who survive to an average life expectancy will develop Alzheimer's disease

          (3) Gradual onset

          (4) Senile plaques and neurofibrillary tangles seen on autopsy

      b. Multi-infarct dementia (MID)

          (1) Onset may be sudden

          (2) Generalized symptoms of disorientation, confusion, behavior change

          (3) MID coexists in 15 to 20% of AD

          (4) Risk factors include high blood pressure, vascular disease, diabetes, or previous stoke

      c. Parkinson's disease (P.D.)

          (1) Lack of dopamine which controls muscle activity

          (2) Symptoms include tremors, stiffness, and slow speech

          (3) Late in the course, some individuals develop dementia

      d. Other related disorders include Huntington's disease, Creutzfeldt-Jakob disease, Pick's disease, and normal pressure hydrocephalus

      e. Other causes of dementia are alcohol, drugs, nutritional and metabolic disorders; rarely a tumor

3. Effective treatment

      a. Good preventive health practices may impact the risk of developing dementia

      b. Use of lists to assist with memory impairment

      c. Correct vision and hearing deficits

      d. Use of day hospital and outpatient day care centers

      e. Make little environmental changes to avoid confusion

      f. Drug therapy shows limited success at present

- Depression—psychiatric condition which is an affective disorder characterized by physical, cognitive and emotional symptoms; frequently under diagnosed in the elderly and less likely to be treated than in younger adults; decrease in cognitive functioning may be falsely attributed to dementia when the underlying cause is actually depression

  1. Definitive diagnostic features

      a. Regular markedly depressed mood

      b. Cognitive symptoms worsen; inability to concentrate

      c. Loss of interest in life, vegetative symptoms

      d. Lack of pleasure in almost all activities

      e. General feeling of worthlessness

      f. Significant unintentional weight loss or weight gain

      g. Insomnia or hypersomnia

      h. Improvement in mentation seen with treatment

      i. Past and family history more likely

  2. Marked depressive symptoms noted with the following medical conditions

      a. Endocrine/metabolic disorders (thyroid disease, diabetes mellitus, hypokalemia, anemia)

      b. Brain tumors

      c. COPD

      d. Vitamin deficiencies

      e. Neurological disorders (Parkinson's disease, stroke, multiple sclerosis, seizure disorder)

      f. Drug therapy used to treat medical conditions

      g. Alcohol abuse

      h. Chronic pain

      i. Cancer

  3. Complications in diagnosing in the elderly

      a. Behavioral and cognitive changes of the aging central nervous system (CNS) make the differential diagnosis of depression versus dementia challenging

      b. Presence of other major medical conditions

      c. Common complaints of insomnia, awakening during sleep or sleepy during day

  4. Effective treatment

    a. Counseling, psychotherapy

    b. Exercise, diet, rest

    c. Cautious trial of pharmacologic interventions—in most cases, the dosage should be reduced 30 to 50%

- Suicide—increasing rates in this population, higher than at younger ages; multiple losses and decreased internal and external resources contribute to incidence; perceived intolerable psychological distress, frustration and unmet needs

  1. Risk factors

    a. Sex (male-rate is seven times higher than for older women)

    b. Race (white)

    c. Marital status (divorced, separated or single)

    d. Economic status (low, unemployed)

    e. Mental illness (depression, schizophrenia and individuals in early stages of dementia who are aware of their deficits are at highest risk)

    f. Health, pain (cancer, AIDS, dialysis patients)

    g. Alcohol abuse, dependence

    h. Bereavement (especially within one year of a loss, retirement)

    i. Social isolation

    j. Previous attempts

  2. Types

    a. Overt suicide—specific act which terminated life (weapon, hanging, poison, toxic fumes)

    b. Covert suicide—destructive behaviors that erode health and lead to death

      (1) Alcohol abuse, drug abuse

      (2) Medication misuse (overdosage or omission)

      (3) Smoking

      (4) Poor dietary habits, self-starvation

      (5) Ignoring disease symptoms

  3. Treatment—prevention depends on prompt recognition of signs; autonomy and confidentiality do not take priority over one's safety

    a. May be difficult

    b. Close observation during acute phase

    c. Identify and treat underlying depression

    d. Excellent listening skills and willingness to listen

    e. Ensure safe environment; determine if hospitalization is indicated

Pharmacotherapy and the Elderly

Age-related physiological changes result in elderly being at high risk for side effects and toxic effects; compounded when chronic diseases are present

- Important Issues

  1. Cost of prescription medications for elderly account for 30% of all prescription medications, and 40% to 50% of all non-prescription medications in United States

  2. More than $3 billion a year are spent by elderly on prescription and nonprescription drugs

  3. Majority of elderly have one or more chronic conditions such as arthritis, hypertension, heart disease and diabetes which are treated with multiple medications

  4. Increased number of adverse drug reactions (ADR); ADR have occurred in 30% of elderly outpatients and account for up to 10% of hospital admissions

     a. Reflective of number and type of medications taken

     b. Frequent use of over-the-counter, self-prescribed medication, home remedies

     c. Multiple health care providers with lack of coordination of care

     d. Multiple pharmacies used with lack of ability to identify potential drug interactions

     e. Do not assume that behavior change is age-related

  5. Common ADR in the elderly include edema, nausea, vomiting, anorexia, dizziness, diarrhea, constipation, confusion, and urinary retention; should not be misinterpreted as signs and symptoms of illness or due to the aging process

- Physiological Changes—may lead to increased plasma concentrations of drugs

  1. Decreased tolerance of standard dosages; toxic reactions occur at lower doses

  2. Decreased metabolism—usually occurs in the liver which is decreased in sized with decreased blood flow

  3. Decreased absorption—decreased liver enzyme activity and gastric emptying time; gastric pH increased

  4. Variable distribution—lean muscle mass decreases and fat tissue increases; fat soluble drugs have longer duration; water soluble drugs have smaller volume of distribution and higher plasma concentrations; increased adipose tissue can cause increased storage of lipid-soluble drugs

  5. Decreased ability to excrete drugs due to decreased glomerular filtration rate (GFR); results in decreased excretion time for medication; GFR declines 50% between third and ninth decades of life

- Potential Side Effects of Commonly Prescribed Drugs
    1. Confusion—digoxin, cimetidine, dopamine agents, antihistamines, hypnotics, sedatives
    2. Anorexia—digoxin
    3. Fatigue/weakness—diuretics, antidepressants, antihypertensives
    4. Ataxia—sedatives, hypnotics, anticonvulsants, antipsychotics
    5. Forgetfulness—barbiturates
    6. Constipation—anticholinergics
    7. Diarrhea—oral antacids
    8. GI upset—iron, nonsteroidal anti-inflammatory drugs (NSAID), salicylates, corticosteroids, estrogens, alcohol
    9. Tinnitus—analgesics
    10. Urinary retention—anticholinergics
    11. Orthostatic hypotension—antihypertensives, sedatives, diuretics, antidepressants
    12. Depression—benzodiazepines
    13. Delirium—corticosteroids, sedatives, antihistamines
    14. Dizziness—sedatives, antihypertensives, anticonvulsants, diuretics
- Problems With Use of Medication
    1. Overuse—elderly feel when they seek care from a health care provider, they should receive a prescription
    2. Misuse—self-prescribing habits, changing dosages, use of old prescriptions, use of friend's medication, poor history given to provider, out-dated prescriptions
    3. Knowledge deficit—difficulty understanding due to educational level *or* misunderstanding due to hearing deficits, *or* inadequate information provided by health care professional
    4. Memory deficit—forget purpose, dosage, frequency of taking medication, may accidentally repeat dosage
    5. Cost—may not purchase medication due to limited financial resources
    6. Visual deficit—inability to properly read label, may take wrong medication
    7. Mobility problems—difficulty opening bottles, small tablets hard to handle, splitting pills in half is sometimes necessary, difficulty manipulating inhalers
    8. Multiple providers/multiple pharmacies—conflicting/duplicate medications prescribed by various health care practitioners; generic and brand name prescriptions being taken concurrently
- Recommendations for drug use in the elderly—identify factors that predispose the elderly to ADR, e.g., multisystem disease, greater severity of disease, female gender, small body

size, hepatic or renal disease, previous drug reactions; proceed cautiously with the following:

1. Clear indication for use

2. Reliably effective drug

3. Shortest duration appropriate

4. Lowest dosage, "start low, go slow"

5. Cost effective

6. Will it enhance quality of life

7. Avoid adverse outcomes

8. Evaluate patient compliance

9. Identify resource person to assist in administering if necessary

10. Use calenders, pill boxes, and large print to assist

11. Use of devices to aid administration such as spacers for inhalers

Preventive Health Care Recommendations (U.S. Preventive Services, 1996)

The focus is to prevent disease or injury and promote health. Life expectancy has improved, but chronic diseases remain the major causes of death. The elderly have a greater absolute risk of disease and respond positively to preventive measures. Implement the following by using a tracking system such as a checklist or flowsheet.

- History—annual review and recommendations for persons over age 65

   1. Dietary intake—protein-calorie malnutrition is common

   2. Functional status—identify issues

   3. Substance abuse

      a. Tobacco—directly and negatively affects both health and financial status

      b. Alcohol—heavy use is more than two drinks/day

      c. Illegal drug use

      d. Abuse of prescription medications

   4. Physical activity—exercise and physical fitness improve multiple physiological functions such as cardiorespiratory capacity, muscle strength, endurance, range of motion, sleep and cognitive function; reduces falls and injury

- Physical Examination

   1. Height and weight, blood pressure

   2. Clinical breast exam

   3. Complete skin exam

4. Thyroid nodules (if history of irradiation), auscultation for carotid bruits (if risk factors for cerebrovascular, cardiovascular, or neurological disease)

5. Oral cavity examination

- *Recommended* screening tests by U.S. Preventive Services

    1. Fasting glucose if marginally obese, or family history of diabetes

    2. Papanicolaou smear—perform if no previously documented screen is consistently negative or hysterectomy was performed because of cervical cancer or its precursors; otherwise there is insufficient evidence for routine Pap testing over age 65

    3. Dipstick urinalysis

    4. Mammography—every one to two years

    5. PPD—if at high risk for close/personal contact with disease

    6. Fecal occult blood/sigmoidoscopy—annual fecal occult blood and flexible sigmoidoscopy every three to five years

    7. Electrocardiogram with two or more risk factors (high blood cholesterol, hypertension, smoking, diabetes mellitus, family history of coronary artery disease)

    8. Thyroid function tests

    9. Glaucoma and visual acuity testing

    10. Hearing impairment testing

    11. Total cholesterol in older persons with major coronary heart disease risk factors (smoking, hypertension, diabetes)

- Immunizations

    1. Influenza vaccine—annually

    2. Pneumococcal vaccine

        a. Once

        b. Revaccination is not recommended for healthy persons 65 years and older

        c. A one-time revaccination is recommended by the Centers for Disease Control and Prevention (CDC) for adults at highest risk for serious pneumococcal infection

            (1) As long as a minimum of five years has passed since first vaccinated

            (2) Were less than 65 years old at the time

            (3) Risk groups include, but are not limited to, adults with leukemia, lymphoma, Hodgkin's disease, malignancy, HIV infection, chronic renal failure, nephrotic syndrome, asplenia, and other conditions associated with immunosuppression and immunosuppressive chemotherapy

    3. Tetanus - diphtheria toxoids (Td) should be completed for adults who have not received the primary series; periodic Td boosters

- Routine screening—data does **not** yet indicate *for or against* routine screening for the following:

  1. Depression in asymptomatic patients

  2. Dementia in asymptomatic patients

  3. Osteoporosis with bone densitometry in postmenopausal women, but women should be counseled about hormone prophylaxis

  4. Controversy over whom and how to screen for colon and prostate cancers; digital rectal exams and serum tumor markers such as PSA are not routinely recommended for prostate cancer screening; should be limited to males with a greater than 10 years life expectancy

  5. Total cholesterol in asymptomatic patient

Questions
Select the best answer

1. Since the turn of the 20th century, the population over age 65 has increased by:

    a. 3-fold
    b. 5-fold
    c. 11-fold
    d. 20-fold

2. By the year 2050, the elderly population will:

    a. Begin to decrease
    b. Level off at 50 million persons
    c. Include those persons 55 and over
    d. More than double to 80 million

3. Elderly women outnumber elderly men:

    a. Three to two
    b. Twenty million to ten million
    c. Five to two
    d. Two to one

4. Which of the following elderly groups have lower income levels:

    a. African-American males over age 65
    b. Elderly African-Americans and Hispanics
    c. Middle and oldest-old Asians
    d. Oldest-old Whites

5. Better education has proven to improve one's life. The following statement is true:

    a. Half of the elderly have completed high school
    b. The elderly are as likely to have only completed 8th grade as persons under 75 years old
    c. Middle-old have the highest percentage of college degrees
    d. Lack of education increases with age

6. Racial and ethnic differences in the aging population exist. It is predicted that:

    a. The African-American population will double
    b. The Asian population will triple
    c. The Hispanic population will quadruple
    d. The White population will decrease by 20%

7. When performing a health history on the elderly, which of the following should the nurse practitioner avoid?

    a. Standing near the window so the patient can see the interviewer more clearly

   b. Implications of cultural differences and social mores
   c. Asking open-ended questions, but keeping conversation focused
   d. Observing for signs of fatigue

8. A common cause of weight loss in the elderly is:

   a. Hypothyroidism
   b. Hyperthyroidism
   c. Delirium
   d. Hemophilia

9. Which statement is most accurate about the sleep patterns of older persons?

   a. Sleep apnea of 10 seconds or more may occur awakening the elderly
   b. The elderly fall asleep quickly but awaken frequently during the night
   c. The elderly have difficulty falling asleep, but then sleep soundly
   d. There are shorter stages 3 and 4 and longer stage 1 sleep cycles

10. Elder abuse is presently a problem in the United States. Which of the following statements regarding elder abuse is not true?

   a. The most common abusers are the family or caregivers
   b. Physical abuse is four times more common than psychological abuse
   c. It is a common form of domestic violence
   d. Up to 10% of the elderly may be subjected to one type of abuse

11. Which of the following is not included in the Patient Self Determination Act of 1990?

   a. Durable power of attorney for health care
   b. Living will
   c. Organ donation
   d. Indication of patient's intent for medical care

12. In performing activities of daily living:

   a. The elderly overrate their own abilities
   b. The family members overrate their loved one's ability
   c. The elderly cannot manage their finances well
   d. The elderly frequently pay for services such as cooking and cleaning

13. When observing general physical findings, the nurse practitioner is aware that:

   a. The elderly lose one to two inches in height due to the thickening of the cartilage
   b. The fat distribution shifts from the trunk to the extremities
   c. Weight is constant
   d. Fat increases as water decreases

14. Anatomical and physiological changes of the integument system include:

    a. Decreased heat tolerance
    b. Increased wrinkles, folds and sagging
    c. Coarse body and facial hair
    d. Rapid nail growth with easy breaking of nails

15. Which of the following clinical implications related to the skin do not occur in the elderly?

    a. Risk of infection decreases
    b. Decreased wound healing
    c. Sun exposure changes
    d. Pruritus

16. Which of the following is a normal age-related change of the cardiovascular system?

    a. Slightly increased heart size
    b. Decreased exercise tolerance
    c. Decreased peripheral vascular resistance
    d. Presence of S_3 heart sound

17. Coronary artery disease may present with the following abnormal changes and/ or disease?

    a. Dyspnea and palpitations
    b. Isolated systolic hypertension
    c. Congestive heart failure
    d. Arrhythmias

18. Which of the following aging changes of the respiratory system is not found in the elderly?

    a. Decreased vital capacity and tissue elasticity
    b. Increased residual volume
    c. Decreased anterior-posterior diameter of the chest
    d. Less efficient cough and clearance of congestion

19. Normal age-related changes frequently result in atypical presentation of illness in the elderly client. Which of the following signs and symptoms of pneumonia is frequently not found in the elderly?

    a. High fever
    b. Tachypnea
    c. Confusion
    d. Chest pain

20. The elderly have breast-related variations. Which statement is true?

    a. Elderly men have a decrease in breast size
    b. There is atrophy of the fatty tissue and a nodular appearance

c. Significantly unequal breast size is a normal variation
d. Dimpling and bloody discharge are often seen

21. Which of the following is not a normal age related change of the GI tract?

    a. Decreased gastric acid secretions
    b. Decreased response to alcohol, caffeine and nicotine
    c. Constipation and indigestion
    d. Weakening of the esophageal sphincter

22. Which of the following is a result of normal age-related changes of the GU system?

    a. Asymptomatic urinary tract infections
    b. Urinary incontinence
    c. Urinary retention
    d. Urgency, frequency and nocturia

23. Which of the following is not a result of endocrine changes?

    a. Decreased sweat gland activity
    b. Decreased glucose metabolism
    c. Increased ability to perspire
    d. Response to insulin is delayed

24. Abnormal disease processes of the musculoskeletal system include:

    a. Osteoporosis, degenerative joint disease
    b. Bony growths at joints
    c. Decreased strength and endurance
    d. Decreased muscle mass

25. Which of the following is not a normal physiological change of the eyes?

    a. Decreased visual acuity
    b. Poor color discrimination
    c. Yellowing, clouding and stiffening of the lens
    d. Degeneration of the macula

26. Aging results in a variety of normal, non-pathological changes in the body. Which of the following is a normal, age-related change in the structure or function of the ear?

    a. Decreased discrimination of pitch and acuity
    b. Increased sensitivity to low-pitched sounds
    c. Decreased hair growth in the canals
    d. Increased mobility of the tympanic membrane

27. Variations in the elderly's ability to taste are related to:

    a. Decreased taste buds
    b. Increased ability to distinguish specific tastes
    c. Development of new taste buds
    d. Difficulty swallowing

28. Mrs G. is an 86-year-old female who lives alone. She has been functionally independent until two days ago when her daughter found her to be disheveled, incontinent of urine, and "talking nonsense." When evaluating Mrs. G. to rule out causes of delirium, the nurse practitioner knows that which of the following is not typically a cause?

    a. Infection
    b. Polypharmacy
    c. Hyponatremia
    d. Depression

29. Alzheimer's disease is characterized by:

    a. Long-term memory loss more dramatic than short term
    b. Acute onset
    c. Plaques and tangles
    d. Affects elderly men and women equally

30. Which of the following is not a diagnostic feature of depression?

    a. Inability to concentrate
    b. Short-term memory impairment
    c. Mood swings
    d. Unintentional weight loss or gain

31. Risk factors for suicide in the elderly include:

    a. Elderly, married females
    b. Dementia, depression
    c. Limited educational background
    d. Minority ethnic groups

32. It is important to remember that physiological changes in the elderly affect drug therapy. Which of the following statements is true?

    a. Metabolism of drugs usually occurs in the kidneys
    b. The liver increases in size in relation to the number and types of drugs used
    c. Gastric pH is decreased
    d. Decreased ability to excrete drugs is due to the decreased GFR

33. The U.S. Preventive Services Task Force made the following recommendation for routine screening of all individuals over 65 years old:

    a. Total cholesterol annually

b. Prostatic specific antigen annually
c. Complete skin exam annually
d. Papanicolaou smear annually on all females

34. Controversy exists for routine screening. The following is not recommended for screening of the elderly?
    a. PPD if at high risk
    b. Bone densitometry for osteoporosis
    c. Td boosters periodically
    d. Fasting glucose with a positive family history

Answers

1. c	12. a	23. c
2. d	13. d	24. a
3. a	14. b	25. d
4. b	15. a	26. a
5. d	16. b	27. a
6. c	17. a	28. d
7. a	18. c	29. c
8. b	19. a	30. c
9. d	20. b	31. b
10. b	21. b	32. d
11. c	22. d	33. c
		34. b

Bibliography

Cassel, C. K., Cohen, H. J., Larson, E. B., Meier, D. E., Resnick, N. M., & Rubenstein, L. Z. (Eds.). (1997). *Geriatric medicine.* New York: Springer Publishing Company.

Cassidy, K. (1996). Health assessment of the elderly. In C. Kopac & V. Millonig (Eds.), *Gerontological nursing certification review guide for the generalist, clinical specialist, and nurse practitioner* (pp. 42-67). Potomac, MD: Health Leadership Associates.

Duthie, E., & Katz, P. R. (1998). *Duthie: Practice of geriatrics* (3rd ed.). Philadelphia: W. B. Saunders.

Fitzpatrick, T. B., Johnson, R. A., Polano, M. K., Suurmon, D., & Wolff, K. (1997). *Color atlas of synopsis of clinical dermatology* (3rd ed.). NY: McGraw-Hill.

Folstein, M. F., Folstein, S. E., & McHugh, P. R. (1975). Mini-mental state: A practical method for grading the cognitive state of patients for the clinician. *Journal of Psychiatric Research, 12,* 189-198.

Gallo, J. J., Busby-Whitehead, J., Rabins, P. V., Selleman, R. A., Murphy, J. B. (Eds.). (1999). *Reichel's care of the elderly: Clinical aspects of aging* (5th ed.). Philadelphia: Lippincott Williams & Wilkins.

Gallo, J. J., Fulmer, T., Paverza, G. J., Reichel, W. (2000). *Handbook of geriatric assessment* (3rd ed.). MD: Aspen Publishers.

Green, J. (2000). *Neuropsychological evaluation of the older adult, a clinician's guidebook.* San Diego: Academic Press.

Guide to clinical preventive services. US preventive services task force (2nd ed.). (1996). Baltimore: Williams & Wilkins.

Hazzard, W. R., Blass, J. P., Ettinger, W. H., Halter, J. B., & Ouslander, J. G. (Eds.). (1999). *Principles of geriatric medicine and gerontology* (4th ed). NY: McGraw Hill.

Katz, S. (1983). Assessing self-maintenance: Activities of daily living, mobility, and instrumental activities of daily living. *Journal of the American Geriatric Society, 31,* 721-727.

Kopac, C. A. (1994). Care of the aging adult. In V. L. Millonig (Ed.), *Adult nurse practitioner certification review guide* (pp. 574-613). Potomac, MD: Health Leadership Associates.

Smith, S. F., Duell, D. J., Martin, B. C. (2000). *Clinical nursing skills, basic to advanced skills* (5th ed.). NJ: Prentice-Hall, Inc.

Swanson, E. A., Tripp-Reimer, T. (Eds.). (1997). *Advances in gerontological nursing, chronic illness and the older adult.* NY: Springer Publishing Co.

U.S. Census Bureau (1995). (Revised May 13, 1997). *Statistical briefs.* Economics and Statistical Administration, U.S. Department of Commerce.

Multisystem and Genetic Disorders Infancy Through Adolescence

Alison W. Schultz

Introduction

All disorders addressed in this chapter occur relatively rarely, but for the involved child, family, and caregivers, each presents life-long challenges in health care, adaptation, and coping. In general, when one of these disorders is suspected or diagnosed, the FNP should refer the child and family to the most appropriate specialty center for consultation and collaborative management. Knowledge about each condition and its management is rapidly expanding, and personnel at such centers are most current in this essential practice foundation.

The Family Nurse Practitioner (FNP), however, remains responsible for assisting the child and family with all primary care issues, some of which will be disorder specific. The FNP also is a central contact for the child and family for issues of care coordination and community based interventions, advocacy, assistance with stress management and promotion of positive adaptation and coping. FNPs working with children who have any of these disorders must become familiar with the issues commonly confronting such children and their families, legislation protecting the rights of individuals who have chronic illness or disability, and support organizations and agencies that can be helpful to caregivers and families. Among the most helpful are the 65 University Affiliated Programs (UAPs) for Developmental Disabilities in the United States and territories, and the Federal, State and local divisions of the Maternal Child Health Bureau (MCHB). Information about UAPs can be obtained by calling the American Association of UAPs at 301-588-8252. Information about MCHB programs is usually available in your local telephone book, or can be obtained by calling 301-443-2350. Also, many support organizations and other information about these disorders can be found on the Internet, using the disorder's name as the key word. The Alliance of Genetic Support Groups, (800) 336-4363 and http://www.geneticalliance.org is a comprehensive resource for conditions with genetic basis.

Where possible, information about disorder specific support organizations is included in the management sections of this chapter. *Exceptional Parent* magazine, 1170 Commonwealth Avenue, Boston MA 02134-4645, (617) 730-5800, provides a wealth of information for parents of children who have various special health care needs. The March of Dimes Birth Defects Foundation, 1275 Mamaroneck Avenue, White Plains NY 10605, (888) 663-4637 provides information about congenital diseases and disorders, and the National Information Center for Children and Youth with Disabilities (NICCHY), PO Box 1492, Washington DC 20013, provides information on all disabling conditions.

Congenital Diseases

Acquired Immune Deficiency Syndrome (AIDS)

- Definition: Advanced stage of illness in individuals infected with the Human Immunodeficiency Virus (HIV); CDC case definition of HIV classifies children according to presence or absence of clinical signs and symptoms and according to status of immune function and clinical findings. Refer to most current edition of the *AAP Red Book* for details.

- Etiology/Incidence

  1. In children, primarily (90%) maternal to infant perinatal HIV transmission; breast feeding is primary postnatal vertical maternal to infant transmission route

  2. National infant cord blood seroprevalence of HIV 0.17%; rates vary widely, up to 8%; most seroprevalence is maternal antibody; 13% to 40% of perinatally exposed infants acquire disease if mother is untreated during pregnancy and with no chemoprophylaxis during labor or for the newborn

- Signs and Symptoms: Median onset for infants with perinatal infection is 12 to 18 months; HIV, however, can be latent for years

  1. Prematurity

  2. Low birth weight

  3. Recurrent serious bacterial or viral infections—especially oral thrush

  4. Failure to thrive

  5. Recurrent fevers

  6. Chronic diarrhea

  7. Diminished activity

  8. Developmental delays

- Differential Diagnosis

  1. Infectious disease or other associated conditions without underlying HIV

  2. Other immune deficiencies of infancy

- Physical Findings

  1. Falling ratio of head circumference to height and weight, due to encephalopathic direct effect on brain growth

  2. Lymphadenopathy—≥ 0.5 cm at more than 2 sites; bilateral at one site

  3. Hepatosplenomegaly

  4. Parotitis, nephropathy, CNS disease

- Diagnostic Tests/Findings

  1. Detection of HIV—DNA from anticoagulated whole blood or by Polymerase Chain Reaction (PCR) from peripheral blood mononuclear cells

2. For adolescents ≥ age 13, documentation of HIV infection with one or more of 26 clinical conditions such as multiple or recurrent serious bacterial infections (AAP, 2000, p. 327)

3. Cases of HIV meeting AIDS criteria are reportable

- Management/Treatment

    1. Risk reduction through prevention of maternal infection, assuring clean blood and tissue supplies, prevention of STD and needle sharing

    2. Reduction of risk of perinatal HIV—through treatment of pregnant mother and perinatal chemoprophylaxis of mother and infant

    3. Monitoring of CD4$^+$ lymphocyte count and percentage, CBC, differential, platelet count

    4. Antiretroviral therapy in consultation with HIV management specialists

    5. Treatment of infections and other associated conditions

    6. Early intervention for developmental delay

    7. Maximum supportive care for child and family

    8. *CDC National Prevention Information Network*
       P.O. Box 6003
       Rockville MD 20849-6003
       (800) 458-5231
       http://www.cdcnpin.org

Chlamydia (Refer to Gu/Gyn chapter)

- Definition: A group of intracellular parasites with three known species, *C. trachomatis, C. psittaci* and *C. pneumoniae*

- Etiology/Incidence

    1. 40% to 70% of infants born to women infected with chlamydia will develop infection at one or more sites

    2. Transmission occurs from cervical maternal infection to infant during vaginal delivery

    3. Prevalence among sexually active women about 5%; among adolescents may be as high as 20%

    4. *Chlamydia trachomatis*—most prevalent sexually transmitted disease in the U.S.

- Signs and Symptoms: *Chlamydia trachomatis* in the neonate

    1. Neonatal conjunctivitis—mild to severe

        a. 5 days to several weeks after delivery, usually vaginal

        b. Conjunctival injection

        c. Mucoid eye discharge, ocular edema

2. Neonatal pneumonia

    a. 2 to 19 weeks of age

    b. Persistent "staccato" cough with congestion

- Differential Diagnosis

  1. Nonchlamydia conjunctivitis

    a. Chemical reaction to silver nitrate

    b. Infections due to gonorrhoeae, *Staphylococcus aureus, Haemophilus influenzae,* streptococcus, herpes simplex, enteric bacteria

  2. Bronchitis/Pneumonia—respiratory syncytial virus, other viral, bacterial causes

- Physical Findings

  1. Neonatal conjunctivitis

    a. Injected conjunctiva with exudate within first weeks of life

    b. Pseudomembrane

    c. Friable conjunctiva

  2. Neonatal pneumonia

    a. Afebrile

    b. Tachypnea

    c. Rales, but rarely wheezes

- Diagnostic Tests/Findings

  1. Chest radiograph shows hyperinflation, no consolidation, bilateral diffuse infiltrates

  2. Peripheral eosinophilia (> 300 cells/mL)

  3. Elevated serum immunoglobulins

  4. Isolation of organism by tissue culture; culture must contain epithelial cells

    a. In addition to eye and respiratory tract, *Chlamydia trachomatis* may be found in rectal, vaginal and nasopharyngeal secretions of infants born to infected mothers; infants often not symptomatic, but may shed organism for up to three years

    b. Frequently isolated from vagina, and sometimes from rectum of children who have been sexually abused; sometimes difficult to know whether infection related to child abuse or congenital transmission

- Management/Treatment: Infants, oral erythromycin suspension, 50 mg/kg/ day for 10 to 14 days, repeated once if needed; approximately 20% of infants need second course of treatment

Gonococcal Infection (Refer to Gu/Gyn chapter)

- Definition: Infections caused by acquisition of *Neisseria gonorrhoeae*
- Etiology/Incidence: Maternal transmission to neonate from contact with vaginal secretions during birth
- Signs and Symptoms
    1. Ophthalmia; injected, swollen conjunctiva with exudate
    2. Fever, irritability, rapid respiration, rapid heart rate
    3. Purulent exudate or secretions from any orifice
- Differential Diagnosis
    1. Conjunctivitis
        a. Chemical reaction to silver nitrate
        b. Infections due to chlamydia, *Staphylococcus aureus, Haemophilus influenzae,* streptococcus, herpes simplex, or enteric bacteria
    2. Bronchitis/pneumonia—respiratory syncytial virus (RSV), other viral, bacterial causes
    3. Skin, oropharyngeal, arthritic, vaginal, urethral, rectal, systemic infection
    4. Other causative organisms
    5. Allergy
- Physical Findings
    1. Gonococcal ophthalmia neonatorum—conjunctivitis, appearing 2 to 5 days after birth, occasionally up to 25 days
        a. Thin, clear discharge from eye that becomes thick, mucoid, sometimes bloody
        b. Edema of lids, conjunctiva
        c. Untreated, may progress to edema and ulceration of cornea, globe perforation and blindness, and/or may become systemic infection
    2. Other—scalp abscesses (neonate); purulent vaginal, urethral, or rectal secretions; exudative pharyngitis or tonsillitis; cough; rales; fever; rash; multiple joint swelling
- Diagnostic Tests/Findings:
    1. Initial evaluation—microscopic identification of gram-negative intracellular diplococci in smears of exudate
    2. Culture in approved laboratory against strict CDC standards
- Management/Treatment: **Follow current CDC guidelines**
    1. Ophthalmia neonatorum prophylaxis—silver nitrate 1% aqueous; erythromycin ophthalmic ointment 0.5%; tetracycline ophthalmic ointment (1%)
    2. Hospitalize infected neonates

3. Ceftriaxone IM or IV is drug of choice for gonococcal infections in children; dose varies by age of child and site of infection; ceftriaxone given as prophylaxis to asymptomatic infants of mothers with untreated gonococcal infections

Congenital Syphilis (Refer to Gu/Gyn chapter)

- Definition: Systemic infection of transplacental or perinatal acquisition resulting in a non-random association of clinical findings

- Etiology/Incidence
    1. *Treponema pallidum*—mother with history of syphilis whose treatment is not documented as complete with full follow-up
    2. Incidence rising, especially among children of women of lower socioeconomic status; often coexistent with HIV

- Signs and Symptoms
    1. 60% of infants with congenital infection have no symptoms in the first week of life, but will develop symptoms if not immediately treated; initial presentation up to 2 years of age
    2. Low birth weight/prematurity
    3. Bone pain or tenderness; decreased movement
    4. Rhinitis, coryza
    5. Syphilitic rash (maculopapular, bullous, followed by desquamation)

- Differential Diagnosis
    1. Any of the "TORCH" congenital conditions
    2. Rash stage—pityriasis rosea, scabies, tinea

- Physical Findings
    1. May be asymptomatic at birth
    2. Hepatomegaly
    3. Splenomegaly
    4. Lymphadenopathy

- Diagnostic Tests/Findings
    1. Direct visualization of spirochete by dark field microscopy; direct fluorescent antibody test for *Treponema pallidum*
    2. Nontreponomel tests—Venereal Disease Research Laboratory microscopic slide test (VDRL); Rapid plasma reagin (RPR)
    3. Treponemal tests—fluorescent treponemal antibody absorbed; microhemagluttination assay for antibody to *Treponema pallidum*
    4. Elevated LFT; positive VDRL in CSF

5. Anemia, thrombocytopenia

6. Radiographic changes (''moth eaten'' metaphysis)

- Management/Treatment

   1. Prevention of sexually transmitted diseases; treat all infected individuals, especially sexually active women and partners

   2. Screen serum of all mothers before infant is discharged; treat all neonates ≤ 4 weeks of age of seropositive mothers, who meet criteria, with aqueous penicillin G 100,000 to 150,000 U/kg/day IV for 10 to 14 days (AAP, 2000, p. 555)

   3. Older infants and children—aqueous penicillin G 200,000 to 300,000 U/kg/day IV for 10 days

   4. Follow-up to determine appropriately falling titers

Herpes (Refer to Gu/Gyn chapter)

- Definition: Group of infectious diseases caused by the Herpes simplex virus (HSV) Type I or II

- Etiology/Incidence

   1. Infection through direct contact of virus with host mucous membrane or abraded skin

   2. Neonatal incidence—1:3000 to 1:20,000 live births

- Signs and Symptoms

   1. Neonatal skin-eye-mouth (SEM) disease

      a. Usually presents in first two weeks of life

      b. Blisters, most often on presenting part, frequently at site of abraded skin

   2. Neonatal CNS disease

      a. Ill infant in second to third week of life

      b. Seizures

      c. Apneic episodes

   3. Neonatal disseminated disease

      a. Acutely ill infant during first week of life

      b. Seizures, lethargy, appears ill

      c. Unresponsive to antibiotic therapy

- Differential Diagnosis: ''TORCH'' diseases—toxoplasmosis, other agents (HIV, *listeria,* syphilis, gonococcus, group B streptococcus, varicella-zoster, malaria), rubella, cytomegalovirus inclusion disease, herpes simplex

- Physical Findings

  1. Neonatal skin-eye-mouth (SEM) disease

     a. Vesicles with erythematous base, clear or cloudy fluid, sometimes appearing pustular, limited to skin, eyes and mouth

     b. Transient fever, malaise (low acuity)

  2. Neonatal CNS disease

     a. Herpetic skin lesions in 60% of cases

     b. Cranial nerve abnormalities

     c. Bradycardia

  3. Neonatal disseminated disease

     a. Seizures, lethargy, often on first day of life

     b. Fever, tachypnea, labored breathing with onset of HSV pneumonitis

     c. Clinical signs of hepatitis—hepatomegaly

- Diagnostic Tests/Findings

  1. Virus isolation from skin, mucous membranes, urine, blood, stool or CSF

  2. Detection of fluorescent antibodies (especially when skin lesions are active)

  3. Polymerase chain reaction (PCR)—helpful in CNS infection

  4. Serology rarely useful in acute HSV infection

  5. Increased CSF protein and pleocytosis

  6. Pulmonary radiograph reveals bilateral, patchy infiltrates from 3 to 10 days of neonatal disseminated disease

  7. Abnormal liver function test results

- Management/Treatment:

  1. Parenteral acyclovir treatment of choice for neonatal HSV infection

  2. Infants with ocular involvement add topical ophthalmic drug treatment.

  3. Refer to APA, 2000, p. 675

Cytomegalic Inclusion Disease (CMV)

- Definition: Congenital infectious disease caused by prenatal infection with cytomegalovirus, a member of herpes virus family

- Etiology/Incidence

  1. During maternal infection with CMV, virus crosses placenta and spreads via fetal blood stream, mainly affecting CNS, liver and eyes

  2. Most common intrauterine infection, affecting 1% of newborns; approximately 10%

are symptomatic; about half present with classic cytomegalic inclusion disease; remainder can shed virus for months, but may never show sequelae

- Signs and Symptoms
    1. Early global developmental delay
    2. Mental retardation
    3. Growth retardation
- Differential Diagnosis
    1. Congenital toxoplasmosis
    2. Rubella
    3. Herpes
- Physical Findings: Classic congenital CMV manifestations are: (Stamos & Rowley, 1994)
    1. Small for gestational age (SGA)
    2. Petechiae, purpura, thrombcytopenia
    3. Hepatosplenomegaly
    4. Jaundice
    5. Microcephaly
    6. Chorioretinitis
    7. Intracranial calcification
    8. Hearing impairment
    9. Intrauterine growth retardation
- Diagnostic Tests/Findings: Isolation of CMV from infant urine, pharynx or peripheral blood leukocytes within first three weeks of life
- Management/Treatment
    1. Primary prevention in women of child-bearing age and younger, since both initial infection and reactivation during pregnancy can cause fetal infection
    2. Congenitally affected infants—refer to developmental disabilities center for interdisciplinary management of complex disabilities
    3. Asymptomatic infants with congenital CMV
        a. Refer to audiology for periodic sensorineural hearing evaluation
        b. Screen frequently for growth retardation and emerging developmental delays
        c. Refer to ophthalmology—emerging chorioretinitis
        d. Refer to dentistry—defective tooth enamel
        e. Monitor for hepatosplenomegaly

4. Neonatal acquisition—often presents as afebrile pneumonia after 8 week incubation period; test suspect infants

5. Seek specialist consultation regarding use of anti-viral drugs; use is not routinely recommended at this time

Congenital Rubella Syndrome (CRS) (Refer to Infectious Disease chapter)

- Definition: Non-random association of congenital abnormalities associated with maternal infection with rubella virus during first 16 weeks of fetal gestation

- Etiology/Incidence

  1. Maternal to fetal transmission of rubella virus

  2. 1:10,000 births in areas where vaccination rates are high; higher in areas of low vaccination; serologic surveys reveal 10% of young adults are susceptible

- Signs and Symptoms

  1. Intrauterine growth retardation

  2. Developmental delays/mental retardation

  3. Deafness

  4. Blindness

  5. Failure to thrive, related to heart defects

- Differential Diagnosis

  1. Congenital CMV

  2. Syphilis

  3. Toxoplasmosis

- Physical Findings

  1. Congenital heart defects

  2. Cataracts, retinopathy, glaucoma

  3. Petechial or purpuric rash

  4. Sensorineural defects

  5. Microphthalmia

- Diagnostic Tests/Findings

  1. Viral culture of nasopharyngeal secretions; laboratory must be notified of suspected rubella

  2. Serology

- Management/Treatment

  1. Isolate infants with CRS from pregnant/potentially pregnant women for one full year

2. Two-thirds of infants with CRS show no symptoms at birth; if maternal infection known or suspected, obtain cultures to determine if infant is shedding virus

3. Early intervention for developmental stimulation

4. Refer to cardiology, ophthalmology, audiology for evaluation

5. Psychosocial support to child and family

6. Ensure appropriate school placement and supports

7. Rubella is a reportable disease

Hepatitis B (Refer to Gastrointestinal Disorders chapter)

- Definition: Incurable infectious disease affecting the liver resulting in chronic carrier state; can cause serious complications such as hepatocellular carcinoma or chronic liver disease; complications fatal for 4000 to 5000 people annually in U.S.

- Etiology/Incidence

  1. Person to person transmission of hepatitis B virus via close personal contact, saliva and other secretions, blood and blood products through wound exudates or sexual contact with infected individuals; perinatal vertical transmission from infected/carrier mother to infant

  2. 22,000 carrier mothers deliver annually; 70% to 90% of newborns infected, 80% if mother had clinical hepatitis during third trimester; chronic carrier state ensues for up to 90%; approximately 25% die of chronic liver disease as adults

- Signs and Symptoms

  1. Long incubation period—50 to 180 days

  2. Skin rash

  3. Arthralgia

  4. Moderate fever, nausea, vomiting in some cases

  5. Loss of appetite

- Differential Diagnosis

  1. Hepatitis A, Hepatitis C, Hepatitis D, Hepatitis E

  2. Cystic fibrosis, Wilson disease, metabolic liver disease

  3. Infectious causes such as CMV, toxoplasmosis, echovirus, Epstein Barr virus

- Physical Findings

  1. Neonatal infection usually results in ''healthy'' chronic carrier state

  2. Later, progression to liver disease with:

     a. Liver enlargement, tenderness

     b. Jaundice

    c. Arthralgia or arthritis

    d. Rash or urticaria

- Diagnostic Tests/Findings

    1. Presence of surface antigen HBsAg, HBeAg antigen, or antibodies to either of these or HBcAg (core antigen)

    2. Aminotransferase elevation—peaks at about one month

    3. Bilirubin elevation

    4. Elevated WBC; elevated serum alpha-fetoprotein concentration

- Management/Treatment

    1. No specific therapy for HBV infection yet available

    2. Perinatal exposure—HBIG 0.5 mL + vaccination in first 12 hours of life

    3. Prevention—universal child HBV immunization, with adolescent "catch up"

    4. Supportive care during acute phase

    5. Monitor for hepatic failure (rare), hospitalize if occurs, restrict protein intake

Toxoplasmosis

- Definition: Communicable parasitic infection

- Etiology/Incidence

    1. Placenta to fetus transmission of *Toxoplasma gondii* in mother with primary infection during pregnancy

    2. 1:1000 to 1:10,000 live births; about 40% of infants of mothers with primary infection will become infected

- Signs and Symptoms

    1. Severe

        a. Immediate—microcephaly, seizures, jaundice, fever

        b. Later—developmental delays, cerebral palsy, visual problems, hearing impairment/deafness

    2. Subclinical (later signs)

        a. Visual impairment

        b. Hearing impairment

        c. Poor coordination

        d. Developmental delays

- Differential Diagnosis

    1. Cytomegalovirus

2. Syphilis

3. Rubella

4. Hemolytic disease of the newborn

- Physical Findings

    1. Severe

        a. Retinal lesions on fundoscopic examination

        b. Splenomegaly, hepatomegaly

        c. Lymphadenopathy

        d. Jaundice

        e. Thrombocytopenia

        f. Growth failure

    2. Subclinical (later signs)—retinal lesions on fundoscopic examination

- Diagnostic Tests/Findings

    1. Pre-natal—fetal blood or tissue analysis; ultrasonography for bilateral, symmetrical ventriculomegaly

    2. Polymerase chain reaction assay (PCR)—detection of genomic material

    3. Visual detection of tachyzoites in newborn CSF, ventricular fluid, blood, bone marrow, brain or placental tissue, or detection 1 to 6 weeks after mouse innoculation

    4. Detection of antitoxoplasma IgM in umbilical cord or newborn serum

    5. Persistent high IgG titers

    6. Ventricular dilitation

    7. Cerebrospinal fluid abnormalities

    8. Intracerebral calcifications

- Management/Treatment

    1. Congenital—one year treatment with pyrimethamine with sulfadiazine and folinic acid supplement; corticosteroids for acute inflammation

    2. Spiramycin for primary infection during pregnancy if no evidence of fetal infection; pyrimethamine and sulfonamide after fetal infection has occurred

    3. Offer consideration of selective termination of pregnancy if evidence of severe effects on fetus early in pregnancy

Fetal Alcohol Syndrome (FAS)

- Definition: Non-random grouping of congenital anomalies in persons whose mothers ingested alcohol during pregnancy

- Etiology/Incidence

1. Dose related (*dose necessary to cause FAS unknown*) teratogenic effect of maternal prenatal alcohol ingestion; alcohol and its metabolite acetaldehyde cross placenta and are believed to:

    a. Decrease protein syntheses

    b. Impair cellular growth and migration

    c. Decrease production of neurotransmitters

    d. Inhibit nerve myelination

2. Differential effects according to trimester

    a. First trimester—physical defects and mental retardation

    b. Second trimester—growth retardation and mental retardation

    c. Third trimester—mental retardation without physical defects or growth retardation

3. Most common cause of mental retardation in U.S.

4. Incidence of FAS 2:1000; incidence of fetal alcohol effects (FAE) at least 2 to 3 times higher

- Signs and Symptoms

    1. Alcoholic mother

    2. Infant alcohol withdrawal symptoms (irritability, hyperactivity, jitteriness) and alcohol odor to amniotic fluid if alcohol abuse during last days of pregnancy

    3. Term birth, but small for gestational age

    4. Slow growth

    5. Mental retardation

- Differential Diagnosis: Other congenital disorders causing atypical appearance and mental retardation (e.g., Down syndrome, Fragile X syndrome)

- Physical Findings

    1. Small head circumference

    2. Widely spaced eyes with narrow lids and epicanthal folds

    3. Short, upturned, or beak like nose with broad nasal bridge

    4. Thin upper lip-vermilion border

    5. Absent or flattened philtrum

    6. Micrognathia

    7. Dental malocclusion

    8. Congenital heart defects

    9. Hip subluxation or dislocation

10. Seizure disorder

11. Attention deficit disorder

12. Ophthalmologic disorders—myopia/strabismus

13. Hearing impairment

14. Below average height and weight for age

15. Cleft palate

- Diagnostic Tests/Findings

    1. IQ usually in 60 to 80 range, stable throughout life

    2. History of maternal alcohol abuse during pregnancy

- Management/Treatment

    1. No known treatment to reverse primary defects

    2. Promote stable, supportive home environment

    3. Ensure appropriate education with necessary support services

    4. Identify and treat associated health conditions (e.g., seizures, congenital heart defects, vision problems)

    5. Prophylactic antibiotics for subacute bacterial endocarditis (SBE), if cardiac effects present

    6. National Organization on Fetal Alcohol Syndrome
       216 G Street N.E.
       Washington, DC 20002
       (800) 666-6327

Genetic Syndromes

Trisomy 18 (Edwards' Syndrome)

- Definition: Autosomal chromosomal disorder with karyotype 47 XY or XX + 18, trisomy of chromosome 18; associated with severe mental retardation and other congenital defects; 5% to 10% survive beyond first year of life

- Etiology/Incidence

    1. Nondisjunction during meiotic division resulting in trisomy of chromosome #18

    2. Second most common autosomal chromosome disorder

    3. 1:3500 to 8000 live births; 3:1 female predominance

    4. 90% die by 1 year

- Signs and Symptoms

    1. Small for gestational age

2. Severe global developmental delays

3. Feeding problems/growth failure

- Differential Diagnosis: Trisomy 13; other rare chromosomal aberrations
- Physical Findings

  1. Apnea

  2. Microcephaly

  3. Low set ears

  4. Heart murmur

  5. Clenched hands with over-riding fingers and crossed thumb

  6. Severe failure to thrive (FTT)

- Diagnostic Tests/Findings

  1. Karyotype

     a. Fluorescent in-situ hybridization (FISH) analysis

     b. Results usually available within 48 hours

  2. Echocardiogram to detect congenital cardiac defects

  3. Chorionic villi sampling or amniocentesis with subsequent pregnancies

- Management/Treatment

  1. Genetic counseling

  2. Psychosocial support to parents and family

  3. Refer to cardiology

  4. Support nutritional needs; may require gastric feedings

  5. Prophylactic antibiotics to prevent subacute bacterial endocarditis (SBE), if cardiac effects present

  6. Enroll in early intervention program for habilitative therapies

  7. Assist family with management of special needs child—may require in-home nursing

  8. Support Organization for Trisomy 18, 13, and Related Disorders (SOFT),
     2982 S. Union Street
     Rochester, NY 14624
     (800) 716-SOFT (7638)

Down Syndrome (DS) (Trisomy 21)

- Definition: A recognizable grouping of congenital physical malformations, coupled with mental retardation and karyotype 47 XY or XX + 21; also known as Trisomy 21

- Etiology/Incidence
    1. Presence of critical lower region of a third #21 chromosome, usually contributed due to nondisjunction in maternal zygote formation
    2. 1:700 births
    3. Affects males and females equally
    4. Increased risk with advanced maternal age, though most infants with DS are born to younger mothers due to higher birth rates among younger women
- Signs and Symptoms
    1. Mental retardation, mild to severe
    2. Typical phenotypic signs at birth
        a. Flattened, hypoplastic mid-face
        b. Small mouth with high, narrow palate
        c. Tongue large for mouth
        d. Small ears
        e. Inner epicanthal folds
        f. Upward slanting palpebral fissures
        g. Hypotonia
        h. Sometimes brachydactyly, single transverse palmar crease
        i. Flattened occiput
        j. History of seizures—up to 13%
- Differential Diagnosis: Other genetic or chromosomal syndromes
- Physical Findings
    1. Phenotype as above
    2. Signs of congenital heart disease—50%, e.g., murmur, abnormal heart rate, rapid respiratory rate, labored respirations, cyanosis
    3. Signs of hypothyroidism and other endocrine problems—15%
    4. Signs of esophageal or duodenal atresia—12%
    5. Ligamentous laxity—100%
    6. Vision or hearing impairments—up to 90%
    7. Obesity—50% by early childhood
- Diagnostic Tests/Findings
    1. Pre or postnatal chromosome analysis reveals 47 XY or XX + 21 karyotype
    2. CBC with differential to identify those with leukemia; 10 to 15 fold increased risk

3. Radiographic finding of atlantoaxial instability—10%

- Management/Treatment

    1. Primary prevention via education re: risk factors; secondary prevention via prenatal diagnosis

    2. Early intervention by PT, OT, speech therapists

    3. Genetic counseling for parents and older siblings

    4. Periodic full history and physical with sensory and developmental evaluations

    5. Nutritional support

    6. Prophylactic antibiotics to prevent SBE, if cardiac effects

    7. Prompt consultation and referral for specialist treatment of associated conditions

    8. Association for Children with Down Syndrome
       2616 Martin Avenue
       Bellmore, NY 11710

       National Down Syndrome Congress
       7000 Peachtree-Dunwood Road N.E.
       Lake Ridge 400 Office Park Bldg 5
       Suite 100
       Atlanta, GA 30328
       (800) 232-NDSC

       National Down Syndrome Society
       666 Broadway, Suite 800
       New York, NY 10012
       (800) 221-4602
       http://www.ndss.org

Fragile X Syndrome

- Definition: Nonrandom association of clinical signs and symptoms including recognizable phenotype of subtle physical abnormalities, mental retardation of varying degrees, behavioral abnormalities, and karyotype showing fragile site on X chromosome

- Etiology/Incidence

    1. Genetic anomaly, labeled FMR1, on X chromosome at Xq27.3, the same position as the fragile site

    2. Atypical X-linked recessive inheritance pattern

    3. Affected individuals—1:1000 males; 1:2000 to 1:2500 females

    4. Carrier females—1:700

    5. Approximately 20% of males asymptomatic, but can transmit gene resulting in symptomatic offspring

6. Most common inherited cause of mental retardation (MR); second most common genetic cause of MR

- Signs and Symptoms
    1. Developmental delay
    2. Hyperactivity
    3. Speech delay; perseverative speech; echolalia
    4. Poor gross motor coordination
    5. Stereotypies, e.g., talking to self, spinning, hand flapping
    6. Gaze aversion
    7. History of seizures—17% to 50%

- Differential Diagnosis
    1. Autism, Asperger syndrome, or pervasive developmental disorder
    2. Mental retardation with nonspecific etiology
    3. Klinefelter syndrome, Sotos syndrome
    4. Attention deficit hyperactivity disorder

- Physical Findings
    1. Macrocephaly
    2. Prominent forehead with long thin face and prominent jaw, especially in adolescence
    3. Macro-orchidism in adolescent males; may be seen as early as age 5
    4. Protuberant, large ears, long or wide
    5. Soft, smooth skin
    6. Heart murmur or apical midsystolic click
    7. Serous otitis media
    8. Strabismus—40%
    9. Joint laxity (especially fingers), hip subluxation, occasionally club foot

- Diagnostic Tests/Findings
    1. DNA analysis from whole blood in approved laboratory to confirm diagnosis
    2. Prenatal testing from chorionic villus or amniocentesis sample

- Management/Treatment
    1. Psychosocial support to parents, child and family

2. Genetic counseling—no spontaneous mutations have been found for Fragile X syndrome; all family members should undergo genetic testing to identify transmitting males, carrier females, and affected individuals

3. Regular well-child examination with attention to:

    a. Cardiac auscultation—if click or murmur heard, obtain echocardiogram, consider referral to cardiologist for possible mitral valve prolapse

    b. Otoscopic evaluation—serous otitis media

    c. Ophthalmologic evaluation—strabismus (40%), myopia

    d. Developmental evaluation—mild to severe delays, (usually moderate)

    e. Anticipatory guidance

4. Enroll in early intervention as soon as delays are recognized; speech/language therapy and sensory/motor integration therapy thought to be most helpful

5. Ensure appropriate educational placement with necessary supports

6. Prophylactic antibiotics with dental care and all surgeries for SBE, mitral valve prolapse

7. National Fragile X Foundation
P.O. Box 190488
San Francisco, CA 94119
(800) 688-8765
http://www.nfxf.org

Turner's Syndrome (XO Karyotype)

- Definition: Chromosomal anomaly resulting in 45,XO (female) karyotype, with predictable associated signs and symptoms

- Etiology/Incidence

1. Nondisjunction during meiotic division, usually maternal; more than half have a mosaic chromosomal complement (45,XO/46,XX)

2. 1:1500 to 1:2500 live births; most common sex-chromosome anomaly affecting females; many affected embryos do not survive to term

- Signs and Symptoms

1. Short stature with "square" appearance

2. Low hairline

3. Chronic ear infections

4. Learning disabilities

5. Lack of development of secondary sexual characteristics

- Differential Diagnosis

1. Congenital lymphedema without Turner's karyotype

2. Coarctation of aorta without Turner's karyotype

- Physical Findings

    1. Neonatal—lymphedema, webbed neck, low hairline, swelling of hands and feet

    2. Widely spaced, often inverted nipples with "shield" shaped chest

    3. Heart murmur

    4. Ear deformities

    5. Strabismus, amblyopia, ptosis

    6. Scoliosis (10%)

    7. Nail dysplasia

    8. Defective dentition

    9. High blood pressure

- Diagnostic Tests/Findings

    1. Cytogenetic testing for Karyotype 45 XO

    2. Cardiac ultrasonography or MRI for:

        a. Coarctation of aorta (20%)

        b. Bicuspid aortic valve (50%)

    3. Renal ultrasound to detect renal anomalies

    4. Thyroid function tests to detect low T_4, high TSH indicating hypothyroidism

    5. Abdominal and pelvic ultrasound to detect gonadal dysgenesis

    6. Plasma gonadotropin studies to detect low levels of normal female hormones

- Management/Treatment

    1. Refer to endocrinology

        a. Growth hormone therapy beginning when growth falls below 5th percentile on normal female child growth chart

        b. Hormone (estrogen) replacement therapy beginning about 14 years of age

        c. Monitor for hypothyroidism

    2. Genetic counseling

    3. Psychosocial support

    4. Assistance in school for learning disabilities

    5. Referral to cardiology for cardiac anomaly diagnosis and treatment

    6. Prophylactic antibiotics for SBE if cardiac effects present

    7. Referral to ENT, orthopedics, urology, ophthalmology, pediatric dentist as needed

8. Turner's Syndrome Society of the U.S.
   14450 T. C. Jester
   Suite 260
   Houston, TX 77014
   (800) 365-9944

Klinefelter Syndrome (XXY Karyotype)

- Definition: Nonrandom association of physical characteristics and learning and behavioral disorders seen in males with the 47,XXY karyotype

- Etiology/Incidence

  1. Maternal meiotic nondisjunction resulting in contribution of two X chromosomes to maternal zygote (ova); when ova is fertilized by sperm containing one Y chromosome, resulting embryo has Klinefelter karyotype

  2. 1:1000 live births

  3. Most common cause of hypogonadism and infertility in men

- Signs and Symptoms

  1. Tall male, especially at adolescence and beyond

  2. Slow, incomplete pubertal development

  3. Behavioral and psychiatric disorders (shy, immature, anxious, aggressive, anti-social)

  4. Thin child, often overweight as adolescent

  5. Language impairment

- Differential Diagnosis

  1. Marfan syndrome

  2. Sotos syndrome

  3. Trisomy 8p

- Physical Findings

  1. Tall for age, with disproportionate lower limb length

  2. Gynecomastia

  3. Small, firm testes

  4. Cryptorchidism

  5. Small phallus

  6. Hypospadias

- Diagnostic Tests/Findings

  1. Chromosome analysis yields 47, XXY karyotype

  2. High FSH, LH and low testosterone levels

- Management/Treatment

    1. Early intervention for learning disorders

    2. Counseling/therapy for behavioral disorders

    3. Psychosocial support for family

    4. Genetic counseling

    5. Refer to endocrinology for consideration of testosterone therapy at age 11 or 12

    6. Screen for breast cancer (4%)

    7. Reduction mammoplasty for severe gynecomastia

    8. American Association for Kleinfelter Syndrome
       Information and Support
       2945 W. Farwell Ave.
       Chicago, IL 60645-2925
       (888) 466-5747

Tay-Sachs Disease

- Definition: Inborn error of metabolism resulting in neurologic degenerative disease and death, usually by 3 years of age

- Etiology/Incidence

    1. Autosomal recessive single gene disorder; deficiency of hexosaminidase A (hex A) which is necessary for breakdown of ganglioside G_{m2}; as glycoside accumulates in neurons, axons degenerate and demyelination occurs

    2. 3:10,000 live births; mainly in Ashkenazic Jewish population; gene carrier frequency in U.S. 1:27 among Jews and 1:380 among non-Jews

- Signs and Symptoms

    1. Normal development until age 3 to 6 months, then progressive deterioration

    2. Listlessness

    3. Muscle weakness

    4. Slow neurological development, loss of developmental milestones

    5. Feeding problems

    6. Frequent upper respiratory infections

    7. Apathy, irritability

    8. Seizures

    9. Deafness/blindness

- Differential Diagnosis

    1. Other inborn errors of metabolism

    2. Leukodystrophies

    3. Muscular dystrophy

- Physical Findings

    1. Hypotonia, followed by spasticity and paralysis

    2. "Cherry red" spot on retina

    3. Translucent skin, delicate pink coloring

    4. Abnormal increase in head size due to cerebral gliosis

    5. Dysphagia

    6. Decerebrate posturing

    7. Eventual vegetative state

- Diagnostic Tests/Findings: Serum enzymatic assay yields deficiency of hexosaminidase A

- Management/Treatment

    1. Genetic counseling

    2. Primary prevention via carrier screening

    3. Secondary prevention via prenatal diagnosis and elective termination of pregnancy

    4. No known treatment for underlying metabolic deficiency

    5. Supportive/comfort care for child; assist to obtain home nursing services as disease progresses and care burden increases

    6. Psychosocial support for parents and family

    7. The National Tay-Sachs and Allied Diseases Association
       2001 Beacon Street, #204
       Brookline, MA 02146
       (617) 277-4463

Marfan Syndrome

- Definition: Inherited disorder of connective tissue; affects the skeletal, cardiovascular and ocular systems

- Etiology/Incidence

    1. Autosomal dominant inheritance of defective fibrillin gene (FBN1 mapped to chromosome 15 [15q21.1]); 15% sporadic mutation

    2. Incidence is 1:20,000

- Signs and Symptoms

    1. Skeletal—tall stature; long, thin extremities, long fingers, narrow facies

2. Rapid heart rate, chest pain; palpitations or syncope suggestive of mitral valve prolapse

3. Vision impairment

4. Normal intelligence with learning disorders, attention deficit hyperactivity disorder (40%)

- Differential Diagnosis

    1. Beals syndrome (congenital contractural arachnodactyly)

    2. Homocystinuria

- Physical Findings

    1. Skeletal

        a. Loose joints

        b. Scoliosis (60%)

        c. Pectus excavatum or carinatum

        d. Narrow palate

        e. Dolichomorphism—elongation of tubular bones, as evidenced by increased upper limb span, low upper to lower segment ratio, hand length exceeding 11% of height, foot length exceeding 15% of height

    2. Murmur indicative of mitral valve prolapse

    3. Ocular—upwardly dislocated lens, retinal detachment

    4. Myopia

- Diagnostic Tests/Findings

    1. Diagnosis based on clinical manifestations; must document involvement of at least one of the three systems—cardiovascular, ocular, skeletal

    2. Positive family history plus one or more systems(as above) conclusive

    3. Cardiac evaluation (chest radiograph, electrocardiogram, echocardiogram)—mitral valve prolapse common; signs of dilatation of aortic root or dissecting aortic aneurysm

    4. Ocular evaluation—slit-lamp examination

    5. Skeletal evaluation—scoliosis screening; trunk/extremities ratio

- Management/Treatment

    1. Refer to cardiology for periodic echocardiogram to detect dissecting aortic aneurysm, mitral valve prolapse; severe cases; surgical graft repair of the ascending aorta and aortic valve has been successful

    2. Propanolol to reduce effect of ventricular ejection on ascending aorta

3. Refer to ophthalmology for treatment of myopia, lens subluxation, cataracts, glaucoma, retinal detachment

4. Refer to endocrinology for hormonal treatment to curtail height, valuable psychological effect; prevention of scoliosis and kyphosis; prevention of secondary problems of feet

5. Psychosocial support for patient and family

6. Genetic counseling

7. Ensure mainstream or inclusive school placement with any necessary supports, with attention to physical activity limitations if cardiovascular involvement

8. National Marfan Foundation (NMF)
   382 Main Street
   Port Washington, NY 11050
   (800) 862-7326
   http://www.marfan.org

Hurler Syndrome (MPS IH)

- Definition: Inborn mucopolysaccharidosis metabolic disorder in which dermatan and heparan sulfate accumulate and are excreted in urine; typically, death occurs by 10 years of age

- Etiology/Incidence

  1. Deficiency of enzyme α-L-iduronidase; autosomal recessive inheritance

  2. 1:100,000 incidence

- Signs and Symptoms

  1. Coarse facial features with enlarged tongue, full lips, flat nasal bridge; mild at birth, progressing with growth

  2. Developmental peak at age 2, followed by deterioration

  3. Recurrent upper respiratory tract infections

  4. Recurrent inguinal hernia

  5. Vision and hearing impairments

  6. Joint limitations and contractures

  7. Short stature

- Differential Diagnosis: Other progressive neuropathies and inborn errors of metabolism, particularly other mucopolysaccharidoses and thyroid deficiency

- Physical Findings

  1. Skeletal abnormalities, including spinal anomalies/gibbus formation

  2. Macrocephaly, scaphocephaly

  3. Hepatosplenomegaly

4. Clouded corneas

5. Inguinal/umbilical hernia

6. Valvular heart disease; coronary artery disease

- Diagnostic Tests/Findings

    1. Prenatal diagnosis with amniocentesis or chorionic villus sampling and enzyme analysis

    2. Postnatal via serum and urine enzyme analysis

- Management/Treatment

    1. Genetic counseling

    2. Psychosocial support

    3. Anticipatory guidance

    4. Early intervention; appropriate school placement with supports as needed

    5. Bone marrow transplantation in selected cases, especially after early diagnosis and with human leukocyte antigen (HLA) matched sibling donor

    6. Refer to audiology and opthalmology for evaluation and treatment, as indicated

    7. To date, enzyme replacement therapy not effective

    8. National MPS Society, Inc.
       102 Aspen Drive
       Downingtown, PA 19335
       (601) 942-0100

Prader-Willi Syndrome

- Definition: Congenital disorder characterized by voracious, uncontrollable appetite, and obesity

- Etiology/Incidence

    1. Usually sporadic mutation; when detectable (about 50%) mutation at same location of Chromosome 15 as the mutation for Angelman syndrome, although conditions are very dissimilar due to phenomenon of genetic imprinting

    2. 1:10,000 to 1:15,000 incidence

- Signs and Symptoms

    1. Voracious appetite during childhood and beyond, resulting in severe obesity

    2. Mental retardation

    3. Behavior problems

    4. Hypontonia, poor suck and feeding problems in infancy; resolution with time

- Differential Diagnosis: Other neurological and musculoskeletal disorders with early hypotonia (including cerebral palsy) and developmental delay

- Physical Findings

  1. Obesity

  2. Small hands and feet

  3. Small genitalia

  4. Cryptorchidism

  5. Short stature

  6. Scoliosis

- Diagnostic Tests/Findings

  1. In 50% of cases, chromosome analysis detects aberration of chromosome 15 section 15q11 to 15q13

  2. Remainder of cases are diagnosed on clinical signs and symptoms

  3. Growth Hormone deficiency frequent, but not universal

- Management/Treatment

  1. Behavioral therapy for control of eating and other problem behaviors

  2. Genetic counseling

  3. Early intervention and appropriate school placement with supports

  4. Psychosocial support for child and family

  5. Refer to endocrinology for evaluation and management of Growth Hormone deficiency

  6. Prader Willi Syndrome Association
     5700 Midnight Pass Road
     Sarasota, FL 34242
     (800) 926-4797
     http://www.pwsausa.org

Multisystem Disorders

Cerebral Palsy (CP)

- Definition

  1. Disorders of motion and posture related to static injury to the developing brain

  2. Types

     a. Spastic (diplegia, tetraplegia, hemiplegia) **most frequent**

     b. Dyskinetic

     c. Ataxic

     d. Mixed

- Etiology/Incidence
    1. CNS insult may be congenital, hypoxic, traumatic or ischemic; may occur prenatally, perinatally, postnatally
    2. Birth asphyxia associated with only 3% to 13% of cases
    3. High association with prematurity and very low birth weight
    4. Apgar score of 3 or less at 20 minutes associated with 250 times increased risk
    5. Tetraplegia associated with serious intrauterine infections, fetal encephalopathies and perinatal hypoxia
    6. Prevalence 2.7:1000 at school entry; most common pediatric physical disability
    7. Hereditary spastic type CP—rare
- Signs and Symptoms
    1. Movement or posture abnormality that evolves with growth, but is not itself progressive
    2. Delays in reaching developmental milestones, especially motor
    3. Infancy
        a. Abnormal or retained primitive reflexes
        b. Poor muscle tone in first few weeks
        c. Some irritability, lethargy
        d. Weak suck, difficulty swallowing
        e. Oral hypersensitivity
        f. Fisted hands, even at rest
    4. Later infancy/toddler
        a. Scissoring
        b. Toe to toe gait if ambulatory
        c. "W" sitting
        d. "Bottom scoot" in place of crawl
        e. Resistance to spoon feeding/table foods
        f. Tonic bite, tongue thrust
        g. Early hand preference
    5. Vision impairment (50%)
    6. Hearing impairment (10%)
    7. Seizures (35% to 50%)
    8. Mental retardation (50% to 75%); more common with greater physical disability

- Differential Diagnosis

  1. Neurodegenerative disorders such as Duchenne muscular dystrophy

  2. Inborn errors of metabolism

  3. Spinal cord tumor/syrinx

  4. Brain tumor

  5. Hydrocephalus

  6. Subdural hematoma

  7. Dystonias

- Physical Findings

  1. Abnormal muscle tone (hypo or hypertonia)

  2. Infancy—retained primitive reflexes

  3. Hyperactive tendon and heightened stretch reflexes; positive Babinski

  4. Restricted joint range of motion

  5. Hip click or clunk on Barlow maneuver or Ortolani test

  6. Movement related muscle spasms

  7. "Clasp-knife" limb muscle stretch response

  8. Low weight for height

  9. Neuromuscular scoliosis

- Diagnostic Tests/Findings

  1. Developmental evaluation—delays in gross motor, fine motor, speech, according to type of CP and presence of mental retardation

  2. Brain MRI—periventricular leukomalacia

- Management/Treatment

  1. Coordinate interdisciplinary management to promote optimum health and function

  2. Enroll in early intervention services

  3. Identify and treat associated conditions (e.g., seizures, visual impairment, hearing impairment, gastroesophageal reflux)

  4. Prevent secondary conditions (e.g., failure to thrive, skin breakdown, dental caries)

  5. Functional therapies to build on strengths and promote compensation for physical impairments

  6. Parent/family support for positive coping and stress relief

  7. Spasticity relief

a. Enteral medication—lioresal, diazepam, dantrium sodium, tizanidine hydrochloride

b. Botulinum toxin IM to major affected muscles, or nerve block injections

c. Intrathecal lioresal

d. Selective dorsal root rhizotomy

8. Nutritional support

9. Ensure appropriate education with supportive services and therapies

10. United Cerebral Palsy Association, Inc.
1660 L Street, N.W.
Suite 700
Washington, DC 20036-5602
(800) USA-5UCP
(800) 872-5827

Spina Bifida

- Definition: Congenital multisystem defect resulting from failure of neural tube closure during early embryonic development; one of several "neural tube defects"

- Etiology/Incidence

  1. Multifactorial inheritance pattern; environmental contribution not well understood, although addition of folic acid to dietary intake reduces occurrence probability by one-half

  2. Spina bifida occulta—incidence up to 10% of population

  3. Myelomeningocele—1:1000; decreasing, probably due to folic acid supplementation and prenatal diagnosis with selective termination, (not proven)

- Signs and Symptoms

  1. Urinary "dribbling", unable to achieve urinary continence

  2. Frequent urinary tract infections

  3. Chronic constipation, difficulty with bowel continence

  4. Motor developmental delays, especially lower extremity related gross motor delays

  5. Intelligence in normal range, but with learning disorders, often with attention deficit hyperactivity disorder (AD/HD)

- Differential Diagnosis: Syndromes of which spina bifida is associated, e.g., Meckel-Gruber syndrome

- Physical Findings

  1. Spina bifida occulta—usually benign; may have sacral dimple, hairy patch at base of spine, uneven gluteal folds

2. Arnold-Chiari Type II CNS malformation (nearly 100%)—associated with progressive hydrocephalus, difficulty swallowing, hypoventilation, apnea

3. Meningocele or Myelomeningocele—signs at birth include lesion at some point along thoraco-lumbar-sacral spine, often with a cyst like structure protruding; neural elements may be apparently absent or may be easily visualized within the sac

4. Widely spaced cranial sutures, bulging fontanel, macrocephaly (with hydrocephalus)

5. Lack of typical lower extremity function, sometimes with orthopedic deformity (club foot, dislocated or subluxed hip, tibial torsion)

6. Abnormal deep tendon reflexes in lower extremities

7. Abnormal neonatal reflexes in lower extremities

8. Decreased or absent anal wink

9. Atrophied lower extremity/hip muscles

10. Scoliosis, kyphosis

11. Obesity in older children and adolescents (> 50%)

12. Neurogenic bowel and bladder

13. Latex sensitivity (> 40%)

- Diagnostic Tests/Findings

  1. Prenatal diagnosis possible by maternal serum screening for elevated alpha-fetoprotein, followed by ultrasound diagnostics for spinal anomaly and head "lemon sign"

  2. Postnatal diagnosis made on clinical basis

  3. Hydrocephalus after birth, increasing head circumference out of proportion to other growth parameters

- Management/Treatment

  1. Infants diagnosed prenatally should be referred to tertiary center with appropriate supports for birth (possible planned C-section) and immediate neonatal intensive care

  2. Refer to multidisciplinary treatment center for specialty management—assistance from orthopedist, urologist, neurosurgeon, developmental pediatrician, orthotist, physical and occupational therapists, nutritionist, advanced practice nurse and social worker

  3. Enroll infant in early intervention program as soon as medically stable

  4. Monitor for urinary tract infections; expect less common organisms

  5. Monitor for shunt malfunction if presence of shunted hydrocephalus; baseline head CT scan; follow-up if increased intracranial pressure suspected; refer to neurosurgeon for evaluation of suspected shunt malfunction or tethered card

  6. Monitor for development of orthopedic problems, especially scoliosis and unilateral hip subluxation or dislocation; baseline and follow-up radiographic studies

7. Monitor for skin breakdown

8. Nutritional and behavioral intervention to prevent obesity

9. Test for latex sensitivity (skin or RAST); latex precautions

10. Anticipatory guidance for development, safety

11. Psychosocial support to family and child

12. Assistance finding least restrictive school placement and other community supports—restrict from heavy contact sports only; otherwise full inclusion should be encouraged

13. Genetic counseling

14. All women of child-bearing age should consume 0.4 mg folic acid daily to help prevent neural tube defects; women at high risk should consult obstetrician for higher dose, 4.0 mg/day recommended

15. Spina Bifida Association of America (SBAA)
    4590 MacArthur Blvd., Suite 250
    Washington, DC 20007-4226
    (202) 944-3283
    (800) 621-3141

Toxic Shock Syndrome (TSS)

- Definition: Acute, life-threatening, multisystem infectious disorder leading to shock and multiple organ failure; CDC case definition (Sagraves, 1995)

- Etiology/Incidence:

  1. *Staphylococcus aureus; Streptococcus pyogenes* (Group A streptococci); association with staph or strep infections and use of tampons during menstruation

  2. 0.5:100,000 with wide geographic variations

- Signs and Symptoms:

  1. Headache

  2. Sore throat

  3. Abdominal cramps

  4. Vomiting

  5. Watery, non-bloody diarrhea

  6. Muscle tenderness, weakness

  7. Confusion, disorientation

  8. Generalized erythroderma

- Differential Diagnosis:

  1. Stevens-Johnson syndrome

2. Kawasaki disease

3. Scarlet fever

4. Measles

5. Leptospirosis

6. Rocky mountain spotted fever

7. Septic shock

8. Systemic lupus erythrematosus

- Physical Findings

   1. Inflamed mucous membranes

   2. Erythroderma or scarlitinaform rash

   3. Edematous hands and feet

   4. Hyperemic conjunctiva, non-purulent drainage

   5. CDC diagnostic criteria for *S. aureus* TSS include:

      a. Fever at least 38.9° C (102° F)

      b. Hypotension

      c. Rash

      d. Desquamation of rash

      e. Involvement of at least three major organ systems

- Diagnostic Tests/Findings:

   1. Culture *S. aureus* from nasopharynx, vagina, or wound; or isolation of Group A streptococci

   2. Other findings include:

      a. Leukocytosis

      b. Anemia, thrombocytopenia

      c. Abnormal renal, liver, metabolic and musculoskeletal findings as condition progresses to affect many organ systems

      d. Negative blood, CSF cultures

- Management/Treatment

   1. Hospitalization

   2. Maximum supportive care

   3. Aggressive treatment of hypotension and fluid and electrolyte imbalances

   4. Remove infected foreign bodies (tampons); drain, irrigate infected wounds

5. IV antibiotics at maximum dose for age/weight for *S. aureus* or *S. pyrogenes* as appropriate

6. Surgical consult for necrotizing fasciitis

7. Intravenous immune globulin (IVIG) for nonresponding illness

Sudden Infant Death Syndrome (SIDS)

- Definition—''The sudden death of an infant under 1 year of age that remains unexplained after a thorough case investigation, including performance of a complete autopsy, examination of the death scene, and review of the clinical history'' (Brooks, 1997, p. 1622)

- Etiology/Incidence

  1. Unknown cause

  2. 1.1:1000 live births, twofold greater incidence in African-American infants; somewhat higher in Native-Americans; lower in Asians

  3. Peak incidence 2 to 4 months; uncommon before 2 weeks and after 6 months

- Signs and Symptoms: Infant unexpectedly found lifeless after a period of sleep

- Differential Diagnosis

  1. Meningitis

  2. Intracranial hemorrhage

  3. Myocarditis

  4. Accidental trauma

  5. Child abuse

- Physical Findings

  1. Full cardiorespiratory arrest

  2. Unresponsive to resuscitation

- Diagnostic Tests/Findings: Diagnosis of exclusion, with autopsy and investigation failure to find adequate cause of death

- Management/Treatment

  1. Risk reduction

     a. Promote excellent prenatal care

     b. Supine or side sleeping position for normal healthy infants

     c. Avoid maternal and passive smoking

     d. Separate sleeping place for infants

     e. Avoid soft bedding

     f. Maintain comfortable room temperature

      g.   Avoid heavy blankets, over bundling

      h.   Apnea monitoring for high risk infants

         (1)   Premature with persistent apnea

         (2)   Infant born after two previous siblings with SIDS

         (3)   Post-apparent life threatening event (ALTE) requiring stimulation

         (4)   Infants with central hypoventilation syndrome

2.   After infant's death

      a.   Maximum support to family, others

      b.   Provide factual information

      c.   Assist with necessary tasks

      d.   Assist nursing mother with abrupt cessation of breast feeding

3.   National SIDS Resource Center
2070 Chain Bridge Road
Suite 450
Vienna, VA 22182
(703) 821-8955
http://www.circsol.com/SIDS/

Reye's Syndrome

- Definition: Acute, noninflammatory hepatic encephalopathy, which often follows a viral infection

- Etiology/Incidence

  1. Unknown; association with viral infection (especially varicella and influenza) and aspirin use, but not universal

  2. Decreased occurrence with increased education regarding danger in use of aspirin with viral illness

- Signs and Symptoms

  1. Sudden development of protracted vomiting, delirium, stupor, inappropriate behavior 5 to 7 days after onset of viral infection; often after signs of recovery

  2. Progressive neurological deficit, leading to coma

  3. Headache

  4. Confusion

  5. Lethargy

- Differential Diagnosis

  1. Inborn errors of metabolism

  2. Infections of the CNS

3. CNS effects of poisoning, especially with aspirin, acetaminophen, valproic acid, antiemetics

- Physical Findings
    1. Hepatomegaly without jaundice
    2. Papilledema
- Diagnostic Tests/Findings
    1. Fatty infiltration in liver, CNS tissues, heart, pancreas, kidneys
    2. Elevation of liver enzymes
    3. Low serum glucose
    4. Elevated ammonia
- Management/Treatment
    1. Usual cause of death is cerebral edema and herniation
    2. Hospitalization for maximum supportive therapy to decrease cerebral edema, maintain serum glucose, correct electrolyte imbalances, and correct significant coagulopathy
    3. National Reye's Syndrome Foundation, Inc.
       P.O. Box 829
       Bryan, OH 43506-0829
       (800) 233-7393

Questions
Select the best answer

1. Which of the following is not among the physical signs of Fragile X syndrome in adolescent males?

   a. Protruding ears
   b. Macro-orchidism
   c. Hypertonia
   d. Prominent jaw

2. Which of the following physical stigmata are common in newborns with Down syndrome?

   a. Microcephaly, large ears and mouth, flattened philtrum
   b. Hypotonia, large appearing tongue and small mouth, upward slant to eyes
   c. Fair mottled skin, large hands and feet, broad stocky neck
   d. Funnel or pigeon-breasted chest, brushfield spots, extra digits

3. Two month-old-Kathleen, who had a small sacral myelomeningocele repaired shortly after birth, is brought in by her mother for her well-child check. Her head circumference, which had been along the 75th percentile, was measured and plotted to be at the 97th percentile today. Your most appropriate *first* action would be to:

   a. Order a head CT scan
   b. Refer Kathleen to neurosurgery for placement of VP shunt to manage hydrocephalus
   c. Discount that measurement as a "fluke" and recheck it at the next well-child visit
   d. Recheck and replot the child's head circumference yourself at this visit

4. The diagnosis of Down syndrome in the newborn nursery:

   a. Can be made on the basis of clinical findings, making other studies unnecessary
   b. Indicates concern for associated Wilm's tumor
   c. Indicates need for confirmatory chromosomal studies
   d. Always means the child will have a heart defect

5. Mr. and Mrs. Smith's second child recently died of Edwards' Syndrome (Trisomy 18). While you are seeing their first child, they ask about their chances of having another child with Edwards' syndrome. Your best response is:

   a. They should not worry, since Edwards' syndrome is so rare
   b. They have a 1 in 4 chance, since this condition has an autosomal recessive inheritance pattern
   c. They should seek genetic counseling for the best answer to this question
   d. They should not have more children

6. Your 20-month-old-patient has a confirmed diagnosis of Hurler's syndrome, and is being seen for an upper respiratory illness. Anticipatory guidance should include:

   a. Recurrent upper respiratory infections are common in children who have Hurler's syndrome

   b. Development will progress well until at least age 6, and then deteriorate
   c. Genetic counseling is not advisable, since the chances of these parents having another child with Hurler's are extremely small
   d. Vision and hearing evaluation is unnecessary

7. Young infants with cerebral palsy often show:

   a. Voracious appetite and weight gain
   b. Increased muscle tone in the first weeks of life
   c. Hypotonia in the first weeks of life
   d. Unusually severe reactions to their first immunizations

8. Jeremy, age 2, was born at 28 weeks gestation and now has mild spastic diplegia. He is under the care of a pediatric orthopedist, but does not attend an early intervention program, nor does he attend a referral center for the care of children with cerebral palsy. Which evaluations are especially needed for Jeremy before he enters a mainstreamed preschool in the Fall?

   a. The Stanford Binet IQ Test
   b. Vision and speech
   c. CBC with differential
   d. Chromosome studies

9. Children with Marfan syndrome:

   a. Rarely have ophthalmologic problems
   b. Should be closely evaluated for scoliosis throughout childhood and adolescence
   c. Should not be mainstreamed due to fragile medical status
   d. Usually are retarded

10. Which of the following is a *conclusive indicator* for the use of an infant apnea monitor?

   a. Symptomatic premature infants
   b. Infants of opiate or cocaine abusing mothers
   c. A child who has had one sibling die of SIDS
   d. A child who required no stimulation to recover from parent reported episode of child with apnea

11. Which of these factors is not closely associated with SIDS?

   a. Infants between 12 to 14 months of age
   b. Infants who sleep prone
   c. Infants of mothers who smoke
   d. Infants who are over bundled

12. Congenital HIV infection:

   a. Is diagnosed through finding maternal antibodies in infant serum
   b. Does not respond to antiretroviral therapy
   c. May be latent for years before clinical signs develop
   d. Does not include lymphadenopathy as a physical finding

13. Usual features of Fetal Alcohol Syndrome do not include:

    a. Widely spaced eyes with narrow lids
    b. Strabismus
    c. Taller and heavier than other children, beginning at about age 4
    d. Broad nasal bridge

14. It is known that Fetal Alcohol Syndrome (FAS) is caused by maternal alcohol ingestion during pregnancy. Which of the following statements is true?

    a. There is no concern for FAS in infants of mothers who report having only one or two drinks during their first trimester
    b. FAS is dose dependent. Therefore, if a woman drinks only once a day during her pregnancy, she should not be worried
    c. Heavy maternal drinking during the third trimester places the baby at greatest risk for the most abnormalities
    d. The ''dose'' of alcohol that causes FAS is not known

15. HIV infection must be diagnosed by:

    a. Antigen antibody detection
    b. Detection of HIV DNA from whole blood or by PCR of DNA from peripheral blood mononuclear cells
    c. Diagnosis of one or more conditions in the CDC AIDS definition
    d. Diagnosis of AIDS in the mother

16. Several infectious and chemical agents have similar effects on the developing fetus. These must be differentiated, however, in order for effective management to occur. Which of the following infant diseases is not associated with exposure in the first trimester of pregnancy?

    a. Cytomegalic inclusion disease (CMV)
    b. Chlamydia conjunctivitis
    c. Toxoplasmosis
    d. Rubella

17. Hepatitis B is a serious chronic disease which:

    a. Is curable with acyclovir therapy
    b. Is transmitted only by blood and blood products
    c. Results in recognizable disease in the first six weeks of life
    d. Can be prevented in perinatally exposed infants by giving HBIG and hepatitis immunization

18. Through prenatal diagnosis, Mr. and Mrs. Anderson have learned that their expected infant will have Turner's syndrome. Which of the following facts does not apply to Turner's syndrome?

    a. Their child will be a daughter, but will not develop secondary sexual characteristics without medical intervention
    b. Their child will be mentally retarded

    c. With appropriate growth hormone treatment by an endocrinologist, their daughter will show improved growth approximating more typical stature

    d. Their daughter has a relatively high chance of having a congenital heart defect

19. Joshua is the infant son of Mr. and Mrs. Abrahamson, who are of Askenazic Jewish descent. At his 9 month well-child check, his parents express concerns because he has stopped rolling over, seems listless, and is becoming quite irritable. Within your work-up to rule out Tay-Sachs disease, which of the following would not indicate probable Tay-Sachs?

    a. Hypotonia

    b. Retinal detachment

    c. ''Cherry red'' spot on retina

    d. Transluscent appearance and delicate pink coloring to skin

20. Prader-Willi Syndrome is a congenital genetic disorder characterized by:

    a. Failure to thrive

    b. 100% detection rate with chromosome analysis for a 15q deletion

    c. Emergence of spasticity during toddler years

    d. Voracious appetite and development of obesity

21. Stephanie, age 16, is brought to your office having suddenly become acutely ill with headache, sore throat, abdominal cramps, vomiting, watery, non-bloody diarrhea, and confusion. Her skin is clear. She is menstruating. Which of the following would immediately be a high priority in your differential diagnosis?

    a. Rotavirus

    b. Irritable bowel syndrome

    c. Toxic shock syndrome

    d. Marfan syndrome

22. Reye's syndrome is an acute illness that mainly affects the:

    a. Renal system

    b. Musculoskeletal system

    c. Liver and CNS

    d. Gastrointestinal system

23. Individuals who have spina bifida are at high risk for allergy to:

    a. Eggs

    b. Pollens

    c. Latex

    d. Dust mite feces

24. Gonococcal infections in children are best treated with:

    a. Penicillin

    b. Doxycycline

c. Quinolones
d. Ceftriaxone

25. Which of the following does not apply to neonatal disseminated herpes disease?

    a. Hyperactive newborn with apparent spasticity
    b. Clinical picture consistent with sepsis
    c. Infant acutely ill during the first week of life
    d. Unresponsive to antibiotic therapy

Answers

1. c	10. a	18. b
2. b	11. a	19. b
3. d	12. c	20. d
4. c	13. c	21. c
5. c	14. d	22. c
6. a	15. b	23. c
7. c	16. b	24. d
8. b	17. d	25. a
9. b		

Bibliography

American Academy of Pediatrics. (2000). In L. K. Pickering (Ed.). *Red Book 2000: Report of the committee on infectious diseases (25th ed).* Elk Grove Village, IL: Author.

American Academy of Pediatrics committee on pediatrics AIDS. (1999). *Pediatric human immunodeficiency virus (HIV) infection—a compendium of AAP guidelines on pediatric HIV infection.* Elk Grove Village, IL: Author

American Academy of Pediatrics committee on substance abuse and committee on children with disabilities. (2000). Fetal alcohol syndrome and alcohol related neurodevelopmental disorders. *Pediatrics, 106*(2), 358–61.

American Academy of Pediatrics task force on infant sleep position and sudden infant death syndrome. (2000). *Pediatrics, 105*(3), 650–6.

Bass N. (1999). Cerebral palsy and neurodegenerative disease. *Current Opinions in Pediatrics, 11*(6), 504–7.

Hoekelman, R. A., Adam, H. M., Nelson, N. M., Weitzman, M. L., & Wilson, M. H. (Eds.). (2001). *Primary pediatric care* (4th ed.). St. Louis: Mosby Year Book.

Lashley, F. R. (1998). Clinical genetics in nursing practice. (2nd ed.). NY: Springer Publishing.

Monto, A. S. (1999). The disappearance of Reye's syndrome—a public health triumph. *New England Journal of Medicne, 340*(18), 1423–1424.

Head, Eye, Ear, Nose, Mouth and Throat Disorders Infancy Through Adolescence

Connie Paczkowski

Head

Microcephaly

- Definition: Head circumference (HC) 2 to 3 SD or more below the mean for age and sex or HC percentiles that drop with increasing age
- Etiology/Incidence
    1. Variety of dysmorphic syndromes produced by genetic/chromosomal disorders
    2. Intrauterine infections, e.g., TORCH—toxoplasmosis, other agents [HIV, listeria, syphilis, gonococcus, group β streptococcus, varicella-zoster, malaria], rubella, cytomegalovirus, inclusion disease, herpes simplex
    3. Fetal exposure to toxic substances including alcohol, phenylketones (maternal PKU)
    4. Fetal exposure to radiation in first and/or second trimesters
    5. Placental insufficiency, prenatal hypoxia, trauma, maternal hypoglycemia, degenerative diseases, e.g., Tay Sachs
    6. Extremely poor nutrition during the first six months of life
- Signs and Symptoms
    1. In full term birth and up to six months of age, chest circumference surpasses head circumference (unless child is very obese)
    2. Delayed developmental milestones; neurological problems, e.g., seizures, spasticity
    3. Family history of microcephaly
- Differential Diagnosis
    1. Craniosynostosis
    2. Endocrine disorders, e.g., hypopituitary function, hypothyroidism
    3. Severe malnutrition
- Physical Findings
    1. Early closure of fontanel; prominent cranial sutures
    2. Marked downward sloped forehead with narrowed temporal diameter and occipital flattening (familial microcephaly)
    3. Skull asymmetries, high arched palate and dysplastic teeth (dysmorphic and chromosomal disorders)
- Diagnostic Tests/Findings
    1. Karyotyping for chromosomal disorders, e.g., Fragile X syndrome
    2. Antibody titers for TORCH infections
    3. Test infant serum and urine for amino and organic acids
    4. CT or MRI to detect calcification, malformations or atrophy

- Management/Treatment

    1. Complete history and physical findings crucial to finding treatable disorders, e.g., hypopituitarism, severe protein-calorie malnutrition

    2. Premature closure of sutures may be surgically corrected

    3. Most disorders are untreatable; accurate diagnosis is essential for appropriate genetic and family counseling (Behrman, 2000)

    4. Management is supportive

Macrocephaly

- Definition: Head circumference greater than 2 to 3 SD from the mean for age, sex and gestation or one that increases too rapidly

- Etiology/Incidence

    1. Most likely causes of excessive head growth include hydrocephalus, extra-axial fluid collections, metabolic/genetic disorders and neoplasms

    2. Normal head growth with large heads include:

        a. Familial macrocephaly (benign)

        b. Megalencephaly (large brain) found with neurofibromatosis

- Signs and Symptoms

    1. Excessive head growth

    2. Dependent on cause, e.g., hydrocephalus

- Differential Diagnosis

    1. Benign macrocephaly—familial or catch up growth in thriving premature infant

    2. Pathological macrocephaly

- Physical Findings

    1. Progressive excessive head growth greater than 2 to 3 SD above the mean for age/sex as delineated on growth chart

    2. Transillumination of skull may reveal chronic subdural effusions, hydrocephaly or large cystic defects

    3. May have extensive findings depending on underlying cause

- Diagnostic Tests/Findings: CT, MRI or ultrasonography of anterior fontanel (if not closed) can:

    1. Define structural cause; determine if operable disorder

    2. If benign, provide more accurate diagnosis, prognosis, guide to management and genetic counseling

    3. Provide basis of comparison if future study is necessary

- Management/Treatment
  1. CT, MRI or ultrasound of head if any signs/symptoms of increased intracranial pressure
  2. Surgical correction of premature closure of sutures
  3. Genetic counseling

Caput Succedaneum

- Definition: Diffuse swelling of soft tissue of the scalp which usually crosses suture lines with possible bruising
- Etiology/Incidence: Trauma to scalp while baby descends through birth canal causing edema of scalp, skin and muscles; associated with molding
- Signs and symptoms: Swelling of scalp with some ecchymosis involving the presenting portion of occiput during vertex delivery
- Differential Diagnosis: Cephalohematoma
- Physical Findings: Swelling and bruising of parietal region of the scalp; edema crosses suture line
- Diagnostic Tests/Findings: None
- Management/Treatment
  1. Usually unnecessary with spontaneous resolution within a few days
  2. If extensive ecchymosis, may require phototherapy for hyperbilirubinemia

Cephalohematoma

- Definition: Subperiosteal collection of blood bound by suture lines
- Etiology/Incidence
  1. Slow subperiosteal bleed from trauma due to difficult delivery
  2. Coagulopathy or intracranial hemorrhage
  3. 25% overlie linear skull fracture—not depressed
- Signs and Symptoms
  1. Presents hours to days after delivery; limited to periosteum at suture margins
  2. Occasionally prolongs neonatal jaundice
- Differential Diagnosis
  1. Caput succedaneum
  2. Cranial meningocele
- Physical Findings: Nonecchymotic swelling of parietal area that does not cross suture lines

- Diagnostic Tests: None
- Management/Treatment
    1. Usually unnecessary with resolution within a few weeks/months
    2. Calcification of hematoma possible; may be felt as bony prominence
    3. Observance for hyperbilirubinemia

Hydrocephalus

- Definition: Increased production, impaired absorption or obstruction in flow of cerebrospinal fluid (CSF), leading to dilatation of cerebral ventricles
- Etiology/Incidence
    1. Obstruction of CSF flow anywhere along its route
    2. Origin may be:
        a. Congenital, due to primary cerebral malformation
        b. Acquired postnatally, secondary to tumor, hemorrhage or infection
    3. Obstructive or noncommunicating hydrocephalus
        a. Major cause of hydrocephalus
        b. Obstruction of CSF within ventricular system before CSF reaches subarachnoid space
        c. Sites include aqueduct of Sylvius and obstruction of fourth ventricle (Arnold-Chiari and Dandy-Walker)
    4. Nonobstructive or communicating hydrocephalus
        a. Impairment of CSF within subarachnoid space
        b. Impairment of absorption
        c. Usually caused by scarring due to subarachnoid hemorrhage or meningitis
        d. Most commonly occurs over convexities
    5. Choroid plexus papilloma
        a. Overproduction of CSF
        b. Rare cause of hydrocephalus
- Signs and Symptoms: Presentation is variable depending on age and etiology
    1. Birth to 12 months—apparent large head, sluggish feeding, vomiting, piercing cry and irritability
    2. 12 months through adolescence—signs of increased intracranial pressure (ICP), headache following sleep, lethargy or irritability; confusion, personality changes; possible decline in academic performance; signs and symptoms related to specific focal lesion or tumor

- Differential Diagnosis
  1. Macrocephaly
  2. Megalencephaly
  3. Benign large head
  4. Macrocrania
  5. Meningitis
  6. Sepsis
  7. Tumor
- Physical Findings
  1. Infancy—bulging anterior fontanel, scalp vein distention, bossing, "setting sun sign", separated skull sutures, slow PERRL, hypertonia, hyper-reflexia, spasticity
  2. Childhood—strabismus, extrapyramidal tract signs (ataxia), papilledema, optic atrophy, growth failure from endocrine dysfunction
- Diagnostic Tests/Findings
  1. Cranial radiograph—separated sutures
  2. CT scan/ultrasound—impaired CSF circulation causing ventricular enlargement
  3. Ventriculography—obstruction detection
- Management/Treatment
  1. Most cases require extracranial shunts, particularly ventriculoperitoneal types (Behrman, 2000)
  2. Treatment of underlying cause, e.g., mass or lesion, inflammation, infection, vasogenic edema
  3. Anticipatory guidance for families and caregivers throughout child's life
     a. Referral to support groups
     b. Teaching signs and symptoms of ICP
     c. Daily head circumference measurements
     d. Management of psychomotor challenges

EYE

Conjunctivitis of the Newborn (Ophthalmia Neonatrum)
- Definition: Infection and/or inflammation of conjunctiva in first month of life
- Etiology/Incidence

1. Chemical—irritation from use of silver nitrate or other ophthalmic preparations (occurs in 10% of newborns); erythromycin ophthalmic ointment commonly used in place of silver nitrate with less irritation

2. Gonocococcal—perinatal transmission of *Neisseria gonorrhoeae;* prophylactic treatment with erythromycin ophthalmic ointment 0.5%, topical silver nitrate 1%, tetracycline 1%, or povidone-iodine 2% (AAP, 2000)

3. Inclusion—perinatal transmission of *Chlamydia trachomatis* during vaginal birth; occurs in 50% of infants born to infected mothers (AAP, 2000)

4. Other pathogens after first week of life include *Haemophilus influenzae, Staphylococcus aureus,* enterococci and herpes simplex virus (HSV)

- Signs and Symptoms

  1. Chemical—mild injection of conjunctiva, presents several hours following ophthalmic drop/ointment instillation lasting no longer than 3 to 4 days

  2. Gonococcal—acute purulent discharge 2 to 4 days after birth

  3. Chlamydia—usually presents with mild mucopurulent discharge a few days to several weeks after birth

  4. Other bacteria—purulent discharge normally seen on 5th day

  5. Virus—serous discharge

- Differential Diagnosis

  1. Dacryostenosis

  2. Foreign body

  3. Corneal abrasion

- Physical Findings

  1. Chemical—conjunctival hyperemia, minimal lid edema, scanty discharge

  2. Gonococcal—chemosis, significant lid edema; purulent discharge

  3. Chlamydia—minimal lid edema, conjunctival hyperemia, chemosis, concomitant pneumonia (afebrile, repetitive staccato cough, tachypnea and rales)

  4. Other bacteria—lid edema and chemosis

  5. Herpes simplex—possible serous discharge

- Diagnostic Tests/Findings

  1. Gram and Giemsa stain—gonococci revealed as intracellular gram negative diplococci; chlamydia is revealed as basophilic intracytoplasmic inclusions in the conjunctival epithelial cells

  2. Cultures—positive for specific organism

  3. Direct fluoroscent antibody staining or enzyme immunoassay—detection of HSV antigens

4. Immune fluorescent antibody testing for chlamydia organisms

- Management/Treatment

    1. Chemical—no treatment necessary; resolves spontaneously without sequelae; decreased incidence with use of erythromycin ophthalmic ointment in place of silver nitrate

    2. Gonococcal—hospitalization is necessary; eye should be irrigated initially with normal saline every 10 to 30 minutes gradually decreasing to every 2 hour intervals until purulent discharge is cleared; ceftriaxone 25 to 50 mg/kg/day, IV or IM not to exceed 125 mg given as a single dose; cefotaxime 100 mg/kg/day, IV or IM given as a single dose is an alternative; topical treatment alone is inadequate and unnecessary when systemic therapy is given (AAP, 2000)

    3. Chlamydia conjunctivitis and pneumonia—oral erythromycin 50 mg/kg/day in four divided doses for 10 to 14 days; oral sulfonamides may be used after immediate neonatal period for infants intolerant to erythromycin; topical treatment ineffective and unnecessary; efficacy of erythromycin therapy is 80%, second course sometimes required (AAP, 2000)

    4. Other bacteria—organism dependent; erythromycin ointment every six hours for gram positive organisms; gentamicin ophthalmic solution every six hours for gram negative organisms; moist compresses

    5. Stress thorough hand washing, no sharing of wash cloths or towels

    6. Herpes simplex—treat with idoxuridine, trifluridine, or vidarabine topical ophthalmic preparations in addition to parenteral therapy, under ophthalmologists direction (AAP, 2000)

    7. Mothers and sexual partner(s) should also be treated appropriately

Conjunctivitis of Childhood

- Definition: Inflammation and/or infection of palpabral (lining of eye lids) and bulbar (layer of tissue over the sclera) conjunctiva in children one month or older

- Etiology/Incidence

    1. Most frequent ocular disorder in children; may be associated with otitis media indicating bacterial infection with beta-lactamase resistant organism

    2. Very contagious especially in day care and school age children

    3. Bacterial conjunctivitis—most common pathogens include *Staphylococcus aureus, Haemophilus influenzae* and *Streptococcus pneumoniae* (Graham & Uphold, 1999; Behrman, 2000)

    4. Viral conjunctivitis primarily due to adenovirus 3, 4 and 7; also caused by herpes simplex and varicella zoster

    5. Allergic and vernal (chronic allergic) conjunctivitis—often with unidentified cause; commonly associated with seasonal allergens

- Signs and Symptoms
    1. Pruritus, foreign body sensation, tearing
    2. Headache
    3. Possible sensitivity to light
    4. Discharge
        a. Viral, allergic—watery or thick/stringy mucoid
        b. Bacterial—purulent
- Differential Diagnosis
    1. Nasolacrimal duct obstruction
    2. Blepharitis in older children
    3. Keratitis (can be seen with herpes simplex conjunctivitis)
    4. Systemic infection presenting with conjunctivitis, e.g. rubella, rubeola, Kawasaki
    5. Periorbital cellulitis
- Physical Findings
    1. Discharge, rhinitis
    2. Eyelid edema
    3. Moderate to severe erythema of conjunctiva; chemosis
    4. Preauricular adenopathy commonly seen with viral pathogens
    5. Malaise, pharyngitis and fever may be present
    6. Cobblestone-like papillary hypertrophy along inner aspect of upper lid (vernal conjunctivitis)
- Diagnostic Tests/Findings
    1. Cultures and sensitivities usually unnecessary unless pseudomonas, neisseria or other virulent organism suspected (Graham & Uphold, 1999)
    2. Rule out corneal infiltration with fluorescein stain
- Management/Treatment
    1. Bacterial—most respond readily to topical ophthalmic antibiotics, e.g., tobramycin, erythromycin (used if gram negative bacteria suspected), sulfacetamide, or poly-myxin B sulfate-trimethoprim, one drop each eye every 4 to 6 hours; if concomitant otitis media, also treat with oral antimicrobials
    2. Viral—artificial tears for lubrication, topical steroids (only by ophthalmologist) if keratitis present
    3. Herpes—initial infection self limited, virus remains latent; can recur in children

with recurrent keratitis, ophthalmologist referral necessary; **any child with a history of a herpes ocular infection who presents with red eye, lid vesicles or corneal staining with fluorescein should be referred immediately;** treatment includes topical and systemic antivirals

4. Allergic—avoidance of known allergens, cold compresses, systemic or topical antihistamines, nonsteroidal anti-inflammatories or topical mast cell stabilizers (e.g., cromolyn sodium), refer to ophthalmologist for chronic conjunctivitis

5. Good hand washing and hygiene; stress control of cross contamination, avoid shared linen; cleanse eye lashes with warm sterile water wiping from inner canthus outward

6. Ophthalmologist referral needed:

   a. If conjunctivitis is unresponsive to treatment within 2 to 3 days

   b. If associated with loss of vision, pain, photophobia

   c. If severe conjunctivitis or with corneal/orbital cellulitis involvement

Dacryostenosis

- Definition: Unilateral or bilateral obstruction of the nasolacrimal duct, usually at nasal punctal opening

- Etiology/Incidence

   1. Due to failure of duct canalization during gestation

   2. May also occur secondary to trauma or infection

   3. 90% spontaneous resolution by 12 months

   4. Most common lacrimal disorder in infants

- Signs and Symptoms: Continuous or intermittent tearing (wet look in the eye) with crusting of lashes

- Differential Diagnosis

   1. Ophthalmia neonatorum, conjunctivitis

   2. Dacryocystitis—inflammation/infection of obstructed nasolacrimal duct

   3. Glaucoma

   4. Intraocular inflammation

   5. External irritation

- Physical Findings

   1. Tearing

   2. Expression of thin mucopurulent exudate from lacrimal sac

   3. Inflammation/infection of conjunctiva

4. Signs of dacryocystitis—fever, erythema and edema of lid and/or over lacrimal sac or duct, excoriation of surrounding tissue

- Management/Treatment

    1. Gently massage lacrimal sac and nasolacrimal duct by frequently stroking skin from brow area along lateral aspect of nose

    2. For conjunctivitis or purulent discharge, administration of sodium sulfacetamide or erythromycin ointment

    3. Referral to ophthalmologist by six months of age or earlier for evaluation and treatment if no improvement with antibiotics and massage

    4. Persistent obstruction and recurrent purulent drainage beyond six to twelve months, may require surgical probing of duct

    5. Severe dacryocystitis requires referral to ophthalmologist and systemic antibiotics

Chalazion

- Definition: Obstruction of meibomian glands lining posterior margins of upper or lower lids; usually involves midportion of tarsus resulting in an inflammatory lipogranuloma

- Etiology/Incidence: Unknown cause

- Signs and Symptoms

    1. Progressive swelling of lid

    2. Slight discomfort

    3. Minimal redness

- Differential Diagnosis

    1. Blepharitis

    2. Hordeolum

    3. Sebaceous cell carcinoma (rare)

- Physical Findings

    1. Firm, nontender, nonmovable nodule often on palpebral surface of lid

    2. Large chalazions may cause chronic pressure on cornea leading to astigmatism

- Diagnostic Tests/Findings: None indicated

- Management/Treatment

    1. Small chalazions may resolve without treatment

    2. Warm compresses 2 to 3 times a day for 20 minutes for 2 to 3 days

    3. Treat large, recurrent or infected lesions with local antibacterial drops or ointments (sulfacetamide sodium 10%) q.i.d. for one week

4. If unresponsive to treatment, refer to opthalmologist for surgical excision or cortico-steroid injections

Blepharitis (Granulation of Eyelids)

- Definition:

    1. Common acute or chronic inflammation of eyelash follicles and meibomian glands of eyelid margins

    2. Types

        a. Seborrheic, ulcerated or combination of both

        b. Bacterial infection of lash follicles

- Etiology/Incidence

    1. Seborrheic blepharitis may be associated with seborrheic dermatitis, psoriasis, eczema or allergies; chemicals, smoke, air pollution and cosmetics can aggravate condition

    2. *Staphylococcus aureus* is primary causative pathogen

    3. Common in early childhood; associated with Down Syndrome; eczema

- Signs and Symptoms

    1. Irritation, burning

    2. Sensation of foreign body

    3. Erythema of eyelid margins

    4. Pruritus

    5. Loss of eye lashes

- Differential Diagnosis

    1. Chalazion, conjunctivitis, superficial keratitis

    2. Hordeolum

    3. Seborrhea, pediculosis of eyelashes

- Physical Findings

    1. Seborrheic form—hypertrophy and desquamation of epidermis adjacent to eye lid margin

    2. Loss of eye lashes

    3. Translucent, easily removable scales

    4. Ulcerative form—purulent inflammation with ulcer formation on lid margins with erythema and bleeding; if condition progresses, leads to eyelid margin distortion and possible ectropion

    5. May be associated with conjunctivitis and superficial keratitis

- Diagnostic Tests/Findings: None indicated
- Management/Treatment: Similar for both forms
  1. Warm moist compresses to lid margins several times/day
  2. Daily mechanical scrubbing and cleansing of lid margins with cotton tipped applicator or soft cloth, dipped in dilute baby shampoo
  3. Application of topical antibiotic ointment massaged into lid margins (sulfacetamide sodium 10% or polymyxin B-bacitracin)
  4. When seborrheic dermatitis of the scalp is present, frequent shampooing with selenium sulfide recommended
  5. Continue treatment for several weeks if necessary; recurrences are common

Hordeolum (Stye)

- Definition: An acute localized inflammation of one or more sebaceous glands (meibomian or zeisian) of eyelids
- Etiology/Incidence: Most common infectious pathogen is *Staphylococcus aureus;* highest incidence in children/adolescence
- Signs and Symptoms
  1. Sudden onset of tenderness, redness and swelling of affected lid
  2. Foreign body sensation
- Differential Diagnosis
  1. Chalazion
  2. Blepharitis
  3. Inclusion cyst
- Physical Findings
  1. Painful erythematous swelling on either skin (external stye) or conjunctival (internal stye) surface
  2. May suppurate and drain spontaneously
- Diagnostic Tests/Findings: Culture not necessary
- Management/Treatment
  1. Warm moist compresses for 15 minutes three to four times a day
  2. Sulfacetamide sodium 10% or polymyxin B-bacitracin drops or ointment
  3. Cleanse eye lids with baby shampoo once a day
  4. Refer for incision and drainage if unresponsive to treatment
  5. Dispose of old eye makeup; discourage use of eye makeup until hordeolum is resolved; stress good hand and eye hygiene

Orbital/Periorbital Cellulitis

- Definition
    1. Orbital—inflammation of the orbital contents posterior to orbital septum
    2. Periorbital—inflammation/infection of the skin and subcutaneous tissue surrounding eye; often associated with trauma, septicemia, sinusitis and bacteremia or local infection near the eye
- Etiology/Incidence
    1. Orbit or preseptal areas are infected from local trauma or spread from proximate structures or body parts
    2. Most common causes of bacterial orbital cellulitis in children are paranasal sinusitis and ethmoiditis
    3. Other causes include insect stings or bites, impetigo, foreign body
    4. Most common organisms are *Staphylococcus aureus, Streptococcus pneumoniae, Haemophilus influenzae*
    5. Periorbital cellulitis much more common than orbital cellulitis
- Signs and Symptoms
    1. Orbital cellulitis
        a. Insidious onset
        b. Orbital pain, headache
        c. Decreased vision
        d. Fever
    2. Periorbital cellulitis
        a. Acute onset of unilateral eyelid swelling
        b. Warmth, swelling and tenderness of overlying skin
        c. Eye itself and vision are usually normal
    3. Rhinorrhea, fever (102° to 104° F)
- Differential Diagnosis
    1. Differentiate between orbital (within true orbit), periorbital or preseptal (surrounding orbital septum) cellulitis
    2. Edema secondary to trauma
    3. Allergic periorbital edema
    4. Insect bite
- Physical Findings
    1. Orbital cellulitis

a. Lid edema

b. Chemosis

c. Proptosis

d. Decreased ocular mobility

e. Decreased visual acuity

f. Ophthalmoplegia (paralysis of eye muscles) and proptosis (protrusion of eyeball)—classic findings and distinguish orbital from periorbital cellulitis

2. Periorbital cellulitis

a. Unilateral eyelid edema

b. Erythema

c. Tenderness of overlying skin

d. Visual acuity usually normal

- Diagnostic Tests/Findings

1. Visual acuity exam—decreased vision with orbital cellulitis only

2. Sinus roentgenograms or CT scan—determine sinus involvement

3. Orbital sonography—determine orbit involvement

4. CBC with differential—leukocytosis

5. Blood and/or eye cultures—determine pathogen

6. Lumbar punctures with infants—rule out sepsis

- Management/Treatment

1. Prompt assessment, treatment and referral

2. Systemic antibiotic therapy, primarily IV

3. Moderate to severe cases or children under 1 year old may need hospitalization

4. Complications may include loss of vision, subperiosteal or orbital abscess, meningitis, epidural and subdural abscess, thrombosis in the retina or sinus

Cataracts

- Definition: Partial or complete opacity of the lens

- Etiology/Incidence: May be congenital or acquired during childhood; unilateral or bilateral; can result in significant amblyopia

1. Congenital—results from genetic anomalies, prematurity and/or drug exposure, hypocalcemia, or maternal rubella during first trimester

2. Acquired cataracts due to:

a. Trauma to the orbit

b. Systemic disease—diabetes mellitus, Trisomy 21, hypoparathyroidism, galactosemia, atopic dermatitis, hypocalcemia, Marfan's syndrome

c. Ingestion of poisons found in moth balls/crystals, insecticides

d. Long term use of systemic corticosteroids or ocular corticosteroid drops

e. Complications from other ocular abnormalities, e.g., glaucoma, uveitis, strabismus, pendibular nystagmus with severe amblyopia

- Signs and Symptoms: Severity of visual acuity deficits depends on location and degree of opacity; no pain

- Differential Diagnosis
   1. Retinoblastoma
   2. Glaucoma

- Physical Findings
   1. Strabismus—may be initial sign of cataract in child
   2. Absent red reflex, black dot(s) surrounded by red reflex, or white plaque-like opacities
   3. Signs of other systemic diseases and ocular abnormalities as noted in etiology

- Management/Treatment
   1. Prompt referral to ophthalmologist for diagnosis/treatment
   2. Surgical measures indicated if vision unable to develop due to extent of cataract; visual correction
   3. Determine etiology; any positive family history of congenital cataracts; question if an isolated disorder or part of systemic disorder

Glaucoma

- Definition: Increased intraocular pressure from disruption of aqueous fluid circulation involving one or both eyes resulting in optic nerve damage with loss of visual acuity and eventual blindness

- Etiology/Incidence
   1. Congenital—present at birth and up to 3 years of age
   2. Primary—isolated anomaly of drainage apparatus; 50% of infantile glaucoma is primary; occurs in only 0.03% (Behrman, 2000)
   3. Secondary or juvenile (3 to 30 year olds) from various causes, e.g., trauma, intraocular hemorrhage, intraocular tumor
   4. Possible complication of corticosteroid therapy, ocular injury or disease
   5. May be associated with other developmental anomalies, e.g., Marfan's, neurofibromatosis, congenital rubella syndrome, Pierre Robins syndrome

- Signs and Symptoms
    1. Classic triad ($\frac{1}{3}$ of infants demonstrate these)—photophobia, abnormal overflow of tears (epiphora), blepharospasm (eyelid spasm) (Behrman, 2000)
    2. Decreased vision (peripheral first) leading to tunnel vision
    3. Persistent, extreme pain (occasionally)
- Differential Diagnosis: Cataracts
- Physical Findings
    1. Corneal and ocular enlargement demonstrated as linear white opacities; corneal haziness and edema; firm to pressure
    2. Stretching of corneal and scleral tissues (in primary); thin, bluish sclera with pupillary dilation
    3. Deep cupping of optic disc
    4. Moderate injection or erythema (frequently unilateral) usually bulbar near limbus
- Diagnostic Tests/Findings: Glaucoma pressure test will show increased pressure
- Management/Treatment
    1. Immediate referral to ophthalmologist to confirm diagnosis and initiate therapy
    2. Topical beta blockers and carbonic anhydrase inhibitors; surgery indicated to relieve intraocular pressure (75% success rate)
    3. Enucleation may be necessary
    4. Glaucoma progresses slowly; blindness is highly probable without treatment

Strabismus

- Definition: Ocular misalignment; eyes may deviate outward (exotropia), inward (esotropia), downward (hypotropia) or upward (hyperopia)
- Etiology/Incidence
    1. Intermittent alternating esotropia or exotropia normal in first four to six months of life
    2. Suppression is an adaptation to diplopia; without correction permanent loss of vision is probable
    3. Acquired strabismus occurring after 6 months of age usually from cataracts, retinoblastoma, anisometropia or high refractive errors
    4. Strabismus occurs in 4% of children under 6 years (Behrman, 2000)
    5. Pseudostrabismus—eyes appear to be crossed due to epicanthal folds on either side of bridge of nose; no ocular deviation
- Signs and Symptoms
    1. Varies with age

2. Squinting

3. Decreased vision

4. School problems

5. Head tilting

6. Face turning

7. Over pointing

8. Awkwardness

- Differential Diagnosis

  1. Cataracts

  2. Retinoblastoma

  3. Anisometropia

  4. High refractive errors

  5. Amblyopia

  6. Head trauma

  7. Other congenital eye muscle syndromes

- Physical Findings

  1. Misalignment of eye(s)

  2. Intermittent, alternating or continuous esotropia, exotropia, hypertropia or hypotropia

- Diagnostic Tests/Findings

  1. Abnormal Hirschberg (corneal light reflex unequal) and/or cover/uncover test (movement of covered eye)

  2. Vision screen—may reveal refractive errors, amblyopia or anisometropia

- Management/Treatment

  1. Referral to ophthalmologist

     a. Any children over 6 months with fixed or continuous strabismus

     b. Earlier if other developmental delays are present or deviations are continuous or fixed

     c. Signs of differential diagnosis present

     d. Suspicious history

     e. Immediate if hypotropia or hypertropia is present at any age

  2. Acquired—appropriate treatment depending on pathology and/or refractive errors

3. Patching of fixing eye forces use of deviating eye; orthoptic exercises, corrective lenses may or may not be indicated; surgical alignment may be considered

Nystagmus

- Definition: Involuntary, horizontal, vertical, rotary, or mixed rhythmic movement of eyes
- Etiology/Incidence
  1. Caused by abnormality in one of three basic mechanisms—fixation, conjugate gaze or vestibular mechanisms (Behrman, 2000)
  2. May be familial
  3. Associated with albinism, refractive errors, central nervous system (CNS) abnormalities and various diseases of inner ear and retina
  4. Classified according to direction of movement
- Signs and Symptoms
  1. Irregular eye movements
  2. Abnormal head movements; may be rhythmic
- Differential Diagnosis: Underlying cause
- Physical Findings
  1. Involuntary rhythmic eye movements
  2. Vision screen may be abnormal
- Diagnostic Tests/Findings: Abnormal visual acuity test
- Management/Treatment
  1. Refer to ophthalmologist and neurologist (as necessary)
  2. Treat underlying cause
  3. Monitor child closely

Retinoblastoma

- Definition: Congenital malignancy of retina
  1. Most common malignant intraocular tumor of childhood
  2. See discussion in chapter on Hematologic/Oncologic/Immunologic Disorders

Refractive Errors

Hyperopia (Farsightedness)

- Definition: Alteration in refractive power when visual image is focused behind the retina; ability to see objects clearly at a distance, but not at close range
- Etiology/Incidence

1. Axial length of eye too short and/or due to insufficient convexity of the refracting surfaces of the eye especialy the cornea

2. Familial pattern common

- Signs and Symptoms

   1. Often asymptomatic due to children's ability to easily accommodate for hyperopia

   2. Headache and eye strain during prolonged periods of close work in older children

   3. Strabismus often seen with severe hyperopia

- Differential Diagnosis

   1. Astigmatism

   2. Myopia

   3. Anisometropia

   4. Amblyopia

- Physical Findings: Abnormal vision screen

- Diagnostic Tests/Findings: Vision screen shows hyperopia

- Management/Treatment

   1. Refer to ophthalmologist or optometrist

   2. If strabismus present, see previous section for management

   3. Annual eye examinations

Myopia (Nearsightedness)

- Definition: Alteration in refractive power when visual image is focused in front of retina; ability to see objects clearly at close range, but not at a distance

- Etiology/Incidence

   1. Axial length of eye too long and/or increased curvature of the refracting surfaces of the eye, especially the cornea

   2. Familial pattern common; frequently associated with prematurity

   3. Myopia may be present at birth; usually appears around 8 to 10 years of age

- Signs and Symptoms

   1. Distant objects blurred

   2. Squinting forms physiologic pinhole to improve acuity

   3. Difficulty reading blackboard

- Differential Diagnosis

   1. Hyperopia

   2. Astigmatism

3. Anisometropia

4. Amblyopia

- Physical Findings: Abnormal vision screen

- Diagnostic Tests/Findings: Abnormal vision screen

- Management/Treatment

    1. Refer to ophthalmologist or optometrist

    2. Importance of annual eye examinations

Astigmatism

- Definition: Refractive error due to an irregular curvature of the cornea or changes in the lens causing light rays to bend in different directions

- Etiology/Incidence

    1. Familial developmental variations in the curvature of the cornea

    2. Depending on severity of curvature variation, retina can't focus regardless of distance

    3. Increased risk secondary to injury, periorbital or eyelid hemangiomas or ptosis (Behrman, 2000)

- Signs and Symptoms

    1. Commonly found in conjunction with other refractive errors

    2. Pain in and around eyes, headache, fatigue, reading problems, frowning

- Differential Diagnosis

    1. Myopia

    2. Hyperopia

    3. Amblyopia

    4. Anisometropia

- Physical Findings: Possible abnormal vision screen

- Diagnostic Tests/Findings: Vision screen with possible abnormality

- Management/Treatment

    1. Refer to ophthalmologist or optometrist

    2. Corrective lenses or contacts may be prescribed; patching may be recommended

Blindness (Amaurosis)

- Definition

    1. Varies from inability to distinguish light from darkness to partial vision

2. Best corrected visual acuity between 20/70 to 20/200

3. Legal blindness is distant acuity 20/200 in better eye or visual field; includes an angle of no greater than 20 degrees

4. Primary blindness—present at birth

- Etiology/Incidence

  1. $\frac{1}{3}$ of blindness in children from trauma

  2. Variety of pathological causes—cataracts, glaucoma, retinopathy of prematurity (ROP) (most common cause of severe visual impairment); retinoblastoma, trauma, detached retina, cranial nerve II problems, infection, hydrocephalus, genetic problems

- Signs and Symptoms: Varies with age and mode of onset, abilities of child, laterality and severity of deficit

  1. Developmental delays, e.g., gross motor, walking often delayed to 18 to 24 months

  2. Social skills—increased passivity, increased anxiety around strangers

  3. Decreased social communication and school performance

  4. Increased self-stimulating behavior, e.g., hand flapping, rocking, rubbing eyes

  5. Language delay; cognitive delays, understanding of object permanence; cause/effect

  6. Delay in development of conversational skills

  7. Photophobia, chronic tearing, wandering eyes

  8. Lack of smiling response to visual stimuli

- Differential Diagnosis: If primary or from birth

  1. Developmental malformations

  2. Damage consequent to gestational/perinatal infection

  3. Anoxia, hypoxia, perinatal trauma

  4. Genetically determined diseases

- Physical Findings: In primary blindness

  1. Nystagmus (may be first clue)

  2. Enlarged or cloudy cornea; abnormal or absent red reflex

  3. Lack of pupillary reflex; optic disc pallor; pigmentary deposits

  4. Fixed or intermittent strabismus beyond 6 months of age

  5. History of prematurity with retinopathy of prematurity (ROP)

  6. Possible neurological disorder

- Diagnostic Tests/Findings

  1. Ophthalmologic examination—abnormal as described above

2. Developmental testing—delays as outlined

3. CT or MRI—rule out physiological abnormalities

- Management/Treatment

    1. Obtain complete family genetic visual impairment history

    2. Address family issues; social and emotional needs of child

    3. General medical and development history

    4. Metabolic and genetic studies

    5. Prompt referral to ophthalmologist, neurologist and developmental specialist

Amblyopia (Lazy Eye)

- Definition: Decreased visual acuity in one or both eyes with no apparent abnormality on physical examination, despite correction of any refractive error; suppression of retinal image in affected eye to avoid diplopia

- Etiology/Incidence

    1. Organic—trauma, organic lesion, cataract, diseases of the eye or visual pathways, ptosis

    2. Nonorganic—sensory stimulation deprivation or disuse; abnormal binocular interaction during infancy and early childhood (greatest risk between 2 to 3 years of age but can continue until 9 years of age); large difference in refractive errors between both eyes (anisometropia)

    3. Rarely bilateral; associated with strabismus

    4. Occurs in 2% to 5% of general population

    5. Five types—deprivation (ptosis, opacities), strabismic, anisometropic, occlusion (patching good eye too much), ametropic (both eyes large refractive errors, typically hyperopic and/or astigmatism)

- Signs and Symptoms: Wandering eye

- Differential Diagnosis

    1. Cataracts

    2. Blindness

    3. Ptosis

- Physical Examination

    1. Negative red reflex

    2. Ptosis

    3. Strabismus

- Diagnostics Tests/Findings

1. Abnormal vision and/or ophthalmic examination—abnormal red reflex, positive cover/uncover test, unequal corneal light reflex

2. Abnormal ocular movements

- Management/Treatment

    1. Early detection, prompt intervention, referral to ophthalmologist

    2. Effective vision screening before 3 years of age

    3. Corrective lenses

    4. Occlusion therapy forcing stimulation of amblyopic eye (patching good eye)

    5. Close monitoring of occlusion therapy

    6. Reassurance and support throughout treatment

Eye Injuries

General information regarding corneal abrasion, foreign body, hyphema, ecchymosis and chemical injuries

- Definition/Incidence/Etiology

    1. $\frac{1}{3}$ of blindness in children < ten years of age is due to trauma

    2. Sports and activities in which ocular trauma is common include BB guns (most common), archery, darts, motorcycling, bicycling, racquet sports, boxing, basketball and baseball

- Physical Examination

    1. Steps in proper evaluation include:

        a. Recognizing life threatening nonocular conditions, e.g., chemical injuries

        b. Taking adequate history to assess potential risk of injury

        c. Examining in detail (visual acuity, external ocular motility unless ruptured globe suspected), pupil, anterior segment and fundus

        d. Referral for signs and symptons or history of severe ocular injury

    2. Use caution—severe intraocular injury may be concealed behind minimal external trauma

    3. Examine lids, lacrimal system, adnexa, sclera and conjunctiva for lacerations, foreign body or perforation

    4. Palpate orbital rim for crepitus; CT scan when orbital fracture suspected; can be associated with significant intracranial and ocular injuries

    5. A dislocated lens presents with a quivering iris

    6. Topical anesthetic recommended for examination only; slows healing of cornea

- Management/Treatment

1. Ocular injuries requiring immediate referral include:

   a. Chemical injuries

   b. Globe lacerations, severe lacerations of lid

   c. Hyphemas

   d. Penetrating intraocular injury

2. Avoid pressure to globe by placing a protective shield over injured eye

3. Nonaccidental trauma or child abuse should be considered with presence of lid ecchymosis, conjunctival hemorrhages, hyphema or retinal hemorrhages; ideally injuries should be photographed when possible

4. Acetaminophen for pain, no acetylsalicylic acid (ASA)

5. Injury prevention (e.g., protective eyewear)

6. Date of last tetanus vaccine

7. Rabies prophylaxis if trauma from animal bite

8. Refer to ophthalmologist for further assessment

Corneal Abrasion

- Definition: Loss of epithelial lining from corneal surface of one or both eyes
- Etiology/Incidence—abrasion, trauma or foreign bodies in upper lid leading to corneal injury, e.g., paper, brushes, toys or fingernails, contact lenses, ultraviolet light exposure
- Signs and Symptoms

   1. Possible evidence of foreign body

   2. Severe pain and tearing

   3. Blepharospasm

   4. Injection of sclera

   5. Photophobia

- Physical Findings: Epithelial injury visible with use of fluorescein stain and Wood's lamp
- Management/Treatment

   1. Topical anesthetic for evaluation only

   2. Remove foreign body via irrigation with normal saline

   3. Place eye shield for 24 to 48 hours for protection until re-evaluation and/or referral

   4. Refer to ophthalmologist if no improvement after patching

   5. Acetaminophen for discomfort

Foreign Body Eye Injury

- Definition: Foreign body in the eye
- Etiology/Incidence
    1. Surface—nonadherent/loosely adherent to cornea or conjunctival epithelium (most likely sources dirt, sand, grass)
    2. Penetrating—into but not through cornea or sclera
    3. Perforating—through cornea or sclera and into globe
- Signs and Symptoms
    1. Foreign body sensation
    2. Pain
    3. Sensitivity to light
    4. Tearing
    5. Eye rubbing
- Differential Diagnosis
    1. Corneal abrasion
    2. Chemical injury
- Physical Findings
    1. Foreign body may be visualized
    2. Positive fluorescein examination if corneal abrasion present
    3. Epiphora
    4. Possible visual acuity abnormality
- Diagnostic Tests/Findings
    1. Visual acuity—to determine any deviation from normal
    2. Fluorescein test—to determine presence of corneal abrasion
    3. Possible radiographs to visualize foreign body
- Management/Treatment
    1. All intraocular foreign bodies require referral to ophthalmologist
    2. Topical ophthalmic anesthetic drops for examination unless perforating wound suspected
    3. If persistent corneal abrasion after 24 hours with treatment, penetrating or perforation wound, refer to ophthalmologist
    4. Thoroughly examine lashes, lids, cornea and conjunctival surfaces

5. Remove foreign body via irrigation with normal saline

6. After removal, examine for corneal abrasion, treat appropriately

Hyphema

- Definition: Accumulation of blood in anterior chamber
- Etiology/Incidence

    1. Due to blunt or perforating trauma (e.g., balls, fists and sticks) leading to rupture of iris or ciliary body blood vessels; increased risk of rebleeding and glaucoma with traumatic hyphema (Behrman, 2000)

    2. May also occur with bleeding disorders, e.g., sickle cell disease

    3. Usually lasts 5 to 6 days

- Signs and Symptoms

    1. History of ocular injury

    2. Drowsiness

    3. Pain

    4. Light sensitivity

- Physical Findings

    1. Blood in anterior chamber

    2. Visual acuity changes

- Management/Treatment

    1. Refer to ophthalmologist

    2. Reduce activity for several days, bed rest in supine position with head of bed elevated 30 to 40 degrees to promote reabsorption of blood; hospitalization often necessary; eye patch for 5 days on injured eye; no aspirin or reading

    3. Surgery may be necessary to remove blood

Ecchymoses ("Black Eye")

- Definition: Bruising of periorbital region
- Etiology/Incidence: Blunt contusion injury; due to isolated periorbital injury or other orbital/ocular injury
- Signs and Symptoms

    1. Pain

    2. Visual impairment due to occlusion from edematous eyelid

- Differential Diagnosis: Other orbital/ocular injury (e.g., lens dislocation, globe rupture, retinal detachment)

- Physical Findings
    1. Edema
    2. Ecchymosis
- Diagnostic Tests/Findings
    1. Ophthalmic examination—determine other orbital/ocular injuries
    2. Visual acuity
- Management/Treatment
    1. Uncomplicated—cold compresses for 24 to 48 hours; then warm compresses until swelling resolves; elevate head; inform parents/patient that ecchymosis and edema may spread
    2. Refer to ophthalmologist—closed head injury, damage to skull, facial bone fracture

Chemical Injuries

- Definition: Burns of the eye lids, conjunctiva and/or cornea
- Etiology/Incidence
    1. Steam, intense heat and common household agents
    2. Severe alkali injuries characterized by corneal opacification
    3. Amount of damage directly related to duration of exposure
- Management/Treatment
    1. **Acute ocular emergency**
    2. Copious irrigation with normal saline for 20 to 30 minutes—patch and refer to ophthalmologist immediately to rule out corneal or other ocular trauma
    3. Severe chemical injury to eye(s) requires hospitalization
    4. Topical anesthetic may reduce pain from injury and irrigation
    5. Pseudomonal contamination common with any burn possibly leading to corneal ulceration; prevention—antibiotic preparation containing polymyxin B, gentamicin, tobramycin or colistin should be instilled into the injured eye(s) 3 to 4 times a day

Ear

External Otitis Media (EOM)

- Definition: Acute infection and/or inflammation of external auditory canal; "swimmer's ear"
- Etiology/Incidence
    1. More common in summer months due to excessive wetness (swimming, bathing or

increased environmental humidity) which changes the acidic environment and promotes bacterial/fungal growth due to abnormal neutral or basic environment

2. Common organisms are *Pseudomonas aeruginosa* (most common), *Staphylococcus aureus, Streptococcus pyogenes, Enterobacter aerogenes, Proteus mirabilis, Klebsiella pneumoniae, Staphylococcus epidermis,* and fungi, e.g., candida, aspergillus, trichophyton (Graham & Uphold, 1999)

3. Loss of protective cerumen or chronic irritation

4. Trauma disrupting lining of auditory canal, e.g., foreign body, digital irritation

5. Excessive dryness (eczema, psoriasis); contact dermatitis, e.g., poison ivy, medications, hair spray, perfumes

- Signs and Symptoms

  1. Itching of ear canal (early symptom)

  2. Acute and possibly severe ear pain upon manipulation of pinna/tragus, or performance of otoscopic examination; mastoid pain

  3. Pressure/fullness in ear, possible hearing loss (conductive or sensorineural) (Graham & Uphold, 1999)

- Differential Diagnosis

  1. Acute otitis media with perforation

  2. Dental infection

  3. Mastoiditis, furunculosis

  4. Foreign body

  5. Eczema

- Physical Findings

  1. May be difficult to visualize tympanic membrane (TM), however usually normal

  2. Edematous/erythematous external canal

  3. Black spots on TM indicative of fungal infection

  4. Furuncle may be noted with localized infection

  5. Otorrhea (rare), occasional regional lymphadenopathy

  6. Observe for signs of mastoiditis or cellulitis beyond external canal

- Diagnostic Tests/Findings: Culture of discharge unnecessary unless unresponsive to treatment

- Management/Treatment

  1. Withdraw any foreign bodies or debris from external canal by gentle irrigation with warm water or normal saline

2. Topical antibiotic otic drops containing combinations of neomycin, polymyxin, propylene glycol and corticosteroids, 3 to 4 drops, 3 to 4 times/day for 7 to 10 days

3. If significant swelling, insert cotton wick saturated with antibiotic solution for first 24 to 48 hours

4. Systemic analgesic often required for severe pain

5. Re-examine 1 to 2 weeks for evaluation of TM and removal of any debris

6. Prevention—instillation of white vinegar and rubbing alcohol (50/ 50) in both ear canals after swimming; avoid water in canals, vigorous cleaning, scratching or prolonged use of cerumenolytic agents

7. Incision and drainage (I + D) of furuncle if present

8. Fungal infection treated with 5% boric acid in ethanol solution for 5 to 7 days

Acute Otitis Media (AOM)

- Definition: Inflammation of the middle ear with fluid and associated signs and symptoms of ear infection (suppurative otitis media)

- Etiology/Incidence

    1. Fluid/pathogen accumulation in middle ear due to eustachian tube malfunction secondary to obstruction caused by allergies, viral infections, decreased patency and/or other mechanical factors

    2. Common pathogenic agents

        a. *Streptococcus pneumoniae* (most common, 40%)

        b. *Haemophilus influenzae* (25% to 30%)

        c. *Moraxella catarrhalis* (10% to 20%)

        d. Less common pathogens—*Staphylococcus aureus,* group A beta hemolytic streptococcus and *Pseudomonas aeruginosa,* (more common in chronic otitis media)

        e. Viruses—Influenza, RSV (most common), adenovirus, parainfluenza and coronavirus

        f. Prevalence of β-lactamase producing strains highest in past 15 years

        g. Increase in drug resistant bacteria, especially in children younger than 24 months; those who recently were treated with β-lactamase antibiotics and children exposed to large numbers of children

        h. No growth found in 16% of AOM

    3. Predisposing factors

        a. Physiological considerations—eustachian tube of child under 6 years of age is short, wide, and horizontal allowing access of pathogens from nasopharynx to reach middle ear

   b. Possible hereditary factors

   c. Common occurrence with/following upper respiratory infection

   d. Bottle feeding in supine position and/or no breast feeding

   e. Craniofacial abnormalities, e.g., cleft palate

   f. Allergic rhinitis

   g. Tobacco smoke exposure

   h. Children in group day care centers at higher risk than those in home care

  4. One of the most common pediatric diagnoses—highest prevalence between 6 to 36 months

  5. Highest incidence in winter/spring; males, Caucasians, American Indians, Eskimos and lower socioeconomic groups

  6. Children who develop OM early in life are prone to recurrent OM and chronic otitis media with effusion (OME); recurrent OM rose from 18.7% in 1981 to 26% in 1988 with greatest increase among infants in day care

  7. Natural history of untreated otitis media—70% to 90% spontaneous resolution

- Signs and Symptoms

  1. Fever in $\frac{1}{3}$ to $\frac{1}{2}$ of cases

  2. Complaints of ear fullness, pain or discomfort 50% of the time

  3. Poor appetite/feeding, irritable with sleep disturbances (especially in infants)

  4. Nausea/vomiting

  5. Runny nose

  6. Tugging on ears

- Differential Diagnosis

  1. Crying child with normal erythematous tympanic membranes

  2. Damage to TM

  3. Tympanosclerosis

  4. Cholesteatoma

  5. Otitis externa

  6. Possible complications—mastoiditis rare; sepsis in young infant; hearing loss, developmental/speech delay

- Physical Findings: Diagnosis is determined by changes in color, contour, vascularity and mobility of TM

  1. Color is erythematous or yellow and opaque

  2. Contour may be dull or bulging; light reflexes usually distorted

Table 1
Antibiotic Therapy for Management of Otitis Media

Drug Category	Dosage
First line therapy	
1. Amoxicillin	40–90 mg/kg/d, bid, 10 days
2. Trimethoprim-sulfamethoxazole	8/40 mg/kg/d, bid, 10 days
Second line therapy	
1. Amoxicillin-clavulanate	45 mg/kg/d, bid, 10 days
2. Cefprozil	30 mg/kg/d, bid, 10 days
3. Ceftibuten	9 mg/kg/d, qd, 10 days
4. Cefuroxime	30 mg/kg/d, bid, 10 days
5. Azithromycin	10 mg/kg day 1, 5 mg/kg days 2–5
6. Clarithromycin	15 mg/kg/d, bid, 10 days
7. Loracarbef	30 mg/kg/d, bid, 10 days
8. Cefpodoxime	10 mg/kg/d, qd, 10 days
Third line therapy	
1. Clindamycin	8–12 mg/kg/d, tid, 10 days
2. Ceftriaxone	50–75 mg/kg/d, qd, 1-5 days, IM
Prophylactic therapy	
1. Amoxicillin	20 mg/kg/d, qd, 1 to 6 months
2. Sulfisoxazole	50–75 mg/kg/d, bid, 1 to 6 months

q.d. = once a day; b.i.d. = every 12 hours; t.i.d. = every 8 hours

    3. Distinct vascularity

    4. Mobility decreased or absent via tympanometry or pneumatic otoscopy

    5. Conductive hearing loss

- Diagnostic Tests/Findings: Use depends on age of child, and stage of middle ear disease

    1. Pneumatic otoscopy—visualize degree of mobility impairment

    2. Tympanometry using electroacoustic impedance bridge to measure compliance of the TM—identifies middle ear effusion, perforation, patent ventilation tubes, or excessive hard packed cerumen

    3. Audiometric tests—to rule out conductive hearing loss, especially for otitis media with effusion in children 3 months and older

    4. Language screen—assess degree of possible speech delay

- Management/Treatment

    1. Judicious use of antimicrobials due to increased bacterial resistance

    2. Select appropriate antibiotic—see Table 1

    3. Maintain realistic expectations—90% to 95% symptom relief within 48 to 72 hours; if no better, change antibiotic

    4. Re-treat if signs/symptoms persist—use second line antibiotic; prophylaxis for children with frequent or severe infections not enrolled in day care

5. Use tympanocentesis sparingly; only used for retreatment failures with severe symptoms

6. Monitor residual OME—may last for several months; persistent OME for 6 to 8 weeks, consider treatment with second line antibiotics (see Table 1)

7. Pain and fever control

   a. Analgesics—acetaminophen, ibuprofen

   b. Local anesthetic otic drops (contraindicated in acute/chronic perforations and ventilation tubes)

8. Decongestant use is controversial; usefulness unproven

9. Recheck AOM after 10 to 21 days

10. Prevention

    a. Proper feeding techniques for infants

    b. Encourage breast feeding—shown to be protective against otitis media

    c. Eliminate exposure to tobacco smoke

    d. Antibiotic prophylaxis—see Table 1

    e. Immunization with pneumococcal and influenza vaccines

11. Referral to otolaryngologist

    a. Persistent AOM resistant to treatment over 1 to 2 months

    b. Frequent recurrent OM—3 in 6 months, 4 to 5 episodes in one year, 6 episodes by 6 years of age

    c. Persistent/chronic OME > 3 months

    d. Evidence of hearing deficit and/or language delay

    e. Determine need for tympanostomy tube placement

Otitis Media with Effusion (OME)

- Definition: Inflammation/fluid accumulation in middle ear with decreased TM mobility on pneumatic otoscopy but without signs and symptoms of ear infection; also referred to as serous, secretory, mucoid, and allergic otitis media or "glue ear"

- Etiology/Incidence

  1. Caused by eustachian tube malfunction as frequent sequelae of acute otitis media; negative pressure in middle ear results in fluid accumulation by effusion

  2. OME accounts for 25% to 35% of all cases of OM

  3. 30% to 40% have OME associated with allergic rhinitis

  4. Majority (50% to 80%) clear within 2 to 3 months

  5. Mild to moderate hearing loss with concomitant language delays may occur with

OME contributing to subsequent behavioral difficulties including poor attention and school performance

- Signs and Symptoms

    1. Sometimes none or mild discomfort

    2. Behavioral changes, e.g., hearing loss, decreased attention span

- Differential Diagnosis: Same as AOM

- Physical Findings

    1. Color—opaque or translucent TM; possible presence of air, fluid levels or bubbles

    2. Contour—appears retracted due to negative pressure in middle ear

    3. Vascularity—none visible

    4. Mobility—decreased, tympanometry reveals high negative pressure

- Diagnostic Tests/Findings: Same as AOM

- Management/Treatment:

    1. Most cases resolve without antibiotics

    2. Limit use of antibiotic prophylaxis due to marginal benefit

    3. Limit passive smoking exposure, treat other infections, control allergies

    4. Audiogram after 3 months; referral to otolaryngologist

    5. Consider surgery for chronic OME accompanied by pain, recurrent AOM; speech or hearing problems (Graham & Uphold, 1999)

    6. Decongestants and antihistamines not recommended

    7. Follow up every 3 to 4 weeks

    8. Prevention, education and referral recommendations, same as AOM

Tympanostomy Tubes

- Definition

    1. Surgical incision of ear drum (myringotomy with placement of ventilation tube) to relieve pressure which drains pus/fluid from middle ear

    2. Two types

        a. Short term—intended to remain in TM 8 to 15 months

        b. Long term—intended for more than 15 months

- Etiology/Incidence

    1. One million tubes inserted annually

    2. Indicated for children with failed antibiotic prophylaxis of 4 months or longer;

those allergic to penicillin or sulfonamides; those with associated hearing loss of 20 dB or other complications

3. With increasing number of resistant bacteria, possibility of more frequent use of tubes

- Management/Treatment

  1. Fitted ear plugs with swimming

  2. If drainage occurs from tubes, treat with antibiotic otic suspension, e.g. polymyxin B with neomycin and hydrocortisone

Chronic/Acute Perforations

- Definition: Spontaneous perforation of tympanic membrane during episode of AOM

- Etiology/Incidence

  1. Chronic—perforation lasts longer than one month

  2. Chronic suppurative O.M.—associated with discharge

  3. Chronic sites of perforation

     a. Central—relatively safe from cholesteatoma formation

     b. Peripheral—especially in pars flaccida, increased risk of cholesteatoma

- Signs and Symptoms: Painless ear discharge if infection present

- Differential Diagnosis

  1. Cholesteatoma

  2. Mastoiditis

  3. Extradural, subdural or brain abscess

  4. Meningitis

  5. Labrynthitis

  6. Lateral sinus thrombophlebitis

- Physical Findings

  1. Thickened, inflamed middle ear mucosa

  2. May contain granulation tissue or polyps

  3. Conductive hearing loss dependent on size of perforation

  4. Site of perforation important to note

- Diagnostic Tests/Findings

  1. Culture discharge—*Pseudomonas aeruginosa* and *Staphylococcus aureus* most often seen

  2. PPD—rule out tuberculosis

3. CT scan of mastoid—rule out mastoiditis

- Management/Treatment

    1. Oral antibiotics (see Table 1) for 14 days plus antibiotic ear drops (3 to 4 drops four times a day, for 7 days); if not responsive, suspect mastoiditis or cholesteatoma

    2. Patients with central nervous system sequelae, refer immediately

    3. Hospitalization may be necessary

    4. Follow up every week to 3 months; most heal within 2 weeks

    5. Refer to otolaryngologist

        a. Unresolved perforation after 1 year duration

        b. Surgical repair delayed until 9 to 12 years of age

- Prevention of recurrent infection

    1. Cotton plugs with petroleum jelly (on outer surface) when bathing and hair washing

    2. Discourage swimming (use fitted earplugs if unavoidable)

    3. Diving, jumping into water, and underwater swimming forbidden

    4. Exposure to air is helpful

Mastoiditis

- Definition: Infection of the mastoid antrum and air cells with potential destruction of the mastoid airspaces, a suppurative complication of otitis media

- Etiology/Incidence

    1. Uncommon, due to successful antibiotics for AOM

    2. Develops secondary to OM leading to periostitis and osteitis with abscess formation

    3. Unusual before two years of age

    4. Common pathogens

        a. Most common—*Streptococcus pneumoniae, Streptococcus pyogenes, Staphylococcus aureus*

        b. Less common—*Haemophilus influenzae*

        c. Other agents—Pseudomonas (chronic mastoiditis), *Mycobacterium tuberculosis* (rare), *Moraxella catarrhalis,* enteropathic gram negative rods

- Signs and Symptoms

    1. Pain, tenderness behind ear

    2. Fever or irritability

- Differential Diagnosis

1. Meningitis

2. Extradural abscess

3. Subdural empyema

4. Focal otic encephalitis

- Physical Findings

    1. Severe tenderness over mastoid bone

    2. Mastoid area often edematous with erythema

    3. Presence of AOM

    4. Pinna displaced downward and outward (late finding)

    5. Narrowing of ear canal in posterior superior wall due to pressure from mastoid abscess

    6. Purulent drainage and debris may be present in ear canal

- Diagnostic Tests/Findings

    1. CBC—elevated WBC

    2. Blood culture—rule out sepsis

    3. PPD—rule out exposure to tuberculosis

    4. Radiography or CT scan of mastoid(s)—diffuse clouding of mastoid cells; later in disease, bony destruction and resorption of the mastoid air cells; CT also done if brain abscess is suspected

    5. Tympanocentesis—identify pathogen

    6. Lumbar puncture—rule out meningitis

- Management/Treatment

    1. Prompt referral to ENT and hospitalization

    2. Incision and drainage of abscess; systemic intravenous antibiotics

    3. Complications—meningitis, brain abscess, cavernous sinus thrombosis, acute suppurative labrynthitis, facial palsy

    4. Oral systemic antibiotics for 4 to 6 weeks after discharge

Cholesteatoma

- Definition: Cyst like mass with lining of stratified squamous epithelium filled with desquamated debris; most common in middle ear and mastoid area

- Etiology/Incidence

    1. Congenital or acquired

    2. Varied theories explaining formation, e.g., inflammatory process; perforation or failure of desquamated tissue to clear from middle ear

3. Incidence unknown

4. If surgery delayed, it can invade and destroy other structures of the temporal bone and possibly spread to intracranial cavity

5. If untreated, may lead to facial nerve paralysis, intracranial infection

- Signs and Symptoms
    1. Dizziness
    2. Hearing loss

- Differential Diagnosis: Aural polyps

- Physical Findings
    1. Pearly white, shiny, greasy lesion on or behind tympanic membrane
    2. History of chronic OM with foul smelling purulent otorrhea

- Diagnostic Tests/Findings: Audiogram to rule out hearing deficit

- Management/Treatment
    1. Referral to ENT for surgical excision
    2. Complications
        a. Irreversible structural damage
        b. Permanent bone damage
        c. Facial nerve palsy
        d. Hearing loss
        e. Intracranial infection

Hearing Loss

- Definition: A deficit in hearing process; classified as conductive, sensorineural or mixed; can range from mild to severe; may be congenital or acquired; quantified by measured hearing threshhold
    1. Conductive loss—normal bone conduction and reduced air conduction due to obstruction of transmission of sound waves through external auditory canal and middle ear to the inner ear; usual range of 15 to 40 dB loss
    2. Sensorineural loss—cochlea hair cells and/or auditory nerve damage; may range from mild to profound
    3. Mixed—components of conductive and sensorineural hearing loss present
    4. Hearing loss criteria in children differs from adults since children are in the process of speech and language development (Behrman, 2000)
        a. Mild—15 to 30 dB
        b. Moderate—30 to 50 dB

   c. Severe—50 to 70 dB

   d. Profound—70 dB and above

- Etiology/Incidence

   1. Hearing loss can be classified in five ways

      a. Age of onset

      b. Type—conductive, sensorineural, mixed or central

      c. Degree—ranging from mild to profound

      d. Configuration—decibel (dB) loss

      e. Hearing status of parent(s)

   2. Congenital

      a. Sensorineural—moderate to profound loss; 1–2:1000 live births (Behrman, 2000)

         (1) Genetic—autosomal dominant (80%), autosomal recessive (20%)

         (2) In utero infections—TORCH, CMV and rubella most common causes in newborn (Grover, 1996)

         (3) Erythroblastosis fetalis

         (4) Anoxia

         (5) Birth trauma

         (6) Birth weight < 1500 g

         (7) Exposure to ototoxic drugs

         (8) Prolonged mechanical ventilation

      b. Conductive—congenital atresia, deformities or stenosis of ossicles

   3. Acquired

      a. Sensorineural

         (1) Meningitis

         (2) Mumps, measles

         (3) Labyrinthitis, ototoxic drug exposure

         (4) Severe head trauma

         (5) Noise induced hearing loss (NIHL) from loud music, firecrackers, firearms, toy cap pistols, squeaking toys, recreational vehicles, farm equipment, lawn mowers, inappropriate hearing aids

      b. Conductive

         (1) Otitis media with middle effusion—75% of children have one episode of AOM with conductive hearing loss

(2)   Cerumen impaction; foreign bodies in external canal

(3)   Perforated/damaged tympanic membrane; severe head trauma

(4)   Cholesteatoma, otosclerosis

- Signs and Symptoms
    1. Infants

        a.   Failure to elicit startle or blink reflex to loud sound

        b.   Failure to be awakened by loud sounds

        c.   General indifference to sound

        d.   Lack of babbling by 7 months

    2. Children

        a.   Substitution of gestures for words, especially after 15 months

        b.   Failure to develop intelligible speech by 24 months

        c.   Asking to have statements repeated

        d.   Inappropriate response to questions

        e.   Markedly inattentive

- Differential Diagnosis
    1. Mental retardation
    2. Profound deprivation
    3. Communication disorder—articulation disorders, expressive language delay, global language disorder, autism

- Physical Findings
    1. Careful evaluation of TM, e.g., decreased mobility, bulging, opacity
    2. Congenital abnormalities—external canal abnormalities, craniofacial malformations, structural abnormalities of external ear

- Diagnostic Test/Findings
    1. Audiogram appropriate for age to rule out hearing loss
    2. CT Scan—rule out physiologic abnormalities
    3. Weber and Rinne tests—abnormal response

- Management/Treatment
    1. History screening at two week old visit—family history of hearing loss, perinatal infections (TORCH), anatomic malformations involving head or neck, birth weight < 1500 g, hyperbilirubinemia, bacterial meningitis, asphyxia
    2. Detect hearing loss as young as possible; take parental suspicions seriously; many

tests available for all age groups including newborn (otoacoustic emissions-OAE, auditory brainstem response-ABR)

3. Referral for full audiological testing and language evaluation as soon as deficit is strongly suspected

4. Psychosocial considerations—rehabilitation, hearing aids, educational programs

5. Prevention

   a. Early identification and intervention; periodic hearing and language screening; (birth to 4 months—responds appropriately to loud noises; 4 to 24 months—responds to noise out of field of vision; older children—pure tone audiometry)

   b. Appropriate management and treatment of auditory canal obstruction and middle ear disease

   c. Avoid repeated exposure to loud noises to prevent NIHL

   d. Control erythroblastosis with use of RhoGAM; hyperbilirubinemia with phototherapy and exchange transfusions

   e. Prevent mumps and measles with immunization

   f. Avoid ototoxic medications

Nose

Allergic Rhinitis

- Definition: IgE mediated response to inhaled allergens or irritants producing nasal mucosa inflammation

- Etiology/Incidence

  1. Types—seasonal or perennial depending on exposure/sensitization to allergen

     a. Seasonal—inhaled pollens, e.g., trees, grasses; more common after age 6

     b. Perennial—house dust mites, mold spores, animal dander; may occur in children under age of 6

  2. Most common pediatric atopic disease; commonly associated with conjunctivitis, sinusitis, OME and/or atopic dermatitis

  3. Strong genetic predisposition

- Signs and Symptoms

  1. Chronic, clear nasal discharge

  2. Episodes of sneezing with itching of eyes, ears, nose, palate, pharynx

  3. Open mouth facies, snoring with sleep

  4. Excessive tearing

  5. Purulent secretions indicate secondary infection (e.g., sinusitis, foreign body)

6. Symptoms year-round with perennial rhinitis

- Differential Diagnosis

    1. Bacterial or viral upper respiratory infection, e.g., strep pharyngitis, influenza, OM, sinusitis

    2. Vasomotor rhinitis

    3. Congenital or anatomical abnormalities leading to obstruction, e.g., nasal polyps, foreign body

- Physical findings

    1. Allergic "shiners" and "salute" with nasal crease

    2. Hypertrophied turbinates; halitosis

    3. Nasal mucosa pale blue, boggy, and edematous with watery or mucoid secretions

- Diagnostic Tests/Findings

    1. Nasal smear for eosinophils—10% considered confirmatory

    2. RAST and skin testing—elevations or reactions to specific allergens

    3. CBC differential—elevated eosinophils and total IgE

- Management/Treatment: Referral to allergist may be necessary

    1. First line of therapy—identify and avoid allergen(s)

    2. Environmental controls—removal of carpets, drapes, and stuffed animals; plastic covers for mattresses and pillows; decrease humidity with air conditioner, use of air purifiers, and avoidance of tobacco smoke

    3. Drug therapy—antihistamine H_1 receptor antagonists

        a. Fexofenadine hydrochloide—(> 12 years) 60 mg every 12 hours; nonsedating

        b. Loratadine—(> 6 years and 30 kg) 10 mg daily; nonsedating

        c. Diphenhydramine—(5 mg/kg/day) every 6 hours; sedating

        d. Oral sympathomimetic (e.g., pseudoephedrine) for short term relief by producing vasoconstriction of respiratory tract mucosa

        e. Mast cell stabilizer nasal spray to prevent allergic response— cromolyn sodium (> 2 years) one spray intranasally 4 times/day

        f. Topical nasal corticosteroids to decrease immediate and late phase allergic reactions with reduction of influx of inflammatory cells; start about 1 to 2 weeks before allergy season

            (1) Beclomethasone—(> 6 years) by nasal inhalation

            (2) Flunisolide—(> 6 years) by nasal inhalation

    4. Referrals if symptoms not responsive to avoidance and/or medication

        a. Allergist for skin testing for possible long-term immunotherapy

    b. Immunotherapy effective in relieving symptoms due to dust mites, animal dander, pollens, molds, insect stings and drug sensitivities

    c. HEENT specialist for consultation and possible surgical interventions, e.g., myringotomy tubes

Chronic Rhinitis

- Definition: Chronic nasal discharge with or without acute exacerbations
- Etiology/Incidence

    a. May reflect underlying disorder e.g., nasal polyps, chronic sinusitis, chronically infected tonsils, cystic fibrosis, allergy, foreign body, deviated septum, congenital malformation, syphilis

    b. May result from prolonged topical nasal decongestant use

- Signs and Symptoms: Variable

  1. Foul smelling, nasal discharge

  2. Possible bloody discharge, e.g., with foreign body, syphilis

  3. Disturbances in taste and smell

  4. Fever with superimposed infection

- Differential Diagnosis: Allergic rhinitis
- Physical Findings

  1. Excoriation of anterior nares and upper lip

  2. Nasal discharge—usually clear

- Management/Treatment: Directed at underlying cause

  1. Antibiotic for bacterial infection

  2. Environmental controls to minimize exposure to allergens

  3. Special attention to nutritional status, rest and prevention of exposure to new infections

Foreign Body in Nose

- Definition: Foreign body in either nostril
- Etiology/Incidence: Common items include food, crayons, small toys, erasers, paper wads, beads, beans and stones, alkaline button batteries
- Signs and Symptoms

  1. Initial—sneezing, mild discomfort, rarely pain; can increase with time

  2. Infection usually follows—unilateral purulent, malodorous or bloody discharge is always suggestive of a foreign body

- Differential Diagnosis

1. Nasal polyps, nasal tumors

2. Purulent rhinitis, sinusitis

- Physical Findings

    1. Unilateral foul smelling nasal discharge

    2. Visualization of foreign body

- Diagnostics Tests/Findings: None usually; head mirror or light will provide visualization of object

- Management/Treatment

    1. Remove promptly with forceps or nasal suction

    2. Generally infection resolves after removal

    3. Referral to otolaryngologist if unable to remove

Epistaxis

- Definition: Bleeding from the nose

- Etiology/Incidence

    1. Most cases are benign and frequent in childhood due to increased vascularity of nasal mucosa

    2. Trauma and inflammation of mucosal lining (sudden onset) most common cause—nose picking, foreign body insertion, direct blunt trauma, violent sneezing

    3. Nasal mucosal drying (intermittent bleeding) from poorly humidified air, e.g., heating systems

    4. Chronic infection of nasal tissue viral or bacterial

    5. Substance abuse, e.g., cocaine, cannabis

    6. Systemic diseases—consider with bleeding that is severe, prolonged or recurrent

        a. Hypertension—exacerbates problem

        b. Clotting abnormalities, e.g., hemophilia, aplastic anemia, leukemia, idiopathic thrombocytopenia, platelet dysfunction

        c. ASA and NSAID overuse, neoplasms (gradual onset), cancer treatments, hormonal influences, e.g., menses, birth control pills (BCP), pregnancy

- Signs and Symptoms

    1. Bleeding from nares—usually unilateral

    2. Tarry stools—occasionally with frequent bleeds

- Differential Diagnosis

    1. Foreign bodies

    2. Infection

3. Substance abuse

4. Allergies

5. Chronic rhinitis

6. Chronic nasal spray use

- Physical Findings

    1. Determine location of bleeding

        a. Anterior bleed—most common site (90%) Kesselbach's plexus

        b. Posterior bleed—can see only if nose is normal, no inflammation and with special instruments; may see posterior oropharynx blood flow

        c. High nasal bleed—may represent nasoethmoid or orbit fracture

        d. Recurrent—consider bleeding disorder or chronic irritation

- Diagnostic Tests/Findings

    1. Stool for occult blood—determine if child is swallowing blood

    2. Roentgenograms, CBC with differential, platelets, PT, PTT; coagulation profile (if bleeding disorder is suspected)

- Management/Treatment

    1. Complete history including—recurrent or acute; unilateral or bilateral; duration; recent URI, allergic rhinitis; ASA or NSAID use; signs of underlying disease

    2. Monitor vital signs, especially blood pressure

    3. Apply pressure to anterior nasal septum with patient sitting in upright position with head tilted forward, (most stop within 10 to 15 minutes); application of ice; increase humidity of home; avoid nose blowing

    4. Antibiotics (topical and oral) may be indicated if infection is suggested

    5. Topical nasal vasoconstrictor drops (phenylephrine $\frac{1}{4}$% to $\frac{1}{2}$%) and packing may be needed

    6. Recurrent or severe cases—refer to otolaryngologist

Sinusitis

- Definition: Acute, subacute or chronic inflammation of mucosal lining in one or more of paranasal sinuses

- Etiology/Incidence

    1. Common pathogens (also commonly found in AOM)

        a. Predominately in acute sinusitis—*Streptococcus pneumoniae, Haemophilus influenzae* and *Moraxella catarrhalis*

        b. Prevalent in chronic sinusitis are anaerobes (e.g., Group A beta hemolytic streptococcus and *Staphylococcus aureus*) due to low oxygen content and low pH of fluid

    c. Viruses—less common

2. 5% to 10% of URIs in children develop into sinusitis

3. May be secondary to allergies, adenoidal hypertrophy, anatomical abnormalities, dental abscess, diving and swimming

4. Higher incidence in boys affecting maxillary and ethmoid sinuses

5. Maxillary and ethmoid sinuses most frequently involved

6. Acute sinusitis—persistent symptoms > 10 days and < one month

7. Chronic sinusitis—> 30 days

- Signs and Symptoms: Children have less specific complaints; adolescents usually present with classical symptoms

  1. Persistent URI (beyond 7 to 10 days) with purulent or watery drainage

  2. Cough, low grade fever

  3. Facial pain, toothache, headache or tenderness over involved sinus

  4. Postnasal drip, bad breath, sore throat

  5. Increased pain with cough, bending over or abrupt head movement

  6. Fatigue, malaise, anorexia

  7. Periorbital swelling in morning

- Differential Diagnosis

  1. Dental infections, cleft palate, foreign bodies, tumors and polyps, nasal trauma, malformations

  2. Allergic and purulent rhinitis, common cold

  3. Cystic fibrosis, immunodeficiency states, allergy, or asthma

- Physical Findings

  1. Clear or mucopurulent rhinorrhea and/or postnasal drainage

  2. Erythema of nasal mucosa and/or throat

  3. Pain on percussion with possible erythema/edema in area of affected sinus

  4. OME common finding—especially in younger child

- Diagnostic Tests/Findings

  1. Nasal scrapings—eosinophils present with allergy

  2. Roentgenography—rule out cysts, polyps, abscess

  3. CT scan—used in complicated sinusitis, intraorbital and intracranial involvement, abscess and sinonasal neoplasms

- Management/Treatment
    1. Antibiotic therapy—same as used in AOM (see Table 1)
        a. To penetrate sinuses, need 14 to 21 days of treatment; up to 6 weeks in chronic cases
        b. Trimethoprim/sulfamethoxazole should not be used if group A streptococci is suspected
    2. Decongestants/antihistamines not proven effective except with concomitant allergic manifestations
    3. Comfort measures—analgesics, increased humidity, increase oral fluids
    4. Inflammation control with topical steroid nasal spray, e.g., beclomethasone
    5. Diving/swimming in moderation; consider elimination of activity with chronic cases
    6. Complications
        a. Intracranial complications—subdural empyema, brain abscess, sinus thrombosis
        b. Orbital cellulitis secondary to ethmoiditis (medical emergency)
    7. Refer to otolaryngologist and/or allergist for chronic sinusitis and allergy control

Nasal Polyps

- Definition: Benign pedunculated tumors
- Etiology/Incidence
    1. Originate from edematous, chronically inflamed nasal mucosa in ethmoid sinus
    2. Common in children with cystic fibrosis; 25% develop nasal polyps
- Signs and Symptoms
    1. Nasal obstruction
    2. Mouth breathing
- Differential Diagnosis
    1. Chronic sinusitis
    2. Cystic fibrosis
    3. Chronic allergic rhinitis
    4. Asthma
- Physical Findings
    1. Hyponasal obstruction
    2. Profuse mucoid/mucopurulent rhinorrhea
    3. Shiny grey, grape like mass(es) between nasal turbinates and septum

- Diagnostic Tests/Findings: Sweat test to rule out cystic fibrosis on every child with polyps
- Management/Treatment
    1. Care in distinguishing swollen turbinates from polyps
    2. Antihistamines if allergy related
    3. Local/systemic decongestants/corticosteroids not helpful
    4. Refer for surgical removal in those with complete obstruction or uncontrolled deformity

Mouth

Oral Candidiasis (Thrush)

- Definition: Common fungal infection of oral cavity
- Etiology/Incidence
    1. *Candida albicans* (monilial)
    2. More common in neonate and infant than in other age groups; (transmission during vaginal delivery)
    3. Predisposing factors
        a. Steroid therapy
        b. Antibiotic therapy
        c. Compromised immune system
- Signs and Symptoms: White patches in mouth
- Physical Findings
    1. Characteristic white, curd like adherent plaques that are not easily removed; found on the buccal mucosa, tongue, pharynx and/or tonsils
    2. Bleeding occurs with attempts to remove plaques
- Diagnostic Tests/Findings: Systemic/immune status evaluation if persistent or resistant to treatment
- Management/Treatment
    1. Antifungal therapy—nystatin oral suspension applied to oral mucosa 4 times/day for 10 days; if not responding, consider gentian violet application or fluconazole systemically in severe cases
    2. If breast feeding consider examining and treating mother for candidiasis of breast (cross-infection)
    3. Check diaper area for concurrent diaper rash

4. Sterilize nipples, pacifiers if bottle fed; apply nystatin to nipples if breast feeding; if recurrent, look for other causes, e.g., H.I.V.

Cleft Lip/Palate

- Definition:
    1. Cleft lip—failure of embryonic structures surrounding oral cavity to join
    2. Cleft palate—failure of palatal shelves to fuse
    3. Occurs in various degrees
- Etiology/Incidence
    1. Genetic influence with cleft lip more than palate
    2. Both can occur sporadically
    3. More common to have combination of both than one without the other
    4. Cleft lip with or without palate—1:800 births
    5. Cleft palate alone—1:1,750 births
    6. More common in males, Asians and with maternal drug exposure
    7. Lower incidence in African-Americans
    8. Increase in middle ear/nasopharyngeal/sinus infections with associated hearing loss
    9. Recurrent otitis media is common
- Signs and Symptoms: Separation of lip and/or palate
- Differential Diagnosis: None
- Physical Findings
    1. Degree of cleft varies from small notch to complete separation
    2. Unilateral or bilateral
    3. Involves soft and/or hard palate
    4. Bifid uvula indicates submucosal cleft palate
- Diagnostic Test/Findings: Audiogram to rule out hearing deficit
- Management/Treatment
    1. Surgical repair; timing individualized—lip usually by 2 months, palate by 9 to 12 months
    2. Teach feeding techniques (breast or bottle) before and after repair
    3. Referral for dental restoration if needed
    4. Referrals to otolaryngologist, plastic surgeon, pediatric dentist, prosthodontist, orthodontist, speech therapist, psychiatrist, social worker and genetic counselors
    5. Support family adjustment and management

Dental Caries

- Definition: Demineralization of tooth surface secondary to production of organic acids by bacterial fermentation of dietary carbohydrates (Behrman, 2000)
- Etiology/Incidence
    1. Mutans streptococci are primary etiological organism responsible for human dental caries
    2. Rate of formation depends on frequency of acid environment in mouth; availability of fluoride for remineralization; oral hygiene
    3. Nursing bottle tooth decay (nursing caries)
        a. Tooth decay resulting from repeated/prolonged contact with milk, formula, or juice
        b. Children put to bed with bottle or sleep at the breast or use either the breast/bottle as pacifier are at increased risk
    4. Most pediatric dental caries occur on the occlusal surfaces of posterior and lingual aspect of the maxillary incisors, molars and cuspids
    5. New teeth are at greater risk for caries than established teeth
    6. Fluoride is critical in the process of remineralization
- Signs and Symptoms
    1. Sensitive or painful tooth
    2. Severe decay—pain, edema and infection
    3. Weight loss
    4. Feeding problems
- Physical Findings: Initial decalcification of enamel appears as opaque white spots that turn light brown progressing to dark brown with destruction of tooth
- Management/Treatment
    1. Prevention of dental caries/periodontal disease
        a. Well balanced diet with appropriate feeding practices; low sugar and complex carbohydrate consumption
        b. Wean from bottle, pacifier and breast at one year of age
        c. Brush/clean/wipe teeth as soon as they appear
        d. Daily brushing and flossing of teeth; for children under 8 years, parental involvement needed
        e. Fluoride supplement, dental sealants to occlusal surfaces of the posterior teeth

f. Early dental visits—American Academy of Pediatric Dentists recommend starting dental visits at 12 to 18 months of age for initial discussion of oral hygiene, weaning and fluoride supplementation; routine dental checkups starting at 3 years

2. Dental referral for identified caries

Aphthous Ulcers (Canker Sores)

- Definition: Shallow, painful mouth ulceration
- Etiology/Incidence
    1. Usually affects oral mucosa on ventral surface of tongue, soft palate, buccal mucosa or floor of mouth; occasionally may affect other body tissues
    2. Idiopathic
    3. Precipitated by trauma, stress, sun, allergies, endocrine or hematologic disorders
    4. Onset often in adolescence (20%) and recurrent
    5. "Minor"—1 to 5 lesions, 1 cm, lasting 7 to 14 days
    6. "Major"—10% of cases greater than 1 cm, lasting 6 weeks
- Signs and Symptoms
    1. Burning or tingling before appearance of lesion
    2. Pain at lesion site
    3. Afebrile
- Differential Diagnosis
    1. Herpetic lesions (simplex zoster)
    2. Herpangina (coxsackievirus A)
    3. Trauma
    4. Chemical burns
    5. Hand, foot and mouth disease (coxsackievirus A5, A10, A16)
- Physical Findings
    1. Single or multiple, small, oval, indurated papules with erythematous halo, develops pale center that erodes into ulcers
    2. No systemic symptoms
- Diagnostic Test/Findings: None
- Management/Treatment
    1. Oral analgesics, e.g., 6 to 12 years use chloraseptic spray; greater than 12 years use viscous xylocaine solution

2. Antibacterial (tetracycline) rinses may shorten disease course in children > 9 years of age

3. Referral pediatric dentist if condition lasts more than 14 days

Herpes Labialis (Cold Sore, Fever Blister) and Herpes Simplex Stomatitis

- Definition
    1. Ulceration and inflammation of oral mucosa
    2. Acute primary herpetic gingivostomatitis (APHGS) occurs in previously unexposed children
- Etiology/Incidence
    1. Virus acquired from individual who has mouth sore or herpetic whitlow on a finger or toe; caused by Herpes Simplex Virus 1 (HSV1)
    2. Illness starts 5 to 10 day after exposure
    3. Spontaneous recovery in 7 to 10 days
    4. 50% develop subsequent cold sore episodes after primary acute episode
    5. Oral recurrence—one to several lesions with local pain for 3 to 7 days
- Signs and Symptoms
    1. May be asymptomatic especially cold sores/fever blisters
    2. Fever and chills, mimics "viral syndrome" (initial symptom)
    3. Sore throat, burning in mouth and throat
    4. Anorexia from pain; could lead to dehydration
- Differential Diagnosis
    1. Aphthous ulcers
    2. Hand, foot and mouth syndrome
    3. Herpangina
- Physical Findings
    1. Cold sores—grouped vesicles on erythematous base; commonly found on mucocutaneous border of lips
    2. Primary gingivostomatitis—vesicles on oral mucosa, gingiva, tongue, and lips; ulcer formation following vesicle stage
    3. Cervical adenopathy with gingivostomatitis
    4. May spread to perioral skin
- Diagnostic Tests/Findings: None
- Management/Treatment

1. "Over the counter" (OTC) cold sore treatment

2. Pain management—acetaminophen or ibuprofen; topical relief with occlusive gels, e.g., infant oral anesthetic agents; 1:1 mixture of diphenhydramine combined with antacid preparations consisting of magnesium and aluminum hydroxide *or* anti-diarrheal preparations to provide a protective coating for the oral mucosa (severe cases add 2% viscous lidocaine sparingly)

3. Spontaneous recovery

Hand, Foot, and Mouth Disease

- Definition: Acute viral illness presenting with vesicular enanthem on tongue, gums, palate, oral mucosa; papulovesicular exanthem on hands, feet, legs and occasionally the buttocks

- Etiology/Incidence

  1. Coxsackievirus A16 (most common), A5 and A10

  2. Enterovirus 71—severe illness (aseptic meningitis, encephalitis, paralytic disease common)

  3. Seasonal, predominant in summer and fall

  4. Incubation 4 to 6 days

  5. Spontaneous resolution in one week

- Signs and Symptoms

  1. Fever

  2. Anorexia

  3. Dysphagia

  4. Vomiting

- Differential Diagnosis

  1. Acute primary herpetic gingivostomatitis

  2. Aphthous stomatitis, herpangina

  3. Trauma, burns

- Physical Findings

  1. Small vesicles erode to ulcers on buccal mucosa, hard palate, tonsils, and tongue

  2. Vesicular lesions appear as blanching red lesions on arms, legs, palms, soles and occasionally buttocks

- Diagnostic Tests/Findings: Unnecessary

- Management/Treatment: See Herpangina

Herpangina

- Definition: Acute viral illness presenting with ulceration and inflammation of oral mucosa
- Etiology/Incidence
  1. Coxsackievirus, group A (most common)
  2. Coxsackie B viruses and echoviruses (less common)
  3. Seasonal in U.S.—predominant in summer months
  4. Resolves spontaneously in 3 to 5 days
- Signs and Symptoms
  1. Fever in moderate range
  2. Headache, myalgia, malaise
  3. Dysphagia, vomiting (25%), anorexia, significant oral discomfort, drooling
- Differential Diagnosis
  1. Acute primary herpetic gingivostomatitis
  2. Aphthous stomatitis
  3. Trauma or burns
  4. Hand, foot and mouth disease
- Physical Findings: Small vesicles or punched-out ulcers, especially on soft palate and tonsillar pillars
- Diagnostic Tests/Findings: Unnecessary
- Management/Treatment
  1. Fever and/or pain control—acetaminophen, ibuprofen
  2. Topical relief with 1:1 mixture of diphenhydramine combined with antacid preparations consisting of magnesium and aluminum hydroxide *or* anti-diarrheal preparations to provide a protective coating for the oral mucosa (severe cases add 2% viscous lidocaine; use sparingly)
  3. Encourage fluids to ensure adequate hydration

Throat

Pharyngitis and Tonsillitis

- Definition: Acute inflammation and infection of the throat; when tonsils are main focus of inflammation, tonsillitis is more appropriate term to use
- Etiology/Incidence

1. Causes vary by geographic location, season, age, and amount/time of exposure; most common in 5 to 15-year-olds

2. Viruses

   a. Virus is probable cause in conjunction with nasal congestion and rhinorrhea

   b. Adenovirus (12 types) account for 23% of cases

   c. Epstein-Barr virus

   d. Influenza A and B, RSV, parainfluenza virus, cytomegalovirus, rotavirus

   e. Enteroviruses (e.g., coxsackievirus A and echovirus) seen in summer and fall

3. Bacteria

   a. Group A beta hemolytic streptococcus (GABHS) account for 10 to 15% of all pharyngitis cases; typically occurs in winter and spring

   b. *Haemophilus influenzae*—less common with use of HIB vaccine

   c. *Neisseria gonorrhoeae*—in sexually active adolescents or sexually abused children

   d. *Corynebacterium haemolyticum* and *Corynebacterium diphtheriae*—characteristic presence of grey pseudomembranous exudate on pharynx and tonsils which bleeds with attempts at removal; quite rare in U.S.; still seen in undeveloped countries

4. Other causes

   a. *Mycoplasma pneumoniae*—5% of cases in school age children

   b. Fungal—*Candida albicans*

   c. Parasites

   d. Streptococcal toxin postulated as cause of Kawasaki

5. Noninfectious causes (nearly 50% of cases)

   a. Trauma from tobacco smoke, heat, alcohol

   b. Allergic rhinitis or postnasal drainage

6. Transmission—through exposure to infected respiratory secretions, shared silverware and occasionally household pets

7. Complications

   a. Peritonsillar or retropharyngeal abscess or cellulitis

   b. Cervical adenitis, AOM, sinusitis, pneumonia

   c. Acute rheumatic fever in untreated group A beta hemolytic streptococcal pharyngitis—prevented if treatment started within 9 days of initial complaints of sore throat

   d. Glomerulonephritis—host/immune response to nonrenal infection with

GABHS; not all strains are nephritogenic; manifests in 1 to 3 weeks after pharyngeal or skin infection of GABHS; unrelated to treatment

- Signs and Symptoms: Common symptomatology with some variability by causative organism

    1. Sudden or gradual onset of symptoms

    2. Sore throat

    3. Fever, variable

    4. Headache, anorexia, occasional nausea, vomiting, abdominal pain and malaise

    5. Viral pharyngitis—hoarseness, conjunctivis, runny nose, cough, cold symptoms

    6. GABHS pharyngitis—usually seen at 2 years of age and older, sudden onset of fever with complaints of headache, abdominal pain and vomiting; rash, "strawberry tongue" may be present

- Differential Diagnosis

    1. Stomatitis

    2. Peritonsillar or retropharyngeal abscess, epiglottitis

    3. Allergic rhinitis, postnasal drainage

- Physical Findings

    1. Erythema of pharynx, petechial lesions with or without ulcer formation; petechial lesions on uvula and soft palate common with GABHS

    2. Enlarged tonsils with exudate (occurs in $\frac{1}{3}$ of those with GABHS)

    3. Erythema of nasal mucosa with coryza

    4. Cervical nodes usually enlarged with possible tenderness

- Diagnostic Tests/Findings

    1. Rapid strep test to determine presence of GABHS

        a. 70% to 85% sensitivity; 95% specificity

        b. Treat if positive; throat culture to confirm negative test

    2. CBC—WBC elevated with bacterial infection; decreased with viral agent

    3. Consider other studies—dependent on history, age and clinical presentation, e.g., mono spot, EBV, culture for gonorrhoeae, diphtheria culture

- Management/Treatment

    1. Viral pharyngitis/tonsillitis—symptomatic/supportive care

        a. Saline gargles, throat lozenges

        b. Analgesics for fever/pain (acetaminophen, ibuprofen)

        c. Encourage fluids for maintaining hydration

2. Bacterial pharyngitis/tonsillitis

    a. GABHS—penicillin drug of choice, 125 to 250 mg every eight hours for 10 days or IM Penicillin G Benzathine (600,00 U for less than 60 pounds, 1.2 million U for greater than 60 pounds); erythromycin or first generation cephlosporin for those with penicillin allergy; communicability is eliminated after 24 hours of antibiotic therapy

    b. Second line therapy include macrolides, cephalosprins, or clindamycin

    c. Gonococcal pharyngitis—one IM injection of ceftriaxone

    d. Diphtheria—hospitalization and treatment with erythromycin or penicillin G

    e. *Mycoplasma pneumoniae*—erythromycin for 10 days

Acute Nasopharyngitis (Common Cold)

- Definition: Acute viral infection of upper respiratory tract with potential involvement of nasal passages, sinuses, eustachian tubes, middle ears, conjunctiva and nasopharynx

- Etiology/Incidence

  1. Causative pathogens

    a. Over 100 infectious pathogens—respiratory syncytial virus (RSV) most common

    b. Other common pathogens include parainfluenza viruses, corona viruses, adenoviruses, enterovirus, influenza viruses, *Mycoplasma pneumoniae,* reoviruses (Behrman, 2000)

  2. Pathogen shed in large amounts through nasal secretions and easily spread through self-inoculation from fingers and hands to objects (clothing, environmental surfaces)

  3. Universal susceptibility; children average 5 to 8 infections/year with a peak incidence during first 2 years

  4. Increased susceptability associated with active/passive smoke exposure

  5. More frequent in crowded situations

  6. Occurrence in cooler months in temperate climates—peaks in early fall, late January and early April

- Signs and Symptoms: Generally last one week; dry cough with mild runny nose, may persist up to 3 weeks

  1. Infants

    a. Irritability, restlessness, fever (100° to 102° F)

    b. Rhinorrhea

    c. Occasional diarrhea

    d. Changes in feeding and sleep patterns

  2. Older children

   a.   Afebrile or low grade fever, stuffy nose, watery nasal discharge

   b.   Sore throat, sneezing, cough, chills

   c.   Occasional headache, malaise

- Differential Diagnosis

   1.   Underlying secondary bacterial infection—sinusitis, O.M., pharyngitis, lower respiratory tract disease

   2.   Allergic rhinitis

   3.   Foreign body

   4.   Substance abuse in older children and adolescents, or overuse of medicated nasal spray

- Physical Findings

   1.   Coryza

   2.   Inflamed, moist nasal mucosa and oropharynx

   3.   Chest clear

- Diagnostic Tests/Findings

   1.   Viral cultures expensive; generally unnecessary

   2.   If suspicious of differential diagnosis, consider throat and nose culture, drug screen

- Management/Treatment: Symptomatic/supportive care

   1.   Analgesics for sore throat, muscle aches and fever > 101° F

   2.   Relief of nasal congestion

   a.   Saline nose drops ($\frac{1}{4}$ tsp. table salt with 6 oz water); 3 drops each nostril, wait several minutes, gentle aspiration with nasal bulb syringe

   b.   Cool mist humidification

   c.   Antibiotics, antihistamines and decongestants not recommended in the young child and infant

   d.   Older children and adolescents receive symptomatic relief with decongestant and antihistamine use

   3.   If symptoms persistent beyond 7 to 10 days, consider secondary infection

   4.   Maintain hydration; also helps to liquefy secretions

   5.   Prevention

   a.   Good hygiene and cleaning of clothes, toys and play areas

   b.   Limited exposure to crowded situations

Retropharyngeal Abscess

- Definition: Inflammation of posterior aspect of pharynx with suppurative retropharyngeal lymph nodes
- Etiology
    1. Causative pathogens—GABHS (most common), anaerobic organisms; *Staphylococcus aureus*
    2. In older children—usually superinfection from penetrating injury to posterior wall of oropharynx
    3. Possible complication of bacterial pharyngitis
    4. Relatively rare infection; most common in children under 4 years of age secondary to untreated pyogenic adenitis
- Signs and Symptoms
    1. Acute onset of high fever with persistent severe throat pain
    2. Drooling due to difficulty in swallowing
    3. Tachypnea, dyspnea, stridor
    4. Neck and head hyperextension
- Differential Diagnosis
    1. Epiglottitis
    2. Peritonsillar abscess
    3. Laryngotracheobronchitis (croup)
    4. Acute infectious mononucleosis
    5. Acute pharyngitis
    6. Bacterial tracheitis
    7. Meningitis
- Physical findings
    1. Toxic appearing child; neck and head in hyperextension
    2. Noisy, gurgling respiration
    3. Drooling, meningismus
    4. Stridor, airway obstruction
    5. Prominent swelling of posterior pharyngeal wall—confirms diagnosis
- Diagnostic Tests/Findings
    1. Lateral neck radiography—retropharyngeal space wider than C4 vertebral body
    2. CBC—elevated WBC

3. Computed tomography (CT) scan to visualize abscess

- Management/Treatment

  1. **Immediate and emergency referral to ENT**

  2. Emergency hospitalization necessary

     a. Admission to pediatric ICU for continuous monitoring for airway obstruction and possible respiratory arrest

     b. Surgical incision and drainage necessary

     c. Intravenous (IV) antibiotics—penicillin, clindamycin

Peritonsillar Abscess

- Definition: Infection of tonsils spreading to tonsillar fossa and surrounding tissues (peritonsillar cellulitis); if left untreated, tonsillar abscess forms

- Etiology/Incidence

  1. GABHS (most common)

  2. *Staphylococcus aureus,* anaerobic microorganisms

  3. Can occur at any age; more common in preadolescent or adolescent age groups

  4. Complication of untreated peritonsillar abscess—lateral pharyngeal abscess leading to possible airway obstruction; aggressive early treatment will prevent suppuration

- Signs and Symptoms

  1. Severe sore throat with high fever

  2. Toxic appearance, muffled voice, spasms of jaw muscles

  3. Difficulty swallowing and drooling in severe cases

  4. Bad breath

- Differential Diagnosis

  1. Retropharyngeal abscess

  2. Epiglottitis

- Physical Findings

  1. Unilateral enlargement of tonsil(s), bulging medially with anterior pillar prominence (most common)

  2. Soft palate and uvula edematous, erythematous, displaced towards unaffected side

  3. Extreme tonsillar tenderness on palpation

- Diagnostic Tests

  1. CBC—increased WBC

  2. Rapid strep test to rule out GABHS

- Management/Treatment
    1. **Immediate referral to ENT**
    2. Surgical incision and drainage often necessary
    3. Possible need for hospitalization
    4. Antibiotics (Penicillin), IM, IV or by mouth
    5. If not hospitalized, daily follow up visits until stable

Cervical Lymphadenitis

- Definition: Inflammation affecting one or more cervical lymph nodes
- Etiology/Incidence
    1. Pathogens
        a. *Streptococcus pyogenes* and *Staphylococcus aureus* account for approximately 80% of cases
        b. *Mycobacterium tuberculosis*
        c. Other organisms (e.g., viral, fungal or parasitic)
    2. Secondary to local infections of the ear, nose and throat (most common)
    3. Prevalent among preschool children
- Signs and Symptoms
    1. Complaints of swollen neck or face
    2. Fever
    3. Stridor, hoarseness, drooling if adenopathy impinges on airway
- Differential Diagnosis
    1. Bilateral cervical adenitis—mononucleosis, tularemia, diphtheria
    2. Subacute or chronic adenitis—cat scratch fever, nonspecific viral infections
    3. Atypical mycobacterium—tuberculosis
    4. Cervical node tumors, e.g., leukemia, neurofibromatosis
    5. Mumps, cyst, hematoma
- Physical Findings
    1. Large unilateral cervical mass, greater than 2 to 6 cm
    2. Erythema may be present
    3. Extreme tenderness on palpation
- Diagnostic Tests/Findings
    1. CBC—moderate to marked WBC

2. Mantoux test—rule out tuberculosis

3. Mono spot—rule out mononucleosis

4. Throat culture—rule out GABHS

5. Serology tests if not resolving (e.g., EBV, toxoplasmosis, CMV, histoplasmosis)

6. Aspiration of node if fluctuant—aerobic/anaerobic culture

- Management/Treatment

    1. With no evidence of sepsis, treat empirically with oral antibiotics— dicloxacillin, amoxicillin clavulanate, or cephalexin for a minimum of 10 days and no less than 5 days after resolution of symptoms

    2. Measure and follow size of node

    3. Analgesics for fever and pain; application of cold compresses

    4. Re-evaluation after 36 to 48 hours; if no improvement, possible hospitalization for IV antibiotics, especially with infants and young children

    5. Referral to otolaryngologist if not improving

    6. Surgical aspiration may be necessary

    7. Persistent unexplained, symptomatic node, increasing in size despite treatment, refer for biopsy

Epiglottitis (Supraglottitis)

- Definition: Severe, rapidly developing inflammation and swelling of the supraglottic structures leading to life threatening upper airway obstruction

- Etiology/Incidence

    1. Pathogens—group A beta-hemolytic streptococci, pneumococci, *H. parainfluenzae*

    2. Can occur at any age, highest incidence 2 to 7 years of age

    3. Decreasing incidence from *Haemophilus influenzae* with use of HIB vaccine

- Signs and Symptoms

    1. Acute, sudden onset of high fever, severe sore throat, muffled voice, drooling, poor color, labored breathing in a previously well child

    2. Choking sensation, refuses to speak

    3. Restless, irritable, anxious, apprehensive, frightened

    4. Hyperextension of neck, leaning forward and chin thrust out, prostration; ''sniffing dog'' or tripod position—provides best possible airway

- Differential Diagnosis

    1. Acute laryngeal edema, croup syndrome, foreign body aspiration

    2. Pertussis, diphtheria, Kawasaki syndrome

3. Bacterial tracheitis, retropharyngeal abscess

- Physical Findings

    1. Rapidly progressive respiratory distress—suprasternal and subcostal, soft inspiratory stridor, nasal flaring leading to possible respiratory arrest

    2. Toxic, distressed appearance

    3. Beefy erythematous epiglottis

    4. If epiglottitis suspected, do not attempt to visualize

- Diagnostic Tests/Findings: Often deferred to minimize distress

    1. CBC—WBC (greater than 18,800); laboratory examination is low priority in child with severe respiratory distress

    2. Cultures of blood, tracheal or epiglottis secretions—50% of cases, positive for *Haemophilus influenzae* type b

    3. Radiograph—lateral neck shows a thickened/swollen epiglottis (''thumb sign''); may elect not to perform radiograph due to possibility of airway obstruction and respiratory arrest; airway can be safely visualized in surgery

- Management/Treatment

    1. **Requires prompt recognition and treatment; represents a true medical emergency; death can occur within hours**

    2. While waiting for emergency transport, provide oxygen, keep child calm, be prepared for emergency cardiopulmonary resuscitation

    3. Following diagnosis, airway must be established by nasotracheal or endotracheal intubation or elective tracheotomy immediately; usually extubated within 24 to 48 hours after reducing epiglottis and afebrile

    4. IV antibiotic therapy for 2 to 3 days

        a. Third generation cephalosporins until initial pathogen identified

        b. In areas with penicillin and cephalosporin resistant pneumococci, vancomycin is drug of choice

    5. Oral antibiotic to follow IV to complete 10 day course

    6. Coricosteroid therapy to reduce swelling

    7. Prevention—*Haemophilus influenzae type b* vaccine at 2, 4, 6 or 12 and 15 months of age; no vaccines against other pathogens

Questions
Select the best answer

1. Which of the following would not alert you to microcephaly?

    a. Prominent sutures
    b. Early closure of anterior fontanel
    c. Normocephalic skull
    d. Severe malnutrition

2. When diagnosing an infant with microcephaly, an inappropriate differential diagnosis may be:

    a. Craniosynostosis
    b. Hyperthyroidism
    c. Hypopituitarism
    d. Severe malnutrition

3. At the 6 month well-child visit, you note another increase of 2 SD on the head circumference growth chart which is similar to the increase at the 4 month visit. Which of the following would not be considered a possible cause?

    a. Hydrocephalus
    b. Metabolic/genetic disorder
    c. Benign familial macrocephaly
    d. Hypothyroidism

4. Appropriate treatment of this 6-month-old would not consider:

    a. Waiting until 9 month visit to see if intervention is needed
    b. Ultrasound through anterior fontanel
    c. Referral to neurologist
    d. Referral for genetic counseling

5. At the 2 week visit, the newborn presents with swelling of soft tissue of the scalp which crosses the suture lines with bruising. You suspect:

    a. Cephalohematoma
    b. Child abuse
    c. Caput succedaneum
    d. Hydrocephalus

6. In treating this infant you will need to order:

    a. Nothing, as it will resolve spontaneously
    b. Phototherapy to prevent hyperbilirubinemia
    c. Referral for drainage of lesion
    d. Skull radiographs to rule out fracture

7. Which of the following would not be included in management of cephalohematoma?

    a. No intervention needed
    b. Explain to parents, the hematoma may calcify but will eventually resolve
    c. Observe for hyperbilirubinemia
    d. May need to tap and drain hematoma

8. Which of the following would not be included in the management of hydrocephalus on an infant with macrocephaly, bulging anterior fontanel and separated suture lines?

    a. Complete history with referral for surgical treatment ASAP
    b. Treatment of underlying cause
    c. Order ultrasound of head
    d. Monitor head circumference every day for 1 to 2 weeks, then consider referral if needed

9. The appropriate time to refer an infant for continuous esotropia would be:

    a. At four weeks
    b. At six months or just over
    c. Not until nine months
    d. Not until twelve months

10. Which of the following would not be included in treatment of a hordeolum?

    a. Warm moist compresses for 15 minutes throughout the day
    b. Incision and drainage
    c. Topical antibiotic eye drops
    d. Diphenhydramine for 72 hours

11. Joey (30-months-old) presents with headache, rhinorrhea, fever of 103.8° F, erythema, edema of the right eye lid, conjunctival chemosis, proptosis and decreased ocular movements. You would suspect:

    a. Periorbital cellulitis
    b. Orbital cellulitis
    c. Insect bite or trauma
    d. Acute bacterial conjunctivitis

12. Astigmatism is defined as:

    a. Nearsightedness
    b. Each eye has different refractive errors
    c. Curvature variation of the optical system
    d. Decreased vision in an eye from disuse

13. Which of the following eye disorders would not need a referral to an ophthalmologist?

    a. Pseudostrabismus
    b. Nystagmus in a 9-month-old infant
    c. Nasal lacrimal duct stenosis in a 6-month-old
    d. Cataracts

14. Signs and symptoms of bacterial conjunctivitis would not include:

    a. Mucopurulent discharge
    b. Foreign body sensation
    c. Cobblestone appearing conjunctiva
    d. "Fire red" palpebral conjunctiva

15. Absence of the red reflex usually indicates:

    a. Cataract
    b. Glaucoma
    c. Astigmatism
    d. Iritis

16. The cover/uncover test is used for detecting:

    a. Nystagmus
    b. Cataracts
    c. Strabismus
    d. Astigmatism

17. Which of the following ocular injuries would not need immediate referral?

    a. Chemical burns
    b. Corneal abrasions
    c. Hyphema
    d. Perforation wound to orbit

18. The drug of choice for the treatment of chlamydial conjunctivitis in the newborn is:

    a. Systemic penicillin G 50,000 U/kg/day for 10 days
    b. Ceftriaxone 25 to 50 mg/kg/day given once
    c. Sodium sulfacetamide 10% ophthalmic solution 4 times a day for 21 days
    d. Erythromycin 50 mg/kg/day 4 times a day for 14 days

19. Unilateral or bilateral purulent discharge and erythema of conjunctiva is most likely indicative of:

    a. Chemical conjunctivitis
    b. Bacterial conjunctivitis
    c. Herpes simplex keratoconjunctivitis
    d. Vernal conjunctivitis

20. A 10-year-old child presents with a non-tender, irritating mass in the left upper eye lid. This best describes a:

    a. Hordeolum
    b. Chalazion
    c. Foreign body
    d. Corneal abrasion

21. Which of the following is not included in this child's treatment?

    a. Immediate referral for surgical removal
    b. Warm compresses 2 to 3 times a day for 3 days
    c. Local antibiotic eye drops
    d. Corticosteroid injections

22. The most effective way to prevent spread of conjunctivitis among children and staff in day care settings is to:

    a. Cleanse eye secretions with sterile cotton balls
    b. Disinfect toys
    c. Isolate the infected child until antibiotic therapy is completed
    d. Use good hand washing technique

23. When performing the corneal light reflex assessment in a 12-month-old, the light reflected in the left eye is at 2 o'clock; light in right eye is at 12 o'clock. You would not:

    a. Consider this a normal finding
    b. Refer for further evaluation
    c. Perform the cover/uncover test
    d. Document this as an abnormal finding

24. The refractive error that occurs when light is focused in front of the retina is known as:

    a. Astigmatism
    b. Hyperopia
    c. Myopia
    d. Anisometropia

25. Which of the following clinical findings would not be seen in children with strabismus?

    a. Head tilting
    b. Face turning
    c. School problems
    d. Rhythmic eye movements

26. The following statement is false about glaucoma:

    a. Anomaly of ocular drainage system
    b. May follow eye disease
    c. Occurs bilaterally in 25% of cases
    d. Associated with congenital rubella

27. Which of following are not included in the classic triad of symptoms in glaucoma?

    a. Photophobia
    b. Epiphora
    c. Blepharospasm
    d. Persistent pain (most of the time)

28. Which of the following would not be included in the primary management of glaucoma?

    a. Instillation of anti-glaucoma drops
    b. Warn parents that blindness is inevitable
    c. Immediate referral to an ophthalmologist for diagnosis and treatment
    d. Enucleation

29. The first clue a child may have primary blindness would be the presence of:

    a. A history of prematurity
    b. Strabismus beyond 6 months
    c. Nystagmus
    d. Pigmented deposits on pupil

30. Based on your knowledge of amoxicillin oral suspension which is supplied in 400 mg/5 ml concentration with recommended dose being 40 mg/kg/day divided 2 times a day, you would order the following for Jeremy (45 pounds)?

    a. 1 tsp. orally b.i.d. for 10 days
    b. 1-$\frac{1}{4}$ tsp. orally b.i.d. for 10 days
    c. 1-$\frac{3}{4}$ tsp. orally b.i.d. for 10 days
    d. 2 tsp. orally b.i.d. for 10 days

31. Why are infants and young children predisposed to development of otitis media?

    a. Immaturity of immune mechanisms and eustachian tube is short and horizontal
    b. Eustachian tubes are long, narrow and curved
    c. The cartilage lining of the ear is undeveloped making the eustachian tube less expandable
    d. The lack of lymphoid tissue in pharynx increases vulnerability to infection

32. Sarah, age 6 years, weighing 50 pounds, presents with a history of URI and is complaining of pain in the left ear. On exam, the left ear reveals thickened bulging erythematous TM, absent light reflex, and poor mobility with pneumatic otoscopy. She has a history of penicillin allergy. Your first line antibiotic would be:

    a. Azithromycin
    b. Amoxicillin
    c. Trimethoprim-sulfamethoxazole
    d. No antibiotic is indicated with these findings

33. A tympanogram provides direct information on:

    a. Conductive hearing function
    b. Tympanic membrane mobility
    c. Semicircular canals fluid levels
    d. Pressure in the inner ear

34. Which of the following is not a characteristic of "swimmer's ear"?

    a. Erythema and exudate of the ear canal

b. Pruritus of ear canal

c. Pain upon movement of the tragus

d. Decreased hearing secondary to TM perforation

35. Your management of external otitis media would be:

   a. Neomycin/polymyxin/corticosteroid otic suspension

   b. Amoxicillin 40 mg/kg/day b.i.d. for 10 days

   c. Nothing at this time; recheck in 2 to 4 weeks

   d. Vinegar and alcohol (1:1) solution, 3 to 4 drops before and after swimming until the infection is resolved

36. The most common bacteria found with otitis media is:

   a. *Haemophilus influenza*

   b. *Streptococcus pneumoniae*

   c. *Moraxella catarrhalis*

   d. *Streptococcus pyogenes*

37. Which of the following should not be taught as preventive ear hygiene?

   a. Encouragement of supine positioning during feedings

   b. Encouragement of breast feeding

   c. Weaning off bedtime bottles

   d. Cessation of smoking around children

38. Which of the following ear disorders does not need an otolaryngologist referral?

   a. Cholesteatoma

   b. Persistent/acute O.M. unresponsive to treatment

   c. Persistent chronic O.M.E. for 8 weeks

   d. Evidence of hearing loss and/or language delay

39. A language delay is noted in a 5-year-old child who has had repeated episodes of middle ear effusion. Among the following, the most likely cause of the delay is:

   a. Attention deficit hyperactivity disorder

   b. Conductive hearing loss

   c. Mental retardation

   d. Sensorineural hearing loss

40. Which of the following would not be associated with acquired conductive hearing loss?

   a. Perforated T.M.

   b. Otitis media with effusion

   c. Impacted cerumen

   d. Meningitis

41. Which of the following is not a common complication of acute nasopharyngitis?

    a. Otitis media
    b. Sinusitis
    c. Nasal polyps
    d. Allergic rhinitis

42. A 4-year-old presents with seasonal symptoms of allergic rhinitis. Which of the following is likely to be among the most common allergens for this child?

    a. Dust mite
    b. Mold
    c. Inhaled pollens
    d. Animal dander

43. Which of the following is not a common physical finding with this 4-year-old with allergic rhinitis?

    a. Allergic ''shiner's''
    b. Hypertrophy of gingival mucosa
    c. Purulent nasal discharge
    d. Edema of nasal mucosa

44. The most common cause of epistaxis is:

    a. Trauma
    b. Mucosal irritation (e.g. nose picking)
    c. Mucosal drying
    d. Foreign body

45. Which of the following is not a common cause of sinusitis?

    a. *Haemophilus influenzae*
    b. Adenovirus
    c. *Streptococcus pneumoniae*
    d. *Staphylococcus aureus*

46. A 15-year-old presents with rhinorrhea for 14 days, headache, halitosis, cough, fever and some facial pain. You suspect:

    a. Acute nasopharyngitis
    b. Sinusitis
    c. Seasonal allergies
    d. Cocaine use

47. Which of the following would not be included in the care of the adolescent with chronic sinusitis?

    a. Nasal cultures
    b. Local steroid nasal spray
    c. Referral to allergist and/or otolaryngologist
    d. Prophylactic antibiotic for 1 to 2 months after infection is resolved

48. Which of the following would not support the diagnosis of herpangina?

    a. Vesicles and/or ulcers present on the posterior oral cavity
    b. Fever
    c. Blisters on the lips
    d. Headache and backache

49. A common opportunistic fungal infection of the oral cavity is known as:

    a. Oral candidiasis
    b. Herpangina
    c. Hand, foot and mouth disease
    d. Herpes labialis

50. Which of the following disorders of the mouth does not present with vesicles?

    a. Herpangina
    b. Hand, foot and mouth disease
    c. Oral candidiasis
    d. Herpes labialis

51. Destruction of tooth enamel occurs from:

    a. Acid demineralization
    b. Alkaline demineralization
    c. Fluoride treatments
    d. Hypercalcification

52. In counseling a new mother about her infant with a cleft lip, which of the following choices would not be included?

    a. Surgical repair by 9 to 12 months
    b. Feeding techniques
    c. Referral to otolaryngologist
    d. Referral to pediatric dentist

53. Which statement is true about cleft lip and palate?

    a. Genetics has no influence on either condition
    b. It is more common to have both than one without the other
    c. They are more common in females
    d. There is a higher incidence in African-Americans

54. Shallow, painful ulcers in the mouth that can be brought on by stress and/or trauma and considered idiopathic are:

    a. Herpetic lesions
    b. Aphthous ulcers
    c. Herpangina
    d. Coxsackievirus

55. The most common cause of pharyngitis in the young child is:

    a. Influenza virus, serotypes A + B
    b. Epstein-Barr virus
    c. Adenovirus
    d. Enterovirus

56. Group A beta hemolytic streptococcus accounts for _____ of all pharyngitis cases.

    a. 75%
    b. 50%
    c. 10 to 15%
    d. 5%

57. A 7-year-old male presents with an abrupt onset of high fever, stridor, drooling and hyperextension of the neck. Which of the following would you not suspect:

    a. Epiglottitis
    b. GABHS pharyngitis
    c. Peritonsillar abscess
    d. Retropharyngeal abscess

58. With examination of the throat, one tonsil is much larger than the other with marked erythema and displaced uvula. You suspect:

    a. Epiglottitis
    b. Peritonsillar abscess
    c. Retropharyngeal abscess
    d. Sinus abscess

59. Which of the following would not be included in the differential diagnosis for cervical lymphadenitis?

    a. Infectious mononucleosis
    b. Cat scratch fever
    c. Mumps
    d. Measles

60. One of the most common organisms found in cervical adenitis is:

    a. *Haemophilus influenzae*
    b. *Staphylococcus aureus*
    c. *Mycobacterium tuberculosis*
    d. Anaerobic organisms

61. To avoid the complications of GABHS including rheumatic fever and glomerulonephritis, the antibiotic of choice is:

    a. Penicillin
    b. Cephalosporins

    c. Cyclosporins
    d. Sulfatrim

62. Which of the following would not be appropriate management of epistaxis?

    a. Local compression of nares, position in upright position with head held forward
    b. Local compression of nares, position in supine position
    c. Local nasal phenylephrine HCL
    d. Referral to otolaryngologist for persistent profuse bleeding

Answers

1. c	21. a	42. c
2. b	22. d	43. c
3. d	23. a	44. b
4. a	24. c	45. b
5. c	25. d	46. b
6. a	26. c	47. d
7. d	27. d	48. c
8. d	28. b	49. a
9. b	29. c	50. c
10. d	30. a	51. a
11. b	31. a	52. a
12. c	32. c	53. b
13. a	33. b	54. b
14. c	34. d	55. c
15. a	35. a	56. c
16. c	36. b	57. b
17. b	37. a	58. b
18. d	38. c	59. d
19. b	39. b	60. b
20. b	40. d	61. a
	41. c	62. b

Bibliography

Abzug, M. (1999). Meeting the challenge of antibiotic resistance: An evidence based approach to treatment. *Pediatric Annals, 28*(7), 460–467.

American Academy of Pediatrics. In L. K. Pickering (Ed.). *Red Book 2000: Report of the Committee on Infectious Diseases* (25th ed.). Elk Grove Village, IL.: Author

Adderson, S. (1998). Preventing otitis media: Medical approaches. *Pediatric Annals, 27*(2), 101–107.

Ahmed, S., & Ayoub, E. (1998). Severe, invasive group A streptococcal disease and toxic shock. *Pediatric Annals, 27*(5), 287–292.

Behrman, R. E., Kliegman, R. M., & Jenson, H. B. (Eds.). (2000). *Nelson textbook of pediatrics* (16th ed.). Philadelphia: W. B. Saunders.

Byington, C. (1998). The diagnosis and management of otitis media with effusion. *Pediatric Annals, 27*(2), 96–100.

Chartrand, S., & Pong, A. (1998). Acute otitis media in the 1990s: The impact of antibiotic resistance. *Pediatric Annals, 27*(2), 86–95.

Conrad, D. (1998). Should acute otitis media be treated with antibiotics? *Pediatric Annals, 27*(2), 66–74.

Dajani, A. (1998). Current therapy of Group A streptococcal pharyngitis. *Pediatric Annals, 27*(5), 277–280.

Daly, K., Hunter, L., & Giebink, G. (1999). Chronic otitis media with effusion. *Pediatrics in Review, 20*(3), 85–93.

Gerber, M. (1998). Diagnosis of group A streptococcal pharyngitis. *Pediatric Annals, 27*(5), 269–273.

Graham, M. V., & Uphold, C. R. (1999). *Clinical guidelines in child health (2nd ed.).* FL: Barmarrae Books, Inc.

Hoberman, A., & Paradise, J. (2000). Acute otitis media: Diagnosis and management in the year 2000. *Pediatric Annals, 29*(10), 609–619.

James, J. (1999). The mechanisms and the spread of antibiotic resistance. *Pediatric Annals, 28*(7), 446–452.

Linsk, R., Gilsdorf, J., & Lesperance, M. (1999). When amoxicillin fails. *Contemporary Pediatrics, 16*(10), 67–88.

Nash, D., Schochat, E., Roaycki, A., & Musiek, F. (1997). When loud noises hurt. *Contemporary Pediatrics, 14*(6), 97–109.

Nash, D. (1998). Allergic rhinitis. *Pediatric Annals, 27*(12), 788–808.

Nyquist, A. (1999). Antibiotic use and abuse in clinical practice. *Pediatric Annals, 28*(7), 453–459.

Ogle, J. (1999). Antimicrobial therapy for ambulatory pediatrics. *Pediatric Annals, 28*(7), 434–444.

Family Nurse Practitioner

Pichichero, M. (2000). Acute otitis media: Part I. *American Family Physician, 61*(7), 2051–2056.

Pichichero, M. (2000). Acute otitis media: Part II. *American Family Physician, 61*(8), 2110–2115.

Roddey, O., & Hoover, H. (2000). Otitis media with effusion in children: A pediatric office perspective. *Pediatric Annals, 29*(10), 623–628.

Siberry, G., & Iannone, R. (2000). *The Harriet Lane Handbook* (15th ed.). St. Louis: Mosby.

Tanz, R., & Shulman, S. (1998). Streptococcal pharyngitis: The carrier state, definition and management. *Pediatric Annals, 27*(5), 281–285.

Todd, J. (1999). Principles of antibiotic use for the treatment of bacterial infection. *Pediatric Annals, 28*(7), 423–430.

Turner, R. (1998). The common cold. *Pediatric Annals, 27*(12), 790–795.

Wald, E. (1998). Sinusitis overview. *Pediatric Annals, 27*(12), 787–788.

Wald, E. (1998). Sinusitis. *Pediatric Annals, 27*(12), 811–818.

Wetmore, R. (2000). Complications of otitis media. *Pediatric Annals, 29*(10), 637–645.

Eye, Ear, Nose, and Throat Disorders In Adults

Margaret Hadro Venzke

Conjunctivitis

- Definition: Inflammation of palpebral and/or bulbar conjunctiva; classic description "red eye" or "pink eye"
- Etiology/Incidence
  1. Bacterial
     a. *Staphylococcus aureus*
     b. *Streptococcus pneumoniae*
     c. *Haemophilus influenzae*
     d. *Neisseria gonorrhoeae*
     e. Proteus species
  2. Viral
     a. Adenoviruses (most common)
        (1) Adenopharyngeal conjunctivitis (APC)—"swimming pool"
        (2) Epidemic keratoconjunctivitis (EKC)—highly contagious, corneal involvement
     b. Herpes simplex
     c. Herpes zoster
  3. Allergic
     a. Seasonal allergies—pollen, grass, trees
     b. Hypersensitivity
     c. Chemical irritants
  4. Chlamydia/trachoma
  5. Other
     a. Trauma
     b. Contact lens wearer—more susceptible than general population
     c. Foreign body
     d. Drug induced—preservative in eye drops, antimicrobials
     e. Systemic illness
        (1) Measles
        (2) Varicella
        (3) Rocky Mountain spotted fever
        (4) Reiter's syndrome
     f. Contaminated contact lens solution

g. Mascara/eyeliner, makeup

6. Mode of transmission—direct contact with contagion or allergen

7. Most common eye disease in primary care; usually benign, self-limiting disorder

- Signs and Symptoms

1. Mild to moderate redness and irritation

2. No acute change in visual acuity

3. Absence of photophobia

4. Mild discomfort/pain, often associated with itching, burning sensation or excessive tearing

5. Watery to purulent discharge

6. Bacterial conjunctivitis

    a. Mucopurulent discharge (profuse exudate suggests *Neisseria gonorrhoeae*)

    b. Thick purulent crust of material on eyelids after night's sleep

    c. Unilateral (initially)

    d. Self limiting—10 to 14 days without treatment, resolves in 2 to 4 days with treatment

7. Viral conjunctivitis

    a. Redness, general discomfort, profuse watery discharge

    b. Preauricular adenopathy common

    c. Association with upper respiratory illness, fever, pharyngitis

    d. Bilateral presentation

    e. Symptoms last 2 to 3 weeks (contagious, viral shedding in tears for approximately 2 weeks)

8. Allergic

    a. Moderate to severe bilateral itching

    b. Clear to stringy mucoid discharge

    c. Chronic hypersensitivity—vernal conjunctivitis associated with corneal ulceration

9. Chlamydial conjunctivitis

    a. More often unilateral than bilateral

    b. Moderate exudate

    c. Enlarged, tender preauricular nodes

    d. Symptoms persist 3 to 9 months without treatment

Table 1

	Conjunctivitis	Iritis	Acute Glaucoma
Pain	mild	moderate	severe
Vision	normal	slightly blurred	blurred
Discharge	mucopurulent	clear	clear
Cornea	clear	clear	cloudy
Pupil	normal	small irregular	oval dilated
Light Response	normal	poor	poor
Conjunctival injection	diffuse toward fornices	circumcorneal	corneal/ conjunctival hyperemia

- Differential Diagnosis

    1. Urgent ophthalmic conditions—prompt referral to avoid compromised eyesight. See Table 1

        a. Acute uveitis/iritis

        b. Acute glaucoma

        c. Corneal trauma/infection

        d. Orbital cellulitis

- Physical Findings

    1. Injected conjunctiva

    2. Discharge (see signs and symptoms)

    3. Cornea—clear

    4. Pupillary response—equal and reactive to light

    5. Visual acuity (Snellen)—no acute change

    6. Preauricular adenopathy—often viral etiology

- Diagnostic Tests/Findings

    1. Fluorescein uptake staining—dye uptake suggests corneal involvement

    2. Culture—only if chronic problem or gonococcal conjunctivitis suspected

    3. Gram stain of discharge/scrapings—rarely done unless gonococcal conjunctivitis suspected

- Management/Treatment

    1. Pharmacologic

        a. Bacterial conjunctivitis

            (1) Sodium sulfacetamide 10% ophthalmic solution, one to two drops every 4 hours while awake or q.i.d. for 5 to 7 days

      (2)   Bacitracin/polymyxin ophthalmic ointment, apply thin layer in lower conjunctival sac b.i.d. for 7 days

      (3)   Erythromycin ophthalmic ointment, apply thin layer in lower conjunctival sac q.i.d. for 5 to 7 days

   b.   Gonococcal conjunctivitis—refer to ophthalmologist

      (1)   Topical antibiotics—erythromycin

      (2)   Intravenous (IV) antibiotics

         (a)   Ceftriaxone

         (b)   Aqueous penicillin

   c.   Chlamydia conjunctivitis

      (1)   Doxycycline 100 mg orally b.i.d. for 21 days

      (2)   Erythromycin 250 mg 6 times/day for 21 days

   d.   Viral conjunctivitis

      (1)   Self-limiting

      (2)   Topical antibiotics—to prevent secondary bacterial infection

      (3)   Corticosteroids contraindicated

   e.   Allergic conjunctivitis

      (1)   Topical vasoconstrictors/antihistamines

         (a)   Naphazoline HCL/pheniramine maleate—1 to 2 drops q.i.d.

         (b)   Oral antihistamines

         (c)   Allergen avoidance

2.   General measures

   a.   Cool/warm compresses

   b.   Frequent gentle eye wash to remove discharge

   c.   Artificial tears

   d.   Strict handwashing

   e.   Use separate towels; avoid handshaking

   f.   Contact lens care—clean contacts, use new solutions, avoid ''homemade'' tap water solutions

   g.   Avoid eye cosmetics during infection; change eye products frequently

   h.   Refer if no improvement in 48 hours or if vision is impaired

Blepharitis

- Definition: Inflammation of eyelid margins and eyelashes

- Etiology/Incidence
    1. Commonly affects elderly persons
    2. Associated with seborrheic dermatitis and acne rosacea
    3. Often a chronic condition
    4. Seborrheic blepharitis
        a. Erythematous lid margins
        b. Dry flakes, oily secretions
        c. Cosmetics and chemicals aggravate the condition
    5. Staphylococcal (ulcerative) blepharitis
        a. Acute/chronic inflammation of glands of lid margins
        b. *Staphylococcus aureus* and *Staphylococcus epidermidis* are causative organisms
        c. Mild ulceration of lid margin
        d. Loss of lashes
    6. Mixed blepharitis—most common (seborrheic with secondary staphylococcal infection)
    7. Infestation of eyelashes with lice
- Signs and Symptoms
    1. Gritty, burning sensation
    2. Crusted material on eyelids upon awakening
    3. Redness
    4. Swelling of lid margins
    5. Dry or greasy scales on lashes
    6. Mild conjunctival irritation and erythema
- Differential Diagnosis
    1. Conjunctivitis
    2. Chronic chalazia
    3. Sebaceous cell carcinoma (rare)
    4. Keratitis
- Physical Findings
    1. Erythematous eyelid margins
    2. Scaly lesions on lashes
    3. Sclera—white

4. Conjunctivae—usually clear

5. Masses on lids/lid margins (palpate with gloves)

6. Preauricular adenopathy

7. Visual acuity (no change)

- Diagnostic Tests/Findings—none usually indicated
- Management/Treatment

1. Warm water compresses

2. Eyelid margin scrubs 2 to 4 times a day

   a. Use washcloth or cotton tip applicator, moisten with dilute solution of water and baby shampoo or commercial lid cleaner

   b. Rinse well

3. Antibiotic ointment q.i.d. to lid margins for 7 days (erythromycin, sulfacetamide sodium)

4. Systemic antibiotics for severe infection—doxycycline 100 mg b.i.d. for 6 weeks

5. Co-existing seborrhea of face/scalp—treat with selenium sulfide shampoo

6. Maintain hygiene (lid washes) to prevent recurrence of seborrheic and mixed blepharitis

7. Infestation of lice

   a. 1% permethrin creme rinse, following shampoo of head, which kills both lice and eggs; requires one application whereas others require more than one

   b. Apply thick petrolatum to eyelashes b.i.d.

   c. Remove nits from lashes and hair

Foreign Body in Eye

- Description: Object or debris in eye causing irritation
- Etiology/Incidence

1. Most common ocular injury in primary care

2. Foreign body (FOB) often lodges in conjunctiva or cornea

- Signs and Symptoms

1. Unilateral, acute onset

2. Sensation of ''something in my eye''

3. Photophobia

4. Redness

5. Mild pain

      6. Mild decrease in visual acuity

- Differential Diagnosis
    1. Intraocular foreign body (penetrates eye globe)
    2. Corneal laceration
    3. Corneal abrasion
    4. "Contact lens wearer" keratitis
- Physical Findings
    1. Diagnosis based on physical findings
    2. Visual acuity may be normal
    3. Cornea—examine under magnification and bright light, FOB may show up as a dark speck
    4. Ring-shaped orange stain—embedded iron or steel body
    5. Observe for laceration, hyphema, irregular pupil or absent red reflex—immediate ophthalmic referral
    6. Conjunctiva—instruct patient to look down, grasp lashes, evert eyelid, inspect upper eye and lid
- Diagnostic Tests/Findings—fluorescein stain highlights presence of foreign body and corneal abrasion
- Management/Treatment
    1. Remove simple (non-penetrating) foreign body with moistened cotton applicator with water or sterile normal saline; re-evaluate visual acuity
    2. Irrigation of eye—use only for chemical splash to eyes
    3. Antibiotic ophthalmic ointment
    4. Eye pad
    5. Follow-up in 24 hours to evaluate
    6. Patient education:
        a. Caution—no rubbing of eye
        b. Advise protective eye wear
    7. Refer
        a. Intraocular foreign body
        b. Change in visual acuity
        c. Acute ocular pain
        d. Large corneal abrasion

Corneal Abrasion

- Definition: Disruption in the epithelial surface of the cornea by mechanical or chemical factors
- Etiology/Incidence
    1. Common eye injury
    2. Direct trauma to eye; most commonly a scratch from contact lens, fingernail or piece of paper
    3. Chemical splash
- Signs and Symptoms
    1. Unilateral severe eye pain
    2. Redness
    3. Tearing
    4. Photophobia
    5. Scratchy sensation that worsens with blinking
    6. Decreased visual acuity
    7. Difficulty keeping eye open
- Differential Diagnosis
    1. Keratitis (viral, bacterial, or acanthamoeba)
    2. Foreign body
    3. Corneal laceration
- Physical Findings
    1. Document visual acuity—often decreased
    2. Visualization of corneal lesion following fluorescein stain illuminated with cobalt blue light
- Diagnostic Tests/Findings: Fluorescein dye—abraded or ulcerated areas will become stained and fluorese yellow-green color
- Management/Treatment
    1. Antibiotic ointment or sulfonamide drops to affected eye
    2. May use pressure patch to decrease movement of eye
    3. Oral analgesics or short acting cycloplegic agent for pain relief
    4. Follow-up eye evaluation in 24 hours to assess healing—refer immediately if no improvement
    5. Topical antibiotics q.i.d. for 24 to 48 hours
    6. Avoid topical anesthetic drops; retard healing

7. Topical steroids contraindicated; retard healing and increase risk of infection

8. If chemical or thermal injury to eye, refer immediately to ophthalmology

Glaucoma

- Definition: Increased intraocular eye pressure resulting in atrophy of optic nerve, loss of visual fields and acuity

- Etiology/Incidence

    1. Inadequate drainage of aqueous fluid in the anterior chamber of the eye

    2. Most common type is chronic open angle (wide angle)

    3. Chronic open angle glaucoma

        a. Accounts for 90% of all cases

        b. Predominately seen over age 40

        c. Blacks are affected more frequently

        d. Positive family history

        e. Diabetes mellitus is a risk factor

    4. Primary angle closure (closed angle or narrow angle)

        a. Positive family history

        b. African-Americans and Asians more affected than Caucasians

        c. Predominately age 55 to 75 years

        d. Females more than males

        e. Less common than "open angle" but more severe in presentation

        f. May be precipitated by stress, anxiety, darkness, increased fluid intake or medications

    5. Congenital glaucoma (developmental) in young children

    6. Approximately 0.5% of total population

- Signs and Symptoms

    1. Chronic open angle glaucoma—obstruction to aqueous outflow

        a. Asymptomatic at onset

        b. Mid-peripheral vision affected in early stages

        c. Frequent change of glasses

        d. Central vision loss is a late sign

        e. Gradual, painless visual loss and ultimate blindness

    2. Primary angle closure—mechanical obstruction of flow of aqueous humor; iris may obstruct the trabecular meshwork at canal of Schlemm resulting in elevated

intraocular pressure

    a. Acute ocular pain

    b. Nausea, vomiting

    c. Photophobia

    d. Blurred vision

    e. Halos around lights at night

    f. Unilateral frontal headache

    g. Tearing

    h. Erythema

- Differential Diagnosis

  1. Uveitis

  2. Conjunctivitis

  3. Ocular trauma

  4. Neurological disease

- Physical Findings

  1. Visual acuity—decreased

  2. Cornea is clear

  3. Change in peripheral vision as measured by direct confrontation

  4. Chronic open angle glaucoma

     a. Cupping of optic disc

     b. Normal or elevated intraocular pressure (IOP)

  5. Primary angle closure

     a. Lid edema

     b. Injected conjunctiva

     c. Fixed mid-dilated pupil

     d. Shallow anterior chamber, often cloudy

- Diagnostic Tests/Findings

  1. Tonometry (normal range 10 to 20 mm Hg)

  2. Pressure reading 20 mm Hg or greater requires further evaluation

  3. U.S. Preventive Task Force recommends glaucoma testing after age 65, no consensus on frequency of screening

- Management/Treatment

  1. Refer all patients with

a. Elevated IOP

b. Decreased visual acuity

c. Visual field loss

2. Goal of therapy to stabilize IOP to prevent optic nerve damage and visual loss

3. Pharmacological—chronic open angle glaucoma

a. Parasympathomimetics—topical miotics (pilocarpine) facilitates aqueous outflow

b. Beta blockers decrease aqueous (timolol, betaxolol) production

c. Carbonic anhydrase inhibitors (acetazolamide)—reduces aqueous production

d. Hyperosmotics—reduces formation of fluid (mannitol)

4. Pharmacological—primary angle closure

a. Emergency treatment with IV acetazolamide, mannitol and oral glycerol

b. Maintenance therapy with additional miotic agents and corticosteriods

5. Laser and surgical intervention may be indicated after maximizing medication therapy

6. General measures

a. Encourage frequent follow-up with ophthalmology

b. Monitor side effects of medications

c. Avoid over the counter cold preparations that may exacerbate glaucoma

Cataracts

- Definition: Clouding/opacity of crystalline lens, causing disruption of visual acuity
- Etiology/Incidence
  1. Single largest cause of blindness
  2. 90% of cataracts due to aging process (senile cataract)
  3. Congenital cataract (rubella)
  4. Systemic disease (diabetes and thyroid)
  5. Drug induced, especially steroid use
  6. Ocular trauma
  7. Chronic uveitis
  8. Ultraviolet B light exposure
- Signs and Symptoms
  1. Painless

2. Cloudy, fuzzy, blurred vision

3. Change in refractive error

4. Glare associated with bright lights (night driving)

5. Alteration in color perception

6. Unilateral or bilateral development

- Differential Diagnosis

1. Senile macular degeneration (loss of central vision)

2. Retinal detachment

3. Diabetic retinopathy

4. Ocular tumor

- Physical Findings

1. Lens opacity

2. Disruption of red reflex

3. Visual acuity decreased

4. Reduced color discrimination

- Diagnostic Tests/Findings—refer to ophthalmology

- Management/Treatment

1. Refer to ophthalmologist

2. Surgical intervention—lens implant is preferred treatment

3. Follow-up post operatively to observe for hemorrhage or infection

4. Non-surgical treatment—frequent changes in glasses, bifocals, or contacts

5. Optimize the environment of the inoperable patient with increased light sources, decreased glare, reorganize living space to prevent accidents/falls

6. Prevention with protective eyewear to filter ultraviolet B exposure

Impaired Vision

- Definition: Decreased/blurred visual acuity

- Etiology/Incidence

1. Associated with lens opacity, damage to photoreceptor cells, damage to optic nerve, visual cortex or refractory error

2. Legal blindness—20/200 or less in best eye with correction

3. Presbyopia—loss of accommodative capacity of lens with age; inability to focus on objects at normal reading distance

- Signs and Symptoms

1. Decreased vision

    a. Sudden or gradual

    b. Unilateral or bilateral

2. Pain

3. Floaters

4. Peripheral vision loss

5. Association with systemic symptoms

- Differential Diagnosis

    1. Refractive error

    2. Cataract

    3. Macular degeneration

    4. Glaucoma

    5. Retinal vascular occlusion/detachment

    6. Temporal arteritis

    7. Optic neuritis—often first sign of multiple sclerosis

    8. Cerebrovascular accident (CVA) or tumor

- Physical Findings—vary according to etiology

    1. Decreased visual acuity

    2. Unilateral visual loss, often seen in retinal detachment, temporal arteritis, or optic neuritis

    3. Conjunctiva—clear or injected (glaucoma)

    4. Cornea—clear or cloudy (cataracts)

    5. Visual field deficit—associated with glaucoma, cerebrovascular disease, or tumor

    6. Pupils—small, irregular size, with poor response to light, common in iritis or glaucoma

    7. Extraocular movements—nystagmus associated with neurological disease

    8. Funduscopic examination may reveal

        a. Absent red reflex (cataracts)

        b. Hemorrhages, exudates (diabetes)

        c. Optic disc swelling/cupping (glaucoma, papilledema)

- Diagnostic Tests

    1. Tonometry

    2. Slit lamp

- Management/Treatment—based upon cause of visual loss
  1. Refer to ophthalmologist
     a. Sudden loss of vision—requires emergency consultation
     b. Abnormal physical examination findings
     c. Complaints of flashing lights
     d. Visual loss associated with systemic disease
     e. Diabetics
  2. Prevention
     a. Visual disorders in the elderly often lead to trauma from falls and motor vechicle accidents
     b. U.S. Preventive Task Force recommends screening for glaucoma after age 65; no consensus on routine visual acuity screening

Acute Otitis Media (AOM)

- Definition: Inflammation of middle ear
- Etiology/Incidence
  1. Eustachian tube dysfunction (ETD) or obstruction secondary to viral nasal pharyngitis—major pathogenic factors causing ineffective drainage of middle ear
  2. Bacterial pathogens
     a. *Streptococcus pneumoniae* (most common)
     b. *Haemophilus influenzae*
     c. *Moraxella* (branhamella) *catarrhalis*
     d. Occasional streptococcus or *Staphylococcus aureus*
  3. More frequent in young children (under age 7) than adults
  4. Risk factors include:
     a. Recent URI
     b. Congenital disorders—cleft palate, Down syndrome
     c. Active or passive smoking
     d. Native American/Eskimo heritage
     e. Family history of otitis media
- Signs and Symptoms
  1. Earache
  2. Fever
  3. Hearing loss (conductive)

4. Otorrhea (if perforated eardrum)

5. Intense pain, followed by popping sound; acute relief indicative of perforated tympanic membrane (TM)

6. Vertigo

- Differential Diagnosis

    1. Otitis externa

    2. Referred pain from jaw/teeth

    3. Dental abscess

    4. Mastoiditis

    5. Ear canal furuncle

- Physical Findings

    1. May see bulging tympanic membrane

    2. Distorted light reflex/obscured landmarks

    3. Pneumatic otoscopy may show decreased TM mobility

    4. Erythema—inconsistent finding

    5. Bullae may form on TM—associated with *Mycoplasma pneumoniae* organism

    6. Preauricular or cervical adenopathy

- Diagnostic Tests/Findings

    1. Usually no tests ordered

    2. Needle aspiration of middle ear fluid for culture—only in immunosuppressed patients and severe mastoiditis

    3. Tympanometry—for recurrent infections; indicator of fluid posterior to TM

    4. CBC with differential—if patient appears toxic; elevated WBC count

- Management/Treatment

    1. Antibiotics

        a. Amoxicillin 250 to 500 mg orally t.i.d. for 10 days; alternative is amoxicillin 500 mg b.i.d. for 10 days

            (1) Advantage—inexpensive

            (2) Disadvantage—ineffective against Beta lactamase producing pathogens

            (3) Avoid in those with penicillin allergy

        b. Trimethoprim/sulfamethoxazole (TMP/SMX)—(160 mg TMP/ 800 mg SMX) every 12 hours for 10 days

        c. For recurrent otitis media with resistant pathogens:

> (1) Amoxicillin clavulanate
>
> (2) Cephalosporins—such as cefixime, cefaclor

2. If perforation is present, combined therapy of oral antibiotic and topical cortisporin otic suspension—4 drops in each ear t.i.d. or q.i.d. for 10 days

3. Pain management

   a. Acetaminophen

   b. Codeine

   c. Topical local anesthetic otic solution—pain reliever

4. Refer/consult with MD or otolaryngologist

   a. No response to treatment after 48 to 72 hours

   b. Persistent hearing loss after adequate treatment

   c. Complications

      (1) Mastoiditis

      (2) Facial nerve palsy

      (3) Chronic perforation

      (4) Recurrent infections

   d. Surgical procedures—myringotomy, tympanostomy tubes for recurrent infection

Serous Otitis Media (SOM)

- Definition: Effusion in middle ear (also known as chronic otitis media with effusion)
- Etiology/Incidence

  1. Patency of eustachian tube is impaired; prevents equalization of pressure

  2. Associated with:

     a. Subacute infection

     b. Allergic manifestations

     c. Barotrauma

     d. Deviated septum

     e. Hypertrophic adenoids

     f. Benign or malignant neoplasms

  3. More common in children than adults

- Signs and Symptoms

  1. Hearing loss

2. Popping sensation with yawning/swallowing

3. Fullness in ear

4. Occasional dizziness

5. Often asymptomatic

- Differential Diagnosis

  1. Acute otitis media

  2. Conductive hearing loss

  3. Meniere's disease

- Physical findings

  1. Tympanic membrane—retracted

  2. Air fluid level present, often with yellow/blue tinged fluid posterior to TM or bubbles of air may be seen through tympanic membrane

  3. Decreased membrane mobility with insufflation

  4. Conductive hearing loss

     a. Weber Test—lateralize to affected side

     b. Rinne Test—bone conduction greater than air conduction BC> AC

- Diagnostic Tests/Findings

  1. Audiometry—decreased hearing

  2. Tympanometry—shows middle ear effusion

- Management/Treatment

  1. If mild symptoms, may spontaneously resolve in 2 to 3 weeks

  2. Topical decongestants—phenylephrine 1 to 2 sprays to each nostril every 8 to 12 hours for 3 days only

  3. Oral decongestants may be helpful

  4. Antihistamines usually are ineffective

  5. Patient education on Valsalva maneuver or chewing gum—to relieve eustachian tube blockage

  6. Follow-up in 4 to 6 weeks

  7. Refer if persistent hearing loss

Otitis Externa

- Definition: Inflammation of external auditory canal; commonly known as "swimmer's ear"

- Etiology/Incidence

1. Infectious agents include:

   a. *Pseudomonas aeruginosa* (most common)

   b. *Staphylococcus aureus* or streptococcus

   c. *Proteus mirabilis*

   d. Fungi

2. Inflammation develops from:

   a. Frequent exposure to water (most common)

   b. Mechanical trauma from bobby pins, cotton applicators, ear plugs, hearing aids

   c. Eczema, skin disorders

3. Common in summer months, especially in hot, humid climates

4. More common in swimmers than non-swimmers

- Signs and Symptoms

   1. Otalgia—gradual or acute onset

   2. Pruritus

   3. Purulent discharge

   4. Occasional hearing loss ''plugged ear''

- Differential Diagnosis

   1. Furuncle

   2. Otitis media

   3. Mastoiditis

   4. Foreign body

   5. Eczema

   6. Cellulitis

- Physical Findings

   1. Erythema and edema of ear canal

   2. Pain on manipulation of auricle or pressure on tragus

   3. Purulent or white ''cheesy'' exudate may be present

   4. Preauricular adenopathy

   5. Edema may impair visualization of tympanic membrane; TM usually not affected

- Diagnostic Tests/Findings—culture of discharge if no response to treatment or recurrent infection

- Management/Treatment

1. Pharmacologic

   a. Combined antibiotic, hydrocortisone and propylene glycol will effectively treat infection and reduce inflammation—cortisporin otic solution 4 to 5 gtts in ear(s) t.i.d. or q.i.d. for 7 days

   b. Antifungal and antibacterial—acetic acid otic drops

   c. Saturated cotton wick with medication facilitates entry of medication in ear canal; moisten with antibiotic as directed

   d. Severe cases often require systemic antibiotics

   e. Analgesics

2. General measures

   a. Protect ear from additional moisture

   b. Eliminate trauma to ear canal

   c. Prevent recurrences—instill 2% acetic acid 2 to 3 drops in ear canals b.i.d. after contact with water (commercial OTC products also available)

   d. Improvement in 48 hours after initiating treatment

   e. Instruction on proper technique to clean ears

Hearing Loss

- Definition: Diminished ability to detect pure tones in decibels of 30 or greater

- Etiology/Incidence

  1. 10% of U.S. population has hearing problems

  2. Particularly common among the elderly

  3. Hearing loss may result from interference in sound conduction (conduction loss) or impaired transmission through nervous system (sensorineural) or both (mixed hearing loss)

  4. Conductive loss—decreased ability of external and middle ear to conduct sound waves to inner ear due to:

     a. Cerumen impaction

     b. Foreign body

     c. Otitis media

     d. Otosclerosis—hereditary, bony ankylosis of stapes

     e. Scarring or perforation of TM

     f. Congenital problems

     g. Cholesteatoma

5. Sensorineural loss—results from changes to cochlea and/or involvement of the acoustic nerve; causes include:

    a. Acoustic neuroma

    b. Meniere's disease

    c. Presbycusis—hearing loss associated with aging

    d. Excessive noise exposure

    e. Viral syndrome—rubella, mumps

    f. Drugs—ASA, gentamicin, furosemide, erythromycin

    g. Syphilis

    h. Multiple sclerosis

- Signs and Symptoms

    1. Conductive hearing loss—decreased ability to detect low tones and vowels; often history of ear disease, patient speaks softly

    2. Sensorineural—impaired high tone perception, poor speech discrimination, difficulty with background noise, and high pitched female voice; patient speaks loudly

    3. Presbycusis—hearing loss is bilateral; gradual in onset; loss of high frequencies first, then lower frequency sounds; tinnitus is common

- Differential Diagnosis—see Etiology

- Physical Findings

    1. Otoscopic examination of ear—usually normal

    2. Gross hearing/whisper test—diminished (acoustic nerve)

    3. Rinne test—compares air to bone conduction

        a. Normal—AC>BC

        b. Conductive loss BC>AC in affected ear(s)

        c. Sensorineural loss AC>BC

    4. Weber test

        a. Normal—sound midline

        b. Conductive loss—lateralize to affected ear

        c. Sensorineural loss—lateralize to normal ear

    5. Red flags for immediate referral:

        a. Cholesteatoma in conductive loss

        b. Acoustic neuroma in sensorineural loss

- Diagnostic Tests/Findings

1. Pure tone audiometry by audiologist

   a. Intensity is measured in decibels (dB), frequency is measured in hertz

   b. Threshold of normal hearing O-20 dB

      (1) Mild loss—20-40 dB (soft spoken voice)

      (2) Moderate loss—40-60 dB (normal spoken voice)

      (3) Severe loss—60-80 dB (loud spoken voice)

2. Speech discrimination testing

   a. Detects clarity of hearing—impaired in sensorineural loss

   b. Results recorded as percentage correct

   c. 90 to 100% is normal

3. CT scan or MRI—to detect tumors

- Management/Treatment—dependent on etiology

1. Refer for formal audiogram

2. Refer to otolaryngologist—particularly for sensorineural loss and conductive loss unresponsive to treatment

3. Prevention

   a. Avoid loud music, machines (causes loss of high tones)

   b. Monitor ototoxic drugs carefully; if tinnitus or hearing loss discontinue use

   c. U.S. Preventive Task Force recommends routine screening after 65 years of age

4. Hearing aids—hearing amplification, beneficial to patients with correctable hearing loss

Vertigo

- Definition: Abnormal sensation of movement; disturbances of peripheral/ central vestibular system which maintains spatial orientation/posture

- Etiology/Incidence

1. Causative factors include:

   a. Medications—especially aspirin and alcohol

   b. Infections—middle/inner ear, viral illness

   c. CNS disease—multiple sclerosis, syphilis

2. True vertigo is a vestibular disease

3. Diagnosis of exclusion

- Signs and Symptoms

1. "Room spinning"/weaving sensation

2. Nausea, vomiting, diaphoresis

3. Imbalance

4. Tinnitus

5. Hearing loss

6. Vague lightheadedness

- Differential Diagnosis

    1. Acoustic neuroma

    2. Meniere's disease

    3. Benign positional vertigo—in geriatric patient

    4. Cerebrovascular accident (CVA)

    5. Transient ischemic attacks (TIA)

    6. Vestibular neuritis

    7. Acute labyrinthitis—associated with recent URI

    8. Medication toxicity

- Physical Findings

    1. Nystagmus with testing of extraocular movements

    3. Hearing loss

    4. Changes in blood pressure—associated with positional hypotension

    5. Carotid bruits—suggests impaired cerebral flow

    6. Cranial nerves—especially auditory changes, 5, 7, 8

    7. Romberg test—often abnormal

    8. Barany maneuver—stimulates vestibular system, reproduces vertigo

- Diagnostic Tests/Findings

    1. Audiogram if hearing impaired

    2. CT scan/MRI—to rule out tumor/neurological dysfunction

    3. VDRL and FTA—reactive in syphilis

    4. TSH, CBC with differential and glucose—to rule out infections and systemic disease

    5. Serum B_{12} to rule out pernicious anemia

- Management/Treatment

    1. Immediate referral, if abnormal neurological signs

    2. Bed rest

3. Antivertigo medications

    a. Meclizine—12.5 to 25 mg orally t.i.d.; causes dry mouth and sedation

    b. Dramamine 50 mg orally t.i.d.

    c. Scopolamine transdermal patch

4. Antiemetic for nausea/vomiting—promethazine 25 mg q.i.d.; or prochlorperazine 5 to 10 mg q.i.d.

5. Do not perform tests for positional vertigo on geriatric patients

6. Refer if vertigo persists

Epistaxis

- Definition: Bleeding from nostril, nasal cavity or nasopharynx

- Etiology/Incidence

    1. Anterior nosebleed most common, occurring in the vascular plexus of septum (Kisselbach plexus)

    2. Disruption of nasal mucosa due to:

        a. Trauma

        b. Infection

        c. Allergies

        d. Dry environment

        e. Medications

        f. Cocaine use

        g. Neoplasm

        h. Occasionally systemic disease (hypertension, blood dyscrasia)

    3. 10% of population will experience one significant nosebleed

- Signs and Symptoms

    1. Anterior epistaxis

        a. Unilateral bleeding from nostril

        b. Recurrent episodes last few minutes to $\frac{1}{2}$ hour

        c. Venous source of blood

    2. Posterior epistaxis—occurs more in the elderly, often difficult to correct

        a. Intermittent brisk bleeding

        b. Arterial source

        c. Blood flows into pharynx, may cause nausea and coffee ground emesis

- Differential Diagnosis: Epistaxis is a sign/symptom, not a disease; assess for significant pathology
    1. Coagulation disorders
    2. Nasal malignancy
    3. Hereditary telangiectasia
    4. Malignant hypertension
- Physical Findings
    1. Visual site—usually bleeding from one nostril; bilateral bleeding suggests trauma
    2. Skin, mucous membranes and conjunctivae with evidence of the following suggests a pathological condition:
        a. Rash
        b. Pallor
        c. Purpura
        d. Petechiae
        e. Telangiectasis
- Diagnostic Tests/Findings: Dependent on suspected etiology
    1. Hemoglobin and hematocrit are decreased if severe blood loss
    2. Low platelet count and abnormal PT/PTT suggests a bleeding disorder
- Management/Treatment
    1. Position patient sitting up and leaning forward
    2. Apply continuous pinching pressure to anterior nasal septum for 10 to 15 minutes
    3. If inadequate blood clotting, place a small cotton pledget of 1:1000 epinephrine or vasoconstrictor nasal drops (phenylephrine) into vestibule of nose; apply pressure for 5 to 10 minutes; this will stop most anterior venous bleeds
    4. Application of ice may assist with clot formation
    5. Refer to emergency room or otolaryngologist if bleeding persistent/ continuous or if posterior bleed is suspected
    6. General measures/prevention
        a. Warn against habitual nose picking, rubbing nose, forceful blowing
        b. Advise increased humidity, especially in winter months
        c. Use petrolatum based ointment in nostril—promotes hydration
        d. Instruct patient on how to manage simple nosebleeds
    7. Recurrent episodes of epistaxis require additional investigation

Common Cold

- Definition: Minor, self-limiting viral illness of upper respiratory tract mucosa
- Etiology/Incidence
    1. Caused by rhinoviruses or corona viruses
    2. Most common reason for "sick day"
    3. Incidence decreases with age
        a. Children average 6 to 8 colds per year
        b. Adults average 2 to 4 colds per year
    4. Transmission through hand to hand contact and airborne droplets
- Signs and Symptoms
    1. General malaise and fatigue
    2. Coryza
    3. Sore throat
    4. Low grade fever
    5. Nasal congestion/stuffiness
    6. Watery eyes
    7. Headache
    8. Nonproductive cough
    9. Symptoms last approximately seven days
- Differential Diagnosis
    1. Influenza
    2. *Mycoplasma pneumoniae*
    3. Otitis media
    4. Sinusitis
    5. Rhinitis
- Physical Findings
    1. Mildly elevated temperature
    2. Conjunctivae clear, possible erythema
    3. Injected nasal and pharyngeal mucosa
    4. Lungs clear
    5. Clear rhinorrhea
- Diagnostic Tests/Findings—none indicated; throat culture if streptococcal pharyngitis suspected

- Management/Treatment—palliative

    1. Rest, maintain fluid hydration

    2. Acetaminophen or ibuprofen for fever and headache

    3. Topical decongestants for nasal congestion; use 3 to 4 days only to avoid ''rebound congestion''

    4. Oral decongestants for congestion

    5. Antihistamines not indicated for cold symptoms; often included in over the counter medications (OTC); sedation side effect

    6. OTC decongestants are used cautiously in diabetic, hypertensive and glaucoma patients

    7. Antitussive cough medication

    8. Vitamin C—may reduce days of illness

    9. Frequent hand washing to prevent viral spread

    10. Zinc lozenges to decrease symptoms, contraindicated in pregnancy

    11. Symptoms lasting longer than 2 weeks may indicate secondary bacterial infection

Influenza

- Definition: Acute, contagious, febrile respiratory, viral infection

- Etiology/Incidence

    1. Influenza viral type A, B, C

    2. Type A influenza is most virulent, causing increased mortality

    3. Incubation 1 to 5 days

    4. Infections usually occur during epidemics in winter months

    5. Transmitted by airborne droplets

- Signs and Symptoms

    1. High fever, chills, (sudden onset)

    2. Headache

    3. Myalgia (often severe)

    4. Malaise

    5. Sore throat

    6. Nonproductive cough

    7. Nausea and vomiting

    8. Coryza

- Differential Diagnosis

1. Upper respiratory infection (URI)
2. Bronchitis
3. Pertussis
4. Pneumonia
5. Infectious mononucleosis
6. Early HIV infection

- Physical Findings
    1. Elevated temperature, rapid pulse
    2. Skin flushed
    3. Watery eyes
    4. Clear nasal discharge
    5. Occasional tender cervical lymph nodes
    6. Pharyngeal erythema
    7. Lungs—clear (occasional wheezes or rales)

- Diagnostic Tests/Findings
    1. Usually none
    2. Complete blood count (CBC) or white blood count (WBC)—mild leukopenia
    3. Chest radiography—normal

- Management/Treatment
    1. Supportive measures
        a. Increase fluid intake
        b. Humidified air
        c. Salt water gargles
        d. Analgesics and rest (for fever and myalgia)
    2. Antiviral Medications
        a. Amantadine 100 mg orally b.i.d. for 2 to 7 days
            (1) Only effective against influenza A
            (2) Shortens duration of fever, and respiratory/systemic symptoms by 50%
            (3) Needs to be administered within first 48 hours of onset of illness
            (4) Side effects—insomnia, anxiety, lightheadedness, difficulty concentrating
            (5) Prophylaxis for high risk, unvaccinated persons—100 mg orally daily for 2 weeks

b. Rimantadine 100 mg orally b.i.d. for 7 days

   (1) Only effective against influenza type A

   (2) Fewer side effects than amantadine

   (3) Use in patients with renal failure

c. Zanamivir two inhalations every 12 hours for 5 days

   (1) Effective against influenza type A and B

   (2) Administer within 48 hours of onset of symptoms

   (3) Contraindicated in patients with asthma, COPD

d. Oseltamavir 75 mg orally b.i.d. for 5 days

   (1) Effective against uncomplicated cases of influenza type A and B

   (2) For patients 18 years of age and older

   (3) Administer within 48 hours of onset of symptoms

3. Monitor for complications—especially in the elderly

a. Bacterial pneumonia

b. Otitis media

c. Reye's syndrome

d. Myocarditis (rare)

e. Bronchitis

4. Prevention—Trivalent influenza vaccination 0.5cc IM deltoid

a. Administer every fall, prior to winter months

b. Target populations

   (1) Over age 65

   (2) Nursing home patients

   (3) Patients with chronic cardiac/respiratory disorders

   (4) Immunocompromised patients (i.e: asplenic persons, H.I.V. infection)

   (5) Persons living in institutional settings

   (6) Pregnant females in 2nd and 3rd trimesters

   (7) Health care providers

c. Contraindicated in persons allergic to eggs

d. Administer concomitantly with pneumococcal vaccine in high risk patients

Pharyngitis

- Definition: Inflammation of pharynx, tonsils or both (sore throat)

- Etiology/Incidence
    1. Viral pharyngitis (most common)
        a. Respiratory viruses—adenovirus
        b. Rhinovirus
        c. Herpangina—due to Coxsackie virus
        d. Epstein-Barr (EBV), cytomegalovirus (CMV)—causes infectious mononucleosis
    2. Bacterial pharyngitis
        a. Group A and B hemolytic streptococcus
        b. *Neisseria gonorrhoeae*
        c. *Corynebacterium diphtheriae*
        d. *Haemophilus influenzae*
        e. *Neisseria meningitidis*
    3. Other sources
        a. *Chlamydia trachomatis*
        b. *Mycoplasma pneumoniae*
        c. *Candida albicans*
        d. Trauma/irritating substance
        e. Mouth breathing/allergies
    4. Accounts for 10% of all office visits in primary care
    5. Occurs in all age groups
- Signs and Symptoms
    1. Sore throat
    2. Enlarged tonsils
    3. Dysphagia
    4. Fever
    5. Malaise
- Differential Diagnosis (see etiology for pathogens)
    1. Peritonsillar abscess
    2. Pharyngeal abscess
    3. Epiglottitis
    4. Stomatitis
    5. Meningitis

6. Thyroiditis

- Physical Findings

    1. Elevated temperature

    2. Viral presentation (respiratory)

        a. Tonsillar enlargement with or without exudate

        b. Injected "cobblestone" appearance post-pharynx

        c. Rhinorrhea

    3. Bacterial (group A β-hemolytic streptococcus)

        a. Erythema

        b. Often exudative tonsils

        c. Enlarged tender anterior cervical lymph nodes

        d. Occasionally petechiae

        e. Scarlatina rash

    4. *Corynebacterium diphtheriae* (infrequent in immunized patients)

        a. Gray adherent membrane on tonsils and pharynx

        b. Bleeding when membrane removed

- Diagnostic Tests/Findings

    1. Viral (respiratory) pharyngitis—by clinical diagnosis *only*

    2. Throat culture—if suspect:

        a. Group A β hemolytic streptococcus (GABHS)

        b. *Neisseria gonorrhoeae* (request separately)

    3. Rapid Strep Antigen Test—positive result, detects only GABHS (5% to 10% false negatives)

    4. CBC with differential—WBC count elevated in bacterial infection

    5. Heterophil/monospot—negative

- Management/Treatment

    1. General measures

        a. Increase fluids

        b. Gargle with warm salt water

        c. Lozenges

        d. Acetaminophen or ibuprofen for pain relief

    2. Strep throat (GABHS)

        a. Penicillin V 250 mg t.i.d. or q.i.d. for 10 days

b. Benzathine penicillin 1.2 million units IM one time only

(1) Advantage—full treatment completed

(2) Disadvantage—five to tenfold increase in anaphylactic reaction

c. Alternative for penicillin allergy—erythromycin 250 mg orally q.i.d. for 10 days

d. Post treatment cultures—for recurrent strep infection or rheumatic fever

e. Complications—if no or inadequate antibiotic treatment

(1) Scarlet fever

(2) Peritonsillar abscess (immediate referral)

(3) Suppurative adenitis

(4) Rheumatic fever

(5) Acute glomerulonephritis

f. Tonsillectomy—for recurrent severe infections

3. Gonococcal pharyngitis

a. Ceftriaxone 125 mg IM one dose *or* cefixime 400 mg orally one dose *or* ofloxacin 400 mg orally one dose

b. Co-treat for chlamydia—doxycycline 100 mg orally b.i.d. *or* erythromycin 500 mg orally q.i.d. *or* azithromycin 1 g orally, single dose

4. Diphtheria (refer)

a. Equine antitoxin—to prevent myocarditis

b. Penicillin or erythromycin

Infectious Mononucleosis

- Definition: Acute viral syndrome associated with fever, pharyngitis and adenopathy—often known as "kissing" disease

- Etiology/Incidence

1. Epstein-Barr virus (EBV)—herpes type virus causes 90% of cases

2. Cytomegalovirus (CMV)—rare

3. Transmission via saliva

4. Usually occurs in adolescents and young adults (ages 10 to 35 years) in middle and upper socioeconomic populations

5. Prolonged period of communicability—approximately 2 to 6 months after infection

- Signs and Symptoms—variable, but typically include:

1. Fever

2. Fatigue/malaise

3. Nausea/anorexia

4. Swollen lymph nodes

5. Sore throat

- Differential Diagnosis

    1. Streptococcal pharyngitis

    2. CMV

    3. Toxoplasmosis

    4. Hepatitis A or B

    5. Lymphoma/leukemia

    6. HIV infection

- Physical Findings

    1. Marked erythema and edema of pharynx

    2. Tonsillar enlargement with exudate, occasionally palatal petechiae

    3. Enlarged lymph nodes—especially posterior cervical nodes

    4. Splenic enlargement—50% of cases

    5. Hepatomegaly

    6. Occasionally periorbital edema

    7. Maculopapular rash

- Diagnostic Tests/Findings

    1. Complete blood count with differential

        a. WBC—leukocytosis (range of 10,000–20,000/mm^3)

        b. Increased lymphocytes (greater than 50% of leukocyte count)

        c. Atypical lymphocytes—common characteristic

        d. Thrombocytopenia (range 100,000–140,000/mm^3) 2 to 4 weeks after onset of illness

    2. Positive monospot or elevations in heterophil titer—1:224 or greater is diagnostic

    3. Liver function tests—elevations in aspartate aminotransferase (AST), alanine amino-transferase (ALT), bilirubin and LDH

    4. Throat culture—frequently secondary infection with streptococcus (GABHS)

    5. CT scan imaging—may reveal splenomegaly and/or hepatomegaly

- Management/Treatment

    1. Supportive/palliative measures

2. Rest during acute phase of illness

3. Avoidance of contact sports for at least one month with splenomegaly; CT scan to determine resolution of splenomegaly

4. Avoid alcohol (ETOH) with elevated liver enzymes/hepatomegaly

5. Corticosteriods often prescribed for significant pharyngeal edema and obstructive tonsillar enlargement

6. Analgesics for pain relief

7. Antiviral medications not effective

8. Ampicillin/amoxicillin should be avoided, as patients frequently develop a maculopapular rash

9. Existence of chronic EBV infection (chronic fatigue syndrome) is very controversial

Allergic Rhinitis

- Definition: A noninfectious symptom complex which includes perennial, or seasonal manifestations

- Etiology/Incidence

    1. Seasonal allergies—symptoms at same time each year, related to pollens

        a. Trees (April to July)

        b. Grasses (May to July)

        c. Ragweed (August to October)

    2. Perennial allergies—year round symptoms related to molds, animal dander, feathers, dust mites, cockroaches

    3. Most common allergens—pollens, molds, dust mites, animal dander

    4. 8 to 12% of U.S. population affected; onset usually before age 30

- Signs and Symptoms

    1. Nasal congestion

    2. Sneezing

    3. Clear, watery nasal discharge

    4. Itchy nose, throat, eyes

    5. Cough from postnasal drip

    6. Mouth breather/snoring

    7. Loss/alteration of smell

- Differential Diagnosis

    1. Vasomotor rhinitis

2. Foreign body

3. Nasal polyps/tumor

4. Sinusitis

5. Medications—especially overuse of topical decongestants "rebound"; oral contraceptives

6. Deviated septum

7. Hypothyroidism and pregnancy cause nasal congestion

- Physical Findings

    1. Pale, boggy nasal mucosa

    2. Enlarged turbinates

    3. Injected conjunctiva, tearing

    4. "Allergic shiner" under eyes

    5. No sinus tenderness

- Diagnostic Tests/Findings

    1. Nasal smear for eosinophils—elevated

    2. Serum IgE—elevated in 30 to 40% of patients

    3. Allergy testing—identify specific allergens

    4. CBC if infection suspected

- Management/Treatment

    1. Preventive measures

        a. Allergen avoidance

        b. Air conditioning/air filters

        c. Environmental control—vacuum, dust, remove carpeting, feather pillows, stuffed animals

        d. Minimize contact with animals

    2. Pharmacological

        a. Antihistamines—mainstay of treatment

            (1) OTC usually cause sedation, least expensive (diphenhyrdramine)

            (2) Nonsedating antihistamines are prescriptive drugs and expensive

                (a) Fexofenadine 60 mg orally b.i.d.

                (b) Loratadine 10 mg orally once a day on an empty stomach

                (c) Cetirizine 5 to 10 mg orally once a day

(3) Terfenadine (no longer available) and astemizole (no longer available)—potential drug interaction with erythromycin and ketoconazole; cause of cardiac dysrhythmias

b. Decongestants (oral or topical)—vasoconstriction; decrease mucosal edema

c. Topical corticosteriods

(1) Beclomethasone dipropionate—2 sprays each nostril b.i.d.

(2) Flunisolide—2 sprays each nostril b.i.d.

(3) Steroid sprays (slow onset) up to 2 weeks before significant results appear

d. Cromolyn sodium—one spray each nostril up to 6 times per day

e. Immunotherapy desensitization for management failures; patients receiving desensitization must know signs/symptoms of anaphylaxis

Sinusitis

- Definition: Inflammation of one or more paranasal sinuses
- Etiology/Incidence
  1. Bacterial infections
     a. *Haemophilus influenzae*
     b. *Streptococcus pneumoniae*
     c. *Moraxella catarrhalis*
  2. Viruses
  3. Allergies
  4. Exposure to pathogen following viral URI, often a precipitating factor
  5. Deviated septum
  6. Classified as acute or chronic based upon duration of infection
  7. Maxillary sinuses most common site of infection, followed by ethmoid, sphenoid and lastly frontal involvement
- Signs and Symptoms
  1. Nasal congestion and pressure
  2. Mucopurulent nasal discharge/postnasal drip
  3. Choking cough at night
  4. Malaise and fever
  5. Headache
  6. Pain—dull to throbbing

   a. Over cheeks, worse with bending (maxillary sinus)

   b. Above and behind eye—ethmoid sinus

   c. Above eyebrows—frontal sinus

   7. Periorbital edema

- Differential Diagnosis

   1. Rhinitis—viral or allergic

   2. Dental abscess

   3. Nasal polyp/tumor

   4. URI

   5. Migraine/cluster headache

- Physical Findings

   1. Mild to moderate elevated temperature

   2. May have purulent discharge in nasal cavity

   3. Percussion/palpation over frontal and maxillary sinuses—may exacerbate pain/tenderness

   4. Transillumination of sinuses—may show impaired light transmission

   5. Percussion of maxillary teeth—may reveal dental root infection

- Diagnostic Tests/Findings

   1. None for typical presentation

   2. CT scan—is preferred to conventional radiography sinus films

      a. Equal in cost to sinus films

      b. More sensitive to inflammatory changes and bone destruction

   3. Sinus radiography will demonstrate opacity, air fluid levels, thick mucosa

   4. Nasal culture—sinus fluid to determine actual organisms

   5. CBC with differential, if patient appears toxic—elevated WBC

- Management/Treatment

   1. Antibiotics

      a. Amoxicillin—500 mg orally t.i.d. for 14 days

      b. Trimethoprim/sulfamethoxazole—1 double strength tablet b.i.d. for 14 days (penicillin alternative)

      c. Several cephalosporin options for 14 days

      d. If no response to treatment, suspect Beta lactamase producing strain—consider amoxicillin and clavulanic acid

2. General measures

    a. Increase fluids

    b. Steam inhalation

    c. Avoid smoking

    d. Analgesics for pain relief

    e. Nasal decongestant—improves sinus drainage

3. Topical steroids—reduce mucosal inflammation

4. Refer to MD if no improvement after 48 hours of treatment

5. Instruct patient to report symptoms of complications

    a. Stiff neck (meningitis)

    b. Periorbital edema (orbital cellulitis)

    c. Severe dental pain (abscess)

QUESTIONS
Select the best answer

1. The common cold is caused by:

    a. *Haemophilus influenzae*
    b. Rhinoviruses
    c. Streptococcus
    d. Herpes virus

2. Nasal congestion is a characteristic of upper respiratory infection (URI). It is best treated with:

    a. Antihistamines
    b. Nasal corticosteroids
    c. Topical decongestants
    d. Antibiotics

3. Prevention of influenza epidemics is best achieved by administration of annual "flu" vaccine. Contraindications to administering the vaccine include:

    a. Immunosuppressed patients
    b. Allergy to eggs
    c. Chronic respiratory disease
    d. Allergy to aspirin products

4. Amantadine and rimantadine are used in the treatment of influenza. Which of the following statements is true about these drugs:

    a. No significant side effects
    b. Effective against Type B influenza
    c. Decreases the duration of symptoms
    d. Best if given within 72 hours of illness onset

5. β hemolytic group A strep (GABHS) is a common pathogen in bacterial pharyngitis. It is also an infectious agent in which of the following medical conditions:

    a. Acute pyelonephritis
    b. Rheumatic fever
    c. Viral meningitis
    d. Acute mononucleosis

6. The most common physical finding associated with strep pharyngitis is:

    a. Unilateral tonsillar edema
    b. Exudative tonsils
    c. Ulcerations on buccal mucosa
    d. Injected uvula

7. Infectious mononucleosis is caused by:

    a. Coxsackie virus
    b. Herpes simplex
    c. Viral hepatitis A
    d. Epstein Barr virus

8. Earl Thomas, an 18-year-old college student, presents with fever of 101° F, sore throat, dysphagia and fatigue. Physical exam reveals periorbital edema, exudative tonsils, enlarged tender posterior cervical nodes, no hepatosplenomegaly. Your preliminary diagnosis is infectious mononucleosis. What diagnostic tests would you order to confirm your diagnosis:

    a. Throat culture
    b. Hetrophil antibody
    c. Electrolytes
    d. CMV titer

9. A 40-year-old male accountant presents with a three day history of left eye irritation. On physical examination, there is moderate conjunctival injection, watery discharge, palpable preauricular lymph nodes and visual acuity, 20/20 both eyes. The most likely diagnosis is:

    a. Acute glaucoma
    b. Bacterial conjunctivitis
    c. Blepharitis
    d. Viral conjunctivitis

10. In the history of a patient presenting with red eye, it is important to ask about:

    a. Photophobia
    b. Itchiness
    c. Cold symptoms
    d. Myopia

11. The two most important tests in assessment of a corneal abrasion are:

    a. Pupillary reaction and extraocular movements
    b. Funduscopic exam and peripheral vision
    c. Visual acuity and fluorescein stain
    d. Cover/uncover test and accommodation

12. Miss Shell presents with sinus pain, pressure and yellow nasal discharge. Your examination of this patient would include palpation and transillumination of the:

    a. Ethmoid and frontal sinuses
    b. Maxillary and sphenoid sinuses
    c. Frontal and maxillary sinuses
    d. Sphenoid and ethmoid sinuses

13. Which of the following conditions may predispose a patient to sinusitis:

    a. Tumor, gingivitis, deviated septum
    b. Nasal polyps, allergies, upper respiratory infection

   c. Temporomandibular joint syndrome, rhinitis, otitis

   d. Common cold, pharyngitis, meningitis

14. Ototoxic drugs are a potential cause of sensorineural hearing loss. Which of the following drugs may cause hearing loss:

   a. Gentamicin

   b. Penicillin

   c. Cephalexin

   d. Minocycline

15. A 60-year-old male suddenly develops headache, blurred vision and severe eye pain upon entering a dark movie theater. The most likely diagnosis is:

   a. Angle closure glaucoma

   b. Uveitis

   c. Giant cell arteritis

   d. Open angle glaucoma

16. Absent red reflex may indicate which of the following ophthalmologic conditions:

   a. Foreign body

   b. Cataracts

   c. Glaucoma

   d. Uveitis

17. Presbycusis—hearing impairment associated with aging, is characterized by:

   a. Acoustic nerve damage

   b. Cerumen impaction

   c. High frequency sensorineural loss

   d. Low frequency conductive loss

18. Macular degeneration is manifested by:

   a. Loss of peripheral vision

   b. Irregular pupils

   c. Loss of central vision

   d. Excessive tearing

19. Which condition is most likely associated with conductive hearing loss?

   a. Syphilis

   b. Meniere's disease

   c. Acute otitis media

   d. Hypothyroidism

20. A physical characteristic which differentiates otitis externa from otitis media is:

   a. Hearing loss

b. Pain with movement of pinna
c. Excessive cerumen
d. Enlarged submaxillary node

21. The most common pathogen of acute otitis media in adults is:

a. *Pseudomonas aeruginosa*
b. *Streptococcus pneumoniae*
c. *Mycoplasma pneumoniae*
d. *Escherichia coli*

22. A 30-year-old housewife presents with long standing nasal stuffiness, clear watery nasal discharge and annoying sneezing. The most likely diagnosis is:

a. Chronic sinusitis
b. Nasal polyps
c. Common cold
d. Allergic rhinitis

23. Microscopic examination of nasal secretions of a patient with allergic rhinitis may reveal:

a. Lymphocytes
b. Neutrophils
c. Eosinophils
d. Basophils

24. Allergic rhinitis is primarily treated with:

a. Allergy avoidance and antihistamines
b. Systemic steroids and decongestants
c. Topical nasal sprays and antibiotics
d. Humidified air and cough suppressants

25. An antibiotic that is used in treating otitis media and is effective against B-lactamase producing pathogens is:

a. Amoxicillin
b. Erythromycin
c. Tetracycline
d. Trimethoprim/sulfamethoxazole

26. Topical steroids are contraindicated in patients with corneal abrasions because:

a. They inhibit tearing
b. They increase risk of bacterial infection
c. They increase intraocular pressure
d. They may lead to iritis

27. Which of the following in not a cause of epistaxis?

a. Hypertension
b. Diabetes mellitus
c. Neoplasms
d. Trauma

28. A special diagnostic test/procedure for vertigo is:

a. Tonometry
b. Barany maneuver
c. Pneumatic otoscopy
d. EEG

29. Mr. Jones a 32-year-old salesman presents with a complaint of frequent nosebleeds for the last 2 months. He states they occur spontaneously 3 times a week and usually stop within ten minutes. He denies any other acute or chronic medical problems. Which of the following diagnostic tests is indicated at this time?

a. CBC
b. Hemoglobin electrophoresis
c. Prothrombin time
d. Clotting time

30. Upon further evaluation of Mr. Jones, you find he has nasal congestion, postnasal drip and scratchy throat. He uses an antihistamine at night for nasal symptoms and sleep. Your initial treatment plan for Mr. Jones should be:

a. Add a decongestant to alleviate nasal congestion
b. Increase humidity to moisten nasal mucosa
c. Have patient elevate head of bed to promote sleep
d. Discontinue antihistamine due to drying effect on nasal mucosa

31. Kyle Smith, a 21-year-old law student, presents with fatigue for 3 to 4 months, low grade fever and intermittent sore throat. You order a complete blood count. The result of the CBC is as follows: Hgb and Hct normal, elevated WBC and atypical lymphocytes. The most likely diagnosis is:

a. Hepatitis A
b. Infectious mononucleosis
c. Herpangina
d. Toxoplasmosis

32. Which of the following is *not* commonly a cause of bacterial conjunctivitis:

a. *Neisseria gonorrhoeae*
b. *Proteus mirabilis*
c. *Haemophilus influenzae*
d. *Pseudomonas aeruginosa*

33. An antibiotic which is "the drug of choice" in the treatment of gonococcal pharyngitis is:

a. Erythromycin
b. Ampicillin
c. Ceftriaxone
d. Amantadine

34. Hearing loss caused by cerumen impaction is considered:

    a. Conductive loss
    b. Sensorineural loss
    c. "Mixed" loss
    d. Congenital loss

35. Zeke Gilbert, a 72-year-old retired factory worker has hearing loss in his right ear due to excessive noise exposure. When performing a Weber Test, you would expect to find:

    a. Sound lateralizes equally to both ears
    b. Sound lateralizes to the left ear
    c. Sound lateralizes to the right ear
    d. Sound laterizes to neither ear

36. The most sensitive test for diagnosing sinusitis is the:

    a. CBC
    b. Nasal culture
    c. CT scan
    d. Sinus radiography

37. The most common cause/pathogen in otitis externa is:

    a. Fungi
    b. *Staphylococcal epidermidis*
    c. Alpha streptococcus
    d. *Pseudomonas aeruginosa*

38. A physical finding which differentiates conjunctivitis from glaucoma is:

    a. Injected conjunctiva
    b. Excessive tearing
    c. Clear cornea
    d. Nystagmus

39. When prescribing topical corticosteriods for patients with allergic rhinitis, it is important to discuss that:

    a. Topical steroid use may predispose to infections
    b. It may take up to two weeks before they experience significant reduction in symptoms
    c. Steroids must be taken with antihistamines to be effective
    d. After 48 hours of use, patient will experience reduction in symptoms

40. It is important to highlight the short term use of topical nasal decongestant because of this adverse effect:

    a. Rhinorrhea
    b. Confusion
    c. Somnolence
    d. Rebound congestion

ANSWERS

1. b	14. a	28. b
2. c	15. a	29. a
3. b	16. b	30. d
4. c	17. c	31. b
5. b	18. c	32. d
6. b	19. c	33. c
7. d	20. b	34. a
8. b	21. b	35. b
9. d	22. d	36. c
10. a	23. c	37. d
11. c	24. a	38. c
12. c	25. d	39. b
13. b	26. b	40. d
	27. b	

BIBLIOGRAPHY

Andreoli, T. E., Carpenter, C. J., Griggs, R.C., & Loscalzo, J. (Eds.). (2001). *Cecil essentials of medicine* (5th ed.). Philadelphia: W. B. Saunders.

Barker, L. R., Burton, J. R., & Zieve, P. D. (Eds.). (1999). *Principles of ambulatory medicine.* Baltimore: Lippincott Williams & Wilkins.

Bickley, L. S., & Hoekelman, R. A. (Eds.). (1999). *Bates guide to physical examination and history taking* (7th ed.). Philadelphia: J. B. Lippincott.

Chin, J. (Ed.). (2000). *Control of communicable diseases manual* (17th ed.). Washington, DC: American Public Health Association.

Godshall, S. E., & Kirchner, J. T. (2000). Infectious mononucleosis. *Post Graduate Medicine, 107*(7), 175-186.

Hsu, R., & Levine, S. C. (1998). Sudden hearing loss: How to identify the cause promptly. *Consultant, 38*(1), 23-32.

Institute for Clinical Systems Integration. Healthcare Guidelines Series. (1998). Viral upper respiratory tract infections in adults. *Post Graduate Medicine, 103*(1), 71-80.

Lynch, J. S., & Nettina, S. M. (Eds.). (2000). Ear, nose, and throat problems. *Lippincott's primary care practice. A peer reviewed series. 4*(5), 455-545.

Palay, D. A., & Krachmer, J. H. (1997). *Ophthalmology for the primary care physician.* St. Louis: Mosby Year Book.

Tierney, L., McPhee, S. J., & Papadakis, M. A. (Eds.). (2001). *Current medical diagnosis and treatment* (40th ed.). NY: Lange Medical Books/McGraw-Hill.

Uphold, C. R., & Graham, M. V. (1998). *Clinical guidelines in family practice* (3rd ed.). Gainesville: Barmarrae Books.

Youngkin, E. G., Sawin, K., Kissinger, J., & Israel, D. (1999). *Pharmacotherapeutics: A primary care clinical guide.* Stamford, CT: Appelton & Lange.

Lower Respiratory Disorders Infancy Through Adolescence

Janet Johnston

Croup (Laryngotracheobronchitis)

- Definition: An acute upper airway obstruction typically caused by a viral infection of the larynx
- Etiology/Incidence
    1. Parainfluenza type 1 (most common organism), parainfluenza type 2 and 3, respiratory syncytial virus (RSV), influenza A and B, common organisms; bacterial causes very rare
    2. Most common in children 6 months, to 5 years of age; peak prevalence 2 years
    3. Males more often affected than females
    4. Peak incidence during autumn
    5. Spasmodic croup can recur
- Signs and Symptoms
    1. Prodrome of coryza, low grade fever, sore throat, rhinitis for 3 to 4 days
    2. Rapid onset of ''barky'' cough, inspiratory stridor, hoarseness
    3. Symptoms worse at night
    4. Usually, rapid improvement with cool night air or increased ambient humidity
- Differential Diagnosis
    1. Bacterial infections of the upper respiratory tract, e.g., epiglottitis, tracheitis etc.
    2. Laryngotracheomalacia
    3. Foreign body aspiration
    4. Extrinsic compression of airway from trauma, tumor, abscess, or congenital malformations
    5. Acute laryngeal edema (anaphylaxis, angioneurotic edema)
    6. Severe asthma
- Physical Findings
    1. Inspiratory stridor
    2. Brassy, barky cough
    3. Dyspnea, expiratory stridor if severe
    4. Chest sounds are usually clear
- Diagnostic Tests/Findings
    1. White blood cell count—normal or elevated
    2. Pulse oximetry—hypoxia indicates severe disease
    3. Radiographic image of airway—classic narrowing of the trachea to a sharp point (''steeple sign'')

4. Viral cultures of nasopharyngeal secretions—rapid identification with immunofluorescent; enzyme immunoassay less sensitive

- Management/Treatment

    1. Mild disease—no dyspnea, hypoxia or dehydration

        a. Outpatient care—adequate oral hydration, antipyretics, calm nonintrusive care

        b. Family education regarding worsening respiratory distress

    2. Moderate to severe disease—stridor at rest, dyspnea, hypoxemia, or dehydration

        a. Hospitalize for supportive care, oxygen supplementation, medications, and intravenous fluids if indicated

        b. Less than 1% require intubation

    3. Medications

        a. Nebulized racemic epinephrine—observe for 6 hours after a dose for rebound swelling

        b. Parenteral dexamethasone in doses greater than 0.3 mg/kg, oral dexamethasone (0.15–0.6 mg/kg), and nebulized corticosteroids will lessen the severity and duration of symptoms in moderate to severe disease; oral dexamethasone doses of 0.15 mg/kg are effective for mild disease (AAP, 2000)

        c. Antibiotics are not indicated unless a bacterial infection is present

    4. Isolation—contact precautions during hospitalization (AAP, 2000)

    5. Prevention—hand washing and avoid touching face to prevent spread

Foreign Body Aspiration

- Definition: Inhalation of a foreign body that lodges in the upper trachea or lower airways, resulting in total or partial airway obstruction with local injury and inflammation

- Etiology/Incidence

    1. Food or objects with pliable, slick, or cylindrical surface; peanuts, other nuts, hot dogs, candy, grapes and latex balloons most common

    2. 80% are < 3 years of age

    3. Two-thirds of cases are males

- Signs and Symptoms

    1. Sudden, violent cough with gagging, choking, and subsequent stridor, wheezing and possible cyanosis

    2. History of witnessed choking in 80% to 90% of cases

    3. May be asymptomatic if object is not obstructing or irritating airway

- Differential Diagnosis

    1. Acute phase—laryngotracheitis, epiglottitis, laryngeal edema, pertussis, status asthmaticus, croup, retropharyngeal abscess

    2. Chronic phase—asthma, pneumonia, bronchitis, tuberculosis, and tracheal stenosis

- Physical Findings

    1. Presentation dependent on substance aspirated as well as size and location of foreign body

    2. Rarely (6%) still coughing during examination

    3. Unilateral wheezing and decreased breath sounds on side of aspiration; may also be bilateral

    4. Voice changes, stridor, dyspnea, sputum production, and emesis possible

    5. If foreign body persists, bronchiectasis and abscess formation is likely; may present with recurrent pneumonia and/or hemoptysis

- Diagnostic Tests/Findings

    1. Pulse oximetry—decreased O_2 saturations with significant obstruction

    2. Chest radiograph—10% of aspirated objects are radiopaque; unilateral changes in aeration from obstruction

    3. Expiratory chest, lateral soft tissue neck, decubitus, or fluoroscopy (imaging throughout the complete respiratory cycle)—obstructive emphysema (failure to deflate) or atelectasis typical

    4. Rigid or flexible bronchoscopy may aid diagnosis; delay in diagnosis increases rate of complications

- Management/Treatment

    1. Institute cardiopulmonary resuscitation if needed—unnecessary first aid maneuvers are dangerous

    2. Immediate transport to hospital for evaluation and removal

    3. Refer to an expert pediatric endoscopy team for rigid bronchoscopy evaluation and removal (if convincing history of foreign body aspiration, regardless of radiographic findings)

    4. Humidification, bronchodilators and anti-inflammatory medications may be useful after removal

    5. Antibiotics if evidence of pneumonia or bronchitis

    6. Chest radiograph in six to eight weeks to evaluate resolution of previous findings, or sooner if child is not improving

    7. Prevention

        a. Remove small items from environment of small child

        b. Sit while eating and provide adult supervision

c. Cut food in small pieces for young children

d. Avoid commonly aspirated foods and objects (no latex balloons etc.) in children under three years of age

Bronchitis

- Definition

    1. Acute bronchitis is transient inflammation of the larger lower airways

    2. Chronic bronchitis symptoms persist for more than two weeks; chronic bronchitis is rarely an isolated entity in children, but rather a symptom of some other condition

- Etiology/Incidence

    1. Most commonly viral—adenovirus, influenza A and B, parainfluenza type 3, RSV and rhinovirus

    2. Bacterial causes—*Mycoplasma pneumoniae, Bordetella pertussis, Chlamydia pneumoniae,* and *Corynebacterium diphtheriae*

    3. Acute bronchitis occurs most frequently in the winter and early spring; rates are higher among males

- Signs and Symptoms

    1. Initial phase includes symptoms of an upper respiratory illness

    2. Cough is the hallmark symptom; is initially dry and brassy but may become productive as illness progresses

    3. May have retrosternal pain with cough

- Differential Diagnosis

    1. Asthma

    2. Allergic disease/posterior nasal drainage

    3. Gastroesophageal reflux and/or aspiration

    4. Inhalation of irritants such as cigarette smoke

    5. Cystic fibrosis

    6. Immune deficiency

    7. Chronic sinusitis

    8. Immotile cilia syndrome

    9. Foreign body aspiration

    10. Airway deformity

- Physical Findings

    1. Brassy cough

    2. Coarse, bronchial breath sounds in periphery of lungs

3. May have tracheal tenderness on examination

- Diagnostic Tests/Findings

    1. Diagnosis primarily based on history and physical

    2. Chest radiograph may be normal or show peribronchial thickening

    3. Pulmonary function tests (PFT) may be normal or may indicate an obstructive pattern; PFT may or may not improve after bronchodilator

- Management/Treatment

    1. Avoidance of irritants

    2. Expectorants, increase fluid intake; avoid cough suppressants

    3. Bronchodilators

    4. Inhaled steroids may be indicated for chronic bronchitis

    5. Antibiotics are not usually helpful for viral illnesses; however, antibiotics (with efficacy against mycoplasma and chlamydia species) are useful if bacterial etiology is suspected

Bronchiolitis

- Definition: An acute viral infection of the smaller airways

- Etiology/Incidence

    1. Primarily caused by RSV

    2. Parainfluenza, adenovirus, rhinovirus, influenza less common

    3. Almost all children will have had one episode of bronchiolitis before age three

    4. Those requiring hospitalization include infants < 6 months of age and those with cardiorespiratory disease or immunodeficiency

    5. Most commonly occurs in mid-winter to early spring

- Signs and Symptoms

    1. Initial symptoms—rhinorrhea, congestion, cough, and low-grade fever

    2. Progresses to increased work of breathing, tachypnea, decreased appetite or poor suck; change in level of consciousness or activity level

    3. May present as apnea in very young infants

- Differential Diagnosis

    1. Bacterial or chlamydia pneumonia

    2. Aspiration pneumonia

    3. Asthma

    4. Foreign body aspiration

5. Retropharyngeal abscess

6. Salicylate poisoning

- Physical Findings

    1. Symptoms of rhinorrhea, otitis, conjunctivitis, and/or pharyngitis

    2. Often afebrile, or low-grade fever

    3. Tachypnea, retractions, nasal flaring, prolonged expiratory phase

    4. Wheezing, crackles

    5. Hypoxia

- Diagnostic Tests/Findings

    1. Diagnosis primarily based on history and physical

    2. Chest radiograph—peribronchial thickening, air trapping, patchy or segmental atelectasis

    3. Pulse oximetry—O_2 saturations decreased with significant disease

    4. White blood cell count with differential—may or may not be increased

    5. Viral culture with rapid diagnostic techniques—may be positive for RSV

- Management/Treatment

    1. Oxygen therapy—mechanical ventilation if necessary

    2. Fluid and nutritional support

    3. Bronchodilators

    4. Corticosteroids for those with underlying chronic conditions

    5. Ribavirin use is controversial; use based on clinical condition and physician experience (AAP, 2000)

    6. Prevention

        a. Palivizumab (preferred) or RSV-Immune Globulin Intravenous (RSV-IGIV) given to children younger than 2 years of age with chronic lung disease receiving medical intervention in the last 6 months; also for infants 28 to 32 weeks gestational age (GA) and less than 6 months, infants less than 28 weeks GA and less than 12 months, or infants 32 to 35 weeks GA and other risk factors (AAP, 2000)

        b. Strict contact precautions in hospitalized children, limit exposure to contagious settings for high-risk infants, and careful hand washing

Pneumonia

- Definition

    1. Infectious pneumonia—infection which usually involves small airways in children, but may also infect the larger airways and/or the alveoli

2. Aspiration pneumonia—caused by the ingestion of food, saliva, gastric contents, or other substances into air passages

- Etiology/Incidence

  1. Common viral agents—RSV; parainfluenza types 1, 2, and 3; influenza A and B; and adenovirus types 1, 2, 5, and 6

  2. Newborns—most common bacterial causes include group B streptococcus, gram-negative enteric bacilli, *Chlamydia trachomatis*, ureaplasma, and rarely syphilis

  3. Infants and young children ≤ 6 years of age—*Streptococcus pneumoniae* is primary cause of bacterial pneumonia; incidence of *Haemophilus influenzae* pneumonia has dramatically decreased since introduction of HIB vaccine

  4. Older children and adolescents—*Streptococcus pneumoniae* most likely, more rarely *Staphylococcus aureus*, anaerobes

  5. Mycoplasma and chlamydia may be most common nonviral organisms in children from preschool age to young adulthood

  6. Immunocompromised or malnourished children—opportunistic organisms, such as *Pneumocystis carinii*, yeasts and dimorphic soil fungi should be considered

  7. Aspiration pneumonia occurs in specific settings—most frequently in children with upper airway abnormalities or neurologic deficits; severe gastroesophageal reflux and other esophageal problems; may also occur subsequent to the inhalation of smoke or hydrocarbons; following near drowning, or ethanol ingestion by adolescents

  8. Incidence—4% preschool children and 1% to 2% in school age years

- Signs and Symptoms

  1. Cough, occasionally productive or associated with emesis

  2. Fever

  3. Chest pain or abdominal pain

  4. May have tachypnea, retractions, expiratory grunting, nasal flaring, cyanosis

  5. May have change in level of consciousness and/or activity

- Differential Diagnosis

  1. Atelectasis

  2. Foreign body aspiration

  3. Asthma

  4. Cystic fibrosis

  5. Tuberculosis

- Physical Findings

  1. Fever

2. May have tachypnea; substernal, supraclavicular, and intercostal retractions; grunting, nasal flaring; pallor or cyanosis

3. May have wheezing, crackles, and/or diffuse or localized decrease in breath sounds

4. Localized dullness to percussion

- Diagnostic Tests/Findings

  1. Chest radiograph

     a. Atelectasis (frequently misread as pneumonia)—opacification, intrathoracic structures will shift toward the atelectatic area; hemidiaphragm on affected side will be elevated and intercostal spaces on that side will be narrow

     b. Viral pneumonia usually begins with scattered perihilar and peribronchial infiltrations; in later stages, more localized infiltrations

     c. Bacterial pneumonias—characterized by patchy infiltrates in infants; lobar consolidation is most common with *Streptococcus pneumoniae* or *Haemophilus influenzae;* hilar adenopathy is most common with *Haemophilus influenzae* or *Staphylococcus aureus;* pleural effusion may be present

     d. Acute aspiration pneumonia usually develops in portion of lung that is dependent at time of aspiration; otherwise, radiograph typically shows diffuse or localized mottled infiltrates with or without atelectasis

  2. White blood cell count may or may not be elevated with increased number of neutrophils or lymphocytes

  3. Viral cultures of nasopharyngeal secretions; rapid identification with immunofluorescent; enzyme immunoassay less sensitive

  4. Blood cultures—if bacterial pneumonia is suspected (frequently negative); positive in 10% to 15% of cases

  5. Sputum cultures—warranted if cough is productive; rarely beneficial in younger children

  6. Positive cold agglutinin screen or titer > 1:32 suggestive of *Mycoplasma pneumonia*

  7. Pulse oximetry—decreased O_2 saturations with severe disease

- Management/Treatment

  1. Antimicrobial treatment based on etiology

     a. Currently no antiviral medication for treatment of pneumonia

     b. Antibiotics—penicillin for *Streptococcus pneumoniae,* macrolides or azalides for *Mycoplasma* and *Chlamydia pneumoniae;* amoxicillin/cephalosporin for *Haemophilus influenzae;* high risk of complications with staphylococcal pneumonias; treat with appropriate IV antibiotics

  2. Bronchodilators and chest physiotherapy may improve airway clearance

  3. Flu vaccine for those with chronic illness

Lower Respiratory Disorders —— **417**

4. Other supportive therapy may include additional fluids and/or oxygen

5. Pneumonia in immunocompromised hosts can progress rapidly; should be managed in a monitored setting, with aggressive diagnostic measures (bronchoalveolar lavage) and appropriate broad-spectrum antimicrobial coverage

Pleurisy, Pleural Effusion, and Empyema

- Definition
  1. Pleurisy (pleuritis)—inflammation of the pleural lining
  2. Pleural effusion (pleurisy with effusion)—accumulation of fluid in pleural space
  3. Empyema—inflammation and purulent exudate
- Etiology/Incidence
  1. Inflammation of pleural lining—often caused by a disease process elsewhere in body; most commonly infection; malignancy; trauma; pulmonary vascular obstruction; systemic granulomatous disease, or other inflammatory conditions may precipitate inflammation
  2. Parapneumonic effusions (inflammation of pleural space resulting from infection of lung) may complicate pneumonia
- Signs and Symptoms
  1. Chest pain, particularly with inspiration or cough; chest tightness; dyspnea
  2. High fever, chills, vomiting, anorexia, lethargy
  3. Effusions which abut the diaphragm may cause abdominal pain
- Differential Diagnosis
  1. Tuberculosis
  2. Neoplasm
  3. Connective tissue or collagen disorders
  4. Sarcoidosis
- Physical Findings
  1. Unilateral decrease in chest expansion during inspiration
  2. Pleural rub or decreased breath sounds over affected area
  3. Splinting toward the affected side
  4. Dullness to percussion
- Diagnostic Tests/Findings
  1. Chest radiograph—obliteration of the costophrenic space; supine films may show increased radiodensity of a hemithorax; decubitus films reveal layering of fluid exudate

2. Thoracentesis for evaluation of the pleural liquid—varies according to type of effusion or exudate

3. Mantoux test—positive if tuberculosis

4. Blood cultures—if sepsis suspected

5. Pulse oximetry—evaluate hypoxemia

- Management/Treatment: May involve treatment of any underlying systemic illness; parapneumonic effusions often resolve with appropriate treatment of pneumonia; suspected empyema should be referred to subspecialist, may require tube drainage or surgical management, prolonged antibiotics

Cystic Fibrosis (CF)

- Definition: Defective epithelial chloride transport results in dehydrated, viscous secretions which obstruct the exocrine ducts (with subsequent destruction and scarring) in the respiratory, hepatobiliary, gastrointestinal, and reproductive tracts

- Etiology/Incidence

1. Caused by mutations in a single gene on the long arm of chromosome 7 which directs the production of cystic fibrosis transmembrane regulator (CFTR)

   a. CFTR acts as a chloride channel and may stimulate other chloride channels and inhibit sodium channels

   b. Defective CFTR results in increased sodium reabsorption; decreased chloride secretion; and dehydrated, highly viscous secretions

2. Incidence—most common fatal, autosomal recessive genetic disorder affecting Caucasian population; less frequent among other racial groups

   a. 1:3,100 live Caucasian births

   b. 1:14,000–17,000 live African-American births

   c. 1:11,500 live Latino births

   d. 1:90,000 Asian infants in Hawaii

3. Median life expectancy—29 to 30 years

- Signs and Symptoms

1. Extremely viscid meconium (newborns)

2. Weight loss despite voracious appetite

3. Recurrent respiratory infections

4. Liquid, large, bulky, foul-smelling, greasy stools

5. Frequent flatulence or abdominal pain

6. Recurrent or persistent wheezing

7. Salty-tasting skin

8. Heat prostration

- Differential Diagnosis

    1. Asthma

    2. Immunologic deficiencies

    3. α_1-antitrypsin deficiency (rare)

    4. Airway abnormalities, e.g., airway stenosis, vascular ring, etc.

    5. Gastroesophageal reflux with or without aspiration

    6. Other causes of malabsorption and/or failure to thrive

- Physical Findings

    1. Respiratory

        a. Chronic cough, varies in character but usually productive

        b. Altered lung examination with crackles and/or wheezing

        c. Increased work of breathing; retractions

        d. Increased anteroposterior diameter of chest (barrel chest)

        e. Dyspnea on exertion

        f. Recurrent otitis media

        g. Chronic rhinorrhea

        h. Nasal polyps

    2. Gastrointestinal

        a. Meconium ileus

        b. Failure to thrive—weight (or height : weight ratio) $< 5^{th}$ percentile for age

        c. Abdominal distention

        d. Abdominal pain

        e. Enlarged liver and spleen

        f. Rectal prolapse

        g. Evidence of vitamins A, E, and/or K deficiences

    3. Other—digital clubbing

- Diagnostic Tests/Findings

    1. Pilocarpine iontophoresis sweat test—two tests with a sweat chloride in excess of 60 mEq/L from at least 75 mg of collected sweat; test should be performed by a Cystic Fibrosis Foundation-approved laboratory

    2. Genetic testing from buccal mucosa

3. Chest radiograph—hyperexpansion, increased peribronchial markings, cystic lesions, atelectasis

4. Pulmonary function tests—demonstrates obstructive pattern and decreased flow rates and vital capacity as disease progresses

5. Sputum culture—mucoid *Pseudomonas aeruginosa* is most common organism; non-mucoid *Pseudomonas aeruginosa* and other related organisms, e.g., *Haemophilus influenzae, Staphylococcus aureus* may also be present

6. Oximetry—decreased oxygen saturation with exacerbation and worsening disease

7. Hyponatremia, hypochloremic alkalosis

- Management/Treatment

  1. Referral to Cystic Fibrosis Care Center for long-term care

     Cystic Fibrosis Foundation
     6931 Arlington Road
     Bethesda, Maryland 20814
     (301) 951-4422
     Fax: (301) 951-6378
     1-800-FIGHT CF (1-800-344-4823) for list of approved centers
     www.cff.org.

  2. Interdisciplinary management involving intensive education, airway clearance techniques, replacement of pancreatic enzymes, nutritional support, prevention and treatment of infection, and psychosocial support

Asthma

- Definition: Chronic lung disease characterized by:

  1. Airway inflammation

  2. Airway hyper-responsiveness to a variety of stimuli

  3. Variable airway obstruction that is partially or completely reversible either spontaneously or with treatment

- Etiology/Incidence

  1. Airway inflammation plays a central role

     a. Inflammation causes airway narrowing and increased airway secretions

     b. Inflammation contributes to airway hyper-responsiveness

     c. Broad variety of factors trigger inflammation

     d. Causes recurrent acute episodes

  2. Triggers—factors that provoke airway inflammation and acute episodes

     a. Indoor allergens—dust mites, roaches, mold, animal saliva/ dander

    b. Outdoor allergens—seasonal trees, grasses, weeds, pollens, molds

    c. Respiratory infections/allergies (viruses, sinusitis, allergic rhinitis)—viral respiratory infections most common trigger for young child

    d. Weather/humidity changes

    e. Exercise (cold, dry air)

    f. Gastroesophageal reflux

    g. Irritants—tobacco smoke, pollution, strong odors

    h. Food allergies—nuts, shellfish, sulfites (shrimp, dried fruit, beer or wine)

    i. Medications—aspirin, beta-blockers, nonsteroidal anti-inflammatory drugs

3. Airway obstruction caused by bronchoconstriction, airway edema, chronic mucus plug formation, and airway remodeling

4. Approximately 5% to 6% of children affected—incidence and mortality increasing worldwide

    a. Increased incidence in childhood among males, lower socio-economic groups, African-Americans, and family history of asthma or allergies

    b. Leading cause of hospitalization and school absenteeism

    c. Asthma changes over time—never truly "out grow", although some children have recurrent wheezing associated with viral infections in infancy and early childhood, subsequently normal airway function

5. Under-diagnosis and inappropriate treatment are major contributors to morbidity and mortality

- Signs and Symptoms

  1. Recurrent episodes of cough, wheezing, chest tightness, breathlessness, and decreased endurance

  2. Symptoms often display an initial response (bronchospasm) to a trigger, then a late (inflammatory) phase response in 4 to 8 hours that is more severe and prolonged than the earlier response

  3. Symptoms often worse at night, early morning or after exercise

  4. Some patients may have severe, life-threatening exacerbations separated by long periods of normal lung function and no symptoms

  5. A subset of patients present with chronic (usually nighttime) cough without wheezing or exercise intolerance

- Differential Diagnosis

  1. Aspiration

  2. Cystic fibrosis

  3. Cardiac or anatomical defects

4. Lower respiratory tract infections

- Physical Findings

    1. Cough

    2. Diffuse wheezes (initially expiratory) with decreased air flow

    3. Prolonged expiratory phase

    4. Respiratory distress and hypoxia increases as severity increases

    5. Allergic appearance—allergic ''shiners'', nasal crease, mouth breathing, and nasal edema; polyps (rare)

    6. Skin—atopic dermatitis

    7. Concurrent respiratory infection—viral respiratory illness, sinusitis

    8. Barrel chest—chronic hyperinflation

- Diagnostic Tests/Findings

    1. Thorough history is vital to diagnosis and management, with special emphasis on triggers, severity of previous episodes, response to medications, and family history

    2. Spirometry

        a. Lower airway obstruction—forced expiratory volume in 1 second (FEV_1) < 80% predicted

        b. Reversibility—FEV_1 increases at least 12% after using a short-acting inhaled $beta_2$ agonist

        c. May also challenge with exercise, histamine, or methacholine if symptomatic, but spirometry normal

    3. Chest radiograph

        a. Bilateral hyperinflation with peribronchial thickening

        b. Plate-like atelectasis (often misread as pneumonia)

        c. May be normal

        d. Unnecessary on each acute episode once diagnosis established and responding to therapy

    4. Evaluation of other factors contributing to asthma severity

        a. Allergy testing

            (1) Complete blood count—eosinophilia

            (2) Immunoglobulin E—elevated, values age dependent

            (3) Nasal smear for eosinophilia— > 10% significant

            (4) Radioallergosorbent test (rast)—serum test which identifies possible allergic responses to various environmental substances

(5) Refer for allergy evaluation and skin testing as indicated to improve allergy/asthma control

b. Nasal and sinus evaluation—identify allergic rhinitis, sinusitis

c. Gastroesophageal reflux assessment

5. Pulse oximetry—evaluate hypoxemia during an acute episode

- Management/Treatment: National Asthma Education and Prevention Program: Expert Panel Report II (National Heart, Lung and Blood Institute [NHLBI], 1997) and Pediatric Asthma Promoting Best Practice (American Academy of Allergy, Asthma, and Immunology [AAAAI], 1999)

1. Diagnose asthma and initiate partnership with family

2. Classify severity of asthma

    a. Mild intermittent

    b. Mild persistent

    c. Moderate persistent

    d. Severe persistent

3. Medication classification

    a. Long-term control medicines—taken daily

        (1) Cromolyn sodium or nedocromil (inhaled)

        (2) Inhaled corticosteroids (beclomethasone, budesonide, flunisolide, fluticasone, triamcinolone)—delivered by nebulizer, dry powder inhaler, or meter dose inhaler

        (3) Long-acting beta$_2$ agonists—salmeterol, inhaled

            (a) Effect lasts 12 hours, helps nocturnal symptoms

            (b) Not to be used for exacerbations

            (c) Prevent exercise-induced bronchospasm

        (4) Methylxanthines

        (5) Leukotriene modifiers (montelukast, zafirlukast, zileuton)

        (6) Oral corticosteroids (if severe, chronic asthma)

    b. Quick relief medications—taken as needed to provide prompt reversal of acute airflow obstruction and relief of bronchoconstriction; not for daily long-term use

        (1) Inhaled short-acting beta$_2$ agonists (albuterol)

        (2) Anticholinergics (ipratroprium bromide, inhaled)

        (3) Short course systemic corticosteroids (oral or parenteral)

4. Prescribe medications according to severity (refer to NHLBI, 1997 and AAAAI, 1999)

    a. Anti-inflammatory medications to all patients with persistent asthma

        (1) Symptoms > 2 times a week

        (2) Nocturnal symptoms > 2 times a month

        (3) FEV_1 below 80% predicted (off medication)

    b. Give all patients an inhaled short-acting $beta_2$ agonist for as-needed use to relieve acute symptoms

    c. Increase medication according to severity of asthma and response to therapy

    d. Decrease medication as tolerated once good control maintained

    e. Minimize side effects, use lowest dose of anti-inflammatory that maintains good control

5. Identify and reduce child-specific triggers

6. Provide clear written instructions; problem solve with family for appropriate solutions for trigger control and medication options

7. Educate child/family to monitor and treat symptoms early

    a. Moderate and severe persistent asthma—should monitor peak expiratory flow (PEF) at home; before morning medication and with acute symptoms

    b. Develop a written ''action'' plan for acute episodes for all patients

        (1) 20% drop in PEF—increase medication

        (2) 50% drop in PEF—severe exacerbation

    c. Treat mild exacerbations with inhaled short-acting $beta_2$ agonist every 4 to 6 hours

    d. Add short course of oral corticosteroids early in course of moderate to severe exacerbations

8. Long-term care (every 1 to 6 months, depending on severity)

    a. Review attainment of treatment goals

        (1) Prevent chronic, nocturnal, and troublesome symptoms

        (2) Maintain (near) normal pulmonary function

        (3) Maintain normal activity levels (including exercise)

        (4) Prevent recurrent exacerbations and minimize the need for emergency department visits, hospitalizations, or school absenteeism

        (5) Provide optimal pharmocotherapy with minimal or no adverse side effects

        (6) Meet family's expectations of asthma care

   b.   Adjust medication use

   c.   Review management plan (including trigger control and acute episodes)

   d.   Check child's technique with metered dose inhaler and peak flow meter

   e.   Provide asthma action plan for school or day care

9.   Provide smoking cessation counseling as needed

   a.   Identify all tobacco smokers in child's environment

   b.   Strongly advise all smokers to quit

   c.   Identify all smokers willing to attempt to quit

   d.   Assist cessation by:

       (1)   Clinician delivered social support

       (2)   Nicotine replacement therapy

   e.   Arrange follow-up contact

10.   High risk for asthma related deaths—refer to specialist

   a.   History of severe exacerbations—intensive care admission or intubation

   b.   ≥ 2 hospitalizations/year

   c.   ≥ 3 emergency department visits/year

   d.   Overuse of inhaled short-acting beta$_2$ agonist (> one canister/ month)

   e.   Poor adherence to treatment plan

Bronchopulmonary dysplasia (BPD)

- Definition: Any child at 32 weeks or greater (post-conceptual age) requiring supplemental oxygen for 28 to 30 days following mechanical ventilation with radiographic changes of chronic lung disease

- Etiology/Incidence

   1.   Multifactorial—lung immaturity, oxygen toxicity, barotrauma, infections, nutrition, fluid overload, family history of atopy

   2.   Mild to severe disease possible from decreased lung compliance and increased airway resistance

   3.   Leading cause of chronic lung disease in infants

   4.   Birth weight single most predictive factor; increased incidence in infants < 1000 g at birth

   5.   90% following respiratory distress syndrome; others chronic aspiration, persistent pulmonary hypertension, meconium aspiration, or severe lower respiratory infection

- Signs and Symptoms
    1. Respiratory distress; may have cough and wheeze
    2. Poor growth and poor feeding skills
    3. Fussy with decreased endurance
- Differential Diagnosis
    1. Congenital cardiac or pulmonary defects that result in supplemental oxygen requirement
    2. Upper airway obstruction
    3. Lower airway structural abnormalities
    4. Pulmonary hypertension
    5. Hypermetabolic conditions
    6. Respiratory infections
    7. Chronic gastroesophageal reflux with aspiration
- Physical findings—vary with severity of disease
    1. Tachypnea with retractions
    2. Diffuse inspiratory or expiratory crackles and/or wheezes
    3. Pale with cyanotic episodes
    4. Failure to thrive (FTT)
    5. Fluid sensitivity
    6. Associated findings consistent with sequelae of prematurity and/or chronic lung disease (Loughlin and Eigen, 1994)
- Diagnostic Tests/Findings
    1. Oximetry on room air—hypoxemia
    2. Overnight oxygen saturation monitoring—identifies significant, prolonged desaturations (< 90%) with sleep and assists with weaning schedule
    3. Plot growth patterns—often FTT even after corrected for prematurity
    4. Serum electrolytes
        a. Carbon dioxide retention
        b. Chloride and potassium depletion, metabolic alkalosis—with diuretic use
    5. Arterial blood gases (on room air) -- compensated respiratory acidosis
        a. pH—low/normal
        b. $PaO_2 < 70$ mm Hg
        c. $PaCO_2 > 45$ mm Hg

6. Chest radiograph—increased interstitial markings; cystic changes or fine, lacy densities; hyperinflation common

7. Other studies as indicated to monitor and manage associated findings

- Management/Treatment

    1. Maintain adequate oxygenations (92% or greater) to prevent cor pulmonale and promote growth

        a. Wean as tolerated—gradual improvement with growth

        b. Desaturation commonly occurs during sleeping and feeding

        c. More severe BPD may need long-term mechanical ventilation and tracheotomy

    2. Adequate nutrition and fluids

        a. Achieve 15 to 30 g of growth per day

        b. High calorie formulas with additives often needed; nutrition referral

        c. Occupational therapy intervention for feeding skills

        d. Gastrostomy or supplemental tube feedings as needed

    3. Medications

        a. Bronchodilators—inhaled albuterol as needed

        b. Diuretics—as needed

            (1) Furosemide—acute

            (2) Spironolactone and chlorothiazide—long-term

        c. Anti-inflammatories

            (1) Long-term daily use of cromolyn, nedocromil or inhaled corticosteroids

            (2) Oral prednisone (high dose, short course) needed in acute exacerbations

            (3) Ipratropium bromide may be useful during acute illness or in chronic management

    4. Protective care to avoid lung re-injury

        a. Immunizations

        b. Smoke free environment

        c. Avoid elective procedures

        d. RSV precautions—administer Palivizumb (Impact—RSV Study Group, 1998) or RSV intravenous immunoglobulin in high risk population (AAP, 1997)

        e. Avoid high density day care settings

        f. Good hand-washing

        g. Higher incidence of Sudden Infant Death in this population

5. Family education, support, and follow-up

    a. Rooming in prior to discharge to demonstrate caregiver competency with home equipment and infant care

    b. Close follow-up (every 1 to 3 months), to determine if child requires supplemental oxygen, diuretics, or has poor growth

    c. Monitor for associated findings, manage/refer as needed—airway disorders, gastroesophageal reflux, heart failure, neurodevelopmental problems

    d. Referrals

        (1) Early intervention for developmental assistance and monitoring

        (2) Financial assistance and counseling

        (3) Home nursing and equipment companies

        (4) Family counseling and support groups

        (5) Community rescue services

        (6) Case management

6. Prevention—reduce incidence of premature births

Apnea

- Definition

    1. Respiratory pause lasting > 20 seconds or associated with cyanosis, bradycardia, marked pallor, or hypotonia; may be central, obstructive or mixed

    2. Central apnea—cessation of airflow and respiratory effort

    3. Obstructive sleep apnea (OSA)—cessation of airflow at the nose and mouth with continued respiratory effort; usually caused by upper airway obstruction

    4. Mixed—central apnea followed by respiratory movement without airflow

    5. Apnea of infancy—pathologic apnea in infants that are > 37 weeks gestation at onset

    6. Apnea of prematurity—periodic breathing with pathologic apnea in a premature infant < 37 weeks gestation

    7. Apparent Life Threatening Event (ALTE)—an episode that an observer believes is life-threatening, characterized by some combination of apnea, change in skin color, marked change in muscle tone, choking or gagging and requires significant intervention to restore normal breathing

- Etiology/Incidence

    1. Apneas vary significantly depending on underlying etiology

    2. ALTE occurs in 3% of population

        a. When etiology unidentified, sudden infant death risk increases significantly

   b. Subsequent episodes commonly occur

  3. Obstructive sleep apnea occurs in approximately 2% of children

   a. 3 to 6 years peak age (peak adenotonsillar hypertrophy)

   b. Familial tendency

   c. Increased risk with craniofacial anomalies, obesity, Down syndrome

- Signs and Symptoms

  1. During event, respiratory pause accompanied by marked pallor, cyanosis, hypotonia, and bradycardia

  2. OSA—loud, habitual snoring; apnea followed by gasping, choking, and arousal; restless sleep, and diaphoresis

  3. Behavioral changes, poor school performance, daytime sleepiness, growth delay may be signs of chronic OSA

- Differential Diagnosis (ALTE)

  1. Sepsis/meningitis

  2. Respiratory syncytial virus

  3. Seizures

  4. Metabolic defects

  5. Cardiac defects

  6. GER

  7. Munchausen syndrome by proxy (MSP)

- Physical Findings

  1. Often normal at time of examination

  2. OSA—mouth breathers; upper airway narrowed/obstructed from inflammation or structure; allergic stigmata; congestive heart failure; obese, normal weight, or failure to thrive

  3. Lungs usually clear

- Diagnostic Tests/Findings

  1. Complete history—emphasize circumstances surrounding the event, medical and family history

  2. Complete physical examination with detailed neurodevelopmental assessment

  3. Based on history, examination, and age of child

   a. Arterial blood gas—indicate severity of event and current stability

   b. Pulse oximetry—likely normal; may show hypoxemia

   c. Electroencephalogram—seizure disorder

    d. Viral respiratory panel—RSV infection

    e. Complete blood count, blood culture—indicative of sepsis, polycythemia (chronic hypoxemia), anemia

    f. Fluid balance profile—metabolic status, elevated bicarbonate (chronic respiratory insufficiency)

    g. Lumbar puncture—meningitis

    h. Electrocardiogram—cardiac arrythmias

    i. Chest radiograph—evaluate structure and anatomy, heart size

    j. Sleep study (pneumocardiogram or polysomnogram)—definitive test to identify significant apneas and differentiate type of apneas

- Management/Treatment (based on history and physical findings)

    1. Admit to hospital for close observation and monitoring for ALTE

    2. Institute treatment and referrals based on diagnostic findings, history, and physical examination

    3. If cause unclear; decisions more complex, but should include:

        a. Frequent follow up visits with serial measurements of:

            (1) Height, weight, and head circumference

            (2) Developmental assessment

        b. Emotional support and parental counseling

        c. No specific guidelines for apnea monitor use

            (1) Monitor only detects episodes of central apnea

            (2) Monitoring does not prevent all deaths

            (3) Monitoring is stressful (false alarms, child safety, travel cumbersome, and financial burden)

            (4) Requires close supervision and plan for monitor termination

        d. CPR instruction for family and other caregivers

Tuberculosis (TB)

- Definition: A chronic, granulomatous infection which may cause pulmonary, extrapulmonary, or disseminated disease

- Etiology/Incidence

    1. Caused by *Mycobacterium tuberculosis*

    2. Primary mode of transmission is inhalation of aerosol droplets through person to person contact; virtually all cases of pediatric TB are acquired through contact with an infected adult (Berti, 1996)

3. Tuberculosis is classified as primary infection or tuberculosis disease

   a. Latent tuberculosis infection (LTBI)—positive tuberculin skin test without clinical, radiographic, or laboratory evidence of active disease

   b. Tuberculosis disease

      (1) Pulmonary—hilar adenopathy with or without parenchymal lesion; children younger than 4 years of age increased incidence of miliary disease; pneumonia and pleural effusion may occur in older children; cavitary disease rare in children (Berti, 1996)

      (2) Extrapulmonary—miliary tuberculosis may involve any organ of the body, most frequently seen in lymph nodes and central nervous system (Berti, 1996)

4. TB rates for all ages in U.S. are highest in urban, low-income areas and in nonwhite racial and ethnic groups (AAP, 2000)

5. Increased TB risk associated with

   a. Contacts of persons with confirmed or suspected infectious TB

   b. Minority groups—immigrants from high-risk countries in Asia, Africa, Latin America, and The Middle East; children with travel to these countries; significant contact with persons from these countries

   c. Homeless, migrant, institutionalized, or prison populations

   d. Other—recent skin test conversion, immunodeficiency (HIV) or immunosuppression, IV drug use, certain diseases or some chronic illnesses (AAP, 2000)

- Signs and Symptoms

  1. Usually asymptomatic

  2. Cough, wheezing, dyspnea

  3. Abdominal pain, diarrhea, poor weight gain or weight loss, anorexia or poor suck

  4. Fever, lethargy, night sweats, chills

  5. May present with clinical symptoms of meningitis

  6. Late clinical presentations include symptoms of TB of middle ear and mastoid, bones, joints, skin, and kidneys (AAP, 2000)

  7. Drug resistant TB is indistinguishable from drug-susceptible disease (AAP, 2000)

- Differential Diagnosis

  1. Histoplasmosis

  2. Atypical mycobacteria

  3. Pneumonia

  4. Lung abscess

  5. Foreign body aspiration

6. Sarcoidosis

7. Neoplasm

- Physical Findings

  1. Usually asymptomatic

  2. Dry, hacking, or brassy, paroxysmal cough

  3. Localized wheezing or crackles

  4. Lymphadenopathy

  5. Failure to thrive

  6. Low-grade fever

- Diagnostic Tests/Findings

  1. Tuberculin skin test (TST)—Mantoux test recommended, multiple puncture test lacks adequate specificity and sensitivity

     a. All children should have a routine assessment of their risk of exposure to TB. Skin test only those children with increased risk

     b. Skin test immediately any child identified as a contact of a person with confirmed or suspected infectious TB; any child with clinical or radiographic findings suggestive of TB, any child immigrating from an endemic area or traveling in endemic areas or having significant contact with persons from endemic areas

     c. Skin test annually any child with HIV or living with an HIV-infected person; an incarcerated adolescent

     d. Skin test every 2 to 3 years any child exposed to high-risk persons (refer to #5 etiology/incidence section)

     e. Skin test should be considered at 4 to 6 and 11 to 16 years of age for any child living in high-prevalence areas, travel to high-prevalence areas, or with household contacts from high-prevalence areas

     f. A positive TST indicates likely infection—a reaction of 15 mm or greater is considered positive in any population; reactions of 5 to 14 mm may be considered positive in certain high risk groups

  2. Chest radiograph with lobar or segmental parenchymal lesion, lymphadenopathy, pleural effusion, or miliary disease (characterized by snowflake appearance)

  3. Positive acid fast bacillus culture obtained from sputum or early morning gastric aspirate

- Management/Treatment

  1. Diagnosing a child with TB infection or disease represents recent transmission of TB in the community; every effort should be made to identify and treat the source case and others infected by the source case; all cases should be reported to local

health department. Epidemiological investigation, isolation, compliance with therapy, and evaluation of the resolution of disease are crucial in controlling spread of disease

2. Referral to appropriate specialist

3. Guidelines for chemotherapy vary widely depending on the sensitivity of the organism, the condition of the patient, and the location of disease; refer to most recent edition of AAP *Red Book* for a complete list of drug dosages and side effects as well as therapeutic regimens; commonly used medications are isoniazid, rifampin, ethambutol, pyrazinamide, streptomycin

4. For LTBI, 9 months treatment with isoniazid is regimen of choice; prolonged therapy with immunocompromised conditions

5. For newborns exposed to household contact infected with TB, recommendations vary based on categorization of infection of household contact; refer to most recent edition of AAP *Red Book*

6. Directly observed therapy is recommended for treatment of people with tuberculosis disease

7. Children younger than 12 with primary pulmonary disease are usually not contagious; older children and adults suspected of having TB require TB isolation until proved noncontagious (AAP, 2000)

8. Bacillus Calmette-Guerin (BCG) vaccine—live vaccine from attenuated strains of *Mycobacterium bovis;* recommended only in limited and select circumstances in U.S.; recommended internationally by World Health Organization for administration at birth to help prevent disseminated and other life-threatening diseases caused by *Mycobacterium tuberculosis;* indications, adverse reactions, contraindications, and interpretations of Mantoux skin tests in persons who have received BCG described in AAP *Red Book*

Questions
Select the best answer

1. Shelby, a 4 week old, presents to your office in mid-January with a one week history of nasal congestion and occasional cough. On the evening prior to this visit Shelby developed a temperature of 102° F; refused to breast-feed; had paroxysmal coughing, and noisy, labored breathing. On exam, you note an ill-appearing infant who is lethargic with tachypnea and intercostal retractions. Shelby does not attend day care but has a 3-year old sibling who is in day care and who recently had a "cold". Considering the clinical presentation, what is the most likely cause of Shelby's illness?

    a. Mycoplasma pneumonia
    b. RSV bronchiolitis
    c. Aspiration pneumonia
    d. Streptococcal infection of the pharynx

2. In the above scenario, which of the following would be the treatment of choice?

    a. Antihistamine, decongestant and cough suppressant
    b. Oral antibiotics and follow up chest radiograph in two weeks
    c. Bronchoscopy with lavage, chest physiotherapy, and respiratory isolation
    d. Bronchodilators, supplemental oxygen, and nutritional support

3. Of the following children, which one should not have tuberculin skin testing?

    a. Richard, a 14-year-old, whose uncle was recently granted parole after five years in prison and is currently living with Richard's family
    b. Theresa, a 2-year-old who was infected with RSV three months ago and is currently asymptomatic
    c. Han, a 3-month-old whose family immigrated to the U.S. from Cambodia one month ago
    d. Chris, an 18-month-old whose mother is infected with HIV

4. Which of the following clinical presentations least warrants sweat chloride testing?

    a. 10-year-old female sibling of a patient newly diagnosed with cystic fibrosis; sibling is without pulmonary problems and growth parameters are at 50% for age
    b. 2-year-old male with recurrent pneumonia and growth parameters at 5% for age
    c. 4-year-old female with nocturnal cough which resolves after treatment with bronchodilators and short-term steroids; growth parameters at 10% for age
    d. 14-year-old female with nasal polyps, mildly hyperexpanded lungs, growth parameters at 25% for age

5. Of the following diagnostic findings, which one should be referred to a specialist immediately?

    a. Suspected foreign body aspiration
    b. Sweat chloride results of 30 mEq/L
    c. Pulmonary function tests of 80% predicted
    d. Chest radiograph with hyperexpansion

6. What is the most common etiologic agent for bacterial pneumonia from preschool to young adulthood?

    a. *Mycoplasma pneumoniae*
    b. *Staphylococcus pneumoniae*
    c. *Ureaplasma*
    d. *Haemophilus influenza*

7. Which one of the following diagnoses would not be part of the differential for recurrent lobar pneumonia in a 2 year old?

    a. Cystic fibrosis
    b. Foreign body aspiration
    c. Atelectasis
    d. Bronchitis

8. The most common clinical presentation of pneumonia includes:

    a. Cough, fever, tachypnea, and abdominal pain
    b. Hemoptysis, putrid breath, and weight loss
    c. Sudden chest pain, cyanosis
    d. Retractions, stridor

9. In addition to airway hyper-responsiveness and reversible airway obstruction, asthma is a chronic lung disease characterized by:

    a. Bronchiectasis
    b. Inflammation
    c. Pleural effusion
    d. Pulmonary edema

10. The most common trigger for an acute asthma episode in the young child is:

    a. Respiratory infections
    b. Exercise
    c. Tobacco smoke
    d. Outdoor allergens

11. Luke has mild persistent asthma. Appropriate daily medication should include:

    a. An inhaled low-dose corticosteroid
    b. Short-acting beta$_2$ agonists
    c. An oral systemic corticosteroid
    d. A cough suppressant

12. Which of the following is not a goal of appropriate asthma management?

    a. Limited activity and exercise
    b. Prevent recurrent exacerbations
    c. Prevent chronic troublesome symptoms

d. Maintain near normal pulmonary functions

13. Deon is a 4-year-old African-American male with a history of atopic dermatitis and recurrent pneumonias according to his mother. He presents with a persistent night time cough. His most likely diagnosis is:

    a. Asthma
    b. Foreign body aspiration
    c. Croup
    d. Cystic fibrosis

14. The most typical chest radiographic finding consistent with the diagnosis of asthma is:

    a. Normal chest film
    b. Diffuse airway edema
    c. Right upper lobe infiltrate
    d. Hyperinflation

15. When providing asthma education regarding the use of a long-acting beta$_2$ agonist, it is important to stress:

    a. It should not be used to treat acute exacerbations
    b. May be given every 30 minutes times three for rescue therapy
    c. May be most beneficial for exercise-induced asthma
    d. Should never be taken while also using inhaled corticosteroids

16. Claire is an 8-year-old with moderate persistent asthma who is still having mild symptoms. She reports three times a day use of a short-acting inhaled beta$_2$ agonist and cromolyn sodium at her clinic visit. Your management plan should be altered to include:

    a. Broad spectrum antibiotics and recheck in two weeks
    b. Addition of systemic corticosteroids for five days
    c. Replace cromolyn sodium with inhaled cortiocosteroids and when symptoms resolve reduce short-acting beta$_2$ agonist to as-needed use
    d. Addition of an inhaled anticholinergic

17. Ben is a 10-year-old who has recently been diagnosed with mild intermittent asthma. Which of the following is not a routine part of his clinic management?

    a. Spirometry evaluation
    b. Metered dose inhaler technique demonstration
    c. Environmental triggers and control methods review
    d. Allergy skin testing

18. Major contributors to asthma morbidity and mortality are:

    a. Under-diagnosis and inappropriate treatment
    b. An increase in indoor allergens
    c. Overuse of anti-inflammatory medications
    d. An increase in air pollution

19. The primary treatment for bronchopulmonary dysplasia is:

    a. Pancreatic enzymes
    b. Surgical repair
    c. Adequate oxygenation
    d. Chest physiotherapy

20. The single most predictive factor in the development of bronchopulmonary dysplasia is:

    a. Birth weight
    b. Maternal age
    c. Maternal educational level
    d. Respiratory infections

21. The classic radiographic finding in croup is:

    a. Hyperinflation
    b. Perihilar lymphadenopathy
    c. Thumb sign
    d. Steeple sign

22. Unilateral wheezing is a finding suggestive of:

    a. Croup
    b. Asthma
    c. Foreign body aspiration
    d. Pneumonia

23. Which of the following is not characteristic of an apparent life-threatening event (ALTE):

    a. Change in muscle tone
    b. Fever
    c. Change in skin color
    d. Apnea

24. Following an ALTE, management and treatment are based on findings from:

    a. A thorough history and physical exam
    b. An electroencephalogram
    c. A chest radiograph
    d. A sleep study

25. The predominant characteristic of a young infant with bronchopulmonary dysplasia is:

    a. Prolonged fevers
    b. Hypoxemia on room air
    c. Recurrent pneumonias
    d. Chronic hypoinflation

Answers

1. b		11. a		19. c	
2. d		12. a		20. a	
3. b		13. a		21. d	
4. c		14. d		22. c	
5. a		15. a		23. b	
6. a		16. c		24. a	
7. d		17. d		25. b	
8. a		18. a			
9. b					
10. a					

Bibliography

American Academy of Allergy Asthma & Immunology (AAAAI). (1999). *Pediatric asthma promoting best practice: Guide for managing asthma in children.* Milwaukee: AAAAI.

American Academy of Pediatrics. (2000). *Red book 2000: Report of the committee on infectious diseases* (25th ed.). Elk Grove Village, IL: Author

Berti, L. C. (1996). Childhood tuberculosis. *Journal of Pediatric Health Care, 10*(3), 106–114.

Bressler, K., Green, C., & Holinger, L. (1999). Foreign body aspiration. In L. Taussig, L. Landau (Eds.), *Pediatric Respiratory Medicine* (pp. 430–435). St. Louis: Mosby.

Cohn, D. L., & O'Brien, R. J. (2000). Targeted tuberculin testing and treatment of latent tuberculosis infection. *American Journal of Respiratory and Clinical Care Medicine, 161,* 5221–5247.

Goodman, M. H., & Brady, M. A. (1996). Respiratory disorders. In C. E. Burns, N. Barber, M. A. Brady & A. M. Dunn (Eds.), *Pediatric primary care: A handbook for nurse practitioners* (pp. 646–650). Philadelphia: W. B. Saunders.

Harvey, K. (1996). Bronchopulmonary dysplasia. In: P. H. Jackson & J. A. Vessey (Eds.), *Primary care of the child with a chronic condition* (pp. 172–192). St. Louis: Mosby.

Hilman, B. C. (Ed.). (1993). Infectious diseases and noninfectious disorders of the respiratory tract. In *Pediatric respiratory disease* (pp. 185–590). Philadelphia: W. B. Saunders.

Loughlin, G. M., & Eigen, H. (Eds). (1994). Common pulmonary diseases. In *Respiratory disease in children: Diagnosis and management* (3rd ed., pp. 223–559). Baltimore: Williams and Wilkins.

National Heart, Lung, and Blood Institute (NHLBI). (1997). *Expert panel report II: Guidelines for the diagnosis and management of asthma.* National Asthma Education and Prevention Program. (NIH Publication No. 97-4051). Washington, DC: U.S. Government Printing Office.

Montgomery, M. (1998). Air and liquid in the pleural space. In V. Chernick & T. F. Boat (Eds.), *Disorders of the respiratory tract in children* (6th ed., pp. 389–411). Philadelphia: W. B. Saunders Company.

The Impact—RSV Study Group, (1998). Pavlizumab, a humanized respiratory syncytial virus monoclonal antibody, reduces hospitalization from respiratory syncytial virus infection in high-risk infants. *Pediatrics, 102*(3), 531–537.

U. S. Department of Health and Human Services. (1996). *Clinical practice guidelines Number 18: Smoking cessation* (AHCPR Publication No. 96-0692). Washington DC: U.S. Government Printing Office.

Appreciation is extended to LaCrecia Britton, MSN, CRNP
Pediatric Pulmonary Nurse Practitioner
Children's Hospital, Birmingham, Alabama for her contribution to this chapter

Respiratory Disorders In Adults

Margaret Hadro Venzke

Pulmonary Function Tests

Proper assessment of most patients with pulmonary disease requires the use of pulmonary function testing. Understanding these tests is important in interpretation of results in relationship to the patient's diagnosis. Pulmonary function tests objectively measure the respiratory system's ability to perform gas exchange via assessment of ventilation, diffusion and mechanical properties.

- Indications for Use of Pulmonary Function Tests (PFT)

  1. Evaluation of dyspnea, cough, pulmonary dysfunction

  2. Early detection of lung dysfunction

  3. Disability assessment, including evaluation of risk factors in work settings

  4. Evaluation of response to therapy

  5. Re-evaluation of progress of restrictive or obstructive disease

  6. Pre-operative evaluation

- Types of Pulmonary Function Tests

  1. Spirometry—measure air flow rates and forced vital capacity (FVC)

     a. Forced vital capacity (FVC)—volume of air forcefully expelled from lungs after maximal inhalation

     b. Forced expiratory volume (FEV_1)—the volume of air expelled in the first second of FVC

     c. Forced expiratory flow 25-75 (FEF_{25-75})—maximal midexpiratory airflow rate

     d. Peak expiratory flow rate (PEFR)—the maximum air flow rate on forceful expulsion after maximum inspiration

     e. Maximum voluntary ventilation (MVV)—maximum volume of gas that can be breathed in one minute

  2. Lung volumes

     a. Total lung capacity (TLC)—volume of air in the lungs after maximum inspiration

     b. Functional residual capacity (FRC)—air left in lungs after a normal unforced expiration

     c. Residual volume (RV)—air remaining in lungs after maximum expiration

     d. Slow vital capacity (SVC)—volume of gas slowly exhaled after maximal inspiration

     e. Expiratory reserve volume (ERV)—the gas volume difference between the FRC and RV

- General Relationship of PFT to Pulmonary Disease

1. Obstructive pulmonary disease is characterized by reduced air flow rates; examples include:

   a. Asthma

   b. Emphysema

   c. Chronic bronchitis

   d. Cystic fibrosis

2. Restrictive pulmonary disease is associated with reduced lung volumes; examples include:

   a. Pulmonary infiltrate

   b. Lung resection

   c. Chest wall disorders

   d. Neuromuscular disease

Acute Bronchitis

- Definition: Acute inflammation of trachea, bronchi and bronchioles

- Etiology/Incidence

  1. Common causes

     a. Rhinovirus, coronavirus—usually short course of afebrile illness

     b. Adenovirus, influenza, *Mycoplasma pneumoniae*—more severe febrile bronchitis

     c. *Chlamydia pneumoniae*

     d. *Moraxella catarrhalis*

  2. Associated with secondary bacterial infections

     a. *Streptococcus pneumoniae*

     b. *Haemophilus influenzae*

  3. Mucous membranes become hyperemic, edematous with increased bronchial secretions

  4. Frequency and severity increase with cigarette smoking

- Signs and Symptoms

  1. Cough (hallmark symptom)

     a. Initially dry

     b. Later productive with mucopurulent sputum

  2. Fever

  3. Fatigue, malaise

4. Chest burning or substernal pain

5. Headache

6. Occasional dyspnea

7. Wheezing

8. Generally self-limiting illness

- Differential Diagnosis

    1. Pneumonia

    2. Asthma

    3. Influenza

    4. Pertussis

    5. Upper respiratory infection

    6. Allergies

    7. Cystic fibrosis

    8. Tuberculosis

- Physical Findings

    1. Temperature less than 101° F

    2. Chest and lungs

        a. Clear to auscultation

        b. Resonant to percussion

        c. Wheezes

        d. Diffuse rhonchi (often clear with coughing)

        e. Occasional crackles

- Diagnostic Tests/Findings

    1. Diagnosis based on clinical presentation

    2. If diagnosis uncertain or symptoms severe

        a. Chest radiograph—normal in acute bronchitis

        b. Sputum cultures—not helpful in the diagnosis

        c. CBC/WBC—normal or slightly elevated

    3. PPD—if patient at risk for tuberculosis

- Management/Treatment

    1. No treatment with antibiotics in otherwise healthy persons

    2. Palliative measures

a. Rest

b. Increase fluid intake to thin secretions

c. Humidity/steam

d. Expectorants—questionable efficacy

e. Cough suppressants—dextromethorphan or codeine for night cough

f. Avoid antihistamines—dry out secretions

g. Decrease environmental irritants

h. Analgesics for pain/fever

3. Smoking cessation

4. Bronchodilator for wheezing/cough

5. Recovery usually in 7 to 14 days

6. Follow-up visit if no improvement or worsening symptoms after 72 hours

7. Secondary bacterial infections associated with high fever, productive cough with purulent sputum; treat with antimicrobial therapy

a. Erythromycin—250 to 500 mg orally q.i.d. for 10 days for *Mycoplasma pneumoniae*, *Streptococcus pneumoniae* organisms

b. Amoxicillin 250 mg orally t.i.d. for 10 days for *Streptococcus pneumoniae*, *Haemophilus influenzae* organisms

c. Doxycycline 100 mg b.i.d. for 10 days for coverage of chlamydia, *Mycoplasma pneumoniae* organisms

d. Trimethoprim/sulfamethoxazole—one double strength tablet orally b.i.d. for 10 days for coverage of *Haemophilus influenzae*, *Moraxella catarrhalis* organisms

8. Refer/consult with MD if no improvement after 4 to 6 weeks

Pneumonia

- Definition

1. Acute inflammation of lung parenchyma including alveoli and interstitial tissues; usually secondary to infection

2. Categorized as either hospital acquired (nosocomial) or community acquired regardless of causative organism

a. Hospital acquired occurs > 48 hours after admission

b. Community acquired encompasses all others occurring as an outpatient or within first 48 hours of hospitalization

- Etiology/Incidence

1. Aspiration of secretions, inhalation of pathogens and/or hematogenous dissemination

2. Common pathogens

    a. Viruses (4 to 39% of adult pneumonias, more prevalent in children)

        (1) Influenza

        (2) Parainfluenza

        (3) Adenovirus

        (4) Varicella

    b. Bacteria

        (1) *Streptococcus pneumoniae* (pneumococcus)—most common

        (2) *Haemophilus influenzae*—ranked 2nd to streptococcal pneumonia

        (3) *Staphylococcus aureus*

        (4) *Klebsiella pneumoniae*

        (5) *Legionella pneumophila*—1 to 4% of community acquired pneumonia

        (6) *Moraxella catarrhalis*

        (7) *Chlamydia pneumoniae*

        (8) *Mycoplasma pneumoniae* (most common in adolescents/ young adults)

        (9) *Pseudomonas aeruginosa*

        (10) *Escherichia coli*

3. Hospital acquired pneumonia (nosocomial)—occurs more than 48 hours after hospital admission, more common in patients requiring intensive care and mechanical ventilation

    a. Rickettsia

    b. Protozoans

    c. Parasites

    d. Fungi

    e. *Pneumocystis carinii*—immunosupressed and HIV patients

4. Increasingly common in the elderly and patients with co-existing illness or disease

5. First ranked cause of death from infectious disease

6. Sixth leading cause of death in the U.S.

- Signs and Symptoms

    1. Fatigue, malaise

2. Pleuritic chest pain—worsens with inspiration

3. Fever

4. Chills

5. Dyspnea

6. Cough

7. Purulent mucus production—more common in hospital acquired

- Differential Diagnosis

    1. Types of pneumonia (see Etiology)

    2. Atelectasis

    3. Pneumothorax

    4. Lung abscess

    5. Congestive heart failure

    6. Neoplasms

    7. Chronic obstructive pulmonary disease (C.O.P.D.)

    8. Tuberculosis

- Physical Findings

    1. Elevated temperature and pulse

    2. Observe respiratory status, may have

        a. Cyanosis

        b. Nasal flaring/grunting

        c. Tachypnea

        d. Intercostal retractions

    3. Diminished localized breath sounds

    4. Evidence of consolidation

        a. Dullness to percussion

        b. Increased fremitus

        c. Egophony ''e to a'' changes

        d. Whispered pectoriloquy

        e. Rales

    5. Fine crepitant rales—do not clear with cough

- Diagnostic Tests/Findings

    1. Chest radiograph may show any variety of abnormalities—findings lack specificity and are not pathognomonic

2. CBC with differential—WBC often elevated

   a. WBC differential with left shift—bacterial origin

   b. Differential useful in evaluating severity and prognosis

3. Gram stain and sputum culture—consider when atypical pathogen suspected or patient is immunocompromised

   a. Gram positive—*Streptococcus pneumoniae, Staphylococcus aureus*

   b. Gram negative—*Haemophilus influenzae,* klebsiella

4. Serum electrolytes, hepatic enzymes—important in severe cases (when considering hospitalization); hyponatremia

5. Blood cultures—severely ill, toxic patients

6. Refer for thoracentesis if pleural effusion

7. PPD to rule out tuberculosis

8. Serum cold agglutinins—for mycoplasma

- Management/Treatment

1. General Measures

   a. Increase fluid intake

   b. Analgesics for fever and headache

   c. Avoid cough suppressants and cigarettes

   d. Humidification

2. Empiric antimicrobial treatment of community acquired pneumonia

   a. Patients without comorbidity *and* less than 60 years old

      (1) Erythromycin 500 mg orally q.i.d. for 14 days *or*

      (2) Clarithromycin 250 mg orally b.i.d. for 7 to 14 days *or*

      (3) Azithromycin 500 mg orally day 1 then 250 mg orally daily for 4 days *or*

      (4) Tetracycline 500 mg orally q.i.d. for 14 days for macrolide allergic patients

   b. Patients with comorbidity or over 60 years old

      (1) Cefuroxime axetil 250 to 500 mg orally b.i.d. for 10 days or

      (2) Trimethoprim/sulfamethoxazole (TMP/SMX) 160 mg TMP/800 mg SMX orally b.i.d. for 14 days or

      (3) Amoxicillin-potassium clavulanate 500 mg orally t.i.d. for 10 days

      (4) Macrolides (in doses shown for patients without

co-morbidity and less than 60 years old) if Legionnaire's disease suspected

   c. Patients hospitalized with community acquired pneumonia

     (1) Cefuroxime sodium 0.75 to 1.5 grams intravenously every 8 hours for 5 to 10 days or

     (2) Ceftriaxone sodium 1 to 2 grams intravenously every 12 to 24 hours for 5 to 10 days

     (3) Macrolide (in doses shown above) intravenously if Legionnaire's disease suspected

   d. Severely ill hospitalized patients require combination antibiotic therapy

3. Empiric treatment of hospital acquired pneumonia

   a. Combination antibiotic therapy required

   b. Pharmacologic selection dependent upon suspected organism

4. Discuss potential side effects of medication and stress importance of completing antibiotic treatment regimen

5. Follow-up within 24 hours by telephone

6. Schedule return visit in 3 to 4 days to evaluate progress

7. Follow-up chest radiograph in 4 to 6 weeks in patients over age 40 and all smokers

8. Prevention

   a. Pneumococcal 23 valent vaccine (pneumovax) 0.5 cc IM—indicated for patients over age 65 and those with immunosuppression or chronic disease

   b. Influenza vaccine annually—may administer with pneumovax at the same time, at different sites

9. Refer/consult with MD regarding:

   a. Seriously ill, toxic patients

   b. Persons with coexisting chronic disease

Asthma

- Definition: A reversible, episodic lung disorder characterized by increased responsiveness of the trachea and bronchi and manifested by widespread narrowing of the airways

- Etiology/Incidence

1. Caused by a single or multiple triggers such as:

   a. Allergies

     (1) Airborne pollens

     (2) Molds

        (3)   House dust

        (4)   Animal dander

        (5)   Food additives/preservatives

        (6)   Feather pillows

   b.   Nonallergic factors

        (1)   Smoke and other pollutants

        (2)   Infections

        (3)   Medications—ASA, NSAID, beta-blockers

        (4)   Exercise

        (5)   Gastroesophageal reflux

        (6)   Emotional factors

        (7)   Menses, pregnancy

        (8)   Thyroid disease

  2.   Affects men and women equally, approximately 5% of the U.S. population

  3.   Chronic disease with acute exacerbations

- Signs and Symptoms

  1.   Cough—often the only symptom

  2.   Wheezing—may be absent in severe exacerbation

  3.   Dyspnea

  4.   Chest tightness

  5.   Exercise intolerance

  6.   URI symptoms

  7.   Conditions associated with asthma

    a.   Rhinitis

    b.   Sinusitis

    c.   Nasal polyps

    d.   Eczema/atopic dermatitis

- Differential Diagnosis

  1.   Heart disease—congestive heart failure

  2.   Foreign body aspiration (FOB)

  3.   Chronic obstructive pulmonary disease (C.O.P.D.)

  4.   Acute infection—bronchitis/pneumonia

5. Pulmonary embolism

6. Cough secondary to beta-blockers or ACE inhibitors

7. Anaphylaxis due to allergen

- Physical Findings

    1. General appearance—note distress or decreased responsiveness

    2. Nasal flaring

    3. Use of accessory respiratory muscles, retraction

    4. Lungs

        a. Tachypnea

        b. Prolonged expiration

        c. Expiratory wheezing—unilateral wheezing suggests mechanical obstruction

        d. Generalized decreased or distant breath sounds

    5. Red flags—indicate potentially life threatening severe exacerbation requiring immediate emergency treatment

        a. Pulsus paradoxus—an exaggerated fall in systolic blood pressure during inspiration

        b. Diaphoresis

        c. Inaudible breath sounds

        d. Inability to lie flat

        e. Cyanosis

- Diagnostic Tests/Findings

    1. Pulmonary function tests/spirometry

        a. Peak expiratory flow rate < 80% of predicted norm for age, gender, height

        b. Vital capacity reduced

        c. Increase of 15% in FEV_1 or FVC after bronchodilator treatment confirms diagnosis

    2. CBC

        a. Slight increase in WBC during acute attack

        b. Eosinophil increase related to allergic response

    3. Chest radiograph—normal, rarely hyperinflation

    4. Arterial blood gases (ABG)

        a. Hypoxia in severe cases

        b. Hypocapnia

      c. Normal pCO_2 indicates very ill patient

      d. Hypercapnia is a medical emergency

  5. Sputum examination—positive for eosinophilia

  6. Nasal secretion—positive for eosinophilia

  7. Allergy testing

  8. Broncho-provocation with methacholine, histamine, or exercise challenge induces symptoms

- Management/Treatment

  1. Indications for referral to MD or asthma specialist

      a. Newly diagnosed patients

      b. Elderly patients

      c. Lack of response to therapy

  2. Indications of acute severe exacerbations requiring emergency hospitalization

      a. Pulsus paradoxus

      b. Cardiovascular disease

      c. Nonresponse to emergency treatment

      d. Persistently low PEFR

      e. Respiratory acidosis

  3. Monitor measures of lung function with peak flow meter—establish patient's "personal best" and treat based on percent of "personal best"; "personal best" is the highest PEFR measurement after a period of maximum therapy

      a. 80 to 100%—maintain on treatment as prescribed

      b. 50 to 80%—acute exacerbation; contact clinician, adjust maintenance program

      c. Below 50%—medical alert identification; emergency treatment

  4. Goals of treatment

      a. Activity without symptoms; sleep through the night

      b. Prevention of chronic troublesome symptoms

      c. Sports and exercise participation

      d. Optimal pharmacotherapy with minimal/no adverse effects

      e. Maintain nearly normal pulmonary function

      f. Meet patient/family's expectations of, and satisfaction with asthma care

  5. A stepwise approach to pharmacologic therapy is recommended to gain and maintain asthma control

6. Classes of medications

    a. Long-term control—used to achieve and maintain control of persistent asthma

        (1) Anti-inflammatory agents—inhaled corticosteroids most potent and effective

            (a) Beclomethasone

            (b) Triamcinolone

            (c) Flunisolide

            (d) Oral corticosteroids—used in severe asthma

        (2) Sympathomimetic agents—relax bronchial smooth muscle; *long acting* β_2 adrenergic agonist agents—use with anti-inflammatory therapy and for prevention of exercise induced bronchospasm (EIB)

            (a) Salmeterol—inhaled medication

            (b) Albuterol—sustained released oral medication

        (3) Antimediators—inhaled anti-inflammatory agents indicated for long-term prevention of symptoms and preventive treatment prior to exercise or allergen exposure; 4 to 6 week trial needed to determine maximal benefit

            (a) Cromolyn—nebulizer delivery may be preferred to metered dose inhaler

            (b) Nedocromil—20% of patients complain of unpleasant taste

        (4) Methylxanthines—often used as adjunct therapy to anti-inflammatory drugs for nocturnal symptoms

            (a) Theophylline—sustained release oral medication, many side effects, drug interactions

            (b) Aminophylline—IV drug, seldom used

        (5) Leukotriene modifiers—new asthma drugs, alternative to inhaled corticosteriods in mild persistent asthma for patients 12 years of age or older

            (a) Zafirlukast—take on empty stomach

            (b) Zileuton—causes elevated liver enzymes

    b. Quick-relief medications treat acute symptoms and exacerbations

        (1) Short acting β_2 adrenergic agonists—drugs of choice for relief of acute symptoms and prevention of E.I.B.

            (a) Albuterol

            (b) Bitolterol

            (c) Pibuterol

            (d) Terbutaline

(2) Anticholinergic—Ipratropium bromide may provide additive benefit when used with inhaled β_2 adrenergic agonist; used alone when β_2 adrenergic agonists not tolerated; more effective as therapy for C.O.P.D. than asthma

(3) Systemic corticosteroids—for moderate to severe exacerbations; prevent progression of exacerbation, speed recovery and reduce rate of relapse

    (a) Methylprednisolone

    (b) Prednisolone

    (c) Prednisone

7. Pharmacotherapy in mild intermittent asthma (step 1)

  a. Characteristics of mild intermittent asthma include one or more of the following:

    (1) Brief symptoms, no more than twice weekly

    (2) Asymptomatic between exacerbations

    (3) Nocturnal symptoms less than twice a month

    (4) PEFR 80% or greater than predicted value; variability less than 20%

  b. Medications

    (1) No daily medication

    (2) Short acting β_2 adrenergic agonist for symptom relief; if used more than twice weekly, consider long term therapy

8. Pharmacotherapy in mild persistent asthma (step 2)

  a. Characteristics of mild persistent asthma include one or more of the following:

    (1) Symptoms > twice a week, but less than once daily

    (2) Exacerbations affect sleep and level of activity

    (3) Nocturnal symptoms more than twice a month

    (4) PEFR 80% with 20 to 30% variability

  b. Medications—one daily medication

    (1) Low dose inhaled corticosteroids (200 to 500 μg) daily divided in 2 to 4 doses; (i.e., beclomethasone 2 to 4 inhalations b.i.d.) *or*

    (2) Inhaled cromolyn or nedocromil 2 inhalations t.i.d. or q.i.d. *or*

    (3) Theophylline, sustained release tablets, 10 mg/kg per day up to 300 mg maximum; monitor theophylline level—not preferred, but may be used as alternative

    (4) Leukotriene modifier—may be considered

(5) Short-acting inhaled β_2 adrenergic agonist agent for *quick relief;* if daily usage, need additional long term therapy

9. Pharmacotherapy in moderate persistent asthma (step 3)

   a. Characteristics of moderate persistent asthma include one or more of the following:

      (1) Daily symptoms

      (2) Daily use of short-acting β_2 adrenergic agonist

      (3) Nocturnal symptoms more than once a week

      (4) Exacerbations affect activity and sleep

      (5) Exacerbations at least twice weekly, may last for days

      (6) PEFR 60% to 80% of predicted value; variability exceeds 30%

   b. Medications—one or two daily medications

      (1) Medium dose inhaled corticosteroids; i.e., beclomethasone 500 to 840 mg daily in 2 to 4 divided doses *and/or*

      (2) Medium dose inhaled corticosteroid plus long acting bronchodilator

      (3) Quick relief—short acting β_2 adrenergic agonist; if increased or daily use, need additional long term therapy

10. Pharmacotherapy in severe persistent asthma (step 4)

    a. Characteristics of severe persistent asthma include one or more of the following:

       (1) Continuous symptoms

       (2) Frequent exacerbations

       (3) Limited physical activity

       (4) Frequent nocturnal symptoms

       (5) PEFR no greater than 60% of predicted value; variability exceeds 30%

    b. Medications—refer to asthma specialist; two or three daily medications

       (1) High dose inhaled corticosteriods (i.e., beclomethasone greater than 840 μg in divided daily doses) *and*

       (2) Long-acting bronchodilator (inhaled or oral $\beta_2$adrenergic agonist or theophylline) *and*

       (3) Oral corticosteroids—make report attempts to reduce systemic steroids and maintain control with high dose inhaled steroids

       (4) Quick relief—short acting β_2 adrenergic agonist as needed for symptoms

11. The stepwise approach is a general guideline to asthma therapy

a. Review treatment every 1 to 6 months

b. Rescue course of systemic corticosteroids may be needed at any time/step

c. Refer to asthma specialist if difficulty maintaining control of asthma

12. Environmental measures to decrease irritants

a. Avoid outdoor allergens

b. Eliminate indoor allergens

c. Use of air conditioners and air filters

13. Educating the patient—key components

a. Signs and symptoms to report

b. Controlling asthma triggers, planning avoidance strategies

c. Correct use of inhalers and/or spacers

d. Use of peak flow meter

14. Written guidelines for patient concerning drug treatment, PEFR measurements, and signs and symptoms of serious exacerbation

15. Discuss adverse effects of oral steroids, including need to taper dose

16. Use of inhaled corticosteriods; rinse mouth after use to avoid oral candidiasis

17. Discuss adverse effects/drug interactions when receiving theophylline

18. Include patient's family in treatment plan

19. Avoid use of ASA and NSAIDS—may cause serious exacerbations

20. Beta-blocker medications are contraindicated

21. Stress management

22. Advise annual influenza vaccine and consider pneumococcal vaccine

Chronic Obstructive Pulmonary Disease (COPD)

- Definition: A disease state characterized by airflow obstruction due to emphysema, chronic bronchitis, or both; may be partially reversible

  1. Emphysema—permanent abnormal distention of the terminal air spaces with destruction of alveolar walls and resultant air trapping

  2. Chronic bronchitis—excessive sputum production with chronic or recurring cough on most days for 3 months or more during 2 consecutive years

- Etiology/Incidence

  1. Occupational exposure to irritants

  2. Heredity—alpha$_1$ protease inhibitor deficiency may cause emphysema; suspect in patients under age 35 who have COPD

3. 10 to 15% of smokers develop COPD

4. Affects 14 million people in the U.S.

5. 4th leading cause of death in the U.S.

6. Predominantly seen over age 40

7. Affects men more than women, but prevalence in women rising

- Signs and Symptoms
    1. Emphysema (Pink Puffer)
        a. Early stage
            (1) Mild dyspnea
            (2) Cough uncommon
            (3) Fatigue
        b. Later stage
            (1) Severe dyspnea
            (2) Dyspnea on exertion
            (3) Pursed lip breathing
            (4) Muscle wasting
            (5) Weight loss
            (6) Flushed appearance
            (7) Mild cough with clear mucoid sputum
    2. Chronic bronchitis (Blue Bloater)
        a. Mild
            (1) Productive cough of mucopurulent sputum, especially in the mornings
            (2) Intermittent dyspnea
            (3) Copious mucus production, causing nocturnal awakening
            (4) Frequent infections
        b. Severe
            (1) Cyanosis
            (2) Edema
            (3) Recurrent respiratory failure
- Differential Diagnosis
    1. Asthma
    2. Congestive heart failure (CHF)

3. Tuberculosis (TB)

4. Acute bronchitis

5. Chronic sinusitis

6. Lung cancer

- Physical Findings

    1. Emphysema

        a. Thin

        b. Hypertrophied accessory muscles

        c. Increased anteroposterior chest diameter (barrel chest)

        d. Lungs

            (1) Hyper-resonance to percussion

            (2) Diminished breath sounds

        e. Absence of cyanosis, clubbing

    2. Chronic bronchitis

        a. Obesity

        b. Central cyanosis

        c. Normal chest diameter

        d. Lungs

            (1) Normal resonance to percussion

            (2) Wheezes, rhonchi

        e. Enlarged heart

- Diagnostic Tests/Findings

    1. Forced expiratory volume greater than 3 seconds in both emphysema and chronic bronchitis

    2. Decreased vital capacity and expiratory flow rates

    3. Increased respiratory volume and total lung capacity in emphysema

    4. 15 to 20% increase in expiratory flow after use of bronchodilator in COPD

    5. Arterial blood gases

        a. Hypoxemia in chronic bronchitis

        b. Hypercapnia in emphysema

    6. Increased hematocrit indicative of polycythemia in advanced chronic bronchitis

    7. Chest radiograph

        a. Hyperinflation, occasional bullae/blebs in emphysema

       b. Increased markings and cardiac enlargement in chronic bronchitis

  8. ECG may show right ventricular hypertrophy

  9. PPD to rule out tuberculosis

- Management/Treatment

  1. Refer patients with signs and symptoms of respiratory failure to MD

  2. Discontinue smoking—consider pharmacologic interventions

  3. Avoid airway irritants and temperature extremes

  4. Maintain hydration and indoor humidity

  5. Bronchodilators

       a. Ipratropium bromide inhaler 2 to 4 inhalations every 4 to 6 hours (drug of choice)

       b. Theophylline

       c. Corticosteriods (oral) during acute exacerbations

       d. Discontinue bronchodilator if no objective improvement in PFT

  6. Chest physiotherapy as needed

  7. Home oxygen therapy

  8. Educate regarding factors that contribute to upper respiratory infections

  9. Exercise training program

  10. Pursed lip breathing, diaphragmatic exercises may be helpful

  11. Prevention of infection with pneumococcal and annual influenza vaccines

  12. Early treatment of recurrent and chronic bacterial infections; common organisms include:

       a. *Haemophilus influenzae*

       b. *Streptococcus pneumoniae*

       c. *Moraxella catarrhalis*

  13. Avoid beta-blockers, cough suppressants, and antihistamines

  14. Review signs and symptoms of respiratory failure and CHF

  15. Teach effective cough technique

Tuberculosis (TB)

- Definition: Chronic bacterial infectious disease most commonly infecting the lungs; may occur in lymph nodes, bones, kidneys, meninges and can disseminate throughout body

- Etiology/Incidence

1. Mycobacteria of "tuberculosis complex," primarily *Mycobacterium tuberculosis,* a gram positive, acid fast bacillus

2. Usually spread by airborne droplet nuclei

3. 10 to 15 million infected in the U.S.

4. Incidence of TB is greatest in Asians, Pacific Islanders, American Indians, Alaska natives, and Hispanics

5. 90 to 95% of primary TB infections remain in a latent or dormant stage

6. High risk populations include:

   a. HIV infected individuals

   b. Close contacts of infected persons

   c. Low income populations

   d. Alcoholics and IV drug abusers

   e. Elderly

   f. Immigrants from Asia and Central/South America

   g. Persons in correctional institutions and in long term care facilities

   h. Individuals with chronic disease

- Signs and Symptoms (90% asymptomatic at the time of primary infection)

  1. Fatigue

  2. Anorexia, weight loss

  3. Fever

  4. Night sweats

  5. Productive cough with purulent sputum

  6. Hemoptysis

  7. Pleuritic chest pain

- Differential Diagnosis

  1. Pneumonia

  2. Malignancy

  3. Pleurisy

  4. Histoplasmosis

  5. Silicosis

  6. COPD

- Physical Findings

  1. Appear chronically ill

2. Weak and cachectic

3. Lungs

    a. Auscultation—apical rales, often a positive whispered pectoriloquy

    b. Palpation—increased tactile fremitus over consolidated areas

    c. Percussion—dull

- Diagnostic Tests/Findings

1. Chest radiograph—pulmonary infiltrates with hilar adenopathy

2. PPD

    a. Positive with active disease or prior exposure

    b. BCG may produce positive PPD for one year; then interpretation is standard

    c. AIDS patients and immunosupressed patients have diminished reactivity

3. PPD Interpretation (record induration, not erythema)

    a. A reaction of 5 mm is considered positive in patients with:

        (1) Recent close contact with infected person

        (2) Evidence of inactive disease

        (3) HIV infection

    b. A reaction of 10 mm is considered positive in patients with:

        (1) Diabetes mellitus, cancer or end stage renal disease

        (2) Immigrants from Asia, Africa, Latin America

        (3) Medically underserved, low income populations

        (4) High risk minorities

        (5) Residents of nursing homes and prisons

        (6) Health care workers

    c. A reaction of 15 mm is considered positive for all populations

    d. False-negative result

        (a) PPD administered after live virus vaccine (e.g., postponed for 4 to 6 weeks following measles vaccination)

        (b) Immunosuppressed

        (c) Elderly

    e. False-positive result

        (1) Recent BCG vaccine

        (2) Nontuberculosis mycobacterium

    f. ''Positive converter''—previous negative PPD, turns positive within a two year period, person is asymptomatic for active disease and has negative chest radiograph

4. Sputum culture

   a. Essential to confirm diagnosis of TB—three specimens advised

   b. Takes 3 to 6 weeks for results to be obtained

5. Gastric aspirate culture

   a. Alternative to bronchoscopy

   b. Use for culture only—not stained smear

- Management/Treatment

  1. Prevention

     a. Bacillus Calmette-Guérin (BCG) vaccine intended for prophylaxis of noninfected persons; not routinely used in the U.S.

     b. Positive PPD converter—prescribe isoniazid 300 mg orally every day for 6 to 12 months

  2. Pharmacotherapy—consult/refer to MD or specialist prior to initiating therapy

     a. Medications (for sensitive organisms)

        (1) Isoniazid daily 5 mg/kg up to 300 mg per day for 2 months, together with

        (2) Rifampin daily 10 mg/kg up to 600 mg per day for 2 months

        (3) Pyrazinamide 15 to 30 mg/kg up to 2 grams per day for 2 months

        (4) After 2 months of triple therapy above, follow with 4 months of daily or twice weekly isoniazid and rifampin

     b. Medication (for resistant bacilli) in addition to above, until sensitivities to drugs are known

        (1) If isoniazid resistance suspected, ethambutol added first 2 months 15 to 20 mg/kg for 2 months or

        (2) Pyrazinamide 15 to 30 mg/kg for 2 months or

        (3) Streptomycin 15 mg/kg IM

  3. Order baseline liver function tests prior to initiating antituberculosis medications

  4. Perform baseline color vision (red-green) test prior to ethambutol therapy

  5. Follow-up on contacts of persons with active disease

  6. Reportable disease—report to state and local health departments

  7. BCG vaccine may be recommended for skin test negative individuals who have repeated exposure

  8. After therapy completion, follow up in one year; monitor for recurrence

9. Stress importance of compliance; Direct Observed Therapy (DOT)—one method of ensuring adherence

10. Review symptoms of drug side effects and toxicity

    a. Isoniazid

        (1) Peripheral neuropathy (prevent with daily pyridoxine)

        (2) Hepatitis

        (3) Hypersensitivity

    b. Rifampin

        (1) Orange discoloration of secretions and urine

        (2) Permanent orange stain to contact lenses

        (3) Nausea

        (4) Vomiting

    c. Pyrazinamide

        (1) Hepatotoxicity

        (2) Hyperuricemia

    d. Ethambutol

        (1) Fever

        (2) Rash

        (3) Optic neuritis

    e. Streptomycin—ototoxicity

11. Stress importance of nutritious diet and education regarding selection of food

Lung Cancer

- Definition: Primary malignant neoplasm of the lung; cell types involved include squamous cell, adenocarcinoma, large cell carcinoma and small cell carcinoma

- Etiology/Incidence

    1. Cigarette smoking accounts for 95% of lung cancer in men and 85% of those in women

    2. Cigarette smoke in combination with other environmental pollutants (e.g., asbestos) influences increased incidence

    3. Most common in 50 to 70 year olds

    4. Occurs in males more frequently than females

    5. Leading cause of cancer death in men and women in the U.S.

- Signs and Symptoms: Depend on the area of tumor location and involvement of nodes or other organs; only 10 to 25% of patients are asymptomatic at time of diagnosis; symptoms occur with advanced disease

1. "Smoker's cough"—most common early symptom
2. Anorexia/weight loss
3. Dyspnea—related to obstruction of major bronchus
4. Hemoptysis—20% of all patients with hemoptysis have lung cancer
5. Wheezing
6. Fever
7. Chest pain—related to extension beyond parenchyma
8. Fatigue
9. Hoarseness
10. Bone pain
11. Neurological deficits

- Differential Diagnosis
  1. Pneumonia
  2. Lung abscess
  3. Bronchitis
  4. Tuberculosis

- Physical Findings
  1. Examination may not reveal significant changes
  2. Tumor obstructing bronchus—may cause atelectasis
  3. Visible or palpable supraclavicular lymph nodes
  4. Hepatomegaly

- Diagnostic Tests/Findings
  1. Chest radiograph
     a. Negative in 15% of patients with lung cancer
     b. Not diagnostic in itself, but indicates need for additional work up
     c. Manifestations—hilar or enlarging mass, infiltrate, atelectasis, cavitation or pleural effusion
  2. Laboratory
     a. CBC
     b. Liver function tests
     c. Serum electrolytes and calcium

3. Definitive diagnosis requires cytologic or histologic evidence

4. Sputum for cytology—positive in 40 to 60% of patients

5. Bronchoscopy with biopsy

6. MRI/CT scan

- Management/Treatment

  1. Surgery—25% of patients with lung cancer are candidates for surgery

  2. Chemotherapy

  3. Radiation therapy—generally palliative

  4. Refer to MD when lung cancer suspected

  5. Encourage patient to stop smoking

  6. Decrease exposure to pollutants

  7. Realistic assessment for patient and family of prognosis, pros and cons of therapy—essential to patient's decision for treatment

  8. Discuss side effects of chemotherapy/radiation

  9. Encourage nutritious diet

  10. Effective pain control

  11. Hospice care

Questions
Select the best answer

1. Which of the following drugs is contraindicated in the treatment of severe asthma?

    a. Propranolol
    b. Theophylline
    c. Amoxicillin
    d. Albuterol

2. The most common organism causing community-acquired pneumonia is:

    a. *Eschericia coli*
    b. *Staphylococcus aureus*
    c. *Streptococcus pneumoniae*
    d. *Klebsiella pneumoniae*

3. Which of the following is not a part of the differential diagnosis of chronic cough?

    a. Tuberculosis
    b. Gastroesophageal reflux disease
    c. Allergies
    d. Pneumonia

4. The most common side effect of isoniazid is:

    a. Idiopathic splenomegaly
    b. Seizures
    c. Gynecomastia
    d. Peripheral neuropathy

5. Alpha$_1$ antitrypsin deficiency is associated with which of the following conditions?

    a. Chronic bronchitis
    b. Asthma
    c. Emphysema
    d. Cystic fibrosis

6. A 25-year-old nurse presents to employee health for her annual physical examination. Her previous PPD, one year ago, is negative. A PPD is repeated and results 3 days later show 14 mm of induration. The nurse is asymptomatic and her chest radiograph is normal. The most appropriate management at this time would be:

    a. Repeat chest radiograph yearly
    b. Prescribe isoniazid for 6 to 12 months
    c. Prescribe ethambutol for 6 to 12 months
    d. Repeat PPD in two months

7. Which of the following statements is true in the treatment of moderate persistent asthma?

    a. Inhaled corticosteroids are the cornerstone of therapy
    b. Beta-blockers should be used vigorously
    c. Cromolyn is used during acute attacks
    d. Theophylline should not be used with steroid therapy

8. Which of the following signs/symptoms are not associated with chronic bronchitis?

    a. Productive cough
    b. Obesity
    c. Dyspnea
    d. Pursed lip breathing

9. The most important measurement of pulmonary function in asthma is:

    a. The total lung capacity
    b. The forced vital capacity
    c. The residual volume
    d. The peak expiratory flow rate

10. The most common cause of pneumonia in adolescents and young adults is:

    a. Pneumococcal
    b. Mycoplasma
    c. Varicella
    d. Chlamydia

11. Outpatient treatment of pneumonia for a 50-year-old healthy male would be:

    a. Amoxicillin
    b. Trimethoprim/sulfamethoxazole
    c. Erythromycin
    d. Cephalexin

12. Physical findings in bacterial pneumonia would include:

    a. Hyper-resonance to percussion
    b. Rales that clear with cough
    c. Decreased fremitus
    d. Positive egophony

13. Max Murphy, a 30-year-old postal worker, presents with malaise, fatigue and dry cough. Physical exam findings include low grade fever 100° F, right tympanic membranes with bullae, lungs clear, no lymphadenopathy. The most likely diagnosis for this patient is:

    a. Influenza
    b. Legionnaire's Disease
    c. Acute bronchitis
    d. Asthma

14. Pneumococcal vaccine is considered a preventive measure to bacterial pneumonia. It is indicated for which populations?

    a. Patients with acute bronchitis
    b. Patients with C.O.P.D.
    c. Adolescents and young adults
    d. Persons over age 45

15. An indicator of a severe asthma attack requiring emergency treatment includes:

    a. Prolonged expiration
    b. Bilateral rales
    c. Chest tightness
    d. Inaudible breath sounds

16. When ordering a CBC in a person with acute exacerbations of asthma, you would expect to see:

    a. Moderate elevation in WBCs and atypical lymphocytes
    b. Decrease in WBCs and lymphocytosis
    c. Increased hematocrit and increased platelets
    d. Mild elevation in WBCs and eosinophilia

17. Albuterol is an example of:

    a. Antihistamine
    b. β_2 adrenergic agonist
    c. Corticosteroid
    d. Antitussive

18. Which of the following is not a risk factor for lung cancer?

    a. Radon exposure
    b. Passive cigarette smoking
    c. Allergen irritant
    d. Asbestos exposure

19. The leading cause of cancer deaths in the U.S. is:

    a. Gastric cancer
    b. Malignant melanoma
    c. Breast cancer
    d. Lung cancer

20. The drug of choice in treatment of chronic bronchitis is:

    a. Theophylline
    b. Erythromycin
    c. Cromolyn sodium
    d. Ipratropium bromide

21. Pulsus paradoxus is:

    a. Increase in diastolic blood pressure on expiration
    b. Decrease in systolic blood pressure on inspiration
    c. Increase in systolic blood pressure on expiration
    d. Decrease in diastolic blood pressure on inspiration

22. Mary is a 44-year-old housewife with mild intermittent asthma since she was age 7. She requests you renew her β_2 adrenergic agonist inhaler and states she has heard how she should test her lung function with a peak flow meter at home. What is the most important rationale for home measurement of peak expiratory flow rate?

    a. It improves total lung capacity
    b. It is the most objective measure of respiratory status
    c. It measures the effectiveness of β_2 adrenergic therapy
    d. It improves the inspiratory/expiratory ratio

23. Which of the following groups are *not* at high risk for tuberculosis?

    a. HIV infected individuals
    b. Asian immigrants
    c. Homeless individuals
    d. College students

24. The serum cold agglutinins test is used to diagnose:

    a. *Haemophilus influenzae* pneumonia
    b. Legionella pneumonia
    c. Rickettsia infection
    d. Mycoplasma pneumonia

25. The problem with diagnosing early stage lung cancer is that:

    a. The CBC lab result is normal
    b. It mimics the symptoms of asthma
    c. Patients are often asymptomatic until late in the disease
    d. Pulmonary function tests are normal

26. Signs and symptoms of COPD correlate with which one of the following:

    a. Emphysema with decreased total lung capacity (TLC)
    b. Asthma and right sided heart failure
    c. Chronic bronchitis and airway obstruction
    d. Hemoptysis and hypoxemia

27. Larry Bates, a 32-year-old accountant with moderate persistent asthma, presents with dyspnea and wheezing for 2 days. His current medications include beclomethasone 2 inhalations b.i.d. and theophylline 300 mg at hs. His PEFR is approximately 60% of his personal best. Based on this information, what treatment would you prescribe for Larry?

   a. Add cromolyn sodium inhaler to regimen

   b. Give albuterol inhaler 2 inhalations q.i.d. for acute symptoms

   c. Add salmeterol inhaler for daytime symptoms

   d. Give antihistamine to decrease symptoms

28. Additional history reveals that Larry's girlfriend has just acquired a kitten. He noticed his asthma got worse after playing with the kitten. The best intervention for Larry to do at this time is:

   a. Wash hands before and after playing with the kitten

   b. Consider allergy shots

   c. Avoid contact with the kitten

   d. Take an antihistamine/decongestant approximately 30 minutes prior to exposure to the kitten

29. Young Chow, an 18-year-old Chinese exchange student, presents to student health for immunization update. He states he had BCG vaccine as a young child and therefore will never get tuberculosis. You administer a PPD and the result is positive. Your next best intervention would be to:

   a. Assume the positive result is due to BCG vaccine, no further evaluation needed

   b. Assume the positive result is related to TB exposure or infection, order a chest radiograph

   c. Begin isoniazid therapy immediately

   d. Repeat PPD test in one month to verify results

30. The most common side effect of the anti-tuberculin drug rifampin is:

   a. Hepatotoxicity

   b. Optic neuritis

   c. Fever

   d. Orange discoloration of secretions

Answers

1. a	11. c	21. b
2. c	12. d	22. b
3. d	13. c	23. d
4. d	14. b	24. d
5. c	15. d	25. c
6. b	16. d	26. c
7. a	17. b	27. b
8. d	18. c	28. c
9. d	19. d	29. b
10. b	20. d	30. d

Bibliography

Abrams, W. B., Beers, M. H., & Berkow, R. (Eds.). (2000). *The Merck manual of geriatrics (3rd ed.).* Whitehouse Station, NJ: Merck & Co.

Chin, J. (Ed.). (2000). *Control of communicable diseases manual* (17th ed.). Washington: American Public Health Association.

Clinician reviews supplement. (2000). The journal of COPD management. (Winter 2000). Clifton, NJ: Partners in Medical Communications.

Dambro, M. R. (Ed.). (1998). *Griffith's 5 minute clinical consult.* Baltimore: Williams & Wilkins.

Davis, A., Kane, G., & Plouffe, J. F. (1999). The changing care of community acquired pneumonia. *Patient Care For The Nurse Practitioner.* (Special issue, March, 1999). 52–63.

Goroll, A. H., & Mulley, A. G., Jr. (Eds.). (2000). *Primary care medicine* (4th ed.). Philadelphia: Lippincott Williams & Wilkins.

Mackin, L., & Nettina, S. M. (Eds.). (1998). Pulmonary health. *Lippincott's Primary Care Practice. A Peer Reviewed Series.* 2(6), 545–653.

National Asthma Education and Prevention Programs. (1997). Expert Panel Report 2: *Guidelines for the Diagnosis and Management of Asthma.* Bethesda, MD: National Institutes of Health, National Heart, Lung and Blood Institute. US Dept of Health and Human Services publication #NIH 97-4051.

Report of U.S. Preventive Services (1998). *Guide to clinical preventive Services* (2nd ed.). http://odphp.osophs.dhhs.gov/pubs/guidecps/

Richman, E. (1997). Asthma diagnosis and management. *Clinician Reviews, 7*(8), 76-112.

Tierney, L., McPhee, S. J., & Papadakis, M. A. (Eds.). (2001). *Current medical diagnosis and treatment* (40th ed.). NY: Lange Medical Books/McGraw-Hill.

Youngkin, E. G., Sawin, K., Kissinger, J., & Israel, D. (1999). *Pharmacotherapeutics: A primary care clinical guide.* Stamford, CT: Appleton & Lange.

Cardiovascular Disorders Infancy Through Adolescence

Karen Uzark

Congenital Heart Disease/Defects

- Definition: Cardiovascular malformations that result from abnormal structural development of the heart and/or vessels; most heart defects occur within first 8 weeks of gestation

- Etiology/Incidence

  1. Etiology of most defects unknown

  2. Probably genetic predisposition interacting with environmental trigger

  3. Chromosomal abnormalities account for nearly 10% of cardiac malformations (Down syndrome, Turner's syndrome, DiGeorge syndrome, others)

  4. Environmental or adverse maternal conditions account for 2% to 4%

     a. Maternal diabetes mellitus, phenylketonuria, systemic lupus erythematosus, rubella or other viruses

     b. Maternal ingestion of thalidomide, alcohol, lithium, anticonvulsant agents, other drugs

  5. Approximately 8 per 1000 live births; about 32,000 new cases of congenital heart disease per year in the U.S.

  6. Ventricular septal defect (VSD) is most common (25% to 30% of all lesions)

- Signs and Symptoms

  1. Cyanosis—usually apparent at oxygen saturation of 85% or less

     a. Central (arterial desaturation)—generalized, mucous membranes

     b. Peripheral

     c. "Spells" characteristic of tetralogy of fallot

        (1) Often in the morning with crying

        (2) Acute increase in cyanosis with hyperpnea

        (3) May be followed by limpness, loss of consciousness, rarely convulsions

  2. Increased respiratory rate and/or effort at rest or with activity

  3. Poor feeding; fatigue during feeding

  4. Excessive sweating in infant, unrelated to the environment, especially while feeding

  5. Recurrent respiratory infections

  6. Decreased exercise tolerance

  7. Squatting with fatigue (rare)

  8. Chest pain (uncommon, usually noncardiac origin)—most common with severe aortic stenosis

  9. Syncope (uncommon)

- Differential Diagnosis
  1. Pulmonary disease
  2. Arrhythmias
  3. Myocardial diseases
  4. Rheumatic fever
  5. Sepsis
  6. Hypoglycemia, anemia, polycythemia, especially in neonates
  7. Central nervous system disorders
- Physical Findings
  1. Cyanosis (central or peripheral); pallor
  2. Clubbing of the fingers or toes (with long-standing arterial desaturation)
  3. Poor growth/weight gain
  4. Abnormal respiratory patterns
     a. Tachypnea
     b. Hyperpnea
     c. Dyspnea
  5. Tachycardia
  6. Hepatic enlargement with some defects
  7. Precordial prominence or increased precordial activity, palpable thrill
  8. Abnormal heart sounds
     a. Increased intensity
     b. Abnormal splitting
     c. Ejection clicks
     d. Fourth heart sound (gallop)
     e. Murmurs (may be absent or soft in spite of serious heart defect)
  9. Abnormal peripheral pulses
     a. Decreased
     b. Bounding
     c. Unequal (decreased lower extremity pulses suggest coarctation of the aorta)
  10. Abnormal blood pressure
     a. Hypotension
     b. Upper extremity blood pressure higher than lower extremity blood pressure suggestive of coarctation of aorta

Cardiovascular Disorders —— 475

11. Peripheral edema, uncommon in infants

- Diagnostic Tests/Findings

  1. Chest radiograph to evaluate heart size and pulmonary vascular markings

  2. Electrocardiogram to evaluate rhythm, chamber enlargement or hypertrophy

  3. Arterial blood gas and hemoglobin in infant with cyanosis—if decreased PO_2 in room air, repeat arterial blood gas after 10 to 15 minutes in 100% inspired oxygen (oxygen challenge) to help differentiate between cardiac and pulmonary cyanosis; if minimal increase in PO_2, cardiac etiology suggested

  4. Echocardiogram for diagnosis of specific congenital heart defect

- Management/Treatment

  1. Referral to pediatric cardiologist

     a. Prompt referral of symptomatic neonate

     b. Prompt referral of infant with cyanotic spells

Table 1

Cyanotic Heart Defects

Defect	Anatomy	Surgical Management
Transposition of the great arteries	The aorta arises from right ventricle; pulmonary artery from the left ventricle	Arterial switch (Jatene) operation in neonatal period or intra-atrial baffle (Mustard or Senning procedure) later in infancy
Tetralogy of Fallot	Combination of four defects: (1) pulmonary stenosis, (2) ventricular septal defect, (3) overriding aorta, and (4) right ventricular hypertrophy	*Palliative:* Blalock-Taussig or other aortopulmonary shunts in infancy *Repair:* patch closure of VSD and resection of infundibular pulmonary stenosis ± pulmonary valvulotomy if necessary
Tricuspid atresia	Complete agenesis of tricuspid valve with no direct communication between right atrium and a hypoplastic right ventricle	*Palliative:* shunt (or pulmonary artery banding if increased pulmonary blood flow via a ventricular septal defect) *Repair:* pulmonary artery connected to right atrium/vena cavae (Fontan procedure)
Total anomalous pulmonary venous connection	Pulmonary veins do not enter left atrium but are connected either directly or indirectly to right atrium	*Repair:* pulmonary venous trunk connected to left atrium in infancy
Truncus arteriosus	Single arterial trunk forms aorta and pulmonary artery, overriding ventricles and receiving blood from them through a ventricular septal defect	*Repair:* closure of ventricular septal defect, removing origin of the pulmonary arteries from trunk, and connecting pulmonary arteries to right ventricle with a conduit in infancy
Pulmonary atresia with intact ventricular septum	Complete atresia of pulmonary valve and varying degrees of hypoplasia of right ventricle	*Palliative:* Blalock-Taussig shunt ± pulmonary valvulotomy *Repair:* right ventricular outflow tract reconstruction or Fontan procedure
Ebstein's anomaly of the tricuspid valve	Redundant tricuspid valve tissue with the septal and posterior leaflets displaced downward into right ventricle for a variable distance	*Repair:* tricuspid valve replacement or modified tricuspid annuloplasty (patients with less severe forms do not require surgery)

Note. From "Alterations in cardiac function" by K. Uzark. In W. Votroubek (Ed.), (1997) *Pediatric Home Care* (2nd ed., p. 135). Frederick, MD: Aspen Publishers. Copyright 1997 by Aspen Publishers. Reprinted with permission.

2. Monitoring and counseling to promote optimal growth and development

3. Primary care, immunizations

4. Endocarditis prophylaxis with dental or surgical procedures

5. Psychosocial support of child and family

6. Surgical management/treatment of most significant congenital heart defects—see Table 1

Congestive Heart Failure (CHF)

- Definition: Clinical syndrome that reflects the inability of the heart to meet metabolic requirements of the body

- Etiology/Incidence

    1. Congenital heart defects with volume or pressure overload (most common cause in pediatric age group)—see Table 2

        a. Hypoplastic left heart syndrome

        b. Coarctation of the aorta

        c. Ventricular septal defect

        d. Atrioventricular septal defect

        e. Patent ductus arteriosus

    2. Acquired heart disease (less common cause)

        a. Myocarditis

        b. Metabolic abnormalities

        c. Endocardial fibroelastosis

        d. Rheumatic heart disease

        e. Cardiomyopathy (idiopathic, doxorubicin toxicity, muscular dystrophy)

    3. Other causes

        a. Tachyarrhythmias, complete heart block in infancy

        b. Severe anemia, hydrops fetalis

        c. Acute hypertension

        d. Bronchopulmonary dysplasia

        e. Acute cor pulmonale

        f. Arteriovenous malformations

    4. Incidence unknown

- Signs and Symptoms

    1. Increased respiratory rate and/or effort at rest or with activity

Table 2

Acyanotic Heart Defects Commonly Causing Congestive Heart Failure In Infancy

Defect	Description
Hypoplastic left heart syndrome	Aortic atresia and underdevelopment of the left ventricle, mitral valve, hypoplastic aortic arch, and/or coarctation
Coarctation of the aorta	Constriction of the aorta usually located slightly distal to origin of left subclavian artery
Ventricular septal defect	Abnormal opening between right and left ventricle that may result in congestive heart failure if left-to-right shunt is large
Atrioventricular septal defect (endocardial cushion defect)	Defect in lower part of atrial septum (ostium primum) and membranous ventricular septum and a single common atrioventricular valve
Patent ductus arteriosus	Connection between pulmonary artery and aorta that fails to close after birth, allowing increased blood flow to lungs

2. Poor feeding

3. Excessive sweating, especially with feeding in infants

4. Decreased exercise tolerance

5. Poor weight gain

6. Orthopnea in older child, chronic cough

- Differential Diagnosis

    1. Pulmonary diseases

    2. Cardiac diseases (see etiology)

- Physical Findings

    1. Tachycardia (common)

    2. Tachypnea (common)

    3. Hepatomegaly

    4. Puffy eyelids common in infants, peripheral edema less common in children

    5. Wheezing, pulmonary rales may be present

    6. Pallor, mottling of extremities

    7. Weakly palpable peripheral pulses; cool extremities

    8. Gallop rhythm with myocardial failure

    9. Cyanosis with alveolar edema

- Diagnostic Tests/Findings

    1. Chest radiograph—cardiomegaly almost always present; pulmonary vascular congestion dependent on etiology

    2. Echocardiogram to assess ventricular function, chamber enlargement, anatomy

    3. Electrocardiogram not diagnostic, may help assess etiology

- Management/Treatment
    1. Referral to cardiologist to determine etiology if heart disease suspected
    2. Drug therapy
        a. Inotropic agents—usually digoxin
        b. Diuretics
        c. Afterload-reducing agents
    3. Other measures
        a. Semi-Fowler position (infant seat, pillows)
        b. Prostaglandin E_1 if systemic perfusion dependent on patency of ductus arteriosus
        c. Caloric supplementation of formula, breast milk fortifier (low sodium formulas not recommended)
        d. Frequent rest periods
    4. Treatment of underlying condition if specific therapy available
    5. Possible referral for cardiac transplantation if refractory, end-stage heart failure

Murmurs (innocent)

- Definition:
    1. Innocent murmurs are murmurs not associated with any anatomic abnormality
    2. Result from turbulence of blood flow, usually at origin of great arteries
    3. Also referred to as functional, normal, benign, or insignificant
    4. Common innocent murmurs
        a. *Still's murmur*—vibratory, groaning, or musical systolic murmur heard best between lower left sternal border and apex, attributed to turbulence in left ventricular outflow tract
        b. *Pulmonary systolic ejection murmur* or *pulmonary flow murmur*—slightly harsh systolic ejection murmur heard best at second to third left intercostal space; attributed to turbulent flow in right ventricular outflow tract
        c. *Supraclavicular arterial bruit*—early systolic murmur heard above clavicles, attributed to turbulence at site of branching of brachiocephalic arteries
        d. *Physiologic peripheral pulmonary stenosis*—low intensity systolic ejection murmur heard best at upper left sternal border, axillae, and back bilaterally in neonates until 3 to 6 months of age, attributed to relative hypoplasia of branch pulmonary arteries at birth
        e. *Venous hum*—humming continuous murmur usually heard best at upper right sternal border in sitting position with marked decrease or disappearance of murmur in supine position

- Etiology/Incidence
    1. Heard in more than 50 percent of normal children from infancy through adolescence
    2. Still's murmur most common; heard most frequently from 3 to 7 years of age
    3. Increased intensity (incidence) associated with increased cardiac output state (fever, acute illness, anemia, anxiety, exercise)
- Signs and Symptoms: Asymptomatic
- Differential Diagnosis
    1. Congenital heart disease
    2. Conditions associated with high cardiac output
- Physical Findings
    1. No cyanosis or other cardiovascular abnormalities
    2. Normal blood pressure, peripheral pulses in upper and lower extremities
    3. Normal heart sounds, including normal splitting (not fixed) of second heart sound
    4. No clicks
    5. Characteristics
        a. Usually systolic with exception of venous hum; never diastolic alone
        b. Usually low intensity (grade 1 to 3); never associated with precordial thrill
        c. Usually short duration, not holosystolic
        d. Well-localized, poorly transmitted except neonatal peripheral pulmonary stenosis
        e. Intensity may vary with position change
- Diagnostic Tests/Findings
    1. Testing not routine
    2. May be indicated to rule out congenital heart defect
        a. Chest radiograph normal
        b. Echocardiogram if recommended by cardiologist
- Management/Treatment
    1. Inform parents of murmur
    2. Provide reassurance that child's heart is normal
    3. Referral to cardiologist if:
        a. Symptomatic
        b. Cardiovascular abnormalities on physical examination

    c.   Uncertainty regarding innocence of murmur

    d.   Persistent parental concern

Hypertension

- Definition: "Average systolic and/or average diastolic blood pressure greater than or equal to the 95th percentile for age and sex with measurements obtained on at least three occasions" (Task Force on Blood Pressure Control in Children)—see Table 3

- Etiology/Incidence

    1.   Primary hypertension

        a.   No known underlying disease present to cause hypertension

        b.   May be related to factors such as heredity, salt intake, stress and obesity

        c.   More commonly recognized in adolescents

    2.   Secondary hypertension

        a.   Etiology varies with age

            (1)   Newborn infants—renal artery thrombosis, renal artery stenosis, congenital renal malformations, coarctation of the aorta, bronchopulmonary dysplasia

Table 3

Classification of Hypertension by Age Group

Age Group	Significant Hypertension (mm Hg)	Severe Hypertension (mm Hg)
Newborn		
7 d	Systolic BP ≥96	Systolic BP ≥106
8–30 d	Systolic BP ≥104	Systolic BP ≥110
Infant (<2 yr)	Systolic BP ≥112	Systolic BP ≥118
	Diastolic BP ≥74	Diastolic BP ≥82
Children (3–5 yr)	Systolic BP ≥116	Systolic BP ≥124
	Diastolic BP ≥76	Diastolic BP ≥84
Children (6–9 yr)	Systolic BP ≥122	Systolic BP ≥130
	Diastolic BP ≥78	Diastolic BP ≥86
Children (10–12 yr)	Systolic BP ≥126	Systolic BP ≥134
	Diastolic BP ≥82	Diastolic BP ≥90
Children (13–15 yr)	Systolic BP ≥136	Systolic BP ≥144
	Diastolic BP ≥86	Diastolic BP ≥92
Children (16–18 yr)	Systolic BP ≥142	Systolic BP ≥150
	Diastolic BP ≥92	Diastolic BP ≥98

Note. From "Task Force on Blood Pressure Control in Children" by Report of the second task force on blood pressure control in children (1987), *Pediatrics,* 79(1) p. 7. Copyright 1987 by American Academy of Pediatrics. Reproduced by permission.

(2) Infancy to 6 years—renal parenchymal diseases, coarctation of the aorta, renal artery stenosis

(3) 6 to 10 year olds—renal artery stenosis, renal parenchymal disease

b. Other causes—endocrine disorders, neurogenic tumors, drugs or toxins, increased intracranial pressure

c. More common in infants and children

3. Prevalence of hypertension in childhood is low (1% to 3%)

- Signs and Symptoms
  1. Primary hypertension—usually no symptoms
  2. Severe hypertension—may complain of headaches, dizziness, visual disturbances, epistaxis
  3. Secondary hypertension—symptoms related to underlying disease and may include:
     a. Congestive heart failure
     b. Respiratory distress (infants)
     c. Failure to thrive
     d. Irritability
     e. Convulsions
     f. Feeding problems

- Differential Diagnosis: Causes of secondary hypertension (see etiology)
- Physical Findings
  1. Elevated blood pressure on at least three occasions (without acute illness)
  2. Related to underlying disease if secondary hypertension—may include edema, pallor, increased sweating, absent or delayed femoral pulses, signs of specific syndrome

- Diagnostic Tests/Findings
  1. Based on history, age, other clinical findings
  2. Complete blood count (to evaluate anemia)
  3. Urinalysis
  4. BUN, creatinine (to evaluate renal function)
  5. Lipid profile
  6. Echocardiogram if hypertension severe or drug therapy considered
  7. Additional tests based on suspected cause

- Management/Treatment
  1. Depends on cause and degree of elevation

2. General counseling regarding cardiovascular risk factors such as family history, obesity, lack of exercise, smoking

3. Nonpharmacologic therapy

   a. Weight reduction if indicated

   b. Regular aerobic exercise programs (especially in adolescents)

   c. Dietary modification—sodium reduction

4. Antihypertensive drugs if significant diastolic hypertension; evidence of target organ injury, or if symptoms related to elevated blood pressure

   a. Thiazide-type diuretic

   b. Adrenergic inhibitor/beta blocking drugs

   c. Vasodilator or angiotensin—converting enzyme inhibitor if blood pressure control not achieved with drugs previously cited

5. If secondary hypertension, therapy for underlying disease

6. Long-term follow-up, referral to subspecialist (cardiologist, nephrologist) if poor blood pressure control

Rheumatic Fever/Heart Disease

- Definition: A post-infectious inflammatory disease, based on standardized clinical (Jones) criteria, which can result in rheumatic valvular heart disease

- Etiology/Incidence

  1. Follows a group A streptococcal infection of the upper respiratory tract

  2. Probably involves abnormal immune response of certain individuals with genetic predisposition to this complication

  3. Incidence of acute rheumatic fever (ARF) approximately 3% of individuals with untreated or inadequately treated group A streptococcal tonsillopharyngitis (greater risk of recurrence)

  4. Most common in children between 6 and 15 years of age; rarely seen before 5 years

  5. Seasonal incidence follows that of streptococcal pharyngitis; peak incidence in spring

  6. Greater frequency of rheumatic heart disease in patients who had severe cardiac involvement during initial attack or recurrence of ARF

     a. Mitral valve regurgitation most common lesion

     b. Tricuspid and pulmonary valve involvement rare

- Signs and Symptoms
    1. Diagnosis of the initial attack of acute rheumatic fever based on evidence of preceding group A streptococcal infection **PLUS** two major or one major and two minor manifestations of the following:
    2. *Major Manifestations*
        a. Cardititis (approximately 50% of patients)
            (1) Valvulitis usually, as evidenced by development of new murmur, especially apical systolic murmur of mitral regurgitation
            (2) Myocarditis in absence of valvulitis rare—evidenced by tachycardia; other signs of congestive heart failure
            (3) Pericarditis rare in absence of valvulitis—evidenced by distant heart sounds, friction rub, chest pain
        b. Polyarthritis (approximately 70% of patients)
            (1) Almost always migratory
            (2) Most frequently larger joints—knees, ankles, elbows, wrists
        c. Chorea (Sydenham's chorea)
            (1) Purposeless, involuntary, rapid movements of trunk and/or extremities
            (2) Often associated with muscle weakness and emotional lability
        d. Erythema marginatum
            (1) Macular, nonpruritic rash with serpiginous erythematous border surrounding normal looking skin
            (2) Lesions most commonly located on trunk and proximal limbs; never on face
        e. Subcutaneous nodules (rare)—firm, painless nodules over the extensor surfaces of certain joints, particularly elbows, knuckles, knees, and ankles
    3. *Minor Manifestations*
        a. Arthralgia without objective evidence of inflammation
        b. Fever usually at least 39° C (102.2° F)
        c. Elevated acute phase reactants
        d. Prolonged PR interval on electrocardiogram
        e. Other clinical features—abdominal pain, malaise, epistaxis
- Differential Diagnosis
    1. Juvenile rheumatoid arthritis
    2. Other connective tissue diseases
    3. Infective endocarditis

4. Septic arthritis

5. Viral myocarditis and pericarditis

6. Reactions to drugs or foreign serum

- Physical Findings: No single specific finding; see manifestations
- Diagnostic Tests/Findings
    1. No specific diagnostic test
    2. Elevated acute phase reactants
        a. Erythrocyte sedimentation rate
        b. C-reactive protein
    3. Elevated streptococcal antibody titer (ASO)
    4. Electrocardiogram may indicate prolonged PR interval, rarely 2nd or 3rd degree heart block
    5. Echocardiogram may show valvular regurgitation
- Management/Treatment
    1. Referral to pediatrician/cardiologist if suspected
    2. Antibiotic treatment of group A streptococcal infection
    3. Anti-inflammatory agents for treatment of arthritis or carditis
        a. Salicylates or nonsteroidal agents
        b. Possible steroids if carditis severe
    4. Bedrest for period of acute carditis
    5. Treatment of congestive heart failure, if present
    6. Prevention of streptococcal infection and recurrence of rheumatic fever
        a. Prompt and adequate treatment of streptococcal pharyngitis
        b. Administration of monthly injections of long-acting benzathine penicillin (most reliable) or daily oral antibiotic regimen
        c. Antibiotics for endocarditis prophylaxis prior to dental work or surgical procedures in patients with rheumatic heart disease

Disturbances Of Rate And Rhythm

- Definition:
    1. A heart rate below the lower limits of normal for age (bradycardia)
    2. A heart rate above the upper limits of normal for age (tachycardia)
    3. An irregularity of heart rhythm, usually related to premature contraction

- Etiology/Incidence
  1. May be congenital or acquired
     a. Congenital complete heart block (CHB); 1 in 25,000 live births, can be associated with maternal systemic lupus erythematosus or other connective tissue diseases
     b. Acquired CHB caused by damage to conduction system during cardiac surgery, severe myocarditis, acute rheumatic fever, mumps, tumors in conduction system, endocrine/metabolic disorders
  2. Other causes
     a. Drugs (theophylline, cocaine, others)
     b. Electrolyte imbalance
     c. Acidosis/hypoxia
     d. Increased intracranial pressure
     e. Cardiomyopathy, long QT syndrome, structural heart disease or surgery
  3. Supraventricular tachycardia (SVT)
     a. Most common symptomatic tachycardia in first year of life
     b. May be associated with Wolff-Parkinson-White syndrome (10% to 20%)
  4. Premature atrial contractions (PAC) and premature ventricular contractions (PVC) common in healthy children
- Signs and Symptoms
  1. Children usually asymptomatic
  2. Symptoms of low cardiac output or congestive heart failure if bradycardia or tachycardia is severe and/or prolonged
  3. Irritability, pallor, poor feeding in infants
  4. Palpitations, syncope, dizziness
  5. Seizures
  6. Rare sudden death (with ventricular tachycardia and fibrillation)
- Differential Diagnosis
  1. Normal sinus arrhythmia (phasic acceleration and deceleration of heart rate with respiration)
  2. Sinus tachycardia and associated causes
  3. Sinus bradycardia and associated causes (normal in athletes)
  4. Conditions associated with heart rate disturbances (see etiology)

- Physical Findings

    1. Bradycardia, tachycardia, or irregular rhythm

    2. Tachypnea, hepatomegaly, poor perfusion especially in infants if rate disturbance severe and/or prolonged

- Diagnostic Tests/Findings

    1. Electrocardiogram

    2. Other tests based on clinical findings and symptoms

- Management/Treatment

    1. Referral to cardiologist for evaluation and treatment if:

        a. Symptomatic

        b. Sustained arrhythmia, or

        c. Recurrent arrhythmia

    2. Treatment of underlying condition if noncardiac cause

Myocarditis

- Definition: Focal or diffuse inflammation of the myocardium in association with myocellular necrosis

- Etiology/Incidence

    1. Precise etiology usually unknown

    2. May be caused by virtually any bacterial, viral, rickettsial, fungal, or parasitic organism—viral infections the most common etiology, especially coxsackie B virus (> 50%) and adenovirus

    3. Other causes include autoimmune or collagen-vascular diseases, or hypersensitivity drug reactions (rare)

    4. Possible genetic predisposition with viral trigger

    5. Incidence unknown, as many mild cases may go undetected

    6. In patients who present with severe congestive heart failure or shock (20% to 30%), approximately one-third will die or require transplantation

- Signs and Symptoms

    1. Great variability—from no distress to severe congestive heart failure or shock

    2. Often fever or history of antecedent "flu-like" viral illness

    3. Suspect if onset of congestive heart failure with no obvious structural or functional etiology

        a. Persistent tachycardia (out of proportion to fever if present)

        b. Tachypnea, dyspnea

      c. Easy fatigue, poor feeding in infant

      d. Gallop rhythm, usually no murmur

      e. Hepatomegaly

      f. Poor perfusion

  4. Can also present as new onset arrhythmias, syncope, or sudden death

- Differential Diagnosis

  1. Carnitine deficiency

  2. Idiopathic dilated cardiomyopathy

  3. Pericarditis

  4. Endocardial fibroelastosis

  5. Hereditary mitochondrial defects

  6. Anomalies of the coronary arteries

  7. Metabolic or endocrine disorders (hyperthyroidism)

- Physical Findings: See section on congestive heart failure

- Diagnostic Tests/Findings

  1. Erythrocyte sedimentation rate and heart enzymes (CPK, LDH) elevated

  2. Viral cultures, antibody titers, and polymeraze chain reaction (PCR) may suggest viral etiology

  3. Laboratory studies to rule out metabolic causes of cardiomyopathy

  4. Echocardiography to assess ventricular function and rule out other cardiac anomalies

  5. Chest radiograph to assess cardiac enlargement which is variable

  6. Electrocardiogram may show ST segment and T wave abnormalities, possible reduced QRS voltage, or arrhythmias

  7. Endomyocardial biopsy for possible confirmation of diagnosis

- Management/Treatment

  1. Immediate referral to pediatrician and/or pediatric cardiologist if suspected

  2. Supportive measures for congestive heart failure

      a. Inotropic agents, including digoxin, at reduced dosage (may be arrythmogenic)

      b. Diuretics, afterload reduction

      c. Bedrest

  3. Treatment of arrythmias

  4. Use of immunosuppressive medication controversial

5. Possible administration of intravenous immunoglobulin—effectiveness not proven; risk of anaphylaxis

6. Psychosocial support of child and/or family—usually sudden onset of illness in previously healthy child

7. Outcome varies from complete resolution and recovery to development of chronic cardiomyopathy or death without cardiac transplantation

Hypercholesterolemia

- Definition: Elevated serum cholesterol level

  1. Total cholesterol of 200 mg/dL or above

  2. Total cholesterol of 170 to 199 mg/dL considered "borderline high"

  3. Low density lipoprotein (LDL) cholesterol of 130 mg/dL or above

- Etiology/Incidence

  1. High tracking correlations for total and LDL cholesterol levels from childhood to adulthood

  2. Potential increased risk for developing atherosclerotic or coronary heart disease as adults, especially in association with other risk factors

     a. Positive family history of premature coronary heart disease (before 55 years of age), peripheral vascular disease, or hypercholesterolemia (above 240 mg/dL)

     b. Diabetes

     c. Hypertension

     d. Obesity

     e. Smoking

     f. Physical inactivity

  3. Among children aged 2 to 11 years in U.S., about 25% with cholesterol levels in borderline high or high range

  4. Familial hypercholesterolemia (autosomal dominant) prevalence rate of heterozygous form 1 in 500, homozygous form 1 in 1,000,000

  5. Secondary causes of hypercholesterolemia

     a. Obesity

     b. Endocrine and metabolic conditions

     c. Obstructive liver disease

     d. Nephrotic syndrome

     e. Anorexia nervosa

     f. Collagen disease

       g. Drugs

          (1) Corticosteroids

          (2) Isotretinoin

          (3) Thiazide diuretics

          (4) Some beta blockers

          (5) Some oral contraceptives

- Signs and Symptoms: Asymptomatic during childhood

- Differential Diagnosis: Causes of secondary hypercholesterolemia (see etiology)

- Physical Findings

    1. Rare xanthomas with familial hypercholesterolemia and very high cholesterol levels

    2. Signs of risk factors (hypertension, obesity)

- Diagnostic Tests/Findings

    1. Measurement of total cholesterol in children over 2 years of age with a positive family history or other risk factors (U.S. Department of Health and Human Services, 1991)

        a. If total cholesterol level acceptable (< 170 mg/dL), repeat measurement within 5 years

        b. If total cholesterol level borderline (170 to 199 mg/dL), repeat measurement, and if average is borderline or high, do lipoprotein analysis

        c. If total cholesterol level high (above 200 mg/dL), do lipoprotein analysis

    2. Additional studies to evaluate causes of secondary hypercholesterolemia, as indicated

- Management/Treatment

    1. Nutrition assessment/diet therapy in children over 2 years of age

        a. If LDL cholesterol ≥ 110 mg/dL, step 1 diet—no more than 30% of total calories from fat, less than 10% of total calories as saturated fat, and less than 300 mg of cholesterol per day; adequate calories to reach or maintain desirable body weight

        b. If LDL cholesterol > 130 mg/dL after 3 months of step 1 diet, step 2 diet is prescribed—saturated fatty acid intake reduced to less than 7% of calories and cholesterol intake to less than 200 mg per day; adequate amounts of nutrients, vitamins, and minerals provided

    2. Drug therapy in children aged 10 years and older if after an adequate trial of diet therapy (6 months to 1 year), LDL cholesterol ≥ 190 mg/dL or LDL cholesterol ≥ 160 mg/dL plus positive family history of premature cardiovascular disease or 2 or more other cardiovascular risk factors are present; bile acid sequestrants recommended

3. Increase exercise

4. Prevention—anticipatory guidance during all well-child maintenance visits to maintain well-balanced diet, encourage daily exercise, and avoid known risk factors

Kawasaki Disease (Mucocutaneous Lymph Node Syndrome)

- Definition: Acute febrile syndrome associated with generalized vasculitis and the leading cause of acquired coronary artery disease in children

- Etiology/Incidence

   1. Etiology uncertain

      a. Epidemiology and clinical presentation highly suggestive of infectious etiology

      b. May be associated with exposure to house dust mites or recently shampooed carpets

   2. Most frequently (80%) affects infants and children under 5 years of age; most less than 2 years

   3. Male to female ratio 1.5:1

   4. All racial backgrounds affected; highest incidence in children of Asian ancestry

   5. Approximately 20% risk of developing coronary artery abnormalities with decreased risk if intravenous gamma globulin therapy instituted before 10th day of illness

- Signs and Symptoms

   1. Vary in severity and over course of illness

   2. Early (acute phase)

      a. Preceding or concurrent respiratory symptoms—runny nose, cough, ear infection

      b. Diarrhea, vomiting, or abdominal pain (common)

      c. Irritability

      d. Persistent fever > 5 days

      e. Reddened eyes

      f. Red tongue and throat

      g. Redness and/or swelling of hands and feet

      h. Rash

      i. Swollen nodes

      j. Fast and/or irregular pulse

      k. Irritability

   3. Mid-course (sub-acute phase)

      a.   Dry, peeling skin on lips, fingers and toes

      b.   Joint pain

   4.   Late (convalescent phase)—resolution of symptoms

- Differential Diagnosis

   1.   Measles

   2.   Scarlet fever

   3.   Drug reactions

   4.   Stevens-Johnson syndrome

   5.   Other febrile viral exanthems

   6.   Rocky mountain spotted fever

   7.   Staphylococcal scalded skin syndrome

   8.   Toxic shock syndrome

   9.   Juvenile rheumatoid arthritis

  10.   Leptospirosis

  11.   Mercury poisoning

- Physical Findings

   1.   Diagnostic criteria includes presence of at least 5 of following clinical features:

      a.   Persistent fever of at least 5 days

      b.   Bilateral, painless bulbar conjunctival injection without exudate

      c.   Lips/oral cavity—erythema and cracking of lips, strawberry tongue, erythema of oropharyngeal mucosa

      d.   Peripheral extremities—acute erythema and/or edema of hands/ feet; membranous desquamation of fingertips during sub-acute and convalescent phases (1 to 3 weeks after onset of fever)

      e.   Polymorphous exanthem of trunk extremeties within 4 days of fever onset

      f.   Cervical nonfluctuant lymphadenopathy; at least one lymph node more than 1.5 cm in diameter; usually unilateral

   2.   Coronary artery abnormalities (usually beyond 10 days of illness onset) with fever and fewer than 5 clinical features is diagnostic

   3.   Other physical findings

      a.   Arthritis or arthralgia

      b.   Tachycardia out of proportion to degree of fever; gallop rhythm (signs of myocarditis); new murmur (less common)

     c.   Sterile pyuria

     d.   Aneurysm of peripheral arteries (less common)

- Diagnostic Tests/Findings

  1.   No specific diagnostic test

  2.   Thrombocytosis, may be marked; frequently seen after first week of illness

  3.   Leukocytosis with left shift

  4.   Erythrocyte sedimentation rate elevated

  5.   C-reactive protein positive

  6.   Mild anemia in acute phase

  7.   Hypoalbuminemia

  8.   Electrocardiogram abnormal in $\frac{1}{3}$ of children

     a.   ST-T wave changes

     b.   Decreased R wave voltage

     c.   Prolonged PR or QT intervals

     d.   Atrial or ventricular arrhythmias

  9.   Echocardiogram—coronary artery aneurysms or ectasia; occasional pericardial effusion or decreased contractility

- Management/Treatment

  1.   Immediate referral to pediatrician and/or subspecialist (immunologist, pediatric cardiologist) if suspected

  2.   Management goals

     a.   Reducing inflammation, particularly in the coronary arterial wall and myocardium

     b.   Preventing coronary thrombosis

  3.   Therapy during acute phase

     a.   Intravenous gamma globulin within 10 days of onset of illness, *PLUS*

     b.   High-dose aspirin (80 to 100 mg/kg/day) until patient is afebrile, then reduced to 3 to 5 mg/kg/day for 6 to 8 weeks

  4.   If coronary arterial abnormalities detected

     a.   Low-dose aspirin continued indefinitely

     b.   Dipyridamole considered if high risk for myocardial infarction

     c.   Long-term follow-up by pediatric cardiologist

  5.   Administration of live virus vaccines delayed at least 5 months after intravenous gamma globulin treatment unless risk of exposure is high

6. Administration of influenza vaccine in patients on long-term aspirin therapy
7. Activity restrictions beyond initial 6 to 8 weeks based on risk for severity of coronary artery involvement

Questions
Select the best answer

1. The most common congenital heart defect in children is:

    a. Tricuspid atresia
    b. Ventricular septal defect
    c. Aortic stenosis
    d. Pulmonary atresia

2. The mother of a 4-month-old infant reports that he turned "blue" and seemed to have fast, labored breathing after vigorous crying soon after awakening. He "fell asleep" and his color and breathing seemed to improve. On physical examination, the mucous membranes of the lips and mouth appear mildly cyanotic. A systolic murmur is heard best at the mid- to upper left sternal border. Vital signs are normal with normal peripheral pulses. There is no hepatomegaly. A likely diagnosis is:

    a. Congestive heart failure
    b. Apnea
    c. Coarctation of the aorta
    d. Cyanotic spell related to Tetralogy of Fallot

3. Management of the infant with suspected heart disease and a reported cyanotic spell should include:

    a. Prompt referral to a cardiologist
    b. An apnea monitor
    c. Instructing the parent to keep a diary of these episodes
    d. Continous administration of oxygen

4. Chest pain in young children is usually:

    a. A symptom of congenital heart disease
    b. Noncardiac in origin
    c. A sign of hypercholesterolemia
    d. A symptom of congestive heart failure

5. A common cause of congestive heart failure in the first year of life is:

    a. Pulmonary stenosis
    b. Ventricular septal defect
    c. Rheumatic fever
    d. Complete heart block

6. The least likely physical finding in a 2-month-old with congestive heart failure is:

    a. Tachypnea
    b. Tachycardia
    c. Hepatomegaly
    d. Pedal edema

7. A vibratory systolic murmur is heard between the lower left sternal and the apex in a healthy 4-year-old at her preschool physical. The cardiovascular exam is otherwise normal. A likely diagnosis is:

    a. Venous hum
    b. Still's murmur
    c. Transposition of the great arteries
    d. Rheumatic heart disease

8. Characteristics of a venous hum include:

    a. A systolic murmur
    b. Radiation over precordium
    c. Marked decrease or disappearance of murmur when child is supine
    d. Heard best at lower left sternal border

9. Which of the following is true regarding innocent mumurs?

    a. The murmur is often holosystolic
    b. Prompt referral to a cardiologist is indicated
    c. A precordial thrill is present
    d. The murmur is low intensity, grade 1–3

10. Primary hypertension with no known underlying disease is most common in:

    a. Infants
    b. Children 3–5 years old
    c. Children 6–9 years old
    d. Adolescents

11. A 12-year-old girl seen at a routine visit has a blood pressure of 140/90. She denies any symptoms. The initial management would include:

    a. Intravenous pyelogram
    b. Return for two repeat blood pressure measurements
    c. No follow-up needed—blood pressure probably related to anxiety
    d. Diuretic therapy

12. A 9-year-old boy presents with a fever of 102° F and complaints of leg pains. His mother reports that he had an upper respiratory infection with a sore throat approximately two weeks ago which subsided without therapy. On physical examination, he has tender, swollen knees bilaterally. His heart rate is 120/min and a blowing systolic murmur is heard at the apex. No murmur was noted at a previous well child visit. The most likely diagnosis is:

    a. Kawasaki disease
    b. Rheumatic fever
    c. Sickle cell anemia
    d. Viral illness

13. The most useful test for evaluation of suspected acute rheumatic fever is:

a. Antistreptolysin-O titer
b. Electrocardiogram
c. Hemoglobin electrophoresis
d. Urinalysis

14. The initial attack of acute rheumatic fever is preceded by:

a. A viral illness
b. A group A streptococcal infection
c. Exposure to mites
d. Exposure to chicken pox

15. A 3-week-old infant has a one day history of irritability, pallor, and poor feeding. He is afebrile. On physical examination, his heart rate is 240/min while asleep. The most likely diagnosis is:

a. Supraventricular tachycardia
b. Premature ventricular contractions
c. Sinus tachycardia
d. Cyanotic heart defect

16. Congenital complete heart block may be associated with:

a. Maternal lupus erythematosus
b. Wolff-Parkinson-White syndrome
c. Maternal myocardial infarction
d. Kawasaki disease

17. The most common cause of myocarditis is:

a. Bacterial
b. Viral
c. Drug reaction
d. Radiation therapy

18. Which of the following is not an expected finding in a child with myocarditis?

a. Persistent tachycardia
b. History of antecedent "flu-like" illness
c. A gallop rhythm
d. A significant heart murmur

19. Hypercholesterolemia in children over 2-years-old is defined as a total cholesterol at or above:

a. 100 mg/dL
b. 130 mg/dL
c. 160 mg/dL
d. 200 mg/dL

20. A potential childhood risk factor for development of atherosclerotic or coronary heart disease as adults is:

    a. Obesity
    b. Tachycardia
    c. Heart murmur
    d. Aerobic exercise

21. Which of the following is not likely to cause secondary hypercholesterolemia?

    a. Nephrotic syndrome
    b. Hypertension
    c. Corticosteroids
    d. Obstructive liver disease

22. Which of the following is a common cause of acquired coronary artery disease during childhood?

    a. Rheumatic fever
    b. Hypertension
    c. Systemic lupus erythematosus
    d. Kawasaki disease

23. Kawasaki disease is most common in:

    a. Neonates
    b. Children less than 5 years of age
    c. Children over 6 years of age
    d. Females

24. A principal clinical feature of Kawasaki disease includes:

    a. Low grade fever for 24 hours and a pruritic rash
    b. Conjunctivitis with exudate and facial rash
    c. Arthritis and chorea
    d. Fever persisting at least five days and acute erythema and/or edema of hands and feet

25. An essential test in the evaluation of a 2-year-old with suspected Kawasaki disease is:

    a. An echocardiogram
    b. Electrolytes
    c. Cholesterol
    d. Streptococcal antibody titer

Answers

1. b	10. d	18. d
2. d	11. b	19. d
3. a	12. b	20. a
4. b	13. a	21. b
5. b	14. b	22. d
6. d	15. a	23. b
7. b	16. a	24. d
8. c	17. b	25. a
9. d		

Bibliography

American Academy of Pediatrics, Committee on Nutrition. (1998). Cholesterol in childhood. *Pediatrics, 101,* 141–147.

American Heart Association, Special Writing Group from the Task Force on Children and Youth. (1994). Cardiovascular health and disease in children: Current status. *Circulation, 89,* 923–930.

American Heart Association, Special Writing Group of the Committee on Rheumatic Fever, Endocarditis, and Kawasaki Disease. (1993). Guidelines for the diagnosis of rheumatic fever: Jones criteria, updated 1992. *Circulation, 87,* 302–307.

American Heart Association, Committee on Rheumatic Fever, Endocarditis, and Kawasaki Disease. (1993). Diagnosis and therapy of Kawasaki disease in children. *Circulation, 87,* 1776–1780.

American Heart Association, Committee on Rheumatic Fever, Endocarditis, and Kawasaki Disease. (1994). Guidelines for long-term management of patients with Kawasaki disease. *Circulation, 89,* 916–922.

Behrman, R. E., Kliegman, R. M., & Jenson, H. B. (Eds.). (2000). *Nelson textbook of pediatrics* (16th ed.). Philadelphia: W. B. Saunders.

Emmanouilides, G. C., Riemenschneider, T. A., Allen, H. D., & Gutgesell, H. P. (Eds.). (1995). *Heart disease in infants, children, and adolescents.* Baltimore: Williams & Wilkins.

Tyler, D. C. (Ed.). (1992). *Nadas' pediatric cardiology.* Philadelphia: Hanley & Belfus, Inc.

National Cholesterol Education Program. (1992). Report of the expert panel on blood cholesterol in children and adolescents. *Pediatrics.* 89, 525–584.

Park, N. (1996). *Pediatric cardiology for practitioners* (3rd ed.). Chicago: Yearbook Medical Publishers.

Task Force on Blood Pressure Control in Children. (1987). Report of the second task force on blood pressure control in children. *Pediatrics.* 79, 1–25.

U.S. Department of Health and Services. (1991). *Report of the expert panel on blood cholesterol levels in children and adolscents* (NIH Publication No. 91-2732). Washington, DC: Author.

Cardiovascular Disorders In Adults

Sally K. Miller

Hypertension (HTN)

- Definition: Persistent elevation of systolic blood pressure (SBP) > 140 mm Hg or diastolic blood pressure (DBP) > 90 mm Hg based upon an average of two or more blood pressure readings at each of two or more visits after an initial screening visit, or persons taking antihypertensive medication; important to perform blood pressure measurements under nonstressful circumstances, i.e., well rested, empty bladder, no immediate psychosocial stressors; hypertension should not be diagnosed based upon one blood pressure measurement unless that measurement is greater than 180/110 or is accompanied by end organ damage (National Heart, Lung, and Blood Institute, 1997)

  1. Blood Pressure Classification Guidelines

Classification	SBP		DBP
Optimal	< 120	and	< 80
Normal	< 130	and	< 85
High-normal	130-139	or	85-89
Hypertension			
Stage 1	140-159	or	90-99
Stage 2	160-179	or	100-109
Stage 3	≥ 180	or	≥ 110

- Etiology/Incidence: 95% due to unknown etiology; currently several proposed theories, including hyperactivity of the sympathetic nervous system (SNS); hypertension of unknown etiology is known as primary, essential, or idiopathic hypertension; remaining 5% of cases are attributable to secondary causes

  1. | Theories of Etiology of HTN | Etiology of Secondary HTN |
     |---|---|
     | SNS hyperactivity | Renal disease |
     | Renin-angiotensin system | Renal vascular disease |
     | Defect in natriuresis | Hyperaldosteronism |
     | Elevated intracellular Na^+ | Cushing's syndrome |
     | | Pheochromocytoma |
     | | Coarctation of the aorta |
     | | Pregnancy |

  2. Incidence

     a. 10% to 15% of Caucasian adults

     b. 20% to 30% of African-American adults

     c. Heredity

     d. Cigarette smoking

     e. Increased salt intake

     f. Obesity

     g. Affects over 50 million Americans

- Signs and Symptoms

  1. Often no symptoms—known as ''silent killer''

2. Symptoms of underlying cause may present in secondary hypertension

   a. Flushing

   b. Palpitations

   c. Pallor

   d. Tremor

   e. Profuse perspiration

3. Suboccipital pulsating headache occurring early in morning and improving throughout the day in severe hypertension

4. Chronic hypertension may result in ventricular hypertrophy and associated symptoms of heart failure

5. Oliguria, nocturia, or hematuria may be present

6. Epistaxis in severe hypertension

7. Severe hypertension may present with signs and symptoms of hypertensive encephalopathy

   a. Nausea and vomiting

   b. Somnolence and confusion

   c. Visual disturbances

- Differential Diagnosis: Secondary causes of hypertension must be ruled out

   1. Renal disorders

      a. Medical renal disease

      b. Diabetic nephropathy

      c. Acute tubular necrosis

   2. Endocrine disorders

      a. Cushing's syndrome

      b. Hyperaldosteronism

      c. Pheochromocytoma

      d. Diabetes mellitus (DM)

      e. Acromegaly

      f. Hyperthyroidism

   3. Structural disorders

      a. Coarctation of the aorta

      b. Carotid artery stenosis

      c. Renal artery stenosis

    4. Pregnancy

- Physical Findings

    1. Most significant is elevated pressure noted in definition

    2. S_4 gallop due to decreased left ventricular compliance is common

    3. Displaced point of maximal impulse (PMI) when left ventricular hypertrophy present

    4. Diffuse anterior chest wall heave when right ventricular hypertrophy present

    5. Peripheral pulses may be abnormal in some secondary cases

        a. Coarctation of the aorta

        b. Stenosis of major arteries

    6. Systolic murmur of aortic stenosis may be heard

    7. Dependent edema in chronic, uncontrolled disease

    8. Renal artery bruit in cases of renal artery stenosis

    9. Neurologic evidence of previous cerebral infarcts may be present

    10. Flame hemorrhages and/or fluffy exudate on ophthalmoscopic examination

- Diagnostic Tests/Findings

    1. Laboratory findings usually normal in uncomplicated essential hypertension

    2. Hematuria and/or proteinuria in secondary renal disease

    3. Rapid sequence intravenous pyelogram (IVP) to rule out renal vascular disease

    4. Chest radiograph

        a. Rule out coarctation of the aorta

        b. Cardiac hypertrophy in chronic, uncontrolled disease

    5. Plasma lipids may be elevated

    6. Hormone levels to evaluate underlying endocrine cause

        a. Elevated serum aldosterone levels—primary hyperaldosteronism

        b. Elevated adrenocorticotropic hormone or serum cortisol—Cushing's syndrome

        c. Low thyroid stimulating hormone and elevated T_3—hyperthyroidism

        d. Elevated serum and urine catecholamines—pheochromocytoma

- Management/Treatment

    1. Nonpharmacologic treatment should be instituted in all patients diagnosed with hypertension according to the definition presented

        a. Weight reduction

        b. Low sodium diet (2 g)

c. Cessation of smoking

d. Avoidance/reduction of alcohol intake

e. Stress management

f. Relaxation/exercise

g. Lipid control

2. Pharmacologic therapy should be instituted in all patients with stage 2 or greater hypertension. The decision to begin pharmacologic therapy in patients with stage 1 hypertension is controversial, but should be considered in all clients with any of the risk factors noted or the presence of end organ damage.

    a. Diuretics are the most widely used antihypertensive medication

        (1) Hydrochlorothiazide 12.5 to 50 mg once daily

        (2) Furosemide 20 to 320 mg in daily or divided daily doses—not ordinarily used in the treatment of hypertension except in the presence of renal dysfunction

        (3) Use cautiously in patients with osteoporosis, gout, and diabetes

    b. Beta-blockers, calcium channel blockers, alpha-adrenergic blockers, and angiotensin converting enzyme (ACE) inhibitors are also first line choices; physiologic responses to medication groups vary in response to demographic factors; accompanying illness is also factor in medication selection

        (1) Beta-blockers

            (a) Atenolol 25 to 200 mg daily

            (b) Labetalol 200 to 1200 mg daily in two divided doses

            (c) Metoprolol 50 to 200 mg daily in one or two divided doses

            (d) Contraindicated in patients with CHF, type 1 DM, and bronchial asthma

            (e) Use cautiously in patients with conduction disorders and hypertriglyceridemia

        (2) Calcium channel blockers widely effective

            (a) Diltiazem 90 to 360 mg daily in two divided doses

            (b) Verapamil 180 to 480 mg daily in two divided doses

            (c) Contraindicated in the presence of disorders of conduction; use cautiously when baseline heart rate less than 50 beats per minute (bpm)

            (d) Contraindicated in the presence of sick sinus syndrome and 2nd or 3rd degree atrioventricular block

            (e) Generally contraindicated in patients with CHF—may be used in specialized cases of mild diastolic failure

  (3) ACE inhibitors

    (a) Captopril 50 to 300 mg daily in two or three divided doses

    (b) Lisinopril 5 to 40 mg once daily

    (c) Agent of choice in patients with type 1 DM or renal dysfunction

    (d) Contraindicated in bilateral renal artery stenosis

    (e) 15% of patients develop cough as side effect

 c. Alpha$_2$ agonists are second line option

 d. Angiotensin II receptor antagonists for patients who cannot tolerate side effects of angiotensin converting enzyme inhibitors

 e. Combination therapy often utilized

3. Counseling regarding medication side effects, compliance, follow-up and lifestyle modifications

4. Consult physician when instituting pharmacologic therapy and when patient does not respond to first-line pharmacotherapy

Coronary Artery Disease (CAD)

- Definition: Clinical syndrome also known as angina pectoris that occurs from atherosclerotic changes to the coronary vasculature; the result is decreased blood flow through vessels either due to partial obstruction (sclerosis) or vasospasm (may happen in a nonsclerotic vessel); when tissue ischemia and pain occur as a result of decreased blood flow, angina occurs

- Etiology/Incidence

 1. Hypertension (two times greater risk than general population)

 2. Tobacco use (2 to 3 times greater risk than general population)

 3. Total serum cholesterol > 260 mg/dL (two times greater risk than general population)

 4. Diabetes mellitus (two times greater risk than non-diabetic population)

 5. Family history with a first degree relative (2 to 5 times greater risk than general population)

 6. Sedentary lifestyle

 7. Use of oral contraceptives

 8. Gender prevalence depends upon age

  a. Overall more prevalent in men by a 4:1 ratio

  b. Under age 40, ratio is 8:1

  c. Over age 70, ratio is 1:1

 9. Obesity

10. Personality type is less certain risk factor

- Types of Angina

  1. Exertional—occurs with activity, generally subsides with rest

  2. Variant threshold occurs at various times, including rest

  3. Prinzmetal's angina occurs only at rest

     a. Chest pain occurs without the usual precipitating factors

     b. Often affects women under age of 50

     c. Characteristically occurs in early morning, awakening patient from sleep

     d. Tends to involve right coronary artery

- Signs and Symptoms

  1. Characteristic chest discomfort

     a. Sensation of tightness, squeezing, burning, pressure

     b. 80% to 90% of cases discomfort is felt behind or slightly to the left of the mid-sternum

     c. Radiates most often to left shoulder and upper arm, traveling down inner aspect of arm to elbow, forearm, wrist, and fourth or fifth finger

     d. May be felt in lower jaw, back of neck, or upper left side of back

     e. Typically lasts 15 to 20 minutes, may resolve more quickly but usually lasts at least several minutes; pain lasting > 30 minutes is unstable angina

  2. Anxiety

  3. Dyspnea

- Differential Diagnosis

  1. Gastroesophageal reflux (heartburn)

  2. Anxiety

  3. Depression

  4. Costrochondral pain

  5. Pneumothorax

  6. Congestive heart failure

  7. Pneumonia

  8. Pericarditis

  9. Asthma

  10. Aortic dissection

  11. Myocardial infarction

- Physical Findings
  1. Systolic and diastolic blood pressures usually elevated during attack
  2. May hear apical systolic murmur due to transient mitral regurgitation
  3. Transient S_3 and/or S_4 may be present
  4. May detect signs of disease that contribute to or accompany CAD
     a. Diabetes mellitus
     b. Hypertension
     c. Aortic stenosis
     d. Hypertrophic cardiomyopathy
     e. Mitral valve prolapse
  5. Pulse and respirations may be elevated
  6. May see tobacco stained teeth or fingers
  7. May see signs of peripheral artery disease
     a. Diminished distal pulses
     b. Pale skin
     c. Poor hair growth
  8. Levin's sign (clenched fist over sternum) highly suggestive of angina
  9. May not have any remarkable physical findings
- Diagnostic Tests/Findings
  1. Serum lipid levels—LDL cholesterol must be lowered to < 100 mg/dL
  2. The electrocardiogram (ECG)
     a. Normal in 25% patients with angina
     b. Characteristic finding is down sloping of S-T segment or T wave peak or inversion during attack; reverses after attack
     c. May show signs of old myocardial infarction or hypertrophy
  3. Exercise electrocardiography (stress testing)
     a. Ischemic changes or angina during exercise test—clinically diagnostic
     b. Markedly positive test is any one of the following
        (1) S-T segment depression after start of exercise
        (2) > 2 mm of new S-T segment depression in multiple leads
        (3) New S-T segment elevation
        (4) Decreased systolic blood pressure with exercise

(5)   Development of heart failure with exercise

(6)   Inability to exercise for > two minutes

(7)   Prolonged interval after exercise for return to normal ECG

4. Nuclear medicine studies to evaluate presence, location and extent of coronary disease

   a. Exercise thallium imaging

      (1)   Especially useful in patients with pre-existing ECG abnormalities and patients taking digoxin

      (2)   Areas of diminished uptake indicate hypoperfusion

      (3)   Should be conducted at experienced center

   b. Radionuclide ventriculography

      (1)   Images left ventricle and measures ejection fraction

      (2)   Resting abnormalities represent infarction

      (3)   Abnormalities with exercise indicate stress induced ischemia

   c. Coronary angiography

      (1)   Definitive test for diagnosis of CAD

      (2)   Indicated in high risk patients

         (a)   With refractory unstable angina

         (b)   With spontaneous or exercise induced ischemia after myocardial infarction

- Management/Treatment (see Table 1)

   1. Treatment of acute attack

      a. Sublingual or buccal spray nitroglycerin

      b. Dose may be repeated three times at five minute intervals

      c. Pain unrelieved after three doses is unstable and should be evaluated in emergency room

   2. Prevention of further attacks

      a. Reduction of risk factors when possible

         (1)   Weight reduction

         (2)   Smoking cessation

         (3)   Exercise program

      b. Lowering LDL cholesterol to < 100 mg/dL is of paramount importance

         (1)   If LDL cholesterol is between 100 to 160 mg/dL—diet modification program may be implemented

Table 1
TREATMENT ALGORITHM FOR STABLE ANGINA

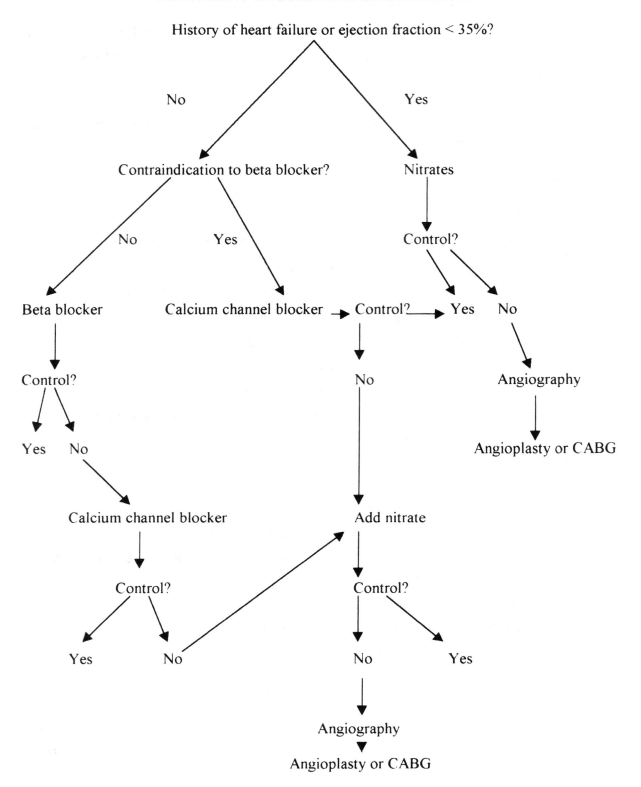

    (2) If LDL cholesterol is > 160 mg/dL or remains > 130 mg/dL after three months of diet modification—pharmacologic therapy should be instituted

        (a) Nicotinic acid

        (b) Bile acid binding resins

        (c) Hydroxymethylglutaryl co-enzyme A (HMG CoA) reductase inhibitors

        (d) All patients whose risk for CAD warrants pharmacologic therapy should also take aspirin daily

c. Beta-blockers prevent angina by reducing myocardial oxygen requirements

    (1) Metoprolol 50 to 200 mg daily in two divided doses

    (2) Atenolol 25 to 200 mg once daily

    (3) Major contraindications are bronchospastic disease, bradydysrhythmias, and heart failure

d. Calcium channel blockers prevent angina by reducing myocardial oxygen demand and inducing coronary vasodilation

    (1) Nifedipine 30 to 120 mg daily

    (2) Verapamil 180 to 480 mg in one or two doses daily

    (3) Diltiazem 360 mg in two daily doses

e. Long acting nitrates prevent angina by inducing coronary vasodilation

    (1) Isosorbide dinitrate 10 to 40 mg three times daily

    (2) Sustained release nitroglycerin 6.25 to 25 mg daily in two to four divided doses

f. Coronary revascularization is indicated in the following:

    (1) Unacceptable symptoms despite medical therapy to its tolerable limits

    (2) Left main coronary artery stenosis greater than 50% with or without symptoms

    (3) Three vessel disease with left ventricular dysfunction

    (4) Unstable angina with ischemia on exercise stress test after symptom control

    (5) Post myocardial infarction with continued angina or ischemia on noninvasive testing

g. Counseling regarding medication side effects

3. Physician consultation

      a.   When pharmacologic therapy initiated

      b.   Failure to respond to pharmacologic therapy

Myocardial Infarction (MI)

- Definition: Myocardial necrosis due to inadequate blood flow, usually a result of atherosclerotic stenosis but may be the result of prolonged vasospasm

- Etiology/Incidence

    1. Risk factors and epidemiology same as for CAD

    2. Leading cause of death in adults in the U.S.; 1.5 million deaths annually

- Signs and Symptoms

    1. One-third of patients give history of alteration in typical pattern of angina

    2. Pain similar to angina but more severe

    3. Diaphoresis, dyspnea, cough and wheeze

    4. Anxiety

    5. Nausea and vomiting

    6. Weakness or light-headedness

    7. Often prefer not to lie quietly—continuously seek comfortable position

    8. Women may present with atypical symptoms, i.e., burning sensation in chest, indigestion, weakness

- Differential Diagnosis

    1. Angina

    2. Gastroesophageal reflux

    3. Pulmonary embolus

    4. Costochondral pain

    5. Pericarditis

    6. Dissecting aortic aneurysm

    7. Anxiety

- Physical Findings

    1. Heart rate may range from bradycardia to tachycardia

    2. Dysrhythmias common

    3. Low grade fever may appear after 12 hours and persist for several days

    4. S_4 and murmur of mitral regurgitation common

    5. S_3 less common—when present indicates severe left ventricular dysfunction

6. Blood pressure may be elevated or abnormally low

7. May see findings consistent with heart failure; jugular vein distention, rales

8. Cyanosis and cold temperature indicate low cardiac output

- Diagnostic Tests/Findings

    1. ECG is essential—most patients have ECG changes

        a. Convex S-T segment elevation with peaked upright or inverted T waves indicative of acute MI

        b. S-T segment depression may indicate non-Q-wave MI

        c. Development of Q waves generally considered diagnostic of MI

    2. Leukocytosis 10,000 to 20,000/μL on second day

    3. Cardiac isoenzymes progressively increase as necrosis evolves

        a. Creatine kinase-muscle brain (CK-MB) increases within 4 to 6 hours of pain onset, peaks in 10 to 20 hours, returns to baseline in 36 to 48 hours

        b. Lactic dehydrogenase (LDH) elevations detectable 12 hours after pain onset, peak in 24 to 48 hours, and remain elevated for 10 to 14 days—LDH_1: LDH_2 ratio > 1.0 consistent with M.I.

        c. Troponin T and Troponin I demonstrate high specificity and sensitivity and remain elevated for 5 to 7 days post M.I.

    4. Echocardiography for assessment of cardiac wall motion and valvular/structural defects post MI

    5. Technetium 99 pyrophosphate scintigraphy used in diagnosis of MI for patients hospitalized late in the course

    6. Radionuclide ventriculography allows assessment of regional wall motion and ejection fraction

    7. Coronary angiography is definitive test to visualize the coronary vasculature

- Management/Treatment: Immediate hospitalization

    1. Immediate goals are to provide oxygen, relieve pain, and treat dysrhythmia

        a. Oxygen by nasal cannula, face mask, or endotracheal tube

        b. Morphine sulfate 2 to 4 mg at 5 to 10 minute intervals p.r.n.

        c. Nitroglycerin sublingual or intravenously

        d. Heparin 5,000 unit bolus followed by intravenous infusion

        e. Chewable aspririn 160 mg

        f. Treat dysrhythmia as indicated

    2. Thrombolytics to reperfuse coronary arteries within 4 to 6 hours of pain onset

    3. Percutaneous transluminal coronary artery angioplasty (PTCA)

4. Other medications have varying levels of effectiveness in the acute setting

    a. Beta blockers

    b. Calcium channel blockers

    c. ACE inhibitors

5. Patient education regarding cardiac rehabilitation and risk factor reduction

6. Physician consultation when acute MI suspected

Congestive Heart Failure (CHF)

- Definition: Clinical syndrome that results when cardiac output is insufficient to meet metabolic demands of body; any condition that affects heart rate or contractile function can precipitate CHF

- Etiology/Incidence

1. Acute myocardial infarction; dysrhythmia

2. Chronic hypertension

3. Valvular stenosis or regurgitation

4. Cardiomyopathy

5. Medication toxicity

6. 2,000,000 estimated cases in the U.S.—400,000 new cases diagnosed annually

- Types of CHF

1. Acute

    a. Abrupt onset usually follows acute MI or valve rupture

    b. Also known as ''left sided failure''

    c. Symptoms are produced by acute diffusion of water into the pulmonary air spaces

2. Chronic

    a. Develops as a result of inadequate compensatory mechanisms that have been employed over time to improve cardiac output

    b. Also known as ''right sided failure''

    c. Symptoms are produced by increased hydrostatic pressure in the venous system and subsequent diffusion of water into the interstitium

3. Systolic—contractile dysfunction results in decreased cardiac output

4. Diastolic—inability to relax and fill with blood results in decreased cardiac output

- Signs and Symptoms

1. Acute CHF

a. Dyspnea at rest

b. Frothy cough worse in the recumbent position

c. Feeling of anxiety and/or impending doom

2. Chronic CHF

a. Dyspena on exertion; easily fatigued

b. Chronic non-productive cough

c. Abdominal fullness

d. Weight gain

e. Paroxysmal nocturnal dyspnea

f. Oliguria, nocturia

g. Peripheral cyanosis

- Differential Diagnosis

1. Acute MI

2. Pulmonary embolus

3. Pneumonia

4. Asthma

5. Chronic venous insufficiency

- Physical Findings

1. Acute

a. Coarse rales over all lung fields

b. Wheezing over all lung fields

c. S_3 gallop very common

d. Appears generally healthy except for the acute event

e. Systolic murmur of mitral regurgitation

f. Usually no edema or systemic signs of fluid overload

2. Chronic

a. Lungs may be clear or may exhibit rales at the bases

b. Dependent edema

c. Appears chronically ill

d. Jugular venous distention

e. Hepatosplenomegaly

f. Point of maximal impulse displaced to the left

g. Diffuse anterior chest wall heave

h. S_3 and/or S_4

i. Any variety of stenotic or regurgitant murmurs

- Diagnostic Tests/Findings

1. Acute

   a. Hypoxemia and hypocapnia on arterial blood gas

   b. Serum multichemical analysis (SMA) 7 (sodium, potassium, chloride, carbon dioxide, blood urea nitrogen, creatinine, and glucose) usually normal

   c. Urinalysis usually normal

   d. Chest radiograph shows pulmonary edema, Kerley's lines, effusions

   e. Echocardiogram will show contractile, relaxation, and valve function

2. Chronic

   a. SMA7 may show electrolyte abnormalities

   b. Mild hypoxemia on arterial blood gas—pCO_2 usually normal

   c. Chest radiograph shows redistribution of flow, enlarged heart

   d. Echocardiogram will show contractile, relaxation, and valve function

- Management/Treatment

1. Of primary importance is identification and treatment of underlying cause

2. Nonpharmacologic

   a. Sodium/fluid restriction

   b. Rest/activity balance

   c. Weight reduction in the obese

3. Pharmacologic

   a. Angiotensin converting enzyme (ACE) inhibitors

      (1) Captopril 6.25 to 50 mg three to four times daily

      (2) Enalapril 2.5 to 40 mg daily in two divided doses

      (3) Lisinopril 2.5 to 10 mg daily

   b. Diuretics

      (1) Hydrochlorothiazide 12.5 to 25 mg daily

      (2) Furosemide 20 to 160 mg daily in one or two daily doses

   c. Beta adrenergic antagonists

      (1) Carvedilol 3.125 mg b.i.d.

      (2) Improve function by blocking excessive adrenergic stimulation

(3) Indicated for refractory to diuretics and ACE inhibitors

d. Inotropic

(1) Beneficial in mild to moderate systolic failure

(2) Digoxin 0.125 to 0.25 mg daily

e. Neurohormonal antagonists

(1) Spironolactone 25 mg daily

(2) Mediate major effects of renin-angiotensin-aldosterone activation, e.g., remodeling

f. Vasodilators—useful as adjunct therapy in heart failure refractory to initial therapies

4. Patient counseling

a. Lifestyle modification

b. Medication toxicities and side effects

5. Physician consultation

a. When pharmacologic therapy initiated

b. When patient unresponsive to initial medications

Peripheral Vascular Disease

- Definition: Narrowing and eventual obstruction of the arterial lumen usually caused by atherosclerosis; occlusion tends to be segmental; result is decreased blood supply to limbs

- Etiology/Incidence: Same as those for coronary artery disease

- Signs and Symptoms

  1. Intermittent claudication usually presenting symptom

  2. Distance patient can walk is indicative of degree of circulatory impairment

  3. Cold and/or numbness of the extremity

  4. Pain or ache at night/rest suggestive of severe disease

- Differential Diagnosis

  1. Sciatica

  2. Myopathies

  3. Acute arterial emboli

- Physical Findings

  1. Reduced or absent pulses distal to obstruction

  2. Dependent rubor

3. Skin pallor or cyanosis

4. Poor hair/nail growth

5. Dry ulceration/gangrene in severe disease

- Diagnostic Tests/Findings

    1. Radiography of affected extremity may show calcification

    2. Doppler ultrasound will demonstrate reduced pressures distal to occlusion

    3. Arteriography will show location and extent of block

- Management/Treatment

    1. Control risk factors as possible

    2. Walk daily to develop collateral circulation—walking to point of pain followed by a three minute rest should be done eight times daily

    3. Aspirin 80 to 325 mg has theoretical value and should be given to all patients with severe disease

    4. Surgical revascularization

Thrombophlebitis

- Definition: Partial or complete occlusion of a vein by a thrombus with secondary inflammation of venous wall—may be superficial or deep

- Etiology/Incidence

    1. Trauma, particularly if venous stasis present

    2. Venous stasis

    3. Prolonged bedrest

    4. Hypercoagulation states

    5. Use of oral contraceptives (particularly in smokers)

    6. Post-operative period

    7. More prevalent in females

- Signs and Symptoms

    1. Sudden onset of pain (superficial)

    2. Pain, tenderness, ache, or tightness especially with activity (deep)

- Differential Diagnosis

    1. Muscle strain or contusion

    2. Cellulitis

    3. Arterial disease

    4. Lymphatic obstruction

- Physical Findings
    1. Localized heat and erythema (superficial)
    2. Edema distal to occlusion (deep)
    3. Distention of superficial venous collateral vessels
    4. Low grade temperature
    5. Cool skin
    6. Palpable cords
- Diagnostic Tests/Findings
    1. Doppler ultrasound and impedance plethysmography to evaluate venous flow
    2. Contrast venography is definitive study to identify location and extent
- Management/Treatment
    1. Elevation of extremity and warm compress (superficial)
    2. Bedrest with extremity elevated (deep)
    3. Anticoagulation therapy for deep thrombosis
        a. Heparin infusion for 7 to 10 days
        b. Coumadin therapy for 12 weeks

Chronic Venous Insufficiency

- Definition: Impaired venous return with resultant chronic lower extremity edema
- Etiology/Incidence
    1. Destruction of valves in deep venous channels of lower legs secondary to deep thrombophlebitis
    2. Neoplastic obstruction of pelvic veins
    3. Leg trauma
    4. Sustained elevation of venous pressure
    5. More common in women than men
- Signs and Symptoms
    1. Aching of lower extremities relieved by elevation
    2. Edema at end of day or after prolonged standing
    3. Night cramps
- Differential Diagnosis
    1. Lymphedema
    2. Congestive heart failure

  3. Renal disease

  4. Liver disease

- Physical Findings

  1. Edema of lower extremities

  2. Trophic changes with brownish discoloration

  3. Cool to touch

  4. Thin, shiny, atrophic skin

  5. Wet ulcerations on the medial or anterior aspect of the leg

- Diagnostic Tests/Findings

  1. BUN/creatinine to rule out renal disease

  2. Liver function tests to rule out liver disease

  3. Chest radiograph to rule out congestive heart failure

  4. Doppler ultrasound to rule out thrombosis

- Management/Treatment

  1. Bedrest with legs elevated to diminish chronic edema

  2. Use of elastic stockings

  3. Weight reduction in the obese

  4. Hydrocortisone cream for stasis dermatitis

Questions
Select the best answer

1. When is it appropriate to diagnose and treat hypertension based upon one blood pressure?

   a. When there is a strong family history
   b. When the diastolic pressure is > 100 mm Hg
   c. When there is end organ damage
   d. When there is suboccipital headache

2. Which of the following is not a cause of secondary hypertension?

   a. Sympathetic nervous system hypersensitivity
   b. Renal vascular disease
   c. Pheochromocytoma
   d. Coarctation of the aorta

3. What is the percentage of Caucasian adults afflicted with hypertension?

   a. < 10%
   b. 10-15%
   c. 20-30%
   d. > 50%

4. The patient with chronic hypertension presents with lower extremity edema, abdominal pain and fatigue. Physical exam findings reveal a diffuse chest wall heave and displaced point of maximal impulse. This makes you suspicious that the patient has:

   a. Biventricular hypertrophy
   b. Renal vascular stenosis
   c. Hypertensive encephalopathy
   d. Malignant hypertension

5. Which of the following endocrine disorders is not a cause of secondary hypertension?

   a. Cushing's syndrome
   b. Diabetes mellitus
   c. Hyperthyroidism
   d. Addison's disease

6. Pharmacologic therapy should be started in any patient who is diagnosed with hypertension and has end organ damage. The most widely used antihypertensive medications are:

   a. Beta blockers
   b. Calcium channel blockers
   c. Diuretics
   d. Angiotensin converting enzyme inhibitors

7. Which of the following medications is the drug of choice for the patient with hypertension and comorbid diabetes mellitus?

    a. Lisinopril 5 mg p.o. q.d.
    b. Furosemide 20 mg p.o. q.d.
    c. Metoprolol 50 mg p.o. b.i.d.
    d. Diltiazem 90 mg p.o. b.i.d.

8. Which of the following risk factors puts a client at greatest risk for coronary artery disease?

    a. Stage 3 hypertension
    b. Serum cholesterol of 300 mg/dL
    c. A parent with history of myocardial infarction
    d. Type I diabetes mellitus

9. Prinzmetal's angina typically occurs:

    a. During periods of emotional stress
    b. Early in the morning
    c. In men under age 50
    d. In extremes of temperature

10. Your patient complains of chest pain just to the left of the midsternal area that occurred while mowing the lawn. As you pursue the history of present illness in an effort to rule out angina, which of the following characteristics of the pain experience makes angina less likely?

    a. The pain was also felt in the back of the neck
    b. The pain felt like a burning sensation
    c. The pain lasted 15 minutes
    d. The pain was a stabbing, knife like sensation

11. Aortic stenosis can be a contributing cause of coronary artery disease. Which of the following heart sounds is suggestive of aortic stenosis?

    a. A systolic murmur loudest at the second intercostal space, right sternal border
    b. A diastolic murmur loudest at the second intercostal space, left sternal border
    c. An extra heart sound heard early in diastole
    d. An extra heart sound heard early in systole

12. Exercise electrocardiography (ECG) is clinically diagnostic for coronary artery disease. Which of the following is not a positive finding on exercise ECG?

    a. > 2 mm of new S-T segment depression in multiple leads
    b. Decreased systolic blood pressure with exercise
    c. S-T segment depression after start of exercise
    d. Inability to exercise for > 5 minutes

13. You diagnosed coronary artery disease in Mrs. J. three months ago. At that time her LDL cholesterol was 160 mg/dL, and so your teaching interventions included ways to lower fat in her diet. Today her LDL cholesterol is 125 mg/ dL. The most appropriate intervention is to:

    a. Begin lovastatin 10 mg q.d. and re-evaluate in one month
    b. Continue diet modification and re-evaluate in three months

c. Begin enteric coated aspirin 325 mg q.d. and re-evaluate in one month

d. Begin cholestyramine 12 gm b.i.d. and re-evaluate in three months

14. Which of the following pharmacological agents prevents angina by reducing myocardial oxygen demand and inducing coronary vasodilation?

a. Diltiazem

b. Isosorbide dinitrate

c. Atenolol

d. Aspirin

15. Mr. L. is a 64-year-old patient with difficult to control angina. His initial therapy was atenolol 25 mg q.d., and increased until his dose was 200 mg daily. When angina persisted diltiazem 180 mg b.i.d. was added to the regimen, but even the combination of medications is not controlling symptoms. At this point the next appropriate step would be to:

a. Recommend cardiac angiography

b. Begin nifedipine 30 mg q.d.

c. Begin isosorbide dinitrate 10 mg. t.i.d.

d. Recommend radionucleide ventriculography

16. Patients having a myocardial infarction (MI) may report that the chest pain they are experiencing is different from their usual anginal pain. Which of the following is also suspicious for MI rather than angina?

a. Pain lasting > 15 minutes

b. Nausea and vomiting

c. Elevated systolic blood pressure

d. Presence of S_3 or S_4 heart sounds

17. Which of the following diagnostic findings is most suggestive of myocardial infarction?

a. 15,000/μL leukocytes

b. Development of Q waves

c. LDH 500 U/L

d. S-T segment depression

18. Acute congestive heart failure produces symptoms as a function of the diffusion of water into the pulmonary air spaces. Acute failure is most commonly caused by:

a. Chronic hypertension

b. Valvular stenosis

c. Medication toxicity

d. Myocardial infarction

19. When increased hydrostatic pressure in the venous system causes water to diffuse into the interstitium, resultant physical findings would most likely include:

a. Weight gain

b. S_3 gallop

    c. Coarse rales in all lung fields

    d. Dyspnea at rest

20. Kerley's lines on chest radiography are suggestive of:

    a. Inadequate compensatory mechanisms when cardiac output fails

    b. Hydrostatic pressure increase in the peripheral vascular system

    c. Diffusion of water into pulmonary air spaces

    d. Prinzmetal's angina

21. Congestive heart failure is a syndrome that results when the cardiac output is insufficient to meet the metabolic demands of the body. This can be either an acute or chronic state. Causes of chronic failure include:

    a. Hypertension

    b. Mitral valve rupture

    c. Myocardial infarction

    d. Cardiac ischemia

22. Typical laboratory findings in acute CHF include:

    a. Red blood cells in urinalysis

    b. Blood urea nitrogen (BUN) 70mg/dL; serum creatinine 2.0 mg/dL

    c. PaO_2 64 mm Hg by arterial blood gas

    d. Redistribution of flow by chest radiography

23. Beta adrenergic antagonists may be useful therapy in congestive heart failure when:

    a. Failure is unresponsive to angiotensin converting enzyme inhibitors

    b. Failure is severe and refractory to digoxin

    c. Failure is due to cardiomyopathy

    d. Failure is severe and refractory to vasodilators

24. Dependent rubor is a physical finding associated with:

    a. Chronic venous insufficiency

    b. Arteriosclerotic occlusive disease

    c. Deep vein thrombosis

    d. Superficial thrombophlebitis

25. Which of the following physical findings is not associated with thrombophlebitis?

    a. Low grade temperature

    b. Cool skin

    c. Heat and erythema

    d. Reduced or absent peripheral pulses

26. Edema of the lower extremities is a physical finding associated with a variety of medical conditions. A diagnosis of chronic venous insufficiency is made when other causes are ruled out. When chronic venous insufficiency is diagnosed, the appropriate treatment includes:

    a. Heparin infusion for 7 to 10 days
    b. Use of elastic stockings
    c. Aspirin 325 mg daily
    d. Surgical revascularization

27. Which of the following blood pressures would be classified as stage 2?

    a. 170/100 mm Hg
    b. 180/95 mm Hg
    c. 200/110 mm Hg
    d. 146/98 mm Hg

Answers

1. c	10. d	19. a
2. a	11. a	20. c
3. b	12. d	21. a
4. a	13. b	22. c
5. d	14. a	23. a
6. c	15. c	24. b
7. a	16. b	25. d
8. c	17. b	26. b
9. b	18. d	27. a

Bibliography

Donaldson, M. C., & Olin, J. W. (1996). Peripheral arterial disease: 5 steps to a better outcome. *Patient Care, 30*(1), 224-6, 226, 231.

Eftychiou, V. (1996). Clinical diagnosis and management of the patient with deep vein thrombophlebitis and acute pulmonary embolism. *Nurse Practitioner: American Journal of Primary Health Care, 21*(3), 50, 52, 58.

Khan, M. G. (1996). *Heart disease diagnosis and therapy: A practical approach.* Baltimore, MD: Williams & Wilkins.

Mancia, G., & van Zweiten, P. A. (1996). How safe are calcium channel antagonists in hypertension and coronary heart disease? *Journal of Hypertension, 14*(1), 13-7.

Massie, B. M., & Amidon, T. A. (2001). Heart. In L.M. Tierney, Jr., S. J. McPhee, & M. A. Papadakis (Eds.). *Current medical diagnosis and treatment* (40th ed., pp. 352–447). NY: Lange Medical Books/McGraw-Hill.

McGovern, P. G., Pankow, J. S., Shahar, E., Doliszny, K. M., Folsom, A. R., Blackburn, H., & Luepker, R. V. (1996). Recent trends in acute coronary heart disease and mortality, morbidity, medical care and risk factors. *New England Journal of Medicine, 334*(14), 884-901.

Miller, S. K. (1997). Clinical assessment and pharmacologic management of congestive heart failure in the acute and chronic phases. *Advance for Nurse Practitioners, 5*(6), 16-26.

National Heart, Lung, and Blood Institute. (1997). The sixth report of the Joint National Committee on Detection, Evaluation and Treatment of High Blood Pressure, (DHHS) (NIH Publication No. 98-4080). Bethesda, MD: National Institutes of Health.

Peters, S. (1997). On the trail of a killer: New developments in heart disease. *Advance for Nurse Practitioners, 5*(5), 45-49.

Sadowski, A. V., & Redeker, N. S. (1996). The hypertensive elder: A review for the primary care provider. *Nurse Practitioner: American Journal of Primary Health Care, 21*(5), 99-100, 105-12.

Hematologic/Oncologic/Immunologic Disorders
Infancy Through Adolescence

Juanita Conkin Dale

ABO/Rh Incompatibility

- Definition: Incompatibility between the ABO or Rh blood group of the fetus and mother that may result in isoimmunization and red cell hemolysis
- Etiology/Incidence
  1. Rh incompatibility—mother rhesus antigen (Rh) negative, baby Rh positive
     a. Occurrence in first born—5%
     b. More severe in subsequent sensitized pregnancies
  2. ABO incompatibility—major blood group antigen of mother (type O) is different from the baby (type A, B or AB); 20% of pregnancies are at risk for ABO incompatibility; about 33% of neonates at risk are Coombs' test positive (usually weakly positive), only 20% of the Coombs' test positive neonates develop clinically significant jaundice requiring phototherapy
- Signs and Symptoms
  1. Mild cases—asymptomatic
  2. Severe cases—yellow discoloration of skin, whites of eyes, and gums or inside of mouth
- Differential Diagnosis
  1. Physiologic jaundice—most common
  2. Infection
  3. Hyperbilirubinemia of prematurity
  4. Metabolic disorder
- Physical Findings
  1. Jaundice usually occurring within first 24 hours of life; may be present or appear up to a week later
  2. May have hepatosplenomegaly
- Diagnostic Tests/Findings
  1. Rh incompatibility
     a. Blood type—mother Rh negative, baby Rh positive
     b. Direct Coombs' test (direct antiglobulin test [DAT])—positive
     c. Hemoglobin—below normal, may be very low; hemolysis often continues up to 3 months
     d. Serum indirect bilirubin—markedly elevated
  2. ABO incompatibility
     a. Blood type—mother usually O, baby A, B, or AB
     b. Coombs' test (DAT)—usually positive (often weakly positive)

    c. Hemoglobin—moderately low; hemolysis occasionally occurs up to 2 to 3 months

    d. Serum bilirubin—variably elevated

- Management/Treatment

  1. Rh isoimmunization

    a. Obstetrical

      (1) Rh isoimmunization screen at first prenatal visit to identify "setups"; prevention if pregnancy at risk

      (2) If mother Rh negative, test father; if pregnancy at risk, follow titers and anti-D; consider Rh immunoglobulin at 28 weeks or within 72 hours of delivery

    b. Neonatal

      (1) Cord blood bilirubin, hemoglobin, and DAT

      (2) Hydration—aggressive oral feeding, IV if indicated

      (3) Phototherapy, if indicated

      (4) Exchange transfusion if indicated based on rate of rise in bilirubin and age of baby

  2. ABO isoimmunization

    a. Monitor unconjugated bilirubin levels

    b. Phototherapy if indicated based on bilirubin, gestational and post-delivery age of neonate

Hyperbilirubinemia

- Definition: An increased amount of unconjugated (indirect) or conjugated (direct) bilirubin in the blood associated with a range of conditions and liver dysfunction

- Etiology/Incidence

  1. Unconjugated (indirect) types—may be caused by overproduction of bilirubin, impaired conjugation, transport or uptake of bilirubin

    a. Physiological hyperbilirubinemia—indirect bilirubin 5 to 7 mg/dL; generally not > 12.7 to 12.9 mg/dL at peak within 3 to 5 days of life; usually resolves within 10 days; 50% full-term infants; higher incidence among preterm infants

    b. Breast-feeding hyperbilirubinemia

      (1) Breast feeding associated with prolonged physiologic hyperbilirubinemia in 30% breast-fed infants

      (2) True breast-milk hyperbilirubinemia

        (a) Begins by 4th day with peak bilirubin of 10 to 30 mg/dL by 10 to 15 days

        (b)   Incidence—1% to 2% breast-fed infants

    c. Prolonged (non-physiologic) neonatal hyperbilirubinemia—associated with breast feeding, maternal diabetes, induced labor, prematurity, oriental ethnicity and male gender

    d. Common in infancy

    e. Less common in older children but associated with:

        (1) Hemoglobinopathies

        (2) Crigler-Najjar syndrome (type 1 glucuronyl transferase deficiency)—autosomal recessive disorder

        (3) Gilbert syndrome—mild congenital defect in conjugation

2. Conjugated (direct) types—caused by range of pathologic conditions (rare in newborns) including biliary obstruction, infection, drugs (aspirin, acetaminophen), and other metabolic disorders

    a. Direct bilirubin > 1.5 to 2 mg/dL

    b. Jaundice in first day of life

    c. Total bilirubin > 12.9 mg/dL (full-term); > 15 mg/dL (preterm)

    d. Persistence > 1 week (full-term); > 2 weeks (preterm)

    e. More common in older children

- Signs and Symptoms: Yellow discoloration of skin, whites of eyes, gums and oral mucosa

- Differential Diagnosis

    1. Transient neonatal hyperbilirubinemia

        a. Physiologic

        b. Breast-milk associated

        c. Breast-milk jaundice

    2. Infection

    3. Hepatic disease

    4. Intestinal obstruction

- Physical Findings

    1. Clinical jaundice varies based on bilirubin level—5 mg/dL appears first on head, progresses down chest/abdomen as bilirubin increases; usually at least 15 mg/dL when noted on distal extremities

    2. Hepatosplenomegaly

    3. Edema

- Diagnostic Tests/Findings

1. Evaluate for pathologic causes for jaundice—sepsis, polycythemia
2. Coombs' test (DAT)
   a. Blood group incompatibilities—DAT usually positive
   b. Membrane disorders, red cell enzyme disorders, bacterial or viral sepsis, drug toxin—DAT usually negative
3. Bilirubin
   a. Indirect hyperbilirubinemia—unconjugated bilirubin increased
   b. Direct hyperbilirubinemia—conjugated bilirubin increased
4. Reticulocyte count—may be increased

- Management/Treatment: Based on etiology and age of child
  1. Indirect (unconjugated) hyperbilirubinemia
     a. Hydration and feeding
     b. Phototherapy
     c. Exchange transfusion
  2. Direct (conjugated) hyperbilirubinemia—treat underlying disease and/or refer as appropriate

Hemoglobinopathies

- Definition: Chronic hemolytic anemia resulting from production of abnormal hemoglobin due to inherited genetic mutation in globin genes
- Etiology/Incidence: Incidence associated with specific ethnic groups
  1. Beta (β) thalassemia
     a. β-chain synthesis decreased in β thalassemia intermedia; absent in β-thalassemia major (Cooley's anemia)
     b. Increased but ineffective erythropoiesis
     c. Shortened red cell life span
  2. Alpha (α) thalassemia
     a. α-chain production is impaired
     b. Increased but ineffective erythropoiesis
     c. Shortened red cell life span
  3. Hemoglobin C and E
     a. Amino acid substitution of lysine for glutamic acid
     b. Hemoglobin C—carrier state in 2% of African-Americans
     c. Hemoglobin E—prevalent in populations from Southeast Asia

4. Ethnic groups—individuals of African, Asian, and Mediterranean descent

- Signs and Symptoms

  1. β-thalassemia major and intermedia

     a. Pale skin or mucous membranes

     b. Weakness

     c. Facial deformities

  2. β-thalassemia minor (trait), α-thalassemia trait, Hemoglobin C, Hemoglobin E—usually asymptomatic

- Differential Diagnosis

  1. Iron deficiency anemia

  2. Lead poisoning

- Physical Findings

  1. β-thalassemia major and intermediate

     a. Splenomegaly, occasional hepatosplenomegaly (HSM)

     b. Jaundice, usually mild

     c. Abnormal facies secondary to extramedullary hematopoiesis— prominence of malar eminences, frontal bossing, depression of bridge of nose, exposure of upper incisors

     d. Growth retardation

  2. β-thalassemia minor, α-thalassemia trait, and hemoglobin C trait— physical examination normal

  3. Hemoglobin C and E—splenomegaly

- Diagnostic Tests/Findings

  1. β-thalassemia

     a. CBC with red cell indices

        (1) Hemoglobin—decreased

        (2) Hypochromia, microcytosis, low MCV, anisocytosis, target cells

        (3) Reticulocyte count—increased

     b. Hemoglobin electrophoresis

        (1) β^+ thalassemia

           (a) Hgb A—present

           (b) Hgb A_2—increased (usually > 3.6%, depending on laboratory)

           (c) Hgb F—normal or slightly increased

(2) β^0 thalassemia

    (a) Hgb A—absent

    (b) Hgb A_2—increased (usually > 3.6%, depending on laboratory)

    (c) Hgb F—normal or slightly increased

2. β-thalassemia (minor or trait)—usually discovered on routine examination or in family investigation

  a. CBC with red cell indices

    (1) Hemoglobin—slightly decreased (9 to 11g/dL)

    (2) Hypochromic, microcytic cells, target cells, anisocytosis, basophilic stippling, low MCV, low MCH, normal RDW

  b. Hemoglobin electrophoresis

    (1) Hgb A_2—increased (usually > 3.6%, depending on laboratory)

    (2) Hgb F—may be mildly elevated

3. α-thalassemia trait

  a. CBC with red cell indices

    (1) Hemoglobin—may be slightly decreased

    (2) Microcytosis, hypochromia

  b. Hemoglobin electrophoresis—Hgb Barts on newborn screen; disappears by 1 to 3 months of age (2 gene deletion ~ 2%, 3 gene deletion ~ 2% to 6%)

4. Hemoglobin C and Hemoglobin E

  a. CBC with red cell indices

    (1) Hemoglobin—may be decreased

    (2) Hemoglobin C—target cells, spherocytes, increased reticulocytes

    (3) Hemoglobin E—target cells, microcytosis

  b. Hemoglobin electrophoresis

    (1) Hemoglobin C (Hgb C)—present

    (2) Hemoglobin E (Hgb E)—present

- Management/Treatment

  1. β-thalassemia major

    a. Refer to hematologist

    b. Chronic transfusion protocol—to maintain hemoglobin, support growth, and prevent extramedullary hematopoiesis

    c. Chelation therapy (desferoxamine) after serum ferritin $\geq$ 2000 ng/mL—to remove excessive intracellular iron

      d.   Splenectomy—may reduce transfusion requirements

          (1)   Conjugate and polysaccharide pneumococcal vaccines as recommended by the American Academy of Pediatrics; should be given at least 2 weeks or longer prior to surgery, if possible, to increase the likelihood of eliciting a protective antibody response

          (2)   Prophylactic penicillin 250 mg b.i.d. life long post-splenectomy

          (3)   After splenectomy, increased risk for bacterial infections—for fever (> 101.5° F), immediate referral for blood cultures, empiric parenteral antibiotics active against encapsulated organisms

2.   β-thalassemia intermedia

    a.   Observe hemoglobin

    b.   Splenectomy may help

3.   β-thalassemia minor, α-thalassemia trait, hemoglobin C and E—no therapy

4.   Genetic counseling

Iron Deficiency Anemia

- Definition: A microcytic, hypochromic anemia caused by inadequate supply of iron
- Etiology/Incidence
  1. Causative factors
     - a. Deficient dietary intake
     - b. Increased demand—growth (low birth weight, prematurity, adolescence, pregnancy), cyanotic congenital heart disease
     - c. Blood loss—GI tract is most common site
     - d. Malabsorption—rare except for intestinal resection
  2. Incidence
     - a. Most common nutritional deficiency in children
     - b. Most common between 8 and 18 months of age and in adolescence
     - c. Higher incidence in lower socioeconomic groups
- Signs and Symptoms: Vary with severity of anemia
  1. Mild anemia—usually asymptomatic
  2. More severe anemia
     - a. Fatigue
     - b. Irritability
     - c. Delayed motor development
     - d. Eating nonnutrient substances such as ice, plaster, clay, paint, fabric (pica)

Table 1
Diagnostic Tests for Iron Deficiency Anemia

Hemoglobin—< 3%tile for age[a]

Peripheral blood smear

- Hypochromic, microcytic red cells, confirmed by RBC indices MCV < 3%tile for age[a]
- Wide red cell distribution width (RDW) > 17

Serum ferritin—decreased

Serum iron and iron binding capacity

- Decreased serum iron
- Increased iron binding capacity (TIBC)
- Decreased iron saturation (16% or less)

Free erythrocyte protoporphyrin (FEP)—elevated

Therapeutic response to oral iron

- Reticulocyte with peak in 3 to 5 days after initiation of therapy
- Following peak reticulocytosis, hemoglobin level rises on average by 0.25 to 0.4 g/dL/day or hematocrit rises 1% per day
- Thereafter, hemoglobin rises more slowly—0.1 to 0.15 g/dL/day

[a] Refer to Dallman-Siimes algorithm on p. 323 of *The Harriet Lane handbook* (15th ed.) by G. K. Siberry & R. Iannone (Eds.), 2000, St. Louis: Mosby.
Note. From *Manual of Pediatric Hematology and Oncology* (2nd ed., p. 45) by P. Lanzkowsky, 1995. Copyright 1995 by Churchill Livingstone. Adapted with permission.

- Differential Diagnosis
  1. Hemoglobinopathy
  2. Lead poisoning
  3. Anemia of chronic disease or inflammation
- Physical Findings: Vary with severity of anemia
  1. Mild—normal physical examination
  2. More severe—pallor, tachycardia, systolic murmur, hepatomegaly, CHF
- Diagnostic Tests/Findings—see Table 1
- Management/Treatment
  1. Nutritional counseling—prevention
     a. Maintain breast feeding for 6 months if possible, supplemental iron drops or iron fortified cereal by 4 to 5 months of age
     b. Use iron fortified infant formula until 1 year of age

    c. Use iron fortified cereals from 6 to 12 months of age

    d. No cow's milk before 1 year of age, then limit to 18 to 24 oz/day

    e. Prescribe 2 to 3 mg/kg/day elemental iron in 1 to 2 doses/day for prophylaxis in low birth weight infants

2. Oral iron medication

    a. Prescribe as elemental iron—3 to 6 mg/kg/day in 1 to 3 doses until hemoglobin normal, then 2 to 3 mg/kg/day for 4 months to replace iron stores

    b. See Table 1 regarding expected therapeutic response

    c. Failure to respond—consider the following reasons in this order

        (1) Failure or inconsistent administration of medication

        (2) Persistent or unrecognized blood loss

        (3) Incorrect diagnosis

        (4) Impaired GI absorption

3. Parenteral iron-dextran—in cases of noncompliance, severe bowel disease, genuine intolerance, chronic hemorrhage, chronic diarrhea

4. Packed red cell transfusion—consider in debilitated children with infection, especially when signs of cardiac dysfunction are present and when the hemoglobin level is ≤ 4 g/dL

Sickle Cell Disease

- Definition: A group of hemoglobinopathies that include inheritance of two hemoglobins that sickle; these hemoglobins include Hgb S, C, O_{Arab}, D, G $_{Philadelphia}$, and α-chain mutant; transmitted as an autosomal recessive gene

- Etiology/Incidence

    1. Hemoglobin S results from a single base pair substitution of valine for glutamic acid at the sixth position of the beta (β) globin gene; this results in red blood cells that become sickle shaped when deoxygenated; sickled shape of the RBCs leads to hemolysis and intermittent episodes of vascular occlusion that can cause tissue ischemia and acute and chronic organ dysfunction

    2. Sickle cell disease occurs in individuals of African, Mediterranean, Indian, and Middle Eastern decent; incidence and clinical severity of sickle cell disease and trait in U.S. African-American population is listed in Table 2

- Signs and Symptoms: Vary with associated problems (see Table 3)

    1. Infection (peak incidence between 1 and 3 years of age)

        a. Fever

        b. Malaise

Table 2

Differential Diagnosis and Incidence of Sickle Cell Disease and Sickle Cell Trait in U.S. African-Americans

Syndrome (Genotype)	Incidence	Clinical Severity	Hgb (g/dL)[a]	MCV (fl)[a]	Reticulocytes (%)[a]	Newborn Screening[b]	Electrophoresis (%)
Sickle cell anemia (SS)	1:400	Usually marked	6.5–9.5	> 80	5–20	FS	S 80–90 F 2–20 $A_2 < 3.6$
Sickle hemoglobin C (SC)	1:1000	Mild to moderate	9.5–13.5	75–95	5–10	FSC	S 45–55 C 45–55
Sickle beta plus ($S\beta^+$) thalassemia	1:4000	Mild to moderate	8.5–12.5	< 75	5–10	FSA or FS[c]	S 65–90 A 5–30 F 2–20 $A_2 > 3.6$
Sickle beta zero ($S\beta^0$) thalassemia	1:10,000	Marked to moderate	6.5–9.5	< 80	5–20	FS	S 80–92 F 2–10 $A_2 > 3.6$
Sickle cell trait (AS)	1:10	Asymptomatic	Normal	Normal	Normal	FAS	S 35–45% A 55–65%

[a] Hematologic values are approximate; results apply to older children
[b] Hemoglobins reported in order of quantity (e.g., FSA = F > S > A); F, fetal hemoglobin; S, sickle hemoglobin; C, hemoglobin C; A, hemoglobin A.
[c] Quantity of Hb A at birth; sometimes insufficient to quantitate
(Lane, 1996, NIH, 1996)

Table 3
Associated Problems of Sickle Cell Disease

Hemolysis

Chronic anemia

Jaundice

Aplastic crises

Cholelithiasis

Delayed growth and sexual maturity

Vaso-occlusion

Recurrent acute pain (e.g., dactylitis, musculoskeletal, abdominal)

Functional asplenia (bacterial infections)

Splenic sequestration[a]

Acute chest syndrome[a]

Stroke[a]

Hyposthenuria and enuresis

Papillary necrosis of kidneys

Chronic nephropathy

Priapism

Avascular necrosis of humeral heads, femoral heads

Proliferative retinopathy

Leg ulcers

[a] Important cause of mortality during childhood. (Lane, 1996)

      c.   Anorexia

      d.   Poor feeding

  2. Acute painful events—''pain crisis'', ''vaso-occlusive crisis''

      a.   Pain—most often in bones; but can occur in any part of body (chest, stomach, hands and/or feet, back, etc.); in children < 2 years of age usually in hands and/or feet (dactylitis)

      b.   Swelling—sometimes seen at site of pain

      c.   Low grade fever—sometimes occurs

  3. Splenic sequestration

      a.   Weakness

      b.   Irritability

      c.   Unusual sleepiness

      d.   Paleness

  e. Large spleen

  f. Fast heart rate

  g. Pain in the left side of the abdomen—does not always occur

 4. Aplastic crisis (is associated with parvovirus B19)

  a. Pale

  b. Malaise

  c. Headache

  d. Fever

  e. Mild upper respiratory infection symptoms

- Differential Diagnosis

 1. Infection

  a. Septicemia

  b. Meningitis

  c. Pneumonia

  d. Osteomyelitis

  e. Viral illness

 2. Acute painful events

  a. Bone pain

   (1) Bone infarct

   (2) Osteomyelitis

   (3) Rheumatoid arthritis

   (4) Leukemia

  b. Abdominal pain

   (1) Cholelithiasis—right upper quadrant

   (2) Splenic infarct—left upper quadrant

   (3) Functional abdominal pain

   (4) Gas pain

 3. Splenic sequestration—chronic splenomegaly

 4. Aplastic crisis—other viral illnesses

- Physical Findings: Sometimes but not always present

 1. Jaundice

 2. Cardiac murmur

3. Splenomegaly

4. Pallor

- Diagnostic Tests/Findings

  1. Prenatal diagnosis—can be done by analysis of DNA obtained through chorionic villus sampling (9 to 11 wks gestation) or amniocentesis (11 to 17 wks gestation)

  2. Usual diagnostic hemoglobin electrophoresis and hematologic results in infants and adults with sickle cell disease are presented in Table 2

  3. "Sickle prep" (metabisulfite solution)—should not be used as diagnostic test; does not distinguish among sickle cell anemia, other forms of sickle cell disease, and sickle cell trait or common interacting hemoglobinopathies such as Hgb C or thalassemia

  4. Splenic sequestration

     a. Hemoglobin—below baseline (steady state)

     b. Platelets—decreased

  5. Aplastic crisis

     a. Hemoglobin—below steady state

     b. Reticulocyte count— < 1.0%

- Management/Treatment

  1. Infection secondary to functional asplenia

     a. Prevention

        (1) Immunizations as recommended by American Academy of Pediatrics including conjugate pneumococcal and HIB vaccines

        (2) Polysaccharide pneumococcal vaccine—at 2 and 5 years of age

        (3) Prophylactic penicillin—in children with sickle cell anemia and sickle β^0 thalassemia; initiate before 3 months of age and continue until at least 5 years of age; oral penicillin VK 125 mg twice daily up to age 3 years, then 250 mg twice daily

        (4) Family education regarding increased risk of infection due to functional asplenia and need to seek medical attention promptly for evaluation of febrile illnesses

     b. Febrile illness (T ≥ 101.5° F) in children with sickle cell anemia, sickle β^0 thalassemia, sickle C disease (> 5 years of age or if spleen surgically removed)—immediate referral for blood culture and empiric parenteral antibiotics active against encapsulated organisms such as *Streptococcus pneumoniae* and *Haemophilus influenzae*

  2. Acute painful events

     a. Prevention—education regarding factors that may precipitate painful events, i.e., dehydration, hypoxia, fever, exposure to extreme temperatures; how to manage mild to moderate pain; and how to recognize signs of serious problems

    b. Home-based management

        (1) Oral intake of at least 150 cc/kg/day of fluids

        (2) For mild pain—acetaminophen or ibuprofen

        (3) For more severe pain—codeine should be alternated with NSAIDs

    c. Emergency department (ED) management—if home trial of oral opiods and NSAIDs fail, parenteral opioids (preferably morphine) may be used

    d. Inpatient management—if pain not reduced by ED management, hospitalization for hydration, parenteral opioids, and concomitant NSAID

    e. Nonpharmacologic measures such as heat, massage to area of pain, and distraction

3. Management of other problems associated with sickle cell disease— consultation with or referral to a pediatric hematologist

4. Frequent reinforcement of education regarding fever and pain management, spleen palpation

5. Anticipatory guidance regarding developmental issues such as toilet training, school attendance, delayed growth and development (SS and $S\beta^0$ thalassemia)

6. Genetic counseling

Lead Poisoning (Plumbism)

- Definition: A chronic disease particularly among young children due to the accumulation of toxic amounts of lead absorbed by the body; expert panel convened by Centers for Disease Control and Prevention (CDC) recommended a cut-off definition of lead poisoning as a whole blood lead level ≥ 10 µg/dL

- Etiology/Incidence

1. Ingestion or inhalation of lead or lead compounds; transplacental transmission may also occur

2. Sources of lead exposure

    a. Lead-based paint in older homes built prior to 1970s

    b. Lead contaminated soil and dust from automobile emissions (decreasing with use of lead-free gasoline)

    c. Lead contaminated drinking water (lead or lead-soldered pipes)

    d. Certain Mexican and Indian lead-containing folk remedies

3. Highest prevalence among poor, inner-city children living in older, deteriorating housing

4. Children between 1 and 3 years of age at greatest risk; 9 out of every 10 children with lead poisoning have history of pica

5. Prevalence estimates have shown progressive declines in elevated blood lead levels (BLL); most recent data reports incidence of elevated BLL among U.S. children 1 to 5 years decreased from 88.2% (1976-1980) to 4.4% (1991-1994) (AAP, 1998)

- Signs and Symptoms: Vary with degree of exposure, usually none

  1. Mild acute lead poisoning—resembles gastroenteritis, e.g., anorexia, nausea, vomiting, constipation or diarrhea, and abdominal pain; other possible symptoms are sleep disturbances, metallic taste in mouth, limb pain, and headaches

  2. Severe lead poisoning—lethargy, difficulty walking, tingling

- Differential Diagnosis

  1. Iron deficiency anemia

  2. Alpha or beta thalassemia

- Physical Findings

  1. May see bluish discoloration of gingival border (Burtonian blue lines)

  2. Bradycardia

  3. Neuropathy

  4. Papilledema

  5. Ataxia

- Diagnostic Tests/Findings

  1. CDC revised guidelines (1997) no longer recommend universal screening

     a. Target screening based on well-child surveillance of risk

        (1) Living or regular contact with housing built before 1950 or built before 1978 and being renovated

        (2) Contact with children who have history of lead poisoning

     b. Universal screening for children living in high risk environments

        (1) Available data indicating areas with ≥ 27% of housing built before 1950

        (2) Available data indicating areas with ≥ 12% of children between 1 and 2 years of age with elevated BLL

     c. American Academy of Pediatrics endorsed new CDC guidelines (AAP, 1998)

  2. Whole blood lead levels by categories of risk (PbB)

     a. Class I—lead level < 10 μg/dL—(normal)

     b. Class IIA—lead level of 10 to 14 μg/dL (borderline)

     c. Class IIB—lead level of 15 to 19 μg/dL (venipuncture confirmation)

    d. Class III—lead level of 20 to 44 μg/dL (requires environmental and medical evaluation; possible treatment)

    e. Class IV—lead level of 45 to 69 μg/dL (high risk, requires environmental and medical interventions including chelation therapy)

    f. Class V—lead level of > 70 μg/dL (urgent risk, immediate treatment)

- Management/Treatment

  1. Class I—no follow-up necessary

  2. Class II—at risk for lead poisoning; more frequent screening, every 3 to 4 months; if lead level between 15 and 19 μg/dL (Class IIB)— include educational and nutritional counseling

  3. Classes III to V—refer for further medical evaluation, interventions and follow-up

     a. Test for iron deficiency

     b. Environmental assessment and removal of known sources of lead in environment

     c. Medical evaluation for symptoms and possible pharmacologic management

        (1) Class III may require pharmacologic management

        (2) Classes IV and V require chelation therapy

  4. Primary prevention

     a. Outreach education regarding nutrition and avoidance of exposure

     b. Assessment of potential risk with specific environmental and health questions during routine well-child visits

Glucose-6-Phosphate Dehydrogenase (G-6-PD) deficiency

- Definition: X-linked autosomal recessive disorder in which activity of red cell enzyme G-6-PD is decreased or absent

- Etiology/Incidence

  1. Lack of G-6-PD decreases the ability to deal with oxidative stress and results in hemolysis; episodes of hemolysis may be induced by the following:

     a. Drugs such as aspirin, sulfonamides, antimalarials

     b. Fava beans, ingestion or exposure to pollen from the bean's flower (occurs in Mediterranean and Canton type deficiencies)

     c. Infection (in more susceptible individuals)

  2. Many genetic variants described with altered enzyme levels which determines the severity of disorder

     a. A Type—enzyme activity decreases with age of cell; hemolyzes only old RBC; occurs in 11% African-American males; 2% African-American females

      b.   Mediterranean Type—associated with severe deficiency of enzyme

      c.   Canton Type—severe disease in Asians

  3.   Most common among individuals of African or Mediterranean descent

- Signs and Symptoms: Symptoms develop 24 to 48 hours after ingestion of substance having oxidant properties

  1.   Weakness

  2.   Pale appearance

  3.   With severe cases

      a.   Blood in the urine

      b.   Yellow discoloration of skin, whites of eyes, and gums or inside of mouth

- Differential Diagnosis

  1.   Other causes of hemolytic anemia

  2.   Hemoglobinopathies

- Physical Findings

  1.   Neonatal jaundice—usually associated with Mediterranean and Canton individuals

  2.   Jaundice during episodes

- Diagnostic Tests/Findings

  1.   G-6-PD fluorescence-based screen (may give false negative)

  2.   Red blood cell indices during or just after hemolytic episode

      a.   Heinz bodies present

      b.   Fragmented cells and blister cells

  3.   Reticulocytosis

  4.   Hemoglobin—usually normal between episodes of hemolysis; may be decreased in Mediterranean or Canton

  5.   Acute self-limiting hemolytic anemia with hemoglobinuria (Type A variant)

  6.   Acute life-endangering hemolysis often leads to acute renal failure (all other variants)

- Management/Treatment

  1.   Generally mild symptoms require minimal intervention

  2.   Identification and avoidance of foods and drugs that cause hemolysis

  3.   Transfusion for severe hemolysis

  4.   Genetic counseling; routine screening not generally recommended

Bleeding Disorders

Hemophilia

- Definition: Bleeding disorder caused by congenital deficiency of either clotting factor VIII or IX
- Etiology/Incidence
    1. Hemophilia A (factor VIII deficiency, classical hemophilia)
        a. Third most common X-linked disorder, but 20% to 30% by spontaneous mutation
        b. Approximately 1:5000 male births
        c. 10% to 15% of patients develop antibodies against the functional activity of factor VIII
    2. Hemophilia B (factor IX deficiency, Christmas disease)
        a. X-linked disorder, but 20% to 30% by spontaneous mutation
        b. Less prevalent than hemophilia A by 15% to 20%
- Signs and Symptoms: Vary based on severity of factor deficiency
    1. Bruising at injection sites
    2. Bleeding following circumcision
    3. Excessive bruising after child begins walking
    4. Prolonged bleeding in any part of the body
- Differential Diagnosis
    1. Thrombocytopenia
    2. von Willebrand disease
    3. Vitamin K deficiency
    4. Disseminated intravascular coagulation (DIC)
    5. Child abuse
- Physical Findings: With acute bleeds, swelling and warmth may be present at the site
- Diagnostic Tests/Findings
    1. Diagnostic test—direct assay of plasma factor activity level for hemophilia A and B—see Table 4
    2. Screening tests
        a. Activated partial thromboplastin time (APTT)—prolonged
        b. Prothrombin time (PT)—normal

Table 4

Relationship of Factor Levels to Severity of Clinical Manifestations of Hemophilia A and B

Type	% Factor VIII/IX	Type of Hemorrhage
Severe	< 1	Spontaneous hemarthrosis and deep tissue hemorrhages
Moderate	1–5	Gross bleeding following mild to moderate trauma; some hemarthrosis; rare spontaneous hemorrhage
Mild	5–25	Severe hemorrhage only following moderate to severe trauma or surgery
Carrier females	30–50	Gynecologic and obstetric hemorrhage

Note. From *Manual of Pediatric Hematology and Oncology* (2nd ed., p. 256) by P. Lanzkowsky, 1995. New York: Churchill Livingstone. Copyright 1995 by Churchill Livingstone. Adapted with permission.

      c. Bleeding time (not indicated)—normal

- Management/Treatment

    1. Collaborative interdisciplinary approach facilitated by regional hemophilia treatment center

    2. Factor replacement therapy

        a. Hemophilia A—factor VIII concentrate intravenously

        b. Hemophilia B—factor IX concentrate intravenously

        c. If development of inhibitor, consultation with hemophilia treatment center regarding factor replacement

    3. Desmopressin intranasally or intravenously—for mild factor VIII deficiency

    4. Antifibrinolytic therapy—for oral mucosal bleeds

    5. Physical therapy—for musculoskeletal bleeds

    6. Surgery—Synovectomy, arthroscopic or with use of isotopes

    7. Anticipatory guidance regarding developmental issues such as discipline, child care, and schooling

    8. Genetic counseling

von Willebrand Disease (vWD)

- Definition: An inherited hemorrhagic disorder characterized by defective primary hemostasis and prolonged bleeding time due to abnormal von Willebrand factor

- Etiology/Incidence:

    1. The most common congenital bleeding disorder

    2. Three variant types

        a. Type I—most common

     b.   Type II/IIA

     c.   Type III—most severe

   3.   Affects at least 1% of the population

- Signs and Symptoms: Great variation in frequency, severity, and bleeding manifestations
    1. Nosebleeds
    2. Bleeding gums
    3. Heavy menstrual bleeding
    4. Prolonged oozing from cuts
    5. Increased bleeding after trauma or surgery

- Differential Diagnosis
    1. Thrombocytopenia
    2. Hemophilia
    3. Vitamin K deficiency
    4. Disseminated intravascular coagulation

- Physical Findings
    1. Easy bruising
    2. Multiple sites of bruising
    3. Oozing or bleeding at trauma or surgical site

- Diagnostic Tests/Findings
    1. Variation in findings by specific type of vWD as well as within same patient over time
    2. Bleeding time—usually prolonged
    3. von Willebrand factor—usually decreased or absent
    4. von Willebrand factor antigen—usually decreased or absent
    5. Blood group—vWD factor decreased in type O

- Management/Treatment
    1. Desmopressin—used to treat bleeding complications or as preoperative preparation for Type I; not used with Types IIA and III
    2. Alternative treatment if desmopressin not indicated or effective—vWD factor with cryoprecipitate or fresh frozen plasma

Idiopathic Thrombocytopenia Purpura (ITP)

- Definition: Immune-mediated disorder characterized by production of antiplatelet antibodies

1. Acute ITP—platelet count returns to normal (> 150,00/mm^3) within 6 months

2. Chronic ITP—platelet count low beyond 6 months; approximately 10% of children with ITP

3. Recurrent or relapsing ITP—the platelet count decreases again after having returned to normal levels (rare)

- Etiology/Incidence

    1. Often appears to be related to sensitization by viral infection

    2. 4 to 8 cases/100,000 children

    3. Most prevalent during early to mid-childhood and in older adults, although it affects all ages

    4. Chronic ITP—more prevalent in females (3:1 ratio)

- Signs and Symptoms

    1. Bruising

    2. Nose bleeds

    3. Bleeding of gums and lips

    4. Except for bleeding, child appears well

- Differential Diagnosis

    1. Thrombocytopenia of other causes

        a. Bone marrow infiltration

        b. Septicemia

        c. Aplastic anemia

    2. Disseminated intravascular coagulation (DIC)

    3. Hemolytic uremic syndrome

    4. Acute leukemia

- Physical Findings

    1. Petechiae, purpura, and ecchymosis

    2. Hemorrhages in mucous membranes

    3. Pallor usually not present (unless there has been significant bleeding)

- Diagnostic Tests/Findings

    1. CBC—generally the only required test

    2. Hemoglobin—normal or slightly reduced with prior bleeding; can drop with bruising only

    3. Platelet count

a. $\leq$ 20,000/mm^3 (diagnostic for acute ITP); often $\leq$ 10,000/mm^3

b. < 100,000/mm^3 for > 6 months (diagnostic for chronic ITP)

4. WBC—normal; if active infection, may have increased neutrophils, lymphocytes, or atypical mononuclear cells

5. Bleeding time test (unnecessary)—always abnormal if platelets < 50,000 mm^3

- Management/Treatment: Controversial

  1. Acute ITP

     a. No treatment indicated if platelet count > 35,000/mm^3 and child is asymptomatic (mild bruising with no evidence of mucous membrane bleeding); family reassurance with a brief physical examination and CBC with platelet count monthly

     b. Below 20,000 to 35,000/mm^3, some would also follow counts weekly; caution family to take precaution to avoid head trauma in child

     c. Pharmacologic management

        (1) Corticosteroids (prednisone 2 to 5 mg/kg/day orally for 1 to 3 weeks) may accelerate recovery in acute ITP but does not change outcome

        (2) Intravenous gamma globulin (IVGG)—regimens of 400, 800, 1000 mg/day for 2 or 5 days will increase platelet count in 2 to 3 days in most patients; total dose 2g/kg; lasts only 21 to 28 days; may require retreatment

        (3) Methylprednisolone 30mg/kg/day for 3 days

  2. Chronic ITP

     a. Referral to a hematologist.

     b. Pharmacologic management—when thrombocytopenia worsens during viral illness or prior to elective surgery, prednisone or IVGG can be administered

     c. Prolonged use of high dose steroids should be avoided

     d. Splenectomy—treatment of choice when severe or symptomatic chronic ITP interferes significantly with child's lifestyle

        (1) Conjugate and polysaccharide pneumococcal vaccines as recommended by the American Academy of Pediatrics; should be given at least 2 weeks or longer prior to surgery, if possible, to increase the likelihood of eliciting a protective antibody response

        (2) Prophylactic penicillin 250 mg b.i.d. for at least 1 to 2 years postoperatively

        (3) After splenectomy, at increased risk for bacterial infections—for fever (T $\geq$ 101.5° F), immediate referral for blood culture and empiric parenteral antibiotics active against encapsulated organisms

3. Patient/family education

    a. Avoid all competitive contact sports that could result in head trauma

    b. Avoid aspirin and aspirin containing medications and ibuprofen

Cancers

Leukemias

- Definition: A malignant neoplasm of bone marrow characterized by proliferation of immature white cells

- Etiology/Incidence

    1. Etiology is usually unknown

    2. Accounts for 25% to 30% of all childhood cancers

    3. Acute leukemia constitutes 97% of all childhood leukemias and includes most common types:

        a. Acute lymphocytic leukemia (ALL)—75%; survival rate is 60% to 80%

        b. Acute myleloid leukemia (AML), also known as acute non-lymphocytic leukemia (ANLL)—20%; survival rate is 40% to 60%

    4. Chronic myelogenous leukemia (CML) constitutes 3% of childhood leukemia

    5. 1 per 25,000 of population up to 14 years of age

    6. Peak incidence between 2 and 5 years of age

- Signs and Symptoms

    1. Fatigue, headache

    2. Bruising

    3. Fever

    4. Nose bleeds

    5. Bone pain, limp

- Differential Diagnosis

    1. Chronic infections such as Epstein-Barr virus (EBV) or cytomegalovirus (CMV)

    2. ITP

    3. Transient erythroblastopenia of childhood

    4. Aplastic anemia

    5. Juvenile rheumatoid arthritis

- Physical Findings

    1. Pallor

2. Purpura, ecchymosis

3. Organomegaly, adenopathy

- Diagnostic Tests/Findings

    1. CBC—presence of blast cells on peripheral blood smear highly suggestive; needs confirmatory bone marrow examination

    2. Bone marrow aspiration/biopsy (required for diagnosis)—bone marrow replaced by > 30% blasts, usually 80% to 100%

- Management/Treatment

    1. Combination chemotherapy

    2. CNS prophylaxis

        a. Radiation therapy (for high risk patients)

        b. Combined intrathecal chemotherapy

    3. Patient/family education regarding side effects of therapy, anticipatory guidance on coping

    4. For relapse following chemotherapy—second course of chemotherapy may provide cure; for AML, bone marrow transplant is treatment of choice

    5. Long term follow-up for delayed effects of chemotherapy and/or radiation

Neuroblastoma

- Definition: Tumor mass along the neural pathway

- Etiology/Incidence

    1. Etiology—possible genetic factors; familial predisposition

    2. Most common malignancy in infancy, accounts for 7% of all childhood malignancies

    3. Metastases at onset in 70% to 75% of cases

    4. 10 per 1 million live births annually

    5. Survival rate for patients < 1 year of age, 82%; for 1 to 2 years of age, 32%; over 2 years, 10%

- Signs and Symptoms: Dependent on primary site, presence of metastases

    1. Listlessness

    2. Poor feeding

    3. Pale

    4. Weight loss

    5. Abdominal pain

    6. Weakness

    7.   Irritability

- Differential Diagnosis
  1. Trauma
  2. Lymphadenopathy
  3. Leukemia
  4. Lymphoma
  5. Wilms tumor

- Physical Findings: Related to site of primary tumor
  1. Lymph node enlargement
  2. Hepatomegaly
  3. Abdominal or flank mass
  4. Periorbital ecchymoses (raccoon eyes)
  5. Scalp nodules

- Diagnostic Tests/Findings
  1. CT and/or MRI scan to determine site and location of any suspected masses
  2. Tissue biopsy to confirm diagnosis
  3. Bone marrow aspiration and biopsy to evaluate for infiltrating tumor
  4. Serum or urine catecholamine levels—increased

- Management/Treatment: Based on stage and site of tumor
  1. Treatment of emergent symptoms
  2. Surgery
     a. Staging excision of tumor
     b. Evaluation of treatment
  3. Radiation therapy
  4. Combination chemotherapy
  5. Bone marrow transplant in some cases
  6. Patient/family education regarding side effects of therapy
  7. Anticipatory guidance on developmental issues such as sleep, toileting, discipline, and child care
  8. Long term follow-up for delayed effects of chemotherapy and/or radiation

Retinoblastoma

- Definition: Congenital malignant intraocular tumor

- Etiology/Incidence
    1. Abnormal fetal neural crest cell maturation
        a. Hereditary—germinal mutation (40%); siblings and subsequent offspring at risk
        b. Acquired—somatic mutations
    2. Most common intraocular childhood tumor
        a. 1:10,000 live births
        b. Slightly higher incidence in males
        c. Accounts for 7% of all childhood cancers; 15% childhood cancer mortality
    3. Majority diagnosed before 5 years
        a. $\frac{1}{3}$ are bilateral—usually diagnosed in first year
        b. Unilateral—usually diagnosed
    4. Prognosis varies with age and tumor staging
        a. Overall survival rates > 90%
        b. Highest survival for children < 1 year and > 6 years
        c. High incidence of secondary malignancies may limit survival into third or fourth decade of life
- Signs and Symptoms
    1. Squinting
    2. Eyes turning inward or outward
    3. Painful red eye
- Differential Diagnosis
    1. Cataract
    2. Retinal detachment
    3. Persistent hyperplastic primary vitreous
    4. Coloboma
    5. Retinopathy of prematurity
- Physical Findings
    1. Leukocoria—yellow-white pupillary reflex
    2. Strabismus
    3. Hyphema may be present
- Diagnostic Tests/Findings
    1. Fundoscopic examination under anesthesia or sedation—findings may include:
        a. Creamy-pink mass

      b.   White avascular tumor mass

   2. CT of the orbits to evaluate extent of tumor and to determine optic nerve or bony structure involvement

   3. MRI to assess for optic nerve invasion

- Management/Treatment: Determined by stage and extent of disease

   1. Surgery

      a.   Resection

      b.   Enucleation

   2. Radiation therapy

   3. Chemotherapy—palliative

   4. Patient/family education regarding side effects of therapy

   5. Anticipatory guidance on developmental issues such as sleep, toileting, discipline, and child care

   6. Long term follow-up for recurrence or delayed effects of chemotherapy and/or radiation

Lymphomas

- Definition: Malignant disorders characterized by proliferation of cells usually restricted to lymphoid cells but may be found in bone marrow; includes Hodgkin's (HL) and non-Hodgkin's (NHL) lymphomas

- Etiology/Incidence

   1. Etiology unknown—possible etiologic factors

      a.   Genetic predisposition

      b.   Environmental exposures

      c.   Epstein-Barr virus

      d.   Immunologic disorders

   2. Third most common childhood cancer—10%

      a.   HL—1:100,000 children

         (1) Peak age—bimodal age incidence curve

            (a) 15 to 35 years

            (b) > 50 years

         (2) Survival—stages I to II, most are cured; stage III, 75% to 90%; stage IV, 60% to 80%

      b.   NHL—15:100,000 children between 5 to 10 years

         (1) Peak age—5 to 15 years

      (2)   Survival—stages I to II ~ 90%; stages III to IV ~ 70%

- Signs and Symptoms
  1. Hodgkin's
     a. Painless swelling of lymph nodes
     b. Fatigue
     c. Decreased appetite and weight loss
     d. Fever
     e. Night sweats
  2. Non-Hodgkin's
     a. Asymptomatic if not disseminated
     b. Difficulty swallowing or breathing
     c. Swelling in neck, face, upper extremities
     d. Abdominal pain
- Differential Diagnosis
  1. Other malignancy
  2. Lymphadenopathy associated with infection
- Physical Findings
  1. Hodgkin's
     a. Affected nodes—firm, non-tender, discrete; cervical and supraclavicular areas most common
     b. Splenomegaly
  2. Non-Hodgkin's
     a. Similar to Hodgkin's
     b. May vary depending on degree of involvement
- Diagnostic Tests/Findings
  1. Hodgkin's
     a. Chest radiograph—to explore possibility of mediastinal involvement and examine airway patency
     b. Biopsy—tumor giant cells (Reed-Sternberg cells)
     c. CBC with red cell indices
        (1) Hemoglobin—decreased
        (2) Normocytic and normochromic or microcytic and hypochromic
     d. Serum copper—increased

    e.   Serum ferritin—increased

    f.   Sedimentation rate (ESR)—increased

  2. Non-Hodgkin's—tissue diagnosis necessary before treatment is started, findings vary based on specific histiologic type

    a.   Isolated peripheral nodes—excisional or fine-needle biopsy

    b.   Mediastinal mass—thoracotomy or mediastinoscopy, parasternal fine-needle biopsy, or thoracentesis (if associated pleural effusion)

    c.   Abdominal mass—open biopsy usually necessary

- Management/Treatment: Plan developed based on stage of involvement

  1. Multiagent chemotherapy

  2. Radiation

  3. Patient/family education regarding side effects of therapy

  4. Long term follow-up for delayed effects of chemotherapy and/or radiation

Wilms' tumor (Nephroblastoma)

- Definition: A primary malignant renal tumor
- Etiology/Incidence

  1. Etiology unknown; predisposing factors

    a.   Genetic factors

      (1)   Associated with aniridia, Beckwith-Wiedeman syndrome

      (2)   Familial predisposition

    b.   Environmental factors—chronic chemical exposure (hydrocarbons, lead)

  2. 6% of all cancer in children; 9:1 million Caucasian children/year

  3. Equal frequency in males and females

  4. 78% diagnosed between 1 and 5 years of age; peak incidence 3 to 4 years of age

  5. Survival rate—70% to 90%

- Signs and Symptoms

  1. May be asymptomatic

  2. Abdominal mass—usually non-painful

  3. Occasionally abdominal pain

  4. Malaise, fever, loss of appetite

  5. Vomiting

  6. Blood in urine

- Differential Diagnosis
    1. Hydronephrosis
    2. Polycystic kidney disease
    3. Neuroblastoma
    4. Rhabdomyosarcoma
    5. Lymphoma
- Physical Findings
    1. Abdominal mass—usually asymptomatic
    2. Hypertension
    3. Associated congenital anomalies—aniridia, hemihypertrophy, genitourinary anomalies
- Diagnostic Tests/Findings
    1. CBC and urine analysis for anemia, hematuria
    2. CT of abdomen to evaluate:
        a. Presence and function of opposite kidney
        b. Evidence of bilateral involvement
        c. Evidence of involvement of blood vessels of tumor
        d. Lymph node involvement
        e. Liver involvement
    3. Abdominal ultrasound—may indicate that the tumor is intrarenal
    4. Chest radiograph, CT of chest to evaluate for metastasis to lung
- Management/Treatment: Plan developed based on stage of involvement
    1. Surgical excision
        a. If unilateral—complete nephrectomy
        b. If bilateral—nephrectomy of more involved site, excision biopsy/partial nephrectomy of smaller lesion in remaining kidney; or no surgery with radiation
    2. Multiagent chemotherapy
    3. Radiation therapy
    4. Patient/family education regarding side effects of therapy
    5. Long term follow-up for disease recurrence and delayed effects of chemotherapy and/or radiation

Osteosarcoma

- Definition: A solid tumor of the bone in which malignant spindle cell stroma produce osteiod; most common form of bone cancer in children

- Etiology/Incidence
  1. Etiology unknown
  2. Associated factors
     a. Genetic factors and family predisposition
        (1) Increased risk with hereditary retinoblastoma
        (2) Increased risk with chromosome 13 abnormalities
     b. Environmental factors—increased risk associated with previously irradiated bone
     c. Increased risk with taller children
  3. Incidence—7 teenagers per one million
     a. Peak incidence during adolescent growth spurt between 15 to 19 years of age
     b. Male incidence slightly higher than females
- Signs and Symptoms
  1. Local pain
  2. Local swelling
  3. Mass at end of long bone
  4. Decreased range of motion
- Differential Diagnosis
  1. Growing pains
  2. Trauma
  3. Osteomylelitis
  4. Tendonitis
  5. Septic arthritis
  6. Leukemia
- Physical Findings
  1. Pain over involved site
  2. Palpable mass
  3. Swelling
  4. Decreased range of motion of affected extremity
- Diagnostic Tests/Findings
  1. Radiograph of affected bone
  2. Computed tomography (CT) or magnetic resonance imaging (MRI) of affected bone
  3. Biopsy of area

- Management/Treatment
    1. Multiagent chemotherapy
    2. Surgery—amputation/limb sparing surgery
    3. Patient/family education regarding side effects of therapy, anticipatory guidance on coping
    4. Long term follow-up for delayed effects of chemotherapy

Immune deficiencies

Definition: A group of immune defects that can be classified according to
1. Deficiency of immunoglobulin
2. Deficiency of cell-mediated immunity
3. Deficiency of both antibodies and cell-mediated immunity

Common Variable Immunodeficiency (CVID, "Acquired" Hypogammaglobulinemia)

- Definition: An immune disorder resulting from deficiency of all immunoglobulin (Igs)
- Etiology/Incidence: Genetic defect
- Signs and Symptoms (specific to manner of presentation): Recurrent or severe bacterial infections of respiratory tract (sinusitis, otitis, pneumonia) or skin (cellulitis, abscesses)
- Differential Diagnosis: Other immune deficiencies
- Physical Findings: Specific to manner of presentation
    1. Sinusitis—fever (T ≥ 101.5° F), periorbital edema, tenderness on percussion over sinuses
    2. Otitis—hyperemic, opaque, bulging tympanic membrane with poor mobility
    3. Pneumonia—retractions, flaring nares, diminished breath sounds, fine and crackling rales on affected side
    4. Cellulitis or abscess—erythema, swelling, purulent drainage
- Diagnostic Tests/Findings: Serum immunoglobulin
    1. IgG—decreased
    2. IgA—decreased
    3. IgM—decreased
- Management/Treatment: Intravenous immunoglobulin G (IgG) replacement (IVIG)

X-linked Agammaglobulinemia (Bruton's Tyrosine Kinase or BTK)

- Definition: Absent or inadequate gammaglobulins caused by B cell defect
- Etiology/Incidence

1. Inherited, X-linked disorder of B lymphocytes

2. Affected male infants usually asymptomatic for 3 to 6 months due to passive transmission of maternal antibodies then show frequent infections and failure-to-thrive

3. Incidence rates unknown

- Signs and Symptoms: (specific to manner of presentation)—recurrent or severe bacterial infections of the respiratory tract (sinusitis, otitis, pneumonia) or skin (cellulitis, abscesses)

- Differential Diagnosis: Other immune deficiencies

- Physical Findings: Specific to manner of presentation

    1. Sinusitis—fever (T ≥ 101.5° F), periorbital edema, tenderness on percussion over sinuses

    2. Otitis—hyperemic, opaque, bulging tympanic membrane with poor mobility

    3. Pneumonia—retractions, flaring nares, diminished breath sounds, fine and crackling rales on affected side

    4. Cellulitis or abscess—erythema, swelling, purulent drainage

- Diagnostic Tests/Findings

    1. Serum immunoglobulins

        a. IgG—decreased

        b. IgA—decreased

        c. IgM—decreased

    2. Blood T and B Lymphocytes—B cells decreased and T cells normal

- Management/Treatment

    1. Intravenous immunoglobulin G (IgG) replacement (IVIG)

    2. Prophylactic antibiotics

    3. Antibiotic therapy for recurrent infections

Thymic Hypoplasia (DiGeorge Syndrome)

- Definition: A syndrome that includes T cell dysfunction secondary to hypoplasia of the thymus

- Etiology/Incidence

    1. Dysmorphogenesis occurs during embryogenosis resulting in hypoplasia of the thymus and parathyroid glands; may also have cardiac defects, abnormal facies, cleft palate, and hypocalcemia

    2. Occurs in males and females equally

    3. Presentation usually results from cardiac failure or, after 24 to 48 hours of age, from hypocalcemia

4. Sometimes diagnosed during cardiac surgery when no thymus is found in mediastinum

5. Increased susceptibility to viral, fungal, and bacterial infections

- Signs and Symptoms: Specific to manner of presentation

- Differential Diagnosis: Other immune deficiencies

- Physical Findings

    1. Characteristic features—hypertelorism; shortened lip frenulum; lowset, notched pinnae; and nasal cleft

    2. Other physical findings—specific to manner of presentation

- Diagnostic Tests/Findings:

    1. Routine chest radiograph may reveal absent thymus

    2. Blood T and B lymphocytes

        a. Lymphopenia

        b. Decreased T cells

        c. B cells normal

- Management/Treatment

    1. Prophylactic antibiotics

    2. Antibiotic therapy for recurrent infections

    3. Thymus transplant if donor available

    4. Bone marrow transplant

Wiskott-Aldrich Syndrome (WAS)

- Definition: X-linked disorder characterized by thrombocytopenia, eczema, and progressive deterioration of thymus-dependent cellular immunity

- Etiology/Incidence

    1. X-linked recessive inheritance; carrier detection is possible

    2. Specific defect unknown

    3. Incidence— ~ 4 per one million male births

- Signs and Symptoms

    1. Neonatal—bloody diarrhea, prolonged bleeding from circumcision

    2. Later—eczema and frequent infections

- Differential Diagnosis: Usually made during neonatal period due to thrombocytopenia

    1. Other causes of chronic diarrhea

    2. Other immune deficiencies

- Physical Findings: Specific to manner of presentation
- Diagnostic Tests/Findings
    1. Serum immunoglobulins
        a. IgG—normal
        b. IgA—increased
        c. IgM—decreased
    2. Blood T and B Lymphocytes
        a. B cells—normal
        b. T cells—decreased
    3. CBC—thrombocytopenia, small platelets
- Management/Treatment
    1. Platelet transfusions for bleeding
    2. IV Immunoglobulins
    3. Prophylactic antibiotics and antibiotic therapy for recurrent infections
    4. Splenectomy—may increase platelet count
        a. Conjugate and polysaccharide pneumococcal vaccines as recommended by the American Academy of Pediatrics; should be given at least 2 weeks or longer prior to surgery, if possible, to increase the likelihood of eliciting a protective antibody response
        b. Prophylactic penicillin 250 mg b.i.d. for at least 1 to 2 years post-splenectomy
        c. Increased risk for bacterial infections post-splenectomy—for fever (T ≥ 101.5° F) immediate referral for blood culture and empiric parenteral antibiotics against encapsulated organisms
    5. Bone marrow transplant if HLA-matched donor is available

Questions
Select the best answer

1. Baseline management of all neonates with ABO incompatibility includes:

   a. Phototherapy
   b. Serial monitoring of bilirubin levels
   c. Exchange transfusion
   d. Simple transfusion

2. Which of the following is not associated with Rh incompatibility?

   a. Mother Rh negative, baby Rh positive
   b. Mother Rh positive, baby Rh negative
   c. More severe in subsequent sensitized pregnancies
   d. Hemolysis may occur up to 6 weeks or more

3. Clinical jaundice of the distal extremities would be noted at a bilirubin level of:

   a. < 5 mg/dL
   b. 5 mg/dL
   c. 10 mg/dL
   d. ≥ 15 mg/dL

4. β-chain synthesis is absent in:

   a. β-thalassemia minor
   b. β-thalassemia intermedia
   c. β-thalassemia major
   d. α-thalassemia trait

5. Which of the following are most often associated with Hemoglobin C

   a. Growth retardation
   b. Hepatosplenomegaly
   c. Usually asymptomatic
   d. Frontal bossing

6. Diagnostic findings consistent with β-thalassemia are:

   a. Hemoglobin—normal
   b. Reticulocytes—normal
   c. Hgb A_2 < 3.6
   d. Hypochromia, microcytosis

7. Asplenic children are at increased risk for which of the following?

   a. Bacterial infections
   b. Fungal infections

    c. Viral infections

    d. Parasites

8. Which of the following is not considered preventive management for iron deficiency anemia?

    a. Iron fortified cereal from 6 to 12 months of age

    b. Iron fortified formula until 6 months of age

    c. No cow's milk until 1 year of age

    d. If breast feeding, supplemental iron drops or iron fortified cereal by 4–5 months of age

9. The expected clinical severity of hemoglobin sickle C disease (Hgb SC) is:

    a. Asymptomatic

    b. Marked to moderate

    c. Mild to moderate

    d. Severe

10. The expected hemoglobin range for sickle cell anemia is:

    a. 6.5–9.5 g/dL

    b. 13.5–16.5 g/dL

    c. 8.5–12.5 g/dL

    d. 9.5–13.5 g/dL

11. Prophylactic penicillin should be initiated in children with sickle cell anemia by:

    a. 3 years of age

    b. 12 months of age

    c. 2–3 months of age

    d. 9 months of age

12. Hemolysis does not contribute to which of the problems associated with sickle cell disease?

    a. Chronic anemia

    b. Splenic sequestration

    c. Aplastic crisis

    d. Delayed growth

13. The following is considered to be a normal blood lead level:

    a. $< 10\ \mu g/dL$

    b. $10\text{–}14\ \mu g/dL$

    c. $\geq 15\ \mu g/dL$

    d. $> 25\ \mu g/dL$

14. Which of the following is not a precipitating factor for hemolysis in G-6-PD deficiency?

    a. Drugs

    b. Exposure to extreme temperatures

    c. Ingestion of Fava beans

d. Infection

15. What percent of Factor VIII/IX is associated with severe hemophilia A and B?

    a. < 1
    b. 1–5
    c. 5–25
    d. 30–50

16. What type of hemorrhage would be expected with severe Factor VIII deficiency?

    a. Severe hemorrhage following moderate to severe trauma
    b. Gross bleeding following mild to moderate trauma
    c. Gynecologic hemorrhage
    d. Spontaneous hemorrhage

17. Which of the following is the most common type of congenital bleeding disorder?

    a. Hemophilia A
    b. Hemophilia B
    c. von Willebrand Disease
    d. Idiopathic thrombocytopenia purpura

18. Which of the following medications should be avoided in a child with ITP?

    a. Decongestants
    b. Aspirin
    c. Acetaminophen
    d. Sulfa drugs

19. The following test is required to diagnose leukemia:

    a. CBC with differential
    b. Bone marrow aspiration/biopsy
    c. Chest radiograph
    d. Biopsy of an enlarged lymph node

20. Which of the following is not included as part of the initial therapy for ALL?

    a. Chemotherapy
    b. Radiation therapy
    c. Bone marrow transplant
    d. Intrathecal chemotherapy

21. Which malignancy is associated with genitourinary anomalies?

    a. Acute lymphocytic leukemia
    b. Chronic myleogenous leukemia
    c. Osteosarcoma
    d. Wilms' tumor

22. The peak incidence of Wilms' tumor is:

    a. 3–4 years of age
    b. 5–8 years of age
    c. 9–12 years of age
    d. 15–19 years of age

23. The peak incidence of osteosarcoma is:

    a. 4–7 years of age
    b. 8–11 years of age
    c. 12–14 years of age
    d. 15–19 years of age

24. The following type of infection is not associated with hypogammaglobulinemia:

    a. Sinusitis
    b. Pneumonia
    c. Urinary tract infection
    d. Cellulitis

25. The following diagnostic finding is consistent with X-linked agammaglobulinemia:

    a. IgG—normal
    b. B cells—decreased
    c. T cells—decreased
    d. IgA—normal

26. The following is not a characteristic feature of DiGeorge syndrome:

    a. Hypertelorism
    b. Cleft palate
    c. Cardiac defects
    d. Frontal bossing

27. The following diagnostic finding is consistent with Wiskott-Aldrich syndrome:

    a. IgG—normal
    b. IgA—decreased
    c. IgM—increased
    d. B cells—decreased

28. Management of a patient with a splenectomy does not include:

    a. Pneumococcal vaccines at least 2 weeks prior to surgery
    b. Prophylactic penicillin
    c. Blood culture and parenteral antibiotics for febrile illnesses
    d. Treating fever with antipyretics only and observing for resolution

Answers

1. b	11. c	20. c
2. b	12. b	21. d
3. d	13. a	22. a
4. c	14. b	23. d
5. c	15. a	24. c
6. d	16. d	25. b
7. a	17. c	26. d
8. b	18. b	27. a
9. c	19. b	28. d
10. a		

Bibliography

American Academy of Pediatrics. In L. K. Pickering (Ed.), *Red Book 2000: Report of the committee on infectious diseases* (25th ed.). Elk Grove Village, IL: Author.

American Academy of Pediatrics (1994). Practice parameters: Management of hyperbilirubinemia in the healthy newborn. (Provisional Committee for Quality Improvement and Subcommittee on Hyperbilirubinemia). *Pediatrics, 94,* 558–565.

American Academy of Pediatrics. (1998). Screening for elevated blood lead levels. *Pediatrics. 101* (6), 1072–1078.

Behrman, R. E., Kliegman, R. M., & Jenson, H. B. (Eds.). (2000). *Nelson textbook of pediatrics* (16th ed.). Philadelphia: W. B. Saunders Company.

Buchanan, G. R. (2000). ITP: How much treatment is enough? *Contemporary Pediatrics, 17,* 112–121.

Castiglia, P. T. (1995). Lead poisoning. *Journal of Pediatric Health Care, 9,* 134–135.

Foley, G. V., Fochtman, D., & Mooney, K. H. (Eds.). (1993). *Nursing care of the child with cancer* (2nd ed.). Philadelphia: W. B. Saunders.

Hay, W. W., Groothuis, J. R., Haywood, A. R., & Levin, M. J. (Eds.). (1997). *Current pediatric diagnosis & treatment* (13th ed.). Stamford, CT: Appleton & Lange.

Hockenberry-Eaton, M. J., (Ed.). (1998). *Essentials of pediatric oncology nursing: A core curriculum.* Glenview, IL: Association of Pediatric Oncology Nurses.

Hoekelman, R. A., Adam, H. M., Nelson, N. M., Weitzman, M. L., & Wilson, M. H. (Eds.). (2001). *Primary pediatric care* (4th ed.). St. Louis: Mosby.

Jackson, P. L., & Vessey, J. A. (Eds.). (2000). *Primary care of the child with a chronic condition* (3rd ed.). St. Louis: Mosby.

Lane, P. A. (1996). Sickle cell disease. *Pediatric Clinics of North America, 43,* 639–664.

Lanzkowsky, P. (1995). *Manuel of pediatric hematology and oncology* (2nd ed.). New York: Churchill Livingstone.

National Institutes of Health (NIH). (1996). *Management and therapy of sickle cell disease* (3rd ed.) (NIH Publication No. 96-2117) Washington, DC: U.S. Government Printing Office.

Siberry, G. K., & Iannone, R. (Eds.). (2000). *The Harriet Lane handbook* (15th ed.). St. Louis: Mosby.

Werner, E. J. (1996). von Willebrand disease in children and adolescents. *Pediatric Clinics of North America, 43,* 683–707.

Hematological and Oncological Disorders In Adults

Sister Maria Salerno

Common Anemias

Anemia describes a symptom of abnormally low red blood cell count, quality of hemoglobin, and/or volume of packed cells. The World Health Organization defines it in terms of peripheral blood hemoglobin < 13.0 grams(g) [hematocrit < 42%] for men and < 12.0 grams [hematocrit < 36%] for women. Anemias are classified on the basis of red cell morphology (microcytic, normocytic, or macrocytic) and amount of pigment they contain (hypochromic, normochromic), or the etiology.

Microcytic Anemias (MCV < 80μ^3)

Iron Deficiency Anemia

- Definition: A microcytic, hypochromic anemia with a mean corpuscular volume (MCV) < 80μ^3 caused by insufficient iron for hemoglobin synthesis; may be normocytic, normochromic in early stage
- Etiology/Incidence
  1. Inadequate iron intake (< 1 to 2 mg/day), e.g., infants on milk only diets, persons on vegetarian diets, alcoholics, pregnant women or adolescents whose demand is increased
  2. Impaired absorption of iron, e.g., after gastrectomy, in Celiac disease
  3. Slow, persistent blood loss, e.g., menorrhagia, gastritis, aspirin ingestion, polyps, GI neoplasms, peptic ulcer disease, esophageal varices, hemorrhoids; in adult males and postmenopausal females acute or chronic hemorrhage is most common cause
  4. One of the most common anemias throughout the world; particularly prevalent in women of childbearing age; estimated 20% of adult women, 50% of pregnant women, and 3% of adult males in the U.S. have iron deficiency
- Signs and Symptoms
  1. Depend on:
     a. Rate at which anemia develops
     b. Age of the individual
     c. Individual's compensatory mechanisms
     d. Activity level
     e. Underlying disease state
     f. Severity of the anemia
  2. General signs and symptoms
     a. Easily fatigued
     b. Dyspnea on exertion
     c. Dizziness

    d. Listlessness

    e. Pallor (conjunctiva, nail beds, mucous membranes)

    f. Faintness

    g. Weakness

    h. Headaches

    i. Tachycardia

    j. Wide pulse pressure

    k. Heart murmurs

    l. Myocardial hypertrophy

    m. Angina

    n. Anorexia

    o. Pica

- Differential Diagnosis
    1. Thalassemia
    2. Sideroblastic anemia
    3. Anemia of chronic disease
    4. Lead poisoning

- Physical Findings
    1. General appearance—pale, lethargic; no overt signs if anemia is mild
    2. Vital signs—pulse and respirations may be increased in moderate to severe anemia; in severe cases postural hypotension may be evident
    3. Integumentary—pallor and dryness of skin and mucous membranes; brittle, flattened, ridged, concave, or spoon shaped nails (koilonychia); brittle, fine hair
    4. HEENT—smooth, shiny, beefy-red appearance of the tongue with atrophy of the papillae; angular stomatitis or cheilitis; pale conjunctiva and gums
    5. Cardiovascular—tachycardia, mild cardiac enlargement; functional systolic murmurs in severe anemias
    6. Abdominal—may be some hepatic enlargement
    7. Neurological—usually within normal limits; in severe anemia confusion may be evident

- Diagnostic Tests/Findings
    1. See Table 1 and 2 for laboratory tests used in diagnosis of common anemias
    2. Routine CBC (with peripheral smear)
        a. Hemoglobin— < 14 g/dL in males; < 12 g/dL in females

b.   Hct— < 42% in males; < 36% in females

c.   Low MCV (microcytic) and MCHC (hypochromic)

d.   Low erythrocyte count (RBC)

e.   Increased red cell distribution width (RDW)

3.   Iron status determinants—serum ferritin is considered the most sensitive and most specific for iron deficiency; bone marrow studies are done if the diagnosis is unclear and/or there is a lack of response to a three week therapeutic trial

Table 1

Common Laboratory Tests Used in Diagnosing Anemia

Hematocrit (Hct)	Relative amount of plasma to total red blood cell mass; measure of RBC concentration. Normal 40-54% males; 38-47% females
Hemoglobin (Hgb)	Basic screening test for anemia. Main component of erythrocytes. Vehicle for transport of O_2 & CO_2 Normal 13.5-18 g/100 mL males; 12.0-15 g/100 mL females
Red Blood Cell Count (RBC)	Measure of number of Hgb carrying red blood cells (RBC, erythrocytes); needed to calculate other RBC indices
Mean Corpuscular Volume (MCV)	Mathematical measure of average RBC size; expressed in micro cubic millimeters; value classifies cells as microcytic, normocytic, macrocytic; normal $80\text{-}100\mu^3$
Mean Corpuscular Hgb (MCH)	Mathematical measure of hemoglobin concentration of average RBC; expressed in picograms; calculated by dividing Hgb in grams by number of RBC; allows for classification of RBC as hypochromic, normochromic; normal 27-31 pg/cell
Mean Corpuscular Hgb Concentration (MCHC)	Mathematical measure of concentration of Hgb in grams per 100 mL of RBC; normal 32-36 g/dL or 32%-36%; little help in identifying hypochromia or microcytosis
Red Cell Distribution width (RDW)	Mathematical coefficient of width variation in red cell size—RDW increase indicates greater variation in cell size
Serum Iron (SI)	Concentration of iron bound to transferrin; inverse correlation with TIBC; normal 50-150 µg/dL in adults; insensitive to early iron deficiency
Total Iron Binding Capacity (TIBC)	Measures amount of iron that transferrin can still bind; inverse correlation with serum iron; normal 250-450 µg/dL in adults
Bilirubin (indirect)	Fractionation of total bilirubin; reflects breakdown of hemoglobin; elevated levels indicate hemolysis
% Transferrin Saturation (% SAT)	100 X SI/TIBC; low sensitivity for iron deficiency Normal 20-50%
Serum Ferritin	Correlates roughly with total iron stores; no diurnal variation; not affected by exogenous ingestion or injection, or specimen contamination; most sensitive and specific for iron deficiency Normal males 16-300 µg/L; females 4-161 µg/L (Nicoll, 1998)
Coombs Indirect	Detects free antibodies in patient's serum and certain RBC antigens
Peripheral Blood Smear	Smear of whole blood stained with Wright's stain; variations in cell morphology and staining characteristics important to diagnosis of hematologic conditions
Bone Marrow	Marrow aspirated for microscopic examination; indicated when anemia not obviously due to iron deficiency; iliac crest preferred to sternum site
NOTE: Laboratory values differ in different labs. Check normals in laboratory where tests are conducted	

Table 2

**Select Morphological and Etiologic Categories
of Anemia and Related Laboratory Findings**

	Macrocytic (MCV> 100)		Microcytic (MCV <80)		Normocytic (MCV 80-100)
	B₁₂ Deficiency	*Folate Deficiency*	*Iron Deficiency*	*Thalassemia*	*Anemia of Chronic Disease*
Reticulocyte Ct	low	low	low	normal/sl. high	normal/low
MCH	normal	normal	low	low	normal
Fe	high	high	normal/low	normal/sl. high	low-high
TIBC	normal	normal	high	normal	normal/low
Bilirubin	sl. high	sl. high	normal	high	normal
Ferritin	high	high	low	normal	normal/high
B₁₂	low	normal	normal	normal	normal
Folate	normal	low	normal	normal/low	normal/low

a. High total iron binding capacity (TIBC)—usually normal or low in anemia of chronic disease (ACD)

b. Low serum ferritin < 12 µg/L—infection, chronic disease, and liver disease may raise ferritin levels and mask coexisting iron deficiency; in these cases a serum ferritin level < 30 µg/L is consistent with iron deficiency

c. Serum iron—low < 50 µg/dL; may be normal in early stages (oral contraceptives may cause false elevation)

d. Low serum transferrin saturation — < 20%

e. Bone marrow studies

(1) Show depletion of iron (on staining), normocytic hyperplasia

(2) Usually not part of initial work up

4. Bilirubin—normal

- Management/Treatment

1. Diagnostic

a. Once diagnosis is established underlying cause must be identified and if possible, corrected; bleeding must be suspected in the absence of clearly identifiable nutritional intake deficiency or increased body need

b. Search for infection, trauma, neoplasm, GI disorders

c. Stool guaiac, bilirubin, and additional studies may be needed to establish etiology

d. Obtain physician consult on any patient with:

(1) Hct < 25%/dL

(2) Positive stool guaiac or history of bleeding

(3) Family history of anemia

(4) Suspected underlying inflammatory, infectious, or malignant disease

(5) Failure to respond to iron supplementation

2. Therapeutic

    a. Oral iron replacement

        (1) Oral is safer and much less expensive than IM or IV

        (2) Begin six month trial of ferrous sulfate tablets, 300 to 325 mg (depending on brand) three times a day after meals

        (3) Determine effectiveness of iron replacement therapy during the first two weeks of therapy (increased reticulocyte count)

        (4) Refer those on oral iron replacement therapy to a physician if 2 g/100 mL increase in Hgb is not seen in 3 to 4 weeks; in uncomplicated iron deficiency, a 1 g per week increase is expected

        (5) Levels return to normal within two months, 3 to 6 months more needed to replace stores

        (6) Response failure usually due to noncompliance

    b. Parenteral iron is indicated if patient can not tolerate or absorb oral iron or if iron loss exceeds oral replacement; IM or IV iron dextran is used (very rarely used)

        (1) More expensive

        (2) Associated with significant side effects

            (a) Anaphylaxis

            (b) Phlebitis

            (c) Regional adenopathy

            (d) Serum-sickness type reaction

            (e) Staining of IM injection sites

        (3) Dose based on the patient's weight

3. Education

    a. Cause of iron deficiency and treatment plan

    b. Purpose, dosage, side effects, toxic effects of iron replacement

        (1) Side effects of nausea, GI irritation, constipation, diarrhea, and black stools

        (2) Food and fluid taken concurrently may interfere with absorption but may be warranted to alleviate gastric distress

(3) Taking with orange juice or other source of vitamin C (ascorbic acid) will enhance absorption

(4) Milk and antacids will interfere with absorption

(5) Monitor and discuss with patients concurrent use of over the counter medications—some products such as urine and stool deodorizers often used by elderly with incontinence problems can lead to iron overdose and heart failure

(6) Therapy should continue for six or more months to replenish tissue stores

c. Medication should be kept out of reach of children as iron overdose can be fatal to them

d. Nutrition—foods high in iron include organ and lean meats, egg yolk, shellfish, apricots, peaches, prunes, grapes, raisins, green leafy vegetables, iron fortified breads and cereals

e. Activity—frequent rest periods as needed

Thalassemia

- Definition: Thalassemia is a group of genetic inherited syndromes of abnormal hemoglobin synthesis

- Etiology/Incidence

  1. Inherited, autosomal recessive disorder that results in impaired synthesis of either the alpha or beta chain of adult hemoglobin; four genes control alpha chain production, two control beta chain production

  2. Second most common cause of microcytic anemia

     a. Alpha Thalassemia more common in Blacks, Chinese, Vietnamese, Cambodians, and Laotians

     b. Beta Thalassemia more common in those of Mediterranean descent (Italians, Greeks, some Arabs and Sephardic Jews)

  3. In U.S. more common than iron deficiency in African-Americans, Asian-Americans, and Italian-Americans

- Signs and Symptoms: The severity of the anemia can range from mild to severe depending on the number of hemoglobin controlling genes involved; forms seen in adults include:

  1. Alpha trait (carrier state) (1 of 4 alpha chain-forming genes affected)—usually asymptomatic

  2. Alpha-Thalassemia Minor (2 of 4 alpha chain-forming genes affected) and Beta-Thalassemia minor (heterozygous form)—both are usually asymptomatic and have mild presentations with mild to moderate microcytic, hypochromic anemia, enlarged liver and spleen, bronze coloring of the skin, and bone marrow hyperplasia

3. Beta Thalassemia Major (homozygous form affecting both beta chain-forming genes) also called Cooley's anemia—severe anemia with significant cardiovascular burden; high output congestive failure is common; fractures related to bone marrow expansion; retarded growth and maturation; in addition to general signs and symptoms presented in section on Iron Deficiency Anemia

4. Hemoglobin H disease (3 of 4 alpha hemoglobin chain-forming genes affected)—occurs predominantly in Chinese; moderate to severe microcytic anemia with splenomegaly

- Differential Diagnosis

  1. Iron deficiency anemia

  2. Sideroblastic anemia

  3. Anemia of chronic disease

  4. Lead poisoning—not common in adults unless occupation related

- Physical Findings: Will generally be within normal limits unless the more severe forms of thalassemia are encountered

  1. General appearance—pallor or bronze appearance; mild listlessness

  2. Abdominal—enlarged liver, enlarged spleen

  3. Cardiovascular—tachycardia, widened pulse pressure, systolic murmur if anemia is moderate or severe

  4. Respiratory—may have increased respiratory rate

  5. Musculoskeletal—some bone deformity of the face (chipmunk deformity) related to expansion of bones caused by hyperplastic marrow

  6. Neurologic—within normal limits

- Diagnostic Tests/Findings

  1. Hgb—decreased

  2. MCV—low

  3. Serum iron—normal or increased

  4. TIBC—normal

  5. Ferritin—normal or increased

  6. RDW—normal

  7. Reticulocyte count—may be normal or increased

  8. Hemoglobin electrophoresis—demonstrates decreased alpha or beta hemoglobin chains

  9. Peripheral smear will show microcytosis, variable hypochromia, target cells (thin, fragile RBC), basophilic stippling

10. Skull and skeletal radiographs—widened marrow spaces in skull and long bones; osteoporosis

- Management/Treatment

    1. No specific treatment for mild to moderate forms

    2. Iron supplementation generally contraindicated in all thalassemias since iron overload can result—patients with alpha trait and co-existing iron deficiency should be referred to physician for iron supplementation

    3. Sometimes chronic folate supplementation is used

    4. Severe forms should be referred to a hematologist for treatment which often includes transfusions and chelation therapy to avoid fatal iron overload (hemochromatosis)

    5. Refer for genetic counseling

    6. Stress overall good nutrition without additional iron supplementation

    7. Discuss signs and symptoms of iron overload

        a. Weakness/lassitude

        b. Loss of body hair

        c. Weight loss

        d. Palmar erythema

        e. Gynecomastia

        f. Loss of libido

        g. Abdominal pain

        h. Thinning, darkening skin

        i. Pain and or stiffness in joints

        j. Blurred vision or other symptoms related to onset of diabetes

        k. Shortness of breath

        l. Swelling in ankles

    8. Document findings to avoid

        a. Unnecessary repeated work-ups

        b. Inappropriate iron supplementation

Macrocytic Anemias (MCV > 100μ^3)

Pernicious Anemia

- Definition: A megaloblastic, macrocytic, normochromic anemia caused by a deficiency of intrinsic factor produced by the stomach which results in malabsorption of vitamin B_{12} necessary for DNA synthesis and maturation of RBC

- Etiology/Incidence
    1. Possibly due to an autoimmune reaction involving the gastric parietal cell that results in nonproduction of intrinsic factor and atrophy of gastric mucosa
    2. Can also occur secondary to other factors which lead to decreased production of intrinsic factor or decreased absorption of B_{12}
        a. Loss of parietal cells post-gastrectomy
        b. Overgrowth of intestinal organisms
        c. Ileal resection or abnormalities
        d. Fish tape worm
        e. Congenital enzyme deficiencies
    3. Common in Caucasians of Northern European descent
    4. Both sexes equally affected
    5. Usually presents around age 60
    6. Increased incidence in those with other immunologic disease
- Signs and Symptoms
    1. Weakness
    2. Sore tongue or glossitis
    3. Peripheral paresthesia—numbness, burning, tingling
    4. Palpitations
    5. Dizziness
    6. Swelling of legs
    7. Anorexia
    8. Diarrhea
    9. Mucositis
    10. Dementia and spinal cord degeneration in advanced stages
- Differential Diagnosis
    1. Folate deficiency
    2. Anemia of liver disease
    3. Myelodysplastic syndromes
- Physical Findings

1. Vital signs—temperature may be slightly elevated, wide pulse pressure, pulse and respirations may be elevated if anemia is severe

2. General appearance—premature aging; premature graying of hair

3. HEENT—smooth beefy red tongue; sclera and skin may be slightly icteric

4. Cardiovascular—systolic flow murmur, tachycardia, and cardiomegaly if anemia is severe

5. Abdomen—hepatomegaly and splenomegaly may be evident

6. Neurological—deep tendon reflexes increased or decreased; diminished position sense; poor or absent vibratory sense in lower extremities; ataxia; poor finger-nose coordination; positive Romberg and Babinski; mental status changes ranging from mild forgetfulness and irritability to psychotic behavior

- Diagnostic Tests/Findings

   1. Hgb and Hct—decreased

   2. RBC—decreased

   3. Reticulocytes—normal or low

   4. MCV—increased > 100 μ^3

   5. MCHC—normal

   6. Serum B_{12}—decreased < 100 pg/mL

   7. Increased LDH

   8. Serum folate and/or RBC level—normal or decreased

   9. Serum bilirubin—increased

   10. Urinalysis—increased urobilinogen

- Management/Treatment

   1. Diagnostic—consult with physician regarding those:

      a. With other immunologic diseases

      b. With a history of B_{12} replacement

      c. Suspected of having pernicious anemia for further testing, e.g., those with neurological symptoms but without macrocytosis or overt anemia; might include:

         (1) GI radiographic studies

         (2) Gastric analysis—absence of free hydrochloric acid after histamine or pentagastrin injection

         (3) Bone marrow aspiration—hyperplastic, megaloblastic marrow

         (4) Schilling test (tests absorption of radiolabeled vitamin B_{12} both with and without administration of intrinsic factor on basis of 24 hour urine excretion) to distinguish between primary and secondary causes

2. Therapeutic

    a. B_{12} (cyanocobalamin) 100 μg IM daily for 1 week; decrease frequency and administer a total of 2,000 μg during the first 6 weeks of therapy; maintenance treatment requires lifelong administration of 100 μg IM monthly

    b. In select cases, oral cobalamin in high doses (1,000 μg per day) can replace parenteral for maintenance, but must be taken daily and consistently

    c. If anemia is severe may need K^+ supplementation to avoid hypokalemia

    d. Follow up elderly and those with cardiovascular symptoms 48 hours after initiating therapy; rapid increase in RBC production can lead to hypervolemia in these persons

    e. Consider concomitant iron supplementation during first month of therapy; rapid blood cell regeneration increases iron requirement and may lead to iron deficiency

3. Education

    a. Teach client about etiology and nature of the disease

    b. Discuss need for lifelong B_{12} replacement by injection

    c. Provide client with information on side effects of B_{12} injections

        (1) Pain and burning at injection site

        (2) Peripheral vascular thrombosis

        (3) Transient diarrhea

    d. CNS symptoms/signs are reversible if present < 6 months prior to treatment

    e. Teach client or family member to administer injections or refer to home care agency to provide injections

    f. Teach comfort and safety measures to clients with neurological involvement (can be arrested but not reversed with treatment)

4. Follow-up—check initial hematologic response in 4 to 6 weeks; then every 6 months for Hct and stool for occult blood; endoscopy every 5 years; incidence of gastric cancer increased in persons with pernicious anemia

Folic Acid Deficiency Anemia

*   Definition: Macrocytic, normochromic, megaloblastic anemia caused by a deficiency of folic acid needed for DNA synthesis, RBC maturation, and maintenance of gastric mucosa

*   Etiology/Incidence

    1. Inadequate intake may be relative to malabsorption syndrome or increased demand as in pregnancy and infancy; body stores depleted more rapidly than B_{12}

2. Drugs that may cause decreased folic acid levels include oral contraceptives, phenytoin, antimalarials, estrogen, chloramphenicol, phenobarbital; trimethoprim/sulfamethoxazole, and sulfasalazine

3. Found in all races and in all age groups

4. More common than pernicious anemia, especially in alcoholics and other chronically malnourished persons, e.g., anorexics, many elderly, and those who do not eat fresh fruits and vegetables (especially green leafy) or overcook them

- Signs and Symptoms
    1. Similar to those of B_{12} deficiency but more severe; neurological signs are absent
    2. General signs and symptoms
        a. Easily fatigued
        b. Dyspnea on exertion
        c. Dizziness
        d. Listlessness
        e. Pallor (conjunctiva, nail beds, mucous membranes)
        f. Faintness
        g. Weakness
        h. Headaches
        i. Tachycardia
        j. Wide pulse pressure
        k. Heart murmurs
        l. Myocardial hypertrophy
        m. Angina
        n. Anorexia
        o. Pica

- Differential Diagnosis
    1. Pernicious anemia
    2. Anemia of liver disease
    3. Myelodysplastic syndromes

- Physical Findings: Similar to those found in most anemias
    1. General appearance—pale, lethargic or no overt signs if anemia is mild
    2. Vital signs—pulse and respirations may be increased in moderate to severe anemia; in severe cases postural hypotension may be evident

3. Integumentary—pallor and dryness of skin and mucous membranes; brittle nails; brittle, fine hair

4. HEENT—glossitis, angular stomatitis or cheilitis; pale conjunctiva and gums

5. Cardiovascular—tachycardia; mild cardiac enlargement; functional systolic murmurs in severe anemias

6. Abdominal—may be some hepatic enlargement

7. Neurological—usually within normal limits

- Diagnostic Tests/Findings

  1. Hct—decreased

  2. Reticulocyte count—normal or decreased

  3. MCV—elevated

  4. MCHC—normal

  5. RBC folate level— < 150 ng/mL and/or RBC level decreased

  6. Serum folate— < 3 ng/mL; less reliable than RBC folate

  7. Schilling test—normal

  8. Serum B_{12}—normal

- Management/Treatment

  1. Diagnostic—consult with physician regarding clients with suspected folate deficiency for differential diagnosis of concurrent B_{12} deficiency and treatment

  2. Therapeutic—folate 1 mg orally or parenterally per day

     a. Duration of treatment dependent on etiology and its elimination

     b. If related to malabsorption (e.g., Sprue) up to 5 mg/day

     c. Large doses of folic acid will correct hematologic abnormalities of B_{12} deficiency but not arrest neurological abnormalities.

  3. Education—especially important for women of childbearing age as deficiency during first trimester is associated with neural tube defects in the fetus

     a. Nature and cause of anemia

     b. Need for and purpose of therapeutic replacement

     c. Teach dietary sources of folic acid which include asparagus, bananas, fish, green leafy vegetables, peanut butter, oatmeal, red beans, beef liver, wheat bran

        (1) Encourage daily intake from these foods

        (2) Instructions in preparation as overcooking can destroy folic acid

        (3) Provide client with list of foods high in folic acid

      d. Need for frequent rest periods until anemia is corrected

      e. Importance of good oral hygiene

  4. Follow-up

      a. Check initial hematologic response with Hct and reticulocyte count in 4 to 6 weeks

         (1) Reticulocyte count should begin to increase within 2 to 3 days after therapy is begun and should peak in 5 to 7 days

         (2) Hct begins to rise after the second week

         (3) Total correction expected within 2 months

      b. Individuals with a good response can be followed every 6 to 12 months if they must continue therapy

Normocytic Anemias (MCV 80–100 μ^3)

- Hypoproliferative—reticulocyte count normal or decreased < 3% secondary to decreased bone marrow production

- Hyperproliferative—reticulocyte count increased > 3% secondary to increased hemolysis or bleeding

Anemia of Chronic Disease (ACD)

- Definition: A chronic, normochromic, normocytic, hypoproliferative anemia associated with chronic inflammatory disease, e.g., systemic lupus, rheumatoid arthritis; infection, e.g., bacterial endocarditis, tuberculosis, AIDS, Crohn's disease, and some malignancies; *often progresses to a hypochromic anemia*

- Etiology/Incidence

  1. Etiology not fully understood but involves decreased erythrocyte life span, ineffective erythropoiesis, and disturbances of the iron cycle

  2. Most common cause of hypoproliferative, normocytic anemia

  3. Exact incidence unknown, however association with so many other disorders probably ranks it second to iron deficiency in incidence

- Sign and Symptoms

  1. General symptoms common to all anemias such as fatigue, weakness, exertional dyspnea, lightheadedness, and anorexia

  2. Usually fewer and milder than most other anemias

  3. Other signs and symptoms are usually related to the specific underlying disease and may be more overt than those of anemia

- Differential Diagnosis

  1. Aplastic anemia

2. Pure red blood cell aplasia

3. Infiltration marrow diseases

4. Exclude reversible causes

- Physical Findings

    1. General appearance—may appear thin, pale, toxic

    2. Vital signs—increased pulse and respirations

    3. Skin—may be pale, jaundiced, moist

    4. HEENT—sclera may be icteric, tongue may be coated

    5. Cardiovascular—cardiomegaly, tachycardia, systolic murmurs

    6. Abdomen—splenomegaly, hepatomegaly

- Diagnostic Tests/Findings

    1. Hct—low

    2. Hgb—low (if < 9g/dL consider other causes)

    3. MCV—normal or slightly low

    4. Serum iron—low

    5. TIBC—normal or low

    6. Serum ferritin—normal or increased

    7. Percentage of iron saturation (FE/TIBC)—30% or more rules out iron deficiency

- Management/Treatment

    1. Treatment of associated disease

    2. Adequate nutritional intake; use of B_{12}, folic acid, and liver extract have not been effective in treatment of this type anemia

    3. Adequate rest

    4. Consult with physician regarding clients with suspected anemia of chronic disease for further testing (bone marrow biopsy), and treatment of underlying disorder

    5. Education—patient education will most likely be centered on etiology and treatment of the underlying chronic disease and its relationship to anemia

    6. Follow-up—will depend on identified etiology

Sickle Cell Anemia

- Definition: A chronic hemolytic anemia characterized by sickle-shaped RBC

- Etiology/Incidence

    1. Autosomal recessive genetic disorder; individual is homozygous for hemoglobin (Hb SS)

2. Abnormal hemoglobin (Hb S) develops in place of hemoglobin A (Hb A)

3. Some individuals may have *sickle cell trait* (heterozygous with about $\frac{1}{4}$ of their hemoglobin in abnormal S form and remainder as normal A

4. Mutation that causes Hb S to develop involves one amino acid; one valine amino acid is substituted for a glutamic acid

5. Prevalent in black persons of African or African-American ancestry; also found at a lower frequency in persons of Mediterranean ancestry

- Signs and Symptoms

  1. Sickle Cell Trait

     a. Essentially asymptomatic except in extreme conditions

     b. Symptoms from vaso-occlusion occur only in cases of severe hypoxia

  2. Sickle Cell Anemia

     a. Manifestations due to anemia, vaso-occlusive events, and to secondary end-organ damage:

        (1) Osteomyelitis

        (2) Retinopathy

        (3) Renal disease—hematuria

        (4) Cardiomegaly

        (5) Nonpalable spleen in adults

     b. Increased susceptibility to infection

     c. Vaso-occlusive crises

        (1) Due to an increased rate of sickling

        (2) Precipitating factors include conditions that cause hypoxia or deoxygenation of the RBC, e.g., viral or bacterial infections, high altitudes, emotional or physical stress, surgery, blood loss, dehydration; occasionally crisis occurs spontaneously

        (3) Episodes characterized by sudden onset of excruciating pain in back, chest, or extremities

        (4) Occasionally low-grade fever may occur 1 to 2 days following attack

        (5) Pain may last from hours to days

        (6) Severe abdominal pain with vomiting may be present

- Differential Diagnosis

  1. Acute pulmonary infarction without sickle β thalassemia

  2. Acute hepatitis

  3. Choledocholithiasis

4. Cholecystitis

- Physical Findings

    1. During vaso-occlusive crises, there may be no external findings such as heat, swelling or tenderness over the affected bones; if bone infarction occurs close to a joint an effusion can develop

    2. Chronic findings

        a. Skin ulcers/jaundice

        b. Mild scleral icterus; retinal hemorrhage or detachment, neovascularization

        c. Cardiomegaly, systolic murmur

        d. Hepatomegaly

        e. Degenerative arthritis

- Diagnostic Tests/Findings

    1. Peripheral smear

        a. Sickle Cell Trait—normal

        b. Sickle Cell Anemia—partially or completely sickled cells

    2. Sickle Cell preparation/Sickledex

        a. Sickle Cell Trait—sickle cells

        b. Sickle Cell Anemia—sickle cells

        c. Used for initial screening

        d. Can not differentiate between anemia/trait

    3. Hemoglobin electrophoresis

        a. Sickle Cell Trait—Hb S and Hb A

        b. Sickle Cell Anemia—Hb S

        c. Used for confirmation and discrimination between anemia/trait

- Management/Treatment

    1. Physician referral for suspected cases and consultation for management

    2. Therapeutic—primarily supportive

        a. Chronic folic acid supplementation

        b. Use of cytotoxic agents to reduce frequency of painful episodes

        c. Antibiotic prophylaxis

    3. In acute painful episodes

        a. Analgesia

        b. Large volume IV fluids

    c.   Oxygen to treat hypoxia

    d.   Antibiotics to treat associated bacterial infections

    e.   Blood transfusions reserved for aplastic or hemolytic crises, and during third trimester of pregnancy

4. Patient education

    a.   Basis of disease and reasons for supportive care

    b.   Methods to avoid crises

    c.   Pain control

    d.   Availability of support groups

5. Referral for genetic counseling of identified heterozygotes (sickle cell trait) and prenatal diagnostic services for pregnancies at risk for sickle cell anemia

Leukemia

- Definition: Acquired, neoplastic, myeloproliferative disorder of hematopoietic stem cells
- Etiology/Incidence
  1. In most cases no known cause can be found
  2. Possible causes include:
     - a. Exposure to ionizing radiation and certain chemicals, e.g., benzene, prior exposure to alkylating agents
     - b. Genetic and congenital factors
  3. Incidence of all leukemias is approximately 13 per 100,000/per year
  4. More frequent in males than females
- General features of the four common forms of leukemia are shown in Table 3
- Differential Diagnosis
  1. Viral induced cytopenia, lymphadenopathy
  2. Immune or drug-induced cytopenia
  3. Aplastic anemia
- Diagnostic Tests/Findings (see Table 3)
  1. CBC/differential—subnormal RBC, neutrophils and occasionally subnormal platelets
  2. Sedimentation rate—elevated
  3. Reticulocyte count— < 0.5
  4. Bone marrow studies—confirmatory for final diagnosis

Table 3

Comparison of Most Common Types of Leukemia

Type	Age of Onset	Signs & Symptoms Physical Findings	Diagnostic Tests/Findings	Prognosis
Acute Lymphocytic	Childhood More gradual rise in frequency in later life; 20% of acute adult	Fever; pallor; bleeding; anorexia; fatigue; generalized lymphadenopathy and infection, joint pain etc.	Cytopenia, pancytopenia WBC—H, L, or N RBC, Hgb, Hct-L Platelets-L Bone marrow-lymphoblasts	Good response to treatment 80% of adults have complete remission
Acute Myelogenous	Increase with age; 50% under age of 50	Fatigue; weakness; headache; mouth sores; bleeding; fever; sternal tenderness; occasional lymphadenopathy	RBC, Hgb, Hct-L Platelet ct—very low WBC—H to L Myeloblasts—many	Remission rates range from 50 to 85%; patients >50 years are less likely to achieve complete remission
Chronic Lymphocytic	Middle and old age	May be asymptomatic; may have fatigue anorexia, weight loss, dyspnea on exertion; splenomegaly; lymphadenopathy; hepatomegaly	Hallmark is sustained absolute lymphocytosis 40,000-150,000/μL; Bone marrow—increased lymphocytes	Median survival— approximately 10 yrs
Chronic Myelogenous	Occurs most often at median age of 42	May be asymptomatic; or insidious onset of nonspecific symptoms, e.g., fatigue, weakness, anorexia, weight loss, fever, night sweats, splenomegaly; blurred vision; resp. distress; priapism, sternal tenderness	RBC, Hgb, Hct-L Platelet count—H early, L later; WBC-H; leukocytosis with immature granulocytes WBC— about 150,000-200,000/μL in symptomatic pt; Bone marrow—Ph[1] chromosome presence is significant	No advantage to early therapy if asymptomatic; 60% of young adults with allogenic bone marrow transplants complete cure; median survival in non-transplanted patients is 3 to 4 years.

L = low; N = normal; H = high

5.   Chest radiograph—identification of mediastinal mass

6.   Ultrasound or CT—organomegaly

- Management/Treatment

    1.   Physician referral for suspected cases

        a.   Goal of treatment is remission

        b.   Chemotherapy

        c.   Bone marrow transplantation

    2.   Assistance in meeting psychosocial needs

    3.   Assistance for patient and families in adjusting to chronic effects of illness, e.g., dependence, withdrawal, changes in role responsibilities, alterations in body image

    4.   Patient education

        a.   Importance of compliance with chemotherapy regimens; side effects and management

b. Disease process and rationale for treatment

c. Adaptation to any physical limitations

Non-Hodgkin's Lymphoma

- Definition: Heterogenous group of lymphocytic malignancies with absence of giant Reed-Sternberg cells characteristic of Hodgkin's Disease

- Etiology/Incidence

    1. Etiology unclear; animal studies have suggested a viral etiology

    2. Other factors associated with increased incidence include:

        a. Ionizing radiation

        b. Hereditary predisposition

        c. Congenital or acquired immunodeficiency

        d. Exposure to pesticides

    3. Approximately 45,000 new cases occur each year in the U.S., and appear to be increasing (Freedman & Nadler, 1997)

    4. Most common neoplasm between ages of 20 and 40; with increased incidence of AIDS, number of cases has sharply increased

- Signs and Symptoms

    1. More than $\frac{2}{3}$ of patients present with persistent painless peripheral lymphadenopathy

    2. Some patients may present with persistent cough and chest discomfort (mediastinal involvement)

    3. If abdominal contents involved, chronic pain, abdominal fullness, early satiety or viscus obstruction may be presenting symptoms

    4. Diffuse disease may present with skin lesions, testicular masses

    5. Fever, night sweats, weight loss.

- Differential Diagnosis

    1. Infectious mononucleosis

    2. Cytomegalovirus infection

    3. Human immunodeficiency virus involvement

    4. Toxoplasmosis

    5. Other malignant tumors

    6. Cat-scratch disease

    7. Tuberculosis

    8. Syphilis

9. Sarcoidosis

- Physical Findings

    1. Painless peripheral lymphadenopathy may be initial finding

    2. May present with abdominal mass, massive splenomegaly

    3. Early systemic findings usually absent

- Diagnostic Tests/Findings

    1. Requires skilled interpretation of adequate tumor tissue to determine tumor architecture and cell type

    2. B cell and T cell typing—complements pathologic interpretation

    3. Bone marrow biopsy—pathologic confirmation of disease process

    4. Staging procedures conducted once diagnosis established—no perfect classification system exists; various types include the Rappaport classification, Luke and Collins classification, the International Panel Working Formulation (NCI), Ann Arbor staging system

    5. Chest radiograph may show mediastinal mass

- Management/Treatment (Based on grade and extent of disease)

    1. Radiotherapy

    2. Chemotherapy

    3. Bone marrow transplantation

    4. Newer modalities include MAbs alone and combined with radionuclides or toxins to produce cytotoxic effects; cytokines, e.g., interferons, tumor necrosis factor and interleukin 2 are currently under study

    5. General considerations

        a. Prognosis not usually as good as with Hodgkin's disease

        b. Both family and patient require supportive therapy during diagnosis and treatment stages

        c. Education and necessity of drug compliance important factor

        d. Increased susceptibility to infection

Hodgkin's Disease

- Definition: Malignant disorder with lymphoreticular proliferation

- Etiology/Incidence

    1. Cause is unknown

    2. Approximately 8,000 new cases are diagnosed each year in the U.S.

    3. Average age is 32 years; peaks at 15 to 35 years and again after age 50

4. More common in males

- Signs and Symptoms

    1. Most patients present with a painless, enlarging mass, most often in the neck or occasionally in axilla or inguinal region; often the only manifestation at time of diagnosis

    2. Older patients may present with:

        a. Fatigue

        b. Weight loss

        c. Persistent fever and/or night sweats

    3. Pruritus—may be mild and localized, but may be progressive; rarely occurs in the absence of fever

    4. An unexplained symptom is immediate pain in diseased areas after consuming alcoholic beverages

- Differential Diagnosis

    1. Infectious mononucleosis

    2. Toxoplasmosis

    3. Cytomegalic inclusion disease

    4. Non-Hodgkin's lymphoma

    5. Leukemia

    6. Bronchogenic carcinoma

    7. Sarcoidosis

    8. Cat-scratch disease

- Physical Findings

    1. Initial findings are usually enlargement of cervical, axillary, or inguinal lymph nodes (movable, nontender)

    2. Other findings may include hepatomegaly and splenomegaly; usually not present unless the disease is advanced

- Diagnostic Tests/Findings

    1. Presence of characteristic Reed-Sternberg giant cell on biopsy of lymph node tissue or other sites (needle aspiration not sufficient)

    2. WBC—polymorphonuclear leukocytosis may be present

    3. CBC—hypochromic, microcytic anemia in advanced disease

    4. Low serum iron, low iron binding capacity

    5. Chest radiologic examinations—to determine mediastinal involvement

- Management/Treatment
    1. Physician referral for suspected cases
        a. Radiotherapy
        b. Chemotherapy
        c. Autologous bone marrow transplant for chemotherapy failures
    2. For treatment to be precise, Hodgkin's disease needs to be staged which involves determining the extent and involvement of the disease
    3. Psychosocial considerations for patient and family
    4. Since prognosis is usually good, patients need to be helped to deal with the disease realistically even though it is a malignant disorder
    5. Once patient is in remission, ongoing maintenance treatment is usually not needed; patients need to be instructed in the importance of returning for follow-up visits
    6. Patient education
        a. Gonadal side effects of treatment
        b. Consideration of sperm banking for males
        c. Risk of secondary malignancy

Questions
Select the best answer

A 50 year old male of Italian descent comes in for a routine work related health assessment. He has no complaints. His history and physical examination are unremarkable. A routine CBC indicates Hgb 11.2 g/100 mL, MCV $72\mu^3$, WBC 5.7×10^3, Hct 35%, MCH 25

1. Based on this information how would his anemia be classified?

   a. Normocytic, normochromic
   b. Microcytic, hypochromic
   c. Macrocytic, hypochromic
   d. Microcytic, normochromic

2. Which aspect of this patient's history would provide the least useful information for diagnostic decision making?

   a. Diet (including alcohol use)
   b. Social history
   c. Family history
   d. Medical history

You find that this patient has a diet with regular daily intake of lean red meats, vegetables, and fruits and he denies alcohol use except once or twice a year. He does use Maalox almost daily for indigestion. He says that weak blood runs in his family, although he has never had this problem. He has no surgical history and has never been treated for any medical problems except high cholesterol which was treated with diet and exercise

3. This information helps rule out which of the following as cause for his anemia?

   a. Folate deficiency
   b. Inadequate dietary intake
   c. GI bleeding
   d. Malabsorption of vitamins and minerals

4. This patient's lack of abnormal physical signs and symptoms:

   a. Probably indicates a lab error in the blood work
   b. Is not unusual given the degree of his anemia
   c. Is not unusual in a patient of this age
   d. May be masked by use of Maalox

5. Your next step would be to:

   a. Order B_{12} and folate serum levels
   b. Order serum iron and TIBC
   c. Obtain a urine culture
   d. Order a Schilling test

6. What other test would be essential at this point?

a. Stool guaiac
b. GI series
c. Bilirubin
d. Liver function tests

7. Which is the most likely etiology of the type of anemia exhibited in this patient?

a. B_{12} or folate deficiency
b. Chronic disease
c. Dehydration
d. GI bleeding

8. If you obtain a negative stool guaiac in a male patient with a microcytic, hypochromic anemia who has a low serum iron and a high TIBC, you would:

a. Begin ferrous sulfate 300 mg orally t.i.d.
b. Order a Schilling test
c. Repeat the stool guaiac
d. Refer to a hematologist

Mrs. M. is a 30-year-old graduate student from Morocco with a family and personal history of "weak blood" who presents with a complaint of abdominal pain, increasing fatigue, and weight loss. She has never needed treatment for her blood problem but has been supplementing her usually well balanced diet with high potency vitamin and mineral supplements because of the increased stress of graduate studies in a foreign country. A routine CBC indicates a mild microcytic, hypochromic anemia.

9. It is likely that this patient's "weak blood" is:

a. Thalassemia Minor
b. Thalassemia Major
c. Related to an unidentified chronic disease
d. Related to an iron deficiency from gastrointestinal bleeding

10. You need to consider which of the following as a strong etiology for her current symptoms?

a. Iron deficiency
b. Folate deficiency
c. Peptic ulcer
d. Iron overload

11. If further blood studies indicate a decreased TIBC and increased serum iron your next step should be which of the following?

a. Tell Mrs. M. to discontinue her vitamin/mineral supplements; obtain hematologic consult
b. Refer her for genetic counseling
c. Refer for hemoglobin electrophoresis
d. Begin chelation therapy and refer for a GI consult

Ms. Z is a 26 year old, black female who comes in complaining of fatigue, shortness of breath, and lightheadedness. Her history reveals no significant medical problems but several years of fad dieting without vitamin supplementation. Physical findings are unremarkable except for pallor of the mucous membranes, tachycardia, and a systolic flow murmur

12. Your next step would be to:

    a. Start B_{12} injections
    b. Order a CBC, reticulocyte count
    c. Order a TIBC and serum iron
    d. Start on multivitamins with iron

13. Further testing of Ms. Z. reveals a low reticulocyte count and macrocytic cells. Your next step should be to:

    a. Start B_{12} injections
    b. Order serum iron and TIBC
    c. Order RBC-folate and B_{12} levels
    d. Order a Schilling test

14. Which of the following would help in your differential diagnosis?

    a. Patient's history of ice pica
    b. Patient's use of oral contraceptives
    c. A confirmed diagnosis of sickle cell trait
    d. Family history of iron deficiency

15. The anemias most often associated with pregnancy are:

    a. Folic acid and iron deficiency
    b. Folic acid deficiency and Thalassemia
    c. Iron deficiency and Thalassemia
    d. Thalassemia and B_{12} deficiency

16. Neural tube defects in the fetus have been primarily associated with which type deficiency in the mother?

    a. Iron
    b. Folic Acid
    c. Vitamin B_{12}
    d. Vitamin E

17. Most common causes of megaloblastic, macrocytic anemia are:

    a. Folate and or B_{12} deficiency
    b. Chronic disease
    c. Iron deficiency and infection
    d. Hemolysis of blood cells

18. Patients with iron deficiency anemia should be instructed that:

    a. Return of normal blood values will occur within a week of oral iron supplementation

    b. Iron supplements will need to be taken for the rest of their life

    c. Taking iron preparations with milk will enhance absorption

    d. Iron preparation may be taken with meals

19. Elderly persons with pernicious anemia should:

    a. Be instructed to increase their dietary intake of foods high in B_{12}

    b. Be told they will not need to return for follow-up for at least a month after initiation of treatment

    c. Be told that oral B_{12} is safer and less expensive than parenteral replacement

    d. Be told that diarrhea can be a transient side effect of B_{12} injections

20. Which of the following would be included in a diet rich in iron?

    a. Peaches, eggs, beef

    b. Cereals, kale, cheese

    c. Red beans, enriched breads, squash

    d. Legumes, green beans, eggs

21. A woman taking folic acid supplements for Folic Acid Deficiency will need to know that:

    a. It will take several months before she will feel better

    b. Folic acid should not be taken with meals and may cause diarrhea

    c. Iron supplements are contraindicated while one is on folic acid

    d. Oral contraceptives, pregnancy and lactation increase dietary requirements for folic acid

22. In alcoholics with anemia:

    a. Pernicious anemia is more common than folic acid deficiency

    b. Iron deficiency, folic acid deficiency may coexist

    c. The alcohol interferes with iron absorption

    d. Oral vitamin replacement is contraindicated

23. Hypoproliferative normocytic anemia:

    a. Is marked by a normal or decreased reticulocyte count

    b. Is usually secondary to hemolysis or bleeding

    c. Is relatively rare and usually only associated with malignancies

    d. Is only associated with chronic infections

24. In normocytic anemia of chronic disease:

    a. Treatment is purely symptomatic

    b. Long term supplementation of folic acid and B_{12} is needed

    c. Treatment is focused on the associated disease

    d. Serum iron and TIBC are the most specific and sensitive diagnostic tests

25. Which of the following is true of anemia of chronic disease?

a. A Hgb of < 9 g/dL confirms the diagnosis
b. Symptoms associated with the anemia may be masked by the symptoms of the underlying disease
c. Is manifested by more severe signs than most of the other common anemias
d. Is never associated with reversible causes

26. Sickle Cell Anemia is caused by:

    a. Replacement of hemoglobin A with hemoglobin CS
    b. Transposition of glutamic acid on hemoglobin A molecule
    c. Abnormal hemoglobin S in place of hemoglobin A
    d. Sickle cell trait

27. The test used to differentiate sickle cell anemia/sickle cell trait is:

    a. Sickle cell preparation
    b. Peripheral smear
    c. Sickledex
    d. Hemoglobin electrophoresis

28. Chronic myelogonous leukemia usually presents with the following:

    a. Increased platelets and leukocytosis
    b. Presence of Reed-Sternberg cells in bone marrow aspirate
    c. Ph^1 chromosome in bone marrow
    d. With typical fatigue, weakness, anorexia and frequent nosebleeds

29. A 32-year-old male presents in the office with concerns about a lump in the area of his collar bone. He states that someone told him that it might be a sign of some kind of cancer. Your best response at this time would be to:

    a. Examine him and tell him to come back in two weeks to be re-evaluated
    b. Inquire whether he has any cats which might cause Cat Scratch fever
    c. Work him up for a possibility of infectious mononucleosis
    d. Examine him with referral to physician for possible Hodgkin's disease work-up

30. Diagnosis of Hodgkin's disease is based upon:

    a. Hepatomegaly with fatigue, weight loss, pruritus, and night sweats
    b. Presence of Ph^1 chromosome in lymphoid tissue
    c. Extensive lymphadenopathy with elevated WBC count
    d. Presence of Reed-Sternberg cells in lymph node tissue

Answers

1.	b	16.	b
2.	b	17.	a
3.	b	18.	d
4.	b	19.	d
5.	b	20.	a
6.	a	21.	d
7.	d	22.	b
8.	c	23.	a
9.	a	24.	c
10.	d	25.	b
11.	a	26.	c
12.	b	27.	d
13.	c	28.	c
14.	b	29.	d
15.	a	30.	d

Bibliography

Abramsen, N., & Melton, B. (2000). Leukocytosis: Basics of clinical assessment. *American Family Physician, 62,* 2053–2060.

Brill, J. R., & Baumgardner, D. J. (2000). Normocytic anemia. *American Family Physician, 62,* 2255–2263.

Clinical guidelines. (1997). Adult screening for anemia and hemoglobinopathies. *The Nurse Practitioner, 20*(12), 48, 50–51.

Davenport, J. (1996). Macrocytic anemia. *American Family Physician, 53,* 155– 162.

Freedman, A. S., & Nadler, L. M. (1997). Malignancies of lymphoid cells. In A. S. Fauci, E. Braunwald, K. J. Isselbacher, J. D. Wilson, J. B. Martin, D. L. Kasper, S. L. Hauser & D. L. Longo (Eds.). *Harrison's principles of internal medicine* (14th ed., pp. 695–712). NY: McGraw-Hill.

Green, R. (1996). Macrocytic anemias. In J. W. Hurst, M. Markman, & A. E. Lichtin (Eds.). *Medicine for the practicing physician* (4th ed., pp. 821–828). Stamford, CT: Appleton & Lange.

Linker, C. A. (2000). Blood. In L. M. Tierney, S. J. McPhee, & M. A. Papadakis (Eds.). *Current medical diagnosis and treatment* (39th ed., pp. 499–552). Stamford, CT: Appleton & Lange.

Morrison, C., Gordon, S., & Yeo, T. P. (2000). Hodgkin's disease in primary care. *The Nurse Practitioner, 25*(7), 44–62.

Newton, W. (1995). Laboratory diagnosis of iron deficiency anemia. *Journal of Family Practice, 41,* 404–405.

Nicoll, C. D. (2000). Appendix: Therapeutic drug monitoring & laboratory reference ranges. In L. M. Tierney, S. J. McPhee, & M. A. Papadakis (Eds.). *Current medical diagnosis and treatment* (39th ed., pp. 1617–1625). Stamford, CT: Appleton & Lange.

Richer, A. (1997). A practical guide for differentiating between iron deficiency anemia and anemia of chronic disease in children and adults. *The Nurse Practitioner, 22*(4), 82, 85–98.

Gastrointestinal Disorders Infancy Through Adolescence

Victoria A. Weill

Gastroesophageal Reflux In Infancy (GER)

- Definition: Reflux of gastric contents into esophagus due to dysfunction of lower esophageal sphincter
- Etiology/Incidence
    1. Etiology unclear
    2. Begins in early infancy
    3. Physiologic GER
        a. 80% to 90% of healthy infants
        b. Often caused by overfeeding or incomplete burping
    4. Pathologic GER
        a. 5% of infants
        b. Males > females
- Signs and Symptoms
    1. Physiologic GER
        a. Occasional, effortless, painless spitting often within 40 minutes of eating
        b. 40% show improvement by 3 months
        c. 85% resolve between 6 to 12 months with more erect posture and introduction of solids
    2. Functional GER
        a. Frequent, large volume, effortless, nonprojectile regurgitation; no choking or color changes
        b. 70% asymptomatic by 18 months of age
        c. Normal growth—growth chart is key
        d. For functional and physiologic GER—feeding history may indicate excessive intake; burp heard during vomiting may indicate incomplete burping
    3. Pathologic GER
        a. Reflux may cause other physical complications, such as:
            (1) Failure to thrive (FTT)—caused by long term, forceful regurgitation
            (2) Esophagitis—causing irritability, anemia and guaiac positive stools or hematemesis; dysphagia
            (3) Aspiration—pneumonia, wheezing, apnea
            (4) Sandifer syndrome—abnormal posturing of head and neck
        b. May be "silent GER"—no overt vomiting, but complications may be presenting symptom

     c. 60% show improvement by 16 months; 30% may remain symptomatic up to 4 years

   4. Secondary GER

     a. Handicapped, especially neurologically impaired child

     b. Pre-existing condition

- Differential Diagnosis

   1. Pyloric stenosis

   2. (Partial) anatomical obstruction

   3. Formula intolerance

   4. Gastroenteritis

   5. Infections—urinary tract infection (UTI); otitis media (OM); pneumonia

   6. Increased intracranial pressure (ICP)/neurological disorder

- Physical Findings

   1. May have wheezing or respiratory symptoms with aspiration

   2. Abdominal examination normal—no masses, olive or peristaltic waves

   3. Neurological examination normal—no signs of increased ICP

- Diagnostic Tests/Findings

   1. Diagnosis often made by observation and history; testing only to determine if reflux is causing problems since vomiting indicates reflux

   2. Barium swallow/UGI to ligament of Treitz—only evaluates anatomy; to rule out anomalies sensitive to reflux; nearly all babies will show reflux; should be done if using prokinetic medication

   3. pH probe—indicates amount of reflux occurring; does not confirm diagnosis; not good postprandial because food acts as buffer; can be outpatient procedure

   4. Upper endoscopy—especially good for esophagitis and inflammation due to *Helicobacter pylori*

   5. Manometry—research tool

   6. Scintigraphy—''Milk scan''; evaluates motility and aspiration

   7. Guaiac stool/emesis—positive for occult blood if abnormal

- Management/Treatment

   1. Conservative therapy

     a. Positioning—postprandial, prone position for 1 to 2 hours; infant seats/swings worsen by increasing intra-abdominal pressure; caution with diapering/playing postfeeding

b. Breast feed or use predominately whey formula; adding 1 tablespoon rice cereal/ounce to formula may or may not help; change formula only for signs of milk protein intolerance/allergy (bloody diarrhea, eczema, wheezing)

c. Avoid over-feeding—age in months plus 3 equals number of ounces every 3 to 4 hours for most infants.

d. Small feedings with frequent burping

e. Reassure parents with growth charts

f. Decrease anxiety in mother-infant interaction

g. Monitor for problems—aspiration/esophagitits

h. Lateral position for sleep rather than supine position

2. Medications: (if conservative therapy has failed)

a. Antacids/H_2 blockers if irritable from esophagitis

b. Cisapride has been removed from market for most patients

c. Metoclopramide may be cautiously considered for severe reflux under the supervision of a physician or gastroenterologist

3. Surgery—Nissen fundoplication

Pyloric Stenosis

- Definition: Obstruction due to thickening of circular muscle of the pylorus
- Etiology/Incidence

  1. Unknown cause, possibly hereditary

  2. Occurs in 1:500 infants; male > female; unclear if more likely in first born

  3. Familial predisposition—25% chance if mother had pyloric stenosis, 15% chance if other family member, 22% if identical twin

  4. More common in Caucasians than African-Americans or Asians

  5. Symptoms occur later in breast fed infants; greater muscle thickness required to obstruct smaller-sized breast milk curd

  6. Delayed timing in premature infants

- Signs and Symptoms

  1. Not present at birth; may occur in first week; average age of presentation from 3 to 6 weeks through 3 to 4 months of age

  2. Vigorous, non-bilious vomiting after eating; with time becomes projectile with brownish color

  3. "Hungry" after emesis; progressing to lethargy and irritability

  4. Weight loss or poor weight gain

5. Constipation

6. Dehydration develops over time

- Differential Diagnosis

    1. Overfeeding

    2. Gastroesophageal reflux

    3. Milk protein allergy

    4. Gastroenteritis

    5. Malrotation/volvulus if bilious emesis

- Physical Findings

    1. Visible peristaltic waves progressing from left to right across abdomen—darken room, shine bright light on abdomen of naked, supine baby; feed bottle of sugar water; peristaltic waves visible

    2. Palpable pyloric "olive" after vomiting—palpate epigastrium in RUQ deep under liver edge; need very relaxed abdomen; hard, smooth, mobile, non-tender mass may be palpable

    3. Dehydration as obstruction increases

- Diagnostic Tests/Findings

    1. Abdominal ultrasound to determine size of pylorus—preferred test

    2. Upper GI—avoid due to risk of barium aspiration; shows "string sign"; elongated pyloric channel and delayed gastric emptying

    3. Electrolytes to determine dehydration status

- Management/Treatment:

    1. Surgical treatment after correction of fluid and electrolyte deficits

    2. Post-operative monitoring for hypoglycemia

    3. Excellent prognosis

Acute Infectious Gastroenteritis

- Definition: Illness of rapid onset, includes diarrhea with possible nausea, vomiting, fever, or abdominal pain

- Etiology/Incidence

    1. 70% to 80% caused by viral agents; 25% by rotavirus

    2. < age 3 years 1.3 to 2.3 episodes/year; higher if in day care

    3. Predisposing factors (see Table 1)

        a. Day care

        b. Poor sanitation—improper hand washing, food preparation or water quality

      c.   Recent travel especially to endemic areas

      d.   Ill contacts—animals or humans

      e.   Immunocompromised children at risk

      f.   Recent antibiotic use

- Signs and Symptoms

    1.   Rotavirus—URI symptoms, low fever, frequent vomiting, mild to profuse watery diarrhea

    2.   Adenovirus—low fever; vomiting, diarrhea severe enough to cause dehydration, rare respiratory symptoms

    3.   Norwalk—nausea, fever, abdominal pain; vomiting more frequent than diarrhea

    4.   Shigella—high fever, headache, abdominal pain and tenderness; large, watery stools in which blood and mucus may be seen; can lead to dehydration

Table 1

Most Common Causative Agents in U.S.

Agent	Source/Transmission	Risk Factors	Incubation	Duration
VIRUS				
Rotavirus	Infected persons; contaminated toys, hard surfaces	< 3 years; day care; low SES* winter	1-3 days	5-10 days
Adenovirus	Infected person; contaminated toys; hard surfaces	< 4 years; daycare; winter months	3-10 days	5-12 days
Norwalk	Infected persons; contaminated food or water	older children & adults	12 hrs-4 days	12-48 hrs
BACTERIA				
Shigella	Infected persons; contaminated food, water, objects; houseflies	1-4 years; daycare; crowding; poor sanitation; summer/ fall months	1-7 days	4-5 days even without treatment
Salmonella	Contaminated foods (poultry, red meat, eggs, milk, fruits); contaminated water; infected persons or animals	< 5 years; especially first year	6-72 hrs	2-7 days
Campylobacter jejuni	Contaminated poultry; unpasteurized milk; pets	All ages; summer months	1-7 days	5-7 days

Table 1 (*Continued*)

Most Common Causative Agents in U.S.

Agent	Source/Transmission	Risk Factors	Incubation	Duration
PARASITIC				
Giardia lamblia	Infected persons, animals, contaminated food or water	Daycare, institutions; campers, CF	1-4 weeks	May be long-term
Cryptosporidium	Infected persons, animals, contaminated water supplies	Parasite is chlorine-resistant	2-14 days	10-14 days
Entamoeba histolytica	Amebic cysts; contaminated food and water	Tropical areas; crowding; poor sanitation	1-4 weeks	May be long-term
TOXIN				
S. Aureus	Ingestion of contaminated food products: ham, poultry, salads (egg and potato), cream filled pastries	Inadequate cooking, refrigeration	½-6 hrs	12 hours
E. coli	Infected persons or carriers; contaminated foods (undercooked ground beef), apple cider, raw vegetables, salami, yogurt	Day care; poor sanitation; inadequate cooking; poor handwashing; travel to developing countries	3-4 days, up to 8 days	Varies
Clostridium difficile	Infected persons or hospital environment	Hospitals, daycare, normal intestinal flora altered—antibiotics; enema, prolonged NG tube; intestinal surgery; Rare < 12 months	Unknown	May improve with discontinuation of antibiotic if cause

*SES—socioeconomic status

5. Salmonella—fever, abdominal pain and cramps; watery, mucoid or bloody stools

6. *Campylobacter jejuni*—fever, malaise, appendicitis-like abdominal pain, bloody stools

7. *Giardia lamblia*—flatulence, abdominal pain, failure to thrive, anorexia, range of stools, e.g., asymptomatic carrier to foul, steatorrhea

8. *Cryptosporidium parvum*—frequent watery stools most common symptom with abdominal pain, anorexia and weight loss

9. *Entamoeba histolytica*—asymptomatic, mild symptoms, e.g., abdominal distention, constipation, occasionally loose stools; *or* severe abdominal pain with bloody and mucoid diarrhea

10. *Staphylococcus aureus*—abrupt onset of nausea, vomiting, abdominal pain, watery stools

11. *Escherichia coli* (EHEC 0157:H7)—fever $< \frac{1}{3}$ of cases, severe abdominal pain, hemolytic uremic syndrome (HUS), stools usually progress to bloody, or occult

12. *Clostridium difficile*—abdominal pain; pseudomembranous colitis, stools bloody with leukocytes, mucus, pus

- Differential Diagnosis
    1. Urinary tract infection (UTI)
    2. Other infections—otitis media, streptococcal pharyngitits
    3. Inflammatory bowel disease
    4. Malabsorption (lactose intolerance, celiac disease, cystic fibrosis)
    5. Milk protein allergy
    6. Chronic diarrhea
    7. If only vomiting:
        a. Trauma
        b. Congestive heart failure
        c. Toxic ingestion
        d. Metabolic disorder
        e. Increased intracranial pressure

- Physical Findings
    1. Assess hydration—see Table 2
    2. Recent weight (wt) very helpful, but often not available

$$\frac{\text{Pre-illness wt minus wt today}}{\text{Pre-illness wt}} \times 100 = \text{fluid deficit as \% body wt loss}$$

- Diagnostic Tests/Findings
    1. Testing not necessary unless:
        a. Blood or mucus in stools—test for specific organism
        b. No improvement in symptoms > 5 to 6 days
        c. Signs of severe dehydration—BUN, specific gravity, electrolytes

TABLE 2

Assessment of Dehydration

Variable	Mild, 3%-5%	Moderate, 6%-9%	Severe ≥ 10%
Blood pressure	Normal	Normal	Normal to reduced
Quality of pulses	Normal	Normal or slightly decreased	Moderately decreased
Heart rate	Normal	Increased	Increased*
Skin turgor	Normal	Decreased	Decreased
Fontanel	Normal	Sunken	Sunken
Mucous membranes	Slightly dry	Dry	Dry
Eyes	Normal	Sunken orbits	Deeply sunken orbits
Extremities	Warm, normal capillary refill	Delayed capillary refill	Cool, mottled
Mental status	Normal	Normal to listless	Normal to lethargic or comatose
Urine output	Slightly decreased	< 1 mL/kg/hr	<<1 mL/kg/hr
Thirst	Slightly increased	Moderately increased	Very thirsty or too lethargic to indicate

Note. From ''Practice Parameters: The management of acute gastroenteritis in young children'', by Provisional Committee on Quality Improvement, Subcommittee on Acute Gastroenteritis, 1996, *Pediatrics*, 97(3), p.427. Copyright 1996 by the American Academy of Pediatrics. Reprinted with permission.

The percentages of body weight reduction that correspond to different degrees of dehydration will vary among authors. The critical factor in assessment is the determination of the patient's hemodynamic and perfusion status. If a clinician is unsure of the category into which the patient falls, it is recommended that therapy for the more severe category be used.

*Bradycardia may appear in severe cases

    2. Test for specific organism

        a. Virus—EIA, rarely necessary

        b. Bacterial—stool culture; specific testing for *E. coli* 0157:H7 if bloody stools

        c. Giardia—giardia antigen (more specific); stools for ova and parasites

        d. Cryptosporidium—stools for ova and parasites, specify cryptosporidium

        e. *Clostridium difficile—Clostridium difficile* toxins

    3. Persistent vomiting as only sign; diarrhea lasting longer than 10 days or with failure to thrive (FTT) need more extensive testing

- Management/Treatment:

    1. Self-limiting in most healthy children

    2. Increased risk associated with dehydration with fever; prematurity, infancy and adolescent mothers

    3. Assess degree of dehydration and correct deficit following the guidelines suggested by the AAP Subcommittee on Acute Gastroenteritis (1996)

a. Oral rehydration therapy (ORT) can safely and effectively treat mild to moderate dehydration in otherwise healthy child

b. Maintenance solutions have 45 to 50 mmol/L of sodium, suitable for rehydration; continue for a maximum of 24 hours

c. Determine replacement volume; give over 4 hour period

    (1) 50 cc/kg for mild dehydration

    (2) 80 to 100 cc/kg for moderate to severe

    (3) Plus replace ongoing losses:

        (a) 5 to 10 cc/kg for each diarrheal stool

        (b) 2 cc/kg for each episode of emesis

d. Small frequent feedings are key—1 teaspoon every 1 to 2 minutes initially; if tolerated amount may be advanced; do not allow child to drink large amounts quickly; process is labor intensive; parent or staff needs to be available to administer

e. Home remedies such as juice or sports beverages are non-physiologic and should be avoided in the treatment of young children with dehydration

f. Once rehydrated or in children with diarrhea but no dehydration, feeding with age-appropriate diet should be encouraged; rice, wheat, potatoes, bread, cereals, lean meats, yogurt, fruits and vegetables; early refeeding promotes healing of the GI mucosa and decreases stool output; old practice of "bowel rest" may worsen condition

g. In a change from earlier recommendations, once dehydration is corrected, full strength formula or milk can be given; monitor for the 20% of patients who develop transient (4 to 8 weeks) lactose intolerance.

h. Breast milk may be continued

i. Antidiarrheal medications are not appropriate and may be dangerous

j. UA and CBC to monitor E. coli (0157:H7) infection; may develop microangiopathic hemotologic changes and/or nephropathy

4. Antimicrobials only in select cases, (AAP, 2000)

a. Shigella—TMP/SMX for 5 days especially if in daycare; check sensitivity, if resistant, may need parenteral medications; decreases diarrhea and length of shedding of organism

b. Salmonella—only for infants < 3 months with suspected sepsis or immunosuppressed since antibiotics can prolong excretion; amoxicillin, TMP/SMX, cefotaxime or ceftriaxone

c. *Campylobacter jejuni*—only helpful if caught in early stages; erythromycin or azithromycin 5 to 7 days; tetracycline > age 8

d. *Giardia lamblia*—metronidazole (drug of choice) 15mg/kg/day in 3 divided doses for 5 days; furazolidone 6 mg/kg/day in 4 divided doses for 7 to 10 days is less effective, but available in liquid form for children; contraindicated with G6PD deficiency and neonates; albendazole (available as liquid) for children > age 2, 400 mg every day for 5 days; all giardia treatments are potential teratogens in pregnant teens; paromomycin (less effective) useful in pregnancy, 25 to 35 mg/kg/day in 3 doses for 7 days

e. *Entamoeba histolytica*—metronidazole 35 to 50 mg/kg/day in 3 divided doses for 7 to 10 days followed by iodoquinol or paromomycin

f. *E. coli* (0157:H7)—antibiotics may not prevent hemolytic uremic syndrome (HUS)

g. *Clostridium difficile*—stop causative antibiotics: if no improvement; metronidazole 30 mg/kg/day in four divided doses for 7 to 10 days.

5. Severe dehydration/HUS requires physician referral

6. Prevention

   a. Teach children importance of frequent, thorough hand washing

   b. Encourage mothers to breast feed

   c. Day care centers need strict policies for hand washing and food preparation; surfaces and fomites need frequent cleaning with chlorine based disinfectant

   d. Careful food preparation and storage

   e. *E. coli* (0157:H7) requires public health involvement particularly for day care attendees

   f. Teach parents signs/symptoms of dehydration and early at home measures

Pinworms (*Enterobiasis vermicularis*)

- Definitions: Nematode parasite with infestation of intestines and rectum

- Etiology/Incidence

  1. Human pinworm is ubiquitous; adult worm lives in rectum, comes out at night to lay eggs on perianal skin and dies causing pruritus; scratching and finger to mouth contact transfers eggs to intestine; these develop into mature worms and repeat cycle (approximately 2 weeks)

  2. Found in children of all socioeconomic classes

  3. Eggs float easily in air and can be swallowed by others

- Signs and Symptoms

  1. Nocturnal anal itching

  2. Vaginal itching (pinworm crawls into vagina)

  3. Insomnia (itching)

4. Worm like-"threads"—seen in toilet or on underwear

- Differential Diagnosis

  1. Vulvovaginitis secondary to local irritation

  2. Poor hygiene

- Physical Findings

  1. Excoriation of perianal and perineal area

  2. Thread-like worms will be seen on visualization of anus (early morning using flashlight)

- Diagnostic Test/Findings: Adhesive cellophane tape "paddle" with kits available for parental use; or can be made with clear scotch tape and glass slide; prior to arising and bathing, paddle is pressed against anus and then examined for eggs

- Management/Treatment

  1. Medication (over age 2)

     a. Pyrantel pamoate 11 mg/kg one dose (maximum dose 1g); repeat in 2 weeks

     b. Mebendazole 100 mg single dose (same dose for all ages and weights); repeat in 2 weeks

  2. Reassure parents ubiquitous nature of organism; reinfection likely

  3. Test other family members and treat at same time if infected

  4. Prevention

     a. Keep nails clean and short

     b. Bathing will remove eggs from skin and decrease pruritus

     c. Excellent hand washing

Inflammatory Bowel Disease (IBD)

- Definition: Chronic intestinal inflammation with two specific entities of ulcerative colitis (UC) and Crohn's disease; may have extraintestinal symptoms and acute or insidious onset

  1. Location of inflammation in GI tract—Crohn's occurs any part of GI tract, terminal ileum typical; UC more likely in colon

  2. Pattern of inflammation—Crohn's skip pattern; discrete areas of inflammation interspersed with normal; UC mucosal and submucosal inflammation, diffuse and continuous

- Etiology/Incidence (for both types of IBD)

  1. Etiology unclear

  2. Unclear genetic link; 10% to 20% positive family history

3. Occurs more often in Caucasians than African-Americans and Asians; highest in descendents of Ashkenazic Jews

4. Age of onset 10 to 20 years; of these 20% to 40% < 12 years of age

- Signs and Symptoms

    1. Symptoms may be acute or unrecognized for years, dependent on location of lesions; more variability with Crohn's disease since any part of GI tract can be involved

    2. Diarrhea

        a. Crohn's—loose with blood if colon involved, or can have pain but no diarrhea

        b. UC—mild to profuse bloody diarrhea

    3. Weight loss/delayed pubertal maturation—often due to inadequate food intake because eating causes cramps, bloating, diarrhea

        a. Growth failure may be presenting problem especially in Crohn's

        b. Weight loss and delayed puberty more common with Crohn's

    4. Abdominal pain

        a. Crohn's —located in right lower quadrant sometimes as fullness or mass; food related

        b. UC—left lower abdomen

    5. Severe cramps, low grade fevers, anorexia

- Differential Diagnosis (based on area of bowel involved)

    1. Ulcerative Colitis

        a. Enteric infection (particularly those involving bloody diarrhea)

        b. Irritable bowel syndrome

    2. Crohn's (particularly if manifested as extraintestinal symptoms)

        a. Rheumatoid arthritis

        b. Acute appendicitis

        c. Lupus erythematosus

        d. Lactose intolerance

        e. Celiac disease

- Physical Findings (common to both UC and Crohn's unless noted)

    1. Weight deceleration

    2. Diffuse abdominal pain or no tenderness

    3. Extraintestinal symptoms

        a. Fever of unknown origin (FUO)

      b.   Short stature

      c.   Uveitis/iritis

      d.   Aphthous stomatitis

      e.   Arthritis/arthralgias

      f.   Inflammatory lesions of skin

      g.   Liver disease

      h.   Perianal fissures/tags/abscesses especially with Crohn's disease

- Diagnostic Tests/Findings

  1. Blood studies—CBC with differential shows microcytic anemia, increased WBC; sedimentation rate (ESR) elevated; chemistry panel shows low serum total protein and albumin; findings suggest IBD and indicate the need for further studies for both Crohn's and UC

  2. Stool studies—infectious agents that cause bloody diarrhea for both Crohn's and UC

  3. Colonoscopy with biopsy—to differentiate Crohn's vs. UC

  4. Upper GI with small bowel—shows IBD changes and extent of disease

  5. Endoscopy with biopsy

- Management/Treatment

  1. Refer to pediatric gastroenterologist

  2. Nutritional therapy to ensure adequate growth and pubertal development; total parenteral nutrition (TPN) or elemental formula may be necessary and can improve clinical symptoms; in milder cases high protein, high carbohydrate, normal fat diet providing 75 to 90 kcal/ kg/day; avoid overly restrictive diets

  3. Anti-inflammatory agents—short term corticosteroids, sulfasalazine

  4. Long term patients may need colectomy/ostomy; curative for UC

  5. At higher risk for colorectal cancer

  6. Need emotional support to deal with chronic illness with reassurance that emotional factors are not primary cause

Malabsorption

- Definition: Impaired intestinal absorption of nutrients and electrolytes

- Etiology/Incidence: Classified according to stage of digestion affected

  1. Intraluminal phase—maldigestion; need enzymes (cystic fibrosis, see Lower Respiratory Disorders chapter)

  2. Abnormalities of mucosal surface area—absorption; infections can damage mucosa

     a. Secondary lactose malabsorption

(1) Most common cause of malabsorption in children

(2) Can be up to 20% post-gastrointestinal infection

(3) Primary lactose intolerance rare < age 4; 80% Asian, African-American adults

    b. Infectious—bacterial, viral, parasites, e.g., *Giardia lamblia*

    c. Celiac disease—intestinal intolerance to gluten; rate in population 1:1000; more common in children with Irish, Swedish heritage

  3. Decreased conjugated bile acids

    a. Biliary atresia

    b. Hepatitis

    c. Short bowel syndrome

- Signs and Symptoms:

  1. Failure to thrive

  2. Adequate intake per dietary history

  3. Severe, chronic diarrhea

  4. Bulky, foul, pale, steatorrhea stools

  5. Abdominal distention

- Differential Diagnosis

  1. Renal disease

  2. Poor dietary intake

  3. Failure to thrive

- Physical Findings: Disease specific findings

  1. Lactose intolerance—persistent diarrhea after infectious diarrhea

  2. Cystic fibrosis—recurrent pulmonary infection, "salty" taste to skin; nasal polyps; rectal prolapse

  3. Celiac disease—vomiting, abdominal pain, irritability, anorexia, pallor; protuberant abdomen

- Diagnostic Tests/Findings

  1. Stool—(most important) inspection, culture, microscopic examination

    a. Hemoccult test—intestinal mucosa damage

    b. Ova and parasite; giardia antigen to test for giardia and other parasites

    c. pH reducing substances—to rule out carbohydrate malabsorption

    d. Sudan stain for fat (microscopic examination of stool for fat)

2. Urinalysis/culture

3. CBC, electrolytes, ESR

4. Sweat test > 60 mEq/L chloride—cystic fibrosis

5. Hydrogen breath test—increased with lactose intolerance

- Management/Treatment:

    1. Refer to gastroenterologist

    2. Lactose intolerance—avoid lactose containing foods

    3. Celiac disease—gluten free diet; no wheat, oats, rye, barley

    4. Cystic fibrosis—pancreatic enzyme replacement

Intussusception

- Definition: Acute episode of prolapse of one portion of intestine into the lumen of the adjoining part

- Etiology/Incidence

    1. Unknown cause—95% idiopathic; may be caused by adenovirus, Henoch Schönlein purpura, celiac disease, CF; Meckel diverticulum of small intestine, no abdominal pain, but causes bleeding; primary cause in older children

    2. Greater incidence in males than females

    3. 60% occur before first birthday; 80% by 2 years

- Signs and Symptoms

    1. Healthy infant/child presents with sudden cycle of inconsolable screaming, flexing of legs; colicky abdominal pain

    2. 90% have nonbilious vomiting after pain

    3. Periods of quiteness or sleepiness between episodes; lethargy if intussusception not reduced

    4. Eventually shocklike state develops

    5. Within 12 hours of onset, ''current jelly'' (blood with mucus) stool is passed; late presentation

- Differential Diagnosis

    1. Gastroenteritis

    2. Incarcerated hernia

    3. Volvulus/obstruction

- Physical Findings

    1. Abdomen soft between episodes; may palpate sausage shaped mass RUQ

    2. Distention and tenderness increased as obstruction increases

3. Guaiac positive or grossly bloody stool

4. If not reduced, develops perforation and peritonitis leading to fever and shock.

- Diagnostic Tests/Findings

    1. Radiography only to clarify diagnosis—no gas RLQ, air fluid levels consistent with obstruction

    2. Barium enema—diagnostic and results in reduction

    3. CBC and electrolytes—dehydration and anemia

- Management/Treatment

    1. Reduction via barium/air enema

    2. Emergency surgery

    3. Can recur; fatal if untreated

Appendicitis

- Definition: Acute inflammation of the appendix

- Etiology/Incidence

    1. Cause—obstruction of lumen by fecaliths or parasites

    2. Most common in late childhood and early adolescence with average age of 12 years

    3. Preadolescent period—equal male and female rates

    4. Most common cause of pediatric abdominal surgery

- Signs and Symptoms

    1. Young child may not appear ill or have severe pain particularly in early phase

    2. Abdominal pain—earliest symptom

        a. Vague, possibly midline, constant pain for several hours

        b. Pain eventually localized in RLQ; in some, pain may begin in RLQ

        c. Can wake at night over time with increasing severity of pain

        d. Pain on ambulation

    3. Anorexia, nausea and vomiting

    4. Variable changes in bowel patterns—constipation or diarrhea may be noted

    5. Afebrile to very low-grade fever in early phase

- Differential Diagnosis

    1. Gastroenteritis—especially if high fever (early stage) and/or diarrhea

    2. Mittelschmerz

    3. Ovary cyst/ovary torsion/ruptured follicle

4. Pelvic inflammatory disease (PID)

5. Constipation

6. UTI/pyelonephritis

7. Ruptured ectopic pregnancy

8. Inflammatory bowel disease

9. Intussusception

10. Perforated peptic ulcer

- Physical Findings: Depends upon the stage of appendicitis

    1. Observe child—may be motionless, with legs flexed

    2. Tenderness localized to RLQ; intense at McBurney's point halfway between umbilicus and anterior superior iliac crest

    3. Rebound tenderness

    4. Local, right-sided tenderness or mass on rectal examination

    5. Won't jump/difficulty ambulating

    6. Obturator sign—rotating thigh may produce pain in RLQ

    7. Perforation and peritonitis within 24 to 48 hours

        a. Rigidity

        b. Higher fever

        c. Pain improves

        d. Generalized tenderness

        e. Increased vomiting

        f. 40% incidence in young children

- Diagnostic Tests/Findings

    1. Diagnosis based on history and physical; tests often not helpful

    2. CBC with differential—may have a mild leukocytosis with left shift

    3. Ultrasound—if ovarian condition part of differential or findings unclear

    4. Radiography of abdomen to rule out constipation

    5. UA to rule out UTI

- Management/Treatment: Immediate surgical referral

Recurrent Abdominal Pain

- Definition: At least 3 episodes of abdominal pain for three or more months, interfering with routine activities; separated by pain free periods

- Etiolgy/Incidence

  1. Unclear mechanism of pain; may be visceral

  2. Multifaceted problem that includes predisposition aggravated by life events or personality

  3. Most common cause of chronic pain in school-aged and young adolescent; 10% to 15% of school-aged population

  4. Onset before age 3 and after 14 years is very unusual

  5. Greater incidence in girls than boys; average age for females 9 to 10 years, males 10 to 11 years

  6. Family history of GI complaints and somatization disorders; e.g., migraines, peptic ulcers

  7. Cause of pain

     a. Organic—approximately 10%, e.g., inflammatory bowel disease

        (1) With the increased use of endoscopy more dyspepsia disease (peptic ulcer/esophagitis) identified; positive family history; occurs 12 to 18 years; may be caused by *Helicobacter pylori*

        (2) Pancreatitis—more common if positive family history; corticosteroid use

        (3) Cholecystitis—rare < 9 years of age; increased with obesity; positive family history gall stones; birth control pills

     b. Psychogenic—clear psychological component, e.g., school phobia

     c. Nonspecific—80%; interplay between environment and physiology, e.g., irritable bowel; 50% identified as functional abdominal pain

  8. Psychological component unclear; clearly more stress during pain episode; may be a stress reaction

- Signs and Symptoms

  1. Certain personality traits (anxious, high achiever) and family characteristics (protective parents) more frequent; may affect school performance

  2. No mucus or blood in stool or emesis; no diarrhea with functional pain

  3. Nature of pain

     a. Onset of crampy or dull ache; no radiation of pain

     b. Periumbilical, occasionally suprapubic

     c. Lasts less than one hour; nothing relieves pain

     d. Interferes with activities, but no night wakening; unrelated to meals

     e. Resolves between episodes; not constant nor daily

     f. Related symptoms—nausea, sweating, flush, dizziness, pallor, headache

g. Occasionally constipation or mild vomiting

h. If constant, localized, or night pain, or occurs in preschool child, more likely organic

(1) Peptic ulcer or esophagitis—epigastric pain 1 to 3 hours after eating, or awakens child; sour burps; blood in stools or vomitus

(2) Irritable bowel—crampy lower abdominal pain, mucous stools alternating with constipation or diarrhea

(3) Pancreatitis—dull epigastric, postprandial pain with radiation to back; persistent vomiting; fever; flexion of hips and knees provides relief

(4) Cholecystitis—RUQ and vague epigastric, postprandial pain, radiating to right shoulder; history of high fat diet

- Differential Diagnosis:

1. Constipation/chronic stool retention

2. Inflammatory bowel disease

3. Irritable bowel

4. Dysmenorrhea

5. School phobia

6. Depression

7. Peptic ulcer/dyspepsia

8. Malabsorption/lactose intolerance

9. Trauma

10. UTI

11. Abdominal migraine

12. Parasites

13. Pancreatitis/cholecystitis

14. PID

15. Sexual abuse

- Physical Findings: Indicate nonorganic cause

1. Normal weight

2. Afebrile, may have slight temperature increase during episode

3. Abdomen may have diffuse or LLQ tenderness, but no guarding

4. Normal findings on complete examination

- Diagnostic Tests/Findings: Diagnosis of exclusion

1. Excellent history and physical examination key to diagnosis

2. Guaiac stool—negative; rule out inflammatory bowel disease

3. Blood tests—CBC with differential; ESR to rule out infection/inflammation

4. Urinalysis/culture—rule out UTI

5. Ova and parasites; giardia antigen

6. Additional/selected studies may be warranted depending on symptoms

    a. Pelvic examination of adolescent female

    b. Endoscopy for esophagitis, peptic ulcer—dysphagia, chest pain, weight loss present

    c. Upper gastrointestinal (UGI) with small bowel—if recurrent vomiting, stool blood to rule out obstructive lesions, Crohn's disease

    d. Hydrogen breath test—increased with lactose intolerance

    e. Pregnancy test

    f. Endoscopy or serology—rule out *Helicobacter pylori*

    g. Abdominal ultrasound—rule out cholecystitis

    h. Amylase/lipase—increased with pancreatitis

- Management/Treatment

1. Emphasize to child and family—pain is real even though no organic cause can be found; work up should reassure them child is healthy

2. Reinforce normal behavior; go to school, don't allow secondary gain; may go to school nurse briefly if symptoms severe; if too sick to attend school, follow-up with provider required

3. Decrease hectic life style and hurried meals

4. Increasing fiber intake may help

5. Avoid medications if nonorganic

6. Try to identify source of stress in patient or family; stress reduction techniques may help

7. Keep pain diary to identify situations associated with symptoms

8. Treat identified organic disease

Constipation

- Definition: Alteration in frequency, passage, size or consistency of stool

- Etiology/Incidence

1. Functional—5% to 10% of children; stool moves slowly through colon, excess water is absorbed, leading to hard, dry stools; can be caused by family tendencies, diet, drugs or change in routine; painful stools can lead to withholding, creating a cycle

2. Encopresis (fecal soiling)—chronic withholding leads to impaction and soiling; eventually loses urge to stool and results in megacolon; psychological problem not primary cause

3. Anatomical abnormalities—anal or rectal abnormalities; problems often seen in immediate newborn period

4. Intrinsic motor disorder—Hirschsprung's disease (most common), congenital absence of ganglion in segments of colon; 1: 5000 births; 4:1 male to female ratio; increased with positive family history or Down syndrome

5. Metabolic, e.g., hypothyroidism

6. Neurologic, e.g., tumors, spinal injury, myelomeningocele

- Signs and Symptoms
  1. Onset
     a. Functional—during infancy, particularly after change from breast milk to formula or starting solids; 1 to 3 years of age after life change, e.g., new sibling, home, introduction of toilet training; most improve by age 4

     b. Encopresis—4 to 7 years, male > female

     c. Hirschsprung's—constipation from birth; often no meconium in first 24 hours; history of failure to have bowel movement without aid of laxative or enema; "partial" or incomplete Hirschsprung's may manifest itself beyond the newborn period

  2. Stools
     a. Functional—hard, dry stools, "pellets"; occasionally stool caliber very large/wide; may be dark or have strong odor

     b. Encopresis—soiled underwear, may appear to be diarrhea; may occur daily

     c. Hirschsprung's—small, ribbon like stools; no leakage

  3. Complaints
     a. Functional—abdominal pain, blood streaked stools, straining or "dancing around" indicates withholding

     b. Hirschsprung's—no stooling

- Differential Diagnosis
  1. Tumor

  2. Anatomical deficit

  3. Metabolic

  4. Infantile botulism-(recent onset)

- Physical Findings
  1. Functional—rectal examination may show fissure, ampulla full of stool, normal

tone; may have no palpable abdominal mass, may have abdominal pain or cramping, but no distension; normal growth and development

2. Encopresis—may have impacted stool and/or large, dilated rectal vault, normal tone; abdominal distention with sausage-shaped mass in left pelvis or mid-line

3. Hirschsprung's—unable to admit finger for rectal examination due to long tight internal sphincter; empty rectum; stool may be guaiac positive; abnormal bowel sounds; abdominal distention

4. Anal wink, neurological examination, muscle strength and tone should be normal

- Diagnostic Tests/Findings:

  1. Radiograph of abdomen to examine for stool

  2. Unprepped barium enema—rule out Hirschsprung's disease

- Management/Treatment:

  1. Emphasize to parents the definition of constipation; straining with soft stool in infancy is normal

  2. Ensure proper preparation of formula

  3. Mild constipation can be treated with dietary changes; avoid constipating foods, e.g., rice cereal, bananas, apple sauce; introduce more juice and fluids; decrease excessive milk consumption; increase fiber; increase exercise in older child

  4. Infants > 6 months of age—prune juice; malt soup extract $\frac{1}{2}$ to 3 teaspoons twice per day for maximum of 3 days

  5. Constipation causing abdominal pain or encopresis needs more aggressive treatment; withheld stool causes intestinal muscle stretching; multifaceted treatment involves emptying intestines, leading to a return of sensation; preventing recurrence of painful stools and bowel training

  6. Plan for otherwise healthy child

     a. If impacted—day 1 mineral enema to soften stool

     b. No impaction or day 2—sodium phosphate enema one time per day for two to three days

     c. May choose oral medications for impaction

     d. After intestines emptied, keep stool soft to prevent recurrence of withholding cycle—emulsified mineral oil 1 to 3 mL/kg per day (Baker, 1999); may need to treat for 6 months or more; do not use in children < 1 year, with GER, or vomiting due to risk of aspiration; needs daily multivitamin

     e. Prevent pain cycle—emphasize to child that medicine will prevent painful stools

     f. Bowel retraining—child should sit on toilet for one minute per year of age twice per day; don't expect bowel movement every sitting

g. Goal—soft bowel movement every day or every other day; leaking orange oil indicates need to cut back on amount of emulsified mineral oil

7. Hirschsprung's—GI/surgery referral

Hepatitis:

- Definition: Inflammation of the liver
- Etiology/Incidence

1. Hepatitis A virus (HAV)

   a. Most common form of viral hepatitis in children

   b. Highest rates of symptomatic infection 5 to 14 years; less than 10% of infected children under 6 years are symptomatic

   c. Transmission—fecal/oral, raw shellfish, contaminated water; in U.S. HAV shed from asymptomatic, infected children to adults

   d. Incubation—15 to 50 days, average 25 to 30 days; can infect others up to 2 weeks before onset of illness and 1 week after

   e. High risk populations—Native-Americans, Alaskan natives, homosexuals, IV drug users; some Hasidic, Hispanic communities; travelers to developing countries; children in day care

2. Hepatitis B virus (HBV)

   a. Most common form of hepatitis in world

   b. Transmission—blood or body fluids; virus can survive more than one week on inanimate objects

   c. Incubation—45 to 160 days, average 120 days

   d. 5% to 10% of infected people become chronic carriers; inverse relationship between age of infection and carrier state; majority of perinatally infected infants become carriers

   e. High risk populations—sexually active; institutionalized; IV drug users; patients with clotting disorders; household contacts of HBV carriers; hemodialysis patients; infants of Alaskan natives or Pacific Islanders; travelers to China, Southeast Asia

3. Hepatitis C virus (HCV)

   a. Very low rates in children under 12 years of age

   b. Transmission—blood and blood products, occasionally blood transfusion

   c. Incubation—6 to 7 weeks, range of 2 weeks to 6 months

4. Hepatitis D (HDV)

   a. Co or super infection with HBV

   b. Transmission—blood or blood products, IV drug use, sexual contact

    c. Incubation—2 to 8 weeks, if simultaneous with HBV average is 120 days

  5. Hepatitis E (HEV)

    a. Endemic to Asia, Africa, Mexico; U.S. travelers to those areas at risk

    b. Transmission—fecal/oral route especially contaminated water

    c. Incubation—40 days, range 15 to 60 days

    d. More common in adults than children

- Signs and Symptoms

  1. HAV

    a. Infants and young children—asymptomatic or nonspecific symptoms, e.g., nausea, vomiting, diarrhea; no jaundice; misdiagnosed as gastroenteritis

    b. Adults—fever, malaise, anorexia, nausea, abdominal pain, jaundice; later pruritus

    c. Self-limiting disease—several weeks to occasionally 6 months; no chronic or carrier state

  2. HBV and HDV

    a. Children often asymptomatic—mild to severe disease; macular rash and arthritis (early sign); anorexia, nausea, malaise, arthralgia

    b. Up to 90% of perinatally infected infants can develop carrier state

    c. Chronic carrier state can lead to chronic liver disease or cancer

  3. HCV

    a. Children often asymptomatic; those with symptoms have mild disease; < 25% become icteric; gradual onset of headache, fever, nausea, fatigue, anorexia

    b. 50% to 85% become chronic carriers; can lead to chronic liver disease or cancer

  4. HEV

    a. Acute illness with arthralgia, abdominal pain, jaundice, malaise, anorexia and fever

    b. No carrier state

- Differential Diagnosis

  1. Viral gastroenteritis

  2. Hemolytic-uremic syndrome

  3. Reye's syndrome

  4. Cytomegalovirus illness

  5. Toxin/medication exposure

      6.   Fitz-Hugh Curtis syndrome with gonorrheal PID

- Physical Findings

      1.   Possible hepatosplenomegaly; RUQ tenderness

      2.   If jaundiced, may develop dark urine and light stools, sceral icterus

- Diagnostic Tests/Findings

      1.   Non-specific findings

          a.   Elevated liver enzymes—AST, ALT

          b.   Elevated serum bilirubin

          c.   Elevated erythrocyte sedimentation rate (HAV)

      2.   Specific serologic antigen/antibody testing

          a.   Hepatitis A (HAV)

              (1)   AntiHAV IgM—current or recent infection; usually disappears within 4 months

              (2)   AntiHAV-IgG—resolved infection and immune status; may last for years following infection; 40 to 45% general population carry Anti-HAV-IgG

          b.   Hepatitis B (HBV)

              (1)   HBsAg (surface antigen)—earliest marker of acute infection; persistence beyond 6 months indicates carrier status

              (2)   AntiHBc-IgM—current or recent acute infection; usually disappears within 6 months

              (3)   AntiHBc-IgG—chronic infection of at least 6 months duration

              (4)   AntiHBs—immune status following resolved infection or immunization (Heptavax)

              (5)   AntiHBe—recovery phase of infection

          c.   Hepatitis C (HCV)

              (1)   AntiHCV (ELIZA)—may need serial testing due to false negatives up to 5 or more weeks following onset of symptoms

              (2)   AntiHCV (RIBA)—positive after several weeks; confirms infection sooner than AntiHCV

          d.   Hepatitis D (HDV)—AntiHDV from reference laboratory

          e.   Hepatitis E (HEV)—serologic and Polymerase Chain Reaction assays are available experimentally at this time; diagnosis by exclusion of acute hepatitis A, B, C, D and other causes of viral hepatitis

- Management/Treatment
  1. Treatment is supportive, good nutrition, decreased activity, monitor hydration and chronic state
  2. HAV—immunoglobulin (IG) available for decreasing course of disease in early stages or prevention in exposed individuals; not recommended for HCV or HEV; defer measles or MMR immunization for 3 months following administration of immune globulin
  3. Interferon alpha-2B treatment for chronic HBV and HCV infections
     a. Limited improvement (30% to 40% HBV; 10% to 20% HCV)
     b. Expensive
     c. Side-effects
  4. Report to State health department
  5. Prevention
     a. HAV—two inactive HAV vaccines available for use in children > age 2 (see Health Maintenance and Health Promotion chapter); not routinely recommended for children in day care, only if endemic area; Hepatitis A (IG) prophylaxis available for international travelers < age 2
     b. HBV—vaccine available and highly recommended for all newborns and adolescents (See Health Maintenance and Health Promotion chapter)
     c. Cautious intake of food and water when traveling to endemic area
     d. Avoid unprotected sex and drug use
        Source

Hernia

- Definition: Abnormal protrusion of abdominal tissue/structures through umbilical ring in umbilical hernia or external inguinal ring in inguinal hernias
- Etiology/Incidence:
  1. Umbilical—due to imperfect closure or weakness of umbilical ring; common in infancy, reported in up to 60% of African-American infants; many umbilical hernias resolve by age 2, but in the African- American population closure can occur as late as 11 years of age
  2. Inguinal—failed closure of processus vaginalis
     a. Congenital defect—can be noticeable at birth
     b. Four to nine times more frequent in males
     c. Greater risk with premature births
     d. Hydrocele can increase risk; indicates opening present

- Signs and Symptoms

  1. Intermittent or constant bulge of abdominal wall or inguinal region that may worsen with crying or straining

  2. Uncomplicated hernias—asymptomatic

  3. Umbilical—incarceration or strangulation extremely rare

  4. Inguinal

     a. Incarcerated—cranky, anorexia, nausea, vomiting; groin discomfort, constipation

     b. Strangulated—area becomes tender, swollen and progressively reddened in addition to above symptoms, possible fever

- Differential Diagnosis

  1. Hydrocele

  2. Lymphadenopathy

  3. Undescended testes

- Physical Findings:

  1. Umbilical hernia—size of defect varies from 1 to 5 cm in diameter

  2. Inguinal hernia

     a. Maneuvers that increase intra-abdominal pressure (sitting up, crying, coughing) will increase visibility of hernia

     b. May be bilateral, if unilateral, right side more common

     c. "Silk" sign can be diagnostic; elicited by palpation of the spermatic cord over the pubic tubercle, the layers of the peritoneum rubbing together will have a "silky feel"

     d. Transillumination of scrotal sac will highlight the presence of bowel

- Diagnostic Tests/Findings: None may be needed; ultrasound if unclear

- Management/Treatment:

  1. Monitor umbilical hernias; reassure parents.

  2. Refer inguinal for surgical correction

  3. Emergency referral if incarcerated/strangulated

Questions
Select the best answer

1. A ten-month-old child has been diagnosed with gastroenteritis. He attends day care. What is the most likely cause of his illness?

   a. *Clostridium difficile*
   b. Rotavirus
   c. Salmonella
   d. Cryptosporidium

2. In a healthy, eight-month-old with diarrhea, but no dehydration, what would be the most appropriate advice to give parents?

   a. Encourage $\frac{1}{2}$ strength formula for 12 hours
   b. Give oral rehydration solution (ORT) for 12 hours
   c. Give only fluids until stools return to normal
   d. Give bananas and cereal as tolerated

3. When evaluating the abdominal pain in a child with recurrent abdominal pain (RAP) what symptom would lead to a likely organic etiology?

   a. Night waking
   b. Pallor
   c. Suprapubic pain
   d. Sweating

4. Vomiting in infancy has a long list of differential diagnoses. Which accompanying symptom would most likely point to pyloric stenosis?

   a. Diarrhea
   b. Appropriate growth
   c. Acts hungry after vomiting
   d. Sausage shaped mass in abdomen

5. Which of the following is the appropriate regimen for pinworm medication?

   a. Daily times 7 days, repeat as needed
   b. Three times a day for 10 days, repeat as needed
   c. Twice daily for 3 days, repeat in 2 weeks
   d. 1 dose/1 time, repeat in 2 weeks

6. Mrs. Doyle is upset. Two-month-old John's frequent vomiting has her convinced that "something serious is wrong." Which of the following is most suggestive of physiologic GER (gastroesophageal reflux)?

   a. He's gained 5 ounces this month
   b. He has a slight wheeze today
   c. He eats hungrily after vomiting
   d. He drinks 7 to 8 ounces every 3 to 4 hours

7. John's vomiting worsens despite conservative measures. Prokinetic medication might be considered. What diagnostic test should be done first?

    a. pH probe
    b. Milk scan
    c. Endoscopy
    d. Upper GI

8. Baby Sally was in your office last week for her 6-month check up. Her weight was 7 kg. Today she presents with diarrhea and vomiting for four days. Today her weight is 6.5 kg. What is her percentage of dehydration?

    a. 5%
    b. 7%
    c. 10%
    d. < 1%

9. What clinical signs would you expect to see in Sally on your examination?

    a. Normal capillary refill
    b. Normal fontanel
    c. Cool mottled skin
    d. Dry mucous membranes

10. Sally's vomiting and diarrhea has stopped. If she needs oral replacement therapy (ORT) today, what would be the appropriate amount to recommend?

    a. 325 - 350 cc over 4 hours
    b. 600 - 700 cc over 4 hours
    c. 600 - 700 cc over 12 hours
    d. 325 - 350 cc over 8 hours

11. Pinworms can cause which of the following?

    a. Constipation
    b. Anal itching
    c. Abdominal pain
    d. Diarrhea

12. In evaluating Billy, a child with bloody diarrhea, which of the following would not be an appropriate first action?

    a. Check growth chart
    b. Stool culture
    c. Upper GI
    d. Hemoccult test stools

13. Billy's family eats at fast food restaurants 4 to 5 times each week. If the you suspect the diarrhea is infectious in nature, what is a likely causative organism?

    a. Adenovirus
    b. *E. Coli*
    c. *Giardia lamblia*
    d. *S. aureus*

14. Which of the following conditions would be most likely to occur in a four-year-old boy?

    a. Pyloric stenosis
    b. Recurrent abdominal pain
    c. Intussusception
    d. Giardia infection

15. Which of the following findings could be expected to occur in a baby with intussusception?

    a. Inconsolable screaming
    b. Olive shaped mass
    c. Left to right peristaltic waves
    d. Weight loss

16. Which of the following may occur with suspected appendicitis?

    a. Pain not relieved with ambulation
    b. Young children appear very ill in the early phase
    c. Fever is 102 - 103° F
    d. Leukocytosis with left shift

17. In the U.S., parasitic gastroenteritis is most commonly caused by which organism?

    a. *Enterobius vermicularis*
    b. *Entamoeba histolytica*
    c. *Cryptosporidium parvum*
    d. *Giardia lamblia*

18. Which of the following serological findings indicates a carrier state for HBV?

    a. HBs Ag negative for 6 months
    b. IgM anti-HBc negative and HBsAg positive
    c. Anti-HBc positive
    d. Anti-HBs positive

19. Children in day care run the greatest risk of being exposed to which of the following infections?

    a. HAV
    b. HBV
    c. HCV
    d. HDV

20. Infant immunization for hepatitis B often raises many parental questions about the disease. Which of the following is not true about hepatitis B virus?

a. It can survive for more than 1 week on fomites.
b. It is the most common form of hepatitis in the world.
c. Contaminated water and shellfish are the major source
d. Perinatally infected infants are likely to become carriers

21. Two-day-old baby Jamie is in the hospital nursery and still has not passed meconium. This is a red flag for what condition?

    a. Intussusception
    b. Hemolytic uremic syndrome
    c. Pyloric stenosis
    d. Hirschsprung's disease

22. Consistent with the condition in question 21, Jamie's findings on rectal examination would be which of the following?

    a. Tight anal ring with no stool in vault
    b. Impacted stool with fissure
    c. Large, dilated rectum
    d. Soft stool, normal tone

23. What treatment would be appropriate for Jamie's condition?

    a. Emulsified mineral oil $\frac{1}{2}$ tablespoon per day
    b. Referral to gastroenterologist/surgeon
    c. Malt soup extract 2 teaspoons for 3 days
    d. Rectal dilatation with thermometer

24. When evaluating a child with suspected IBD which of the following diagnostic tests would not be helpful?

    a. Amylase and lipase
    b. ESR
    c. Serum total protein and albumin
    d. CBC with differential

25. Your patient has inflammatory bowel disease. Which finding is most consistent with ulcerative colitis?

    a. Occult blood
    b. Perirectal abscess
    c. Aphthous ulcers
    d. Left sided abdominal pain

26. Antimicrobials will improve the condition of a four-year-old child with diarrhea caused by which of the following organisms?

    a. Salmonella
    b. Rotovirus

    c. Shigella
    d. *E. coli* (0157:H7)

27. Katie has functional abdominal pain. When counseling her family on management of painful episodes, you would recommend which of the following?

    a. Take ibuprofen 200 mg for pain
    b. Stay home from school during episode
    c. Decrease milk products
    d. Go to school during episode

28. Which of the following would not be consistent with a diagnosis of functional constipation in an infant?

    a. Vomiting
    b. Anal fissure
    c. Straining
    d. Starting solids

29. A child has developed her second perirectal abscess in six months. She should be evaluated for which condition?

    a. *Giardia lamblia*
    b. Crohn's disease
    c. Ulcerative colitis
    d. Enterobiasis

30. Which of the following symptoms are most common in the early phase of appendicitis?

    a. Abdominal pain after eating
    b. Fever and diarrhea
    c. Severe localized RLQ pain with pallor and sweating
    d. Anorexia, vague, diffuse pain

31. Steatorrhea is not consistent with which of the following?

    a. *C. difficile*
    b. *Giardia lamblia*
    c. Celiac disease
    d. Cystic fibrosis

32. Jamil continues with the third day of diarrhea. His mother calls concerned. Which of the following would not be helpful advice?

    a. Monitor stool for blood or mucus
    b. Encourage solid food
    c. Avoid milk products
    d. Monitor for urination at least every 6 hours

33. Of the following advice, which would be most helpful for the parents of a baby with gastro-esophageal reflux?

    a. Most babies continue to vomit until they are walking; at around one year of age
    b. Laying prone after eating will decrease the amount of vomiting
    c. Increase the interval between feedings to a minimum of four hours
    d. Medications are generally necessary to prevent further problems

34. Which of the following foods would be appropriate for a child with celiac disease?

    a. Oatmeal for breakfast
    b. Boiled rice with butter
    c. Commercially baked bread
    d. Cream of wheat

35. A parent requests that her child receive immunoglobulin (IG) as protection against hepatitis A prior to international travel. Which of the following does this parent need to know?

    a. After IG administration, a 3 month interval is needed prior to the next measles vaccine
    b. There is no impact on future immunizations
    c. No immunizations can be given for 1 year
    d. Since children do not have symptoms with hepatitis A, IG is not necessary

Answers

1. b	13. b	25. d
2. d	14. d	26. c
3. a	15. a	27. d
4. c	16. a	28. a
5. d	17. d	29. b
6. d	18. b	30. d
7. d	19. a	31. a
8. b	20. c	32. c
9. d	21. d	33. b
10. b	22. a	34. b
11. b	23. b	35. a
12. c	24. a	

Bibliography

American Academy of Pediatrics. (2000). *Red Book 2000: Report of the Committee on Infectious Diseases* (25th ed.). Elk Grove Village, IL: Author.

American Academy of Pediatrics. Committee on Quality Improvement, Subcommittee on Acute Gastroenteritis. (1996). Practice parameter: The management of acute gastroenteritis in young children. *Pediatrics, 97*, 424–435.

Baker, S. S., Liptak, G. S., Colletti, R. B., Croffie, J. M., DiLorenzo, C., Ector, W., & Nurko, S. (1999). A medical position statement of the North American Society for Pediatric Gastroenterology and Nutrition. Constipation in infants and children: Evaluation and treatment. *Journal of Pediatric Gastroenterology and Nutrition, 29*, 612–626.

Buzby, M. (1997). Differential diagnosis. Acute diarrheal illness in children. *Lippincott's Primary Care Practice, 1*(3), 252–269.

Caty, M. G., & Azizkhan, R. G. (1994). Acute surgical conditions of the abdomen. *Pediatric Annals, 23*, 192–201.

Fishman, L. N., Jonas, M. M., & Lavine, J. E. (1996). Update on viral hepatitis in children. *Pediatric Clinics of North America, 43*, 57–74.

Gremse, D. A., & Sacks, A. (1997). Evaluation of dyspepsia. *Pediatric Annals, 26*, 251–259.

Hillemeier, A. C. (1996). Gastroesophageal reflux. Diagnostic and therapeutic approaches. *Pediatric Clinics of North America, 43*, 197–209.

Hoekelman, R. A. (1994). Pyloric stenosis is a pediatrician's diagnosis. *Pediatric Annals, 23*, 181–182.

Hofmann, A. D., & Greydanus, D. E. (1997). *Adolescent Medicine* (3rd ed.). Stamford, Ct: Appleton & Lange.

Markowitz, J. F. (1996). Inflammatory bowel disease: The pediatrician's role. *Contemporary Pediatrics, 13*(5), 25–46.

Preud'Homme, D. L., & Mezoff, A. G. (1996). Helicobacter pylori: A pathogen for all ages. *Contemporary Pediatrics, 13*(11), 27–49.

Talusan-Soriano, K., & Lake, A. M. (1996). Malabsorption in childhood. *Pediatrics in Review, 17*, 135–142.

Winesett, M. (1997). Inflammatory bowel disease in children and adolescents. *Pediatric Annals, 26*, 227–234.

Gastrointestinal Disorders In Adults

Sister Maria Salerno

Peptic Ulcer Disease (PUD)

- Definition: Ulceration of the GI mucosa in areas bathed by acid pepsin; stomach, duodenum, and esophagus are common sites

- Etiology/Incidence

  1. Infection with *Helicobacter pylori* leading to imbalance between mucosal protective factors and corrosive effects of acid and pepsin is considered primary cause

  2. Steroidal and nonsteroidal anti-inflammatory drug (NSAID) therapy, particularly aspirin, or other processes or factors leading to

     a. Hypersecretion of gastric mucosa

     b. Increased parietal cell mass

     c. Increased secretion of gastrin and hydrochloric acid

     d. Increased gastric emptying time

  3. Precipitating or aggravating factors include:

     a. Steroidal and nonsteroidal anti-inflammatory drug therapy, particularly aspirin

     b. Physiologic stress—severe trauma, burns, shock

     c. Psychological stress

     d. Alcohol and nicotine use; caffeine, coffee

     e. Presence of alcoholic liver cirrhosis, chronic pancreatitis, chronic lung disease, hyperparathyroidism, rheumatoid arthritis

  4. Lifetime prevalence about 10% for adult population

     a. Duodenal

        (1) 80% are duodenal

        (2) Higher incidence in males

        (3) Without antibiotic treatment 80% recur in year following initial healing

        (4) Incidence decreasing in U.S.

        (5) Familial disposition—more frequent in persons with type O blood

        (6) Peak incidence between 30 and 55 years of age

     b. Gastric

        (1) Occur with about the same incidence in males and females

        (2) About 5% are malignant

        (3) Peak incidence—age 55 to 65 years of age; rare < 40 years of age

- Signs and Symptoms

  1. Intermittent epigastric pain—gnawing, burning, boring, nagging

2. Pain begins 1 to 3 hours after eating, frequently awakens person at night

3. Pain relieved by food or antacids

4. Food sometimes aggravates pain of gastric ulcer

5. Weight loss frequent in persons with gastric ulcer

6. Dyspepsia (bloating, nausea, anorexia, excessive flatulence)

- Differential Diagnosis

    1. History of typical pain-food-relief pattern is most important criterion for diagnosis of duodenal ulcer

    2. History not helpful in distinguishing gastric from duodenal

    3. Rule out other causes of epigastric pain

        a. Pancreatitis

        b. Biliary tract disease

        c. Neoplasms

        d. Liver disease

        e. Gastritis

        f. Pneumonia

        g. Functional problems

        h. Cardiovascular disease, e.g., angina

- Physical Findings

    1. Usually none

    2. Epigastric tenderness in advanced disease

- Diagnostic Tests/Findings

    1. Barium radiograph of the upper GI tract will detect 90% of peptic ulcers—indications include:

        a. Diagnosis of atypical cases

        b. Typical presentations with failure to respond to treatment in 3 to 4 weeks; cases of recurrence

        c. Differentiating gastric from duodenal

        d. Differentiating malignant from nonmalignant gastric ulcers

        e. Documentation of healing

    2. Endoscopy

        a. Expensive but more sensitive and specific than barium radiographs; becoming test of choice in many settings

      b.   Indicated if clinical symptoms persist despite negative barium studies

      c.   Rule out malignancy in gastric ulcers

      d.   For those with diagnosed or suspected blood loss, perforation, vomiting, early satiety, or weight loss

3.   Stool for occult blood—positive if bleeding is present

4.   CBC

      a.   Hgb and Hct may be decreased

      b.   With chronic slow bleeding—hypochromic, microcytic anemia is likely

      c.   If bleeding is acute—normocytic, normochromic anemia

5.   Tests for helicobacter

      a.   Urea breath test

          (1)   95% to 98% sensitivity and specificity; results comparable to endoscopic biopsy

          (2)   Ingested drugs can cause false negatives; perform four weeks after last antibacterial treatment

      b.   Serological tests

          (1)   IgA, IgG antibodies, ELISA

          (2)   Inexpensive; sensitivity and specificity about 95%

          (3)   Not useful for follow up testing because of slow decline after treatment

          (4)   High serum lipid levels can interfere with results

      c.   Histological evaluation

          (1)   Requires endoscopic biopsy

          (2)   Invasive and expensive

      d.   Culture of biopsy

          (1)   Grows slowly and requires selective medium and environment

          (2)   Primary use in research

- Management/Treatment

   1.   Goals

      a.   Relief of symptoms

      b.   Healing

      c.   Prevention of recurrence

      d.   Eradication of bacteria

   2.   Nonpharmacological

a. Stop smoking

b. Avoid ASA and nonsteroidal anti-inflammatory drugs

c. Reduce stress

d. Reduce use of alcohol and caffeine (conflicting data, but still recommended until healing is documented)

3. Pharmacological

a. Antimicrobials to eradicate *H. pylori*

(1) Options include:

(a) Standard triple therapy—metronidazole 250 to 500 mg q.i.d. plus amoxicillin or tetracycline 500 mg q.i.d, with bismuth subsalicylate 4 cc or 2 tablets q.i.d. and omeprazole for 7 to 14 days

(b) MOC—metronidazole 500 mg b.i.d., omeprazole 20 mg b.i.d., with clarithromycin 250 to 500 mg b.i.d.

(c) RBC—ranitidine and bismuth citrate 400 mg b.i.d. for 28 days with clarithromycin for first 14 days

(d) Dual therapy—omeprazole 40 mg once a day for 4 weeks with clarithromycin 500 mg for 2 weeks

(2) Bismuth compounds act as topical antimicrobial, complementing antibiotics

(3) Compliance with combination therapies a problem

(4) Acquired resistance of microbe to metronidazole, and to lesser extent, clarithromycin often occurs with either if given alone

(5) Standard therapy currently least expensive

(6) Side effects of antimicrobial treatment

(a) Candida

(b) Rash

(c) Pseudomembranous colitis

(d) Photosensitivity

(7) No one ''right'' regimen

b. Proton pump inhibitors

(1) Omeprazole 20 mg per day for 4 to 8 weeks

(a) Not approved for maintenance therapy

(b) Short term use with duodenal ulcers, esophagitis

(2) Lansoprazole

(a) Long-term management of hypersecretory conditions

        (b)   Short term use with duodenal ulcers, esophagitis

        (c)   Inactivated by acid: enteric coated, take with food

    (3)   Like H_2 antagonists interfere with cytochrome P450 with similar drug interactions/precautions

    (4)   Create less acidic environment suppressing but not eradicating *H. pylori*

    (5)   Particularly useful in prevention/treatment of NSAID induced ulceration

c. H_2 receptor antagonists

    (1)   Cimetidine—300 mg orally t.i.d. with meals and at bedtime for 4 to 6 weeks (more recent studies indicate similar healing with 400 mg b.i.d. or 800 mg at bedtime)

        (a)   May be given IV in inpatient settings

        (b)   Side effects

            (i)   Frequently associated with acute confusional states in elderly or very ill patients.

            (ii)   Muscular pain; mild, transient diarrhea; impotence; gynecomastia; leukopenia; mildly elevated creatinine and transaminase levels are rare and tend to be seen only with long-term use

        (c)   Interferes with metabolism and increases blood levels of benzodiazapines, lidocaine, metronidazole, phenytoin, theophylline, and warfarin

        (d)   Should not be taken within an hour of taking antacids

    (2)   Ranitidine—150 mg orally b.i.d. or 300 mg orally at bedtime for active PUD; 150 mg orally at bedtime for maintenance

        (a)   Also available for IV use

        (b)   Side effects—rise in transaminase levels (ALT, formerly SGPT); dizziness; headache; tachycardia; malaise; constipation; diarrhea; rash; and rarely confusion

        (c)   No significant drug interactions

        (d)   May cause false-positive protein on urinary dip-stick analysis

    (3)   Famotidine—20 mg orally twice a day or 40 mg at bedtime

        (a)   As efficacious as ranitidine

        (b)   Least risk of drug interaction

    (4)   Nizatadine—150 mg orally twice a day or 300 mg at bedtime for up to 8 weeks

        (a)   No safer than cimetidine

Table 1

Antacids

Content Comments	Brand Name	Dose required for 80–100 mEq of acid neutralizing effect per dose	mEq of sodium per dose
Low Buffering Capacity			
CaCO$_3$ Rebound hyperacidity	Tums Alka II Chooz	8–10 tablets	0.5–0.6
Al(OH)$_3$ Constipating; high sodium	Amphogel	60–75 mL	1.2–1.5
Al(OH)$_3$ & Mg(OH)$_3$ Only for esophageal reflux	Gaviscon	94–118 mL	10.6–13.2
Moderate Buffering Capacity			
Al(OH)$_3$ & Mg(OH)$_3$ Low Sodium	Gelusil Mylanta Maalox Plus Riopan	35–44 mL 32–40 mL 30–38 mL 30–38 mL	0.23–0.29 0.20–0.25 0.36–0.45 0.08–0.1
High Buffering Capacity			
Al(OH)$_3$ & Mg(OH)$_3$ Liquid more effective than tablets.	Geluxil II Maalox TC Mylanta II	17–21 mL 14–18 mL 16–20 mL	0.2–0.25 0.1–0.13 0.15–0.2

Note: Sodium Bicarbonate, Alka Seltzer have a very short duration of action; acid rebound, systemic alkalosis are problems

    (b)   More expensive than cimetidine

  d. Antacids

    (1)   Should give dose equivalent to 80 to 100 mEq acid neutralizing capacity; for most, 30 to 40 mL given 1 and 3 hours after each meal; see Table 1 for comparison of various antacid preparations

    (2)   Primarily aluminum, calcium, or magnesium containing agents; sodium bicarbonate very short acting and systemic absorption can cause alkalosis (not recommended)

    (3)   Length of effect dependent on gastric emptying time; 30 minutes on an empty stomach, longer when taken with meals

    (4)   Side effects

        (a)   Diarrhea with magnesium hydroxide based agents

        (b)   Constipation with aluminum hydroxide containing agents

        (c)   Hypophosphatemia in aluminum containing agents due to aluminum phosphate binding and decreased GI absorption

        (d)   Osteopenia with long-term use of agents containing aluminum

        (e)   Rebound acid secretion and hypercalcemia with calcium containing agents

    (5)   Drug interactions

(a) Interfere with taste; absorption of iron, digoxin, and some antibiotics, e.g., tetracyclines

(b) Interfere with effectiveness of oral contraceptives

e. Anticholinergics

(1) Rarely used in contemporary treatment and only with advice of physician

(2) Primarily for relief of refractory pain

(3) High dosage with severe side effects required to achieve antisecretory effect

f. Sucralfate (mucosal protectant)—1 g orally q.i.d. on an empty stomach

(1) No significant side effects

(2) Drug Interaction

(a) Decreases absorption of digoxin, tetracycline, phenytoin, cimetidine, theophylline and other drugs

(b) Antacids interfere with effectiveness and should not be given within 1 hour of sucralfate administration

g. Treatment with antacids, H_2 receptor antagonists, or sucralfate results in 90 to 95% cure rate in 8 to 12 weeks

4. General considerations

a. Consult with physician regarding:

(1) Additional diagnostic studies for persons with suspected underlying disease or failure to respond to treatment in 2 to 4 weeks

(2) Persons with concurrent weight loss

(3) Persons with indications of peritonitis (rigidity, rebound tenderness, fever)

b. Refer to physician persons with confirmed or suspected complications

(1) Bleeding occurs in about 10% to 15% of persons with PUD

(a) Immediate medical emergency with possible surgical intervention required

(b) Signs and symptoms—heartburn, belching, epigastric discomfort, vomiting of bright red or coffee ground liquid

(c) Sudden relief of epigastric pain may be related to bleeding as blood acts as an acid buffer

(d) Diarrhea may also be evident; blood is a cathartic

(2) Perforation occurs in about 5% to 10% of persons with duodenal and 2% to 5% of those with gastric ulcers

      (a) Surgery is the indicated treatment

      (b) Signs and symptoms include acute pain, fever, leukocytosis, hypotension, peritoneal irritation

      (c) Peritoneal irritation is evidenced by abdominal rigidity, guarding, rebound tenderness, decreased or absent bowel sounds

(3) Gastric outlet (pyloric) obstruction is seen in less than 5% of all patients diagnosed with PUD and is most often associated with duodenal ulceration

      (a) Surgical intervention may be indicated

      (b) Signs and symptoms include worsening pain; vomiting of undigested food; dehydration; hypokalemia; and metabolic alkalosis

c. Patient education

(1) Disease and therapeutic management

(2) Purpose, dosage, side effects of medications

(3) Diet

      (a) No evidence to support need for bland diet or small frequent meals

      (b) Encourage avoidance of known gastric acid stimulants, e.g., coffee, cola, and other caffeine containing beverages

      (c) Avoidance of any foods or beverages which aggravate symptoms

      (d) Avoid eating within three hours of bedtime to avoid nocturnal stimulation of acid secretion

(4) Stress reduction

(5) Need to report to health care provider lack of response to medications, rectal bleeding, weight loss, increased weakness or dizziness, increasing pain

d. Follow up

(1) In 2 to 4 weeks to review:

      (a) Symptom response to medications

      (b) GI bleeding

      (c) Side or toxic effects of medications

(2) For those with gastric ulcers document healing with upper GI barium radiograph or endoscopy—in 6 weeks for small ulcers; 12 weeks for large; imperative in gastric ulcers; unnecessary in uncomplicated duodenal

Table 2

Foods And Other Substances That Decrease Lower Esophageal Sphincter Tone

Anticholinergics
Benzodiazepines
Calcium channel blockers
Diazepam
Meperidine
Narcotics
Progesterone
Alcohol
Caffeine
Nicotine
Chocolate
Fatty foods
Peppermint
Yellow onions

Gastroesophageal Reflux Disease

- Definition: Reflux of stomach and duodenal contents into the esophagus leading to a spectrum of clinical manifestations predominated by inflammation of the esophagus; classified with gastric and duodenal ulcers as a peptic ulcer disease

- Etiology/Incidence

    1. Most often related to inappropriate relaxation of the lower esophageal sphincter (LES) which allows reflux of gastric acid and pepsin into the distal esophagus

        a. Idiopathic

        b. Foods and other agents (see Table 2)

    2. Inflammation can also be caused by ingestion of caustic agents such as lye, or infectious agents such as candida, herpes simplex, or cytomegalovirus which directly attacks esophageal mucosa

    3. Infectious agents most often noted in immunosupressed individuals, e.g., persons with AIDS, diabetes, and persons receiving chemotherapy

    4. Incidence not known, however, a daily prevalence rate of heartburn, the major symptom of esophagitis, has been estimated to be 7% in a normal adult population

- Signs and Symptoms

    1. Retrosternal aching or burning heartburn (pyrosis) occurring 30 to 60 minutes after eating; associated with large meals, and aggravated by lying down or bending over

    2. Chest heaviness, pressure radiating to neck or jaw, or shoulders

    3. Regurgitation of fluid or food particles

    4. Nocturnal aspiration

    5. Recurrent pneumonia or bronchospasm

    6. Pain or difficulty swallowing

- Differential Diagnosis
    1. Myocardial infarction/angina
    2. Esophageal spasm
    3. Cholelithiasis
    4. Neoplasms
    5. Chemical or infectious esophagitis
    6. Conditions leading to gastric dysmotility, e.g., scleroderma, diabetes
- Physical Findings—generally insignificant
- Diagnostic Tests/Findings
    1. Usually only needed in atypical or severe cases
    2. Barium radiograph of upper GI tract
        a. To rule out strictures or other acid-peptic disease indicated in patients with:
            (1) Dysphagia
            (2) Painful swallowing
            (3) Significant weight loss
            (4) Occult blood loss
        b. Usually normal, but may show inflammation, ulcer, or stricture
    3. Endoscopy becoming more routine than barium radiography in most settings—is indicated in same instances as barium radiography; may show visible mucosal damage which can be confirmed by biopsy; in cases of caustic ingestion or suspected infectious etiology endoscopy is usually first diagnostic test
    4. Bernstein acid perfusion—rarely needed with classic history; requires alternating infusion of 0.1 N hydrochloric acid and normal saline into the esophagus; positive reproduction of symptoms with the hydrochloric acid infusion and not the saline is usual in esophageal reflux
    5. Esophageal motility and 24 hour esophageal pH tests are more specialized and reserved for atypical cases; consult with or refer patient to gastroenterologist
- Management/Treatment
    1. Phase I—implement general measures
        a. Weight reduction if obese
        b. Elevation of head of bed
        c. Avoid large meals and carbonated beverages particularly three hours prior to going to bed; no indication that fruit juices aggravate the problem
        d. Limit fats and carbohydrates
        e. Avoid straining at stool

  f. Avoid agents that decrease LES tone—nicotine, alcohol, chocolate, caffeine, theophylline, calcium channel blockers, anticholinergics

  g. Antacids—(see Table 1)

    (1) Mainstay of therapy

    (2) 80 to 100 mEq of neutralizing activity (30 cc for most agents) after meals and at bedtime

    (3) Liquid preferred to tablet forms

2. Phase II—if general measures are ineffective add H_2 antagonist cimetidine or ranitidine in same dosages as in peptic ulcer disease

3. Phase III—if Phase II measures are ineffective consult with physician regarding further testing and use of more aggressive therapies which might include:

  a. Higher dose of H_2 blockers or omeprazole

  b. H_2 blocker and a prokinetic to increase LES tone, esophageal motility, and gastric emptying

    (1) Metoclopramide—10 to 15 mg before meals and at bedtime

      (a) High frequency of side effects

      (b) Include fatigue, anxiety, confusion, and extrapyramidal reactions

    (2) Cisapride—10 mg before meals and at bedtime

      (a) Works synergistically with H_2 receptor antagonists to promote healing

      (b) Fatal cardiovascular events may occur when taken with drugs that inhibit the cytochrome P450 3A4 enzymes and/or when co-morbidities that predispose to dysrhythmias

    (3) Bethanechol 25 mg 30 minutes before meals

      (a) To date has shown limited effectiveness

      (b) Contraindicated in asthma, ischemic heart disease, or urinary retention

4. Phase IV—surgical intervention reserved for patients with stricture, bleeding, pulmonary aspiration, or severe refractory symptoms

5. General considerations

  a. Consult with physician regarding persons

    (1) With atypical presentation

    (2) Refractory to simple treatment

    (3) With dysphagia and or weight loss in addition to heartburn

  b. Education

(1) Mechanism of esophageal reflux and goals of management

(2) Aggravating factors

(3) Correction of misconceptions regarding causes (hiatal hernia seldom a cause) and treatment

(4) Proper use, dosage, side effects of pharmacologic agents

Cholecystitis

- Definition: Acute or chronic inflammation of the gallbladder

- Etiology/Incidence

  1. About 90% related to presence of pigmented or cholesterol calculi which can vary in diameter from 1 mm to 4 cm; when a stone becomes impacted in the cystic duct, inflammation develops behind the obstruction; if not relieved, pressure builds up in the gallbladder and leads to distension, ischemic changes, gangrene, and perforation with subsequent abscess formation and less frequently generalized peritonitis

  2. Occurs subsequent to bile stasis, bacterial infection, or ischemia

  3. Most common form of gallbladder disease; affects more than 15 million Americans

  4. Being 50 to 70 years old, female over 40 years old and obese are all risk factors

  5. Pregnancy, sedentary lifestyle, low fiber diet, use of oral contraceptives or antilipemics also associated with the development of cholecystitis

- Signs and Symptoms

  1. Episodic occurrences of postprandial fullness, heartburn, nausea, flatulence, regurgitation of bitter fluid, vomiting often precipitated by a large or fatty meal

  2. Anorexia (inability to finish an average size meal)

  3. Recurrent episodes of biliary colic—sudden appearance of severe pain in the epigastrium or right hypochondrium which subsides relatively slowly (12 to 18 hours)

     a. Tenderness of the same area may persist for days

     b. Accompanied by vomiting in 75% of the cases

  4. Constant aching pain or pressure in the right upper quadrant or epigastrium that radiates to the back or right shoulder

- Differential Diagnosis

  1. Perforated peptic ulcer

  2. Acute pancreatitis

  3. Appendicitis

  4. Salpingitis

  5. Diverticulitis

  6. Perforated hepatic carcinoma

7.   Liver abscess

8.   Hepatitis

9.   Pneumonia with right sided pleurisy

10.   Myocardial infarction

- Physical Findings

    1.   General appearance—unremarkable between attacks; ill during attack

    2.   Vital signs—mild temperature elevation, tachycardia, and increased respiratory rate during acute attack

    3.   Integument—mild jaundice occurs in about 20% of cases

    4.   Abdomen—guarding, rebound tenderness in right hypochondrium; palpable, tender sausage shaped mass in RUQ during acute attack in 20% to 30% of cases

    5.   Positive Murphy's sign—inspiratory arrest secondary to extreme tenderness when subhepatic area is palpated during deep inspiration

- Diagnostic Tests/Findings

    1.   CBC—mild leukocytosis with increased bands (shift to the left)

    2.   ECG—normal, important in ruling out myocardial infarction as cause of symptoms

    3.   Chest radiograph—normal, important in ruling out pneumonia as cause of symptoms

    4.   Flat plate radiograph of abdomen—gallstones

    5.   Ultrasound (study of choice with 95% sensitivity 98% specificity for stones)—gallstones, thickened gallbladder wall stones

    6.   Technetium T_c99_m PIPIDA (HIDA) scan—cystic duct occlusion and nonvisualized gallbladder

    7.   Alkaline phosphatase—elevated

    8.   Serum amylase—elevated, > 1,000 suspect concomittant pancreatitis

    9.   Serum aspartate aminotransferase (AST, formerly termed SGOT) and serum alanine aminotransferase (ALT, formerly SGPT) may be transiently elevated

    10.   Bilirubin—mildly increased

    11.   Old age, lymphoma, malnutrition, and immunosuppression may alter laboratory tests

    12.   CT scan has no advantage over ultrasound in diagnosis of acute attack

    13.   Oral cholecystography not used for acute attack

- Management/Treatment

    1.   Elective cholecystectomy recommended for:

    a.   Symptomatic patients with radiologic or ultrasound evidence of gallbladder disease

    b.   Those at high risk for complications such as those with:

        (1)   A calcified gall bladder

        (2)   Gallstones > 2 cm in diameter

        (3)   Diabetes

2. Conservative treatment for those who are asymptomatic

    a.   If on clofibrate (an antilipemic) or oral contraceptives stop or decrease dosage

    b.   Avoid foods that seem to precipitate symptoms, otherwise no need to alter diet or restrict fats

    c.   Anticholinergics not helpful

    d.   Treat dyspeptic symptoms with antacids (25% to 50% of patients will respond)

    e.   Some patients may be put on a trial of chenodiol 750 mg orally per day

        (1)   Best results are obtained in patients with small floating cholesterol stones

        (2)   Contraindicated in patients with inflammatory bowel disease or peptic ulcer disease

        (3)   Approximately 50% recurrence rate within five years after treatment

        (4)   Side effects—hepatotoxicity, diarrhea, and increased LDL cholesterol

        (5)   Expensive

3. Lithotripsy or destruction of stones with extracorporeal shock waves has limited application at present

4. General considerations

    a.   Refer all persons with suspected cholecystitis to physician for further evaluation, possible hospitalization, and possible surgery

    b.   Patient education

        (1)   Disease course, expected outcomes, and treatment

        (2)   Changes in symptoms which necessitate contact of health professional, e.g., change in pain pattern or pain accompanied by fever, chills

        (3)   Teach purpose, dosage, side effects of medications

        (4)   Nutrition

            (a)   If fatty foods seem to precipitate symptoms a low-fat diet may be helpful

          (b)   Some research has shown that increased fiber in the diet reduces incidence of gallstone formation

          (c)   If obese, a reducing diet is indicated; avoid rapid weight loss and fad diets which may actually increase risk of gallstone formation and precipitate acute symptoms

      (5)   Encourage regular physical exercise; sedentary life style is associated with stone formation as well as obesity

   c.   Follow-up annually and for acute attacks

   d.   Complications include empyema, gangrene, and perforation

Appendicitis

- Definition: Inflammation of the vermiform appendix

- Etiology/Incidence

   1.   Obstruction of the appendix with hardened feces (fecalith), stricture, inflammation, foreign body, or neoplasm

   2.   Occurs in all age groups, but more common in males between 10 and 30 years of age

   3.   Higher mortality rate due to complications in children, adolescents, and person over 55 years of age

   4.   One of the leading causes for abdominal surgery

- Signs and Symptoms

   1.   Acute onset of periumbilical or epigastric pain which ranges from mildly diffuse to severe

   2.   Anorexia, nausea, and vomiting (usually subsequent to pain onset)

   3.   Shifting of pain to right lower quadrant (McBurney's point) after several hours; aggravated by walking or coughing

   4.   Occasional radiation of pain into the ipsilateral testicle or labia

   5.   Spasm of abdominal muscles

   6.   Constipation usual; diarrhea rare

   7.   Elderly clients may present with mild symptoms of unexplained weakness, anorexia, tachycardia, and abdominal distention with little pain

   8.   After 24 hours may progress to perforation with sudden cessation of pain and subsequent peritonitis manifested by

      a.   Abdominal rigidity

      b.   Generalized abdominal tenderness

      c.   High fever

      d. Vomiting

      e. Dehydration

      f. Decreased bowel sounds

      g. Shock

- Differential Diagnosis

  1. Gastroenteritis

  2. Pneumonia

  3. Ruptured ovarian cyst

  4. Tubal pregnancy

  5. Acute cholecystitis

  6. Neoplastic perforation of the colon

  7. Renal calculi

  8. Pyelonephritis of the right kidney

- Physical Findings

  1. General appearance—may or may not appear ill

  2. Vital signs—fever 100 to 102° F

  3. Slight tachycardia related to pain and fever

  4. Abdominal—point and rebound tenderness in RLQ; decreased or absent bowel sounds

  5. Positive psoas and obturator signs

  6. Rectal/pelvic exams—tenderness in the right perirectal area

  7. Musculoskeletal—abdominal pain (RLQ) with hip extension and with straight leg raise

- Diagnostic Tests/Findings

  1. CBC with differential—leukocytosis with increased band cells (shift to the left); in the elderly shift may be present without leukocytosis

  2. Radiograph of the abdomen may show fecalith

- Management/Treatment: All persons with suspected or diagnosed appendicitis should be immediately referred to a physician for hospitalization and surgery. Appendicitis that has progressed to perforation or peritonitis will be associated with longer morbidity and higher mortality

Diverticulitis

- Definition: Inflammation of one or more diverticula in the bowel wall with microperforation and abscess formation in the pericolic fat

- Etiology/Incidence
    1. Inflammatory process similar to etiologic agents in appendicitis
    2. Occurs in about 33% of persons with diverticula (estimated to be 5% to 20% of the adult population)
        a. Incidence increases over age 40
        b. More frequent in females than males
        c. Higher incidence in persons with low fiber dietary habits
        d. Diverticula found most often in the sigmoid colon but may occur anywhere in the GI tract
    3. Free perforation with signs of peritonitis is rare
- Signs and Symptoms
    1. Acute left lower quadrant pain—steady and severe lasting for several days or crampy and intermittent
    2. Constipation more usual than diarrhea
    3. Pain increased with defecation
    4. Flatulence
    5. Nausea
    6. Low grade fever
- Differential Diagnosis
    1. Appendicitis
    2. Carcinoma of the colon
    3. Crohn's disease
    4. Ischemic colitis
    5. Gynecologic disorders, e.g.,
        a. Ectopic pregnancy
        b. Ovarian abscess
- Physical Findings
    1. Vital signs—mild fever, tachycardia
    2. Abdomen—guarding, rebound tenderness, rigidity especially over LLQ; if abscess has formed, a tender palpable mass may be noted
    3. Rectal examination—tender painful mass may be present
- Diagnostic Tests/Findings
    1. CBC—slight leukocytosis

2. Sed rate—elevated

3. Stool guaiac—positive in about 25% of cases

4. Urine—normal unless colovesicular fistula present then bacteriuria, leukorrhea, hematuria

5. Barium enema will confirm presence of diverticulosis and help rule out other etiologies, however not indicated during acute phase

6. Proctoscopic examination—negative

7. Sigmoidoscopy—inflamed mucosa

8. Stool for ova/parasites—negative

- Management/Treatment: For most patients with mild disease outpatient treatment will be indicated and includes:

  1. Clear liquids for 1 to 2 days followed by a bland diet once symptoms have subsided

  2. Antibiotic therapy with one of the following:

     a. Ampicillin 500 mg orally every 6 hours

     b. Tetracycline 500 mg orally every 6 hours

     c. Amoxicillin/clavulanate potassium 500 mg every six hours

     d. A combination of ampicillin and an aminoglycoside is common

  3. Bedrest to promote colon rest recommended until symptoms subside

  4. General considerations

     a. Consult with physician regarding

        (1) Those who fail to improve in 72 hours

        (2) Those with a temperature > 102° F

        (3) Need for additional testing

     b. Patients with severe disease require hospitalization, antibiotics, bowel rest, and IV hydration

     c. Patient education

        (1) Etiology/incidence and usual clinical course of the disease and rationale for recommended treatment

        (2) Instruction on recommended dietary guidelines

           (a) After acute phase, high fiber diet to include foods such as bran, whole grains, cereals, raw, cooked or died fruit, raw vegetables, cooked high residue vegetables

           (b) High fiber diet may cause bloating and flatulence during the first two weeks of use; this resolves with continued high fiber intake

(3) Avoid laxatives, enemas, antidiarrheal agents and uncooked high residue foods

(4) Report fever, bleeding, increasing pain to health care provider immediately

(5) Bulk forming agents such as psyllium hydrophilic muciloid and use of stool softeners such as docusate sodium may help prevent frequent recurrence

d. Follow-up—return visit or phone follow-up in 24 to 48 hours to verify relief with initiating therapy; and then again after completion of antibiotic therapy

Viral Hepatitis

- Definition: Inflammation of the liver
- Etiology/Incidence
  1. Type A (infectious)
     a. Infection with hepatitis A virus (HAV), a small RNA enterovirus
        (1) Spread primarily by fecal-oral route; also parenterally
        (2) Found in infected water, food, shellfish
        (3) Intimate contact and poor sanitation and personal hygiene seem to be contributing factors
        (4) Incubation period 2 to 6 weeks
        (5) Infectivity—2 to 3 weeks in late incubation and early clinical phase
     b. Common in crowded situations such as low income housing, school, military, and prison dormitories; can occur in any age group; common in immigrants from under developed countries, school age children, and young adults
        (1) Self limiting in > 99% of cases
        (2) No carrier state or chronic infection
        (3) Severity increases with age
        (4) In U.S. seroprevalence of Anti-HAV in adults indicates 40% to 50% have had the disease
  2. Type B (Serum)
     a. Infection with hepatitis B virus (HBV), a DNA virus with core and surface components
        (1) HB_sAg (Hepatitis B surface antigen) found in serum, saliva, semen, stool, and urine
        (2) Core contains HB_cAg (Hepatitis B core antigen) and when present, HB_eAg (secretory form of HB_cAg present only in HB_sAg positive sera); HB_eAg associated with high virus titer and high infectivity

    (3)   Incubation period 6 weeks to 6 months

    (4)   Transmission by blood, blood products, and other body fluids, such as saliva and semen

    (5)   Mother-infant transmission if mother infected during 3rd trimester

    (6)   Approximately 10% of infected individuals become chronic carriers

  b. Common in drug addicts, homosexual males, those with multiple sexual partners and densely populated urban neighborhoods; higher risk individuals include persons exposed to needle punctures and blood products such as IV drug abusers; those on hemodialysis; those requiring blood transfusions, or IV chemotherapy; and health care personnel such as nurses, laboratory workers, surgeons, and hemodialysis personnel

    (1)   Considered to be a sexually transmitted disease

    (2)   Accounts for about 40% of acute hepatitis cases/annually

3. HDV (hepatitis delta virus) incomplete RNA virus

  a. Requires antecedent or simultaneous HBV infection

  b. Common in IV drug users and recipients of multiple transfusions

  c. Concomitant infection usually results in more severe manifestations than HBV alone

  d. Immunity to HBV protects against HDV

4. Type C (parenteral non-A, non-B)

  a. Infection with Hepatitis C Virus (HCV), an RNA virus.

    (1)   Incubation variable—2 weeks to 6 months

    (2)   Chronic liver disease develops in 70%

    (3)   Related to development of hepatocellular carcinoma in 10%

  b. Leading cause of post transfusion hepatitis

  c. High risk population—IV drug users, hospital personnel, male homosexuals, and those receiving multiple transfusions

5. Type E (enteral or epidemic non-A, non-B)

  a. Infection with Hepatitis E Virus (HEV), a single stranded RNA virus

    (1)   Viral particles found in stool of infected persons

    (2)   Does not progress to chronic liver disease

    (3)   Incubation—2 to 9 weeks

    (4)   Usually mild disease in adults > 15 yrs

    (5)   Mortality as high as 10% to 20% in pregnant woman

  b. Rare in the U.S.

6. Type G (HGV)

    a. Infection with a flavivirus

        (1) Transmitted percutaneously

        (2) Most infections asymptomatic

        (3) May result in chronic viremia but chronic disease rare

    b. Risk groups include transfusion recipients, IV drug users

    c. Frequent co-infection with HCV

- Signs and Symptoms: Clinical manifestations for all types are similar and can vary from a minor flu-like illness to fatal liver failure.

1. HAV may present with nonspecific or "flu" syndrome

2. HBV clinical course more variable than HAV and associated with extrahepatic manifestations, e.g., urticaria, other rashes, arthritis

3. HCV acute illness variable, flu-like and subsides spontaneously (60% to 70% are asymptomatic)

4. Prodromal phase or preicteric phase (lasts approximately two weeks)

    a. Fatigue, malaise

    b. Anorexia

    c. Nausea/vomiting

    d. Headache

    e. Hyperalgia

    f. Cough, coryza, pharyngitis

    g. Changes in taste with aversion to alcohol and smoking

    h. Right upper abdominal pain

    i. Weight loss of 2 to 4 kg

5. Active or icteric phase (lasts 2 to 6 weeks)

    a. Jaundice—sclera and skin (never manifested in some patients)

    b. Dark urine

    c. Clay-colored stools; often precedes jaundice

    d. Enlarged tender liver

    e. Pruritus, urticarial rash more often associated with HBV

6. Post-icteric or recovery phase

    a. Resolving jaundice, increasing sense of well-being, and decrease in symptomatology

    b. Chronic active hepatitis in those with HBV may begin at this point and is manifested by persistence of symptoms

- Differential Diagnosis
    1. Infectious mononucleosis
    2. Choledocholithiasis
    3. Hepatotoxic drugs, e.g., chloramphenicol, acetaminophen, methyldopa
    4. Carcinoma of the head of the pancreas
    5. Alcoholic cirrhosis
    6. History and serological tests assist in differentiating type

- Physical Findings
    1. General appearance—mildly ill to generally debilitated
    2. Vital signs—mild fever
    3. Integumentary—slight jaundice; rash
    4. HEENT—yellow sclera, lymphadenopathy
    5. Abdomen—enlarged, tender liver; splenomegaly (in about 10% of cases); normal bowel sounds

- Diagnostic Tests/Findings
    1. CBC with differential—WBC low to normal
    2. Urinalysis—proteinuria; bilirubinuria
    3. Abnormal liver function tests
        a. Elevated AST (formerly SGOT), ALT (formerly SGPT) typically 500 to 2000 IU/L
        a. Rise 7 to 10 days before jaundice
        b. Begin to fall shortly after onset of jaundice; should return to normal after 6 months
        c. Degree of increase does not necessarily parallel disease severity
        d. LDH, serum bilirubin, alkaline phosphatase, prothrombin time normal or slightly increased
    4. Serology tests—refer to Table 3

- Management/Treatment
    1. Consult with physician regarding patient management
    2. Approach is primarily supportive in uncomplicated cases
        a. Activity/rest

Table 3

Serology Tests for Viral Hepatitis

IgM antibody to HAV — appears during acute or early convalescent phase and disappears in about 8 weeks; implies recent infection with HAV
IgG antibody to HAV implies previous infection with HAV; confers immunity
HB$_S$Ag (Hepatitis B surface antigen) — positive throughout the active phase of illness; first test to obtain if acute HBV infection is suspected; will remain positive in asymptomatic carriers and in chronic hepatitis
Anti-HB$_S$ (Antibody specific to HB$_S$Ag [Hepatitis B surface antigen])—positive indication of non-infectious state and recovery, and immunity; appears after HB$_S$Ag disappears
Anti-HB$_C$ (Antibody to HB$_C$Ag [Hepatitis B core antigen])—present at onset of acute illness; remains present for years, and is found in asymptomatic carriers; in many patients there is a period (window) between the disappearance of HB$_S$Ag and the appearance of Anti-HB$_S$ Antibody, usually during late stages of acute phase or early convalescence; during this period, Anti-HB$_C$ will be the only serological marker of the infection
Anti-HDV (Antibody to Hepatitis D) — marker of co/or superinfection by hepatitis D in persons with Hepatitis B; appears late and is short lived
HB$_e$Ag (Protein derived from HBV core) — indicates circulating HBV and highly infectious sera
Anti-HB$_e$ (Antibody to HB$_e$Ag) — appears weeks-months after HB$_e$Ag and HBV are no longer detecable in blood; presence indicates substantially less infectious sera
Anti-HCV (Antibody to HCV) — appears 6 months after initial infection, remains elevated indefinitely, considered infectious and capable of transmission
HCV-RNA (Hepatitis C RNA) can detect circulating virus in 1–2 weeks after infection; becoming the gold standard for HCV detection.

      (1)   Rest recommended during active phase

      (2)   Resumption of full activities during the recovery period does not appear to prolong illness, cause relapse or development of chronic disease

      (3)   Avoidance of activity that might cause trauma to liver or spleen

   b.   Adequate fluid and dietary intake

      (1)   3,000 to 4,000 mL fluid per day; high carbohydrate fluids such as fruit juices, carbonated beverages are encouraged but not always well tolerated

      (2)   Foods high in protein, carbohydrates, and calories

      (3)   Low fat diet not shown to be beneficial

      (4)   Most important to eat whatever is tolerated

   c.   Antiemetics may be prescribed 30 minutes before meals to control nausea and vomiting; rectal administration may be better tolerated than oral

   d.   Patients with elevated PT may be given vitamin K

   e.   Symptomatic relief of pruritus with colloidal baths, soaps, and lotions

   f.   Avoid alcohol and other drugs detoxified or metabolized by the liver

   g.   Avoid birth control pills and C-17 alpha alkyl-substituted androgenic steroids during acute phase; may increase bilirubin levels

 3.   For HCV—interferon alfa-2B (Intron A) 3 million units SC or IM three times a week for six months

a. Exact mechanism of action unknown

b. Produces clinical remission in 40% to 60%

c. 70% to 80% of those with remission have recurrence of active disease in 6 to 12 months post-treatment

d. Most positive response with:

    (1) Low serum titer HCV RNA

    (2) Younger age

    (3) Female

    (4) Absence of cirrhosis

e. No data to date showing better survival rates or inhibition of progress to chronic active hepatitis

4. General considerations

    a. Refer for possible hospitalization and further testing

        (1) Complicated cases

        (2) Severely ill patients

        (3) Persons with signs of fulminating hepatitis or encephalitis

        (4) Dehydrated persons

        (5) Those with a PT > 15 seconds

        (6) Those suspected of having another underlying disease process

    b. Newly diagnosed cases reported to health department

    c. Patient education

        (1) Disease course and expected outcomes

        (2) Verify any drug use including over the counter medications and vitamin supplements with the healthcare provider until completely recovered

        (3) Maintain proper hygiene; proper hand-washing, disposal of all body wastes

            (a) Should not donate blood

            (b) Close personal contacts, family members, and sexual contacts should be evaluated for active disease and may receive immune serum globulin for passive immunity (not useful once disease is clinically evident)

    d. Follow-up

        (1) Follow weekly for the first 2 to 3 weeks; monthly thereafter if symptoms subside and liver function tests improving

        (2) Closer follow-up in those > 40 years of age

e. Complications

(1) HBV infection tends to be longer and more severe than HAV

(2) Carrier states and chronic hepatitis are associated with HBV and HCV, but not with HAV

(3) Fulminant liver failure occurs in less than 1% of those with HAV and in about 5% of those with HBV

(4) Chronic hepatitis can be associated with hepatic cancer

(5) 70% of patients with Hepatitis C will develop chronic hepatitis

f. Prophylaxis—see Table 4

Table 4
Adult Prophylaxis for Viral Hepatitis

Time of Exposure	Agent	Dose	Time
PRE-EXPOSURE			
Hepatitis A			
Persons traveling to or working in endemic areas; men who have sex with men; drug users; those who work with non-human primates with HAV infection or in labs with HAV; persons with chronic liver disease; those with clotting factor disorders; and some food handlers.	HA vaccine (preferred over serum)	1 mL IM	2 doses separated by 6–12 months depending on brand; protection begins 4 weeks after first dose; both doses needed for long-term protection.
If travel or exposure expected in less than 4 weeks after 1st HA vaccine dose.	Immune serum globulin	0.02mL/kg once	
Hepatitis B			
Recommended for health care personnel especially laboratory personnel; surgeons; dialysis personnel. Also recommended for adolescents in areas with high incidence of HBV, drug abuse, STD, teen pregnancies and for homosexually active men	HB vaccine × 3	1 mL IM	Usually given in 3 doses; 2nd & 3rd given approximately 1 mo & 6 mo after the 1st dose; need all 3 doses for adequate protection
POST EXPOSURE			

Hepatitis A
   Close contacts;
   Family members;
   Sexual partners
	Immune serum globulin	0.02 mL/kg	Once, not more than 2 weeks post exposure

Hepatitis B			
Percutaneious needle stick or mucosal exposure if unvaccinated and source HB$_S$Ag +	HB immune globulin & HB vaccine × 3	0.06 mL/kg 1 mL IM	Within 24–48 hours of exposure; at same time as HBIg, then at 1 & 6 mo
Sexual exposure	Globulin & HB vaccine × 3	0.6 mL/kg 1 mL IM	Within 14 days of last sexual contact; at same time as HBIg, then at 1 & 6 mo

Contact Center for Disease Control Hotline for most current and more specific information (404) 332-4555 or URL http//www.cdc.gov

Acute Gastroenteritis

- Definition: Acute inflammation of the gastrointestinal mucosa
- Etiology/Incidence
    1. Commonly due to infectious agents—viruses, bacteria, and parasites (*Giardia*, amoebae)
        a. Exotoxins produced by some organisms, (e.g., staphylococcus) induce hypersecretion or increased peristalsis resulting in diarrhea or vomiting
        b. Bacteria such as *E. coli* and salmonella penetrate and invade the gastric mucosa and lead to diarrhea accompanied by fever and fecal leukocytes
        c. See Table 5 for characteristics of some etiologic agents in gastroenteritis
    2. Second leading cause of morbidity in the U.S.
        a. Occurs universally in all age groups
        b. Epidemic outbreaks of bacterial enteritis occur in groups of persons who have ingested contaminated food
        c. Viral gastroenteritis occurs more frequently in the winter months
        d. Primarily a self-limiting disease
        e. The very young, elderly, and those with concomitant chronic debilitating disease are at higher risk for mortality
- Signs and Symptoms
    1. Abrupt onset of nausea, vomiting
    2. Explosive flatulence
    3. Crampy abdominal pain

Table 5
Characteristics of Select Etiologic Agents in Gastroenteritis

	Incubation or Onset	Fever	Fecal leukocytes	Other
E. coli	24–72 hr	+	+	Common cause of travelers' diarrhea; doxycycline, bismuth subsalicylate used preventively
Campylobacter	2–5 days	+	+	Erythromycin & tetracycline used in treatment
Staphylcoccus	1–6 hr	–	–	Grows in meats; dairy foods
Shigella/Salmonella	8–24 hr	+	+	Highly infectious
Botulism	12–36 hr	–	–	Neuro. signs—diplopia, vertigo, dysphagia; respiratory support may be needed
Giardia lamblia	7–21 days	–	–	Doxycycline, trimethoprim/ sulfamethoxazole, and fluoroquinolones used in treatment; cause of travelers' diarrhea

    4. Frequent, watery diarrhea

    5. Myalgia

    6. Headache

    7. Fever

    8. Generalized weakness/malaise

- Differential Diagnosis

    1. Acute appendicitis

    2. Cholecystitis

    3. Inflammatory bowel disease, e.g., colitis

    4. Fecal impaction with overflow

    5. Pelvic inflammatory disease

- Physical Findings

    1. General appearance—ill

    2. Vital signs—fever moderate to high 101 to 102° F in bacterial; up to 103° F in viral

    3. Abdomen—diffuse tenderness; no spasm or rebound tenderness except with salmonella infection; hyperactive bowel sounds; slight distention; absent or hypoactive bowel sounds common with botulism

    4. Neurological—dizziness, difficulty in swallowing and other neurological deficits are indication of botulism and require emergency intervention; with other etiologies findings are expected to be normal

- Diagnostic Tests/Findings

    1. CBC—normal indices

    2. Stool guaiac—usually negative in viral infections; positive with invasive bacterial infections

    3. Stool examination—if etiologic agent is an invasive bacteria, leukocytes will be present

    4. Stool culture—diagnostic for bacteria

        a. Done in suspected cases of bacterial infection, food poisoning, and if symptoms do not begin to abate in 48 hours

        b. Special cultures needed for suspected campylobacter, cholera

- Management/Treatment

    1. Immediately refer to a physician those with:

        a. Dehydration

        b. Rebound tenderness

    c.   Severe abdominal pain

    d.   Neurological symptoms

    e.   Concomitant debilitating illness

2. Most can be treated for 24 to 48 hours without laboratory testing with:

    a.   Bedrest as needed progressing to regular activity

    b.   NPO except for cracked ice while nausea and vomiting are present, then restriction to clear liquids for 24 hours; follow with addition of toast and crackers, proceeding to a bland then regular diet

    c.   Antiemetics and antidiarrheals are usually not indicated and may prolong the problem; treatment of salmonella has been noted to prolong the carrier state

    d.   Provide for parenteral administration of prescription medications if necessary

3. General considerations

    a.   Consult with physician if major symptoms do not abate in 48 hours; approach may include stool for ova and parasites, specialized stool cultures and proctosigmoidoscopy

    b.   Report bacterial infections and food poisoning to the health department

    c.   Patient education

        (1)   Disease course and expected outcome; symptoms usually resolve in 24 to 48 hours but mild diarrhea may persist for a week or two

        (2)   Explain proper food preparation and storage

        (3)   Appropriate dosage and side effects of medications

        (4)   Proper methods of hygiene including hand washing and disposal of stool and emesis

        (5)   Signs of dehydration; neurological involvement that require contacting health care professional

    d.   Follow-up

        (1)   Usually self-limiting; return visit warranted if symptoms (other than mild diarrhea) do not abate in 48 to 72 hours or worsen

        (2)   Diarrhea may continue for 1 to 2 weeks with salmonella infection

Irritable Bowel Syndrome (IBS) (Functional Bowel Syndrome)

- Definition: Functional disturbance of intestinal motility marked by a common symptom complex which includes abdominal pain and alternating bouts of constipation and diarrhea

- Etiology/Incidence

1. Disturbance in bowel motor activity thought to include a normal response to severe stress and learned visceral response to stress leading to:

   a. Nonpropulsive colonic contractions which lead to constipation

   b. Increased contraction in the small bowel and proximal colon with diminished activity in the distal colon leading to diarrhea

  2. Influenced by emotional factors

  3. Common GI disorder

   a. Accounts for about 50% of most GI complaints seen by health care professionals and a major cause of morbidity in the U.S.

   b. Onset usually occurs before age 35

   c. Women affected more often than men

- Signs and Symptoms

  1. Aching or cramping periumbilical or lower abdominal pain often precipitated by meals and relieved by defecation; does not awaken patient at night

  2. Pain may radiate to left chest or arm (gas in splenic flexure)

  3. Changes in bowel function

   a. Diarrhea

    (1) 4 to 6 movements/day

    (2) Small watery stools with clear mucus

    (3) Nocturnal diarrhea (rare)

   b. Constipation with irregular passage of small hard stools

   c. Alternating episodes of diarrhea and constipation

  4. Flatulence

  5. Exaggerated response to and preoccupation with bowel symptoms

  6. Bleeding, weight loss, and nocturnal diarrhea are not characteristic of IBS

- Differential Diagnosis

  1. Inflammatory bowel disorder, e.g., ulcerative colitis

  2. Viral or bacterial gastroenteritis

  3. GI neoplasms

  4. Parasitic infections

  5. Lactose deficiency

  6. Laxative abuse

  7. Side effects of drugs affecting bowel motility

  8. Rome criteria (Harris, 1997) for diagnosis require at least three months of continuous or recurrent symptoms that include:

a. Abdominal pain relieved by defecation or pain with change in frequency or consistency of stool

b. Disturbance in defecation at least 25% of time including at least two of the following

    (1) Altered frequency

    (2) Altered passage

    (3) Altered consistency

    (4) Passage of mucus

    (5) Abdominal distention

- Physical Findings

  1. General appearance—"worried well," anxious, depressed

  2. Vital signs—normal

  3. Abdomen—mild abdominal tenderness, normal or mildly hyperactive bowel sounds

  4. Rectal examination—normal

- Diagnostic Tests/Findings

  1. Stool examination—negative for blood, ova, parasite, pathogenic bacteria, and giardia specific antigen

  2. CBC, thyroid screen, chemical analysis—normal

  3. Barium enema—decreased motility, otherwise normal

  4. Proctosigmoidoscopy—normal

- Management/Treatment

  1. Confer with physician before ordering barium enema or proctosigmoidoscopy

  2. Provide emotional support, reassurance, information on stress reduction

  3. High fiber diet

  4. Pharmacologic agents

    a. Bulk laxatives—psyllium hydrophilic mucilloid

    b. Narcotics, depressants, and long term pharmaceutical use to be avoided

    c. Consult with physician regarding

      (1) Anticholinergics

        (a) Dicyclomine hydrochloride 20 to 40 mg orally q.i.d. or propantheline 15 mg orally q.i.d.

        (b) Usually given only after nonpharmacologic measures have failed

        (c) Side effects—dry mouth, tachycardia, orthostatic hypotension

(d) Contraindicated if history of glaucoma, urinary retention, cardiac arrhythmia

(2) Loperamide or other opiate derived antidiarrheals are reserved for only very severe cases; potential for abuse in these patients is great

(3) Tricyclic antidepressants

5. Patient education

    a. Disease course and expected outcomes

    b. Rationale for treatment

    c. High fiber diet

6. Planned exercise (may help in stress reduction)

7. Need for annual rectal examination and sigmoidoscopy after age 40

8. Some patients may benefit from psychological counseling and/or relaxation techniques

Colorectal Cancer

- Definition: Malignancy of gastrointestinal tract primarily colon or rectum

- Etiology/Incidence

  1. Causes remain unclear

  2. Risk factors include history of colonic polyps, breast or female genital tract cancer, chronic inflammatory bowel disorders, positive family history; high fat, low fiber, high-caloric diet

  3. Second most common cancer in western world, more common over the age of 50; peaks in the eighth decade

- Signs and Symptoms: Vary by location

  1. Right sided colon cancer

    a. Usually asymptomatic

    b. Vague or crampy, colicky abdominal pain

    c. Unexplained weight loss, fatigue, weakness

    d. Occult blood in stool

    e. Anemia

  2. Left sided colon cancer

    a. Alternating constipation with diarrhea

    b. Change in stool caliber (narrow, ribbon-like)

    c. Lower abdominal pain

    d. Red blood in stool

    e. Sensation of incomplete evacuation

  3. Rectal cancer

    a. Tenesmus

    b. Rectal bleeding (bright red)

    c. Mucous discharge

- Differential Diagnosis

  1. Diverticular disease

  2. Lymphoma

  3. Irritable bowel syndrome

  4. Inflammatory bowel disease

- Physical Findings

  1. Palpable mass primarily in right colon

  2. Lymphadenopathy

  3. Rectal mass found on rectal examination

  4. Stools positive for occult blood

- Diagnostic Tests/Findings

  1. Barium enema radiograph—air contrast preferable to single contrast, may see an apple core lesion or mass

  2. Colonoscopy—may allow for biopsy of lesion found by barium enema

  3. Fiberoptic sigmoidoscope—may find distal tumors

  4. Testing of stools for occult blood—cancers detected with this technique are usually early stage and have a high cure rate

  5. Carcinoembryonic antigen (CEA) test—often performed, although not specific for colon cancer; normal level of CEA does not exclude possibility of malignancy

  6. CBC can demonstrate an anemia

  7. Chest radiograph may reveal metastases

- Management/Treatment

  1. Referral for surgical excision or resection depending upon the depth of invasion of tumors

  2. Patients with metastatic lesions, noted at the time of diagnosis, have a poor prognosis; palliative treatment is then indicated

  3. Patients with a resection often require a temporary colostomy

  4. General considerations

    a. Screening for colon cancer

        (1)   Test stools for occult blood annually after age 50

        (2)   Digital rectal examination annually after age 40

        (3)   Sigmoidoscopy every 3 to 5 years after age 50

  b. Monitor for signs of dehydration during colon preps

  c. Instruct patient on possibility of a colostomy after procedure and begin patient teaching on care of colostomy preoperatively

  d. Encourage patient and family to ventilate feelings regarding the diagnosis

  e. Make referrals to pastoral care or mental health liaison as indicated

  f. Refer to community agencies for assistance after discharge, i.e., American Cancer Society, Ostomy Association

Questions
Select the best answer

1. Mr. P., 55-year-old of Irish decent, complains of pain in his chest and stomach for the past two weeks. He has been taking Alka Seltzer which seems to give him temporary relief. The pain is intermittent but has awakened him at night. The pain has a burning quality, and radiates up into his chest. He has hypertension which is controlled with diuretics.

   Which of the following would least likely be the cause of his pain?

   a. Coronary artery insufficiency
   b. Diverticulitis
   c. Duodenal ulcer
   d. Esophageal reflux

2. Your next step would be to:

   a. Start Mr. P. on antacids
   b. Discontinue his diuretic and switch to another class of antihypertensive
   c. Order an endoscopy
   d. Obtain additional medical history data

3. The fact that Mr. P.'s pain is not increased with activity and is unrelieved by rest makes it less likely that his problem is:

   a. Coronary artery insufficiency
   b. Gastric ulcer
   c. Duodenal ulcer
   d. Esophageal reflux

4. Which fact favors a diagnosis of gastric ulcer in this case?

   a. The patient's gender
   b. The patient's age
   c. The patient's ethnic origin
   d. The use of diuretics

5. Which of the following would be most beneficial in distinguishing a duodenal from a gastric ulcer in this patient?

   a. A history of a confirmed healed duodenal ulcer in the past year
   b. Reported unexplained weight loss in the past six months
   c. Pain aggravated by food intake
   d. An endoscopy or upper GI barium radiograph

6. Predisposing factors for duodenal ulcer include all of the following except:

   a. Genetic factors
   b. Stress
   c. Frequent laxative use

    d. Use of anti-inflammatory drugs

7. Bleeding from a duodenal ulcer:

    a. Usually causes increased pain
    b. In large amounts can cause diarrhea
    c. Is associated with constipation
    d. Indicates perforation

8. If Mr. P. has a peptic ulcer and his physical exam is unremarkable except for mild epigastric tenderness, it:

    a. Would not be unusual
    b. Indicates further diagnostic testing is unnecessary
    c. Is evidence that neoplastic disease is not present
    d. Rules out bleeding

9. A 55-year-old male with a peptic ulcer and mild anemia has a negative stool guaiac. You need to:

    a. Start iron supplementation
    b. Start H_2 antagonists and reschedule for return visit in 2 to 4 weeks
    c. Repeat the stool guaiac
    d. Refer for hematologic work up

10. After two weeks of treatment with omeprazole and clarithromycin all symptoms of a small non-bleeding duodenal ulcer have abated in your 35-year-old female. You:

    a. Need to confirm healing with an upper GI barium radiograph or endoscopy
    b. Instruct her to continue the omeprazole for two more weeks
    c. Instruct her to stop all medication and get a urea breath test
    d. Stop these medications and put her on H_2 antagonists

11. A major side effect of cimetidine that would be of special concern when prescribing for an elderly patient is:

    a. Confusion
    b. Decreased digoxin levels
    c. Hypophosphatemia
    d. Osteopenia

12. Mr. J. is an overweight 38 year old who has had intermittent heartburn for several months. He has been taking Tums which do provide temporary relief. During the past week he has been awakening during the night with a burning sensation in his chest. He is on no medication and has had no other major health problems.

    Which additional information would lead you to believe that gastroesophageal reflux is the cause of his pain?

    a. The pain seems better when he smokes to relieve his nerves

b. Constipation has been a chronic problem and he uses over-the-counter laxatives at least weekly

c. He often awakens at night with coughing and a bad taste in his mouth

d. Coffee and fried foods never bother him

13. Mr. J. had no weight loss or dysphagia and his physical examination is unremarkable. Your next step would be to:

a. Order an endoscopic exam
b. Refer him to a gastroenterologist
c. Start him on liquid antacids
d. Tell him to eat a snack before bedtime

14. If you had decided his problem was esophageal reflux, you should tell him:

a. He probably has a hiatal hernia causing the reflux
b. He will probably require surgery
c. He should avoid all fruit juices
d. Smoking, alcohol, and caffeine can aggravate his problem

15. The most definitive test for LES incompetence and gastroesophageal reflux is:

a. Stool guaiac
b. Upper GI barium radiograph
c. Cardiac and abdominal examination
d. Bernstein test

16. Mary L. is 26 years old, slightly overweight, and 2 months post partum. She is complaining of heartburn, flatulence, and anorexia. During her pregnancy she had experienced similar symptoms but they have become more severe in the last week and she vomited twice. She has an intermittent pain in her right hypochondrium. She also thinks she pulled a shoulder muscle as she has an almost constant dull ache there. Your first step is to:

a. Order liver function tests
b. Obtain a more detailed history
c. Refer her back to her obstetrician
d. Refer her to a gastroenterologist

17. Mary's physical examination is unremarkable except for RUQ tenderness and a positive Murphy's sign. Which of the following could be excluded from your diagnosis at this point?

a. Appendicitis
b. Salpingitis
c. Diverticulitis
d. Cholecystitis

18. Which would be the most helpful diagnostic test at this point?

a. CBC and liver function studies
b. Ultrasound

    c. Liver scan

    d. Chest radiograph and ECG

19. On further testing Mary is diagnosed with cholecystitis and in consultation with a physician is put on a conservative treatment plan. Which of the following would be included in this plan?

    a. Encourage her to undertake a rapid weight reduction plan

    b. Put her on oral contraceptives if she isn't already on them

    c. Decrease fiber in her diet and eliminate all fats

    d. Direct her to contact a health provider if her pain increases or fever or chills develop

20. A 22-year-old male student comes to the student health service complaining of generalized abdominal pain and nausea. He had been out with a group of friends the night before and had been eating pizza and drinking beer. He awoke with generalized abdominal pain this morning and took some Alka Seltzer without much effect. The pain has gotten steadily worse throughout the day and he now feels nauseated. He wonders if he might have food poisoning. Examination reveals hypoactive bowel sounds, and some tenderness in the RLQ. There is no guarding or rebound tenderness. His temperature is 100° F.

    The absence of guarding and rebound tenderness:

    a. Suggests a psychogenic cause of his pain

    b. Rules out appendicitis

    c. Makes peritonitis unlikely

    d. Indicates irritable bowel syndrome

21. The next step you would take is:

    a. Refer to the physician

    b. Obtain a WBC and differential

    c. Obtain a stool culture

    d. Continue careful observation

22. Since he does not appear severely ill at this point, absence of vomiting and decreased bowel sounds and mild fever 15 hours after his last pizza and beer makes it highly unlikely that:

    a. Food poisoning is the problem

    b. He has appendicitis

    c. Perforation of the appendix can occur

    d. Surgery will be needed

23. In the meantime you:

    a. Encourage him to walk around to stimulate bowel activity

    b. Have him sip fluids to avoid dehydration

    c. Tell him you suspect appendicitis

    d. Give him an analgesic for pain relief

24. In elderly patients which of the following would not be an expected indication of appendicitis?

a. Mild fever
b. Abdominal distention with little pain
c. Flatulence and hyperactive bowel sounds
d. Shift to the left without leukocytosis

25. Ms. J is a 29-year-old accountant who comes in complaining of frequent crampy abdominal pain after meals. She is often constipated and takes over-the-counter laxatives which are followed by a couple of days of diarrhea. She does feel better after having a bowel movement but only temporarily. She has also been embarrassed by flatulence and has noticed some abdominal distention. She has had no weight loss and has not noticed any blood in her stool. This problem has gone on for at least six months.

    Your next step would be to:

    a. Obtain a complete history
    b. Order a barium enema
    c. Order a Bernstein test
    d. Suggest a trial of antispasmodics

26. Which of the following makes diverticulitis an unlikely diagnosis in this patient?

    a. Her age
    b. Frequent constipation
    c. Flatulence
    d. Crampy, intermittent pain

27. Which of the following might be expected to occur with irritable bowel syndrome?

    a. Rectal bleeding
    b. Nocturnal diarrhea
    c. Pain radiating to the left chest and arm
    d. Leukocytosis

28. Which of the following would be the reason for hospitalizing a patient with acute diverticulitis?

    a. LLQ tenderness
    b. Advanced age
    c. Leukocytosis
    d. Increased pain with defecation

29. Which of the following would not be considered conservative treatment of acute diverticulitis?

    a. Bedrest
    b. Liquid diet
    c. Antibiotics
    d. Colonic irrigations

30. A positive stool guaiac in a person suspected of having diverticulitis is:

    a. A common finding
    b. An ominous sign indicating need for hospitalization
    c. Requires immediate barium enema
    d. An indication of pending perforation

31. Bacturia in persons with acute diverticulosis may indicate:

    a. Abscess formation
    b. Bowel-bladder fistula
    c. Free perforation into the abdomen
    d. Reason for leukocytosis

32. Ms. S., a 19-year-old college freshman has just completed exam week. She comes in complaining of fatigue, headache, anorexia, and a runny nose. Symptoms began about two weeks ago. She has been taking vitamins and over-the-counter cold preparations but feels worse. "Just the smell" of food makes her nauseated. Her boyfriend had mono about a month ago and she wonders if she might have it. Physical examination reveals cervical lymphadenopathy, a slightly enlarged tender liver and enlarged spleen.

    Which laboratory tests in addition to a CBC, throat culture, and mono spot test would be most helpful in the differential diagnosis at this point?

    a. HAV IgG antibody test
    b. Anti-HB$_s$Ag
    c. Liver enzymes
    d. Stool culture

33. There is no indication in Ms. S's history to indicate IV drug abuse or exposure to blood products. Given the duration of her symptoms and a confirmed increase in her liver enzymes which test would be most helpful in confirming your diagnosis.

    a. IgM antibody to HAV
    b. IgG antibody to HAV
    c. Anti-HDV
    d. Anti-HB$_s$

34. A 30-year-old male with a history of acute hepatitis C over one year ago who was treated with interferon still tests Anti-HCV positive. He should be considered:

    a. Infectious
    b. Incapable of transmitting the virus
    c. Fully recovered
    d. To have high serum viral levels

35. Infection with HDV requires antecedent or simultaneous infection with:

    a. HAV
    b. HBV
    c. HCV

d. HGV

36. When jaundice occurs with hepatitis infection it:
    a. Indicates a more severe infection
    b. Increases the risk of acute liver failure
    c. Indicates development of chronic active hepatitis
    d. Usually resolves in 2 to 6 weeks

37. A normally healthy young adult diagnosed as having salmonella food poisoning should be told:
    a. To take doxycycline 100 mg t.i.d.
    b. That antidiarrheal drugs may decrease his diarrhea temporarily but may also prolong the problem
    c. That he should try to force fluids despite his nausea and vomiting to prevent dehydration
    d. The diarrhea should abate in about 24 hours

38. Which is the next laboratory test to obtain if diarrhea and vomiting persist for more than 48 hours?
    a. Stool guaiac
    b. Sigmoidoscopy
    c. Flat plate of the abdomen
    d. Stool culture and microscopic examination

39. Blurred vision and dizziness in a patient with suspected food poisoning requires:
    a. Gastroenterologic consult
    b. Antibiotic therapy
    c. Immediate hospitalization
    d. Follow-up in 24 hours

40. An 18-year-old previously healthy female presents with a case of a sudden onset of nausea, vomiting, generalized crampy abdominal pain followed by explosive diarrhea. The stools are uniformly thin and watery, without blood or pus. Physical exam reveals hyperactive bowel sounds and bilateral lower quadrant tenderness but no guarding or rebound. Rectal exam is negative and she is afebrile.

    The hypothesis that best explains these findings is:
    a. Acute appendicitis
    b. Acute salpingitis
    c. Acute gastroenteritis
    d. Ruptured ovarian cyst

Answers

1. b	14. d	28. b
2. d	15. d	29. d
3. a	16. b	30. a
4. b	17. c	31. b
5. d	18. b	32. c
6. c	19. d	33. a
7. b	20. c	34. a
8. a	21. a	35. b
9. c	22. a	36. d
10. b	23. c	37. b
11. a	24. c	38. d
12. c	25. a	39. c
13. c	26. a	40. c
	27. c	

Bibliography

Benson, L., Binkel, A., Caldwell, L., Stafford-Fox, V., & Casarico, B. (2000). Advances in the treatment of Hepatitis C: Combination antiviral therapy with interferon alfa-2b and ribavirin. *Journal of The American Academy of Nurse Practitioners, 12*(9), 364–373.

Clinical Guidelines. (1997). Hepatitis B immunization/prophylaxis: Recommendations for adults/older adults. *Nurse practitioner, 21*(12), 64–78.

Damianos, A. J., & McGarrity, T. J. (1997). Treatment strategies for *Helicobacter pylori* infection. *American Family Physician, 55*, 2765–2774.

Friedman, L. S. (2000). Liver, biliary tract, and pancreas. In L. M. Tierney Jr., S. J. McPhee, & M. A. Papadakis (Eds.) *Current medical diagnosis and treatment* (39th ed., pp. 658–697). Stamford, CT: Appleton & Lange.

Gauf, C. L. (2000). Diagnosing appendicitis across the lifespan. *Journal of The American Academy of Nurse Practitioners, 12*(4), 129–133.

Harris, M. S. (1997). Irritable bowel syndrome. *Postgraduate Medicine. 101*, 215–226.

Heitkemper, M., & Jarrett, M. (2001). It's not all in your head: Irritable bowel syndrome. *American Journal of Nursing, 101*(1), 26–32.

King, R. R. (1997). Hepatitis C past, present and future issues. *ADVANCE for Nurse Practitioners, 5*(3), 51–52, 55–56.

Larson, R. R. (1997). Gastroesophageal reflux disease. *Postgraduate Medicine, 101*(2), 181–187.

McManus, T. J. (2000). Helicobacter Pylori: An emerging infectious disease. *The Nurse Practitioner, 25*(8), 40–48.

Rodney, W. M., & Pean, C. (2000). Acute abdominal pain in the elderly. *Consultant, 40*(1), 25–39.

Vail B. A. (1997). Management of chronic viral hepatitis. *American Family Physician, 55*, 2749–2756.

Infectious Diseases
Infancy Through Adolescence

Nancy E. Kline

Septicemia (Sepsis)

- Definition: A generalized systemic response to infection; usually severe and associated with presence of pathogenic microorganisms or associated toxins (usually bacterial) in blood stream; neonates are most susceptible due to immature immune system

- Etiology/Incidence
  1. Etiologic agents vary by age, immunologic status and mechanism of transmission
     a. Newborn (< 3 days)—placental transfer of pathogens from infected maternal blood stream or from vaginal mucosa during birth
        (1) Group B streptococcus (GBS)—high mortality
        (2) *Escherichia coli*—most common gram negative organism
        (3) *Listeria monocytogenes*
     b. Postnatal (1 to 3 weeks)—cross-contamination in nurseries or other crowded conditions; poor hand washing and housekeeping
        (1) *Staphylococcus aureus*—most common
        (2) Klebsiella
        (3) Enterococci
        (4) Pseudomonas
     c. Older infants in the community can be at increased risk for sepsis due to inadequate immunization status—*Haemophilus influenzae* type B
     d. Hospitalized immunosuppressed children at risk for nosocomial sepsis—cancer, post-operative, and patients with HIV/AIDS
  2. Leading cause of morbidity and mortality among hospitalized patients due to associated hemodynamic changes affecting tissue perfusion and oxygenation; if not treated, may lead to septic shock
  3. Increased risk of septecemia
     a. High risk, premature infants
     b. Males > females
     c. Invasive procedures—IV, intubation
     d. Bottle feeding—breast milk may be protective
     e. Immunocompromised children and adolescents

- Signs and Symptoms
  1. Neonates—symptoms may be vague and non-specific, e.g., poor feeding, color changes (pallor, mottling), changes in muscle tone, apnea, cyanosis
  2. Other immunosuppressed children—fever may be only sign; reports by caregiver that child ''isn't him or herself''

3. Older children (rarer) with normal immune function—fever, irritability, anorexia, general toxic appearance

- Differential Diagnosis

    1. Viral sepsis

    2. Fungal infection

    3. Rocky mountain spotted fever

    4. Toxic shock syndrome

    5. Non-infectious causes—hemorrhagic, anaphylactic, or neurogenic shock

- Physical Findings

    1. Neonates—hyper or hypothermia; bradycardia or tachycardia; hepatosplenomegaly, jaundice

    2. Older children—irritability, stiff neck

    3. Later phase—lethargy, delayed capillary refill, hypotension and subsequent septic shock

- Diagnostic Tests/Findings

    1. CBC with differential—WBC > 15,000 with increased neutrophils

    2. Chest radiograph to rule out pneumonia

    3. Positive blood cultures identifying source of infection

    4. Cerebral spinal fluid (CSF)—pleocytosis, decreased glucose, increased protein, positive culture

    5. Coagulation studies—prolonged prothrombin time; decreased fibrinogen levels

- Management/Treatment

    1. Medical referral for hospitalization

    2. Close observation, monitoring, and supportive care

    3. IV fluids to maintain hemodynamics

    4. Broad spectrum parenteral antibiotics for gram positive and negative organisms pending culture and sensitivities

    5. Vasoactive medication if septic shock ensues

Diphtheria

- Definition: Highly contagious acute infection of the upper respiratory tract and/or trachea that is relatively rare in the U.S. but may still occur in under-immunized or unimmunized children

- Etiology/Incidence

    1. Caused by *Corynebacterium diphtheriae*

2. Transmission through direct contact with infected person, carrier, or contaminated food/objects

3. Rare in the U.S. due to DTaP/dT immunization; approximately 5 cases reported annually

4. Increased risk among unimmunized children living in crowded conditions

5. Fall/winter incidence most common

- Signs and Symptoms

   1. Sore throat

   2. Low-grade fever

   3. Nasal discharge

   4. Bloody nose

   5. Hoarseness or cough

   6. Difficulty breathing (severe cases)

- Differential Diagnosis

   1. Acute streptococcal pharyngitis

   2. Nasal foreign body

   3. Mononucleosis

   4. Viral croup

   5. Epiglottitis

- Physical Findings

   1. Greyish-white pseudomembrane found at location of infection—nasopharynx, pharynx or trachea

   2. Other findings vary by location of membrane

   3. Toxin-related severe complications include—myocarditis, Guillain-Barré type neuritis and paralysis

- Diagnostic Tests/Findings

   1. Positive culture of *C. Diphtheriae*

   2. CBC—normal or slight leukocytosis and thrombocytopenia

- Management/Treatment

   1. Hospitalization

   2. Evaluation of sensitivity to horse serum; if negative, single dose of equine antitoxin

   3. Antibiotic treatment—erythromycin or penicillin G; antimicrobial treatment is not a substitute for antitoxin

   4. Respiratory isolation

5. Report to State health department

6. Identification of contacts for follow-up care, immunization and treatment according to current American Academy of Pediatrics *Red Book* recommendations

7. Prevention through universal immunization

Pertussis (Whooping Cough)

- Definition: Highly contagious bacterial infection involving the respiratory tract; characterized by prolonged coughing episodes ending in an inspiratory "whoop"

- Etiology/Incidence

    1. Caused by *Bordetella pertussis*

    2. Infection occurs following person to person contact via aerosolized droplets from respiratory tract

    3. 35% of cases occur in infants less than 6 months of age and these children have the highest mortality

    4. Incubation period is 6 to 20 days, usually 7 to 10 days

    5. Infectivity is highest in catarrhal stage

- Signs and Symptoms

    1. Catarrhal stage—mild URI symptoms with cough for approximately two weeks; low-grade fever

    2. Paroxysmal stage—severe coughing episodes with inspiratory "whoops" that may persist for weeks; vomiting, sucking or crying precipitates coughing episodes; poor feeding

- Differential Diagnosis

    1. Pneumonia (bacterial, viral, chlamydial)

    2. Acute bronchitis

    3. Croup

    4. Upper respiratory infection

    5. Foreign body aspiration

    6. Cystic fibrosis

- Physical Findings

    1. Catarrhal stage—mild URI symptoms

    2. Paroxysmal stage—severe coughing episodes with inspiratory "whoops", cyanosis

- Diagnostic Tests/Findings

    1. Chest radiograph—may reveal thickened bronchi and evidence of atelectasis and bronchopneumonia

2. WBC count reveals marked leukocytosis—usually presents during paroxysmal period and persists for 3 to 4 weeks

3. Nasopharyngeal culture of direct fluorescent antibody stain (DFA)—positive in initial phase of illness

- Management/Treatment

  1. Medical referral is necessary

  2. Antibiotic therapy—erythromycin (40 to 50 mg/kg/day divided four times a day for 14 days; maximum 2 g/day)

  3. Hospitalized children should remain in isolation until they have received five days of erythromycin

  4. Children receiving oral erythromycin at home should not attend day care or school until they have received five days of therapy

  5. Supportive treatment for children who cannot tolerate oral intake due to paroxysmal coughing episodes—intravenous hydration, oxygen supplementation, ventilatory support

  6. Report cases of pertussis to State health department

  7. Prevention

     a. Appropriate pertussis immunization according to schedule

     b. Children less than 7 years of age, with close contact with infected individual, who are unimmunized or have received fewer than four doses of pertussis vaccine, should have immunizations started or continued according to schedule

     c. If the third dose of vaccine was received six months or more prior to the exposure, should be given a fourth dose at time of exposure

     d. Children who have not received a vaccine within past three years or those ≥ 6 years of age, should receive a booster dose of pertussis vaccine at time of exposure

     e. Erythromycin (40 to 50 mg/kg/day divided four times a day for 14 days; maximum 2 g/day) is recommended for all household contacts and other close contacts, regardless of vaccination status

Influenza

- Definition: Highly contagious, viral illness characterized by sudden onset of fever, chills, malaise, headache, myalgia and dry cough

- Etiology/Incidence

  1. Epidemic influenza caused by types A and B

  2. Transmission occurs by direct person-to-person contact, via airborne droplet or by articles contaminated with nasopharyngeal secretions

3. During outbreak, school-aged children are most frequently infected and infect household contacts

4. Period of highest infectivity 24 hours prior to onset of symptoms and while symptoms are most severe

5. Incubation period 1 to 3 days

6. Influenza season mid-October through mid-February

- Signs and Symptoms

    1. Fever

    2. Chills

    3. Malaise

    4. Headache, myalgia

    5. Dry cough

    6. Anorexia

    7. Rhinorrhea

    8. Sore throat

- Differential diagnosis

    1. Upper respiratory infections

    2. Pneumonia

- Physical Findings

    1. Listlessness

    2. Nonproductive cough

    3. Rhinorrhea

    4. Rigors

    5. Fever

    6. Conjunctivitis

    7. Pharyngitis

- Diagnostic Tests/Findings

    1. Nasopharyngeal cultures obtained within first 72 hours of illness may reveal influenza

    2. Diagnosis is usually made based on clinical signs and available prevalence data

- Management/Treatment

    1. Management of influenza is primarily supportive

        a. Bed rest

    b.   Acetaminophen or ibuprofen for fever (avoid aspirin-containing products due to risk of developing Reye's syndrome)

    c.   Adequate hydration

  2. Amantadine and rimantadine diminishes severity of influenza A but is not effective in treatment of influenza B

    a.   Not approved for use in infants < 12 months of age

    b.   Dosages—5 mg/kg/day (not to exceed 150 mg/day for children 1 year to 9 years of age; for children ≥ 10 years of age give 5 mg/kg/day if < 40 kg, or 200 mg/day if ≥ 40 kg

  3. Secondary bacterial infection may occur with influenza

  4. Persons in high risk groups (e.g., HIV, cancer, cystic fibrosis, sickle cell disease) should be vaccinated yearly, as should household contacts

Rubella (German Measles)

- Definition: An acute, contagious, viral disease characterized by a minor or absent prodrome, swelling of suboccipital, postauricular and cervical nodes

- Etiology/Incidence

  1. Caused by an RNA virus

  2. Postnatal transmission occurs via contact from nasopharyngeal secretions

  3. Incubation period ranges from 14 to 21 days

  4. Preventable by active immunization

- Signs and Symptoms

  1. History of inadequate immunization

  2. Rash starts on face and spreads over trunk and extremities; disappears by 3rd day

  3. Associated signs and symptoms

    a.   Malaise, low-grade fever

    b.   Transient joint pain

    c.   Bruising (rare)

- Differential Diagnosis

  1. Rubeola

  2. Scarlet fever

  3. Erythema infectiosum

  4. Adenovirus

  5. Rocky mountain spotted fever

  6. Roseola

- Physical Findings
    1. Generalized erythematous, maculopapular discrete rash—usually first indication of illness
    2. Listlessness
    3. Postauricular and suboccipital lymphadenopathy—usually precedes rash
    4. Purpura/petechiae (rare)
    5. Meningeal signs (rare)
- Diagnostic Tests/Findings
    1. Presence of rubella specific IgM antibody indicates recent postnatal infection or congenital infection in newborn
    2. Refer to current American Academy of Pediatrics *Red Book* for further information on available assays for detecting rubella infection
- Management/Treatment
    1. Management of uncomplicated infection is primarily supportive—includes fever and pain (in lymph nodes) control with acetaminophen or ibuprofen
    2. Determine contacts that may require immunization
    3. Infected children should limit contact with susceptible persons, including women of childbearing age
    4. Educate adolescent females regarding teratogenic nature of rubella in pregnancy
    5. Educate caretakers regarding complications of arthritis, and rarely thrombocytopenia and encephalitis

Rubeola (Red measles)

- Definition: An acute, highly contagious viral disease characterized by prodrome of upper respiratory manifestations followed by generalized maculopapular eruptions
- Etiology/Incidence
    1. Caused by a morbillivirus, in *Paramyxovirus* family
    2. Transmitted by direct contact with infected secretions or via airborne droplets
    3. Infected individuals are contagious 3 to 5 days before appearance of rash, to four days after appearance of rash
    4. Increased incidence during winter and spring
    5. Preventable by active immunization
- Signs and Symptoms
    1. History of inadequate immunization
    2. Acute onset of fever, coryza, cough, conjunctivitis, malaise, anorexia

3. Confluent, erythematous, maculopapular rash 3 to 4 days after initial symptoms; progresses in caudal direction

- Differential Diagnosis
  1. Roseola or rubella
  2. Viral infections (e.g., echovirus, coxsackievirus, adenovirus)
  3. Infectious mononucleosis
  4. Scarlet fever
  5. Rickettsial diseases
  6. Serum sickness

- Physical Findings
  1. Confluent, erythematous maculopapular rash; after 3 to 4 days, rash assumes a brownish appearance
  2. Profuse coryza
  3. Conjunctivitis
  4. Pulmonary findings (crackles, rhonchi)
  5. Koplik spots (red eruptions with white centers on buccal mucosa) prior to appearance of rash

- Diagnostic Tests/Findings: Presence of measles specific IgM antibody suggests recent infection

- Management/Treatment
  1. Medical referral necessary
  2. No specific antiviral therapy available
  3. Management of uncomplicated measles is primarily supportive—bedrest, adequate hydration; acetaminophen or ibuprofen for fever; antitussive therapy
  4. Otitis media is most common complication of measles infection— treated with same antibiotics as in standard otitis media
  5. Educate caretakers regarding complications including otitis media, encephalitis and pneumonia

Roseola (Exanthem Subitum)

- Definition: An acute contagious disease characterized by high fever, and appearance of a rash with simultaneous decrease in fever
- Etiology/Incidence
  1. Caused by human herpesvirus 6 (HHV-6)
  2. Mode of transmission not known

3. Incubation period is 5 to 15 days

4. Period of infectivity is thought to be during the febrile episode, prior to appearance of the rash

5. Most commonly occurs in children 6 to 24 months of age

6. Most cases occur in spring and summer

- Signs and Symptoms

  1. Abrupt onset of high fever (102 to 105° F) lasting 3 to 5 days

  2. Appearance of a rash follows resolution of fever

  3. Associated symptoms include irritability and swelling of eyelids

- Differential Diagnosis

  1. Rubeola

  2. Scarlet fever

  3. Rubella

- Physical Findings

  1. Generalized erythematous, maculopapular rash; starts on trunk and spreads to arms, and neck with less involvement of face and legs

  2. Irritability

  3. May have mildly inflamed edematous conjunctiva

- Diagnostic Tests/Findings: Progressive leukopenia during febrile period

- Management/Treatment

  1. Acetaminophen or ibuprofen for fever

  2. Medical referral if meningeal signs appear, or if fever persists

  3. Education

     a. Potential for febrile seizures

     b. Reassurance that appearance of rash is sign of recovery

Fifth Disease (Erythema Infectiosum - EI)

- Definition: A contagious, usually afebrile, exanthematous disease

- Etiology/Incidence

  1. Human parvovirus B19

  2. Typically seen in 5 to 14-year-old children

  3. Outbreaks occur most often during spring months

  4. Incubation period between 4 and 14 days

5. Mode of transmission includes respiratory secretions and blood

- Signs and Symptoms
    1. No prodromal symptoms
    2. Rash
        a. Begins as bilateral erythema on cheeks (''slapped cheek'' appearance)
        b. Spreads to upper arms, legs, trunk, hands and feet
        c. Palms and soles are spared
        d. Lacy-reticular exanthem appears as facial erythema begins to diminish
        e. May reappear when skin is exposed to sunlight, temperature extremes
        f. Rash lasts from 2 to 39 days, average 11 days
    3. Low grade fever may occur
    4. Can cause aplastic crises in young children, and in patients with hemolytic diseases

- Differential Diagnosis
    1. Drug reactions
    2. Rubella, atypical measles
    3. Enteroviral diseases
    4. Systemic lupus erythematosus

- Physical Findings
    1. Early—bilateral erythema on cheeks (''slapped cheek'' appearance)
    2. Late—erythematous rash on upper arms and legs, trunk, hands and feet; palms and soles are spared
    3. Late—lacy-reticular exanthem appears as facial erythema begins to diminish

- Diagnostic Tests/Findings
    1. Parvovirus B19 IgM antibody confirms current infection, or infection within past several months
    2. Parvovirus B19 IgG antibody indicates previous infection and immunity

- Management/Treatment
    1. None indicated
    2. Reassure parent of benign nature of disease
    3. Avoid sunlight as exposure may exacerbate the condition
    4. Period of high infectivity in persons with EI is prior to onset of symptoms; unlikely to be infectious after rash develops; conversely patients with aplastic crises are highly contagious prior to the onset of symptoms and through week of onset, or longer

Varicella-Zoster Virus (VZV) (Chickenpox)

- Definition: An acute contagious disease caused by a herpesvirus; characterized by a short or absent prodrome and usually a sequential rash consisting of papules, vesicles, pustules and crusts

- Etiology/Incidence
    1. VZV is a herpesvirus
    2. Transmission occurs by direct contact with varicella lesions or by airborne droplet infection
    3. Susceptible individuals can contract chickenpox from patients with varicella zoster (shingles)
    4. Incubation period between 10 and 21 days
    5. Infected individual contagious for 24 to 48 hours prior to outbreak of lesions, until lesions have crusted over
    6. Most cases occur between ages of 5 and 10 years
    7. VZV occurs commonly in late winter and early spring

- Signs and Symptoms
    1. Early lesions appear as faint erythematous macules that progress to papules, followed by appearance of vesicles primarily on trunk, scalp, face; lesions eventually crust over
    2. Lesions continue to erupt for 3 to 4 days and may be present in various stages
    3. Associated symptoms may include fever, pruritus, malaise, anorexia, joint pain

- Differential Diagnosis
    1. Herpes zoster
    2. Bullous impetigo
    3. Insect bites
    4. Urticaria

- Physical Findings
    1. Crops of skin lesions that may appear as maculopapular (early), vesicular, pustular with eventual crusts; many maculopapular lesions may progress to vesicular stage and resolve without crusting
    2. Rash usually present on scalp, face, trunk and extremities; most lesions on face and trunk
    3. Hepatomegaly (rare)
    4. Meningeal signs (rare)
    5. Pulmonary findings—crackles, wheezes (rare)

- Diagnostic Tests/Findings: None routinely performed

- Management/Treatment
    1. VZV is a self-limited disease lasting 7 to 10 days
    2. Supportive treatment
        a. Control of pruritus with oatmeal baths, diphenhydramine, calamine lotion
        b. Acetaminophen for fever (*avoid aspirin-containing products due to risk of developing Reye's syndrome*)
    3. Oral acyclovir is beneficial in reducing duration of new lesion formation, and total number of lesions (20 mg/kg/dose, four times a day; maximum 800 mg four times a day); should be started within 24 hours of onset for maximum benefit
    4. Oral acyclovir not usually recommended in healthy children with uncomplicated varicella
    5. Varicella-zoster immune globulin (VZIG) should be given to immune suppressed contacts to provide passive protection
    6. Medical referral necessary for immune suppressed children
    7. Education
        a. Avoid contact with elderly, pregnant women, neonates and immunocompromised children
        b. Live-attenuated varicella vaccine is available in U.S. and is recommended for all healthy children age 12 months to 13 years who lack a reliable history of varicella (AAP, 2000)
        c. Signs and symptoms of complicated varicella infection—meningeal signs, respiratory distress, dehydration, ocular involvement, secondary bacterial infection, thrombocytopenia, pneumonia
        d. Signs and symptoms of Reye's syndrome—persistent vomiting, lethargy, agitation, disorientation, combativeness, coma

Mumps

- Definition: A contagious, systemic, viral disease characterized by swelling of the salivary glands
- Etiology/Incidence
    1. Caused by paramyxovirus
    2. Spread by direct contact via respiratory airborne droplet and fomites contaminated with infected saliva
    3. Incubation period between 12 to 25 days after exposure
    4. Infected individual is contagious for as many as 7 days prior to, and as long as 9 days after onset of symptoms
    5. Infection occurs throughout childhood; rarely during adulthood

6. More common in late winter and spring

- Signs and Symptoms

    1. History of inadequate immunization

    2. Swelling of salivary glands (specifically parotid gland), pain with swallowing

    3. Malaise, fever

    4. Scrotal swelling and pain

- Differential Diagnosis

    1. Submandibular or preauricular lymphadenitis

    2. Salivary duct obstruction

    3. Infectious mononucleosis

    4. Epididymitis

- Physical Findings

    1. Swelling of salivary glands (specifically parotid gland)

    2. Listlessness

    3. Scrotal swelling and pain

- Diagnostic Tests/Findings: Serum for complement fixation (CF)—positive test for complement-fixing antibody against mumps virus suggests recent infection

- Management/Treatment

    1. Acetaminophen for pain and fever

    2. Warm compresses for salivary gland swelling

    3. Soft or liquid diet

    4. Education

        a. Complications include pancreatitis, oophoritis, meningitis, orchitis

        b. May return to day care or school when all symptoms have resolved or 9 days after onset of symptoms

    5. Report cases to State health department

Cat Scratch Disease (CSD)

- Definition: An infection characterized by regional lymphadenopathy in an otherwise healthy person, following a cat scratch or bite

- Etiology/Incidence

    1. Most cases are caused by *Bartonella* spp., which include the former genus *Rochalimaea*

    2. More than 24,000 cases per year occur in the U.S. (Stechenberg, 2000)

- Signs and Symptoms: Mild systemic symptoms
    1. History of cat exposure
    2. Usually do not appear ill
    3. Swollen lymph nodes
    4. May have low-grade fever; general malaise; headache
    5. Anorexia
    6. May have rash
- Differential Diagnosis
    1. Bacterial lymphadenitis
    2. Lymphoma
    3. Tularemia
    4. Lymphogranuloma venereum
- Physical Findings
    1. Papule or pustule at site of cat scratch or bite, followed in 1 to 3 weeks by enlargement of an associated lymph node
    2. Lesion may be present for several days to several months
- Diagnostic Tests/Findings
    1. May have elevated ESR
    2. Immunofluorescence assay (IFA) detects antibody to CSD
    3. Warthin-Starry silver stain used to identify CSD in lymph node, skin or conjunctival tissue
- Management/treatment
    1. CSD is a self-limited disease lasting 2 to 4 months
    2. Supportive Treatment
        a. Analgesics for discomfort and fever
        b. Limited activity
        c. Needle aspiration of painful, suppurative nodes questionable; may result in chronic draining sinus tract
        d. No treatment required for animal that transmitted CSD

Rocky Mountain Spotted Fever (RMSF)

- Definition: A systemic, febrile illness with characteristic petechial or purpuric rash
- Etiology/Incidence
    1. Caused by *Rickettsia rickettsii*

2. Transmitted to humans via tick bites

3. Usually occurs in persons younger than 15 years of age

4. Widespread in U.S.; most prevalent in southern States

5. Incubation period ranges from 1 to 14 days

- Signs and Symptoms

    1. Fever, myalgia, nausea and vomiting precede appearance of rash

    2. Erythematous, macular rash (usually appearing before the sixth day of illness), on wrists, ankles, spreading within hours to the trunk

    3. In some cases rash fails to develop, or develops late in the illness

    4. Disease can last 3 weeks with multisystem involvement (e.g., CNS, cardiac, pulmonary, GI, renal)

- Differential Diagnosis

    1. Rubeola

    2. Rubella

    3. Lyme disease

    4. Septicemia

    5. Meningococcemia

- Physical Findings

    1. Characteristic petechial, erythematous, macular rash

    2. Neurologic deficits

    3. Heart murmur

    4. Pulmonary findings (crackles)

    5. Decreased urine output

    6. Jaundice

- Diagnostic Tests/Findings

    1. Culture is not attempted due to transmission risk for laboratory personnel

    2. Renal failure

    3. Elevated liver enzymes

    4. Increase in antibody titer as established by serologic testing; indirect hemagglutination (IHA) and microimmunofluorescence (micro-IF) are most sensitive

- Management/Treatment

    1. Medical referral

    2. Doxycycline or tetracycline is given until patient is afebrile for 2 to 3 days

3. Tetracycline not routinely given to children less than 8 years of age; doxycycline is drug of choice

4. Education includes preventive measures such as use of tick repellent and protective clothing in tick-infested areas

5. Patients with multisystem organ involvement may require rehabilitative services

6. Report cases to State health department

Lyme Disease

- Definition:
    1. An immune-mediated, inflamatory response
    2. Affects multiple organ systems
    3. Transmitted primarily via the deer tick

- Etiology/Incidence
    1. Caused by a spirochete *Borrelia burgdorferi*; is most often transmitted via the deer tick
    2. Most often seen in Northeast from Massachusetts to Maryland; the Midwest, primarily Wisconsin and Minnesota; and in California; primarily in heavily wooded areas
    3. Persons of all ages and both sexes are affected
    4. Most cases occur during June and July
    5. Incubation period is between 3 to 32 days

- Signs and Symptoms
    1. Appearance of well-circumscribed, erythematous, annular rash with central clearing (erythema chronicum migrans) at site of recent tick bite
    2. Fever, malaise, headache, arthralgia, conjunctivitis, or mild neck stiffness
    3. May initially present as flulike illness if erythema migrans does not occur, or not recognized
    4. Late signs and symptoms (weeks to months later)
        a. Migratory pain in joints, muscles and bones
        b. Transient, but severe, headaches and stiff neck
        c. Poor memory, mood changes, somnolence
        d. Muscle weakness and poor coordination
        e. Chest pain, cardiac abnormalities
        f. Dizziness/fainting
        g. Facial palsies
        h. Joint stiffness

- Differential Diagnosis
    1. Tinea corporis (ringworm)
    2. Insect bite
    3. Cellulitis
    4. Acute rheumatic fever
    5. Influenza
    6. Aseptic meningitis
    7. Juvenile rheumatoid arthritis
    8. Henoch-Schöenlein purpura
- Physical Findings
    1. Well-circumscribed, erythematous, annular rash with central clearing
    2. Malar rash, diffuse erythema or urticaria
    3. Heart murmur
    4. Neurologic findings—seventh cranial nerve palsy
- Diagnostic Tests/Findings
    1. Enzyme-linked immunosorbent assay (ELISA)—detects antibodies against *B. burgdorferi*
    2. Western blot—used to validate a positive or equivocal ELISA
    3. Serum immunoglobulins—IgM, IgG elevated
    4. Culture of erythema migrans lesion—expensive, time to isolation may take four weeks
    5. White blood cell count—normal or elevated
    6. Erythrocyte sedimentation rate (ESR)—elevated
- Management/Treatment
    1. Medical referral is necessary
    2. Early disease
        a. Children > 8 years of age—amoxicillin or doxycycline
        b. Children ≤ 8 years of age—amoxicillin or penicillin V
        c. For penicillin-allergic patients—cefuroxime or erythromycin may be used, although erythromycin may be less effective
    3. Late disease for persistent arthritis, carditis, neurologic disease—parenteral ceftriaxone or penicillin G
    4. Education/prevention
        a. Ticks that carry Lyme disease are 4 to 5 mm in diameter

    b. Prompt removal of ticks from the skin and use of tick repellent decreases the incidence of Lyme disease

    c. Use blunt-end tweezers to grasp tick as close to skin surface as possible; wear rubber gloves

    d. Disinfect skin where tick bite occurred

    e. Early intervention leads to improved prognosis

    f. Wear protective clothing in heavily wooded areas, check skin closely after outdoor activities

    g. Report cases of Lyme disease to State health department

Infectious Mononucleosis (IM)

- Definition: An acute disease characterized by fever, exudative pharyngitis, lymphadenopathy, hepatosplenomegaly and atypical lymphocytosis
- Etiology/Incidence
    1. Caused by Epstein-Barr virus (EBV), a herpesvirus
    2. Contact with infected secretions is required for transmission
    3. Incubation period is 30 to 50 days
    4. Commonly diagnosed in adolescents and young adults
- Signs and Symptoms
    1. Fever, malaise, fatigue
    2. Severe sore throat
    3. Rash especially with administration of ampicillin derivatives
    4. Tender lymph nodes
- Differential Diagnosis
    1. Streptococcal pharyngitis
    2. Hepatitis
    3. Influenza or viral illness
    4. Measles
    5. Blood dyscrasias, especially leukemia
- Physical Findings
    1. Exudative pharyngitis
    2. May have hepatosplenomegaly
    3. Lymphadenopathy
    4. May have jaundice

5. May have erythematous, macular, papular rash

6. Tender posterior cervical nodes

- Diagnostic Tests/Findings

   1. Positive monospot, or positive Epstein-Barr virus titer

   2. WBC count reveals leukocytosis, 10,000 to 20,000 cells/mm^3, with $\geq$ 60% lymphocytes and 20 to 40% atypical lymphocytes

   3. Rapid strep test and throat culture—identifies presence of ß-hemolytic streptococcal infection, if present

- Management/Treatment

   1. IM is a self-limited disease lasting 2 to 3 weeks

   2. Supportive treatment

      a. Bedrest during acute phase

      b. Pain control for pharyngitis and lymphadenitis

      c. Saline gargles for sore throat

      d. Avoid contact sports until spleen is no longer palpable

      e. Antibiotic therapy as needed for pharyngitis—avoid use of ampicillin derivatives such as amoxicillin, and other penicillins; may result in rash (Katz & Miller, 1998)

Infant Botulism

- Definition: A neuroparalytic disorder affecting young infants (< 6 months) resulting from ingestion of *Clostridium botulinum* spores with release of toxins as organism colonizes gastrointestinal tract

- Etiology/Incidence

   1. Etiologic agent is *Clostridium botulinum*; disease is caused by toxins produced by this anaerobic bacillus

   2. Toxin inhibits acetylcholine release at myoneural junction resulting in impaired motor activity

   3. *C. botulinum* spores have been associated with honey, reported association with corn syrup not substantiated (AAP, 2000)

   4. Rural, farm environments associated with increased incidence

- Signs and Symptoms: Evolving symptomatology

   1. May be asymptomatic

   2. Constipation (most common presenting symptom)

   3. Poor feeding

   4. Weak cry

     5.   Weakness

     6.   Loss of head and neck control

     7.   Generalized floppiness

- Differential Diagnosis

     1.   Sepsis

     2.   Benign congenital hypotonia

     3.   Benign constipation

     4.   Hypothyroidism

     5.   Hirschprung's disease

     6.   Other neuromuscular disorders

- Physical Findings

     1.   Generalized weakness

     2.   Diminished deep tendon reflexes

     3.   Cranial nerve deficits

     4.   Swallowing difficulties

     5.   Loss of muscle tone

- Diagnostic Tests/Findings

     1.   Stool culture positive for *C. botulinum*

     2.   Polymerase chain reaction (PCR) assays—detection of organism in stool

     3.   Blood culture—may or may not be positive for *C. botulinum*

- Management/Treatment

     1.   Equine antitoxin not usually recommended for infant botulism

     2.   Hospitalization; possibility of respiratory arrest

     3.   Stool softener

     4.   Prevention/education regarding honey as potential source of botulism; avoid feeding to infants < 12 months of age

     5.   Report to State health department

Poliomyelitis

- Definition: An acute, contagious, potentially paralytic viral disease
- Etiology/Incidence

     1.   Caused by enterovirus (EV)

2. When susceptible person comes in contact with poliovirus, one of three responses occur

    a. Nonspecific febrile illness (most frequent)

    b. Aseptic meningitis (nonparalytic poliomyelitis)

    c. Paralytic poliomyelitis (least frequent)

3. Incubation period to onset of paralysis is 4 to 21 days

4. Preventable by active immunization

5. Occurs more often in infants and young children

6. Occurs more commonly in conditions of poor hygiene

- Signs and Symptoms

1. History of inadequate immunization or recent immunization

2. Fever, weakness

3. Anxiety

4. Urinary incontinence

5. Meningeal signs

6. Respiratory compromise

7. Speech disturbances

8. Headache

9. Nausea, anorexia

- Differential Diagnosis

1. Guillain-Barré syndrome

2. Meningitis

3. Encephalitis

4. Peripheral neuritis or neuropathy

- Physical Findings

1. Meningeal signs

2. Respiratory compromise

3. Inability to speak without frequent pauses

4. Muscle weakness

- Diagnostic Tests/Findings: EV isolated from feces, throat, urine or CSF in cell culture

- Management/Treatment

1. Medical referral necessary

2. Supportive management—bedrest, adequate hydration, pain control, acetaminophen or

ibuprofen for fever, respiratory support if paralysis ensues, physical therapy for deficits associated with muscle weakness and paralysis

3. Education

   a. Educate family regarding potential complications of possible paralysis including respiratory compromise and arrest, hypertension, renal calculi due to immobility

   b. Oral polio vaccine should not be given to persons who reside with immunocompromised individuals; virus is shed in stool and there is risk of contracting poliomyelitis; inactivated poliovirus vaccine (IPV) may be substituted.

Tetanus (Lockjaw)

- Definition: A neurologic disease characterized by severe muscle spasms that can be fatal
- Etiology/Incidence

  1. Caused by neurotoxin produced by anaerobic bacterium *Clostridium tetani* in contaminated wounds

  2. Occurs throughout the world; neonatal tetanus is common in countries where women are not immunized

  3. Incubation period 2 days to 2 months with an average of 10 days; 5 to 14 days in neonates

  4. More common in warmer climates and months

  5. Has dramatically decreased with advent of tetanus vaccine

- Signs and Symptoms

  1. Incomplete tetatus immunization series

  2. History of deep puncture wound, laceration

  3. Insidious onset

  4. Muscle spasms aggravated by stimuli

  5. Muscle rigidity

  6. Increased oral secretions

  7. Respiratory compromise

- Differential Diagnosis

  1. Muscle spasms

  2. Amyotrophic lateral sclerosis (Lou Gehrig's disease)

  3. Hypocalcemic tetany

  4. Phenothiazine reaction

  5. Strychnine poisoning

- Physical Findings

1. Muscle spasms aggravated by stimuli

2. Muscle rigidity

3. Increased oral secretions

4. Respiratory compromise

- Diagnostic Tests/Findings: Diagnosis made clinically

- Management/Treatment

  1. Medical referral

  2. Supportive management—treatment of muscle spasms, intravenous fluids, respiratory support

  3. Minimize external stimuli (e.g., loud noise, bright light) to prevent aggravating muscle spasms

  4. Tetanus immune globulin (TIG) given to prevent circulating toxin from binding to central nervous system sites

  5. Infection with tetanus does not confer immunity; patient should be reimmunized in convalescent period to prevent future infection

  6. Education—educate family regarding potential complications from tetanus including respiratory compromise, inability to speak

Malaria

- Definition: An infectious disease primarily acquired via mosquito bite characterized by high fever, rigors, sweats and headache

- Etiology/Incidence

  1. Caused by *Plasmodium* spp. and transmitted primarily via mosquito bite; although transmission can be congenital; via transfusions or contaminated needles

  2. Infection by *Plasmodium falciparum* is most serious and potentially fatal

  3. Endemic in tropical areas worldwide; most cases in U.S. reported annually, (approximately 1,000) are acquired during foreign travel

- Signs and Symptoms

  1. History of recent travel to endemic area

  2. Classic paroxysmal symptoms—high fever, rigors, diaphoresis and headache

  3. Fever and other symptoms eventually become synchronized, and depending on the infecting species of *Plasmodium*, fever will occur every other, or every third day

  4. Associated symptoms—nausea, vomiting, diarrhea, arthralgia, cough, abdominal and back pain, pallor, jaundice

  5. Multisystem involvement can develop with *Plasmodium falciparum* infection; may be fatal

    a. Neurologic—seizures, signs of increased intracranial pressure, confusion, stupor, coma and death

    b. Pulmonary—coarse breath sounds, pulmonary edema

    c. Renal—decreased urine output, oliguria, hematuria

    d. Cardiovascular—absent peripheral pulses, hypotension

    e. Gastrointestinal—diarrhea

    f. Vascular collapse and shock

- Differential Diagnosis

  1. Influenza

  2. Rocky mountain spotted fever

  3. Septicemia

- Physical Findings

  1. Early findings—listlessness, rigors, muscle weakness, pallor, jaundice, hepatosplenomegaly

  2. Findings seen in *Plasmodium falciparum* infection—neurologic deficits, pneumonia, elevated liver enzymes, renal failure

- Diagnostic Tests/Findings: Diagnosis depends on identification of parasite on stained blood films

- Management/Treatment

  1. Medical referral

  2. Drug therapy based on the infecting *Plasmodium* species; refer to most current American Academy of Pediatrics *Red Book* for varying treatment regimens

  3. Prevention best achieved through prophylactic therapy prior to travel to endemic areas

  4. Education should include natural history of the illness, and specific follow-up or rehabilitation needed after infection with *Plasmodium falciparum*

  5. Report cases to State health department

Questions
Select the best answer

1. Septicemia in the newborn period is most likely caused by which organism?

    a. *Listeria monocytogenes*
    b. *Haemophilus influenzae*
    c. *Neisseria meningitidis*
    d. *Streptococcus pneumoniae*

2. Signs and symptoms of bacterial sepsis in children beyond the neonatal period include:

    a. Cough, fever, abdominal pain
    b. Vesicular rash, pruritus, fever
    c. Irritability, stiff neck, lethargy
    d. Abdominal pain, diarrhea, vomiting

3. Which of the following vaccines provides protection against a common type of sepsis/meningitis?

    a. Smallpox vaccination
    b. Hepatitis B vaccine
    c. *Haemophilus influenzae* vaccine
    d. Inactivated polio vaccine

4. Although relatively rare in the U.S., diphtheria can occur among under-immunized children. Which of the following clusters of signs, symptoms and physical findings would suggest diphtheria in a child presenting with upper respiratory complaints?

    a. Low grade fever, sore throat, nasal discharge, and greyish-white pseudo-membrane in his/her throat
    b. Abrupt onset of high fever, severe sore throat, nasal discharge, and greyish-white pseudo-membrane his/her throat
    c. Low grade fever, abrupt onset of severe sore throat with difficulty swallowing and drooling
    d. Abrupt onset of high fever, severe sore throat, with difficulty swallowing and drooling

5. Infants younger than six-months-of-age with pertussis frequently require hospitalization to manage:

    a. Fever, cough, dehydration
    b. Coughing paroxysms, apnea, cyanosis, feeding difficulties
    c. Coughing paroxysms, dehydration, renal failure
    d. Seizures, fever, pneumonia

6. One of the most appropriate agents used to treat Influenza A is

    a. Acyclovir
    b. Amantadine
    c. Erythromycin
    d. Tetracycline

7. Which of the following symptoms are characteristic of rubella?

    a. Vesicular, crusted lesions and high fever
    b. Postauricular lymphadenopathy and low grade fever
    c. Intense pruritus, usually in finger webs, buttocks, thighs and ankles
    d. Rough textured maculopapular rash that blanches with pressure

8. Although uncommon, a potential sequela of rubella may include:

    a. Pneumonia and chronic otitis media
    b. Arthritis, thrombocytopenia and encephalitis
    c. Oophoritis and infertility
    d. Arthritis, carditis, and neurological involvement

9. Rubeola is:

    a. Preventable by active immunization
    b. Caused by an RNA virus
    c. Treated with intravenous acyclovir
    d. Not associated with severe complications (e.g., encephalitis, pneumonia)

10. You are examining a child who has fever, coryza, cough, conjunctivitis, malaise, and anorexia. During the oral examination, you observe red eruptions with white centers on the buccal mucosa. What are these eruptions called?

    a. Pastia's spots
    b. Rubeola spots
    c. Koplik's spots
    d. Strawberry spots

11. Which of the following best describes the treatment for roseola?

    a. Acetaminophen or ibuprofen for fever, parental reassurance
    b. Warm compresses for salivary gland swelling
    c. Oral acylovir, 20mg/kg/dose, four times a day
    d. Bedrest, saline gargles for sore throat

12. Fifth disease is usually:

    a. Seen in age 5 to 14-year-old children
    b. Transmitted via the deer tick
    c. Treated with oral erythromycin
    d. Characterized by prolonged coughing episodes

13. Which of the following statements is not true regarding the transmission of chickenpox?

    a. Susceptible individuals can contract chickenpox from patients with varicella zoster (shingles)
    b. Children with chickenpox are infectious only during the period of time when skin lesions are present

    c. Children with chickenpox are no longer infectious once crusting of skin lesions has occurred

    d. Varicella-zoster immune globulin (VZIG) should be administered to susceptible immuno-compromised individuals who are exposed to a patient with varicella zoster infection

14. A child with chickenpox and temperature of 102° F should receive which medication for fever?

    a. Aspirin

    b. Amoxicillin

    c. Acetaminophen

    d. Acyclovir

15. The most appropriate agent for use in treating varicella zoster infection in an immunocompromised host is:

    a. Ganciclovir

    b. Acyclovir

    c. Ceftriaxone

    d. Chloramphenicol

16. Varicella zoster infection is most commonly associated with which of the following skin lesions?

    a. Vesicle

    b. Comedone

    c. Nodule

    d. Macule

17. Which of the following is not a complication of mumps?

    a. Meningitis

    b. Pneumonia

    c. Oophoritis

    d. Pancreatitis

18. What recommendation would you make to a parent whose son has been diagnosed with mumps and wants to know when he can return to day care?

    a. He can return once he becomes afebrile and can tolerate eating

    b. He can return 9 days after onset of symptoms

    c. He can return when he is well enough to participate in activities since infectivity is highest prior to symptoms

    d. He can return after a mimimum of 5 days of antibiotic therapy

19. Which of the following are symptoms of cat scratch disease?

    a. Joint pain, conjunctivitis, mild neck stiffness

    b. Irritability, fever, hypotension

    c. Fever, malaise, lymphadenopathy

    d. Severe coughing, vomiting, anorexia

20. The following describes a characteristic rash associated with which disease? Initially erythematous and macular, becoming maculopapular and petechial. The rash first appears on the wrists and ankles, spreading proximally to the trunk. The palms and soles are often involved.

    a. Lyme disease
    b. Roseola
    c. Rubeola (measles)
    d. Rocky mountain spotted fever

21. A 10-year-old child manifests symptoms of fever, sore throat, and swollen lymph nodes. Spleen tip is palpable. Throat culture and Monospot test results are negative. The next logical diagnostic test would involve:

    a. Repeat throat culture
    b. Chest radiograph
    c. Bone marrow examination
    d. Epstein-Barr virus titer

22. Which of the following factors is not associated with increased risk for infantile botulism?

    a. Rural environments
    b. Use of honey
    c. Use of corn syrup
    d. Farm families

23. Which of the following interventions would not be appropriate for a 6-month-old infant with a suspected diagnosis of infantile botulism?

    a. Stool and blood cultures
    b. Immediate administration of equine antitoxin
    c. Stool softeners
    d. Supportive care

24. Which of the following are associated with paralytic poliomyelitis?

    a. Lacy, erythematous, pruritic rash
    b. Respiratory compromise, speech disturbances, urinary incontinence
    c. Abdominal swelling, lymphadenopathy and jaundice
    d. Unlocalized abdominal pain, nausea and vomiting

25. Muscle spasms associated with tetanus are aggravated by which of the following?

    a. Fever
    b. Tetanus immuneglobulin
    c. External stimuli
    d. NSAID

26. Classic symptoms associated with malaria include:

    a. Low grade fever, upper respiratory congestion, cough

b. Annular rash, conjunctivitis, headache, arthralgia
c. High fever, chills, rigors, sweats, headache
d. High fever, jaundice, lethargy, vomiting

27. Lyme disease is most closely associated with which of the following skin lesions?

   a. Erythema migrans
   b. Nodule
   c. Scale
   d. Pustule

28. Many infectious diseases present with rashes along with general complaints of fever, malaise, and headaches. Which of the following clusters of symptoms would make you consider Lyme disease as a likely diagnosis?

   a. Fever, malaise, headache, arthralgia and well-circumscribed, erythematous, annular rash with central clearing
   b. Fever, malaise, headache, transient bone pain, and generalized erythematous, maculopapular rash that began on the face and spread to trunk and extremities
   c. Fever, malaise, anorexia, and confluent, erythematous, brownish maculopapular rash
   d. Fever, malaise, anorexia, and erythematous rash beginning on wrists and ankles then spreading to the trunk

29. Which of the following would be included in patient education regarding Lyme disease?

   a. Educate caretakers regarding complications including hypertension and renal calculi due to immobility
   b. Avoid use of aspirin-containing products for fever control due to association with increased risk for Lyme disease
   c. Protective clothing and tick repellent should be worn in heavily wooded areas
   d. Educate caretakers regarding natural history of the illness, and specific follow-up needed after infection with *Rickettsia rickettsii*

Answer key:

1. a	11. a	21. d
2. c	12. a	22. c
3. c	13. b	23. b
4. a	14. c	24. b
5. b	15. b	25. c
6. b	16. a	26. c
7. b	17. b	27. a
8. b	18. b	28. a
9. a	19. c	29. c
10. c	20. d	

Bibliography

Atkinson, W. (1995). *Epidemiology and prevention of vaccine-preventable diseases* (2nd ed.). Atlanta: Centers for Disease Control and Prevention.

American Academy of Pediatrics. (2000). *Red Book 2000: Report of the committee on infectious diseases* (25th ed.). Elk Grove Village, IL: American Academy of Pediatrics.

Behrman, R. E., Kliegman, R. M., & Jenson, H. B. (2000). Nelson textbook of pediatrics (16th ed.). Philadelphia: W. B. Saunders.

Feigin, R. D., & Cherry, J. D. (1998). *Textbook of pediatric infectious diseases* (4th ed.). Philadelphia: W. B. Saunders.

Hoekelman, R. A., Adam, H. M., Nelson, N. M., Weitzman, M. L. & Wilson, M. H. (Eds.). (2001). *Primary Pediatric care* (4th ed.). St. Louis: Mosby.

Katz, B. Z., & Miller, G. (1998). Epstein-Barr Virus infections. In S. L. Katz, A. A. Gershon & P. J. Hoetz (Eds.). *Krugman's infectious diseases of children* (10th ed., pp. 98–115). St. Louis: Mosby.

Pizzo, P. A., & Poplack, D. G. (1997). *Principles and practice of pediatric oncology* (3rd ed.). Philadephia: J. B. Lippincott.

Stechenberg, B. W. (2000). Bartonella. In R. E. Behrman, R. M. Kliegman & H. B. Jenson (Eds). *Nelson textbook of pediatrics* (16th ed., pp. 872–873). Philadelphia: W. B. Saunders.

Endocrine Disorders
Infancy Through Adolescence

Jacalyn Peck Dougherty

Thyroid Disorders

Hypothyroidism

- Definition

  1. Congenital or acquired metabolic disorder resulting in absent or insufficient production of thyroxin by thyroid gland

  2. May be familial or sporadic; possibly associated with enlargement (goiter) of thyroid gland (Foley, 2001)

  3. Depending on cause, may progress as permanent or transient disorder (Foley, 2001)

  4. Congenital vs. acquired

     a. Congenital—may affect fetus as early as 1st trimester; in children with mild hypothyroidism missed by newborn (NB) screening, symptoms may present in later infancy or childhood

     b. Juvenile-acquired—may have onset within 1st year of life but usually onset occurs in childhood or adolescence

  5. Primary vs. secondary

     a. Primary—disease or disorder of thyroid gland (thyroid gland failure)

     b. Secondary—disease or disorder of hypothalamus or pituitary gland compromises thyroid gland function

- Etiology/Incidence

  1. Congenital hypothyroidism

     a. Absence (athyreosis), underdevelopment (dysgenesis) or ectopic gland most common

     b. Inherent dysfunction in transport or assimilation of iodine or in synthesis or metabolism of thyroid hormone (e.g., thyroid enzyme defects, familial dyshormonogenesis)

     c. Maternal disease adversely affecting fetal thyroid development and function (prenatal exposure to iodine-containing or goitrogenic drugs and agents, e.g., thiouracil, methimazole, iodines; maternal exposure to radioactive iodine; placental crossing of maternal antibodies to fetal thyroid gland)

     d. Iodine deficiency causing endemic goiter and cretinism

     e. Hypothalamic or pituitary disorder (e.g., pituitary agenesis, anencepahly)

     f. Affects 1 infant in every 4000 live births (Foley, 2001; Weinzimer, Lee, & Moshang, 1997)

     g. Higher incidence in Hispanic and Native-American infants (AAP, 1993)

     h. Higher incidence in areas with endemic iodine deficiency

  2. Juvenile-acquired hypothyroidism (Foley, 2001; Rogers, 1994)

a. Chronic lymphocytic thyroiditis (Hashimoto's, autoimmune) most common cause beyond perinatal period

b. Late manifestation of congenital absence, underdevelopment (dysgenesis), or atrophy of thyroid gland

c. Late manifestation of congenital defects in synthesizing or metabolizing thyroid hormone

d. Ablation of thyroid through medical procedures (e.g., surgery, irradiation, radioactive iodine)

e. Exposure to iodine-containing drugs and agents; drug-induced (e.g., antithyroid drugs, excessive iodide, lithium, cobalt); exposure to naturally occurring goitrogens in foods, water pollutants

f. Disease of hypothalamus or pituitary (e.g., pituitary tumors, trauma), rare; child will show other signs of hypothalamic or pituitary disease

g. Endemic goiter from nutritional iodide deficiency—most common thyroid disease worldwide

- Signs and Symptoms

1. Affects multiple systems; many nonspecific, insidious signs and symptoms; severity depends on age of onset and degree of thyroid deficiency; symptoms vary for infants vs. children

2. May be familial history of thyroid and pituitary diseases; may have maternal prenatal history of thyroid disease or ingestion of antithyroid medications or foods

3. May be associated with other autoimmune disease or syndromes (e.g., Down, Turner's)

4. Neonates/infants

   a. Infants may have no obvious symptoms during first month of life

   b. History of lethargy, poor feeding, prolonged elevated bilirubin (>10 mg/dL > 3 days of age)

   c. May be post-mature; increased birth weight (> 4000 g)

5. Older infants, children, adolescents

   a. History of poor growth, intolerance to cold, poor appetite, constipation

   b. Mental and physical sluggishness, developmental delay

- Differential Diagnosis

1. Differentiate primary hypothyroidism due to intrinsic thyroid gland defects from secondary thyroid deficiency caused by pituitary or hypothalamic disorders

2. Congenital thyroxine-binding globulin (TBG) deficiency or ''euthyroid sick syndrome'' seen in small or sick newborns or in children with acute or chronic severe illnesses, surgery, trauma, or malnutrition

- Physical Findings
  1. Affects multiple systems; severity of findings depends on age of onset and degree of thyroid deficiency
  2. Neonates/infants
     a. Prolonged jaundice; poor feeding
     b. Growth deceleration
     c. Hypothermia, skin mottling
     d. Large fontanels, especially posterior; wide sutures; hirsute forehead; coarse facial features; dull expression; facial edema; nasal discharge; macroglossia
     e. Normal, slightly enlarged or goitrous thyroid gland; if thyroid ectopic, may see mass at base of tongue or in midline of neck
     f. Hoarse cry
     g. Axillary, prominent supraclavicular fat pads
     h. Respiratory distress in term infant
     i. Bradycardia (< 100 beats/min.)
     j. Distended or protuberant abdomen, umbilical hernia, constipation
     k. Lumbar lordosis, hypotonia
  3. Infants, children, and adolescents
     a. Increased weight for height, myxedema with hypothyroidism of long duration
     b. Linear growth retardation or growth deceleration; delayed bone maturation, dentition, tooth eruption
     c. Developmental delay; poor motor coordination, dull appearance
     d. Delayed puberty, occasionally precocious puberty or pseudoprecocity; menstrual disorders
     e. Skin cool, pale, gray, mottled, thickened, increased pigmentation, carotenemia
     f. Hair dry, brittle; lateral thinning of eyebrows
     g. Possible enlarged thyroid gland (goiter); may feel cobblestone-like
     h. Galactorrhea, constipation
     i. Myopathy, muscular hypertrophy, poor muscle tone; prolonged relaxation phase of deep tendon reflexes (DTR)
     j. Delayed bone age
     k. If advanced hypothyroidism and myxedema, may be ''chubby'' and have periorbital edema

- Diagnostic Tests/Findings

    1. Newborn screening for congenital hypothyroidism is routine in all 50 states

        a. Abnormal newborn screen—repeat thyroid screen for confirmatory diagnosis with thyroid stimulating hormone (TSH) and thyroxine (T_4)

        b. Elevated serum TSH and low T_4 diagnostic of transient or permanent primary hypothyroidism

        c. Positive TSH receptor-blocking antibodies (TRBAb)—diagnostic for transient congenital hypothyroidism

        d. Additional thyroid function tests—serum thyroxine-binding globulin (TBG); tri-iodothyronine resin uptake (T_3RU) (Weinzimer, Lee & Moshang, 1997)

    2. Acquired hypothyroidism secondary to pituitary or hypothalamic disorders (Foley, 2001; Weinzimer, Lee & Moshang, 1997)

        a. Low free (unbound) thyroxine (free T_4), usually normal TSH; and low thyroxine-binding globulin (TBG)

        b. Abnormal pituitary function tests

    3. Euthyroid sick syndrome (non-thyroidal illness syndrome) secondary to coexisting acute or chronic illness—low T_4 level with normal TBG; low T_3; normal TSH; free T_4 and reverse T_3 levels high normal or elevated

    4. Autoimmune (Hashimoto's) thyroiditis (with goiter present)—normal T_4 and TSH; elevated serum thyroid peroxidase or thyroglobulin antibody titers

    5. Repeat thyroid function tests if clinical suspicion of hypothyroidism, history of thyroid disease in pregnancy; positive history of thyroid dyshormonogenesis (AAP, 1993)

    6. May have abnormal thyroid scan, ultrasound, imaging, or bone age results

- Management/Treatment

    1. Physician consultation or referral to pediatric endocrinologist for suspected or confirmed hypothyroidism

    2. For congenital hypothyroidism, rapid and adequate thyroid hormone replacement critical to avoid irreparable neurologic impairment and mental retardation; treat within first month of life for best prognosis for optimal intellectual development

    3. Drug of choice daily oral levothyroxine (L-thyroxine); after treatment initiated for hypothyroidism in infancy, monitor T_4 and TSH levels monthly during first year of life, every other month during second year, quarterly during third year, and biannually thereafter (Rogers, 1994); monitor additionally as needed whenever dose adjusted

    4. Recommended dosages of levothyroxine (T_4) vary by age; dosage/kg/day decreases over time

5. In older children and adolescents, increase thyroid dose gradually to full replacement dose to avoid undesirable side effects and clinical symptoms of thyrotoxicosis (e.g., headaches, abrupt personality changes)

6. Once older children and adolescents in euthyroid state, monitor adequacy of levothyroxine therapy with regular, periodic T_4 and TSH levels

7. Give levothyroxine an hour before meals to prevent reduced absorption, especially for infants; iron may interfere with absorption

8. Educate parents and child about disease, treatment regimen, and routine monitoring; with thyroid replacement, child will be livelier, less docile, may lose water weight, hair of normal texture will replace dry hair, may have transient stomach or head aches (Weinzimer, Lee, & Moshang, 1997)

9. Genetic counseling may be indicated if familial etiology

10. Trial off of medication may be indicated at age 3, if possibility child had transient congenital hypothyroidism

Hyperthyroidism

- Definition: Excessive production and secretion of thyroid hormone (TH) by thyroid gland (thyrotoxicosis) resulting in increased basal metabolism, goiter, autonomic nervous system disorders, and problems with creatinine metabolism

- Etiology/Incidence

    1. Caused by excess production of thyroid hormone (e.g., Graves' or autoimmune hyperthyroidism, pituitary tumor) or excess release of thyroid hormone (e.g., subacute thyroiditis, Hashimoto's toxic thyroiditis, iodine-induced hyperthyroidism) (Rogers, 1994)

    2. Most common cause is autoimmune response (Graves')—body produces thyroid stimulating immunoglobulins (TSI) which stimulate TSH receptors in thyroid gland, causing overproduction of TH and thyroid hypertrophy; has genetic predisposition

    3. If mother is thyrotoxic prenatally or has history of Graves', infants may have transient congenital hyperthyroidism (neonatal Graves') since thyroid-stimulating immunoglobulins (TSI) cross placenta to fetus; rare

    4. Graves more common in girls than boys (5 or 6:8) (Gotlin & Chase, 1997; Jospe, 2001), highest incidence between 12 and 14 years; rare before 10 years

- Signs and Symptoms

    1. May have family history of thyroid disorder (e.g., Graves') or maternal history of antithyroid drug ingestion for treatment of Graves' during pregnancy

    2. Neonates/infants (Rogers, 1994; Jospe, 2001)

        a. In neonate, signs and symptoms usually present shortly after birth or may present days or weeks later

        b. Prematurity, low birth weight, poor weight gain, weight loss

    c. Restlessness, irritability

    d. Fever, flushing

3. Child/adolescent

    a. Weight loss, although increased appetite; may have accelerated growth and advanced bone age with long-term illness

    b. Nervousness; irritability; decreased attention span; behavior problems; decline in school performance; emotional lability; restlessness; fatigue; weakness; heat intolerance; increased perspiration

    c. Sleeplessness or sleep restlessness, insomnia, nightmares

    d. Visual disturbances, e.g., increased lacrimation, diplopia, photophobia, blurring

    e. Palpitations

    f. Frequent urination and loose stooling, may have enuresis

    g. Amenorrhea

- Differential Diagnosis

1. Neonates—systemic illness, sepsis, and narcotic withdrawal

2. Children and adolescents

    a. Nodular thyroid disease

    b. Thyroid cancer

    c. Euthyroid goiter

    d. Chronic disease, e.g., pituitary disease, severe anemia, leukemia

    e. Thyroiditis

    f. Accidental or deliberate excessive thyroid hormone or iodine ingestion

    g. Chorea

    h. Psychiatric illness, e.g., anxiety disorder, anorexia

- Physical Findings

1. Neonates and infants

    a. May be small for gestational age

    b. Lid retraction, proptosis, periorbital edema

    c. Face may be flushed

    d. Enlarged thyroid

    e. Tachycardia, cardiac problems

    f. Increased gastrointestinal motility

    g. Severely affected neonates may have jaundice, microcephaly, frontal bossing, craniosynostosis, ophthalmopathy, exophthalmia, thrombocytopenia, cardiac problems, hepatosplenomegaly, other signs of severe illness (Zimmerman & Gan-Gaisano, 1990; Jospe, 2001)

2. Children and adolescents (Jospe, 2001)

   a. Warm, moist, smooth, diaphoretic skin; face may be flushed

   b. Eye findings, e.g., proptosis, exophthalmos, upper lid lag with downward gaze, lid retraction, stare appearance, periorbital and conjunctival edema

   c. Variable-size enlarged, tender or nontender, spongy or firm thyroid with palpable border; may have thyroid bruit or thrill

   d. Tachycardia, systolic hypertension, increased pulse pressure

   e. Proximal muscle weakness, diminished fine motor control, tremor, short DTR relaxation phase

   f. Advanced skeletal maturation radiographically

- Diagnostic Tests/Findings

  1. If signs or symptoms of thyrotoxicosis or enlarged thyroid, do confirmatory laboratory thyroid function tests

  2. Thyroiditis indicated by elevated T_4, free T_4, T_3 resin uptake (T_3RU) and low serum cholesterol

  3. Circulating thyroid simulator immunoglobulin (TSI) and other thyroid antibody tests including thyrotropin receptor antibody (TRAb) titers may be positive

  4. May have moderate leukopenia, hyperglycemia, and glycosuria (Gotlin & Chase, 1997)

  5. Graves' Disease—elevated T_4 and low TSH; advanced bone age

  6. Radioactive iodine uptake scan shows increased uptake if excess TH production; if increased release of TH only, will have decreased radioactive iodine uptake

- Management/Treatment

  1. Physician consultation or referral to pediatric endocrinologist for suspected or confirmed hyperthyroidism

  2. Treatment dictated by identified etiology for hyperthyroidism and degree of thyrotoxicity

  3. Prompt diagnosis and treatment especially important in neonates as condition may be life-threatening

  4. Treatment goal is prompt return to euthyroidism with use of:

     a. Antithyroid drugs to inhibit thyroxine (T_4) synthesis and conversion of T_3 to T_4, e.g., propylthiouracil, methimazole

     b. Antithyroid drugs or radioiodine treatment of thyroid gland (ablative therapy)

    c.   Beta-adrenergic receptor blockers to control nervousness and cardiovascular symptoms, e.g., propranolol, atenolol

    d.   Thyroid surgery (Kappy, Steelman, Travers & Zeitler, 2001; Jospe, 2001)

  5. Restricted physical activity if hyperthyroidism severe or in preparation for surgery

  6. Educate parent and child about disease, duration of treatment, side effects of medications or complications if surgery required, adherence to treatment regimen, and, if Graves' disease, need for lifelong monitoring; advise of complications, e.g., thyrotoxicosis

  7. Genetic counseling may be indicated if familial etiology

Thyroiditis

- Definition: Enlargement or inflammation of thyroid gland caused by autoimmune response to the thyroid gland (chronic autoimmune thyroiditis, Hashimoto's); infectious agents (acute suppurative and subacute nonsuppurative), or from exposure to radiation or trauma; occasionally idiopathic

- Etiology/Incidence (Kappy, Steelman, Travers & Zeitler, 2001)

  1. Acute suppurative thyroiditis with bacterial etiology—e.g., group A streptocci, pneumococci, *S. aureas,* and anaerobes; rare

  2. Subacute nonsuppurative thyroiditis caused by viruses—e.g., mumps, influenza, echovirus, coxsackie, Epstein-Barr, adenovirus; rare in U.S.

  3. Chronic autoimmune lymphocytic thryoiditis (Hashimoto thyroiditis)—most common cause of goiter and hypothyroidism in childhood; highest incidence in children 8 to 15 years; more common in females than males (4:1) (Kappy, Steelman, Travers & Zeitler, 2001)

- Signs and Symptoms

  1. May have recent history of or concurrent upper respiratory illness

  2. May have family history of autoimmune thyroid disease

  3. Onset in acute thyroiditis rapid; insidious onset in subacute and chronic lymphocytic

  4. Fever, malaise; may feel quite ill if acute suppurative or subacute thyroiditis

  5. With acute and subacute thyroiditis, pain and tenderness of thyroid with radiation to other areas of neck, ear, chest; with acute suppurative thyroiditis, severe pain with neck extension; no tenderness with chronic lymphocytic thyroiditis

  6. Complaints of unilateral or bilateral swelling of the thyroid, complaints of fullness in anterior neck; sensation of tracheal compression

  7. May have sore throat, hoarseness, dysphagia

  8. May have nervousness, irritability, other symptoms of mild hyperthyroidism

- Differential Diagnosis

  1. Distinguish between infectious toxic thyroiditis and chronic lymphocytic autoimmune thyroiditis; simple goiters due to inborn errors of T_4 synthesis; and thyroiditis associated with adolescence in girls

  2. Goiters induced by drugs—(e.g., from iodine, lithium, para-amino salicylic acid, thionamides, white turnip plants); by transplacental exposure to TH by breast feeding of newborns when mothers on antithyroid therapy (Weinzimer, Lee & Moshang, 1997)

  3. Cancerous or cystic thyroid nodules

- Physical Findings

  1. Findings variable depending on etiology—i.e., infectious vs. autoimmune

  2. May be toxic-appearing if infectious etiology but not necessarily thyrotoxic

  3. In infectious thyroiditis—thyroid gland unilaterally or bilaterally enlarged, tender, firm; in chronic lymphocytic thyroiditis, may have symmetric or asymmetric, nontender, firm, freely moveable, ''pebbly'' goiter

- Diagnostic Tests/Findings (Kappy, Steelman, Travers & Zeitler, 2001)

  1. Laboratory findings variable depending on etiology

  2. In infectious thyroiditis—serum total T_4, free T_4, and T_3RU usually normal or slightly elevated; moderate to marked shift to left in differential; elevated sedimentation rate

  3. In chronic lymphocytic thyroiditis—elevated TSH, thyroid autoantibodies, abnormal thyroid scan

  4. Surgical or needle biopsy diagnostic but rarely indicated

- Management/Treatment

  1. Physician consultation or referral to pediatric endocrinologist for suspected or confirmed thyroiditis

  2. Specific antibiotic therapy required for acute suppurative thyroiditis and may be needed for subacute nonsuppurative thyroiditis since latter is difficult to distinguish from former; acetylsalicylic acid or other anti-inflammatory drugs

  3. Treatment for autoimmune chronic lymphocytic thyroiditis controversial; levothyroxine used to decrease goiter but efficacy in preventing progression of hypothyroidism in long term not supported (Kappy, Steelman, Travers & Zeitler, 2001)

  4. Adolescents with autoimmune chronic lymphocytic thyroiditis need lifelong monitoring since development of hypothyroidism is possible, subacute thyroiditis self-limiting

  5. Genetic counseling may be indicated for familial etiology

Pituitary Disorders

Diabetes Insipidus (DI)

- Definition: Excretion of large amounts of dilute urine due to insufficient function of anti-diuretic hormone (ADH, vaspopressin), disorder in ADH receptors in kidney, primary renal disease, or, rarely in children, to primary polydipsia; compromised ability to concentrate urine

- Etiology/Incidence

    1. Central (hypothalamic, neurogenic, vasopressin-sensitive) DI caused by hypofunction of hypothalamus/posterior pituitary or increased vasopressin metabolism resulting in ADH deficiency

        a. Familial—autosomal dominant trait, rare

        b. Congenital—e.g., anatomic defects in brain

        c. Acquired secondary to accidental or surgical trauma, infection, cerebral anoxia, neoplasm, or infectious disease; trauma following removal of hypothalamic area tumors major cause

        d. Secondary to autoimmune or infiltrative disease, e.g., histiocytosis, lymphocytic hypophysitis

        e. Idiopathic

    2. Nephrogenic (vasporessin-resistant) DI caused by reduced renal responsiveness to ADH (not CNS mediated)

        a. Familial—X-linked inherited disorder of ADH receptor sites in kidney in males primarily; females rarely affected, less common etiology but more severe

        b. Acquired

            (1) Renal failure, e.g., obstructive uropathy, polycystic kidney disease

            (2) Electrolyte disorders (hypercalcemia, hypokalemia)

            (3) Nephrotoxic drugs, e.g., lithium, demeclocycline, amphotericin, methicillin, rifampin

            (4) Other illness, e.g., sickle cell

- Signs and Symptoms

    1. Symptoms variable depending on etiology, age, anterior pituitary function, preservation of normal thirst, diet (Bode, Crawford & Danon, 1996)

    2. Central neurogenic DI

        a. May have family history of congenital ADH deficiency

        b. Generally rapid onset; disease may be masked as failure-to-thrive

        c. History of poor weight gain, deficient growth if long duration

   d. Unexplained fever, irritability

   e. Intense thirst, polydipsia, desire for cold drinks, preference for ice water; irritable when fluid withheld; unable to sleep through night without water intake

   f. Vomiting, constipation

   g. Tendency to avoid diets high in protein and salt

   h. Polyuria, nocturia, enuresis in previously toilet-trained child; clear urine; unable to concentrate urine after fluid restriction

   i. May have symptoms of intracranial tumor (headaches, strabismus, double vision vomiting, precocious puberty)

   j. May follow intracranial surgical procedures or trauma; CNS disease; rarely idiopathic (Goepp & Ackerman, 2001)

3. Nephrogenic DI (Muglia & Majzoub, 1996)

   a. May have family history of congenital nephrogenic DI or maternal history of polyhydramnios; infants may do well on breast feeding until weaning, infection, or introduction of solids, then may fail to thrive; often present with fever, vomiting, dehydration

   b. Female carriers of trait have varying severity of disease

   c. Poor weight gain, deficient growth if long duration; may be malnourished

   d. Increased thirst, polydipsia, history of large water intake, poor food intake because of preference for water over milk or solids

   e. Dehydration, absence of tears, perspiration; if dehydration severe, may have seizures

   f. Irritability; may have poor attention span, poor school performance

   g. Vomiting; polyuria, nocturia

- Differential Diagnosis

   1. Distinguish DI caused by suppression of vasopressin secretion (congenital vs. acquired central DI) from DI caused by reduced renal responsiveness to vasopressin (congenital vs. acquired nephrogenic DI)

   2. Psychogenic polydipsia (compulsive water drinking) and other causes of polyuria (e.g., drug-induced polydipsia [e.g., thioridazine, tricyclics]; hypokalemia; hypercalcemia [including hypevitaminosis D]; primary and secondary renal disease; diabetes mellitus)

- Physical Findings

   1. Central neurogenic DI (Kappy, Steelman, Travers & Zeitler, 2001)

      a. Variable levels of dehydration; if severe, infants may have high fever, vomiting, seizures, circulatory collapse

      b. Poor weight gain, deficient growth if long duration; may be malnourished

    c.   Irritability; may have poor attention span

    d.   May have symptoms of brain tumor (e.g., strabismus, nystagmus)

2.   Nephrogenic DI

    a.   Variable levels of dehydration; dry skin, no tears, no perspiration; if severe, infants may have high fever, convulsions, circulatory collapse

    b.   Failure to thrive, malnourished; if long duration, may have growth retardation, delayed sexual maturation, CNS damage

    c.   Fever, irritability

    d.   Large or distended bladder except immediately after voiding; nonobstructive hydonephrosis, hydroureter

- Diagnostic Tests/Findings (Kappy, Steelman, Travers & Zeitler, 2001)

  1.   Polydipsia and polyuria (> 2 $L/m^2/day$)

  2.   Urine specific gravity (< 1.010; osmolality < 300 mOsm/kg)

  3.   Hyperosmolality of plasma (> 300 mOsm/kg)

  4.   Hypernatremia (> 160 mEq/L) (Bode, Crawford, & Danon, 1996)

  5.   Positive water deprivation test

      a.   Serum osmolality > 300 mOsm/kg, and urine osmolality < 600 mOsm/kg diagnostic of DI

      b.   ADH administration (vasporessin) differentiates central vs. nephrogenic DI

         (1)   Central DI—decreased urine volume and increased urine osmolality

         (2)   Nephrogenic DI—no further changes in urine volume or osmolality

  6.   With MRI, absence or diminished ''bright spot'' in posterior pituitary; diminished blood flow to posterior pituitary (Muglia & Majzoub, 1996)

  7.   Low serum ADH concentration in central DI; high serum ADH level in nephrogenic DI

- Management/Treatment

  1.   Immediate physician consultation or referral to pediatric endocrinologist for suspected or confirmed DI

  2.   Careful adequate rehydration to avoid seizures, intellectual impairment due to CNS damage from hypernatremia and dehydration, particularly in infants who may not be able to make known their need for water or to obtain water necessary to quench thirst (Bode, Crawford & Danon, 1996); early recognition and management needed to avoid sequelae of stunted growth and cognitive impairment

  3.   Treat treatable underlying causes of nephrogenic DI, e.g., hypokalemia, drug-induced, obstructive uropathy

  4.   Treatment of choice for diabetes insipidus—intranasal desmopression acetate

(DDAVP); infants may be given extra free water rather than DDAVP for normal hydration (Kappy, Steelman, Travers & Zeitler, 2001); with nephrogenic DI, may need diuretics, e.g., thiazides, prostaglandin synthesis inhibitors, e.g., indomethacin

5. Breast feeding preferable; adequate calories for growth, restrict sodium intake (Lum, 1997); teach regarding avoidance of severe dehydration (Muglia & Majzoub, 1996)

6. Genetic counseling may be indicated for familial etiology

7. Treat other identified causes, e.g., germinomas, histiocytosis, craniopharyngiomas (Kappy, Steelman, Travers & Zeitler, 2001)

Growth disturbances

Short stature

- Definition

    1. Variation from average pattern of growth (Gotlin & Chase, 1997); height falling $\geq$ 2 standard deviations (SD) below the mean (Tunnessen, 1988) (i.e., $\leq$ 3rd percentile); deviation from previously established growth curve

    2. Growth adequacy determined by consideration of both growth rate and absolute height

- Etiology/Incidence

    1. Multiple etiologies—constitutional, physiologic, genetic, environmental, psychosocial

        a. Normal growth variations (most common)

            (1) Familial or genetic normal variant of average growth pattern which is familial, racial, or genetic; child "constitutionally small" and remains small as adult

            (2) Constitutional delay of growth with delayed growth pattern resulting in delayed physical maturity but normal final adult height

        b. Pathologic growth variations (Kappy, Steelman, Travers & Zeitler, 2001)

            (1) Nutritional—hypocaloric, gastrointestinal disorders

            (2) Endocrine—growth hormone (GH) deficiency; occurs in 1:4000 children

                (a) Hereditary—rare gene deletion

                (b) Idiopathic—about 66% cases caused by suspected deficiency or impairment in hypothalamic secretion of human growth hormone-releasing (hGH) hormone

                (c) Acquired—secondary to pituitary/hypothalamic disease, CNS infection, trauma, intracranial tumors

(3) Other endocrine disturbances—hypothyroidism, hypopititarism, excess cortisol, precocious puberty

(4) Chromosomal defects (Turner's, Down syndrome)

(5) Intrauterine growth retardation (IUGR)—sporadic or associated with syndromes, e.g., De Lange syndrome, Russell-Silver syndrome

(6) Bone development disorders—achondroplasia, skeletal disorders

(7) Metabolic—storage diseases, inborn errors of metabolism

(8) Systemic and chronic diseases and congenital defects— e.g., liver, hematologic, respiratory, cardiovascular, renal, CNS disease or tumors

(9) Associated with birth defects, mental retardation

(10) Psychosocial factors

(11) Chronic drug intake, e.g., glucocorticoids

- Signs and Symptoms

  1. Normal growth variations

     a. Familial short stature—usually small at birth (≤ 3%) but consistent with family pattern

     b. Constitutional growth delay—usually normal size at birth with declining height and weight to < 5% between 1 and 3 years of age; delayed pubesence; family history of similar growth pattern in parents or other family members

  2. Pathologic growth variations

     a. History of poor nutritional intake, malabsorption syndromes

     b. Symptoms of GH deficiency—failure to grow, headaches, delayed dental development, visual field defects, polyuria, polydipsia, delayed sexual maturation, CNS abnormalities, history of trauma, infection, radiation to CNS

     c. Signs and symptoms of other endocrine disorders—fever, lethargy, irritability, developmental delay, dull appearance, FTT, increased weight for height, polyuria, polydipsia, constipation, delayed sexual maturation, CNS symptoms, CNS surgery

     d. Intrauterine growth retardation (IUGR) and low birth weight (LBW); normal BW or normal growth pattern with subsequent onset of decelerated or delayed growth; history of premature aging

     e. Symptoms of other systemic or chronic illness—FTT, congenital defects including intrinsic diseases of bone

     f. Dysmorphism at birth, chromosomal abnormalities, syndromes, congenital skeletal defects or anomalies, e.g., abnormal upper to lower body ratio; abnormal or disproportionate features

g. Signs and symptoms of neglect, emotional maltreatment; abnormalities in psychosocial development; parents may be overwhelmed or disorganized and not intentionally neglectful or abusive

h. Chronic drug intake, e.g., glucocorticoids, high doses of estrogens, androgens

- Differential Diagnosis: Distinguish normal variants of familial short stature and constitutional growth delay from pathologic causes

- Physical Findings

  1. Familial or constitutional short stature—height, weight, occipital-frontal circumference (OFC) growth curve patterns generally consistent, symmetric

      a. Familial—growth chart showing BW ≤ 3% but consistent with family pattern; follows growth curve; normal physical examination; radiographic bone age consistent with chronological age

      b. Constitutional delay—growth chart showing normal size at birth with declining height and weight throughout 1 to 3 years to < 5%; normal physical examination; bone maturation 2 to 3 years behind chronological age

  2. Pathologic short stature

      a. GH deficiency—BW may be normal, birth length 50% that of normal child; height and weight growth deficits; infantile fat distribution; youthful facial features; midfacial hypoplasia; visual field defects; small hands and feet; newborn may have microphallus (stretched penile length of < 2.5 cm vs. normal mean length of 4 cm [Styne, 1996]); may have CNS findings

      b. Primordial short stature

          (1) IUGR—BW and birth length below normal for gestational age, OFC normal or < 3rd percentile; subsequent growth parallel to or < 3rd percentile

          (2) Primordial dwarfism with premature aging—child appears older than age

          (3) Short stature with and without dysmorphism—height, weight < 3rd percentile, may have normal physical examination other than small size or may have various abnormal physical findings, e.g., microcephaly

      c. Short stature associated with chromosomal abnormalities—may have dysmorphism or stigmata of specific congenital or familial disorders, e.g., Turner's syndrome (webbed neck, small jaw, prominent ears, epicanthal folds, low posterior hairline, broad chest, cardiac defects) or Down syndrome

      d. Short stature associated with bone or cartilage development disorders, e.g., skeletal dysplasia, short extremities with normal size head and trunk, frontal bossing, abnormal upper to lower body ratios, abnormal or disproportionate features, rickets, leg bowing

      e. Short stature associated with symptoms of endogenous cortisol excess, e.g.,

Cushing's disease with moon facies, hirsutism, "buffalo hump," striae, hypertension, fatigue, voice deepening, obesity, amenorrhea

    f. Chronic drug intake, e.g., glucocorticoid excess with hypertension, plethora, moon facies, purple striae, interscapular fat pad, truncal obesity, muscle wasting

    g. Abnormalities in psychosocial development; neglectful parents

- Diagnostic Tests/Findings (Weinzimer, Lee, & Moshang, 1997; Kappy, Steelman, Travers & Zeitler, 2001)

    1. Abnormalities in previous sequential, consistent recordings of height, weight, and OFC plotted on age-standardized growth charts

    2. In familial short stature and constitutional delay, height may be < 3rd percentile but growth rate normal; careful family history of familial growth patterns may elucidate familial vs. constitutional delay as etiology of short stature

    3. In growth failure, slower than normal growth rate results in flattened growth curve or decrease in growth parameter percentiles

    4. May have abnormal complete and segmental growth measurements and upper to lower body ratio measurements

    5. Laboratory tests to confirm diagnosis based on clinical findings and to rule out systemic disease or hormonal deficiency; findings depend on etiology

        a. Abnormal CBC—chronic anemia, infection, leukemia

        b. Elevated sedimentation rate—collagen-vascular disease, cancer, chronic infection

        c. Abnormal biochemical profiles—adrenal insufficiency, renal disease

        d. Abnormal stool examination—inflammatory bowel disease, severe parasitism

        e. Abnormal thyroid function studies—hypothyroidism

        f. Low serum human growth hormone (hGH), insulin growth factor (IGF-1), IGF-binding protein—hGH deficiency (Kappy, Steelman, Travers & Zeitler, 2001)

        g. Abnormal urinalysis—renal disease

    6. Delayed maturity on radiographic bone age indicates constitutional delay (generally 2 to 3 years behind chronological age), GH deficiency, hypothyroidism, severe systemic illness; normal bone age found in familial short stature

    7. Nutritional evaluation may show inadequate calories

    8. Abnormal home/social evaluation may suggest psychosocial etiology

    9. Abnormalities on skull radiograph, CT, MRI of cranium if intracranial lesion

    10. Karyotype analysis in short girls with pubertal delay may indicate Turner syndrome

- Management/Treatment
    1. Physician consultation or referral to appropriate pediatric specialists for children with other than familial or constitutional growth delay
    2. If familial or constitutional growth delay, only periodic monitoring of growth pattern needed; reassurance
    3. If marked psychosocial problems arise in boys because of pubertal delay, short-term testosterone may initiate sexual development (Weinzimer, Lee, & Moshang, 1997)
    5. Optimize treatment for other endocrine or systemic or chronic illnesses to minimize compromised growth; adequate calories for growth
    6. GH may be indicated for children with known GH deficiency (controversial)

Excessive growth

- Definition: Variation from average pattern of growth in linear height with height > 2 SD above the mean; excess height for age
- Etiology/Incidence (Frasier, 1996; Gotlin & Chase, 1997)
    1. Normal variation in growth—constitutional tall structure (familial, genetic) most common, familial tendency to mature early
    2. Pathologic variations in growth
        a. Endocrine disorders
            (1) Infant of diabetic mother (IDM)
            (2) GH excess—usually due to pituitary adenoma
            (3) Precocious puberty—androgen or estrogen excess prior to puberty from CNS disorder, adrenal or gonadal disorder, e.g., excess of androgens, estrogens, or both, or idiopathic cause leads to accelerated linear growth, early bone and sexual maturation, and adult short stature; more common in females than males; males have more pathologic etiologies, e.g., CNS disease, females have more idiopathic precocious puberty
        b. Genetic causes
            (1) Marfan syndrome—autosomal dominant, connective tissue disorder
            (2) Chromosomal abnormalities (e.g., Klinefelter syndrome in males with ≥ 2 X chromosomes with usual normal adult stature), XYY, XXYY
        c. Other
            (1) Idiopathic or exogenous obesity—early puberty with accelerated growth; usually adult height not beyond expected genetic potential
            (2) Homocystinuria—inherited inborn error of metabolism
            (3) Cerebral gigantism (Sotos syndrome)—possible hypothalamic dysfunction; adult stature normal to excessive

(4)   Beckwith-Weidemann syndrome

- Signs and Symptoms

    1. Concern about tall stature or excessive growth primarily with adolescent girls/parents

    2. Symptoms accompanying tall stature variable depending on underlying etiology

    3. Familial or constitutional tall stature—length normal at birth, tall stature evident by 3 to 4 years; growth rate slows after 4 or 5 years with curve then parallel to normal curve (Frasier, 1996)

    4. IDM—history of maternal diabetes, large for gestational age (LGA)

    5. Beckwith-Wiedemann—LGA, rapid growth in childhood

    6. GH excess—symptoms vary depending on age when excess GH secretion occurs; concern about height, other symptoms of GH excess (e.g., headache, excessive perspiration, visual impairment, coarsening of facial features, enlargement of nose, ears, jaw, increases in hand and feet, galactorrhea, menstrual irregularity, polyuria, polydipsia, joint pain)

    7. Precocious puberty—concern about height, increase in growth rate, and early development of pubic hair common presenting signs

        a. True precocity of familial or idiopathic origin—causes early secondary sex characteristics with testicular enlargement and spermatogenesis in boys, menarche and mature ova in girls

        b. Incomplete or pseudoprecocity—adrenal or gonadal tumor or dysfunction causes early secondary sex characteristics but no testicular enlargement, no ovulation

        c. CNS disorders/tumors—more common in males, may have seizures

    8. Marfan's—concern about height, vision problems

    9. Klinefelter's syndrome—concern about height, school and behavior problems, lowered verbal IQ, vision problems, delayed adolescent development, testes before puberty normal or small

    10. Obesity—normal height, weight at birth

    11. Homocystinuria—concern about height, mental retardation, vision problems, CNS symptoms, back pain

    12. Cerebral gigantism (Sotos)—concern about height; normal height at birth, rapid growth first year of life (> 97% height at 1 year) to 3 to 4 years, feeding problems, developmental delay

    13. Beckwith-Weidemann—concern about height, large at birth, symptoms of hypoglycemia

- Differential Diagnosis: Normal variants of constitutional tall structure need to be distinguished from pathologic causes; distinguish pseudoprecocity from true sexual precocity;

cause of testicular enlargement may be testicular tumor; ovarian tumor may cause early menarche

- Physical Findings

  1. Constitutional tall stature—2 to 4 SD above average height for age; normal body proportions; normal physical examination and appropriate pubertal development and timing (Frasier, 1996)

  2. Endocrine disorders

     a. IDM—LGA at birth; > 90% for height and weight

     b. GH excess—tall; soft tissue growth; prominent mandible; supraorbital ridge; large nose; space between teeth; hypertension; heart failure; large hands and feet, thickened bones, overgrowth of joints of extremities; visceral enlargement; osteoporosis, kyphosis, may have signs of CNS symptoms

     c. Precocious puberty—tall stature; in males, secondary sexual development before age 9 years (Styne, 1996); in females, breast development before 7.5 years or menses before 9.5 years (Rosenfeld, 1996)

  3. Genetic disorders

     a. Marfan's—tall stature, dolicocephaly, abnormal body proportions, thin extremities, increased arm and leg length, lowered upper/lower segment ratio, increased arm span, arachnodactyly, myopia and other visual abnormalities, external ear abnormalities, pectus excavatum, heart murmur, scoliosis or kyphosis, laxity and hyperextension of joints, hypotonicity

     b. Klinefelter syndrome—tall stature, underweight for height and age, mental retardation, long legs, low upper/lower body segment ratio, gynecomastia, normal penile size and pubic hair but small, firm testes with decreased sensitivity to pressure, cryptorchidism, hypospadias

  4. Other causes of tall stature

     a. Obesity—accelerated height and weight, generally normal examination otherwise

     b. Homocystinuria—tall stature, myopia and other ocular problems, CNS symptoms, possible convulsions, mental retardation, osteoporosis, vertebral collapse

     c. Cerebral gigantism (Sotos syndrome)—large BW and height, dysmorphic features, abnormal body proportions with increased arm span, mental retardation, macrocephaly, dolichocephaly, prominent forehead, hypertelorism with other ocular abnormalities, high arched palate, pointed chin, CNS findings, poor motor coordination

     d. Beckwith-Weidemann syndrome—large BW and height, oomphalocele, umbilical hernia, accelerated growth in childhood, macroglossia, high arched palate, mid-face hypoplasia, hemihypertrophy

- Diagnostic Tests/Findings

  1. Previous sequential, consistent recordings of height, weight, and OFC plotted on age-standardized growth charts show height > 2 SD above mean for age

  2. Careful family history of tall growth patterns may elucidate familial etiology of tall stature; growth rate normal, growth curve parallels normal curve in familial tall stature

  3. Laboratory tests to confirm diagnosis based on clinical findings and to rule out endocrine disease (Weinzimer, Lee & Moshang, 1997)

     a. GH excess—low ACTH, FSH, LH; high or normal GH; abnormal GTT

     b. Cerebral giantism—normal GH secretion

     c. Klinefelter—high pituitary gonadotropin, LH, FSH; azoospermia

     d. True precocious puberty—elevated basal LH, FSH concentrations; pubertal LH response to GnRH

     e. Beckwith-Weidemann—low blood glucose (hyperinsulinemia)

  4. Radiographic bone age not advanced in constitutional tall stature; advanced in cerebral gigantism, obesity, precocious puberty

  5. Abnormal echocardiogram with Marfan's; may have abdominal mass on ultrasound with precocious puberty

  6. Abnormalities on skull radiograph, CT, or MRI of cranium with intracranial lesion

  7. Karyotype analysis may indicate chromosomal abnormalities, syndromes

- Management/Treatment

  1. Physician consultation or referral to appropriate pediatric specialists for children with other than constitutional tall stature

  2. Pharmacologic management controversial; if marked concern about calculated predicted adult height, endocrinologist may accelerate epiphyseal closure with gonadal steroids; if precocious puberty, may slow growth with GnRH agonist

  3. Homocystinuria—restrict dietary methionine, supplement dietary cystine

  4. GH excess from CNS tumor or adrenal or gonadal tumor—surgery as indicated

  5. Management of endocrine disease associated with tall stature

  6. Beckwith-Wiedemann—treat excess insulin production

Adrenal Gland Disorders

Adrenocortical Insufficiency

- Definition: Inadequate production and secretion of adrenal hormones caused by failure of adrenals to secrete glucocorticoids, mineralocorticoids, and adrenal androgen (primary adrenal insufficiency, Addison's) or deficient secretion of ACTH from pituitary (secondary adrenal insufficiency)

- Etiology/Incidence

  1. Primary adrenal insufficiency

     a. Congenital adrenal hyperplasia (CAH)—hereditary

     b. Chronic adrenal insufficiency (hypoadrenocorticism, Addison's disease) with destruction of adrenals from infection or hereditary autoimmune disease or adrenal calcification

     c. Congenital absence or underdevelopment of adrenals; newborn adrenal hemorrhage (with complicated or traumatic delivery)

     d. Malignancy (adrenal tumor)

  2. Secondary adrenal insufficiency

     a. Hypopituitarism—deficient secretion of ≥ 1 pituitary hormones due to congenital brain malformations, head trauma, histiocytosis, infection, tumors, radiation

     b. Cessation of glucocorticoid therapy after prolonged large-dose administration of glucocorticoids (e.g., asthma, nephrosis, leukemia)

     c. Other—post-surgical, infants of steroid-treated mothers, respiratory distress syndrome, anencephaly, pituitary defects

- Signs and Symptoms

  1. Acute adrenal insufficiency (Adrenal crisis)

     a. Known or unknown diagnosis of Addison's—crisis may be first presentation of illness

     b. Recent or concurrent infection or febrile illness; surgery; exposure to excessive heat in susceptible individuals

     c. History of abrupt withdrawal of large-dose steroid therapy

     d. Weight loss, fever, fatigue, nausea, vomiting, diarrhea, dehydration, abdominal pain, anorexia, salt craving despite anorexia, symptomatic hypoglycemia, muscle weakness

  2. Chronic adrenal insufficiency—poor weight gain, weight loss, fatigue, weakness, lethargy, exercise intolerance, headache, anorexia, nausea, vomiting which may be forceful or projectile, diarrhea, dehydration, salt craving, increased pigmentation, hypotension

- Differential Diagnosis

  1. Differentiate acute adrenal insufficiency from acute infections, diabetic coma, CNS disturbances, acute poisoning; in newborn, distinguish from respiratory distress, intracranial hemorrhage, sepsis (Kappy, Steelman, Travers & Zeitler, 2001)

  2. Differentiate chronic adrenal insufficiency from anorexia nervosa, muscular disorders (e.g., myasthenia gravis), nephritis, chronic infection (e.g., TB), recurrent spontaneous hypoglycemia

- Physical Findings

  1. Acute adrenal insufficiency (adrenal crisis)—moribund, fever followed by hypothermia, cachectic, acutely dehydrated, vomiting, hypotension, confusion, coma, weakness, abdominal pain, nausea

  2. Chronic adrenal insufficiency (Addison's)—lethargy, dehydration, poor weight gain, weight loss, vomiting, hypotension, small heart size on radiograph, bronze skin pigmentation, especially of areola, mucous membranes, hand creases, axilla and groin, extensor surfaces of joints, and surgical scars

- Diagnostic Tests/Findings (Kappy, Steelman, Travers & Zeitler, 2001)

  1. Abnormal studies—decreased serum sodium bicarbonate, $PaCO_2$, blood pH, and blood volume; hyperkalemia, and increased BUN; urinary sodium and sodium to potassium ratio elevated relative to degree of hyponatremia; eosinophilia; moderate neutropenia

  2. Confirmatory tests to assess functional capacity of adrenal cortex

     a. Increased baseline serum ACTH in primary adrenal failure

     b. Lack of response to ACTH stimulation testing in primary adrenal failure; inadequate response to ACTH testing in secondary adrenal failure

     c. Decreased urinary free cortisol and other adrenal steroids

     d. Metyrapone test (in hospital)—non-elevation of 11-deoxycortisol level

     e. Corticotropin-releasing-hormone (CRH) abnormal

- Management/Treatment

  1. Immediate treatment of life-threatening acute adrenal crisis

  2. Referral to endocrinologist for suspected or confirmed adrenal insufficiency

  3. Pharmacologic—after initial stabilization, chronic corticosteroid replacement with glucocorticoids (e.g., hydrocortisone), mineralocorticoid, (e.g., fluorocortisone) and/ or sodium chloride (table salt); increased dosages may be needed during severe illness, trauma, stress, or surgery

  4. Monitor for steroid excess, particularly for decreasing height and weight; monitor for insufficient glucocorticoid treatment (headache, weight loss, nausea, hypotension); monitor blood glucose, ACTH, sodium and potassium

  5. Avoid abrupt withdrawal of corticosteroids to avoid adrenal crisis

6. Education regarding risk of acute episodes; Medic Alert tag; consider emergency hydrocortisone injection kit for use in accident or severe stress (New, del Balzo, Crawford & Speiser, 1990)

Adrenocortical Hyperfunction

- Definition: Excessive production and secretion by the adrenal gland of cortisol, adrenocortical androgens, estrogen, and/or aldosterone

- Etiology/Incidence (Migeon & Lanes, 1996)

    1. Hypercortisolism (Cushing's)—excess cortisol (ACTH) secretion by adrenals

        a. Adrenal tumors (Cushing syndrome)—relatively rare but occurs in all ages

        b. Pituitary adenomas (Cushing disease)

        c. Chronic exposure to glucocorticoids to treat inflammation and for immunosuppression

        d. Ectopic ACTH-secreting tumors—nonpituitary tumors stimulate the adrenal cortex, causing excess ACTH secretion, rare; usually seen in children < 12 years

    2. Adrenogenital syndrome—virilizing adrenal tumor causes elevated adrenal androgen secretion

    3. Feminizing adrenal tumors—causes elevated adrenal estrogen secretion

    4. Hyperaldosteronism

        a. Secondary—physiologic attempts to maintain homeostatis with serum electrolytes and fluid volume due to renal compromise or physiologic response to severe illness

        b. Primary—due to adrenal tumor or hyperplasia

- Signs and Symptoms

    1. Ubiquitous effects of adrenal hormones lead to multiple and varied signs and symptoms

    2. Hypercortisolism (Cushing's)—slowed growth and development, obesity, emotional lability (depression and euphoria), delayed pubertal onset, easy bruising, increased appetite, back pain

    3. Adrenogenital syndrome—increase in linear growth rate and muscle development, acne, premature pubarche, development of secondary sex characteristics in boys, enlarged and erectile clitoris in females, menstrual irregularities in older girls

    4. Feminizing adrenal tumors—rapidly increasing height, development of secondary sex characteristics in girls with possible breakthrough vaginal bleeding; gynecomastia in males

    5. Hyperaldosteronism—in infants, FTT, vomiting, weakness; may have history of recent diarrhea, increased sweating, heat exposure; history of renal or liver disease

(e.g., cirrhosis, nephritis, renal ischemia); in primary hyperaldosteronism, muscle weakness, unusual periodic paralysis; paresthesias, tetany; polyuria; polydipsia

- Differential Diagnosis

  1. Distinguish hypercortisolism from exogenous obesity; virilizing adrenal tumors from virilizing gonadal tumors; and feminizing adrenal tumors from premature thelarche and idiopathic sexual precocity

  2. Determine if hyperaldosteronism due to physiologic response to maintain homeostasis in severe illness vs. pathology (e.g., renal disease, adrenal tumor)

- Physical Findings

  1. Ubiquitous effects of adrenal hormones lead to multiple and varied clinical findings

  2. Hyperadrenocorticism—poor growth rate may precede obesity or other symptoms; relatively short stature; obesity; purple striae; truncal obesity; "buffalo type" adiposity of face, neck, and trunk; fat pad in interscapular area; plethoric or "moon" facies; delayed onset of secondary sex characteristics; muscle weakness; may have virilism; may have hemihypertrophy; delayed skeletal maturation; osteoporosis, especially of spine

  3. Adrenogenital syndrome—increase in linear growth rate; hirsutism; acne; deepening voice; increased muscle mass; masculinization of prepubertal children (boys with pubic, axillary, and sometimes facial hair with adult-size penis, frequent erections, pre-pubertal or slightly enlarged testes) (girls with pubic and axillary hair with enlarged and erectile clitoris); advanced bone age

  4. Feminizing adrenal tumor—increase in linear growth rate; gynecomastia in males; prepubertal testes, pubic hair; breast development in females, may have pubic hair; advanced bone age

  5. Primary hyperaldosteronism—in infants, FTT; weakness; dehydration; tetany; hypertensive or normotensive; nocturnal enuresis; muscle weakness, unusual periodic paralysis

- Diagnostic Tests/Findings (Migeon & Lanes, 1996; Kappy, Steelman, Travers & Zeitler, 2001)

  1. Confirmatory tests used to determine specific etiology of adrenal hyperfunction

  2. Plasma cortisol concentrations elevated; may be loss of normal diurnal variation in cortisol secretion

  3. Low serum chloride and potassium levels; may have elevated sodium, pH, CO_2

  4. Serum ACTH slightly elevated with adrenal hyperplasia (Cushing disease); decreased with adrenal tumor and very elevated with ACTH-producing pituitary or ectopic (extra-pituitary) tumors

  5. Low eosinophil counts; leukocyte count with polymorphonuclear leukocytosis with lymphopenia, possibly elevated RBC

6. Elevated urinary free cortisol and urinary 17-hydroxycorticosteroid excretion; abnormal urinary 17-ketosteroid excretion; may have glycosuria

7. Abnormal dexamethasone suppression or CRH stimulation tests

8. Adrenogenital syndrome—androgen secretion not suppressed by dexamethasone administration; advanced bone age

9. Feminizing adrenal tumor—elevated adrenal steroids in urine; elevated urinary and plasma estrogen levels; advanced bone age

10. Hyperaldosteronism—hypokalemia, high aldosterone; may have low or elevated plasma renin level; may have increased chloride, potassium, and prostaglandin excretion in urine

11. CT and MRI to assess for adrenal tumors; pituitary imaging to assess for pituitary tumor

- Management/Treatment

1. Referral to pediatric endocrinologist for management of suspected or confirmed adrenocortical hyperfunction

2. Surgery indicated for adrenal tumors, pituitary adenomas, ectopic ACTH-producing tumors

3. ACTH pre- and postoperatively to stimulate nontumerous contralateral adrenal cortex

4. Discontinuance of excessive glucocorticoid therapy if adrenocorticol hyperfunction

Miscellaneous

Hypoglycemia

- Definition: Symptoms provoked by abnormally low blood glucose levels occurring when child with diabetes receives excessive insulin, fails to eat, or exercises too strenuously; in children without diabetes, blood glucose level must be < 40 mg/dL and < 30 mg/dL in newborns (Gotlin & Chase, 1997)

- Etiology/Incidence

1. Transient neonatal hypoglycemia

    a. SGA infants with decreased production of blood sugar due to physiologic immaturity or inadequate glycogen stores

    b. LGA infants of diabetic mothers (IDM) with hyperplasia of beta cells of pancreas due to chronic intrauterine exposure to elevated maternal blood sugar

    c. Increased glucose use from physiologic stressors secondary to asphyxia, anoxia, respiratory illness, heart disease, infection, cold injury, or starvation

2. Hypoglycemia of childhood

    a. Hyperinsulinism—caused by abnormalities of beta cells (e.g., adenoma, islet cell hyperplasia); most common cause of persistent, recurrent hypoglycemia in first year; peak onset in first year and after age 3 years

b. Functional fasting hypoglycemia (''ketotic hypoglycemia'')— occurs between 1 and 5 years of age; peaks at 2 years; more common in SGA infants, males, and children with BW < 2500 g; associated with fasting in past 24 hours; episodes may occur periodically and with less frequency; rare after 5 years (Orlowski, 2001)

c. Associated with CNS disorders

d. Metabolic disorders and endocrine insufficiency, e.g., deficiency; galactosemia, hypopituitarism, congenital hypothyroidism, adrenal insufficiency; usually apparent in first 2 years of life

e. Severe malnutrition states, e.g., chronic diarrhea, liver disease

f. Other—drug ingestion, drug toxicity (alcohol, aspirin, oral hypoglycemic agents); associated with accidental ingestion or deliberate administration

- Signs and Symptoms

  1. Neonatal hypoglycemia—findings variable depending on degree of hypoglycemia; irritable, jittery, refusal to feed; tend to be small or large for gestational age

  2. Childhood hypoglycemia

     a. Findings variable depending on degree and etiology of hypoglycemia; may have mood changes, nervousness, weakness, hunger, epigastric pain, vomiting

     b. May have history of diabetes with recent history of excessive insulin, failure to eat, strenuous exercise; complaints of hunger; intentional or accidental ingestion of oral hypoglycemic agents, alcohol, salicylate

     c. May have known personal or familial history of inherited metabolic disorder or inherited hormonal deficiency; may have symptoms of metabolic disorder or hormonal deficiency

     d. Functional fasting (''ketotic hypoglycemia'')—history of vomiting, anorexia, failure to eat previous 24 hours, often have URI; may have early morning seizures

- Differential Diagnosis: Distinguish among various possible etiologies of hypoglycemia (e.g., functional ketotic vs. inherited metabolic and endocrine disease) because of underlying implications for management

- Physical Findings

  1. Neonatal hypoglycemia—variable findings

     a. Cachexic or macrosomic infant

     b. Irritability, lethargy, weak cry

     c. Hypothermia, cyanosis, diaphoresis; pallor

     d. Uncoordinated eye movements, eye-rolling

   e.   Apnea, irregular breathing, tachycardia

   f.   Twitching, jitteriness, convulsions, semiconsciousness or coma

   2.   Childhood hypoglycemia

      a.   Signs as above

      b.   May have diminished growth, difficulty talking, signs of other systemic illness, abdominal or pelvic masses, unsteady gait, concurrent illness

- Diagnostic Tests/Findings

   1.   Transient neonatal hypoglycemia—routine Dextrostix on all newborns after birth; if high risk for hypoglycemia, e.g., SGA, IDM, Dextrostix frequently; if Dextrostix ≤ 45 mg/dL, do immediate quantitative blood glucose; hypoglycemic if:

      a.   Whole blood glucose level < 35 mg/dL in first 24 hours or < 40 mg/dL thereafter *or*

      b.   Plasma glucose level < 40 mg/dL in first 24 hours or < 45 mg/dL thereafter (Gilmore & Marks, 2001)

   2.   Low blood glucose levels during hypoglycemic episode; consistent and repeated levels below 40 mg/dL with associated signs and symptoms need further confirmatory tests (Gotlin & Chase, 1997, p. 758)

   3.   In hyperinsulinemia, serum insulin levels may be inappropriately elevated when compared with glucose level obtained at same time (Gotlin & Chase, 1997, p. 758)

- Management/Treatment

   1.   Consultation with or referral to physician or endocrinologist for delineation of etiology and management

   2.   Treat hypoglycemic episodes promptly and adequately to prevent CNS injury; especially important for younger children

   3.   Hypoglycemic reactions in children with diabetes—see diabetes mellitus in this chapter

   4.   Surgery for pancreatic adenoma, partial pancreatomy if insulin secretion suppression unsuccessful

   5.   Children with functional (fasting, ketotic) hypoglycemia—treat with liberal carbohydrate diet with bedtime snacks, moderate restriction on ketogenic foods; avoid prolonged fasting, especially if child ill; parents may need to check urinary ketones

Hyperglycemia

- Definition: Common hereditary metabolic and endocrine disorder characterized by insulin deficiency resulting in abnormal metabolism of carbohydrate, protein, and fat (type 1, formerly termed insulin dependent diabetes mellitus [IDDM]) or may have specific carbohydrate intolerance causing insulin resistance at tissue level (type 2 diabetes, formerly termed Non-insulin Dependent Diabetes Mellitus [NIDDM])

- Etiology/Incidence: Hyperglycemia results from mechanisms that cause failure of pancreatic beta-cell function or other processes not directly involving beta cells; diabetes mellitus (DM) is the third leading cause of serious chronic disease in childhood

  1. Type 1—destruction of beta islet cells of pancreas; uncommon in infancy and toddlerhood, increases until adolescence, then drops sharply; peaks occur between 5 and 7 years and at time of puberty; boys and girls equally affected; more frequently diagnosed in winter, especially with adolescents; environmental factors may increase or decrease expression of diabetes in susceptible individuals; multifactorial, associated with genetic predisposition and environmental factors including viruses (e.g., mumps, coxsackie, congenital rubella), environmental toxins, nutrition, and physical and emotional stress (Drash, 1996a; Sperling, 1996).

     a. Type 1A—immune-mediated (previously termed juvenile diabetes or insulin dependent diabetes); most common type of diabetes in those < 40 years; associated with being overweight, not prone to ketosis, and insensitivity to insulin (Chase & Eisenbarth, 2001)

     b. Type 1B—non-immune-mediated insulin-deficient diabetes; frequently found in overweight teens and in black and Hispanic children who develop diabetes

  2. Type 2—insulin resistance associated with childhood obesity, onset most often > 10 years of age; more likely in children and adolescents of predominantly Native American, Hispanic, African American, and Asian origins; most rapidly increasing form of diabetes; includes Maturity-Onset Diabetes of the Young (MODY) characterized by slow onset, not requiring insulin, having less severe symptoms, and autosomal dominant inheritance pattern (Chase & Eisenbarth, 2001; Stoffers, 2000)

  3. Other—associated with administration of high doses of steroids (e.g., in renal disease, rheumatoid arthritis, asthma, leukemia) or anti-leukemia drugs; excessive endogenous cortisol production; CNS tumors, pheochromocytoma; cystic fibrosis

- Signs and Symptoms

  1. May present with very mild symptoms or in diabetic ketoacidosis

  2. Symptoms of type 1 diabetes mellitus

     a. Polyuria, polydipsia, polyphagia (primary complaints)

     b. Weight loss or failure to gain weight; variable decrease in linear growth

     c. Behavioral changes, headache, emotional lability, fatigue, recent ''flu-like'' illness

     d. Abdominal pain, nausea, vomiting, constipation, nocturia, enuresis

     e. History of recent illness, stress, missed insulin if known diabetic

  3. Symptoms of type 2 diabetes mellitus

     a. Many of the above symptoms but generally less severe than in type 1 diabetes mellitus

     b. Mild to moderate polyuria and polydipsia

    c.   Weight loss

    d.   History of high caloric intake and sedentary lifestyle

    e.   Positive family history of type 2 diabetes mellitus

- Differential Diagnosis

    1.   Diabetes insipidus

    2.   Non-diabetes causes of polyuria, e.g., psychogenic polydipsia, CNS injury, tumors

    3.   Other causes of fatigue, weight loss, behavioral change, e.g., Hashimoto's hypothyroidism, systemic illness

- Physical Findings

    1.   Type 1 diabetes mellitus

        a.   Dehydration, irritability

        b.   Weight loss

        c.   Visual disturbances

        d.   Fatigue, muscular weakness, declining physical performance

        e.   Long-term complications—joint contractures, diabetic retinopathy, compromised renal function

    2.   Type 1 diabetes with diabetic ketoacidosis

        a.   Marked dehydration, irritability, lethargy, drowsiness, stupor, coma

        b.   Tachycardia, cardiac arrhythmias, Kussmaul breathing (long, deep, labored breathing)

        c.   Dry mucous membranes, cherry-red lips, hypotension, rapid and thready pulse, hyperventilation, low temperature, "fruity" acetone breath

        d.   Vomiting, abdominal spasm, tenderness

    3.   Type 2 diabetes mellitus of youth

        a.   Marked obesity

        b.   Acanthosis nigracans

        c.   Vaginal candidiasis in females

- Diagnostic Tests/Findings

    1.   Glycosuria; urinary ketones

    2.   Elevated blood glucose—fasting blood glucose levels > 200 mg/dL or random blood glucose > 200 mg/dL (Chase & Eisenbarth, 2001)

    3.   Elevated plasma glucose—fasting plasma glucose level > 126 mg/dL or plasma glucose level > 200 mg/dL when taken either randomly or two hours after oral glucose load (Chase & Eisenbarth, 2001)

4. Elevated glycosylated hemoglobin (HbA_{1c})

5. In mild diabetic ketoacidosis (DKA) venous blood pH 7.2 to 7.3; moderate DKA venous blood pH 7.10 to 7.19; severe DKA venous blood pH < 7.10 (Chase & Eisenbarth, 1997)

6. Possible positive antibody tests—HLA, islet cell; insulin autoantibody (Gotlin & Chase, 1997); in type 2 diabetes, negative islet cell antibodies

- Management/Treatment

1. Immediate hospitalization if severe diabetic ketoacidosis

2. Consultation with physician or referral to pediatric endocrinology team for diagnostic evaluation, initial care and management and/or for confirmation/management of associated diseases, e.g., hypothyroidism; referral as needed for treatment by ophthalmologist and for emotional/behavioral disorders

3. After initial stabilization, for children with type 2 diabetes, slow gradual weight loss, exercise regimen, education stressing lifestyle changes to achieve weight loss, oral hypoglycemic agents following insulin if insulin initially needed to stabilize blood glucose levels

4. After initial stabilization, children with type 1 diabetes generally treated with combination of short- and long-acting insulin; types, onset, peak action, and duration of insulin varies (see Table 1)

Table 1

Bioavailability characteristics of the insulins

	Human Insulin Type	Onset	Peak Action	Duration
Short-acting	Regular Actrapid,® Velosulin®	30 – 45 min	2 – 4 hr	5 – 7 hr
	Semilente, Semitard®	30 – 60 min	4 – 6 hr	6 – 8 hr
Intermediate-acting	Lente, Lentard,® Monotard®	2 – 4 hr	8 – 10 hr	15 – 18 hr
	NPH, Insulatard,® Protaphane®	2 – 4 h	8 – 10 hr	12 – 14 hr
Long-acting	Ultralente, Ultratard®	4 – 5 hr	8 – 14 hr	15 – 18 hr

From ''Endocrine and metabolic disorders'' by R. W. Gotlin and H. P. Chase (p. 749). In *Handbook of Pediatrics* (18th ed.) by G. B. Merenstein, D. W. Kaplan, & A. A. Rosenberg (Eds.), 1997, Stamford, CT: Appleton & Lange. Copyright by Appleton & Lange. Reprinted with permission.

5. Critical goal of treatment to maintain blood glucose levels at near normal to prevent acute complications (e.g., hypoglycemia and ketoacidosis), intermediate complications (e.g., lipoatrophy and lipohypertrophy, limited joint mobility, growth failure, pubertal delay), and chronic complications (e.g., retinopathy, nephropathy, and neuropathy) (Becker, 1996)

6. Educate child and parents regarding disease; self-monitoring of blood glucose 4 times daily; insulin types, timing, dosages, adjustments; optimal nutrition; need for consistency in meal and snack time and in moderate, regular exercise; need for increased insulin during illness or stress; prompt treatment of infection; signs and symptoms of hypoglycemia and ketoacidosis; urine testing; complications of poor blood glucose management; availability of glucose and glucagon for acute hypoglycemic episodes (0.3 mg for children < 10 years, 0.5 mg sc or IM for older children) (Gotlin & Chase, 1997)

7. Encourage parents to obtain user-friendly resources for helping them to better understand the disease and its management (e.g., *Understanding insulin dependent diabetes* (9th ed.) by H. P. Chase (1999) and coloring books about diabetes available from The Guild of the Children's Diabetes Foundation (1-(800)-695-2873)

8. Supportive care of patient and family through stages of grieving following diagnosis; emphasize normalcy, view of child as "child with diabetes" vs. "diabetic child"

9. Recognize phases of diabetes—development of clinical symptomatology; clinical remission or "honeymoon" period of variable duration due to improved beta cell function after initial therapy started; relapse with progressive increase in insulin requirement

10. Ideal fasting blood glucose level (when without food for 2+ hours) varies with age of child (Chase & Eisenbarth, 2001)

    a. ≤ 4 years, 80 to 200 mg/dL

    b. 5 to 11 years, 70 to 180 mg/dL

    c. ≥ 12 years, 70 to 150 mg/dL

11. Treatment of insulin reactions (Chase, 1999)

    a. Mild reactions (hunger, shakiness, sweatiness, or irritability)—treat with 10 to 15 g carbohydrate (4 oz. juice, 6 oz. milk, 3 to 4 glucose tablets)

    b. Moderate reactions (extreme confusion, pallor, or drowsiness)—treat with Instant Glucose®, cake decorating gel, or some form of simple sugar

    c. Severe reactions (loss of consciousness, seizure or convulsion)—give glucagon; call 911

12. Glycosylated hemoglobin (HbA_{1c}) blood test every 3 months to assess overall blood sugar levels and to help in ascertaining compliance with treatment regimen; gives reliable measurement of long-term glycemic control during preceding 2 to 3 months; normal HbA_{1c} values vary by laboratory but are usually < 6.2%; desired levels for children ≥ 12 years should be < 7.8%, children 5 to 11 years should be < 8.5%,

and children < 5 years should be between 7.5% and 9.3% (Gotlin & Chase, 1997, p. 750; Chase & Eisenbarth, 2001, pp.877–878)

13. Sexually-active adolescents need instruction regarding pregnancy prevention; oral contraceptives are acceptable if blood pressure is normal

14. Explore with parents additional topics such as use of insulin pumps (Chase, 1999) and insulin pens (Fleming, 2000), obtaining medical alert bracelets, communication with extended family and school personnel about child's illness, and the research directed at diabetes prevention research (e.g., The Diabetes Prevention Trial: Type 1, 1-(800)425-8361)

Disorders of Pubertal Development

- Definition: Abnormal development or delay in initiation of secondary sexual characteristics

- Etiology/Incidence: Abnormalities in pubertal development associated with CNS or gonadal disorder or dysfunction; includes temporary and permanent delays of pubertal onset or true (complete) or pseudoprecocious (incomplete) puberty

  1. Intersex—ambiguous genitalia or inappropriate for gonadal sex due to endocrinopathy

  2. Precocious pubertal development—in boys, secondary sexual characteristics before 9 years (Kappy, Steelman, Travers & Zeitler, 2001); in girls, onset of breast development before 7.5 years or menses before the age of 9.5 years (Rosenfield, 1996); however, breast and pubic hair development in females may occur normally for a small percentage of girls between 7 and 7.99 years

     a. True (complete) precocious puberty is mediated by pituitary gonadotropin secretion involving all secondary sex characteristics

     b. Pseudoprecocious (incomplete) puberty involves one type of secondary sexual characteristic (e.g., premature thelarche [breast development] or pubarche [pubic hair development]; mediated by excessive estrogen/androgen stimulation for age from ovaries/testes, adrenal cortex, or exogenous sources

  3. Hypogonadism—causes lack of secondary sexual characteristics (sexual infantilism)

     a. In boys, lack of secondary sexual characteristics after 17 years suggests abnormal testicular maturation; may be due to testicular failure or dysfunction (primary failure due to anorchia, castration, Klinefelter's, mumps, radiation, trauma, tumor, endocrinopathies, etc.) or to pituitary/hypothalamic dysfunction (panhypopituitarism, empty sella syndrome, gonadotropin deficiency, LH, FSH deficiencies, endocrinopathies, etc.)

     b. In girls, may have lack of onset of secondary sex characteristics and amenorrhea due to primary ovarian failure (due to gonadal dysgenesis, enzyme defects, infection, surgery, radiation, chemotherapy, etc.) or to secondary ovarian failure (hypothalamic disorder or dysfunction, CNS irradiation, eating disorders, excessive exercise, chronic illness, etc.)

- Signs and Symptoms

  1. If intersex, history of confusion of sex assignment at birth

  2. May have normal growth and development through childhood; at puberty, may have abnormal sexual development; females may have virilization, primary amenorrhea; males may have incomplete virilization

  3. May have history of underlying disease, dysfunction, or systemic illness causing delay in or premature pubertal onset; history of exposure to radiation, drugs, etc.

  4. May have history of early development of one or all secondary sex characteristics, tall stature, symptoms of endocrine disease (e.g., hypothyroidism, congenital adrenal hyperplasia), intracranial disease (e.g., visual disturbances), abdominal disease (e.g., adrenal or gonadal tumor) or dysfunction (see growth disturbances this chapter)

  5. May have delayed development of secondary sex characteristics and symptoms of metabolic or endocrine disturbances (e.g., constipation); intracranial disease (e.g., failure to grow, seizures); syndrome stigmata (e.g., developmental delays); abdominal disease (abdominal enlargement) or dysfunction (see growth disturbances and adrenal gland disorders this chapter)

- Differential Diagnosis

  1. Ambiguous genitalia or suspected intersex—distinguish true hermaphroditism (both ovarian and testicular tissue present), female pseudohermaphroditism (female genotype, only ovaries), and male pseudohermaphroditism (genotype male, only testes)

  2. Structural abnormalities of genital tract and associated intracranial, endocrine, abdominal, or pelvic disease (Rosenfield, 1996)

  3. Precocious puberty—distinguish between true (complete) precocious puberty mediated by pituitary gonadotropin secretion involving all secondary sex characteristics vs. pseudoprecocious (incomplete) puberty involving one type of secondary sexual characteristics

  4. Premature sexual development—distinguish normal variants of premature thelarche (isolated premature breast development) and pubarche (early pubic hair development) in girls from pathologic causes; distinguish normal variants of premature adrenarche in boys (adrenal maturation with pubic hair and body odor) from pathologic causes

- Physical Findings

  1. May have normal or abnormal physical examination depending on underlying etiology of pubertal disorder (e.g., normal examination in constitutional delay, findings of chronic or systemic illness or midfacial defects in pathologic pubertal delay, tall stature in Klinefelter's, etc.)

  2. May have normal or abnormal genitalia depending on underlying etiology of pubertal disorder and timing (e.g., genitalia may be ambiguous in congenital adrenal hyperplasia; may have cryptorchidism in sexual infantilism or in pituitary insufficiency; may have abdominal mass or testicular mass in gonadal tumor; may have

microphallus in human GH deficiency, may have small testes in testicular failure, may have abnormal pelvic examination, etc.)

3. With precocious puberty, may have tall stature, premature secondary sex characteristics

4. With contrasexual pubertal development may have gynecomastia in males due to hypogonadism from Klinefelter's; excessive virilization of prepubertal girls with pubic hair, oily skin, acne, clitoromegaly, hirsutism

5. With delayed pubertal development for age, may have normal examination except for delayed growth and development (short stature but low normal growth rate) during childhood; delayed bone age; short legs for height or greater upper/lower body ratio, descended testes that are pubertal in size, consistency (Lee, 1996)

6. May have findings consistent with endocrine disorder (e.g., anisomia, the lack of ability to smell, and micropenis in gonadotropin abnormalities; hirsutism and dry hair and skin in hypothyroidism, etc.)

- Diagnostic Tests/Findings

  1. Tanner staging of breast, genitals, pubic hair development

  2. Laboratory findings variable depending on etiology of pubertal disorder; tests may include plasma or serum LH, FSH; GH, electrolytes, thyroid tests; blood and urinary pH, urine specific gravity, sedimentation rates, BUN, creatinine, etc.

  3. Tests of hormonal function as needed (e.g., GnRH to differentiate hypogonadotropic hypogonadism and constitutionally delayed puberty)

  4. CT, MRI, or ultrasound as needed to rule in or rule out central CNS, adrenal, renal, gonadal, or thyroid disease; bone age

  5. Other laboratory tests as needed—karyotype if ambiguous genitalia or Klinefelter's suspected

- Management/Treatment

  1. Physician consultation or referral to pediatric endocrinologist for suspected pathologic cause of pubertal delay or abnormal development

  2. Treatment dictated by identified etiology for pathologic cause of pubertal delay or abnormality in pubertal development (e.g., hormonal therapy may be immediate, as with congenital adrenal hyperplasia, or at puberty with testosterone for testicular failure)

  3. Management of underlying endocrine disorders and diseases and systemic illness (e.g., hypothyroidism, poorly controlled diabetes, anorexia, inflammatory bowel disease, etc.)

Gynecomastia

- Definition: Visible or palpable glandular enlargement of the male breast occurring commonly in healthy adolescent males (pubertal gynecomastia); occasionally indicative of underlying disease (pathologic gynecomastia); seen frequently in newborns (neonatal gynecomastia)

- Etiology/Incidence

  1. Neonatal gynecomastia—due to cross-placental transfer of maternal hormones; usually resolves by 2 to 3 weeks

  2. Pubertal gynecomastia—influence of too little androgen and/or too much estrogen on mammary tissue; transient, may occur in up to 75% of normal boys during puberty (Styne, 1996); onset between 10 and 12 years, peak occurrence 13 and 14 years, usually resolves by 16 to 17 years of age (Braunstein, 1996)

  3. Pathologic gynecomastia—secondary to drug side effects (e.g., cimetadine, digitalis, phenothiazine, treatment with hCG, testosterone, or estrogen), underlying disease or syndromes (e.g., Klinefelter's), injury to the nervous system, chest wall or testes; or, may be idiopathic

- Signs and Symptoms—breast development in other than pubertal females

- Differential Diagnosis:

  1. Transient pubertal gynecomastia from obesity (lipomastia) and pathologic causes—tumor (lipoma, neurofibroma, cancer)

  2. Breast infection

  3. Fat necrosis due to injury

  4. Drugs (estrogens, anabolic steroids, marijuana)

  5. Klinefelter's, gonadal dysfunction

- Physical Findings

  1. Neonatal—usually bilateral, often asymmetric breast tissue enlargement; resolves within 1 to 2 weeks

  2. Pubertal (physiologic) gynecomastia—breast tissue enlargement glandular, movable, disk-shaped, below areola, non-adherent to skin or underlying tissue; typically breasts unequal in size and < 3 cm in diameter; breasts may be tender, nipples irritated due to rubbing on clothing; if tissue ≥ 4 to 5 cm/diameter and breasts dome-shaped, macrogynecomastia present; Tanner stages II to IV pubertal development with testes ≥ 3 cm length (Mahoney, 1990)

  3. Pathologic gynecomastia—malnourishment, lymphadenopathy, delayed sexual maturity with undermasculinization, signs of chronic disease (e.g., goiter, liver or renal disease, endocrinopathies, cancer, colitis, CF, AIDS); breast tissue ≥ 3 cm/diameter, asymmetric, hard, fixed, indurated, not directly beneath areola; may have absent, underdeveloped or asymmetric testes

- Diagnostic Tests/Findings

1. Endocrinology studies as indicated

2. Imaging techniques as appropriate—ultrasonography of testes to identify impalpable testicular tumor; CT, MRI of abdomen to identify adrenal tumors

3. Karyotyping if Klinefelter's suspected

- Management/Treatment

    1. Neonatal—parent education and reassurance about etiology, transience, and normalcy of condition

    2. Pubertal (physiologic) gynecomastia < 4 cm—explanation, reassurance, and observation; regression usually spontaneous, within a few months, rarely beyond 2 years

    3. Physiologic macrogynecomastia (≥ 4 cm mass)—medical or surgical treatment usually required as regression rare, especially if gynecomastia present for > 4 years; pharmacologic therapy (e.g., tamoxifen, danazol, testosterone) sometimes used

    4. Gynecomastia usually very upsetting to adolescent but often not discussed because of embarrassment; reassure about transience and spontaneous regression

Menstrual Disorders: Amenorrhea

- Definition

    1. Primary amenorrhea—failure of onset of menarche in females who are 16 years and have normal pubertal growth and development; 14 years with absence of normal pubertal growth and development; or in girls who have not begun menstruation 2 years after completed sexual maturation (Polaneczky & Slap, 1992)

    2. Secondary amenorrhea—absence of menstruation for > 3 cycles or at least 6 months after menstruation established (Polaneczky & Slap, 1992)

- Etiology/Incidence

    1. Primary amenorrhea

        a. Constitutional/familial (common)

        b. Obstructions of menstrual flow (e.g., fusion or stenosis of labia, imperforate hymen)

        c. Estrogen deficiency

            (1) Primary ovarian insufficiency—organic or functional ovarian failure (e.g., anatomic anomalies, pelvic irradiation, enzyme defects, autoimmune disease, infection)

            (2) Secondary ovarian insufficiency—organic or functional ovarian failure from hypothalamic/pituitary disorders (e.g., decreased gonadotropin secretion, effects of chronic diseases such as DM, CF, anorexia; excessive exercise; endocrine disease)

        d. Androgen excess (e.g., polycystic ovaries, adrenal androgen excess [Cushing's])

e. Ovarian tumors

2. Secondary amenorrhea; many causes same as primary amenorrhea

   a. Pregnancy (most common)

   b. Hypothalamic, pituitary, and adrenal disorders or tumors; chromosomal abnormalities (e.g., Turner's); endocrinopathies; chronic illness, especially those causing severe weight loss or malnutrition; conditions affecting gonadal function

   c. Pharmacologic agents (discontinuance of birth control pills, use of tranquilizers)

   d. Significant emotional stress or strenuous exercise programs, especially with runners, ballet dancers, and gymnasts; major weight loss

   e. Uterine dysfunction after abortion, infection, C-section

   f. Hysterectomy

- Signs and Symptoms

  1. Primary amenorrhea—no history of menses in adolescence; may have symptoms of marked psychosocial stress, adrenal dysfunction or gonadal disease, pituitary or hypothalamic disease, chronic illness including eating disorders, chromosomal abnormalities, pregnancy; may have cyclic abdominal pain without menstruation in pseudoamenorrhea

  2. Secondary amenorrhea—sudden or gradual cessation of menses; symptoms vary depending on underlying etiology; may exercise excessively. See primary amenorrhea in this chapter

- Differential Diagnosis

  1. Determine if underlying etiology due to chronic illness, CNS disease, endocrinopathy

  2. Distinguish primary amenorrhea due to constitutional or familial etiology from pregnancy

  3. Distinguish secondary amenorrhea due to pregnancy, underlying disease or disorder

  4. Determine amenorrhea vs. ''pseudoamenorrhea'' (menstruation occurs but obstruction prevents release of menstrual blood)

- Physical Findings

  1. May have normal physical examination or signs of chronic, systemic illness or syndromes (e.g., underweight, CNS tumor or dysfunction, endocrinopathies, autoimmune disease, anorexia, malnourishment, unusually tall or short stature); may show signs of pregnancy

  2. May have lack of development of secondary characteristics or normal sexual development

3. Pelvic examination may show pregnancy, reproductive system abnormalities (e.g., cervical atresia, imperforate hymen)

- Diagnostic Tests/Findings

    1. Pregnancy test

    2. Careful family history to rule out constitutional/familial delay, then consultation with physician and/or referral to specialists as needed

- Management/Treatment

    1. Constitutional/familial primary amenorrhea—education, reassurance, monitoring

    2. Amenorrhea associated with other etiologies requires further evaluation, physician consultation or referral to appropriate specialist (e.g., reproductive endocrinologist, surgeon, pediatric neurologist, obstetrician, psychologist)

    3. Treatment directed at management or correction of underlying cause of abnormal menstrual processes (e.g., surgery if imperforate hymen, adrenal tumors)

    4. Sensitivity to significant concern of delayed development by child and family very important

    5. Parent and child education regarding amenorrhea and adherence to any treatment regimen

    6. Genetic counseling may be indicated if genetic etiology

Questions
Select the best answer

1. Secondary hypothyroidism results from:

   a. Excess release of thyroid hormone beyond the newborn period
   b. Intrauterine exposure to thyrotoxic drugs
   c. Disease or disorder of the thyroid gland itself
   d. Disease or disorder of the hypothalamus or pituitary gland compromising thyroid function

2. Congenital hypothyroidism has a higher incidence in which of the following populations?

   a. African-Americans
   b. Hispanic and Native-Americans
   c. Asian-Americans
   d. Euro-Americans

3. Which of the following is not a sign or symptom of congenital hypothyroidism?

   a. Hoarse cry
   b. Frequent stooling
   c. Coarse features
   d. Lethargy

4. The most common cause of hyperthyroidism in children and adolescents is:

   a. Graves' (autoimmune) disease
   b. Thyroid cancer
   c. Thyroid nodules
   d. Pituitary tumor

5. Which of the following is not found in an adolescent with untreated Graves' disease?

   a. Behavioral problems
   b. Sleep disturbances
   c. Tendency to gain weight easily
   d. Tachycardia

6. In which one of the following children would you most suspect hyperthyroidism?

   a. A 16-year-old male who complains about restlessness
   b. A 14-year-old adolescent female who is heat intolerant and has amenorrhea
   c. A male pre-teen with behavior problems
   d. A six-year-old female who complains of tiredness

7. The most common thyroiditis is:

   a. Subacute thyroiditis caused by a viral infection of the gland
   b. Acute suppurative thyroiditis caused by bacterial infection
   c. Caused by exposure to radiation or trauma

d. Hashimoto's or chronic autoimmune thyroiditis

8. Nephrogenic, or vasopressin-resistant, diabetes insipidus:

   a. Is caused by anatomic defects in the brain causing hypofunction of the pituitary or hypothalamus
   b. Results from damage to the hypothalamus or pituitary from surgical trauma or infection
   c. Is caused by reduced renal responsiveness to antidiuretic hormone (ADH)
   d. Has oliguria as a primary presenting symptom

9. An infant with polydipsia, polyuria, irritability, and failure to thrive, should be evaluated for:

   a. Diabetes insipidus
   b. Homocystinuria
   c. Growth hormone deficiency
   d. Hyperglycemia

10. Which one of the following is not characteristic of constitutional growth delay?

    a. There is generally no history of a similar growth pattern in other family members
    b. The child usually remains constitutionally small as an adult
    c. Final adult stature tends to be normal
    d. Weight and height at birth are generally in the lower percentiles

11. A newborn or infant with birth length < 50% and microphallus should be suspected of having:

    a. Growth hormone deficiency
    b. Congenital hypothyroidism
    c. Primordial short stature
    d. Down syndrome

12. An adolescent male who fails to develop secondary sex characteristics at puberty and who has small, underdeveloped testes should be suspected of having:

    a. Adrenal hyperplasia
    b. Klinefelter's syndrome
    c. Marfan's syndrome
    d. Cerebral gigantism (Sotos syndrome)

13. Individuals with chronic adrenal insufficiency often have:

    a. Frequent otitis media
    b. High energy levels
    c. Love for physical activity
    d. A craving for salt

14. In the newborn period, infants of diabetic mothers (IDMs) are particularly at risk for:

    a. Small size for gestational age
    b. Intrauterine growth retardation (IUGR)

c. Disorders in bone development

d. Hypoglycemia

15. Which statement is true about true (complete) or incomplete (pseudoprecocity)?

a. True precocity occurs because of hormonal stimulation from the pituitary or hypothalamus causing gonadal maturation and fertility

b. Pseudoprecocity does not involve development of any secondary sex characteristics

c. Incomplete precocity is caused by adrenal or gonadal tumor or dysfunction and results in increased linear growth but no development of secondary sex characteristics

d. Incomplete or pseudoprecocity leads to testicular enlargement and ovulation

16. An adolescent who has tall stature, increased arm span, arachnodactyly, laxity of joints, pectus excavatum, and an abnormal echocardiogram would be suspected of having:

a. Turner's

b. Beckwith-Wiedemann syndrome

c. Marfan's

d. Klinefelter's syndrome

17. Which one of the following is not found in children with growth hormone excess?

a. Tall stature

b. Prominent mandible and supraorbital ridge

c. High or normal plasma growth hormone

d. Short stature

18. A pathognomonic skin finding in children with chronic adrenal insufficiency (Addison's) is:

a. Purple striae

b. Increased pigmentation in the axilla, groin, areola, hand creases and in surgical scars

c. Dry, thickened skin

d. Increased perspiration

19. Which of the following findings is not characteristic of children and infants with hyperadrenocorticism?

a. Advanced skeletal maturation

b. "Moon" facies

c. Delayed onset of secondary sex characteristics

d. "Buffalo type" adiposity of face, neck, and trunk

20. Transient neonatal hypoglycemia is:

a. Most common in AGA infants

b. Low in premature SGA infants

c. Most common in LGA infants

d. Least common in LGA infants

21. Regular insulin:

    a. Has a quicker onset of effect and longer duration than NPH

    b. Has a slower onset of effect and shorter duration than NPH

    c. Has a quicker onset of effect and shorter duration than NPH

    d. Has the longest duration of the insulins available

22. The preferred name now for insulin-dependent diabetes mellitus (IDDM) is:

    a. Maturity-onset diabetes

    b. Type 1 diabetes

    c. Type 2 diabetes

    d. Insulin resistance syndrome

23. Blood glucose levels of children 5 to 11 years with diabetes should be maintained between:

    a. 70 to 180 mg/dL

    b. 100 to 200 mg/dL

    c. 60 to 80 mg/dL

    d. Slightly over 200 mg/dL

24. Blood glucose levels of younger children with diabetes are maintained at slightly higher levels than blood glucose levels of older children because:

    a. Children have a greater need for available glucose in the blood system

    b. Younger children tend to be more active

    c. Younger children become more irritable than do older children

    d. Lowering the risk of hypoglycemia in younger children is particularly important in order to avoid the potential for hypoglycemia with consequent neurological system damage

25. Glucagon should be used to treat:

    a. Children with mild hypoglycemia

    b. Children with moderate hypoglycemia

    c. Children with severe hyperglycemia

    d. Children with severe hypoglycemia

26. Which finding is not a sign or symptom of diabetes onset in children?

    a. Alopecia

    b. Glycosuria

    c. Polydipsia

    d. Polyuria

27. Abdominal pain and vomiting are particularly critical to monitor in children with diabetes because these findings may represent the onset of:

    a. Ketoacidosis

    b. Gastrointestinal infection

    c. Hyperglycemia

    d. Autoimmune response to the pancreas

28. Which of the following statements is not true about type 1 diabetes?

    a. The ''honeymoon'' period post-diagnosis is of variable duration
    b. Diabetes is a relatively common disease in childhood
    c. Children with type 1 diabetes can switch to oral insulin agents once they reach adulthood
    d. Three factors influence a child's potential to develop diabetes—genetic predisposition, autoimmune response, and exposure to viral or chemical agents

29. Precocious pubertal development is defined as the development of secondary sexual characteristics in boys before age ___ years and menses in girls before the age of ___ years.

    a. 10 years; 10 years
    b. 6 years; 8 years
    c. 9 years; 9.5 years
    d. 6 years; 9 years

30. In boys, lack of secondary sexual characteristics after 17 years suggests:

    a. Castration
    b. Abnormal testicular function
    c. True hermaphroditism
    d. Pituitary adenoma

31. The peak incidence for adolescent gynecomastia occurs at age:

    a. 10 years
    b. 13-14 years
    c. 16 years
    d. 18 years

32. The most common cause of primary amenorrhea is:

    a. Obstructions of menstrual flow
    b. Primary ovarian insufficiency
    c. Secondary ovarian insufficiency
    d. Constitutional or familial

Answer key:

1.	d	12.	b	22.	b
2.	b	13.	d	23.	a
3.	b	14.	d	24.	d
4.	a	15.	a	25.	d
5.	c	16.	c	26.	a
6.	b	17.	d	27.	a
7.	d	18.	b	28.	c
8.	c	19.	a	29.	c
9.	a	20.	c	30.	b
10.	c	21.	c	31.	b
11.	a			32.	d

Bibliography

American Academy of Pediatrics (1993). Newborn screening for congenital hypothyroidism: Recommended guidelines. *Pediatrics, 91*(6), 1203–1209.

Becker, D. J. (1996). Complications of insulin-dependent diabetes mellitus in childhood and adolescence. In F. Lifshitz (Ed.), *Pediatric endocrinology* (3rd ed., pp. 583–605). NY: Marcel Dekker, Inc.

Bode, H. H., Crawford, J. D., & Danon, M. (1996). Disorders of antidiuretic hormone homeostasis: Diabetes insipidus and SIADH. In F. Lifshitz (Ed.), *Pediatric endocrinology* (3rd ed., pp. 731–751). NY: Marcel Dekker, Inc.

Chase, H. P. (1999). *Understanding insulin dependent diabetes* (9th ed.). Denver, CO: Hirschfield Press.

Chase, H. P., & Eisenbarth, G. S. (2001). Diabetes mellitus. In W. W. Hay, Jr., A. R. Hayward, M. J. Levin & J. M. Sondheimer (Eds.), *Current pediatric diagnosis and treatment* (5th ed., pp. 874–880). NY: Appleton & Lange.

Drash, A. L. (1996a). Diabetes mellitus in the child: Classification, diagnosis, epidemiology, and etiology. In F. Lifshitz (Ed.), *Pediatric endocrinology* (3rd ed., pp. 555–565). NY: Marcel Dekker, Inc.

Drash, A. L. (1996b). Management of the child with diabetes mellitus. In F. Lifshitz (Ed.), *Pediatric endocrinology* (3rd ed., pp. 617–629). NY: Marcel Dekker, Inc.

Fleming, E. R. (2000). Mightier than the syringe. *American Journal of Nursing,* 100(11), 44–48.

Foley, T. P., Jr. (1996). Disorders of the thyroid in children. In M. A. Sperling, *Pediatric endocrinology* (pp. 171–194). Philadelphia: W. B. Saunders.

Foley, T. P., Jr. (2001). Hypothroidism. In R. L. Hoekelman, H. M. Adam, N. M. Nelson, M. L. Weitzman & M. H. Wilson (Eds.), *Primary pediatric care* (4th ed., pp. 1561–1565). St. Louis: Mosby.

Frasier, S. D. (1996). Tall stature and excessive growth syndromes. In F. Lifshitz (Ed.), *Pediatric endocrinology* (3rd ed., pp. 163–174). NY: Marcel Dekker, Inc.

Gilmore, M. M., & Marks, K. H. (2001). Critical neonatal illnesses. In R. L. Hoekelman, H. M. Adam, N. M. Nelson, M. L. Weitzman, & M. H. Wilson (Eds.), *Primary pediatric care* (4th ed., pp. 600–610). St. Louis: Mosby.

Goepe, J. G., & Ackerman, A. D. (2001). Fluid therapy. In R. L. Hoekelman, H. M. Adam, N. M. Nelson, M. L. Weitzman, & M. H. Wilson (Eds.), *Primary pediatric care* (4th ed., pp. 380–392). St. Louis: Mosby.

Gotlin, R. W., & Chase, P. (1997). Endocrine and metabolic disorders. In G. B. Merenstein, D. W. Kaplan, & A. A. Rosenberg (Eds.), *Handbook of pediatrics* (18th ed., pp. 708–762). Stamford, CT: Appleton & Lange.

Jospe, N. (2001). Hyperthyroidism. In R. L. Hoekelman, H. M. Adam, N. M. Nelson, M. L. Weitzman, & M. H. Wilson (Eds.), *Primary pediatric care* (4th ed., pp. 1554–1557). St. Louis: Mosby.

Kappy, M. S., Steelman, J. W., Travers, S. H., & Zeitler, P. S. (2001). Endocrine Disorders. In W. W. Hay, Jr., A. R. Hayward, M. J. Levin, & J. M. Sondheimer (Eds.), *Current pediatric diagnosis and treatment* (15th ed., pp. 835–873). NY: Appleton & Lange.

Lee, P. A. (1996). Disorders of puberty. In F. Lifshitz (Ed.), *Pediatric endocrinology* (3rd ed., pp. 175–195). NY: Marcel Dekker, Inc.

Lifshitz, F., & Cervantes, C. (1996). Short stature. In F. Lifshitz (Ed.), *Pediatric endocrinology* (3rd ed., pp. 1–18). NY: Marcel Dekker, Inc.

Lum, G. (2001). Kidney & urinary tract. In W. W. Hay, Jr., A. R. Hayward, M. J. Levin, & J. M. Sondheimer (Eds.), *Current pediatric diagnosis and treatment* (15th ed., pp. 609–631). NY: Appleton & Lange.

Mahoney, C. P. (1990). Adolescent gynecomastia - Differential diagnosis and management. *Pediatric Clinics of North America, 37*(6), 1389–1404.

Migeon, C. J., & Lanes, R. L. (1996). Adrenal cortex: Hypo- and hyperfunction. In F. Lifshitz (Ed.), *Pediatric endocrinology* (3rd ed., pp. 321–345). NY: Marcel Dekker, Inc.

Muglia, L. J., & Majzoub, J. A. (1996). Disorders of the posterior pituitary. In M. A. Sperling, *Pediatric endocrinology* (pp. 195–227). Philadelphia: W. B. Saunders.

New, M. I., del Balzo, P., Crawford, C., & Speiser, P. (1990). The adrenal cortex. In S. A. Kaplan (Ed.), *Clinical pediatric endocrinology* (pp. 181–234). Philadelphia: W. B. Saunders.

Orlowski, C. C. (2001). Hypoglycemia. In R. L. Hoekelman, H. M. Adams, N. M. Nelson, M. L. Weitzman & M. H. Wilson (Eds.), *Primary pediatric care* (4th ed., pp. 1985–1991). St. Louis: Mosby.

Polzaneczky, M. W., & Slap, G. G. (1992). Menstrual disorders in the adolescent: Amenorrhea. *Pediatrics in Review, 13*(2), 43–48.

Rogers, D. G. (1994). Thyroid disease in children. *American Family Physician, 50*(2), 344–350.

Rosenfeld, R. G. (1996). Disorders of growth hormone and insulin-like growth factor secretion and action. In M. A. Sperling (Ed.), *Pediatric endocrinology* (pp. 117–169). Philadelphia: W. B. Saunders.

Rosenfield, R. L. (1996). The ovary and female sexual maturation. In M. A. Sperling (Ed.), *Pediatric endocrinology* (pp. 329–385). Philadelphia: W. B. Saunders.

Sperling, M. A. (1996). Diabetes mellitus. In M. A. Sperling (Ed.), *Pediatric endocrinology* (pp. 229–263). Philadelphia: W. B. Saunders.

Stoffers, D. A. (2000). Maturity-onset diabetes of young (MODY): The past, present, and future. *Growth Genetics and Hormones, 16*(3), 37–41.

Styne, D. M. (1996). The testes: Disorders of sexual differentiation and puberty. In M. A. Sperling (Ed.) *Pediatric endocrinology* (pp. 424–476). Philadelphia: W. B. Saunders.

Tunnessen, W. W., Jr. (1988). *Signs and symptoms in pediatrics* (2nd ed., pp. 10–20). Philadelphia: J. B. Lippincott.

Weinzimer, S. A., Lee, M. M., & Moshang, T., Jr. (1997). In M. W. Schwartz, T. A. Curry, A.

J. Sargent, N. J. Blum, & J. A. Fein (Eds.), *Pediatric primary care: A problem-oriented approach*, (3rd ed., pp. 529–541). St. Louis: Mosby.

Zimmerman, D., & Gan-Gaisano, M. (1992). Hyperthyroidism in children and adolescents. *Pediatric Clinics of North America*, 37(6), 1273–1288.

Endocrine Disorders In Adults

Sister Maria Salerno

Diabetes Mellitus (DM)

- Definition: Genetically influenced metabolic disorder of carbohydrate, fat, and protein metabolism characterized by abnormally high blood glucose levels due to inadequate or absent insulin production and/or impaired insulin action

- Etiology/Incidence

  1. Type 1—immune mediated (formerly insulin-dependent, [IDDM] type I, juvenile-onset, ketosis-prone)

      a. Genetic susceptibility (HLA-DR3 gene) with environmental exposure to virus or other infectious processes leading to abnormal autoimmune response and destruction of insulin producing pancreatic beta cells is suspected

         (1) Family history of autoimmune disorders

         (2) Islet cell antibodies

         (3) Insulin autoantibodies

         (4) Absence of C-peptide

      b. Occurs more often in those < 20 years of age; those with European ancestry

      c. 10% to 15% of diabetics are of this type

  2. Type 2 (formerly type II, non-insulin-dependent, [NIDDM] adult or maturity onset, ketosis-resistant)—may range from predominantly insulin resistant with relative insulin deficiency to predominantly insulin secretory defect with insulin resistance

      a. Strong genetic autosomal dominant familial pattern

         (1) Impaired insulin production response of beta cells to increased demands of obese state

         (2) Insulin resistance mediated by decreased insulin receptors in target cells

         (3) Post cell receptor defect impairing glucose transport into the cells

         (4) No specific HLA or islet cell antibodies

      b. Risk factors include:

         (1) Family history of diabetes

         (2) Being previously identified as glucose intolerant

         (3) African-American, Asian-American, Hispanic-American, Native-American, or Pacific Islander race

         (4) Age ≥ 45

         (5) Physical inactivity/obesity

         (6) Having given birth to an infant weighing ≥ 9 lb.

         (7) "Syndrome X"—a cluster of disorders which may include:

            (a) Hypertension

      (b) Abnormal lipid profile

         (1) HDL cholesterol $\leq$ 35 mg/dL

         (2) Triglycerides $\geq$ 250 mg/dL

      (c) Truncal obesity

      (d) Insulin resistance

      (e) Hyperinsulinism

3. Diabetes associated with certain conditions or syndromes

  a. Includes endocrinopathy, infection, drug/chemically induced

  b. Genetic syndromes

4. Impaired fasting glucose (IFG)

  a. Glucose levels fall between normal and overt diabetes

  b. May worsen over time, remain unchanged, or revert to normal

5. Gestational diabetes mellitus (GDM)

6. About 8 million diagnosed cases and estimated 8 million undiagnosed; after thyroid disease and obesity most common metabolic disorder encountered in primary care settings; third leading cause of death in U.S.

- Signs and Symptoms

1. Type 1

  a. Usually sudden and severe in onset

  b. Early

    (1) Polyuria

    (2) Polydipsia

    (3) Polyphagia

    (4) Weight loss with normal or increased appetite

    (5) Blurred vision

    (6) Fatigue/weakness

    (7) Nausea/vomiting

    (8) Vaginal itching/infections

    (9) Skin rashes

  c. With advanced disease and long-term complications

    (1) Loss of appetite

    (2) Bloating

    (3) Dehydration

        (4)   Decreased level of consciousness

        (5)   Neurogenic and microvascular changes

            (a)   Paresthesias

            (b)   Progressive visual impairment

            (c)   Cold extremities

            (d)   Decreased or absent pedal pulses

            (e)   Constipation, nocturnal diarrhea

            (f)   Nocturia, neurogenic bladder, uremia, impotence

2.   Type 2

   a.   Onset more insidious

   b.   Early may not be noticed

        (1)   Polyuria

        (2)   Polyphagia

        (3)   Polydipsia

        (4)   Blurred vision

        (5)   Fatigue

        (6)   Sores that heal slowly

        (7)   Recurrent infections (vaginitis, especially candida; urinary tract, furuncules)

        (8)   Spontaneous abortion

   c.   With advanced disease and long term complications

        (1)   Similar to type 1, but macrovascular changes more prominent than microvascular

            (a)   Atherosclerosis

            (b)   Vascular insufficiency

            (c)   Coronary heart disease

        (2)   Hyperosmolar, hyperglycemic, nonketotic coma

- Differential Diagnosis

1.   Pancreatitis

2.   Cushing's syndrome

3.   Pheochromocytoma

4.   Acromegaly

5.   Cirrhosis

6. Secondary effects of drug therapy

   a. Oral contraceptives

   b. Corticosteroids

   c. Thiazides

   d. Phenytoins

- Physical Findings

   1. Type 1

     a. Early

       (1) Thin, decreased weight

       (2) Ill appearance

       (3) Orthostatic hypotension

       (4) Skin infections

     b. With more advanced disease

       (1) Skin—ulcerations of feet and legs, "shin spots" over tibial bones; loss of hair over lower legs and toes

       (2) Eyes—retinopathy, including microaneurysms; yellow hard or fluffy "cotton wool" exudates; neovascularization, cataracts, glaucoma

       (3) Cardiovascular—diminished or absent pedal pulses; decreased capillary filling, pretibial edema, cool extremities

       (4) Neurologic—sensory loss, absent knee and ankle jerks, deficits in extra-ocular movements

   2. Type 2

     a. Early

       (1) Usually obese

       (2) Hypertension

     b. With advanced disease similar to type 1

- Diagnostic Tests/Findings

   1. Plasma blood sugar—criteria for confirmation

     a. Newer guidelines indicate the oral glucose tolerance test (OGTT) not be used but the diagnosis based on the fasting blood sugar (FBS)

     b. The diagnosis of diabetes will be made if FBS $\geq$ 126 mg/dL and is $\geq$ 126 mg/dL on repeat testing *or*

     c. A random non-fasting glucose level is $\geq$ 200 mg/dL and

       (1) Symptoms of polydipsia, polyuria, and weight loss are present *or*

       (2)   On a subsequent day the FBS is $\geq$ 126 mg/dL or OGTT glucose level at 2 hours is $\geq$ 200 mg/dL

   d.   It is advised that the OGTT not be used routinely

   e.   If fasting glucose level are $\geq$ 110 mg/dL but < 126 mg/dL a diagnosis of ''impaired fasting glucose'' is made

   f.   Pregnant women should be screened for gestational diabetes at 24 to 28 weeks gestation with a 50 g glucose load

       (1)   A 1 hour glucose level < 140 mg/dL is negative

       (2)   A 1 hour glucose level > 200 mg/dL is diagnostic

       (3)   A 1 hour glucose level between 140 mg/dL and 200 mg/dL requires confirmation by a 100 g OGTT—the diagnosis is confirmed if two of four values meet or exceed recommended cutoff points

          (a)   Fasting 105 mg/dL

          (b)   1 hour 190 mg/dL

          (c)   2 hour 165 mg/dL

          (d)   3 hour 145 mg/dL

       (4)   Those with known risk factors such as race/ethnicity do not need the screening level 50 g exam but should receive the diagnostic 100 g exam at the 24 to 28 week point

2.   Urinalysis—presence of glucose, acetone (in type 1), and in advanced stages protein

3.   Blood urea nitrogen and urine creatinine—elevated in acute dehydration and with renal involvement

4.   Serum cholesterol and triglyceride levels—often elevated especially in type 2

5.   Electrocardiogram and chest radiography—for coronary and pulmonary pathology

6.   Hemoglobin A_{1c}—predominately used as a measure of glycemic control; indicates average plasma glucose level for previous 60 to 90 days; tested every 3 to 6 months, 5.5 to 7% considered good control

7.   Glycated serum protein (GSP)

   a.   Index of glycemic status over past 1 to 2 weeks

   b.   Clinical utility still under study

- Management/Treatment

1.   Goals of therapy are to attain best possible metabolic control while avoiding potential side effects—see Table 1

2.   Unless acutely ill treatment can be instituted on an outpatient basis

Table 1
Glycemic Control for Diabetics

Glycemic Index	Target	Non-Diabetic	Therapeutic action suggested
Fasting and preprandial glucose (mg/dL)	80–120	< 115	< 80 > 140
Bedtime glucose (mg/dL)	100–140	< 120	> 160 < 100
HbA$_{1c}$ (%)	< 7	< 6	> 8

3. Consult physician for:

   a. Newly diagnosed

   b. Anyone refractory to treatment

   c. Anyone with a blood sugar > 400 mg/dL

4. Give consideration to work schedule, life style, economic, social, and cultural aspects in management approach, e.g., persons who are homeless, persons working a night shift

5. Diet along with exercise is cornerstone of therapy

   a. Refer newly diagnosed to registered dietician and annually or semi-annually for follow-up

   b. Consistent dietary schedule; ideally 3 meals and 3 snacks; especially important for persons with type 1 diabetes and type 2 on insulin; teach use of exchange lists to those on insulin; for type 2, space meals 5 hours apart with few or no snacks

   c. Avoid refined carbohydrates and simple sugars

   d. Total carbohydrate intake should be 50% to 60% of total caloric intake

   e. Limit fats to 20% to 30% of total calories; saturated at < 8 to 9%

   f. Increase fiber to 25 g/1,000 calories

   g. Moderate protein intake, 0.8 g/kg/day or 20% of total caloric intake

   h. Total caloric intake to maintain or achieve ideal body weight (IBW)

      (1) Calculation of IBW

         (a) Females—allow 100 lb for first 5 feet of height plus 5 lb for each additional inch of height

         (b) Males—allow 106 lb for first 5 feet of height and add 6 lb for each additional inch of height

         (c) Small frame subtract 10%

         (d) Large frame add 10%

      (2) Caloric requirement

      (a) Multiply IBW by 10 = baseline calories

      (b) Add 3 × IBW if activity level is sedentary (most fall in this category); 5 × IBW if moderate; and 10 × IBW if strenuous

      (c) IBW = 125 lb
125 × 10 = 1250 (baseline calories)
125 × 3 = 375 (activity calories)
1250 + 375 = 1625 (total calories needed per day)

      (d) In type 2—obese, where weight reduction is primary treatment, subtract 500 calories from the total number needed per day

6. Exercise

    a. Planned daily exercise is an essential component for all diabetics, at least 30 minutes every other day

    b. Older persons with diabetes may be limited in types of exercise due to other concurrent problems such as arthritis, retinopathy

    c. Diminishes need for insulin by enhancing oxidation of sugar and facilitating absorption of insulin from injection sites

    d. Those on insulin should be instructed to inject insulin furthest from site of intensive exercise, e.g., abdomen rather than arms or thighs

    e. Additional carbohydrate should be ingested prior to exercise

    f. Contributes to weight and lipid control, reduces risks of CVD, improves insulin action

7. Examples of oral pharmacologic agents

    a. Sulfonylureas—see Table 2

      (1) First generation potent with long duration of action, increased risk of hypoglycemia, especially in the elderly

      (2) Contraindicated in pregnancy, for those with sulfa allergy, gestational or type 1 diabetes, or in ketoacidosis

      (3) Few side effects, but special precautions in those with renal, liver, or cardiovascular disease

      (4) Risk of hypoglycemia and weight gain

    b. Insulin resistance reducers

      (1) Biguanide (Metformin) 1.5 to 2.5 g daily in divided doses

        (a) Causes moderate weight loss

        (b) Improved lipid profile regardless of glycemic effect

        (c) Low risk of hypoglycemia

        (d) Side effects of flatulence, diarrhea; metallic taste minimized by taking with meals and increasing doses more slowly

Table 2
Examples of Sulfonylureas

Agent	Daily Dose mg	Doses/day	Onset hours	Duration hours	Metabolism
Chlorpropamide (a) (Diabinese)	100-500	1	1	72	Renal
Glyburide (b) (DiaBeta) (Micronase)	2.5-20	1 or 2	1.5	24	Hepatic
Glimepiride (Amaryl)	1-4	1	1	24	Hepatic
Glipizide (c) (Glucotrol)	2-40	1 or 2	1	12-18	Hepatic
(Glucotrol)	5-20	1	1	24	
(Glucotrol XL)	5-20	1	1	24	Hepatic

(a) Potent; contraindicated for use in elderly and renal desease; disulfiram-like reaction with alcohol; may cause hyponatremia
(b) Take on empty stomach; low toxicity, NO disulfiram reaction; caution in elderly
(c) 50-200 times more potent than other hypoglycemics; no disulfiram-like reaction; low toxicity; caution in the elderly
* See current pharmacology references for additional antidiabetic medications

      (e)   Contraindicated in renal, liver, or advanced cardiovascular disease

      (f)   Rare incidence of lactic acidosis; check pharmacology reference for precautions

   (2)   Thiazolidinediones (Pioglitazone, Rosiglitazone)

      (a)   Used for type 2 diabetes as monotherapy or in combination with insulin, metformin, or a sulfonylurea

      (b)   Pioglitazone 15 to 45 mg/day; Rosiglitazone 4 to 8 mg/day (refer to pharmacology reference for details on dosing)

      (c)   Monitor liver function every 2 months for first 12 months and periodically thereafter

      (d)   Increased risk of hypoglycemia with combination therapy

      (e)   May induce postmenopausal ovulation/risk of unintended pregnancy

      (f)   May cause or potentiate congestive heart failure

      (g)   Potential for multiple drug interactions

      (h)   Adverse reactions include upper respiratory infections, sinusitis, headache, pharyngitis, anemia, and edema

  c. Alpha-glucosidase inhibitor (Acarbose)

   (1)   Lowers postprandial blood glucose levels

   (2)   Low risk of hypoglycemia or weight gain

      (3)   Somewhat less efficacious than sulfonylureas or biguanides

      (4)   Flatulence, bloating, diarrhea frequent but abate with continued use

   d.   Administer angiotensin converting enzyme inhibitor (ACE) if not contraindicated

      (1)   Drug of choice to treat hypertension in those with DM

      (2)   Shown to prevent progression of nephropathy even in normotensives with type 2 DM

8.   Insulin (see Table 3)

   a.   Indicated

      (1)   Confirmed or suspected type 1 or gestational diabetes

      (2)   Type 2 dietary and/or oral agent management fails to control glucose levels, or in times of stress

      (3)   For those for whom oral agents are contraindicated

   b.   Some may need more than three injections per day and or use an insulin pump to maintain control

   c.   Weight gain and need for frequent glucose monitoring can be problems

   d.   Purity

      (1)   Standard beef or pork— > 10 but < 25 parts per million (ppm) proinsulin (immunogenic agent)

      (2)   Purified beef or pork— < 10 ppm proinsulin

      (3)   Human synthetic < 10 ppm proinsulin

Table 3

Insulins

Type	Action	Onset (Hours) (a)	Peak (Hours)	Duration (Hours) (b)
Insulin analog (Lispro)	Very Rapid	0.25	1	3.5–4.5
Regular	Rapid	0.5–1	1–2	5–6
Semilente	Rapid	0.5–2	1–2	12–16
NPH	Intermediate	1–2	2–8	24–48
Lente (isophane)	Intermediate	1–2	2–8	24–48
NPH (70%) with Regular (30%) (Mixtard, Novolin 70/30)	Intermediate	0.5	4–8	24
PZI (protamine zinc)	Long	2–4	8–12	38
Ultralente	Long	2–4	8–12	36

NOTE: Pork, beef-pork, and human synthetic insulin available in rapid, intermediate, long-acting
Long-acting are not currently available in human insulin
(a) Onset depends on site of injection, dose size, brand
(b) Duration is proportional to dose size and is increased in renal failure

          (4)   Beef more antigenic than pork species; human insulin least antigenic of all

    e.   Initiation and adjustment of dosage

        (1)   Exogenous insulin replacement begins with 10 to 30 units of intermediate acting insulin before breakfast each morning

            (a)   Lower doses for thin patients and higher for obese (tend to have more insulin resistance)

            (b)   Change dose no more than every 2 to 3 days

        (2)   As long as plasma glucose is > 140 mg/dL before the evening meal, dose is increased by 2 to 5 units every 2 to 3 days

        (3)   When afternoon postprandial plasma glucose is consistently < 140 mg/dL fasting plasma glucose is checked for sustained effect of single insulin dose; if fasting glucose is elevated, dose will be split with $\frac{2}{3}$ given before breakfast and $\frac{1}{3}$ before the evening meal; doses are adjusted until fasting plasma glucose is 120 to 140 mg/dL

        (4)   Once afternoon and before breakfast regulation is achieved, late morning levels are assessed; if needed, regular insulin can be combined with morning injection to keep late morning plasma glucose levels < 140 mg/ dL

            (a)   THE AMOUNT OF REGULAR INSULIN NORMALLY SHOULD NOT EXCEED 50% OF THE INSULIN GIVEN AT ANY TIME

            (b)   Do not mix lente or ultra lente with regular; zinc in lente precipitates regular, decreasing effective proportion of regular and increasing that of the lente

            (c)   Do not mix lente with velosulin short acting (Nordisk)—phosphate buffer increases concentration of unmodified soluble insulin and diminishes effect of intermediate acting preparation

            (d)   Regular insulin should be drawn up first if mixing regular and NPH in the same syringe

        (5)   Once daily regimen is established, urine and self-monitored plasma glucose levels are tested 3 to 4 times a day as indicated by the insulin schedule and severity of the disease

            (a)   Daily dose requirement decreases with progressive renal failure

            (b)   Control is assessed at 3 to 6 month intervals; glycosylated Hgb which reflects average glucose levels of the preceding 8 to 12 weeks may be helpful

9.   Combination therapy usually instituted if failure of monotherapy in type 2

    a.   Most frequently used—sulfonylurea with insulin or biguanide or alpha-glucosidase inhibitor

    b.   Less frequently used—insulin with biguanide and a sulfonylurea; insulin with biguanide; insulin with alpha-glucosidase inhibitor; or biguanide with alpha-glucosidase inhibitor.

    c.   No evidence of significant adverse interactions

    d.   Increase complexity and cost of treatment regimen

    e.   Morning sulfonylurea and NPH-lente insulin in the evening for select persons with type 2 diabetes

        (1)   Helps control morning hyperglycemia without concomitant hypoglycemia seen with insulin alone

        (2)   May help patient avoid need for multiple insulin injections

        (3)   Seems to work best in those who are less than 150% of Ideal Body Weight and have had the disease for less than 15 years

10.   Patient education—should begin at time of diagnosis and will extend over several weeks

    a.   Cause and general management of diabetes

    b.   Importance of diet and weight control

    c.   Self-monitoring of blood and urine glucose

    d.   Administration of insulin, dosing, action, side effects, and site rotation

    e.   Administration of oral hypoglycemic agents, dosing, action and side effects

    f.   Potential alteration in glucose metabolism with acute illness, exercise, and emotional stress

    g.   Test for and significance of ketonuria

    h.   Recognition and treatment of hypoglycemia

    i.   Proper leg and foot care

    j.   Sick-day guidelines

    k.   Guidelines for economizing with repeated use of needles and splitting glucose test strips

11.   Complications

    a.   Hypoglycemia

        (1)   Causes

            (a)   Insulin overdosage

            (b)   Omission or delay of meals

            (c)   Heavy exercise

(d) Errors in injection technique

(e) Renal failure

(f) Weight loss

(g) Development of hepatitis, pituitary or adrenal insufficiency, or other conditions that cause hypoglycemia

(h) Drugs that affect insulin metabolism/action; see Table 4

(2) Symptoms

(a) Weakness

(b) Sweating

(c) Shakiness

(d) Tremors

(e) Nervousness

(f) Headache

(g) Dizziness

(h) Hunger

(i) Irritability

(j) Convulsions, confusion, coma

(k) Tachycardia, palpitations

b. Somogyi phenomenon

(1) Cause—morning rebound hyperglycemia; occurs in response to nocturnal hypoglycemia with excessive insulin administration

(2) Clues—erratic plasma glucose and urine ketone values; symptoms of nocturnal hypoglycemia (night sweats, nightmares, low serum glucose 2 to 3 a.m.), weight gain in presence of heavy glycosuria

(3) Treatment—reduce insulin dose 10% to 20%

(4) Distinguish from *Dawn Phenomenon* which is early morning fasting hyperglycemia without nocturnal hypoglycemia; thought to be related to circadian rhythm secretion of growth hormone and treated by evening or bedtime dose of insulin

c. Lipodystrophy

(1) Atrophy—subcutaneous fat atrophy at insulin injection sites

(a) Cause—impurities in the insulin, possible autoimmune mechanism

(b) Treatment—switch to purified insulin, inject directly into atrophic areas

Table 4
Medication Effect On Insulin Metabolism/Action

Medication	Action
Alcohol	Decreased half-life of sulfonylureas in alcoholics, can cause severe hypoglycemia in those on hypoglycemics
Beta-adrenergic	Inhibit insulin secretion; block most hypoglycemia symptoms; prolong effect of insulin
Calcium channel blockers	Inhibit insulin secretion
Diazoxide	Inhibits insulin secretion
Glucocorticoids	Insulin antagonism
Nicotinic acid	Insulin resistance
Oral contraceptives	Insulin resistance
Phenytoin	Inhibits insulin secretion
Sympathomimetics	Insulin antagonism Inhibit insulin secretion
Thiazide diuretics	Inhibit insulin secretion
MAO inhibitors	Increase effects of antidiabetic agents
Salicylates	Increase effects of antidiabetic agents
Coumarin	Increase effects of sulfonylureas
Phenylbutazone	Increase effects of sulfonylureas

    (2)   Hypertrophy—over-growth of subcutaneous tissue

        (a)   Cause—growth promoting effects of insulin; improper rotation of injection sites

        (b)   Treatment—prevent by proper rotation of injection sites

  d.   Insulin allergy

    (1)   Rare and usually localized

    (2)   Treatment—change to human synthetic insulin

    (3)   Localized allergies may be treated with antihistamines or corticosteroid; consultation required

  e.   Insulin resistance requiring more than 200 units per day

    (1)   Rare and even less common with increased use of human insulins

    (2)   Cause—over-production of insulin-binding immunoglobulins

    (3)   Treatment—change to less immunogenic pork or human synthetic insulins

    (4)   May require glucocorticoid treatment; consultation required

  f.   Diabetic ketoacidosis (DKA)—hyperglycemia with ketonuria and disruption of the fluid, electrolyte, and pH balance leading to coma and even death; marked by hyperglycemia, metabolic acidosis, and ketonemia; sometimes PRESENTING SIGN in undiagnosed type 1

(1) Cause—infection, trauma, myocardial infarction, other severe stress, and noncompliance with therapeutic regimen

(2) Treatment—emergency fluid replacement, insulin therapy, sodium bicarbonate therapy, and close monitoring of blood chemistries

g. Hyperosmolar nonketotic syndrome—severe hyperglycemia, hyperosmolarity, and dehydration in the absence of ketoacidosis which may lead to coma; most often occurs in elderly on oral hypoglycemics and those with undiagnosed type 2

(1) Precipitating factors—calcium channel blockers, corticosteroids, thiazide diuretics, propranolol, phenytoin

(2) Treatment—similar to ketoacidosis, but need less insulin and more fluid replacement

(3) Prognosis is poor in elderly, particularly those with concurrent renal disease, hypertension, or congestive heart failure

12. Follow-up

   a. Well controlled patients—minimum every 3 to 4 months

   b. Yearly ECG, chest radiograph, creatinine, urinalysis with microprotein analysis, lipid profile, physical examination including fundoscopic, full neurologic examination

   c. Annual ophthalmologic examination by ophthalmologist

   d. Skin inspection, feet inspection, fundoscopic, and evaluation of glycemic control by fasting or postprandial plasma glucose measurements at each visit

   e. Hemoglobin A_{1c} every 3 to 6 months

13. Referrals to local support groups and identification of local chapters of the American Diabetes Association for information, support, and publications

14. Routinely screen all ≥45 years of age, if negative repeat every three years or earlier if risk factors are present.

Hyperthyroidism (Thyrotoxicosis)

- Definition: Excessive secretory activity of the thyroid gland; symptoms produced by excess exogenous or endogenous thyroid hormone; called Graves' disease when associated with ocular signs or ocular disturbances and a diffuse goiter

- Etiology/Incidence

   1. Causes

      a. Autoimmune response (Graves' disease accounts for more than 85% of cases)

      b. Subacute thyroiditis

      c. Toxic multinodular goiter; toxic uninodular goiter (autonomous thyroid adenoma)

      d.   Metastatic follicular thyroid carcinoma

      e.   Thyrotoxicosis factitia

      f.   TSH secreting pituitary tumor (secondary hyperthyroidism)

      g.   hCG secreting tumors (choriocarcinoma, hydatiform mole)

      h.   Testicular embryonal carcinoma

  2. One of the most common endocrine disorders

  3. Highest incidence in women between 20 and 40 years of age

- Signs and Symptoms

  1. Most frequent

      a.   Anxiety

      b.   Diaphoresis

      c.   Fatigue

      d.   Hypersensitivity to heat

      e.   Nervousness

      f.   Palpitations

      g.   Weight loss

      h.   Insomnia, nightmares

  2. Frequent

      a.   Dyspnea

      b.   Weakness

      c.   Increased appetite

      d.   Eye complaints, e.g., difficulty focusing

      e.   Swelling of legs

      f.   Hyperdefecation without diarrhea, hyperactive bowel sounds

      g.   Diarrhea

      h.   Oligomenorrhea or amenorrhea

      i.   Tremors

      j.   Angina

  3. Infrequent

      a.   Anorexia

      b.   Constipation

      c.   Weight gain

     d.   Signs of pseudobulbar palsy

   4.   Elderly patients may present with few signs or symptoms noted in younger patients (apathetic hyperthyroidism); may present with cardiovascular problems unresponsive to digitalis, quinidine, or diuretics

     a.   Atrial fibrillation

     b.   Angina

     c.   Congestive heart failure

- Differential Diagnosis

   1.   Anxiety neurosis, especially in menopause

   2.   Other diseases associated with hypermetabolism, e.g., pheochromocytoma and acromegaly

   3.   Myasthenia gravis (causes the same ophthalmoplegic signs)

   4.   Orbital tumors which can cause exophthalmos

   5.   Psychosis

- Physical Findings

   1.   General—thin, muscle wasting may be evident; nervous; quick motions

   2.   Vital signs—tachycardia, irregular pulse, widened pulse pressure

   3.   Integumentary—skin moist, velvety, may show increased pigmentation or vitiligo; hair thin, fine; spider angiomas and gynecomastia may be evident

   4.   Eyes—prominent; appear to "stare;" lid lag; lack of accommodation, chemosis; proptosis (exophthalmos)

   5.   Neck—enlarged thyroid gland (goiter) smooth or nodular, symmetric or asymmetric; thyroid bruit or thrill; absence of signs does not rule out hyperthyroidism

   6.   Cardiovascular—paroxysmal atrial fibrillation, harsh pulmonary systolic murmur, congestive failure, possible enlargement

   7.   Neurologic—hyperactive reflexes; fine tremors of fingers, tongue; mental changes ranging from mild exhilaration to delirium; in elderly, apathy, lethargy and severe depression may be manifested

   8.   Lymphatic—lymphadenopathy and splenomegaly may be present

- Diagnostic Tests/Findings (see Table 5 for list of thyroid function tests)

   1.   TSH assay best text for thyroid dysfunction—decreased in hyperthyroidism

   2.   Free thyroxine index (FTI) usually elevated; if normal and clinical impression is strong for hyperthyroidism then do

   3. T_3, radioimmunoassay (T_3, RIA)—elevated with a normal T_4 in early hyperthyroidism and T_3 toxicosis

Table 5

THYROID ASSESSMENT TESTS

Thyroxine (T$_4$)	Major hormone secreted by the thyroid gland
T$_4$ (RIA-serum)	By radioimmunoassay (RIA); normal adult is 5 to 12 μg/dL
Free Thyroxine Index (FT$_4$I)	Unaffected by TBG and is a better reflection of the true index hormonal status; serum T$_4$ and T$_3$ resin uptake (T$_3$, RU) used to calculate this index; normal adults 0.9–2.2ng/dL
T$_3$ Resin Uptake (T$_3$RU)	Indirect measure of T$_4$ levels by assessing T$_4$ binding sites; may be thought of as the reciprocal of the T$_4$ RIA; in hyperthyroidism there is a high T$_3$ resin uptake; in hypothyroidism the T$_3$ is low; normal adult is 25 to 35%
T$_3$ RIA (Serum)	Direct measure of triiodothyronine (T$_3$) thyroid hormone; helpful in diagnosing thyrotoxicosis when T$_4$ is normal; in hypothyroidism T$_3$ often normal; T$_4$ more helpful; normal adult is 80 to 200ng/dL (RIA)
Thyroid Antibodies, Thyroglobulin	High titers suggest autoimmune disease, e.g., Hashimoto's thyroiditis; also elevated in carcinoma of the thyroid; normal adult is 1:20, 0–50 ng/mL (RIA)
Throid Stimulating Hormone (TSH)	Direct measure of TSH secreted from the anterior pituitary in response to thyroid-releasing hormone (TRH); normal adult is 2 to 5.4 μU/mL < 10 μU/mL (RIA)
TSH Immunoradiometric Assay (IRMA)	Newer assay replacing TSH (RIA); normal adult is 0.5 to 5.0 μU/mL; more sensitive to suppressed TSH in hyperthyroidism
Radioactive Iodine Uptake (RAIU)	Used primarily to detect hyperthyroidism etiology; radioactive iodine given orally or intravenously; the thyroid is scanned at 3 different intervals to determine iodine uptake of the thyroid gland; an elevated RAIU indicates hyperthyroidism; normal adult is 2 hr., 1 to 13%; 6 hr., 2 to 25%; 24 hr., 15 to 45%

   4. T$_4$ level elevated in later stages

 • Management/Treatment

   1. Refer for hospitalization for suspected "thyroid storm"

      a. High fever

      b. Severe agitation

      c. Confusion

      d. Cardiovascular collapse

      e. Malignant exophthalmus

      f. Difficulty in breathing due to enlarged or tender thyroid gland

   2. Obtain physician consult for clients suspected of/or newly diagnosed with hyperthyroidism for treatment which may include:

      a. Propranolol 10 to 60 mg orally every 6 hours to control symptoms

      b. Radioactive iodine (^{131}I)

         (1) Therapeutic dose is 80 to 120 mCi administered in doses of 5 to 15mCi based on estimated weight of the thyroid gland

         (2) Most become euthyroid after 3 to 6 months

         (3) Hypothyroidism is frequent and can occur anytime after radioactive iodine therapy

(4) Contraindicated in pregnancy

c. Antithyroid drugs—indicated for initial control of thyrotoxicosis especially in pregnant women, those not wanting to take ^{131}I, or in preparation for surgical removal; effective in patients with small goiters

    (1) Propylthiouracil (PTU)—usual dose 300 to 400 mg/day in divided doses

        (a) Preferred for use in pregnant women

        (b) During pregnancy dose kept < 200 mg/day

    (2) Methimazole (MMI)—15 to 60 mg/day orally in three divided doses

    (3) Side effects

        (a) Dermatitis

        (b) Nausea

        (c) Agranulocytosis (most serious)

        (d) Hypothyroidism which can cause a TSH stimulated increase in goiter size

3. Patient education:

    a. Medication is to be taken for about two years and not abruptly discontinued

    b. At first sign of infection or fever drug should be stopped and healthcare professional contacted

    c. Therapeutic effect of medication is not usually evident for about three weeks

4. Surgery

    a. Not used as frequently now

    b. Indicated for children, adolescents, pregnant women unable to tolerate PTU, adults nonresponsive to thiourea treatment who refuse RAI

    c. Usually rendered enthyroid with drugs preoperatively

5. General considerations

    a. Client education

        (1) Rationale for treatment; dosage and side effects of medications; takes at least three weeks before antithyroid medications become effective

        (2) Instructions regarding nutritional needs: high carbohydrate, high caloric diet until medication takes effect; avoidance of stimulants such as caffeine

        (3) Symptoms of ''thyroid storm''

        (4) Symptoms of hypothyroidism

    b. Follow-up

        (1) Periodic examinations until euthyroid

(2) All patients who have been treated for hyperthyroidism should be periodically checked for hypothyroidism which may occur anytime during treatment

Adult Hypothyroidism (Myxedema)

- Definition: Decreased or deficient thyroid hormone—primary (glandular dysfunction) or secondary (pituitary insufficiency); occurs in all age groups
- Etiology/Incidence
    1. Major classifications
        a. Primary—caused by damage to the hormone producing capabilities of the thyroid gland itself
            (1) Most common cause in adults is autoimmune thyroiditis (Hashimoto's, chronic lymphocytic)
            (2) Can also be caused by ablation of the gland by surgery, medication, radiation, and goitrogens (thiocyanates, rutabagas, lithium carbonate)
            (3) More common than secondary
        b. Secondary—often related to destructive lesions of the pituitary gland as with chromophobe adenoma or postpartum necrosis (Sheehan's syndrome); frequently associated with signs of adrenal and gonadal disorders
        c. Tertiary—TRH deficiency arising in the hypothalmus; sometimes grouped with secondary
    2. Occurs in all age groups; more prevalent in women and those
        a. With a history of thyroiditis
        b. With previously treated hyperthyroidism (all modalities)
        c. Being treated with lithium or para-aminosalicylic acid
        d. With coexistent autoimmune disorders (e.g., rheumatoid arthritis, lupus, pernicious anemia)
- Signs and Symptoms
    1. Most frequent
        a. Cold intolerance
        b. Coarse skin
        c. Decreased sweating
        d. Dry skin
        e. Lethargy
        f. Swelling of eye lids
    2. Frequent

a. Anemia (normocytic, normochromic, microcytic, or macrocytic)

b. Anorexia

c. Coarse hair

d. Cold skin

e. Constipation

f. Hair loss

g. Hoarseness or aphonia, thick tongue

h. Hyperlipidemia including hypercholesterolemia

i. Leg edema

j. Menorrhagia

k. Memory impairment

l. Swelling of face

m. Paresthesias

n. Weight change

- Differential Diagnosis

    1. Rule out coexisting autoimmune disease or secondary hypothyroidism

    2. Nephrotic syndrome

    3. Chronic renal disease

- Physical Findings

    1. Vital signs—bradycardia, mild hypotension, or diastolic hypertension

    2. Edema of hands, face, eyelids

    3. Integumentary—dry, scaly skin with carotenemic tone; brittle nails; alopecia; puffy eyelids; temporal thinning of the eye brows

    4. ENT—enlarged tongue, possible hearing decrease, thyroid often enlarged

    5. Cardiovascular—bradycardia, decreased intensity of heart tones, cardiac enlargement (myxedemic heart may be related to pericardial effusion)

    6. Respiratory—pleural effusion

    7. Abdominal—ascites, decreased bowel sounds

    8. Neuromuscular—slow or delayed deep tendon reflexes, cerebellar ataxia, dementia (myxedema madness, manifested with hallucinations, paranoid ideation, and hyperactive delirium), pseudomyotonia, carpal tunnel syndrome

- Diagnostic Tests/Findings

    1. Free thyroxine index (FTI) or T_4; if low a TSH is helpful in determining etiology

2. TSH elevated in primary hypothyroidism

3. If T_4 is normal and TSH is elevated, may be mild hypothyroidism

4. Thyrotropin releasing hormone (TRH) stimulation done if low TSH with low T_4 or low FTI; may indicate secondary hypothyroidism

5. CBC—may demonstrate anemia

- Management/Treatment

   1. Refer for immediate hospitalization any client suspected of developing myxedemic coma—severe hypothyroidism associated with hypothermia, decreased mentation, hypoventilation, respiratory acidosis, relative hypotension, hyponatremia, hypoglycemia

   2. Obtain physician consultation for clients with suspected or newly diagnosed hypothyroidism for further testing and/or initiation of treatment which would include administration of synthetic T_4 (levothyroxine); desiccated thyroid is no longer used due to variability in composition

      a. Average replacement dose of T_4 is thyroxine 0.125 mg/ day in healthy, non-elderly adults and may range from 0.025 to 0.3 mg/day

      b. Dosage starts with 0.1 mg/day for those < 50 years of age, and 0.025 to 0.05 mg/day in those > 50 years of age or with known ischemic heart disease without angina

      c. Dosage is increased by 0.025 mg/day every two weeks until the patient is clinically euthyroid

      d. Patients with coexisting adrenal insufficiency, coronary insufficiency, or angina require particular care

      e. Initial effects of replacement not usually perceptible for at least two weeks after initiation of therapy and are initially demonstrated by decreased facial edema and increased urination

   3. On follow-up visits, after replacement therapy has been instituted:

      a. Check cardiopulmonary status; if pulse is > 100/minute consult with physician

      b. Monitor for symptoms or signs of too vigorous therapy, side effects, and toxic effects of replacement therapy; ask about dyspnea, orthopnea, angina, palpitations, nervousness, insomnia

      c. Be alert to concomitant use of opiates, barbiturates, other central nervous system depressants, digitalis, and insulin; persons with hypothyroidism are particularly sensitive to these agents; as they become euthyroid dosages may have to be increased

   4. Monitor control of clinical symptoms and periodically monitor serum FTI and TSH; persistently high TSH or low FTI may indicate under-replacement; a high T_4 and low TSH with symptoms of hyperthyroidism usually indicates over replacement

   5. Patient education

a. Nature and chronicity of the disease and the need for life long treatment

b. Rationale for treatment—dosage, side effects, and toxic effects of treatment

c. Teach signs of hyperthyroidism

d. Management of symptoms of hypothyroidism until abatement with replacement therapy

   (1) Fatigue

   (2) Dry skin

   (3) Constipation (increased fiber, fluids)

Thyroid Nodule

- Definition: Discrete enlargements within the thyroid gland
- Etiology unknown but nodules are common
  1. Palpable in 5 to 10% of U.S. population
  2. Majority are benign
  3. Risk of nodule malignancy less than 10% in most adults
     a. Men have a higher incidence than women
     b. Papillary and follicular carcinoma are most common types of malignancy
        (1) Papillary tends to spread within the thyroid gland or to cervical lymphatics
           (a) Twice as common in women as men
           (b) Accounts for 80% of thyroid malignancies in adults < 40
        (2) Follicular accounts for approximately 20% of all thyroid cancers
           (a) Incidence somewhat higher in older individuals
           (b) Usually slow growing but more aggressive than papillary; can spread rapidly to lymph nodes and to distant sites via the blood stream, often to lung, bone, brain, or liver
     c. Medullary and anaplastic carcinoma are rarer but tend to metastasize very early; anaplastic carcinoma, because of high invasiveness and early metastasis, results in death in weeks or months regardless of treatment modality
     d. Risk of carcinoma is increased with a history of radiation exposure, particularly during childhood, to the head or neck for acne, tonsils, adenoids; the risk is also increased in those with a family history of thyroid cancer—this is especially true for medullary carcinoma
- Signs and Symptoms
  1. Thyroid mass
  2. Expanding goiter or nodule which is hard and/or tender

   3. Hoarseness or dysphagia

- Differential Diagnosis: Distinguish from non-neoplastic enlargements, e.g., cystic nodules, multinodular goiters

- Physical Findings

   1. Single hard thyroid nodule (or multiple nodules) fixed to overlying tissue

   2. Regional lymphadenopathy

- Diagnostic Tests/Findings

   1. Free thyroxine index (FTI)—usually normal; if elevated chances of malignancy are decreased

   2. RAI scan—nonfunctioning (cold) nodule

   3. Ultrasonography—if cystic, rarely malignant

   4. Thyrocalcitonin—increased in medullary carcinoma

   5. Biopsy (open or needle)—positive cytology if malignant

- Management/Treatment

   1. Any individual with the signs and symptoms or physical findings previously described should be referred

   2. Treatment may include:

      a. Excision of the nodule (complete thyroidectomy in the case of medullary carcinoma) and regional lymph nodes

      b. Ablation of metastasis with large doses of radioactive iodine

      c. Suppression of thyroid function with L-thyroxine

      d. Chemotherapy for anaplastic carcinoma; (thyroid suppression and radioactive ablation of metastasis are not effective in medullary thyroid carcinoma)

   3. Client education related to diagnostic tests

   4. Follow-up for detection of metastasis, recurrence, and subsequent treatment is usually on an annual basis

Cushing's Syndrome

- Definition: A constellation of clinical abnormalities due to an excess of corticosteroids

- Etiology/Incidence

   1. Excessive or prolonged administration of glucocorticoids (most common)

   2. Excessive pituitary ACTH secretion (Cushing's disease)

   3. Secretion of ACTH by a non-pituitary tumor (ectopic tumor), e.g., carcinoma of the lung or other malignant growths

   4. Tumors within the adrenal cortex—adenomas or carcinoma

5. Cushing's disease and primary adrenal tumors more common in females

6. Ectopic corticotropin production more common in males

- Sign and Symptoms

   1. Central obesity with slender extremities

   2. Full face

   3. Muscular weakness

   4. Back pain

   5. Mental changes

   6. Thin fragile skin

   7. Poor wound healing

   8. Acne

   9. Menstrual disorders

- Differential Diagnosis

   1. Hypercortisolism due to alcoholism

   2. Hypercortisolism due to depression

- Physical Findings

   1. Moon face with facial plethora

   2. Hirsutism

   3. Skin—thin and atrophic

   4. Purplish-red striae on abdomen, breast or buttocks

   5. Truncal obesity with wasting of limbs

   6. Prominent supraclavicular and dorsal cervical fat pads ("buffalo hump")

   7. Hypertension

- Diagnostic Tests/Findings

   1. Plasma cortisol—evening cortisol levels and 24 hour total levels are elevated

   2. Urinary cortisol—elevated

   3. Dexamethasone test (most reliable for distinguishing among causes of Cushing's syndrome)

   4. MRI, CT and ultrasonographic imaging for identification of pituitary tumor, non-pituitary ACTH-producing neoplasms

   5. Blood glucose—increased

   6. Hypokalemia but not hypernatremia

- Management/Treatment

1. Treatment of choice for Cushing's disease—surgery

2. Adrenal tumors or hyperplasia—removal

3. If surgery is contraindicated radiation and drug therapy (used to control cortisol excess) may be used which includes ketoconazole 400 to 500 mg b.i.d.; metyrapone 2 g per day; aminoglutethimide 1 g per day

4. For Cushing's syndrome due to prolonged administration of steroids

    a. Discontinuation of therapy gradually

    b. Reduction of steroid dose

    c. Changing to an alternate-day schedule

Addison's Disease (Primary adrenocortical insufficiency)

- Definition: An insidious, usually progressive disease due to destruction of the adrenal cortex

    1. Primary—due to destruction of adrenal cortex

    2. Secondary—lack of corticotropin stimulation

- Etiology/Incidence

    1. Idiopathic autoimmune destruction of adrenal tissue (over 80%); two to three times more common in females; usually diagnosed between ages 30 to 50 years

    2. Tuberculosis—second most frequent cause (common cause in underdeveloped countries)

    3. Acquired immunodeficiency syndrome (AIDS)—becoming a more frequent cause

    4. Less common—hemorrhage, fungal infections, antineoplastic chemotherapy, abrupt withdrawal of exogenous steroids

    5. Primarily a rare disease

- Signs and Symptoms

    1. Chronic primary adrenocortical insufficiency—develops gradually

        a. Weakness and fatigue, orthostatic hypotension may be early symptoms

        b. Anorexia, weight loss

        c. Tan appearance to the skin

        d. Gastrointestinal symptoms

    2. Acute adrenocortical insufficiency—seen more often in patients without previous diagnosis or those with a diagnosis who are exposed to stress with related increased requirement for glucocorticoids; symptoms of chronic are exaggerated especially profound hypotension

    3. Most dangerous feature of Addison's disease is hypotension which may cause

shock, especially during stress AND is nonresponsive to usual treatment; requires glucocorticoid replacement

- Differential Diagnosis
    1. ADH syndrome
    2. Salt-losing nephritis
    3. Hemochromatosis
- Physical Findings
    1. Hyperpigmentation of skin
    2. Hypotension
    3. Black freckles over forehead, face, neck, and shoulders
    4. Areas of vitiligo
    5. Bluish-black discolorations of the areolae and of the mucous membranes of the lips, mouth, rectum, vagina
- Diagnostic Tests/Findings
    1. Sodium levels—low (< 130 mEq/L; normal 135 to 145 mEq/L)
    2. Potassium levels—high (> 5 mEq/L; normal 3.5 to 5 mEq/L)
    3. BUN—elevated
    4. Plasma renin level—increased
    5. ACTH plasma levels—increased
    6. Ratio of serum sodium to potassium (< 30:1)
    7. Low fasting blood glucose (< 50 mg/dL; normal 60 to 115 mg/dL)
    8. Hematocrit—elevated
    9. WBC—low
    10. Eosinophils—increased
- Management/Treatment
    1. In acute crisis referral with hospitalization
    2. Chronic
        a. Lifetime of treatment
        b. Cortisol 15 to 20 mg orally every a.m.; 5 to 10 mg 4 to 6 p.m.
        c. Fludrocortisone acetate 0.05 to 0.3 mg daily or every other day if insufficient sodium retention with cortisol alone
        d. Monitor weight, blood pressure, and electrolytes
    3. General considerations

    a. Education regarding increasing cortisol during times of stress

    b. Education regarding carrying an identification bracelet or card

    c. Salt additives for excess heat or humidity

    d. Prognosis is excellent with continued substitution therapy

Questions
Select the best answer

Mrs. O. is a 46-year-old female whose hypertension has been controlled with hydrochlorothiazide 50 mg every day for the past three years. She is 5'8'' and weighs 220 lb. Although no other abnormal physical findings were noted, blood work done as part of her routine annual physical examination reveals a fasting blood glucose of 300 mg/dL. Other abnormal laboratory tests included elevated serum cholesterol (250) and triglyceride level (170), a K+ of 3.4, and 4+ glycosuria.

1. You should then:

    a. Discontinue her hydrochlorothiazide
    b. Order a glucose tolerance test
    c. Repeat a fasting glucose
    d. Start insulin therapy

2. Mrs. O. is about how many pounds over her ideal body weight?

    a. 80
    b. 105
    c. 140
    d. 154

3. Persons with type 2 diabetes:

    a. Are apt to develop ketosis
    b. Account for less than 10% of persons with diabetes
    c. Tend to be obese and hypertensive
    d. Often present with severe polydipsia, polyuria and polyphagia

4. Mrs. O. has led a fairly sedentary life style and asks if enrolling in an exercise club would help get her sugar down. You would tell her that:

    a. Exercise is an important part of control of her blood sugar
    b. She should start a virgorous exercise program as soon as possible
    c. Exercise at this point won't affect her blood sugar
    d. Exercise will probably increase her appetite

5. Given her sedentary life style and need to lose weight, how many calories/ day should Mrs. O. be consuming? Wt. 220 lb. Hgt. 5'8''
    a. 1,000
    b. 1,300
    c. 1,400
    d. 1,800

6. Mrs. O.'s second fasting blood sugar is 296 and she has been diagnosed with type 2 diabetes. Mrs. O. does not want to take insulin. You tell her:
    a. Most type 2 diabetics never have to take insulin
    b. It is usual to try dietary modification and exercise first
    c. It would be a lot easier if she started insulin as soon possible

d. The value of using insulin to control type 2 diabetes is not clear

7. Dietary recommendations for persons with diabetes do not include:

   a. Strict carbohydrate restriction
   b. Limiting fats and cholesterol
   c. Limiting protein intake
   d. Eating meals at regular intervals

8. Indications for starting a person with diabetes on oral hypoglycemics include:

   a. Allergy to sulfa drugs
   b. Pregnancy in a type 2 diabetes controlled by diet
   c. Diagnosis of type 2 diabetes
   d. Failure to control hyperglycemia with diet in a client with diabetes type 2

9. A person with type 2 diabetes has had good control of his blood glucose with oral hypoglycemics. He is in for a routine three month check. He had a complete work up 6 months ago. Which of the following is LEAST likely to be done at this visit?

   a. Urinalysis.
   b. Blood glucose.
   c. Fundoscopic examination
   d. ECG

10. Mr. P. is on 30 units of NPH and 5 units of regular insulin each morning and 15 units of NPH each evening to control his type 1 diabetes. His blood glucose levels for the past three days have been:

Fasting	Before Lunch	Before Supper	At hs
200–250	95–110	110–120	95–130

He should be instructed to:
   a. Add 2 units of NPH to his p.m. dose
   b. Add 2 units NPH before breakfast
   c. Add 2 units of regular insulin to his pm dose
   d. Do nothing

11. Hemoglobin A_{1c} gives an indication of glucose control over the past:

    a. Week
    b. Four to six weeks
    c. Month
    d. 60 to 90 days

12. When treating diabetes the goal for hemoglobin A_{1c} (normal 4% to 6%) should be:

    a. < 6%
    b. < 7%

    c. < 8%
    d. < 10%

13. Which of the following is an adverse effect of sulfonylureas?

    a. Increased blood pressure
    b. Weight loss
    c. Gastrointestinal distress
    d. Hypoglycemia

14. In addition to controlling glucose levels metformin also:

    a. Causes weight loss
    b. Increases total cholesterol levels
    c. Increases triglyceride levels
    d. Is likely to cause hypoglycemia

15. Synthetic human insulin:

    a. Causes more antibody formation
    b. Contains more impurities than purified pork insulin
    c. Is least antigenic of all insulins
    d. Has a more rapid action onset than pork counterparts

16. Mr. J. is a 50-year-old person with type 2 diabetes who has been on insulin for the past six months. He reports that his fasting blood glucose levels have been running above two hundred but they have been great during the rest of the day. His evening dose of NPH insulin has been increased three times in the last two weeks with no improvement in the fasting values. Currently he is on 30 units NPH/4 units regular in the morning and 18 Units NPH/4 units regular before supper. This is his most recent glucose pattern

B	L	S	hs
250–280	130–144	120–132	100–120

If he has fairly good dietary compliance, you should instruct him to:

    a. Increase the evening NPH by 2 more units
    b. Check his blood glucose between 2 and 3 a.m. for the next 2 days
    c. Increase the morning dose of regular insulin by 2 units
    d. Increase the morning dose of NPH insulin by 2 units

17. High fasting glucose after a nocturnal hypoglycemia in a person with diabetes otherwise in good control with insulin would indicate:

    a. Dawn phenomenon
    b. Somogyi effect
    c. Insulin allergy
    d. Lipodystrophy

18. Which action would counteract this problem?

    a. Increase his morning dose of NPH
    b. Have him use human insulin instead of pork insulin
    c. Decrease his evening NPH insulin dose
    d. Increase his morning dose of regular insulin

19. Mrs. J. is a person with type 2 diabetes who has been on pork insulin for the past two years and she has begun to develop hard lumpy raised areas in her right thigh where she has been placing injections. The only action that will prevent further development of such areas would be to:

    a. Switch to human synthetic insulin
    b. Inject insulin directly into the lumpy areas
    c. Rotate the injection sites
    d. Switch to oral hypoglycemics

20. Ms. W. is a 34-year-old who is seeking care because of increased irritability, weight loss "despite a great appetite" and diarrhea (not watery but 2 to 3 stools a day). She feels exhausted but can't seem to sleep and states she "feels like I could jump out of my skin."

If excess thyroid hormone is the problem which of the following might be noted?
    a. Yellowing skin
    b. Fine tremor
    c. Delayed tendon reflex
    d. Sinus bradycardia

21. Graves' disease is caused by:

    a. Viral infection
    b. Use of lithium
    c. An autoimmune response
    d. Excessive ingestion of thyroid hormone

22. In Graves disease you would expect:

    a. TSH to be decreased
    b. T_3 to be decreased
    c. T_3 resin uptake to be decreased
    d. T_4 to be decreased

23. If Ms. W. is diagnosed with Graves' disease and placed on antithyroid medication you will include which of the following in your initial patient teaching?

    a. The need of life long use of antithyroid medications
    b. Initial signs of the effectiveness of treatment will be increased urination
    c. The possibility of developing myxedemic coma
    d. Signs of hypothyroidism

24. The most serious side effect of both PTU and methimazole is:

a. Skin rash
b. Diarrhea
c. Agranulocytosis
d. Hepatitis

25. The best guide to adequacy of the dosage of antithyroid medication in thyrotoxicosis is:

   a. Thyroid antibodies
   b. T_3 (RIA)
   c. TSH
   d. T_4

26. Sally G. is a 44-year-old who thinks she is beginning menopause because her menstrual periods have become irregular. Her major complaint is a lack of energy and weight gain. Physical examination reveals dry skin, thinning hair, a puffy facial appearance, and an enlarged, nontender thyroid. Her BP is 130/92 with a heart rate of 60. These findings are consistent with:

   a. Graves disease
   b. Hypothyroidism
   c. Plummer's disease
   d. Thyrotoxicosis

27. Which of the following findings would be consistent with a hypothyroid state?

   a. Hyperactive bowel sounds
   b. Lid lag
   c. Insomnia
   d. Parethesias

28. Ms. H. is diagnosed with hypothyroidism and placed on levothyroxine 0.1 mg per day. After a week she calls to tell you she hasn't seen any improvement and wants to discontinue her medication. Your best response would be to:

   a. Add propranolol to her regimen
   b. Change to desiccated thyroid
   c. Increase her dosage 0.125 mg/day
   d. Encourage her to take this dose for at least another week

29. Ms. L. is a 50-year-old female who has been diagnosed as having primary myxedema. An initial dose of 0.15 mg/day of levothyroxine has been prescribed. Patient education would include which of the following?

   a. Discussion of the chronicity of the disease and the life-long medication use
   b. That it will take six months to a year for her fatigue to disappear
   c. Avoidance of foods causing increased peristalsis
   d. Explanation that after two years of therapy this medication may not be needed

30. Your 57-year-old patient has been on prednisone for her rheumatoid arthritis. She has the

typical "moon face," excess weight in her torso area, and is complaining that she bruises easily when she bumps herself. As her primary care provider the best action would be to:

a. Discontinue her prednisone immediately
b. Add a NSAID to her treatment regimen
c. Convert to an alternate-day schedule
d. Discontinue prednisone immediately and start on naproxen 250 mg b.i.d.

31. Skin changes in Addison's disease include:

a. Circumoral pallor
b. Maculopapular eruptions associated with stress
c. Hyperpigmentation
d. Facial plethora and hirsutism

Answers:

1. c	11. d	21. c
2. a	12. b	22. a
3. c	13. d	23. d
4. a	14. a	24. c
5. b	15. c	25. c
6. b	16. b	26. b
7. a	17. b	27. d
8. d	18. c	28. d
9. d	19. c	29. a
10. a	20. b	30. c
		31. c

Bibliography

Bell, D. S., & Alele, J. (1997). Diabetic ketoacidosis: Why early detection and aggressive treatment are crucial. *Postgraduate Medicine, 101*(4), 193–198, 201– 204.

Bohannon, N. J. (1997). Benefits of lispro insulin. *Postgraduate Medicine, 101*(2), 73–80.

Fitzgerald, P. A. (2000). Endocrinology. In L. M. Tierney, S. J. McPhee, & M. A. Papadakin (Eds.), *Current medical diagnosis and treatment* (39th ed., pp. 1079–1151). Stamford, CT: Appleton & Lange.

Flick, M., & Schumann, L. (1997) Continuing education forum. Non-insulin-dependent diabetes mellitus. *Journal of the American Academy of Nurse Practitioners, 9*, 337–343.

Gardner, D. F. (2000). Thyroid disease: When to screen: How to avoid treatment pitfalls. *Consultant, 40*(14), 2397–2401.

Glauser, V. (1998). Diabetes treatment moves forward: New criteria for diagnosis, screening, and classification. *Patient Care Nurse Practitioner, 1*(1), 12–17.

Gurowski, C. (2000). Understanding new pharmacologic therapy for Type 2 Diabetes. *The Nurse Practitioner, 24*(6), 15–47.

Larson, J., Anderson, E. H., & Koslawy, M. (2000). Thyroid disease: A review for primary care. *The Nurse Practitioner, 12*(6), 226–232.

Minchoff, L. E., & Grandin, J. A. (1996). Syndrome X recognition and management of this metabolic disorder in primary care. *Nurse Practitioner, 21*(6), 74–75, 79–80, 83–86.

Mudlair, S. R. (1997). Strategies for preventing type II diabetes. *Postgraduate Medicine, 101*(1), 181–189.

Singer, P. A., Cooper, D. S., Levey, E. G., Ladenson, P. W., Braverman, L. E., Daniels, D., Greenspan, F. S., McDougall, I. R., & Nikolai, T. F. (1995). Treatment guidelines for patients with hyperthyroidism and hypothyroidism. *Journal of the American Medical Association, 273*(10), 808–12.

Skyler, J. S. (1997). Insulin therapy in type II diabetes. *Postgraduate Medicine. 101*(2), 85–90, 92–94, 96.

Stegbauer, C. C. (2000). Diagnosing and treating hypothyroidism. *The Nurse Practitioner, 25*(3), 92–105.

Thyroid Guidelines Task Force (1996). *AACE clinical practice guidelines for the evaluation and management of hyperthyroidism and hypothyroidism.* Washington DC: American Association of Clinical Endocrinologists.

White, J. R., & Campbell, R. K. (1997). Insulin analogues new agents for improving glycemic control. *Postgraduate Medicine, 101*(2), 58–60, 63–70.

Musculoskeletal Disorders Infancy Through Adolescence

Susan Heighway

Torticollis (Wry neck)

- Definition: Abnormal position of head and neck, due to contracture of one of sternoclei-domastoid muscles that may be congenital (most common) or acquired

- Etiology/Incidence
    1. Cause not well-defined, but may be due to:
        a. Compartment syndrome
        b. Soft tissue compression at delivery
        c. Occlusion of venous outflow of sternocleidomastoid muscle
        d. Uterine crowding
        e. Neurogenic myopathy from trauma or ischemia
    2. Neurogenic causes rare
    3. Higher incidence in children with breech presentation and forceps delivery, but occurs with normal births or C-sections
    4. Familial tendency (rare)
    5. 0.4% live births; males more frequently effected

- Signs and Symptoms
    1. Child's head tilted toward side of contracture
    2. Chin rotated away from contracted side (origin of muscle on mastoid process)

- Differential Diagnosis
    1. CNS tumors
    2. Syringomyelia
    3. Arnold-Chiari malformation
    4. Ocular dysfunctions
    5. Paroxysmal torticollis of infancy

- Physical Findings
    1. Contracture of one of sternocleidomastoid muscles
    2. Fusiform, firm mass or "tumor"
        a. In body of contracted muscle
        b. Palpable after 4 weeks of age, then recedes
    3. Plagiocephaly, or asymmetry of face/skull development present with progressive deformity

- Diagnostic Tests/Findings
    1. Cervical radiograph

    a. To rule out congenital spine abnormalities, e.g., hemivertabrae

    b. Normal with muscular torticollis

  2. Other imaging (MRI or CT scan) not indicated—abnormalities not detected unless neurogenic pathology (rare) exists

- Management/Treatment

  1. Conservative measures—initial treatment

    a. Stretching exercises—guided by physical therapist

    b. Encourage infant stretching by placing toys, mobiles, items of interest in infant's line of vision, on the affected side

  2. Surgery recommended when:

    a. Defect persists beyond 1 year of age

    b. Stretching exercises have been unsuccessful

    c. Infant between 1 and 4 years of age; best outcome for surgical release

Developmental Dysplasia of the Hip (DDH)

- Definition: Abnormal development or dislocation of the hip(s), which is congenital, but may not be recognized until ambulation occurs

- Etiology/Incidence

  1. Multifactorial etiology in an otherwise normal child

    a. Intrauterine mechanical factors

      (1) Breech presentation (30% of cases)

      (2) Infants with oligohydramnios

    b. Genetic effects in primary acetabular dysplasia

      (1) Various degrees of joint laxity

      (2) 20% have positive family history

    c. Increased incidence in first born Caucasian infants; tight uterine muscles limit movement

  2. Left hip involved more commonly than right

  3. Sixfold greater incidence in girls (girls more often in breech position)

  4. Incidence 1 to 1.5:1000 live births

- Signs and Symptoms

  1. Newborn

    a. Instability without significant fixed deformity

    b. Detected during newborn examination

2. Sometimes not detected at birth

   a. Untreated dislocation becomes fixed, with less instability, more limitation of movement

   b. Limp noticeable at onset of walking

   c. Afebrile, painless, may have ligamentous laxity

- Differential Diagnosis

1. Leg length discrepancy

2. Innocent hip "click"—not associated with movement of femoral head

3. Arthrogryposis

4. Cerebral palsy

- Physical Findings

1. Galeazzi's sign—knee height comparison with infant in supine position with flexed hips/knees

   a. Asymmetry evident in DDH

   b. Shortening of the femoral segment limits abduction and full extension

   c. Not helpful finding for detecting bilateral dislocation

2. Limited abduction of affected hip in older child

3. Indicators of hip instability in newborn—test each hip individually

   a. Barlow's sign

      (1) Positive when movement of femoral head can be felt as it slips out onto the posterior lip of acetabulum

      (2) Not diagnostic, but indicates need for surveillance

   b. Ortolani's sign (positive findings)

      (1) Newborn period—sometimes a "click" or "clunk" is heard as femoral head enters or exits acetabulum

      (2) After newborn period—"click" is less apparent and decreased abduction of flexed legs (at hip) is more significant

4. Three degrees of hip dysplasia

   a. Subluxation

      (1) First degree, least severe

      (2) Femoral head rests in acetabulum

      (3) Can be dislocated partially by examination

   b. Dislocatable

      (1) Second degree

    (2) Hip can be dislocated fully with manipulation, but is reducible

   c. Dislocated hips

    (1) Third degree, most severe

    (2) Fixed dislocation

- Diagnostic Tests/Findings

  1. Physical examination is most reliable

  2. Radiographs

   a. Not commonly used before 6 months of age

   b. After 6 months of age assess femoral head/acetabulum relationship

  3. Ultrasonography

   a. Occasional use by experienced clinician

   b. Assesses hip stability and acetabular development

- Management/Treatment

  1. Identification during newborn period essential for good prognosis

  2. Goal is to restore contact between femoral head and acetabulum

  3. Subluxation in newborn

   a. High incidence of spontaneous improvement in perinatal period

   b. Observe and re-examine 3 to 4 weeks after birth

  4. Dislocated hips

   a. Treat at time of diagnosis

   b. Before 6 months of age

    (1) If unstable, stabilize with an abduction-flexion device, (e.g., Pavlik harness); triple diapers not effective

    (2) If device is ineffective, surgery is indicated

   c. If diagnosis made after 6 months of age

    (1) Child usually too large and strong to tolerate brace

    (2) Surgical reduction indicated

Talipes Equinovarus Congenita (Clubfoot)

- Definition: Complex congenital anomaly of foot associated with adduction of forefoot, equinus positioning and heel inversion

- Etiology/Incidence

  1. Cause unknown; possibly related to primary defect or very early insult to leg muscles or tarsal bones

2. Abnormal position in utero

3. 50% cases are bilateral

4. 1:700 to 1:1000 live births; more common in males

5. Sometimes associated with neuromuscular problems, e.g., spina bifida or spinal muscular atrophy

- Signs and Symptoms

    1. Toeing-in

    2. No pain

    3. Foot resembles shape of club

- Differential Diagnosis

    1. Internal femoral torsion

    2. Internal tibial torsion

    3. Metatarsus adductus

    4. Neuromuscular disorders

- Physical Findings

    1. Small foot with limited dorsiflexion; usually obvious at birth

    2. Combination of deformities

        a. Results in 90 degree rotation of forefoot in all planes

        b. Leg and foot resemble shape of club

    3. Deep crease on medial border of foot

    4. Calf muscles thin and atrophic (more obvious in older child)

- Diagnostic Tests/Findings: Radiographs

    1. Rule out other conditions

    2. Done serially to evaluate progression of treatment

- Management/Treatment

    1. Refer to orthopedist

    2. Serial casting with manipulation begins at birth; usually 3 to 6 months

    3. If further corrections required, surgery indicated

Metatarsus Adductus/Metatarsus Varus

- Definition: Congenital deformity of forefoot

- Etiology/Incidence

    1. Uncertain etiology; often associated with abnormal intrauterine positioning

2. Most common congenital foot deformity

3. 10% of children with metatarsus also have developmental dysplasia of the hip

- Signs and symptoms

  1. Toeing-in; "pigeon-toed" gait in older child

  2. No pain

- Differential Diagnosis

  1. Internal femoral torsion

  2. Internal tibial torsion

  3. Equinovarus

- Physical Findings

  1. Adductus—forefoot adducted only; full ROM

  2. Varus—forefoot adducted and inverted; limited ROM

  3. Ankle joint has normal dorsiflexion and plantar flexion

- Diagnostic Tests/Findings

  1. Physical examination—usually sufficient to establish treatment plan

  2. Radiographs

     a. Usually unnecessary

     b. Used when:

        (1) Underlying congenital anomalies are suspected

        (2) Foot is unusually rigid

        (3) Failure of spontaneous improvement with growth

     c. Done serially to evaluate effects of stretching treatment

- Management/Treatment

  1. Supple deformity (adductus)

     a. Parents stretch forefoot in all planes of motion with each diaper change for 4 to 6 months

     b. Observe and follow-up

  2. Rigid deformity (varus)

     a. Serial casting or bracing done until age 2 years

     b. Then straight-laced/outflare shoes fitted for daytime until no chance of recurrence

     c. Surgical intervention required for child older than 4 years if significant residual metatarsus adductus persists

Tibial Torsion (Internal)

- Definition: Abnormal bowing (internal or external rotation) of the tibia
- Etiology/Incidence
    1. Combination of genetic factors and intrauterine position
    2. Usually not pathological
    3. Internal tibial torsion—12% at birth; usually resolves by 2 years
    4. External tibial torsion—develops after birth or by 2 years
- Signs and Symptoms
    1. Toeing-in appearance of child's legs when walking/running
    2. Rarely painful
    3. Tripping and falling may be noticed
- Differential Diagnosis
    1. Metatarsus adductus
    2. Femur anteversion
    3. Neuromuscular disorders
    4. Equinovarus
- Physical Findings
    1. No obvious deformity
    2. Full ROM
    3. Internal rotation of affected leg, flat feet, increased lumbar lordosis
- Diagnostic Tests/Findings
    1. Observation
    2. Angle measurement
        a. Between foot and thigh
        b. With ankle and knee position at 90 degree angle
        c. With child lying in prone position
- Management/Treatment
    1. Reassure parents that most children have spontaneous correction with growth and need no treatment
    2. Recommend supine sleeping position

Genu Varum (Bowleg)

- Definition: Lateral bowing of the tibia

- Etiology/Incidence
    1. Joint laxity may contribute to deformity
    2. Considered normal until 2 years
    3. May be related to intrauterine position
- Signs and Symptoms
    1. Parental concern common regarding appearance of legs
    2. Physiologic bowing of up to 20 degrees is normal in children until 18 to 24 months of age
    3. Bowing does not generally increase after walking
- Differential Diagnosis
    1. Rickets
    2. Blount disease (tibia vara)
    3. Injury to medial proximal epiphysis of tibia
    4. Osteogenesis imperfecta
    5. Achondroplasia, and other skeletal dysplasias
    6. Extreme physiologic bowing
- Physical Findings
    1. With child standing
        a. Clinically present—space between knees is greater than 5 cm or 2 inches with apposition of medial malleoli
        b. Resolution usually occurs without treatment
    2. Full range of motion
- Diagnostic Tests/Findings: Radiographs used for extreme and/or unilateral bowing
- Management/Treatment
    1. Observation to verify resolution
    2. Avoid unnecessary treatment of mild to moderate bowing
    3. Further evaluation with radiographs necessary if:
        a. Genu varum is present after 2 years of age
        b. Progressive after 1 year of age
        c. Unilateral involvement
        d. Appears to be severe
        e. Occurs in a high risk group, e.g., obese; African-American children with early ambulation

Genu Valgum (Knock-knee)

- Definition: Deformity in which the knees are abnormally close and space between the ankles is increased
- Etiology/Incidence
    1. A natural shifting occurs from varum to valgus between 30 to 60 months
    2. Normal alignment about 7 years of age
    3. Underlying bone disease can cause marked bilateral valgum
- Signs and Symptoms
    1. Parental concern common regarding appearance of legs
    2. Associated with pronation; more common in overweight children
- Differential Diagnosis
    1. Injury to lateral proximal tibial epiphysis causes unilateral valgum
    2. Rickets
    3. Hurler Syndrome
- Physical Findings
    1. Knees are together and distance between medial malleoli (ankles) is greater than 3 in. (7.5 cm) when standing
    2. Full range of motion
    3. No pain
    4. Child may walk and run awkwardly
    5. Normal knee alignment usually occurs before 8 years of age
- Diagnostic Tests/Findings: Radiographs used for extreme valgum; standing AP and lateral views
- Management
    1. Observation to verify resolution
    2. Further evaluation with radiographs necessary if:
        a. Genu valgum is present after 7 years of age
        b. Unilateral involvement

Transient (Toxic) Synovitis of the Hip

- Definition: Self-limiting inflammation of hip joint
- Etiology/Incidence
    1. Etiology uncertain; possible immune or viral process
    2. Most common cause of irritable hip

3. Males affected more often

4. Occurs most often in 2 to 6 year-olds, but also in 1 to 15 year-olds

- Signs and Symptoms

  1. Painful limp, or hip pain with acute or insidious onset, usually unilateral

  2. Afebrile or low-grade temperature

- Differential Diagnosis

  1. Septic arthritis

  2. Osteomyelitis

  3. Legg-Calve'-Perthes disease

  4. Juvenile monoarthritis

  5. Rheumatoid arthritis

  6. Slipped capital femoral epiphysis

- Physical Findings

  1. Range of motion of hip causes spasm and pain, particularly with internal rotation

  2. No obvious signs on inspection or with palpation

- Diagnostic Tests/Findings

  1. Radiography elicits no abnormal findings

  2. Normal or slightly elevated WBC

  3. Joint fluid aspiration—normal

- Management/Treatment

  1. Hospitalize child

     a. If high fever or severe symptoms are present

     b. To differentiate between transient synovitis and septic arthritis

  2. Analgesics (ibuprofen every 4 to 6 hours)

  3. Bedrest

  4. Benign, self-limiting illness

Legg-Calve'-Perthes Disease (LCPD)

- Definition: Aseptic or avascular necrosis of the femoral head

- Etiology/Incidence

  1. Unknown etiology; possibly due to vascular embarrassment

  2. Generally, slightly shorter stature/delayed bone age compared to peers

  3. Most common in Caucasian boys, ages 4 to 9 years

  4. 15% of cases are bilateral

- Signs and Symptoms

  1. Insidious onset of limp with knee pain

  2. Pain also in groin or lateral hip

  3. Pain less acute and severe than transient synovitis or septic arthritis

  4. Afebrile

- Differential Diagnosis

  1. Transient synovitis

  2. Septic arthritis

  3. Hematogenous osteomyelitis

  4. Various types of hemoglobinopathy

  5. Gaucher's disease

  6. Hypothyroidism

  7. Epiphyseal dysplasias

- Physical Findings

  1. Limited passive internal rotation and abduction of hip joint

  2. May be resisted by mild spasm or guarding

  3. Hip flexion contracture and leg muscle atrophy in long-standing cases

- Diagnostic Tests/Findings

  1. Radiograph studies

    a. Show disease progression and sphericity of femoral head

    b. Used initially for definitive diagnosis

    c. Subsequently used to assess reparative process

  2. Other laboratory studies not indicated

- Management/Treatment

  1. Goal—to restore range of motion while maintaining femoral head within acetabulum

  2. Observation only if full ROM preserved

    a. Children < than 6 years of age

    b. Involvement of < than one-half the femoral head

  3. Aggressive treatment

    a. Indicated when > one-half femoral head involved and in children older than 6 years

    b. Use of orthosis

        (1) Produce abduction with or without internal rotation

        (2) Document containment with radiographs

        (3) Worn until early reossification seen

        (4) Child allowed activity that is possible while in the brace

    c. Surgical treatment

        (1) Femoral osteotomy, shelf procedure

        (2) Used more commonly as alternative to orthosis

4. Patient/family education—inform family that LCPD lasts 1 to 3 years and is potentially serious if not treated properly

Growing Pains

- Definition: A controversial diagnosis of exclusion for (usually intermittent) lower extremity pain
- Etiology/Incidence
  1. Onset at 3 to 5 years of age, or more commonly, 8 to 12 years of age
  2. Related factors
     a. Rapid growth
     b. Puberty
     c. Fibrositis
     d. Weather
     e. Psychological factors
- Signs and Symptoms: Pain/ache localized to lower extremities; usually intermittent
- Differential Diagnosis
  1. Trauma
  2. Infection
  3. Hematologic causes—sickle cell, hemophilia
  4. Slipped capital femoral epiphysis
  5. Osgood Schlatter
  6. Osteochondritis dissecans
- Physical Findings (usually none)
  1. No history of traumatic insult
  2. No loss of ambulation or mobility

    3. No systemic changes

    4. No edema or erythema

    5. Full range of motion

- Diagnostic Tests/Findings

    1. All laboratory studies normal—CBC with differential, ESR

    2. Radiograph of affected area normal

- Management/Treatment

    1. Prescribe anti-inflammatory medication

    2. Massage and heating pad to area

    3. Rest during painful episodes, activity as tolerated

Osgood-Schlatter Disease

- Definition: Inflammation of tibial tubercle from repetitive stresses in athletes with immature skeletal development

- Etiology/Incidence

    1. Tiny stress fractures in apophysis likely etiology

    2. Associated with a rapid growth spurt

    3. Occurs 11 to 14 years of age when immature cartilage susceptible to repeated trauma

- Signs and Symptoms: Pain and tenderness localized to tibial tubercle

- Differential Diagnosis

    1. Osteomyelitis

    2. Osteosarcoma

    3. Patellar tendonitis

- Physical Findings

    1. Point tenderness over tibial tubercle

    2. Prominence/enlargement of tibial tubercle compared with unaffected side

    3. 50% have bilateral involvement

- Diagnostic Tests/Findings

    1. Diagnosis accurate by clinical examination

    2. CT and MRI scans rarely indicated

    3. Radiographs

        a. Used to rule out presence of more serious bone pathology

    b. Lateral view

       (1) May demonstrate ossicle between patellar tendon and tibial tubercle

       (2) For pain which persists after skeletal maturity

    c. Rarely useful at follow-up

- Management/Treatment

    1. Self-limiting condition

    2. Conservative and largely symptomatic treatment

    3. Pain resolves with full ossification of tibial tubercle and closure of apophysis

    4. Activity limitations

       a. Complete avoidance of sports activities not recommended

       b. Limit activity to control pain at tibial tubercle

       c. Stretching exercises before activity, icing helpful afterwards

       d. Use knee immobilizer

          (1) Pain relief—briefly to avoid muscle atrophy

          (2) In combination with thigh muscle strengthening

    5. Corticosteroid injections—not recommended; may aggravate apophysitis

    6. Surgery

       a. Indicated if tubercle pain persists after skeletal maturity

       b. Excision of ossicle may ameliorate symptoms

Scoliosis (Idiopathic)

- Definition: Lateral curvature of spine
- Etiology/Incidence

    1. Multifactorial etiology

    2. 70% cases idiopathic

    3. Most common occurrence during adolescent growth spurt

    4. Female to male ratio of 8:1

    5. Mild curves occur equally between the sexes

    6. Positive family history in about 70% of cases

- Signs and Symptoms (usually asymptomatic)

    1. Infancy to school age—parents may notice alteration in back contour

    2. Adolescence—more likely detected on routine screening

    3. Rarely painful

- Differential Diagnosis
    1. Hip disease
    2. Transient synovitis
    3. Legg-Calve' Perthes disease
    4. Slipped capital femoral epiphysis
- Physical Findings: Inspection in standing position
    1. Asymmetry of shoulder height
    2. Uneven hip level
    3. Waistline uneven
    4. Thoracic spinal curve
    5. Rib asymmetry
    6. Unequal arm length
    7. Asymmetry of scapulae
- Diagnostic Tests/Findings
    1. Adams' forward-bending test
        a. Child bends forward 90° or more, keeping knees straight, dropping head with arms hanging downward, elbows extended, palms together
        b. Observed from caudal aspect to detect abnormal prominence of thoracic ribs
    2. Radiographs evaluate degree of deformity
- Management/Treatment
    1. If pain occurs, further evaluation required
    2. Treatment mode depends on severity of curve and child's age
        a. Curves of 25 degrees
            (1) No further evaluation/treatment if child skeletally mature
            (2) Follow-up for possible progression if child is still growing
            (3) Bracing treatment 80% successful
        b. Curves of 40 to 50 degrees
            (1) Likely to increase even after growth complete
            (2) Surgery required for thoracic curve > 50 degrees or lumbar curve > 40 degrees
    3. Clinical pulmonary restriction may occur with thoracic curves > 75 degrees

Sports Injuries

- Definition: Musculoskeletal injuries occurring as a result of participation in athletic activities; most common include sprains/strains, fractures or overuse injuries

  1. Head and neck injuries

     a. Common in football and ice hockey

     b. Generally not severe

     c. Include brachial plexus injuries

     d. Concussions

  2. Back Injuries—low back pain caused by:

     a. Muscle strain

     b. Spondylolysis—overuse from repetitive hyperextension of back as in gymnastics

  3. Upper extremity injuries

     a. Anterior shoulder dislocation, shoulder separation

     b. Overuse injuries

        (1) Impingement syndrome—"pitcher's shoulder", "swimmer's shoulder" or "tennis shoulder"

        (2) Lateral epicondylitis—"tennis elbow"

  4. Lower extremity injuries

     a. Sprains

        (1) Medial collateral ligament sprain

        (2) Anterior cruciate sprain and tear

     b. Overuse injuries

        (1) Iliac apophysitis

        (2) Femoral stress fracture

        (3) Chondromalacia (chronic patellar pain "runner's knee")

- Etiology/Incidence

  1. Leading causes—trauma, improper training

  2. Contributing factors include fatigue and improper nutrition

  3. 20 million children participate in organized athletics

  4. One out of fourteen adolescents treated for athletic injury

  5. Highest frequency in adolescent boys; football and wrestling cause most injuries

- Signs and Symptoms

1. Fracture
    a. Edema
    b. Erythema
    c. Ecchymosis
    d. Pain
    e. Obvious angulation
    f. Point tenderness
2. Sprain
    a. Various degrees of pain
    b. Swelling
    c. Difficulty weight bearing
    d. Detectable joint laxity
    e. Decreased ROM
3. Overuse—various degree of pain with or without activity limitations
- Differential Diagnosis: Possible underlying disease process of metabolic, neoplastic or infectious origins
- Physical Findings
    1. Fracture
        a. Decreased ROM
        b. Pain
        c. Obvious deformity
        d. Swelling
        e. Evidence of injury seen on radiographs at site of injury
        f. Localized tenderness
    2. Sprains—use subjective grading
        a. Grade I
            (1) Few fibers torn within ligament; does not compromise ligament's strength
            (2) Minimal pain and swelling
            (3) Full ROM
            (4) No increase in joint laxity
        b. Grade II
            (1) Tears portion of the ligament

  (2) Clinically significant pain and swelling

  (3) Impairment of ROM

  (4) Detectable increase in joint laxity

 c. Grade III

  (1) Complete tear of ligament

  (2) Marked laxity evident when ligament is stressed

- Diagnostic Tests/Findings

 1. Physical examination and accurate history to evaluate injury

 2. Radiographs

  a. Injured area and contralateral area

  b. View open growth plate

  c. Rule out fracture or tumor

  d. Compare affected with nonaffected area

 3. MRI—utilized to evaluate torn ligaments or damage to cartilage

 4. Ultrasonography

- Management/Treatment

 1. Encourage sports physical examinations prior to participation in athletic events to identify conditions that may interfere/worsen with athletic participation

 2. Fractures—immobilization, ice, pain management, ROM exercise

 3. Sprain/strain

  a. Minimize hematoma and swelling with rest, ice, compression, elevation (RICE)

  b. ROM exercise

  c. Grade III sprains may require surgery

 4. Overuse Injuries

  a. Usually respond to conservative treatment, rest, ice and gradual return to athletic activities

  b. Nonsteroidal anti-inflammatory drugs prescribed to decrease inflammation and pain

 5. Refer to orthopedist

  a. If complex, open fracture

  b. If sprain/strain or overuse injuries not resolving with conservative treatment measures

6. Child can return to athletic activity based on functional evaluation of actions required during the activity

Slipped Capital Femoral Epiphysis

- Definition: Spontaneous dislocation of femoral head (capital epiphysis) both downward and backward relative to femoral neck and secondary to disruption of epiphyseal plate
- Etiology/Incidence
    1. Etiology unknown—thought to be precipitated by hormone changes related to puberty
    2. Generally occurs without severe, sudden force or trauma; sometimes related to trauma
    3. Usually occurs during growth spurt (ages 10 to 17), and before menarche in girls
    4. Rare condition, 1:100,000 to 8:100,000
    5. More common in males and African-Americans
    6. One-quarter to one-third have bilateral involvement, with one side following the other
    7. Incidence greater among obese adolescents with sedentary lifestyles
- Signs and Symptoms
    1. Varies with acuity of the process
    2. Most children have limp
    3. Varying degrees of aching or pain (in groin, often referred to thigh/ knee)
    4. Some have acute, severe pain and inability to walk or move hip
- Differential Diagnosis
    1. Knee complaint with no obvious cause
    2. Trauma
    3. Septic arthritis
    4. Transient (toxic) synovitis
    5. Juvenile arthritis
    6. Legg-Calve'-Perthes disease
- Physical Findings
    1. Unable to properly flex hip as femur abducts/rotates externally
    2. May observe limb shortening, resulting from proximal displacement of metaphysis
- Diagnostic Tests/Findings
    1. Accurate history combined with knowledge of etiological factors

2. Radiographs

    a. Confirms diagnosis

    b. Shows degree of slipping between femoral head and neck

3. Laboratory studies

    a. Depend on findings from physical examination and history

    b. Done to rule out associated causes of infection or inflammation

- Management/Treatment

  1. Immediate referral to orthopedist

  2. Treatment goal is to prevent further slippage

  3. No ambulation is allowed

  4. Surgery

    a. Pin fixation, open epiphysiodesis using bone graft

    b. Done to stabilize upper femur and cause growth plate to close

  5. Monitor other hip for same problem

Juvenile Rheumatoid Arthritis

- Definition: Chronic, idiopathic arthritis characterized by presence of chronic synovial inflammation with associated swelling, pain, heat and/or limited ROM

- Etiology/Incidence

  1. Cause unknown, possible etiological factors include infections, autoimmunity, genetic predisposition or stress and trauma

  2. Most common rheumatic disease of childhood

  3. Mean incidence 16:100,000; estimated 65,000 to 70,000 children in U.S. affected

  4. Mean age of onset 1 to 3 years; rarely before 6 months

  5. Females affected twice as often as males

- Signs and Symptoms

  1. Range of severity of disease

    a. May be mild in one joint with no symptoms

    b. May have severe disease in many joints with fever, rash lymphadenopathy, and organomegaly

  2. Signs of joint inflammation

    a. Swelling with heat

    b. Redness

    c. Pain

      d. Limited ROM

  3. May also exhibit

      a. Morning stiffness, limp, refusal to walk

      b. Irritability, fatigue

  4. Hallmark of systemic disease is high spiking fever with rash

- Differential Diagnosis

  1. Hip disease

  2. Transient synovitis

  3. Legg-Calve'-Perthes disease

  4. Slipped capital femoral epiphysis

  5. Leukemia

  6. Other rheumatic diseases, e.g., kawasaki, systemic lupus erythematosus (SLE)

- Physical Findings

  1. Diagnostic criteria

      a. Age of onset < 16 years

      b. Joint involvement

          (1) Arthritis (swelling/effusion) in one or more joints, or

          (2) Presence of 2 or more of these signs:

              (a) Range of motion limitation

              (b) Tenderness

              (c) Pain with movement

              (d) Increased heat

      c. Duration of disease 6 weeks or longer

      d. Further classified by onset type during first 6 months

      e. Exclusion of other forms of juvenile arthritis

  2. Polyarthritis (polyarticular disease)

      a. 40% to 50% of all cases

      b. 5 or more inflamed joints

      c. May be acute or gradual onset

      d. Symmetric pattern

      e. Commonly affects large joints, e.g., knees, wrists, elbows, ankles

      f. May not complain of pain

3. Oligoarthritis (pauciarticular disease)

    a. 40% to 50% of cases

    b. 4 or less joints affected

    c. Gradual onset

    d. Can be painless

    e. Often confined to lower extremity joints, knee or ankles

    f. Usually no systemic signs, except for chronic uveitis

        (1) Early onset (< than 5 years of age)

            (a) Asymmetric involvement

            (b) Large joints commonly affected

            (c) Hips and sacroiliac (SI) joint spared

            (d) Systemic symptoms usually not present

        (2) Late onset

            (a) Asymmetric involvement

            (b) Hips and SI joint involvement present

4. Systemic

    a. 10% to 20% of cases

    b. Occurs in late childhood > 8 years of age

    c. Systemic onset may precede arthritis appearance by weeks, months, or years

    d. High, daily intermittent spiking fevers is hallmark symptom

        (1) Temperature elevations occur once or twice/day

        (2) To 39° C (102° F) or higher with quick return to baseline temperature or lower

    e. Discrete rash present

        (1) Salmon-colored nonpruritic macular lesions

        (2) Commonly on trunk and proximal extremities

        (3) Most characteristic feature is transient nature

    f. Painful multiple joint involvement

    g. Associated findings

        (1) Hepatosplenomegaly

        (2) Lymphadenopathy

        (3) Visceral disease, e.g., pericarditis, hepatitis

        (4) Pulmonary involvement

(5) CNS

h. 50% of cases have chronic, destructive arthritis

5. Associated problems

a. Periarticular soft tissue edema

b. Intra-articular effusion

c. Hypertrophy of synovial membrane

6. Synovitis—painful inflammation of synovial membrane, with fluctuating swelling

a. May develop insidiously, existing months to years without joint destruction

b. May cause joint damage in relatively short time

- Diagnostic Tests/Findings

1. No specific laboratory studies, however abnormalities may be found

2. CBC—characteristics of chronic anemia of inflammation

a. Moderately severe anemia; hemoglobin between 7 and 10 g/dL

b. Leukocytosis

3. Synovial fluid WBC count—moderately elevated 10,000/mm^3 to 20,000/mm^3

4. Rheumatoid factor present in:

a. Approximately 15% to 20% of cases

b. Child with later onset, or older child

c. Child with prominent symmetric polyarthritis with:

(1) Involvement of small joints

(2) Subcutaneous rheumatoid nodules

(3) Articular erosions

(4) Poor functional outcome

5. Antinuclear antibodies (ANA)—seropositivity for antibodies

a. Present in about 40% of cases

b. Presence correlated significantly with development of chronic uveitis

c. Less commonly found in older boys or in systemic disease

d. Valuable diagnostic measure for JRA

(1) Usually not positive in other childhood illnesses

(2) Positive in SLE, scleroderma, transient acute viral disease

6. Radiographs

a. Early changes

        (1)   Soft tissue swelling

        (2)   Juxta-articular osteoporosis

        (3)   Periosteal new bone apposition

    b.   Development of ossification centers may be age accelerated

    c.   Stunting of bone growth secondary to premature epiphyseal closure

    d.   Cervical spine disease characteristic feature

  7. Joint disease may be better evaluated with MRI, CT, bone scans

- Management/Treatment

  1. Goal is to control clinical manifestations and prevent/minimize deformity

  2. Suppress inflammation and fever

    a.   Use NSAID (ibuprofen, naproxen) for most children

    b.   In severe, progressive disease resistant to therapy

        (1)   Methotrexate

            (a)   Most successful and safe drug

            (b)   10 to 15 mg/m^2/once a week

            (c)   No oncogenic potential or risk of sterility

        (2)   Hydroxychloroquine—useful adjunctive agent

            (a)   Retinopathy possible adverse reaction

            (b)   Low dose, e.g., 5 mg/kg/day

            (c)   Frequent ophthalmologic examinations required

        (3)   Gold salts—given IM or as oral compound

            (a)   Toxicities are hematologic, renal, hepatic

            (b)   Must be constantly monitored during treatment

        (4)   Glucocorticoid drugs

            (a)   Indicated for resistant or life-threatening disease

            (b)   Ophthalmic administration for chronic uveitis

            (c)   Toxicities, e.g., Cushings syndrome and growth retardation

  3. Maintenance of function and prevention of deformity

    a.   Prescriptions for physical and occupational therapies

    b.   Balanced program of rest and activity

    c.   Selective splinting

    d.   Encourage normal play

e. Avoid high levels of stress on inflamed weight-bearing joints

4. Counsel parents about course of chronic disease with exacerbations

5. Refer to pediatric rheumatologist

Systemic Lupus Erythematosus

- Definition: Multisystem disease characterized by widespread inflammatory involvement of connective tissues with immune-complex vasculitis

- Etiology/Incidence

  1. Unknown, but many factors implicated

     a. Excessive sun exposure

     b. Drug reaction

     c. Infection

     d. Hereditary

     e. Immunogenetic

  2. Can develop at any age

     a. Usually after 5 years of age

     b. More common during adolescent years

  3. Females affected 8 times more often after 5 years of age

  4. Relatively more boys affected at younger ages

- Signs and Symptoms:

  1. Fever

  2. Malaise

  3. Weight loss

  4. Facial rash

- Differential Diagnosis

  1. Juvenile rheumatoid arthritis (JRA)

  2. Other forms of acute glomerulonephritis

  3. Hemolytic anemia

  4. Leukemia

  5. Allergic or contact dermatitis

  6. Idiopathic seizure disorder

  7. Mononucleosis

  8. Acute rheumatic fever with carditis

9. Septicemia

- Physical Findings

    1. Onset is usually acute—three quarters of children usually diagnosed within 6 months of symptoms

    2. Diagnosis delayed for others by 4 to 5 years

    3. Early diagnostic suspicion based on:

        a. Episodic, multisystem constellation of clinical disease

        b. Associated with persistent antinuclear antibody (ANA) seropositivity

    4. Severity of manifestations variable

        a. Rapidly fatal illness

        b. Insidious chronic disability with multisystem exacerbation

    5. Each exacerbation of disease tends to mimic previous episodes

    6. Rash

        a. Characteristic of acute onset or exacerbation

        b. Malar erythematous

        c. Butterfly distribution across bridge of nose and over each cheek

    7. Arthritis

        a. Affects majority of children

        b. Involves small joints

        c. Transient and migratory

        d. Never erosive

        e. No permanent deformity in 95% of cases

    8. Pericarditis is most common manifestation of cardiac involvement

    9. Central and peripheral nervous system manifestations

        a. Recurrent headaches

        b. Seizures

        c. Chorea

        d. Frank psychosis

    10. Kidney involvement in all children

- Diagnostic Tests/Findings

    1. Leukopenia—otherwise unexplained, common at onset

    2. ANA—positive in most children

    3. Coombs test—often positive

4. Rheumatoid factor (RF) and other antitissue antibodies—often positive

- Management/Treatment

  1. Long-term supportive care

     a. Maintain adequate nutrition

     b. Maintain fluid and electrolyte balance

     c. Early recognition and treatment of infections

     d. Control of hypertension

  2. Anti-inflammatory drugs useful for minor manifestations, e.g., myalgia and arthralgia

  3. Counsel parents and child about chronic nature of disease with repeated exacerbations, remissions often prolonged over many years

Osteomyelitis

- Definition: Inflammation of bone caused by a pyogenic organism

- Etiology/Incidence

  1. Causative agents

     a. In all age groups, *Staphylococcus aureus*

     b. Consider also *Streptococcus pneumoniae* and *Haemophilus influenzae*

  2. Peak ages—infancy (less than 1 year) and preadolescence (9 to 11 years)

  3. More frequent in males

- Signs and Symptoms

  1. May appear well

  2. Systemic involvement ranging from malaise to shock

  3. Neonates usually afebrile, swollen or motionless limb early sign

  4. Earliest symptom in child may be refusal to bear weight

- Differential Diagnosis

  1. Neoplasm

  2. Contusion

  3. Non-displaced fracture

  4. Sickle cell crisis

- Physical Findings

  1. Early signs

     a. Fever

    b.   Local bone tenderness

  2. If subperiostal or soft tissue abscess develops, fluctuant mass present

- Diagnostic Tests/Findings

  1. WBC & ESR—elevated, but not diagnostic

  2. Radiographs—at earliest stage may show soft-tissue swelling

  3. Bone scan

    a.   May be initially normal

    b.   Repeated after 48 hours, may show cold/photopenic areas (indicating avascular sites)

  4. Aspiration—always indicated to identify pathogen

- Management/Treatment

  1. Refer to physician

  2. Delivery of antibiotic to all infected tissue

    a.   Broad spectrum antibiotic initially

    b.   Follow with antibiotic

      (1) Most effective against isolated organism

      (2) Least toxic antibiotic

      (3) Used for 4 to 6 weeks

  3. Surgery reserved for:

    a.   Child with systemic illness

    b.   Worsening symptoms under medical treatment

    c.   Abscess present

Duchenne Muscular Dystrophy (DMD)

- Definition: Progressive genetic disorder that affects muscles in lower extremities and eventually muscles of upper extremities, chest wall and heart

- Etiology/Incidence

  1. X-linked recessive genetic disorder which results in absence or severe deficiency of cytoskeletal protein known as dystrophin

  2. Most commonly inherited neuromuscular disease in children

  3. Affects 1:3,500 males; 1:1,750 females are carriers

  4. Average age of diagnosis is 3 to 5 years of age

- Signs and Symptoms

  1. At birth—rarely affected clinically

2. Becomes clinically evident by 3 to 5 years of age

    a. Abnormalities of gait and posture

    b. History of developmental "clumsiness"

    c. Large "muscular" looking calves

    d. Inability to keep up with peers when running

3. Progresses over next 2 decades—weakness more evident in proximal muscles

4. Wheelchair dependent by 10 to 12 years of age

    a. Muscles decrease in size

    b. Contractures progress with loss of joint mobility

    c. Kyphoscoliosis develops with respiratory function problems

5. Complications from:

    a. Cardiac involvement

    b. Nervous system involvement

    c. Musculoskeletal deformities

    d. Compromised respiratory function

6. Eventual death from cardiac or respiratory failure

- Differential Diagnosis

    1. Hypothyroidism

    2. Carnitine deficiency

    3. Spinal muscular atrophy

    4. Fascioscapulohumeral dystrophy

    5. Other types of muscular dystrophies of childhood

- Physical Findings

    1. Preschooler—3 to 5 years of age

        a. Increasing lumbar lordosis

        b. Pelvic waddling

        c. Gowers' maneuver

            (1) Child may "walk" hands up legs to attain a standing position when arising from floor

            (2) Indication of pelvic girdle weakness

            (3) Distinctive in DMD, but seen in other conditions as well

        d. Proximal muscle strength and ankle reflexes may be depressed

        e. Calf hypertrophy present

2. Cardiac involvement in all patients

3. Contractures develop before ambulation is compromised

   a. Iliotibial bands

   b. Hip flexors

   c. Heel cords

- Diagnostic Tests/Findings

  1. Obtain 3-generation family history

     a. May be positive history of muscle disorders, weakness, DMD

     b. Carrier females have symptoms of weakness or cramping of muscles

  2. Laboratory studies

     a. Creatine kinase (CK)—will be markedly elevated in affected males (15,000 to 35,000 IU/L)

     b. EMG—distinctively myopathic

     c. ECG—changes are distinctive

        (1) Tall right precordial R waves

        (2) Deep Q waves in left precordial and limb leads

     d. Muscle biopsy—histopathologic findings

        (1) Groups of necrotic degenerating fibers most prominent

        (2) Variation in fiber size evident

        (3) Dystrophic immunoreactivity confirms DMD

     e. Genetic testing

        (1) Utilizes WBC from blood specimen

        (2) DNA analysis of DMD gene confirms diagnosis

- Management/Treatment

  1. No cure available at present

  2. Goal of treatment is essentially symptomatic aimed at delay of progression and supportive care

  3. Maintenance of strength and mobility

     a. Exercise

     b. Use of ankle/foot orthoses, bracing, spinal support measures and wheelchair as needed

  4. Consultation with neuromuscular disease specialty team for diagnosis and for periodic evaluations

5. Refer family for genetic testing/counseling

6. Counsel family regarding course of disease

7. Refer parents

   a. To other families who have children with DMD

   b. To other community resources for support

Questions
Select the best answer:

1. Which of the following disorders is usually associated with adduction of the forefoot?

    a. Internal femoral torsion
    b. Talipes equinovarus congenita
    c. Genu valgum
    d. Internal tibial torsion

2. The most common rheumatoid disease of childhood is:

    a. Systemic lupus erythematosus
    b. Kawasaki disease
    c. JRA
    d. Legg-Calve'-Perthes disease

3. Radiographic findings of disease progression and sphericity of femoral head is helpful in the diagnosis and follow-up of:

    a. Transient synovitis of the hip
    b. Osgood-Schlatter disease
    c. Legg-Calve'-Perthes disease
    d. Slipped capital femoral epiphysis

4. A 4-year-old boy is brought in by his mother concerned about a sudden onset of a painful limp in his right leg 2 days ago. Today he has a low-grade fever. Which of the following diagnosis is most likely?

    a. Osgood-Schlatter
    b. JRA
    c. Osteomyelitis
    d. Transient synovitis of the hip

5. Which of the following would be the most appropriate initial management of a newborn diagnosed with developmental dysplasia of the hip?

    a. Observe and re-examine at 2 week well-child visit
    b. Triple diapering in nursery
    c. Pavlik harness
    d. Surgical reduction

6. A physical finding not usually associated with talipes equinovarus congenita is:

    a. Contracture of the illiotibial bands
    b. Deep crease on medial border of foot
    c. Atrophy of calf muscles
    d. Small foot with limited dorsiflexion

7. A characteristic feature of polyarticular JRA disease is:

   a. The involvement of 5 or more inflammed joints
   b. Confinement to lower extremity joints, knees and ankles
   c. Asymmetric involvement
   d. High, daily intermittent spiking fevers

8. ANA seropositivity for antibodies is:

   a. A valuable diagnostic marker for JRA
   b. Is not positive in any other childhood diseases
   c. More commonly found in older boys or in systemic disease
   d. Present in over 75% of cases

9. Dislocation in the hip of a child six months or older may typically present with:

   a. Asymmetry of skin folds
   b. Atrophied hip muscles
   c. Positive Galeazzi sign
   d. Negative Trendelenburg sign

10. For a newborn, the correct management of hip dislocation should include:

   a. Use of flexion-abduction device, such as Pavlic harness to stabilize hip
   b. Follow and observe closely for 3 to 4 weeks, then refer to orthopedist
   c. Surgical reduction
   d. Traction for 6 weeks

11. Duchenne muscular dystrophy is characterized by which of the following signs and symptoms?

   a. At birth affected infants are notably hypotonic, ''floppy'' babies
   b. Earliest symptom is often refusal to bear weight
   c. Abnormalities of gait and posture become evident during preschool years
   d. Unable to keep up with peers when running by school-age

12. Most children with Duchenne muscular dystrophy become wheel-chair dependent by what age?

   a. 7 to 9 years of age
   b. 10 to 12 years of age
   c. 14 to 16 years of age
   d. Highly variable depending on response to treatment

13. School-aged children and young adolescents actively involved in athletic activities may not be at increased risk for:

   a. Osgood-Schlatter disease
   b. Chondromalacia
   c. Spondylolysis
   d. Slipped capital femoral epiphyis

14. Management of scoliosis depends on the severity of curve as well as the age of the child. Which of the following would require surgical intervention?

a. Curves of 25 degrees in a child who is still growing
b. Thoracic and/or lumbar curve greater than 25 degrees even if growth is complete
c. Thoracic curve greater than 40 degrees or lumbar curve greater than 50 degrees
d. Thoracic curve greater than 50 degrees or lumbar curve greater than 40 degrees

15. In performing a diagnostic work-up and management plan for a child with osteomyelitis, which of the following is not accurate or recommended?

    a. Elevated ESR confirms diagnosis
    b. Aspiration is always indicated
    c. Antibiotic treatment for 4 to 6 weeks is recommended
    d. Surgery is recommended if abscess is present

16. A 6-year-old child presents with a limp and knee pain. The PNP finds limited passive internal rotation and abduction of the hip joint on physical examination. The most likely diagnosis is

    a. Slipped capital femoral epiphysis
    b. Osgood-Schlatter disease
    c. Transient synovitis of the hip
    d. Legg-Calve'-Perthes disease

17. Which of the following statements is true about acute osteomyelitis?

    a. Occurs more frequently in females than males
    b. Peak ages are infancy (less than 1 year) and preadolescence (9 to 11 years)
    c. Most common sites are radius and ulna
    d. A self-limiting disorder

18. Which of the following statements is not true of slippped capital femoral epiphysis?

    a. Thought to be precipitated by hormone changes during puberty
    b. Unilateral involvement is more common than bilateral
    c. More common among males and African-Americans
    d. Thought to be caused by repetitive stresses in young athletes prior to growth spurt

19. Genu varum is considered an abnormal condition when:

    a. Extreme knock-knees continues after 7 years of age
    b. Extreme bowing continues after 2 years of age
    c. Parents are concerned about their child's appearance
    d. Evident before 2 years of age

20. Tibial torsion is commonly associated with:

    a. Pain
    b. Restricted ROM
    c. Internal rotation of affected leg
    d. Occurrence in adolescents 13 to 16 years of age

21. Which of the following diagnoses is associated with contracture of one of the sternocleidomas-toid muscles?

    a. Lordosis
    b. Torticollis
    c. Scoliosis
    d. Kyphosis

22. Sports injuries are commonly associated with:

    a. Improper training
    b. Higher frequency in females
    c. Scoliosis
    d. Low socioeconomic status

23. Initial treatment of a sprain includes which of the following

    a. Rest, ice, compression, elevation
    b. Heat, ROM exercise, compression, elevation
    c. Rest, heat, compression, elevation
    d. Rest, ice, ibuprofen, compression

24. The most definitive feature(s) for a diagnosis of "growing pains" includes:

    a. Exclusion of other causes of lower extremity pain
    b. Pain, swelling, erythema
    c. Loss of ambulation
    d. Decreased ROM

25. Systemic-onset JRA is most commonly associated with:

    a. High, daily intermittent spiking fevers and rash
    b. Single joint involvement
    c. Positive RF factor
    d. Painless joint involvement

26. Signs and symptoms associated with Duchenne muscular dystrophy are

    a. History of "clumsiness", delayed motor development
    b. Visual-motor disturbance, calf hypertrophy
    c. Delayed motor development, positive Ortolani maneuver
    d. History of "clumsiness", visual-motor disturbance

27. Which of the following are suspected etiologic factors of systemic lupus erythematosis (SLE)?

    a. Excessive sun exposure, drug reaction, infection
    b. Drug reaction, immunogenetic factors, lack of sun
    c. Excessive sun exposure, arthritis, sickle cell crisis
    d. Infection, immunogenetic factors, arthritis

28. Complications of SLE commonly include which of the following?

    a. Pericarditis, arthritis, nephritis
    b. Encephalitis, nephritis, pericarditis
    c. Nephritis, arthritis, rheumatic fever
    d. Nephritis, hemolytic anemia, contact dermatitis

29. Which of the following children need an immediate orthopedic referral?

    a. A 6-year-old with mild bowing of the lower legs
    b. A 6-month-old with internal tibial torsion
    c. A three-week-old with fixed metatarsus adductus
    d. A newborn with a positive Pavlic sign

30. Antonio is a newborn and the NP notes on physical assessment that both his feet turn in. When attempting range of motion, she finds that both feet move relatively freely in all directions. Antonio has:

    a. Clubfoot
    b. Congenital hip dysplasia
    c. Metatarsus adductus
    d. Tibial torsion

31. Which of the following is an appropriate goal for a child being treated for osteomyelitis?

    a. Prohibiting activities
    b. Complete course of antibiotic therapy
    c. Encouraging a high-iron diet
    d. Restricting visitors

32. In a newborn, a diagnosis of hip dislocations is confirmed by:

    a. A longer left leg when both legs are extended
    b. Resistance of the left leg when both legs are flexed and abducted
    c. Flaccidity of the left leg following extension of both legs with return to flexion
    d. Tonic neck reflex in which the left leg is flexed

33. Which of the following statements is true for slipped capital femoral epiphysis?

    a. More common in females
    b. Generally occurs following severe sudden trauma
    c. Incidence more common in athletes
    d. The goal of treatment is to stabilize or improve the position of the femoral head

34. In Legg-Calve'-Perthes disease, which of the following signs and symptoms are seen?

    a. Insidious onset of limp with knee and groin pain
    b. Sudden onset of limp and pain in lateral hip
    c. Fever and insidious onset of limp
    d. Afebrile and sudden onset of limp

35. Which of the following is true for Idiopathic scoliosis which occurs primarily in adolescents?
    a. Mild curves occur equally between the sexes
    b. Generally there is no family history
    c. Back pain is usually associated with curves of 35 degrees or greater
    d. Bracing is indicated for thoracic curves of 10 to 25 degrees

Answers

1.	b	13.	d	25.	a
2.	c	14.	d	26.	a
3.	c	15.	a	27.	a
4.	d	16.	d	28.	a
5.	c	17.	b	29.	c
6.	a	18.	d	30.	c
7.	a	19.	b	31.	b
8.	a	20.	c	32.	b
9.	c	21.	b	33.	d
10.	a	22.	a	34.	a
11.	c	23.	a	35.	a
12.	b	24.	a		

Bibliography

Behrman, R. E., Kliegman, R. M., & Jenson, H. B. (Eds.). (2000). *Nelson's textbook of pediatrics* (16th ed.). Philadelphia: W. B. Saunders.

Berman, S. (1996). *Pediatric decision-making.* (3rd ed.). St. Louis: Mosby.

Cassidy, J. T., & Petty, R. E. (1995). *Textbook of pediatric rhematology* (3rd ed.). Philadelphia: W. B. Saunders.

McIlvain-Simpson, G. (1996). Juvenile rheumatoid arthritis. In P. L. Jackson & J. A. Vessey (Eds.), *Primary care of a child with a chronic condition.* (2nd ed., pp. 530–552). St. Louis: Mosby.

Hoekelman, R. A., Adam, H. M., Nelson, N. M., Weitzman, M. L. & Wilson, M. H. (Eds.). (2001). *Primary pediatric care* (3rd ed.). St. Louis: Mosby-Year Book.

McMillan, J. (1999). *Oski's pediatrics: Principles and practice.* Philadelphia: Lippincott, William & Wilkins.

Mihran, T. (1997). *Clinical pediatric orthopedics.* Stamford, CT: Appleton & Lange.

Morrissy, R., & Weinstein, S. (1996). *Lovell & Winter's pediatric orthopaedics* (4th Ed.). Philadelphia: Lippincott-Raven Publishers.

Oski, F., DeAngelis, C., McMillan, J., Feigin, R., Warshaw, J. (Eds.). (1994). *Principles and practice of pediatrics* (2nd ed.). Philadelphia: J. B. Lippincott Company.

Roberts, K. (1995). *Manual of clinical problems in pediatrics* (4th ed.). Boston: Little, Brown & Co.

Skinner, S. (1996). Orthopedic problems in children. In A. Rudolph, J. Hoffman, & C. Rudolph (Eds.). *Rudolph's pediatrics* (20th ed.). Stanford, Conn.: Appleton & Lange.

Verst, A. (1997). Musculoskeletal system. In J. A. Fox (Ed.). *Primary health care of children* (pp. 628–666). St. Louis: Mosby.

Musculoskeletal Disorders In Adults

Madeline Turkeltaub

Osteoarthritis (OA)

- Definition: Degenerative disorder of movable joints which causes deterioration of articular and new bone formation at joint surfaces

- Etiology/Incidence

    1. Primary osteoarthritis—occurs without obvious cause

        a. Frequency

            (1) Ten times more frequent in females than males

            (2) 85% of cases are in people between 55 to 64 years of age

        b. Familial tendency

        c. Obesity

        d. Postural abnormalities

        e. Joint enlargement

        f. Gait changes

    2. Secondary osteoarthritis—results from underlying abnormality

        a. Trauma—old fracture

        b. Joint disorders—gout, congenital dysplastic hip

        c. Avascular necrosis—post trauma, post sepsis, use of steroids

- Signs and Symptoms

    1. Pain—aggravated by activity and relieved with rest; may become persistent as disease progresses

    2. Joints affected become edematous but not hot or red

    3. Limitation of movement in affected joint

    4. Joints most frequently involved

        a. Weight bearing

        b. Distal interphalangeal joints (DIP), proximal interphalangeal joints (PIP)

        c. Neck, low back, hip, knee, metatarsophalangeal (MTP)

- Differential Diagnosis

    1. Rheumatoid arthritis

    2. Pseudogout

    3. Reiter's syndrome

    4. Arthritis of chronic ulcerative colitis

- Physical Findings

    1. Hands

a. Heberden's nodes—enlargement of DIP joints

b. Bouchard's nodes—enlargement of PIP joints

2. Joints

a. Localized tenderness

b. Crepitus on movement

c. Bony consistency to enlargement

3. Neurologic—pain due to pressure on nerves by affected joints

4. Hips—reduced internal rotation, pain may be referred to knee

- Diagnostic Tests/Findings

1. Radiograph—four cardinal radiologic features

a. Unequal loss of joint space

b. Osteophytes

c. Juxta-articular sclerosis

d. Subchondral bone

2. Synovial fluid aspirate is usually normal

- Management/Treatment

1. Preserving function and decreasing pain are goals of treatment

2. Treating biomechanical factors

a. Weight loss

b. Correct uneven leg length with heel wedge

c. Use canes on opposite side or crutches to decrease weight bearing on affected joint

d. Quadriceps setting for knee involvement

e. Cervical collar for cervical spine pain

f. Isometric exercises for abdominal muscles decreases lumbosacral spine pain

g. Orthotic shoe modification

3. Local measures

a. Ice to improve range of motion (ROM) and exercise performance

b. Moist heat to decrease muscle spasm and relieve morning stiffness

c. Temporary rest such as removable splint to decrease motion

4. Medications

a. Acetaminophen 500 mg to 1 g t.i.d. or q.i.d.

b. Non-steroidal anti-inflammatory drugs (NSAID) e.g., ibuprofen 400 to 800 mg t.i.d.; indomethacin 50 to 200 mg/day up to 1 g q.i.d.

5. Consider H$_2$ blocker when using NSAID

6. Instruction on side effects of NSAID including:

   a. Gastrointestinal intolerance

   b. Fluid retention

   c. Platelet abnormalities

   d. Hepatic and renal dysfunction

7. Surgery—refer to physician for procedures, such as fusion or joint replacement

8. Educate regarding body mechanics, muscle strengthening, range of motion exercises and weight reduction strategies

Rheumatoid Arthritis (RA)

- Definition: Chronic multisystem disease resulting in symmetrical joint inflammation

- Etiology/Incidence

  1. Cause unknown

  2. Affects approximately 1% of the adult population

  3. 30% of patients have mild disease with remissions and little deformity

  4. 10% have a single period of active disease with only occasional exacerbations

  5. About one-half of patients have progressive disease

  6. Affects three times as many women as men

  7. Onset most frequent in fourth and fifth decades; 80% develop disease between 35 and 50 years of age

  8. Other diseases of joints, such as gout and OA may predispose to RA

- Signs and Symptoms

  1. Morning stiffness lasting several hours

  2. Pain—joint pain and/or stiffness develops insidiously over several weeks to months in three or more joints symmetrically

  3. Fatigue, malaise, weakness, low-grade fever

  4. Proximal interphalangeal (PIP) and metacarpophalangeal (MCP) joints are the most commonly affected

  5. The first ROM loss is full extension

- Differential Diagnosis

  1. Ankylosing spondylitis

2. Rheumatic fever

3. Systemic lupus erythematosus

4. Arthritis of inflammatory intestinal disease

5. Psoriatic arthritis

6. Reiter's syndrome

- Physical Findings

    1. Soft tissue swelling

        a. Most frequently in MCP joints, wrists and PIP joints

        b. Usually symmetrical

    2. Tenderness and pain on passive motion

    3. Warmth at site of inflamed joint

    4. Limited range of motion at joint

    5. Permanent deformity in chronic disease

        a. Flexion contractures

        b. Subluxation

        c. Ulnar deviation of fingers at MCP joints or deformities of fingers (swan neck, boutonniere)

    6. Synovial cysts can be visualized and palpated; Baker's cysts (synovial cysts of popliteal space) are common

- Diagnostic Tests/Findings

    1. Erythrocyte sedimentation rate is elevated

    2. Rheumatoid factor can be isolated in 70 to 80% of patients

    3. Antinuclear antibodies are present in 20% of patients

    4. Radiograph findings

        a. Early changes are often limited to periarticular osteoporosis

        b. In time, bony margins of joints show erosion

        c. In late stage, joint space will be narrowed

    5. Joint fluid shows inflammatory changes

    6. CBC—mild to moderate anemia

- Management/Treatment

    1. The goals of treatment are

        a. To relieve pain

        b. To relieve inflammation

    c. To maintain optimal function

    d. To prevent deformity

    e. To educate the patient

2. Conservative management includes:

    a. Education

    b. Rest

    c. Physical therapy

    d. Nonsteroidal anti-inflammatory agents

    e. Cold and heat therapies

3. If patient is unresponsive, additional medications from the following categories may be added

    a. Disease-modifying antirheumatic drugs (DMARDS)—methotrexate preferred, supplemented with Folate 1 mg daily or 7 mg once weekly

    b. Antimalarials, e.g., hydroxychloroquine sulfate

    c. Gold salts—intramuscular or orally

    d. Corticosteroids (not more than 10 mg of prednisone or equivalent per day) on short term basis to relieve disabling symptoms

    e. Intra-articular corticosteroids if medications do not relieve symptoms

4. Education

    a. Explanation of autoimmune disease

    b. Stress management and relaxation techniques

    c. Abstinence from alcohol while taking methotrexate

    d. Methotrexate is contraindicated in pregnancy and in those with impaired renal function

5. Multidisciplinary management

    a. Physical therapy

    b. Occupational therapy

6. Management plan for daily living

Gout

- Definition: Gout is a metabolic disease associated with abnormal accumulation of urates in the body and characterized by recurring acute arthritis; classic gouty attack is podagra, involving the big toe
- Etiology/Incidence
  1. Due to deposition of crystals of monosodium urate (MSU)

2. Related to either excess production or decreased excretion of uric acid

3. Decreased uric acid excretion is present in 90% of patients

4. 90% of patients with primary gout are men over 30 years of age

5. The onset in women is usually at menopause plus 20 to 30 years

6. Rapid fluctuation of serum urate levels may be precipitated by alcohol and food excess; surgery, infection, diuretics or uricosuric drugs

- Signs and Symptoms

   1. Acute onset, frequently monarticular, affecting the first metatarsophalangeal joint, called Podagra

   2. Tophi due to accumulation of urate crystals may be found in ears, hands, feet

   3. Remissions and exacerbations

   4. Involved joint is swollen, tender, warm, red

   5. Temperature elevation to 39° C

   6. May become chronic with progressive loss and disability

- Differential Diagnosis

   1. Diagnosis may be confirmed based on dramatic response to NSAID or colchicine

   2. Acute stage may be confused with cellulitis

   3. Pseudogout presents with similar symptoms but normal serum uric acid

   4. Chronic gout may mimic rheumatoid arthritis

   5. Chronic lead intoxication may result in attacks of gout

   6. See rheumatoid arthritis

- Physical Findings

   1. Limited, painful range of motion in affected joint

   2. Elevated temperature during acute attack

   3. Palpation of tophi in areas indicated above

   4. Affected area hot to touch

- Diagnostic Tests/Findings

   1. Synovial fluid aspirate contains monosodium urate crystals

   2. In later stages of disease, radiograph may show punched-out areas in bone

   3. Erythrocyte sedimentation rate elevated

   4. White cell count elevated

   5. Uric acid elevated

   6. Hyperuricemia—serum urate > 7.5 mg/dL

- Management/Treatment
    1. Acute attack should be treated first, hyperuricemia later
    2. NSAID—indomethacin, 50 mg every 8 hours, continued until symptoms resolve
    3. Colchicine
        a. Most effective during first 24 to 48 hours
        b. Dose—0.5 to 0.6 mg orally, every hour, until pain relieved or GI symptoms occur or maximum dose of 6 mg
    4. Corticosteroids—used for patients who cannot tolerate NSAID
    5. Analgesics—codeine or meperidine may be indicated; ASA is *contraindicated*
    6. Bed rest—for 24 hours after acute attack subsides
    7. Diet to maintain daily output of 2000 cc of urine; avoid obesity and prevent dehydration; low purine diet has little effect on blood levels
    8. Support is needed during remissions for patient to maintain medical regimen, including:
        a. Diet instruction
        b. Prophylactic medication
            (1) Uricosuric drugs—probenecid, 0.5 g/day, with gradual increase to 1 to 2 g/day; avoid use with salicylates
            (2) Allopurinol—100 mg/day for one week initially, then 200 to 300 mg/daily; observe for rash associated with hypersensitivity
    9. Comfort may be obtained with cold or hot compresses and elevation of affected area during acute attack

Osteoporosis

- Definition: Demineralization of bone, resulting in decrease in bone mass with an otherwise normal structural matrix
- Etiology/Incidence
    1. Most common metabolic bone disease in the U.S.
    2. Clinically evident in middle years and beyond
    3. Type I—affects women more frequently than men, especially postmenopausal women
    4. Type II—in men and women older than 75
    5. Caucasians have highest incidence, then Asians, then African-Americans
    6. Most frequently associated with
        a. Lack of estrogen (postmenopausal or postoophorectomy)

   b. Lack of activity (immobilization)

   c. Malabsorption (postgastrectomy, lactase deficiency)

   d. Vitamin D deficiency

   e. Low calcium intake

7. Secondary causes—drug related, endocrine, gastrointestinal, neoplastic, renal, rheumatologic disorders

- Signs and Symptoms

   1. Loss of height

   2. Kyphosis

   3. Backache

   4. Spontaneous fracture or collapse of vertebrae

- Differential Diagnosis

   1. Adrenal cortical excess

   2. Hyperthyroidism

   3. Metabolic bone disease, such as hyperparathyroidism and osteomalacia

   4. Multiple myeloma

   5. Metastatic bone disease

- Physical Findings

   1. There may be no specific physical findings, unless a fracture is present

   2. Loss of height is most common

   3. Kyphosis ("dowager's hump") is evident with vertebral compression fractures

- Diagnostic Tests/Findings

   1. Serum calcium, phosphorus and alkaline phosphatase are within normal limits.

   2. Standard radiography is not a reliable indicator since more than 25 to 30% of bone loss must occur for detection with this method

   3. Lateral radiograph of spine might show:

      a. Anterior wedging of thoracic vertebral bodies

      b. Widening intervertebral bodies

      c. New or old fractures of vertebrae

   4. Dual-energy x-ray absorptiometry (DEXA)—more sensitive to bone loss

   5. Additional laboratory tests may be ordered for older patients, including:

      a. Albumin (to allow interpretation of serum calcium)

      b. Serum and urine protein electrophoresis (differentiate multiple myeloma)

c. BUN and creatinine (to rule out chronic renal disease)

- Management/Treatment: Treatment of established osteoporosis must take into consideration severity of disease, age and coexisting medical problems; prevention is key factor

  1. Prevention and treatment of osteoporosis includes:

     a. Balanced diet—protein not to exceed 20% of total calories; diet counseling to include dietary sources high in calcium and low in fat

     b. Exercise

        (1) Prevention

            (a) Weight-bearing, at least 30 minutes 3 to 4 times per week

            (b) Encourage life style changes related to importance of exercise

            (c) Strength training, e.g., lifting weights, swimming

        (2) Moderate walking for those with diagnosed osteoporosis, depending upon severity

        (3) Active or passive range of motion for bedridden patients

     c. Hormone replacement therapy (HRT) in postmenopausal women or postoophorectomy—decreases rate of bone resorption

        (1) Estrogen and progestin in women with intact uterus

        (2) Estrogen may be used alone in women without uterus

        (3) HRT should be initiated as soon as possible following menopause

        (4) Major role is prevention; effective in mild to moderate disease

     d. Bisphosphonates

        (1) Alendronate—inhibits osteoclast-mediated bone resorption, taken at least one half-hour prior to eating; used for both prevention and treatment

        (2) Risedronate—for prevention or treatment

        (3) Etidronate—not nearly as effective as alendronate

     e. Salmon calcitonin—decreases bone resorption

        (1) Used primarily for treatment

        (2) Alleviates bone pain

     f. Selective Estrogen Receptor Modules (SERMS)—raloxifene

        (1) Antiestrogens

        (2) Increase bone density

        (3) Decrease lipid levels

        (4) Negative effect on breast and uterus

    g.   Adequate calcium intake

       (1)   Ages 11 to 24—1200 to 1500 mg/day

       (2)   Ages 25 to 49—1000 mg/day

       (3)   Ages 50 to 64—1500 mg/day (no HRT)

       (4)   Ages 50 to 64—1000 mg/day (on (HRT)

       (5)   All men and women over 65 years 1500 mg/day

    h.   Calcium may be obtained through dietary sources or through calcium supplements; calcium carbonate—least expensive; calcium citrate—absorbed easily; calcium phosphate—decreased chance of constipation

    i.   400 to 600 IU vitamin D daily

2.   Elderly patients must be protected from falls—educate family regarding safe environment

3.   Alcohol and smoking should be avoided

4.   Judicious use of glucocorticoids

5.   Regular follow-up with mammogram and pelvic examination for women on HRT

6.   Educate teens and young women regarding adequate calcium intake and dangers of excess exercise

7.   Treatment for acute back pain includes:

    a.   Rest

    b.   Analgesia

    c.   External support

    d.   Heat

    e.   Stool softeners

Low Back Pain (LBP)

- Definition: Acute, chronic or recurrent pain occurring in the lumbosacral spine region and associated musculoskeletal areas

- Etiology/Incidence

1.   Most acute neck or back pain is caused by muscle strain and spasm of the paraspinal muscle groups

2.   Low back pain from trauma or mechanical causes is most common from 30 to 40 years of age

3.   80% of the population will experience low back pain sometime during their lifetime

4.   LBP is a self limited condition

    a.   40% remit in one week

        b.   60 to 80% in three weeks

        c.   90% in two months

- Signs and Symptoms

  1. Pain

  2. Numbness

  3. Weakness

  4. Bowel and bladder dysfunction

- Differential Diagnosis

  1. Congenital disorders, e.g., asymmetry

  2. Tumors involving nerve roots or meninges

  3. Trauma

     a. Lumbar strain

     b. Compression fracture

  4. Spondylosis and spondylolisthesis

  5. Metabolic disorders, e.g., osteoporosis

  6. Arthritis of the spine

  7. Degenerative diseases

  8. Herniated nucleus pulposus

  9. Infections

  10. Mechanical causes, e.g., weak abdominal muscles, pelvic tumors, prostate disease

  11. Psychogenic

- Physical Findings

  1. Postural deformity of the spine

  2. Gait and heel-and-toe walking will detect weakness of gastrocnemius and tibialis anterior muscles

  3. Straight leg raising—pain on early arc is associated with L_5-S_1 disc

  4. Flexing thigh on pelvis (femoral stretch test)—associated with L_3 problems

  5. Neurologic testing for motor weakness and sensory deficits

  6. Local tenderness or spasm on palpation

  7. Specific lesion-isolating findings

     a. L_{3-4} disc

        (1) Pain in lower back, hip, anterior leg to great toe

        (2) Numbness in anteromedial thigh and knee

(3) Weakness in quadriceps leading to atrophy

(4) Diminished patellar reflex

b. L$_{4-5}$ disc

(1) Pain over sacroiliac joint, hip, lateral thigh

(2) Numbness of lateral leg, web of great toe

(3) Weakness on dorsiflexion, difficulty walking on heels

(4) Reflexes usually unchanged

c. L$_5$-S$_1$ disc

(1) Pain over sacroiliac joint, hip, back of thigh and leg to heel

(2) Numbness in back of calf and lateral foot to small toe

(3) Difficulty walking on toes

(4) Atrophy of gastrocnemius

(5) Diminished or absent Achilles tendon reflex

8. Complete physical examination to rule out non-musculoskeletal etiology

- Diagnostic Tests/Findings

1. If conservative management is not effective in 4 to 6 weeks then begin with standard radiography—AP, lateral and oblique to determine lumbar alignment, vertebral body size, bone density

2. CT Scan—can detect lateral entrapment of spinal nerve roots

3. MRI—provides early detection of disc degeneration; can be used in pregnant women

- Management/Treatment: Key elements include:

1. Bedrest not indicated—limit select activities that increase pain

2. Analgesia

a. Salicylates or acetaminophen

b. Nonsteroidal anti-inflammatory drugs

c. Occasionally, opiates may be required

3. Muscle relaxants

a. Limit use to 1 to 2 weeks

b. Avoid in older patients

4. Patient education

a. Good body mechanics

b. Diet—weight loss if indicated

      c.   Appropriate exercise

      d.   Sleeping posture

  5. Traction

  6. Back and abdominal exercises for prevention and recurrences; contraindicated during acute episode; walking better than jogging

  7. Back massage

  8. Many times there is a psychosocial overlay—a psychosocial assessment should be conducted for:

      a.   Stress

      b.   Depression

      c.   Domestic violence

      d.   Inadequate coping ability

      e.   Marriage/family problems

  9. Early return to work with limited activity

  10. Stress management

Bursitis

- Definition: Inflammation of the synovial membrane lining of a bursal sac; more than 150 bursae throughout the body

- Etiology/Incidence

  1. Infection in a joint space

  2. Inflammation as part of a systemic process, such as rheumatoid arthritis or gout

  3. Occurs most commonly in middle and old age, following trauma or unaccustomed repetitive use of the part

  4. Most common locations

      a.   Subdeltoid

      b.   Olecranon

      c.   Ischial

      d.   Prepatellar

- Signs and Symptoms

  1. Abrupt onset of pain which increases on motion (superficial)

  2. Local tenderness, erythema, edema

  3. Regional tenderness and limited motion (deep bursitis)

- Differential Diagnosis

    1. Rheumatoid arthritis

    2. Gout or pseudogout

    3. Septic arthritis

- Physical Findings

    1. Restriction of movement

    2. Tenderness over rotator cuff

    3. Swelling and redness (prepatellar/olecranon)

- Diagnostic Tests/Findings: Aspirate fluid with 18 gauge needle and request laboratory analysis

    1. Culture

    2. WBC count—elevation is associated with bacterial infection

    3. RBC count—associated with trauma

    4. Glucose—decreased with bacterial infection

    5. Crystals—associated with microcrystalline bursitis

    6. Mucin clot—poor clot associated with bacterial infection

- Management/Treatment

    1. If bursitis is traumatic

        a. Splint part

        b. Apply heat 30 minutes t.i.d. or q.i.d.

        c. ASA or NSAID—Naproxen 250 mg b.i.d. or t.i.d.

    2. If symptoms recur and fluid reaccumulates inject long acting corticosteroids into bursa

    3. If septic bursitis

        a. Incision and drainage

        b. Parenteral antibiotics

    4. Education regarding care of injured part

        a. Ice for first 24 hours

        b. After swelling is stabilized, warm, moist heat several times daily

Epicondylitis (Tennis Elbow)

- Definition: Inflammation in the region of the lateral epicondyle of the humerus at the origin of the common extensor muscles

- Etiology/Incidence
    1. Specific pathogenesis of tennis elbow is not known
    2. Occurs most frequently in the dominant extremity during mid-life (may be athletic or work related)
- Signs and Symptoms
    1. Pain exacerbated by constant motion of the forearm and twisting motions, aggravated by hand and wrist movements
    2. Gradual onset of dull pain along lateral aspect of elbow
    3. Point tenderness over the epicondyle
    4. Limited motion
- Differential Diagnosis
    1. Rheumatoid arthritis
    2. Localized intra-articular pathology
    3. Radial tunnel syndrome
- Physical Findings
    1. Burning or aching pain with grasping or lifting
    2. Point tenderness present at or just distal to lateral epicondyle
- Diagnostic Tests/Findings: Radiographs usually normal or show small calcium deposits
- Management/Treatment
    1. Pain relief
        a. Mild analgesics
        b. Rest
        c. Ice to tendon
    2. Counterforce brace; wrist splint
    3. Peri-tendon cortisone injection
    4. For continued pain
        a. Immobilize for 6 to 8 weeks in a long arm cast with 90° elbow flexion
        b. Physical therapy to restore strength and motion when cast is removed
    5. Reinforce an exercise program to condition muscle groups in the forearm and wrist
    6. If associated with a sport, evaluate whether improper technique was responsible for injury
    7. If nonoperative management fails surgical intervention recommended

Carpal Tunnel Syndrome

- Definition: Median nerve compression of wrist beneath transverse carpal ligament
- Etiology/Incidence
    1. Related to repeated forceful wrist flexion
    2. More common in women
    3. Frequently involves dominant hand
    4. May be associated with
        a. Pregnancy
        b. Endoneural edema in diabetes mellitus
        c. Thyroid disease
        d. Occupational activities
- Signs and Symptoms
    1. Burning, tingling, numbness sensation along distribution of median nerve
    2. Pain exacerbated with dorsiflexion of wrist
    3. Night pain that interferes with sleep
    4. Clumsiness in performing fine hand movements
    5. May be unilateral or bilateral
- Differential Diagnosis
    1. Compression syndromes of median nerve
    2. Mononeuritis multiplex
- Physical Findings
    1. Decreased two point discrimination on affected side
    2. Positive Tinel's sign—sensation of electric shock on percussion of volar aspect of wrist
    3. Positive Phalen's sign—pain and/or paresthesia when hands are held in forced flexion for 30 to 60 seconds
    4. Decreased sensation and muscle atrophy of thenar eminence
- Diagnostic Tests/Findings
    1. Electromyography—assists in documenting motor involvement
    2. Segmental sensory and motor conduction testing
    3. Abnormal monofilament test—used to determine sensation

- Management/Treatment
    1. Elevate extremity
    2. Splint hand and forearm
    3. Injection of corticosteroids into carpal tunnel, if bursitis is involved
    4. Refer to M.D. for surgical intervention
    5. Notification of health care provider if symptoms increase
        a. Numbness and tingling persists
        b. Sensation in fingers decreases
    6. Take NSAID with food and report any gastric distress
    7. Consideration of occupational changes if appropriate

Knee Pain

- Definition: Knee pain is due to mechanical, inflammatory and/or degenerative problems
- Etiology/Incidence
    1. Trauma
    2. Most frequently exercise related condition
    3. Tears of medial meniscus 10 times more common than lateral meniscus
- Signs and Symptoms
    1. Locking—most frequently indicative of meniscal tear or loose bodies
    2. "Giving way" or "buckling"—related to patella dislocation or ligamentous instability or anterior cruciate tear
    3. Effusions around knee—associated with hemarthrosis and anterior cruciate ligament; fluid under patella noted on ballottement
    4. Crepitus
- Differential Diagnosis
    1. Single painful knee with minimal edema
        a. Dislocated patella
        b. Degenerative joint disease (DJD)
        c. Prepatellar bursitis
    2. Single edematous knee
        a. Baker's cyst
        b. Torn ligaments
        c. Loose bodies

d. Meniscal tears

- Physical Findings—the physical examination is confirmatory, following a careful history

  1. McMurray's test—a palpable or audible click when knee is raised slowly with foot externally rotated; examiner's hand rests on joint line; positive = medial meniscal injuries

  2. Anterior drawer test—positive = anterior cruciate ligament (ACL) tear
     Posterior drawer test—positive = posterior cruciate ligament (PCL) tear

  3. Lachman test—(anterior drawer test for ACL tear) most sensitive and easy to perform test on a swollen, painful knee; place knee in 20° to 30° flexion, grasp leg with one hand with anterior force to proximal tibia (to stress ACL) while opposite hand stabilizes thigh; graded 1+ to 3+ grade of displacement

  4. Pain on resisted knee extension

  5. Appley's grind test—flex knee to 90° with patient prone; put pressure on heel with one hand while rotating the lower leg internally and externally; pain or click = positive = medial or lateral collateral ligament damage

- Diagnostic Tests/Findings

  1. Radiographs of knees—AP and lateral

  2. Laboratory examination indicated if arthritis suspected

- Management/Treatment

  1. Rest, cold pack, immobilization

  2. NSAID

  3. ROM of knee, if possible, to prevent stiffness

  4. Quadriceps setting

  5. Aspirate effusion

  6. Review range of motion and muscle strengthening exercises

  7. ACL/PCL tears not responsive to conservative management should be referred to orthopedic surgeon

Ankle Sprain

- Definition: Stretched, partially torn or completely ruptured ligaments

- Etiology/Incidence

  1. Lateral ankle sprains most frequent sports-related injury

  2. Between 5 to 10 million ankle sprains occur annually

  3. Most commonly involved structures include the anterior talofibular and fibulocalcaneal ligaments

4. 10% of ankle sprains are injuries to the medial ligament, as a result of pronation and eversion of the ankle

- Signs and Symptoms

    1. Sprains are classified on a grading system of 1 through 3; signs and symptoms are associated with each grade as follows:

        a. Grade 1—related to a stretched ligament; mild or minimal sprain

            (1) Mild localized tenderness

            (2) Normal range of motion

            (3) No functional disability

        b. Grade 2—characterized by incomplete or partial rupture of ligament fibers

            (1) Moderate to severe pain with weight bearing; difficulty walking

            (2) Abnormal range of motion

            (3) Swelling and local ecchymosis

            (4) Pain immediately after injury

        c. Grade 3—complete disruption of ligament

            (1) Ambulation is impossible

            (2) Resists any motion of the foot

            (3) Marked pain, edema, hemorrhage

            (4) Egg-shaped swelling within 2 hours of injury

- Differential Diagnosis

    1. Avulsion fractures of the malleoli or tarsal bones

    2. Epiphyseal fractures in young patients

    3. Fracture of the calcaneus

    4. Fracture of the fifth metatarsal base

    5. Injury to the bifurcate ligament

- Physical Findings: Drawer sign determines anterior talofibulor rupture— tibia is stabilized with one hand with foot in neutral and plantar flexed position, force applied to heel with other hand, if positive anterior displacement of talus occurs

- Diagnostic Tests/Findings

    1. Radiograph to detect fractures

    2. Arthrography—determines site and extent of ligamentous injury

    3. MRI

- Management/Treatment: Treatment depends upon the degree of injury
    1. General treatment
        a. Rest
        b. Ice—15 to 20 minutes every 1 to 2 hours for 72 hours, then begin contrast baths
        c. Compression
        d. Elevation
        e. Non-weight bearing
        f. NSAID for 10 to 14 days
        g. Begin ROM when asymptomatic
        h. Reevaluate grades 1 and 2 sprains in 7 to 10 days
        i. Refer grade 3 sprains for casting
    2. Rehabilitation may begin on the first day after injury and is individualized
        a. ROM
        b. Achilles tendon stretching
        c. Isometrics
        d. Manual resistance exercises
        e. Build up ankle strength after healing to prevent subsequent injury

Muscle Strain

- Definition: Overuse of muscle tendons, resulting in inflammation, often associated with repetitive motion; does not include disruption of tissue
- Etiology/Incidence: Strains occur during mild stress by overusing muscle groups not usually used
- Signs and Symptoms: Pain after overuse or injury
- Differential Diagnosis
    1. Sprain
    2. Fracture
- Physical Findings
    1. Pain on range of motion
    2. Edema
    3. Ecchymosis
    4. Pain of muscle strain resolves after 1 to 2 days.

- Diagnostic Tests/Findings: Usually none indicated unless symptoms persist or to rule out suspected fracture
- Management/Treatment
    1. Rest of affected part with assistive devices, if needed
    2. Ice t.i.d. for 20 minutes
    3. Compression
    4. Elevation
    5. Analgesics
    6. NSAID
    7. Education efforts focus on prevention
    8. Increase awareness of repetitive motion
    9. Identify possible changes which will decrease stress on the extremity
    10. Emphasize warm up and stretching before any activity—occupational or sports related

Questions
Select the best answer

1. Mr. Johnson, age 55, has developed a slight limp and pain in his right leg which is worse with weight bearing. These complaints are most frequently associated with:

   a. Rheumatoid arthritis
   b. Osteoarthritis
   c. Gout
   d. Osteoporosis

2. On history, Mr. Johnson indicated that he had suffered a fracture of his right leg in a car accident 10 years ago. Based on this history, it is likely that his present symptoms are:

   a. Unrelated
   b. Related to infection
   c. Secondary to the trauma
   d. Associated with obesity

3. On physical examination, enlargement of an 83-year-old patient's distal interphalangeal joints is noted. Enlargement of these joints is known as:

   a. Heberden's nodes
   b. Bouchard's nodes
   c. Tinel's sign
   d. Tenosynovitis

4. Most frequently, synovial fluid aspirate to diagnose osteoarthritis:

   a. Is high in protein
   b. Has a poor mucin clot
   c. Is normal
   d. Has WBC

5. Osteoarthritis is often associated with:

   a. Systemic symptoms of disease
   b. Restricted joint motion
   c. Elevated temperature
   d. Inflammation of the proximal interphalangeal joints

6. Which of the following is not a radiological feature of osteoarthritis?

   a. Unequal loss of joint space
   b. Subchondral bone
   c. Osteophytes
   d. Osteoporosis

7. Applications of ice to arthritic joints is more frequently done to:

    a. Decrease muscle spasm
    b. Improve range of motion
    c. Numb the affected extremity
    d. Reposition the joint

8. Rheumatoid arthritis is often associated with:

    a. Systemic symptoms
    b. Weight bearing joints
    c. Obesity
    d. High purine diet

9. Nonsteroidal anti-inflammatory medications are frequently used in the treatment of musculo-skeletal conditions. It is important to remind a patient to:

    a. Take antacids one hour after taking NSAID
    b. Exercise at least one-half hour after taking medication
    c. Take the medication at least one time per day
    d. Take NSAID with food

10. The onset of rheumatoid arthritis is most frequent:

    a. During 20s and 30s
    b. During 60s and 70s
    c. During 30s and 40s
    d. During 40s and 50s

11. Mrs. Franklin has been complaining of fatigue and painful, hot, swollen PIP joints. Mrs. Franklin's symptoms occurred six months ago, and recurred one week ago. It would not be unusual for a CBC to show:

    a. Positive antinuclear antibodies
    b. Mild to moderate anemia
    c. Elevated hematocrit
    d. Elevated WBC

12. The joints most commonly affected by rheumatoid arthritis are the:

    a. Proximal interphalangeal and metacarpophalangeal joints
    b. Distal interphalangeal joints
    c. Spinous processes
    d. Elbow and shoulder

13. When diagnosing rheumatoid arthritis, which of the following would not be considered as a potential differential diagnoses?

    a. Reiter's syndrome
    b. Multiple sclerosis
    c. Rheumatic fever
    d. Ankylosing spondylitis

14. Which of the following would not be considered a goal of treatment for rheumatoid arthritis?

    a. Pain relief
    b. Independence
    c. Prevention of deformity
    d. Reversal of deformity

15. Methotrexate is included in which category of medication used to treat rheumatoid arthritis?

    a. Antimalarials
    b. Corticosteroids
    c. Non-steroidal antiinflammatory agents
    d. Disease-modifying antirheumatic drugs

16. Podagra is an example of:

    a. Pseudogout
    b. Gout
    c. Osteosarcoma
    d. Septic arthritis

17. Tophi associated with gout are often found in:

    a. Ear lobes
    b. Kidneys
    c. Fingernails
    d. Ankle and knee joints

18. Mr. Adams, age 55, has a history of chronic exposure to lead. He presents with pain and swelling of his left foot. These facts are both associated with:

    a. Rheumatoid arthritis
    b. Gout
    c. Fracture
    d. Osteoarthritis

19. The most common metabolic bone disease in the U.S. is:

    a. Rickets
    b. Scurvy
    c. Osteomyelitis
    d. Osteoporosis

20. When providing dietary counseling for a patient at risk for osteoporosis, it would be best to recommend:

    a. Baked potato and one ounce of sour cream
    b. A dish of ice cream with whipped cream
    c. A glass of skim milk and an apple
    d. Spinach salad with oil and vinegar

21. When a patient with gout experiences mild pain, the medication indicated is:

    a. ASA
    b. NSAID
    c. Allopurinol
    d. Probenecid

22. Mr. Jones, age 27, is complaining of acute onset lower back pain after helping to move a refrigerator. His pain is on the right and shoots down the back of his thigh. The intervertebral space most likely affected is:

    a. L_4-L_5
    b. L_5-S_1
    c. L_3-L_4
    d. T_{10}-L_1

23. Mr. Jone's pain persists for one week. He has been treated with activity limitation and NSAID with minimal relief. The first diagnostic test to be ordered is:

    a. Anteroposterior and lateral radiograph of the spine
    b. MRI
    c. CT scan
    d. Spinal tap

24. A scan for a patient with back pain would be indicated if:

    a. Spinal nerve entrapment is suspected
    b. The history and physical exam do not suggest a cause
    c. The pain radiates to one or both legs
    d. The patient is pregnant

25. Aspirate from a joint space affected by bursitis may be indicative of a bacterial infection, when:

    a. WBC are decreased
    b. Glucose is decreased
    c. RBC are increased
    d. Glucose is increased

26. Tennis elbow is a type of:

    a. Tenosynovitis
    b. Rheumatic disease
    c. Epicondylitis
    d. Osteoarthritis

27. Mrs. Thomas was seen, complaining of pain and point tenderness in the area of her elbow which has increased since one week ago, following a day of gardening. A physical finding which differentiates the diagnosis of ''tennis elbow'' is:

a. Burning or aching pain with extension
b. Burning or aching pain with lifting
c. Inability to pronate arm
d. Inability to push down against resistance

28. Positive Tinel's and Phalen's signs are associated with:

   a. Carpal tunnel syndrome
   b. Torn medial meniscus
   c. Baker's cyst
   d. Epicondylitis

29. "Loose bodies" in the knee would result in the following symptom

   a. Inflammation
   b. "Click" on extension
   c. "Locking"
   d. Instability

30. Mrs. Abbott, age 32, "turned" her ankle when stepping off a curb. She immediately experienced pain on weight bearing and had limited range of motion on examination. The most likely diagnosis is:

   a. Muscle strain
   b. Grade 2 ankle sprain
   c. Fractured calcaneus
   d. Grade 3 ankle sprain

Answers

1. b	11. b	21. b
2. c	12. a	22. b
3. a	13. b	23. a
4. c	14. d	24. a
5. b	15. d	25. b
6. d	16. b	26. c
7. b	17. a	27. b
8. a	18. b	28. a
9. d	19. d	29. c
10. d	20. c	30. b

Bibliography

Dharmarajan, T. S., & Ugalino, J. T. (2000). Prevention and treatment of osteoporosis. *Family Practice Recertification,* Special Geriatrics Issue, 17–26.

Downs, D. (1997). Non-specific work-related upper extremity disorders. *American Family Physician, 55*(4), 1296-1302.

Fan, P. (1997). An approach to rheumatoid arthritis, evaluation, early management and patient involvement. *Family Practice, 19*(2), 37-51.

Fenstermacher, K., & Hudson, B. (1997). *Practice guidelines for family nurse practitioners.* Philadelphia: W. B. Saunders.

Ham, R., & Sloane, P. (1997). *Primary care geriatrics, a case based approach.* St. Louis: Mosby.

Jones, K., & Patel, S. (2000). A family physician guide to monitoring methotrexate. *American Family Physician, 62*(7), 1607–1612.

Masear, V. (1996). *Primary care orthopedics.* Philadelphia: W. B. Saunders.

Millonig, V. L. (1996). *Today and tomorrow's woman—menopause: Before and after.* Potomac, MD: Health Leadership Associates, Inc.

Noble, J. (Ed.). (1996). *Textbook of primary care medicine.* St. Louis: Mosby.

Ramsburg, K. (2000). Rheumatoid arthritis. *American Journal of Nursing, 100*(11), 40–43.

Ross, C. (1997). A comparison of osteoarthritis and rheumatoid arthritis: Diagnosis and treatment. *The Nurse Practitioner, 22*(9), 20-39.

Santarlasci, P. (2000). Common injuries in recreational athletes. *Advance for Nurse Practitioners, 8*(4), 42–46.

Schmitt, M. (1999). Evaluation of the wrist and hand. *Patient Care for the Nurse Practitioner, 2*(9), 42–48.

Schnare, S. (1995). Evaluating and managing acute low back pain. *Contemporary Nurse Practitioner, 1*(6), 10-16.

Smith, B., & Green, G. (1995). Acute knee injuries: Part I. *American Family Physician, 51*(3), 615-621.

Tierney, L., McPhee, S., & Papadakis, M. (Eds.). (2000). *Current medical diagnosis and treatment* (39th ed.). NY: Lange Medical Books/McGraw-Hill.

Neurological Disorders Infancy Through Adolescence

Susan Heighway

Seizure Disorders/Epilepsy

- Definition
    1. Seizures—disturbances of normal nerve cell function characterized by uncontrolled, spontaneous electrical activity in the brain, that may result in loss of consciousness, altered body movements or disturbances of sensation and behavior
    2. Seizure disorder (epilepsy)—condition of recurrent seizures
    3. Status epilepticus—a series of rapidly, repetitive seizures without any periods of consciousness between them

- Etiology/Incidence
    1. Caused by any event with potential to produce insult to the brain
    2. Multiple causes; specific etiologies remain uncertain for 50% of cases
        a. Genetic component or familial predisposition
        b. Genetic disorders—tuberous sclerosis; neurofibromatosis
        c. Hemorrhage (intracranial)
        d. CNS infection (encephalitis, meningitis)
        e. Head trauma
        f. Developmental defects of brain
        g. Biochemical factors (inborn metabolic errors, electrolyte imbalance)
        h. Intracranial tumors
        i. Toxic ingestions—e.g., alcohol
        j. Poor drug compliance or altered drug metabolism because of illness
    3. Incidence varies greatly with age
        a. 1:1000 during first year of life
        b. 50% of all cases of epilepsy occur before age 25
    4. Variation in clinical manifestations due to location of brain involved

- Signs and Symptoms: International Seizure Classification System (1985) used to group seizures with similar clinical presentations
    1. Partial seizures
        a. Simple partial seizures
            (1) Characterized by seizure activity restricted to one side of body
            (2) No loss of consciousness and no postictal state
            (3) Motor—part of body or entire side (e.g., arm, leg, Jacksonian march, postural, vocalizations)
            (4) Sensory—visual, auditory, olfactory, parasthesias

(5) Autonomic—e.g., tachycardia, pallor, sweating, flushing

(5) Psychic—e.g., fearful or feelings of déjà vu

b. Complex partial seizures—variety of clinical expressions

    (1) Limited to impairment of consciousness, for 30 seconds or longer

    (2) Cognitive symptomatology

        (a) Abrupt alteration in mental state

        (b) Involves disruption of time relationships and memory

    (3) Affective symptomatology—inexplicable feelings, e.g., fear or dread without obvious cause

    (4) Somatosensory disturbances

        (a) Distortions of perception or hallucinations

        (b) May involve taste, smell, vision

    (5) Automatisms

        (a) Occur in 50% to 75% of cases

        (b) Semi-purposeful perseverative movements

        (c) May involve walking, sucking, lip-pursing or picking at clothing

2. Generalized seizures—involve electrical discharges of both hemispheres of the brain usually with some loss of consciousness

a. Absence seizures (petit mal)

    (1) Onset between 4 and 8 years of age, higher incidence in girls

    (2) Brief generalized, nonconvulsive episode with no aura and no postictal state

    (3) Characterized by interruption of activity, staring and unresponsiveness

    (4) Usually lasts between 5 and 15 seconds

    (5) Episode begins and ends abruptly

    (6) Child may be unaware of episode

b. Tonic-clonic (grand mal)

    (1) Consists of motor manifestations with loss of consciousness

    (2) May begin with aura

    (3) Tonic phase

        (a) Sustained contraction of muscles

        (b) Person falls to ground

        (c) Extensor posturing and tonic contraction

        (d) Lasts less than 1 minute

        (4)   Clonic phase

           (a)   Bilateral and rhythmic jerking

           (b)   May bite tongue

           (c)   Bowel or bladder incontinence may occur

           (d)   Stops after several minutes

        (5)   Postictal phase

           (a)   Period of cortical inhibition

           (b)   Vomiting

           (c)   Confusion and lethargy

           (d)   Gradual recovery of consciousness

  c. Myoclonic seizures

      (1)   Brief, sudden muscle contractions

      (2)   May involve only one part of body or be generalized

      (3)   May occur in clusters

      (4)   May be no alteration in consciousness

  d. Infantile spasms

      (1)   Onset during first year of life; usually between 4 and 8 months

      (2)   Brief, symmetric contraction of muscles in neck, trunk and extremities

      (3)   Spasms may be flexor, extensor or mixed

      (4)   Often in clusters up to 100 individual spasms

      (5)   Classified in two groups—infants with cryptogenic spasms have good prognosis whereas those with symptomatic type have a specific etiological factor identified and an 80% to 90% risk of mental retardation

  e. Atonic

      (1)   Also termed "drop" attacks

      (2)   Characterized by sudden loss of muscle tone, which may result in head nodding or mild flexing of legs

      (3)   Usually no alteration in consciousness

  f. Lennox-Gastaut syndrome

      (1)   Severe epileptic encephalopathy

      (2)   Characterized by variety of primary, generalized seizures

      (3)   Onset between 3 and 5 years of age

      (4)   Mental retardation and cerebral palsy common prior to onset

(5) Frequently preceded by infantile spasms

- Differential Diagnosis
    1. Breathholding spells—usually under 6 years of age
    2. Sleep disorders, e.g., narcolepsy
    3. Tics
    4. Complicated migraine headaches
    5. Syncope—more common in adolescence
    6. Gastroesophogeal reflux
    7. Benign paroxysmal vertigo
    8. Pseudoseizures
- Diagnostic Tests/Findings
    1. Clinical versus laboratory diagnosis
    2. Complete history
        a. Detailed description of seizure—onset, type, duration
        b. Previous seizures and frequency
        c. Evidence of infection
        d. Abnormal behavior
        e. Previous static or progressive neurologic/developmental dysfunction
        f. Pica; possible ingestion
        g. Trauma
        h. Birth history
        i. Current medication including anticonvulsants
        j. Family history of febrile and nonfebrile seizure
    3. Laboratory studies—to identify possible underlying etiology
        a. Serum fasting glucose, calcium, magnesium and serum electrolyte levels
        b. Seizures and mental retardation suggestive of metabolic problem
            (1) Plasma amino acids
            (2) Blood ammonia
            (3) Blood lactate and pyruvate
            (4) Urinary organic acids
            (5) Cytogenetic analysis
        c. Other studies as determined by history/physical findings
    4. Lumbar puncture—not routine

5. Neuroimaging studies
   a. Skull radiographs—rarely indicated, but helpful to rule out skull fracture
   b. Cranial CT and MRI
      (1) For detection of structural abnormalities
      (2) Indicated for:
         (a) A changing seizure pattern
         (b) Focal or lateralized abnormalities
         (c) History of trauma
         (d) Focally abnormal EEG
         (e) Evidence of increased intracranial pressure
         (f) Known or suspected specific white or gray matter disease
         (g) First seizure in all adolescents
   c. MRI more sensitive for detection of low grade tumors
   d. CT more sensitive to small foci or calcifications

6. EEG—measures physiologic function of brain
   a. Performed on all children, at least initially, to evaluate seizures
   b. Interpret in context of child's age, history, and physical findings
   c. Recorded for 1-hour, during periods of wakefulness and sleeping
   d. Helps to define seizure type
   e. Epileptiform EEG supports diagnosis; normal EEG does not exclude diagnosis

- Physical Findings
  1. Physical examination can be abnormal with underlying cerebral pathology
  2. Transient abnormal neurologic signs common during and after seizures
     a. Intention tremor
     b. Incoordination
     c. Weakness of one or more extremities
     d. Pathologic exaggeration of reflexes
     e. Confusion
  3. Warning signs of serious neurologic problems
     a. Asymmetric pupils
     b. Signs of increased intracranial pressure
     c. Focal deficits

Table 1
Antiepileptic Drugs and Type of Seizures

Type of Seizure	Drug(s) of Choice	Drugs also Used
Generalized tonic/clonic	Carbamazepine Valproic acid	Phenobarbital Phenytoin
Simple/complex partial	Carbamazepine Valproic acid	Phenobarbital
Absence	Valproic acid Ethosuximide	Clonazepam
Myoclonic	Valproic acid	Clonazepam
Lennox-Gastaut	Valproic acid	Ethosuximide
Infantile spasm	ACTH or corticosteroids	Valproic Acid

   d. Change in seizure pattern

 ● Management/Treatment: Referral to neurologist for initial management

  1. Antiepileptic drugs

   a. Principles

    (1) Utilize least number of medications

    (2) Maintain maximum level of alertness, with fewest number of seizures

    (3) Select drug effective for specific seizure type (see Table 1)

    (4) Use least toxic, least expensive, requiring least amount of laboratory monitoring

    (5) Begin with single drug, easier to assess side effects

    (6) Obtain baseline of child's physical status

     (a) Complete blood count

     (b) Liver function tests

     (c) Blood urea nitrogen and urinalysis

   b. Factors to consider in choice of drug (See Table 2)

    (1) Type of seizure

    (2) Dosage

    (3) Potential side effects

    (4) Half-life

    (5) Age, sex, weight and physical condition of child

  2. Anticipatory guidance

   a. First aid measures

    (1) Protect child from injury, but do not restrain

Table 2
Characteristics of Antiepileptic Drugs

Drug	Oral Dosage (mg/kg/d)	Half-life hours	Side Effects
Carbamazepine	20–40	8–12	Allergic rashes, nausea, lethargy, blurry vision, nystagmus, dizziness, bone marrow suppression, decreased liver function
Valproic acid	20–60	6–12	Nausea, weight gain, tremor, transient alopecia, hepatotoxicity, leukopenia, thrombocytopenia, rash
Ethosuximide	20–40	30	Abdominal discomfort, nausea, rash, hiccups, behavioral problems, drowsiness, dystonias, blood dyscrasias
Phenytoin	4–7	7–42	Rash, hirsutism, nausea, psychomotor slowing, neuropathy, ataxia, gingival hyperplasia, folate deficiency
Phenobarbital	3–6	36–120	Sedation; paradoxical hyperexcitability, rare
Clonazepam	0.01–0.03	18	Ataxia, sedation, drooling, inattention, withdrawal seizures
ACTH	20–40 IU		Cushing syndrome, hypertension, susceptibility to infections, GI bleeding, hypergylcemia

     (2)   Assess for adequate airway, breathing and circulatory status

     (3)   Do not insert items in mouth

     (4)   Note time, duration and activity

     (5)   If seizure persists beyond 10 to 15 minutes, seek medical assistance

  b. Observe for side effects of drugs

  c. Possible drug interactions

  d. Guidelines for activities/activity restrictions

     (1)   Avoid activities where seizures may cause dangerous fall (e.g., high diving, rope climbing)

     (2)   Supervised swimming only

     (3)   Discuss other sports participation with parents and child

  e. Importance of compliance with drug therapy

3. Intractable seizures—15% children with epilepsy

  a. Refer to epilepsy center with interdisciplinary team

  b. Alternative treatments

     (1)   Ketogenic diet—very restricted, high fat/low carbohydrate diet

     (2)   Epilepsy surgery—approximately half of children with intractable seizures are appropriate candidates for surgical procedures

Febrile Seizures

- Definition: Generalized tonic or tonic-clonic seizures which occur as a consequence of an abrupt and steep rise in body temperature in young children

- Etiology/Incidence

    1. 3% to 4% of otherwise healthy children between the ages of 9 months and 5 years of age have one or more febrile seizures; peak onset between 18 and 24 months of age

    2. Exact cause unknown; hereditary influence suspected

    3. Most common non-epileptic seizure disorder

- Signs and Symptoms

    1. Two groups based on clinical features

        a. Simple (benign) febrile seizures

            (1) Duration < 15 minutes

            (2) No focal features

            (3) If occur in series, total duration of less than 30 minutes

        b. Complex febrile seizures

            (1) Duration > 15 minutes

            (2) Focal features or postictal paresis present

            (3) Occur in series with total duration greater than 30 minutes

- Differential Diagnosis

    1. Underlying meningitis or encephalitis

    2. Chills

    3. Underlying metabolic disorder

    4. Epilepsy

- Physical Findings

    1. Often associated with viral or bacterial illness

        a. While fever is rising

        b. Usually above 102° F (39° C)

    2. Associated more frequently with severe constitutional symptoms during illness

- Diagnostic Tests/Findings

    1. Detailed description of seizure

    2. Complete physical assessment with careful neurological examination

    3. Lumbar punctures not routine; but indicated for:

a. Infants < 1 year of age

b. If seizure occurs after second day of illness

c. Rule out meningitis

4. Skull radiographs not routine

5. Blood laboratory studies, EEG, CT or MRI not routine but performed if indicated by history or physical findings

- Management/Treatment

1. Urgent treatment for unabated seizures of ≥ 10 minutes

2. Fever control for temperature > 101° F

a. Sponge baths with tepid water for at least 1 hour; avoid chilling

b. Antipyretic use, e.g., acetaminophen

3. A comprehensive search for cause of fever and treatment of underlying illness

4. Reassurance to parents regarding excellent prognosis

5. Antiseizure drugs

a. Short-term or prolonged anticonvulsant prophylaxis not recommended

b. Oral diazepam safe and effective method of reducing risk of recurrence; at onset of each febrile illness, diazepam 0.3 mg/kg every 8 hours orally is administered for duration of illness (usually 2 to 3 days)

Headaches

- Definition: Head pain

- Etiology/Incidence

1. Exact etiology unknown; pain may be extracranial and/or intracranial

2. Difficult to distinguish tension headaches from migraine headaches in many children

3. Chronic and recurrent headaches are most common neurologic complaints; occur in 3% to 20% of children and adolescents

a. Migraines—account for 50% of chronic or recurrent headaches; 60% of affected children are male

b. Cluster headaches

(1) Briefer in duration and more frequent than migraines

(2) Begin in teenage years

(3) More frequent in males

4. Headache pain is produced by several factors which activate pain fibers

a. Inflammation

    b.   Stretching

    c.   Torsion

    d.   Contraction of innervated structures

        (1)   Large intracranial arteries and veins

        (2)   Dural sinuses

        (3)   Periosteum of bone

        (4)   Muscle/skin of scalp

        (5)   Teeth and gums

- Signs and Symptoms

    1.   Migraine headaches—recurrent headaches with varied frequency, intensity and duration

        a.   Diagnostic criteria: Repeated episodes of headache accompanied by at least 3 of the following symptoms

           (1)   Recurrent abdominal pain (with or without headache) or nausea and vomiting

           (2)   An aura, usually visual, but may be sensory, motor, or vertiginous

           (3)   Throbbing or pounding pain

           (4)   Pain restricted to one side of head (although may shift sides from one headache to next); bilateral before puberty

           (5)   Relief of pain by brief periods of sleep

           (6)   Family history of migraine in one or more immediate relatives

    2.   Tension headaches—headaches occurring with most frequency and intensity during periods of increased stress

        a.   Tend to involve occipital or temporal regions bilaterally and often extend to the neck, or may be diffuse

        b.   Nausea and vomiting may occur, but not as often as with migraine

    3.   Intracranial headaches—may have certain distinguishing factors

        a.   Severe occipital headache

        b.   Exacerbated by straining, sneezing or coughing

        c.   Awakens child from sleep

        d.   Exacerbated or improved markedly by position changes

        e.   Associated with projectile vomiting or vomiting without nausea

        f.   Associated with history of focal seizures

        g.   Increase in intensity and severity if not treated

4. Sinus headache—chronic or recurrent headaches which occur in about 15% of children with chronic sinusitis

   a. Often occur same time each day, build slowly, with throbbing quality

   b. Accompanied by rhinorrhea, postnasal drip, persistent cough, recurrent ear infections; afebrile

   c. Pain or pressure over frontal or maxillary sinuses

- Differential Diagnosis

   1. Acute, severe headache—distinguish between intracranial and extracranial cause by thorough history and physical examination

      a. Intracranial causes

         (1) Intracranial mass

         (2) Infection—meningitis, encephalitis

         (3) Intracranial hemorrhage

         (4) Post-head injury

         (5) Post-seizure

      b. Extracranial causes

         (1) Sinusitis—rare

         (2) Temporomandibular joint problem

   2. Chronic headaches—stress, anxiety, or tension with resulting muscle contractions

- Physical Findings

   1. Chronic migraine or tension headaches—physical examination generally normal

   2. Acute headache—critical indicators of possible intracranial cause

      a. Meningismus

      b. Focal neurologic signs

      c. Papilledema

      d. Split sutures

      e. Evidence of cranial trauma (including blood in or behind ear)

      f. Depressed level of consciousness

- Diagnostic Tests/Findings: Unnecessary unless history/physical examination suggest intracranial etiology, e.g., infection, bleeding or tumors

- Management/Treatment

   1. Specific treatment determined by etiology

   2. Headaches with suspected intracranial etiology need evaluation by physician/neurologist

   3. Cautious use of medications for pain relief

   a. Initial treatment with simple analgesics

   b. Acetaminophen

     (1) Under 1 year—60 mg orally every 4 to 6 hours

     (2) 1 to 3 years—60 to 120 mg orally every 4 to 6 hours

     (3) 3 to 6 years—120 to 180 mg orally every 4 to 6 hours

     (4) 6 to 12 years—240 mg orally every 4 to 6 hours

     (5) Older than 12 years—325 to 650 mg orally every 4 to 6 hours

   c. If mild analgesics ineffective in children older than 11 years, may progress with caution to:

     (1) Midrin

       (a) Combination of isometheptene mucate 65 mg; acetaminophen 325 mg and dichloralphenazone 100 mg

       (b) 1 to 2 capsules immediately; repeat 1 capsule every hour until relieved to a maximum of 3/day or 5/week

     (2) Ergotamine tartrate—2 mg sublingual

   d. Prophylactic treatment:

     (1) With headaches more than once/week and those that interfere with routine activities, e.g., school attendance

     (2) Unresponsive to symptomatic treatment

     (3) Medications used

       (a) Propranolol—.5 to 3.0 mg/kg/day $\geq$ 11 years of age

       (b) Cyproheptadine hydrochloride—0.25 mg/kg/day $\geq$ 3 years of age

       (c) Phenobarbital—3 to 5 mg/kg/day every night (3 to 10 years)

       (d) Phenytoin—5 mg/kg/day in 2 doses

       (e) Amitriptyline hydrochloride—1 to 2 mg/kg/day $\geq$ 11 years of age

4. Stress management and relaxation techniques

5. Eliminate foods which may be triggers, e.g., chocolate, cheese, MSG

6. Refer to specialists for further evaluation if headaches are recurrent, unresponsive, including allergist, psychiatrist, neurologist or pain clinic

Neurofibromatosis (NF)-1 (von Recklinghausen Disease)

- Definition
  1. A neurocutaneous syndrome characterized by multiple café-au-lait spots (CLS) on the body; nerve tumors (neurofibromas present within the body and on skin)
  2. Most common type of NF
  3. Always a progressive disorder
  4. Intelligence is usually normal

- Etiology/Incidence
    1. Inherited autosomal dominant disorder; associated with chromosome # 17
    2. Occurs 1:3000 to 1:4000 persons
    3. High variability and severity among individuals and within families
    4. Penetrance (likelihood that mutant gene will express itself at all if it is present) is virtually 100%
- Signs and Symptoms
    1. Skin lesions and/or freckling
    2. Developmental delays
    3. Seizures
- Differential Diagnosis
    1. Benign condition with < 5 or 6 CLSs
    2. McCune-Albright syndrome
    3. Neurolemmoma
    4. Proteus syndrome
- Physical Findings: A diagnosis of NF is made when two or more of the following diagnostic criteria are met (developed by the 1987 National Institutes of Health Consensus Development Conference on NF) are met:
    1. 6 or more CLSs > than 5 mm diameter in prepubertal child and > 15 mm in postpubertal adolescent; 5 or more in young child < 5 years is highly suggestive
    2. 2 or more cutaneous and/or subcutaneous neurofibromas, or one plexiform neurofibroma
    3. Axillary or inguinal freckling
    4. Optic pathway glioma
    5. 2 or more iris Lisch nodules
    6. Distinctive osseous lesion (e.g., sphenoid wing dysplasia or thinning of long-bone cortex, with or without pseudarthrosis)
    7. First degree relative (parent, sibling or offspring) with NF-1 diagnosed by above criteria
- Diagnostic Tests/Findings: Additional tests to confirm diagnosis and identify complications
    1. Slit-lamp ocular examination to identify ocular abnormalities (e.g., iris Lisch nodules and signs of optic pathway glioma)
    2. Cranial MRI—to identify gliomas
    3. Radiographs of spine, chest, skull—to identify neurofibromas and other tumors

4. EEG—to detect epileptogenic foci

5. Psychological evaluation of school-age child for school—to determine abilities and deficiencies

6. Audiogram/brain stem evoked response testing—baseline for hearing and detection of acoustic neuromas

- Management/Treatment

   1. Problems associated with NF-1 most likely to require medical treatment

      a. Constipation

      b. Seizures

      c. Headaches

      d. Hyperactivity

      e. Learning disabilities

      f. Anxiety

      g. Renovascular hypertension

   2. Surgery

      a. Removing or debulking tumors

      b. Treating skeletal dysplasia

      c. Correcting scoliosis

      d. Treatment of vascular compromise

   3. Frequent consultation with medical and surgical specialists, social workers, and other health care specialists

   4. Genetic counseling

   5. Referral to support group for NF

Tuberous Sclerosis (TS)

- Definition

   1. Neurocutaneous syndrome with a combination of skin abnormalities, seizures, and cognitive deficits

   2. Progressive disorder with deterioration over time including new lesions and complications with increasing patient age

   3. Majority have ongoing debilitation from TS throughout their lives

   4. Mental retardation and seizures are most common problems

- Etiology/Incidence

   1. Autosomal dominant mutant gene

2. Previously negative family history does not exclude diagnosis

3. Incidence—1:10,000 to 1:50,000

4. Recurrence risk for affected person's children is 50%

- Signs and Symptoms

  1. Hypopigmented skin lesions often noted at birth

  2. Developmental delay

  3. Abnormal movements, particularly myoclonic jerking movements

- Physical Findings

  1. Establishing diagnosis of TS depends on detecting presence of two or more specific abnormalities:

     a. Skin

        (1) Hypopigmented macules, of elliptical shape (ash-leaf spots)

        (2) Fibroadenomas—adenoma sebaceum

        (3) Distinctive brown patch on forehead

        (4) Shagreen patch (characteristic)—raised lesion in lumbosacral region

     b. Teeth—characteristic pitting of enamel

     c. Eye

        (1) Choroidal hamartomas

        (2) Hypopigmented defects of iris

     d. CNS

        (1) Periventricular tubers

        (2) Cerebral astrocytomas

        (3) Nonspecific EEG abnormalities, including hypsarrhythmia

     e. Cardiovascular

        (1) Cardiac rhabdomyomas

        (2) Aortic and major artery constrictions

     f. Kidney—renal angiomyolipomas

     g. Lungs—diffuse interstitial fibrosis

  2. Seizures of all types, particularly myoclonic jerks, and mental retardation most common symptoms

- Differential Diagnosis: Seizures, or mental retardation

- Diagnostic Tests/Findings

  1. MRI scan of brain—virtually diagnostic and must be used in suspected TS

2. Once diagnosis is made, close follow-up surveillance is essential using appropriate clinical laboratory and radiographic techniques to monitor progression and identify new lesions

- Management/Treatment

    1. No specific medical treatment available

    2. Treat seizures and other complications (e.g., heart failure, renal failure) the same as if TS were not present, unless surgery on primary lesions is indicated

    3. Genetic counseling

    4. Psychometric testing and psychoeducational techniques for cognitive needs

    5. Family and individual support and counseling

    6. Refer to tertiary care center for specialized treatment, information, and support

Tic Disorders

- Definition

    1. Tic—repetitive, brief, involuntary, stereotypic muscle movement or vocalizations

    2. Severity ranges from mild and transient to more severe and permanent

    3. Types

        a. Transient tic disorder—duration less than 1 year

        b. Chronic tic disorder—duration more than 1 year, simple or complex

        c. Gilles de la Tourette syndrome—most severe chronic tic disorder; symptoms include multiple motor and vocal tics varying in nature and severity over time

- Etiology/Incidence

    1. Uncertain etiology; possible genetic central nervous system disturbance

    2. Occasionally precipitated by stimulant medications

    3. Transient tics

        a. Occur in 25% of normal children

        b. Often begin in school-age children and can be intensified by anxiety, fatigue, or excitement

    4. Gilles de la Tourette syndrome

        a. Onset between 2 and 15 years of age with mean age 6 to 7 years

        b. Incidence—1:10,000 persons

        c. Males 3 times more frequently affected

- Signs and Symptoms

    1. Characteristics of tics

a. Variable expression—frequency, intensity, and severity

b. Exacerbated by stress

c. Some degree of voluntary control often present

d. Typically subside during sleep

2. Simple tics

a. Movements present that resemble nervous habits

b. Facial "twitches", head shaking, eye blinking, shoulder shrugging or throat clearing

3. Gilles de la Tourette syndrome

a. Simple tics

b. Complex sequences of coordinated movements (e.g., bizarre gait, kicking, jumping, body gyrations, scratching, and seductive or obscene gestures)

c. Involuntary vocalizations occur, ranging from simple to complex noises

d. Expression is gender influenced

(1) Motor and vocal manifestations more prevalent in boys

(2) Behavioral problems, such as obsessive-compulsive disorder more common in girls.

- Differential Diagnosis

1. Chronic tic disorder

2. Stuttering

3. Seizures

4. Medication-induced tics

5. Pervasive developmental disorder

6. Psychiatric disorders, e.g., schizophrenia

7. Medical conditions with associated abnormal movements, e.g., post-viral encephalitis, multiple sclerosis

- Physical Findings

1. Usually normal

2. Some degree of voluntary ability to suppress tics is usually present

- Diagnostic Tests/Findings: None

- Management/Treatment

1. Transient tics—support and education for child and family

2. Chronic tics/Gilles de la Tourette syndrome

a. Referral to mental health specialist

b. May involve psychotherapy, behavior management, stress management

c. Pharmacologic management

    (1) Consultation and/or referral—pediatric neurologist

    (2) Medications useful to suppress behavioral symptoms interfering with daily functioning

    (3) Pimoxide—beginning dose of 1 mg at bedtime

        (a) Gradual increases (every 5 to 7 days) until symptoms subside

        (b) Maximum dose of 10mg/day in children; 20mg/ day in adolescents

        (c) Side effects—sedation, lethargy, acute dystonic reactions, tardive dyskinesia

        (d) Less frequent side effects than haloperidol

    (4) Haloperidol—beginning dose of 0.25 to 0.50 mg at bedtime

        (a) Gradual increases (every 4 to 5 days) until symptoms subside

        (b) Side effects similar to pimoxide; tardive dyskinesia more common than with pimoxide

    (5) Clonidine—less effective but with fewer side effects is sometime used

Head Injuries

- Definition: Any injury to the meninges, scalp, skull, or any part of the brain; severity of injury ranges from very mild to severe brain-damaging injury

- Etiology/Incidence

1. Injury resulting from external physical force to the cranium and internal brain structures

2. Approximately 1 in 25 children receives medical attention each year for head injuries

3. Twice as frequent in boys

4. Greatest incidence in children < 1 year and > 15 years

5. Age specific etiology

    a. Infant—child abuse, falls

    b. One to 4 years of age—falls

    c. School age—falls, motor vehicle accidents, sports/recreation

    d. Adolescents—motor vehicle accidents; athletic injuries

- Signs and Symptoms: Important to determine specific circumstances associated with head trauma

  1. Scalp injuries—contusions and lacerations are most frequent complications

  2. Concussion

     a. Head injury sufficient to cause brief loss of consciousness or amnesia for event

     b. Presence and duration of amnesia is indicative of severity

     c. Usually brief loss of consciousness is followed in minutes by complete return to normal mental status and behavior

     d. Recovery usually complete without complications

     e. Few children experience postconcussional syndrome, several hours after concussion, characterized by:

        (1) Headache

        (2) Drowsiness

        (3) Confusion or irritability

        (4) Symptoms may last for several days

  3. Diffuse Axonal Injury (DAI)

     a. Diffuse injury, usually resulting from violent motion, e.g., motor vehicle accidents

     b. Diagnosis of exclusion associated with:

        (1) Unconsciousness $\geq$ 6 or more hours

        (2) No other cause for symptoms, such as seizures or hematoma

     c. More serious diagnosis with less favorable prognosis than concussion

     d. Other symptoms depend on severity of injury

        (1) Abnormal movements with abnormal pupillary reaction

        (2) Difficulty regulating respirations and blood pressure

  4. Contusion

     a. Bruising or tearing of cerebral structures

     b. Common locations include frontal, temporal lobes and orbital area

     c. Focal motor signs related to increased intracranial pressure (ICP) may be diagnostic

  5. Hematomas

     a. Epidural hematoma—blood clot formation between skull and dura of the brain

        (1) Most treatable, but potentially most lethal type of head injury

(2) Classic clinical sign is delayed onset of symptoms

(3) Initial neurological symptoms may be minimal or absent

(4) Secondary injury from increased ICP as hematoma enlarges may result in neurological symptoms

　(a) Headache

　(b) Confusion

　(c) Vomiting

　(d) One-sided weakness

　(e) Agitation

(5) Symptoms may progress to lethargy, coma, and even death if left untreated

(6) Prognosis is favorable if surgery is performed before secondary injury becomes irreversible

b. Subdural hematoma—blood clot formation on brain surface beneath the duramater

(1) Acute presentation

　(a) Symptoms appear within 48 hours of head injury

　(b) Signs of intracranial hypertension including irritability or lethargy, vomiting, headache

(2) Subacute

　(a) Symptoms between 2 and 21 days

　(b) Chronic hematoma with symptoms appearing after 21 days

　(c) Signs include seizures, motor abnormalities (hypertonicity and agitation), systemic (irritability, vomiting, fever, anemia, poor weight gain)

6. Skull fracture

a. Brain damage may not be present, and conversely, brain can be injured without skull fracture present

b. Type, severity, symptomatology depend on area involved, age of child, and force of impact

c. Linear

(1) Fracture in temporoparietal region

(2) Most common

(3) Frequent in children less than 2 years old who fall from low heights

(4) Outcome is usually excellent

      d. Depressed

          (1) Skull is disrupted/depressed at point of impact

          (2) Underlying structures may be bruised or lacerated

      e. Basal

          (1) Diagnosis dependent on recognition of signs including hemorrhage in nose, nasopharynx, middle ear

          (2) Bruising over mastoid bone (Battle sign) or around eyes (raccoon's eye sign)

          (3) Cranial nerve palsy

          (4) Cerebral spinal fluid from ears or nose

- Differential Diagnosis

  1. Seizure disorder

  2. Child maltreatment

- Physical Findings

  1. Alterations in vital signs may indicate shock

  2. Headache, irritability and/or crying may indicate acute pain

  3. Tense anterior fontanel in young child

  4. Alterations in level of consciousness (LOC) vary from irritability, agitation, restlessness to confusion and/or coma

  5. Skull fractures may or may not show bony displacement

  6. Unilateral swelling may present from a possible hematoma

  7. Other signs:

    a. Asymmetry

    b. Focal neurologic deficits

    c. Cranial nerve injuries

    d. CSF rhinorrhea or otorrhea

    e. Ecchymosis

    f. Hearing impairments

  8. With cerebral edema and increasing ICP, may observe:

    a. Changes in level of consciousness

    b. Abnormal respiratory patterns

    c. Loss of protective reflexes (e.g., cough, gag or corneal)

    d. Changes in motor function or posturing

e. Nausea and projectile vomiting.

- Diagnostic Tests/Findings

    1. Skull radiography

        a. Indicated when severity of head trauma includes:

            (1) Loss of consciousness

            (2) Presence of focal neurologic signs

        b. Only 20% of basal skull fractures can be recognized on standard skull radiographs

        c. If depressed skull fracture is suspected, obtain tangential along with standard views

    2. CT scan—useful in detection of intracranial hemorrhage; investigation of localizing neurologic signs

    3. MRI—most useful in evaluation of subacute or chronic rather than acute injuries

- Management/Treatment

    1. For acute injury, rapid, accurate assessment of primary injury and level of severity

    2. Most head trauma is minor, with momentary unconsciousness, then child resumes activity and does not require treatment

    3. Hospital observation may be required for:

        a. More than momentary loss of consciousness

        b. Lethargy, confusion or irritability

        c. Severe headache

        d. Changes in speech or movements in arms and legs

        e. Significant bleeding from wound

        f. Vomiting 1 to 2 hours following injury

    4. Anticipatory guidance

        a. Instructions for home observation

        b. Need to return to health care provider if child exhibits:

            (1) Excessive prolonged sleepiness

            (2) Disorientation

            (3) Confusion

            (4) Persistent vomiting

            (5) Seizure

            (6) Change in swelling of scalp

Meningitis

- Definition—Inflammation of the meninges
- Etiology/Incidence—related to age
  1. Most frequently a result of hematogenous dissemination
  2. Bacterial pathogens—related to age
     a. Newborn
        (1) *Escherichia coli*
        (2) Group B streptococci
        (3) *Listeria monocytogenes* (less frequent)
     b. Etiologic agents responsible for 95% of cases that occur in children over 2 months of age have been:
        (1) *Haemophilus influenzae* type b (decline in incidence with H. influenzae immunization)
        (2) *Streptococcus pneumoniae*
        (3) *Neisseria meningitidis*
  3. Other etiologic agents
     a. Mycobacteria
     b. Fungal infections
     c. Aseptic (viral)
     d. Protozoa
  4. Highest risk—infants between 6 and 12 months of age; 90% of all cases occurr in children between 1 month and 5 years
- Signs and Symptoms
  1. Newborn
     a. Often nonspecific and indistinguishable from those of septicemia
     b. Most frequent signs:
        (1) Temperature instability
        (2) Respiratory distress
        (3) Irritability, lethargy
        (4) Poor feeding
        (5) Vomiting
     b. Seizures present in 40%
  2. Older infants and children

a. Nausea and vomiting

b. Irritability, confusion

c. Anorexia

d. Headache, back pain, nuchal rigidity

e. Hyperesthesia, cranial nerve palsy, ataxia

f. Photophobia

- Differential Diagnosis

1. Brain abscess

2. Spinal, epidural, or intracranial abscess

3. Bacterial endocarditis with embolism

4. Subdural empyema with or without thrombophlebitis

5. Brain tumor

- Physical Findings

1. Newborn

    a. Bulging fontanel (with or without suture diastasis)

    b. Increased ICP

    c. Cardinal signs of meningitis in older children are usually absent in infants

       (1) No stiff neck

       (2) No evidence of Kernig's and Brudzinski's signs

2. Older infants and children

    a. Common clinical signs associated with meningeal irritation are:

       (1) Kernig's sign:

          (a) Flexion of the leg 90° at hip

          (b) Pain on extension of leg

       (2) Brudzinski's sign—involuntary flexion of legs when neck is flexed

    b. Headache is frequent sign of increased intracranial pressure

- Diagnostic Tests/Findings

1. Diagnosis based on examination and culture of cerebrospinal fluid (CSF)

2. Lumbar puncture for CSF analysis

    a. Contraindicated in following conditions

       (1) Cardiopulmonary compromise

       (2) Signs of increased ICP—papilledema

    (3) Infection in area overlying lumbar puncture location

  b. Adverse reactions—pain, headache, bleeding

 3. CSF analysis

  a. Cloudy

  b. Increased cell count (300 to 10,000)

  c. Increased protein

  d. Decreased glucose

- Management/Treatment

 1. Hospitalization for bacterial meningitis—first 3 to 4 days are critical

 2. Initiate antibiotic therapy once diagnosis is confirmed by clinical findings while awaiting specific CSF and blood culture results

 3. Neonates:

  a. Fatality rate is 15% to 30% in neonates

  b. Prognosis depends upon:

   (1) Causative pathogen

   (2) Predisposing risk factors

   (3) Availability of intensive care facilities

  c. Follow-up

   (1) Group B streptococcus

    (a) 15% to 20% have sequelae—spastic quadriplegia; profound mental retardation; hemiparesis; hearing/ visual deficits

    (b) 11% have hydrocephalus

    (c) 13% have seizure disorder

   (2) Gram negative meningitis

    (a) 10% have severe sequelae of developmental delays

    (b) About 25% to 35% have mild to moderate sequelae, which may not interfere with normal development

    (c) Hydrocephalus develops in $\frac{1}{3}$ of infants

  d. Neonatal survivors without major sequelae seem to develop normally

 4. Older infants and children

  a. Prognosis depends on several factors:

   (1) Patient's age at onset

(2) Duration of disease before appropriate antibiotic therapy initiated

(3) Specific microorganism involved and number of organisms

(4) Whether disorder is compromising host response to infection

    b. Mortality rate 1% to 5% beyond the neonatal period

    c. Up to 50% of survivors have some sequelae

        (1) 10% have hearing deficits

        (2) 15% have language disorder/delay

        (3) 2% to 4% have vision impairment

        (4) 10% to 11% have mental retardation

        (5) 3% to 7% have motor problems

        (6) 2% to 8% have seizures

Brain Tumors

- Definition: Expanding intracranial lesion

- Etiology/Incidence

1. Etiology is unknown, may be genetic predisposition, congenital factors, environmental exposures

2. Two most common primary tumors in childhood

    a. Cerebellar astrocytomas (20% of all brain tumors in children)

    b. Medulloblastoma

3. In children between 4 and 11 years, infratentorial (posterior fossa) tumors predominate, including cerebellar and brain stem tumors

- Signs and Symptoms

1. In infants with open sutures

    a. Increased head circumference

    b. Irritability

    c. Head tilt

    d. Loss of developmental milestones

2. Older children

    a. Headache; symptoms usually increase in frequency, becoming more severe in the morning followed by vomiting

    b. 85% of children with malignant tumors have abnormal neurologic or ocular examinations within 2 to 4 months of onset of headaches

c. Certain specific neurologic symptoms may occur later and suggest localization of the CNS tumor

  (a) Ataxia, hemiparesis, cranial nerve palsies

  (b) Somnolence

  (c) Seizures

  (d) Head tilt

  (e) Diencephalic syndrome—failure to thrive (FTT), emaciation

  (f) Diabetes insipidus

- Differential Diagnosis

  1. Brain abscess

  2. Intracranial hemorrhage

  3. Nonneoplastic hydrocephalus

  4. Arteriovenous malformations or aneurysm

  5. Indolent viral infections

  6. Subdural hematoma

- Physical Findings: Directly related to anatomic location, size and to some extent the age of the child; may include:

  1. Tense bulging fontanel at rest (in infant)

  2. Cranial enlargement (present in infants and young children)

  3. Papilledema (edema of optic nerve)

  4. Nuchal rigidity

  5. Incoordination or clumsiness

  6. Poor fine motor control

  7. Hypoflexia or hyperflexia

  8. Positive Babinski sign

  9. Spasticity/paralysis

  10. Behavioral changes—may be earliest symptom in child/adolescent

- Diagnostic Tests/Findings

  1. MRI—superior, sensitive neuroimaging technology

  2. CT scan

    a. Without contrast, can detect:

      (1) Whether lesion is cystic or solid

      (2) Presence of calcifications, hemorrhage, edema, and hydrocephalus

    b.   With contrast can detect:

        (1)   Small tumors

        (2)   Differentiation of areas of edema

3.   Angiography—determines blood supply to affected structures

4.   Lumbar puncture contraindicated in presence of increased ICP

- Management/Treatment: Therapy selected depends on type and site of tumor

   1.   Surgery (usually treatment of choice)

   2.   Radiation therapy

   3.   Chemotherapy

   4.   Follow-up

      a.   EEG for seizures

      b.   VER for visual problems

      c.   BAER for hearing problems

      d.   Multidisciplinary approach for comprehensive health and developmental needs of child/family

Questions
Select the best answer

1. Which of the following children is most likely to experience a typical febrile seizure?

    a. A 1-year-old with otitis media and a fever of 104° F
    b. A 3-month-old with unequal pupils and bulging fontanels
    c. An 11-year-old with fever of 101° F who is on valproic acid for seizure disorder
    d. A 5-year-old with bacterial meningitis

2. Which of the following responses during a tonic-clonic seizure is most appropriate to teach family members of a child who has these seizures?

    a. Restrain the child
    b. Insert an airway into the mouth to prevent tongue biting
    c. Note the time, duration, and activity of the seizure
    d. Protect child from injury

3. Which of the following is an appropriate strategy to instruct the parents of an 18-month-old child who has just been diagnosed with a febrile seizure and who has a fever of 104° F?

    a. Aspirin every 4 hours for temperature over 101° F
    b. Bathe with cold water mixed with alcohol
    c. Dress warmly to avoid chills
    d. Continue sponge baths with tepid water for at least 1 hour

4. What is the primary method of preventing and controlling the incidence of bacterial meningitis in infants and children?

    a. Keeping infants and young children away from crowded places
    b. Administering antimeningitis vaccines during outbreaks
    c. Immediately isolating all children suspected of having meningitis
    d. Routinely giving infants *H. Influenzae* vaccine

5. Which type of seizure is first seen between 4 and 8 months of age, may be confused with myoclonic seizures and may be associated with serious developmental problems?

    a. Febrile seizures
    b. Infantile spasms
    c. Absence seizures
    d. Tonic-clonic

6. Which of the following would not be associated with a concussion?

    a. Focal motor signs
    b. Brief loss of consciousness
    c. Headache
    d. Confusion or irrritability

7. Which of the following factors is not usually associated with migraine headaches?

    a. Complaints of diffuse occipital pain
    b. Positive family history in immediate relatives
    c.. Pain relieved by brief sleep
    d. Recurrent abdominal pain

8. Sarah is a 13-month-old whose parents are very concerned after she experienced a second febrile seizure. At today's visit, they ask you about the use of medications to prevent any further seizures. Which of the following statements is not true regarding febrile seizure prophylaxis?

    a. Short-term anticonvulsant prophylaxis is not indicated
    b. Prolonged anticonvulsant prophylaxis for preventing recurrent febrile convulsions is controversial and no longer recommended
    c. It may be indicated for children < 12 months with recurrent febrile seizures
    d. Oral diazepam may be used at the onset, and for the duration of the febrile illness to reduce the risk of recurrence of febrile seizures

9. Problems associated with NF-1 most likely to require treatment include which of following?

    a. Learning disabilities
    b. Transient tics
    c. Obsessive-compulsive behavior
    d. Progressive mental retardation

10. An 11-year-old girl is brought in by her mother complaining of severe headaches associated with nausea and vomiting. Which of the following signs and symptoms would lead you to consider a brain tumor as part of your differential diagnoses?

    a. Throbbing pain restricted to one side
    b. Bilateral throbbing pain
    c. Visual aura
    d. More severe in the morning followed by vomiting

11. The National Institutes of Health Consensus conference on NF describes guidelines for diagnosis of NF. Which of the following is not among the diagnostic criteria?

    a. Family history of first degree relative with NF-1
    b. 6 or more CLSs > 5 mm diameter in prepubertal child
    c. 6 or more neurofibromas > 15 mm in postpubertal adolescent
    d. Optic glioma

12. Although meningitis related mortality decreases dramatically after the neonatal period, as many as 50% of survivors experience some sequelae. Which of the following is the most frequent post-meningitis sequelae in older infants and children?

    a. Motor deficits
    b. Seizures
    c. Language delays/disorders
    d. Visual impairments

13. A neonate is being worked up for meningitis after experiencing a seizure preceded by fever, irritability, and poor feeding for one day. On physical examination which of the following findings would be most consistent with a diagnosis of meningitis?

    a. Bulging fontanel
    b. Positive Brudzinski's sign
    c. Nuchal rigidity
    d. Positive Kernig's sign

14. Diagnostic criteria for Gilles de la Tourette syndrome includes which of the following?

    a. Must have both motor and vocal tics
    b. Steady pattern of motor tics
    c. Presence of tics for 6 months
    d. Multiple voluntary motor tics

15. Which of the following statements about Tourette's syndrome is not true?

    a. It is the most severe type of tic disorder
    b. It is more common among males than females
    c. Mean age at onset is between 6 and 7 years
    d. Expression is not gender influenced

16. A prominent feature in simple partial seizures is:

    a. Night terrors
    b. Microcephaly
    c. Bilateral tremor
    d. No loss of consciousness

17. Absence seizures:

    a. Often begin in infancy
    b. Appear as altered awareness and blank stare for brief period
    c. More commonly occur in first-born children
    d. Always progress to a more severe seizure disorder beyond childhood

18. The differential diagnosis for seizures includes which of the following:

    a. Poliomyelitis with paralysis
    b. Schizophrenia
    c. Sleep disorders
    d. Multiple sclerosis

19. The most useful diagnostic tool for diagnosing epilepsy is:

    a. MRI
    b. EMG
    c. EEG
    d. ECG

20. Which of the following drugs are used for treatment of generalized tonic/clonic seizures?

    a. Ethosuximide, carbamazepine, valproic acid
    b. Carbamazepine, valproic acid, phenytoin
    c. Clonazepam, carbamazepine, valproic acid
    d. Clonazepam, valproic acid, phenobarbital

21. Which of the following is included in the diagnostic criteria for migraine headache in children?

    a. Recurrent abdominal pain, throbbing head pain not relieved by sleep
    b. Nausea and vomiting, positive family history, aura
    c. Positive family history, nausea and vomiting, pain not relieved by sleep
    d. Aura, positive family history, diffuse head pain relieved by sleep

22. Headache caused by intracranial factors include which of the following distinguishing features?

    a. Severe occipital headache, awakens child from sleep, and vomiting
    b. Not affected by change in position, severe occipital headache
    c. Severe occipital headache, sleep unaffected, nausea and vomiting
    d. Severe occipital headache, aura, exacerbated or improved with change in position

23. Tuberous sclerosis is progressive, neurocutaneous syndrome in which there is a combination of:

    a. Skin abnormalities, blindness and cognitive deficits
    b. Skin abnormalities, seizures, cognitive deficits
    c. Cerebral palsy, cognitive deficits and skin problems
    d. Skin abnormalities, blindness and cognitive deficit

24. Tuberous sclerosis is caused by:

    a. Autosomal dominant mutant gene
    b. Autosomal recessive mutant gene
    c. Autosomal recessive mutant chromosome
    d. Autosomal dominant mutant chromosome

25. Seizures of all types are associated with tuberous sclerosis, but most commonly:

    a. Tonic-clonic seizures
    b. Simple partial seizures
    c. Myoclonic jerks
    d. Absence

26. For children 1 to 4 years of age, the most common cause of head injury is:

    a. Motor vehicle accidents
    b. Falls
    c. Child abuse
    d. Bicycle accidents

27. A concussion can be identified by which of the following:

    a. Brief loss of consciousness or amnesia with complete return to normal
    b. Usually associated with brief loss of consciousness and poor recovery
    c. Usually associated with sequelae of paralysis and seizures
    d. Usually associated with Battle sign

28. A head injury in which bruising or tearing of the brain occurs is:

    a. Contusion
    b. Concussion
    c. Hematoma
    d. Diffuse axonal injury

29. The most common type of skull fracture in children with an excellent prognosis is:

    a. Depressed
    b. Basilar
    c. Linear
    d. Simple

30. Which of the following is most likely to be the etiologic cause of meningitis in the newborn?

    a. *Neisseria meningitidis*
    b. *Escherichia coli*
    c. *Listeria monocytogenes*
    d. *Haemophilus influenzae*

31. Drug therapy commonly used to treat absence seizures, in addition to valproic acid, include:

    a. Phenytoin, phenobarbital
    b. Ethosuximide, clonazepam
    c. Phenobarbital, ethosuximide
    d. ACTH, carbamazepine

Answers

1. a	11. c	22. a
2. d	12. c	23. b
3. d	13. a	24. a
4. d	14. a	25. c
5. b	15. d	26. b
6. a	16. d	27. a
7. a	17. b	28. a
8. c	18. c	29. c
9. a	19. c	30. b
10. d	20. b	31. b
	21. b	

Bibliography

American Psychiatric Association. (1994). *Diagnostic and statistical manual of mental disorders* (4th ed.). Washington, DC: Author

Barkin, R., & Rosen, P. (Eds.). (1997). Pediatric emergency medicine: Concepts and clinical practice (2nd ed.). St. Louis: Mosby

Benitz W., & Tatro, D. (1995). *The pediatric drug handbook* (3rd ed.). St. Louis: Mosby.

Behrman, R. E., Kliegman, R. M., & Jenson, H. B. (Eds.). (2000). *Nelson textbook of pediatrics* (16th ed.). Philadelphia: W. B. Saunders.

Berman, S. (1996). *Pediatric decision-making* (3rd ed.). St. Louis: Mosby

Farley, J. A. (1996). Epilepsy. In P. L. Jackson & J. A. Vessey (Eds.). *Primary care of a child with a chronic condition* (pp. 400–419). St. Louis: Mosby.

Hoekelman, R. A., Adam, H. M., Nelson, N. M., Weitzman, M. L., & Wilson, M. H. (Eds.). (2001). *Primary pediatric care* (4th ed.). St. Louis: Mosby.

Parker, S., & Zuckerman, B. (1995). *Behavioral and developmental pediatrics,* a *handbook for primary care.* Boston: Little, Brown & Co.

Roberts, K. (1995). *Manual of clinical problems in pediatrics* (4th ed.). Boston: Little, Brown & Co.

Neurological Disorders In Adults

Sally K. Miller

Headache

- Definition: Very common complaint in primary care; may be actual product of a disease or syndrome (tension or migraine), or symptom of an underlying disorder (giant cell arteritis, structural lesion); since there are many types of headaches, all with varying degrees of severity, proper assessment of headache and associated symptoms is critical

- Etiology/Incidence

  1. Tension (accounts for 90% of all headaches)

  2. Migraine

     a. Classic (occurs with aura)

     b. Common (no aura)

  3. Cluster headaches

  4. Toxic

     a. Viral infection

     b. Medication induced

  5. Subdural hematoma

  6. Subarachnoid hemorrhage—medical emergency requiring immediate hospitalization

  7. Meningeal irritation

  8. Giant cell arteritis

  9. Structural lesion—infrequently presents as headache but must be considered

  10. Referred pain from eyes, ears, sinuses, teeth

  11. Visual strain

  12. Narrow angle glaucoma

  13. Hypertensive headache

- Components of Headache Evaluation

  1. Chronology is most important item—headache of recent onset that becomes progressively more frequent and/or severe is more ominous than extremely intense headache that has presented in same fashion over a period of time

  2. Location, duration and quality—should be evaluated as they will provide clues to the underlying cause

  3. Associated activity—exertion, sleep, tension, relaxation

  4. Timing of menstrual cycle in women

  5. Presence of associated symptoms such as neurological symptoms, systemic symptoms of illness (rhinitis, pharyngitis), symptoms of anxiety or depression (sleep disturbance, inability to concentrate)

6. Presence of triggers—things that seem to be associated with headache onset such as certain foods, stress, alcohol, weather changes

7. Age of onset

Tension Headaches

- Definition: Single most common type of headache evaluated in primary care
- Etiology/Incidence
  1. Physical or emotional stress
  2. Tension producing circumstances
  3. Most common headache in adults
- Signs and Symptoms
  1. Associated complaints of poor concentration and other vague, nonspecific symptoms
  2. Usually lasts for several hours
  3. Usually described as generalized about the head—may be most intense about the neck or back of head
  4. Described as vise-like or tight in quality
  5. Occur frequently during or following stressful circumstances
  6. No associated focal neurological symptoms
  7. No aura
- Differential Diagnosis
  1. Evaluation of social history very important in differentiating tension headache
     a. Work history
     b. Family circumstances
     c. Recent life changes—birth, death, marriage, divorce
  2. Other syndromes producing similar headache patterns
     a. Common migraine
     b. Toxic headache
     c. Hypertensive headache
     d. Referred pain from other structures in the head
     e. Meningeal irritation
- Physical Findings
  1. Often no physical findings
  2. May find cervical muscle pain/tenderness

3. Other findings depending upon severity

   a. Tremor

   b. Disinterest in appearance

- Diagnostic Tests/Findings

  1. None specific to tension headache

  2. Radiographic imaging of head as appropriate to rule out organic disorder

- Management/Treatment

  1. Over the counter analgesics

     a. Acetaminophen 650 to 1000 mg q.i.d.

     b. Aspirin 650 to 1000 mg q.i.d.

     c. Ibuprofen 400 mg q.i.d.

  2. Relaxation or stress reducing techniques

     a. Biofeedback

     b. Massage

     c. Hot baths

  3. Explore underlying cause of stress

  4. When initial measures fail, a trial of anti-migraine agents is appropriate

Migraine Headache

- Definition: An extremely painful headache syndrome that is disabling during acute attack; commonly divided into two categories:

  1. Classic migraine occurring after an aura—aura precedes pain and may include visual disturbances, auditory, visual or olfactory hallucinations, or other neurological symptoms

  2. Common migraine—not associated with an aura

- Etiology/Incidence

  1. Etiology unknown, but theories include:

     a. Dilation and excessive pulsation of the external carotid artery

     b. Excess release of the neurotransmitter serotonin, leading to an inflammatory process involving the trigeminal nerve

  2. Variety of triggers

     a. Emotional or physical stress

     b. Lack of/or excess sleep

     c. Missed meals

       d.   Specific foods

       e.   Alcoholic beverages

       f.   Menstruation

       g.   Changes in weather

       h.   Nitrate containing foods

   3.   Onset usually in adolescence or early adult years

   4.   Often family history of migraine

   5.   Females more often affected than males

- Signs and Symptoms

   1.   Episodic unilateral, lateralized, throbbing headache

   2.   Builds up gradually and lasts several hours or longer

   3.   Focal neurologic disturbances may precede or accompany migraines

   4.   Visual disturbances frequently occur

       a.   Visual field defects

       b.   Luminous visual hallucinations (stars, sparks, zigzag of lights)

   5.   Aphasia, numbness, tingling, clumsiness or weakness

   6.   Nausea and vomiting

   7.   Photophobia

   8.   Phonophobia

- Differential Diagnosis

   1.   Subarachnoid hemorrhage

   2.   Cluster headaches

   3.   Hypertensive headache

   4.   Cerebrovascular accident

   5.   Space occupying lesion

- Physical Findings

   1.   Physical examination usually normal

   2.   Patient appears acutely ill during migraine

   3.   Thorough neurological examination

       a.   Focal deficits may accompany migraine

       b.   Focal deficits may indicate tumor

- Diagnostic Tests/Findings

1. None available specific to migraine

2. Patients with new onset migraine require baseline studies to rule out organic cause; abnormalities may indicate organic cause of pain

   a. Blood chemistries

   b. Complete blood count

   c. Syphilis screening

   d. Erythrocyte sedimentation rate

   e. Radiographic imaging of the head

   f. Other studies indicated by history and physical examination

- Management/Treatment: Prophylactic

   1. Avoidance of trigger factors very important

   2. Relaxation and stress management techniques described in management of tension headache

   3. Pharmacologic therapy if attacks occur more than 2 to 3 times per month

      a. Aspirin 650 to 1950 mg daily

      b. Propranolol 10 to 20 mg b.i.d. starting dose, gradually increase to effective dose of 80 to 120 mg daily—contraindicated in congestive heart failure, obstructive pulmonary disease, diabetes and severe depression

      c. Amitriptyline 10 to 150 mg daily

         (1) Other tricyclic antidepressants helpful

         (2) Must be taken for 2 to 4 weeks before improvement seen

         (3) Contraindicated in cardiac dysrhythmia, narrow angle glaucoma, and urinary difficulties

      d. Selective serotonin reuptake inhibitors (SSRI)

         (1) Newest category, fewer side effects than tricyclic anti-depressants

         (2) Better choice for geriatric patients and those with cardiac disoders

         (3) Fluoxetine, sertraline, paroxetine and venlafaxine are common choices

            (a) Start 10 mg every day at 7 a.m., build to 20 mg in 7 to 10 days

            (b) Contraindicated in severe depression

      e. Calcium channel blockers widely used but not as effective

         (1) Verapamil 40 mg t.i.d., increased to 80 mg t.i.d. over 2 to 3 weeks; maximum dose 160 mg t.i.d.

         (2) Contraindicated in congestive heart failure, heart block, hypotension

- Management/Treatment: Acute Attack

  1. Rest in dark, quiet room

  2. Simple analgesics (aspirin) taken immediately upon onset may provide some relief

  3. Nonsteroidal agents

     a. Naproxen 250 mg repeat in 1 to 4 hours as needed

     b. Ketorolac 10 mg repeat in 1 to 4 hours as needed

  4. Butalbital-containing medications

     a. Aspirin, caffeine, butalbital combination

     b. Acetaminophen, caffeine, butalbital combination

  5. Opiates—may be effective but should be used with caution

     a. Butorphanol 1 mg every 4 hr

     b. Meperidine 75 to 100 mg with hydroxyzine 50 mg IM every 4 hr

  6. Sumatriptan

     a. 6 mg SQ, may repeat in one hour but no more than three times per day

     b. Also available in 25 and 50 mg oral dose and as nasal spray

     c. Contraindicated in coronary artery disease, Prinzmetal's angina, basilar and hemiplegic migraine, uncontrolled hypertension, history of anaphylaxis, and recent ergotamine use

  7. Ergot alkaloids orally or as suppository—contraindicated in pregnancy, uncontrolled hypertension, peripheral vascular disease, coronary artery disease, liver and kidney disease, and concomitant use of sumatriptan

  8. Migranal 2 mg intranasal spray

  9. Medicate for nausea as indicated

  10. Acetaminophen, aspirin, and caffeine preparation (oral)

Cluster Headaches

- Definition: Among the most painful of all pain inducing conditions

- Etiology/Incidence

  1. Intrinsic histamine-mediated dilation of external carotid artery

  2. Decreased oxygen saturation due to intrinsic hypothalamic abnormality stimulates brainstem causing pain

  3. Episodic (90%); chronic (10%)

  4. Cycles occur the same time each year—most often during fall and spring

  5. Males more often affected than females at 5:1 ratio

- Signs and Symptoms

    1. Severe unilateral, orbital, supraorbital and/or temporal pain occuring in clusters of days or weeks with pain free period in between

    2. Pain lasts 15 minutes to 3 hours

    3. Attacks occur 1 to 8 times daily

    4. May rock, pace, or put fist against the painful eye

- Differential Diagnosis

    1. Migraine headache

    2. Narrow angle glaucoma

    3. Structural lesions

- Physical Findings

    1. May be none

    2. Conjunctival injection

    3. Ipsilateral nasal congestion

    4. Rhinorrhea

    5. Forehead or facial sweating

    6. Miosis

    7. Ptosis

    8. Eyelid edema

- Diagnostic Tests/Findings

    1. None diagnostic of cluster headache

    2. As indicated to rule out organic disorders

        a. Computerized axial tomography (CT) scan of the head

        b. Magnetic resonance imaging (MRI) of the head

        c. Complete blood count

        d. Serum chemistries

        e. Erythrocyte sedimentation rate

        f. Electroencephelogram (EEG)

- Management/Treatment: Prophylaxis

    1. Ergotamine tartrate 2 mg every day, 0.5 to 1.0 mg per rectum, or 0.25 mg SQ t.i.d. 5 days weekly

    2. Prednisone 20 to 40 mg daily or q.o.d. for 2 weeks, then taper

    3. Verapamil 240 to 480 mg every day

4. Methysergide 4 to 6 mg every day

- Management/Treatment: Acute Attack

    1. Oral drugs usually not successful

    2. Sumatriptan 6 mg SQ

    3. Ergotamine tartrate aerosol inhalation may be effective

    4. Inhalation of 100% oxygen—typically only effective in case of cluster headache

Transient Ischemic Attack (TIA)

- Definition: Interruption in the cerebral vascular flow, causing ischemia and resultant temporary focal neurologic deficits; two types of TIA—carotid and vertebrobasilar; treatments are same for either type but presenting signs and symptoms differ

- Etiology/Incidence

    1. Embolization is an important cause

        a. Cardiac dysrhythmia

        b. Rheumatic heart disease

        c. Mitral valve disease

        d. Ulcerated plaque on a major artery

        e. Infective endocarditis

        f. Mural thrombus following myocardial infarction

    2. Fibromuscular dysplasia

    3. Inflammatory disorders

        a. Giant cell arteritis

        b. Systemic lupus erythematosus

    4. Hypotension in clients with extracranial artery stenosis

    5. Hematologic disorders

        a. Polycythemia

        b. Sickle cell disease

        c. Severe anemia

    6. Risk factors for vascular disease are often present

        a. Diabetes mellitus

        b. Tobacco use

        c. Hypertension

        d. Elevated serum cholesterol

7. Patients with acquired immune deficiency syndrome (AIDS) at increased risk

8. 30,000 to 150,000 occur annually (may be under reported)

- Signs and Symptoms (Carotid TIA)

    1. Weakness of the contralateral arm, leg, or face, singly or in combination

    2. Numbness or paresthesia of the contralateral side may occur alone or in combination with motor deficits

    3. Homonymous hemianopsia

    4. Ipsilateral monocular vision loss

    5. Symptoms usually disappear within one hour and must resolve completely within 24 hours for a diagnosis of TIA

    6. Any of the above symptoms may occur singly or in combination with other symptoms

- Signs and Symptoms (Vertebrobasilar TIA)

    1. Unilateral or bilateral weakness

    2. Vertigo

    3. Ataxia

    4. Diplopia

    5. Dysarthria

    6. Perioral numbness

    7. Drop attacks may occur due to bilateral leg weakness

    8. Dysphasia

    9. Hearing loss

    10. Symptoms may occur singly or in any combination

    11. Symptoms usually resolve in < 1 hour, must resolve in < 24 hours to be diagnostic of TIA

- Differential Diagnosis

    1. Focal seizures

    2. Classic migraine

    3. Hypoglycemia

- Physical Findings

    1. Physical findings present only during event

    2. Hyperactive deep tendon reflexes

    3. Slowness of movement

4. Flaccid weakness with pyramidal distribution

5. May identify sensory impairment

6. May see atherosclerotic changes on funduscopic examination

7. Carotid artery bruit

8. Cardiac examination may suggest source

    a. Murmur

    b. Dysrhythmia

9. Physical findings absent if patient examined after resolution of symptoms

- Diagnostic Tests/Findings

    1. Clinical and laboratory evaluation must include assessment of risk factors for vascular disease

        a. Complete blood count

        b. Serum glucose

        c. Serum cholesterol

        d. Syphilis screening

        e. Electrocardiogram

        f. Chest radiograph

    2. Echocardiography if cardiac emboli suspected

    3. Evaluate for hypertension

    4. Holter monitor if transient disturbance in cardiac rhythm suspected

    5. CT scan of the head to rule out small hemorrhage, infarct or tumor

    6. Ultrasound to evaluate cerebral circulation and major vessels to head

    7. Arteriography is definitive study of vasculature—should be considered if patient is good operative risk, CT scan is normal, and no apparent source of cardiac emboli present

- Management/Treatment

    1. Medical management aimed toward preventing further attacks as 30% of patients with cerebrovascular accident have history of TIA

        a. Cessation of tobacco use

        b. Control of underlying medical conditions

            (1) Hyperlipidemia

            (2) Diabetes mellitus

            (3) Hypertension

      (4)   Arteritis

      (5)   Hematologic disorders

  c. Immediate anticoagulation when cardiac emboli is strong possibility—intravenous heparin followed by oral warfarin sodium

  d. Aspirin 325 mg daily when cardiac emboli not strong possibility

  e. Platelet inhibitors in those intolerant of aspirin

      (1)   Dipyridamole/ASA 50 mg daily for patients who have had a TIA or CVA while taking aspirin

      (2)   Clopidogrel bisulfate 75 mg daily for patients with aspirin allergy or intolerance—caution with severe liver disease

      (3)   Ticlopidine 250 mg b.i.d. for patients who can not tolerate first line choices—monitor for neutropenia or agranulocytosis

2. Carotid thromboendarterectomy considered when:

  a. Arteriography reveals a surgically accessible stenosis > 70%

  b. Relatively little atherosclerosis elsewhere

  c. Patient is a good surgical candidate

Seizure Disorder

- Definition

  1. A disorder characterized by transient disturbance of cerebral function due to an abnormal paroxysmal neuronal discharge in the brain

  2. Two main classifications of seizure

    a. Partial seizures

        (1)   Simple partial seizure

        (2)   Complex partial seizure

    b. Generalized seizures

        (1)   Absence (petit mal) seizure

        (2)   Myoclonic seizure

        (3)   Tonic-clonic (grand mal) seizure

  2. Partial seizures result from an activation of part of one hemisphere (unilaterally)

  3. Generalized seizures result from a generalized activation of the brain (bilateral)

- Etiology/Incidence

  1. Congenital abnormalities and perinatal injuries may result in seizures presenting in infancy and early childhood

  2. Metabolic disorders

    a. Hypocalcemia

    b. Hypoglycemia

    c. Hyponatremia

    d. Pyridoxine deficiency

    e. Renal failure

    f. Acidosis

    g. Alcohol withdrawal

3. Infectious diseases

    a. Bacterial meningitis

    b. Herpes encephalitis

    c. Neurosyphilis

4. Trauma an important cause in young adults

5. Tumors and other space occupying lesions

6. Vascular disease, an increasingly frequent cause in the older population—most common cause when seizure onset is after age 60

7. May be due to unknown cause

8. Overall affects approximately 0.5% of the population in the U.S.

- Signs and Symptoms: Simple Partial Seizure

1. No loss of consciousness

2. Lasts approximately one minute

3. Focal motor symptoms (convulsive jerking)

4. Speech arrest or vocalizations

5. Jacksonian march

6. Special sensory symptoms

    a. Light flashes

    b. Buzzing

7. Paresthesias

8. Autonomic symptoms

    a. Flushing

    b. Diaphoresis

    c. Pupillary dilation

9. Dysmnesic symptoms (déjà vu)

- Signs and Symptoms: Complex Partial Seizures—any symptoms of simple partial seizure accompanied by a period of impaired consciousness before, during or after episode

- Signs and Symptoms: Absence (Petit Mal) Seizures

  1. Impairment of consciousness

  2. Mild tonic, clonic, or atonic components

  3. Occasional autonomic components

     a. Flushing

     b. Diaphoresis

     c. Enuresis

  4. Onset and termination very brief, lasting seconds—individual may break off in mid-sentence for a few seconds

  5. Almost always begin in childhood

  6. Frequently cease by age 20, occasionally replaced by other forms of generalized seizure

- Signs and Symptoms: Myoclonic Seizures

  1. Single or multiple myoclonic jerks

  2. No loss of consciousness

- Signs and Symptoms: Tonic Clonic (Grand Mal) Seizure

  1. Sudden loss of consciousness

  2. Patient becomes rigid, falls to the ground

  3. Respiration is arrested

  4. Clonic phase follows tonic phase—jerking of body musculature lasting 2 to 3 minutes followed by stage of flaccid coma

  5. Urinary and/or fecal incontinence may occur

  6. Lips or tongue may be bitten

  7. After one tonic-clonic cycle, patient may:

     a. Recover consciousness

     b. Fall into deep sleep (postictal state)—headache, disorientation, soreness, nausea and drowsiness common upon awakening

     c. More attacks after recovering consciousness (serial seizures)

     d. More attacks without recovering consciousness (status epilepticus)

     e. Display postepileptic automatism

        (1) Behave in an abnormal fashion in immediate postictal period

        (2) No subsequent memory of events

*** AN EYEWITNESSES ACCOUNT OF SEIZURE ACTIVITY IS EXTREMELY
VALUABLE AND SHOULD BE OBTAINED IF AT ALL POSSIBLE ***

- Differential Diagnosis: Partial Seizures

  1. Transient ischemic attacks

  2. Rage attacks

  3. Panic attacks

- Differential Diagnosis: Generalized Seizures

  1. Syncope

  2. Cardiac dysrhythmia

  3. Brain stem ischemia

  4. Pseudoseizures

- Physical Findings

  1. May be none

  2. May show evidence of underlying disorder

     a. Trauma

     b. Focal neurological deficits (brain lesion)

     c. Hyperactive reflexes

  3. Muscle soreness following grand mal seizure

  4. Tongue trauma

- Diagnostic Tests/Findings

  1. As indicated to investigate underlying cause as indicated by history and age of patient

  2. Initial evaluation in patients over 10 years of age should include the following tests in order to investigate cause and provide a baseline for subsequent monitoring of long term treatment

     a. Complete blood count

     b. Serum glucose

     c. Liver function tests

     d. Renal function tests

     e. Serologic test for syphilis

  3. Electroencephelogram (EEG) for paroxysmal abnormalities containing spikes or sharp waves

     a. May help classify disorder

     b. Support clinical diagnosis of seizure

     c. Evaluate candidates for surgical treatment by localizing epileptogenic source

  4. CT scan or MRI to rule out lesion or neoplasm when:

     a. Focal neurological signs and symptoms present

     b. EEG findings suggestive of focal disturbance

     c. Onset after age 30

     d. Seizure disorder is progressive

  5. Chest radiograph to rule out primary or secondary neoplasms

  6. Lumbar puncture (LP)—rule out infectious process

- Management/Treatment: Acute Seizure

  1. Diazepam 5 to 10 mg slow IV

  2. Lorazepam 4 mg slow IV

  3. Treatment not indicated for alcohol withdrawal seizures

- Management/Treatment: Preventive

  1. May need to be reported to Department of Motor Vehicles

  2. Treat underlying problem as appropriate

     a. Infectious process

     b. Metabolic disturbance

  3. Pharmacologic choice depends upon type of seizure

  4. Pharmacologic options for generalized tonic-clonic or partial seizures

     a. Phenytoin 200 to 400 mg daily or in divided doses

        (1) Maintain serum level 10 to 20 μg/mL

        (2) Contraindicated in patients with sinoatrial or atrioventricular block

     b. Carbamazepine 600 to 1200 mg in two divided doses daily

        (1) Maintain serum level 4 to 12 μg/mL

        (2) Contraindicated in patients with known hypersensitivity to tricyclic antidepressants, patients with past or present bone marrow depression, and patients on monoamine oxidase inhibitors

     c. Valproic acid 1500 to 2000 mg in three divided doses daily

        (1) Maintain serum level 50 to 100 μg/mL

        (2) Contraindicated in patients with known hepatic disease

  5. Pharmacologic choices for petit mal seizures

     a. Ethosuximide 100 to 1500 mg in two divided doses daily

        (1) Maintain serum level 40 to 100 μg/mL

        (2)   Use with extreme caution in patients with hepatic or renal disease

    b.   Valproic acid at doses indicated for tonic-clonic seizure

    c.   Clonazepam 0.05 to 0.2 mg/kg in two divided doses daily

        (1)   Maintain serum level 20 to 80 ng/mL

        (2)   Contraindicated in patients with known hypersensitivity to benzodiazepines, hepatic disease, chronic respiratory disorders, and untreated glaucoma

6. Pharmacologic choice for myoclonic seizure

    a.   Valproic acid at doses indicated for tonic-clonic seizure

    b.   Clonazepam at doses indicated for petit mal seizure

7. Newer antiseizure medications for adjunctive therapy of partial or secondary generalized seizures

    a.   Gabapentin 900 to 1800 mg daily in divided doses

    b.   Lamotrigine 100 to 500 mg daily in divided doses

    c.   Topiramate 200 to 400 mg daily in divided doses

8. Patients should be advised to avoid dangerous situations

9. When first drug choice does not provide control, add second drug until therapeutic levels obtained, then first drug gradually withdrawn

10. Prophylactic medication not generally indicated based on one seizure unless further attacks occur or investigation identifies untreatable pathology

11. Withdrawal of medication should only be considered when patient has been free of seizure activity for at least four years

    a.   Dose reduction over a period of weeks/months

    b.   Reinstitution of same drug(s) if seizure recurs

Parkinson's Disease

- Definition: Degenerative central nervous system disorder characterized by any combination of tremor, rigidity, bradykinesia or progressive postural instability

- Etiology/Incidence

    1. Degeneration of the dopaminergic nigrostriatal system leads to dopamine depletion and consequently a dopamine/acetylcholine imbalance

    2. Most commonly idiopathic, but causes may include:

        a. Exposure to toxins

            (1) Manganese dust

            (2) Carbon disulfide

(3)   Carbon monoxide

b.   Postencephalitic parkinsonism

3.   Onset usually between 45 and 65 years of age

4.   Approximately equal gender distribution

5.   Occurs in all ethnic groups

- Signs and Symptoms

  1.   Any combination of:

      a.   Tremor

      b.   Rigidity

      c.   Bradykinesia

      d.   Progressive postural instability

  2.   Wooden facies

  3.   Impaired swallowing

  4.   Decreased automatic movement

  5.   Seborrhea of scalp and face

- Differential Diagnosis

  1.   Side effects of high potency neuroleptics

  2.   Brain tumor

  3.   Depression

  4.   Benign essential tremor

  5.   Dementia

  6.   Huntington's disease

  7.   Creutzfeldt-Jakob Disease

- Physical Findings

  1.   Relatively immobile face with wide palpebral fissures

  2.   Infrequent blinking

  3.   Seborrhea

  4.   Myerson's response—repetitive tapping over bridge of nose produces sustained blinking response

  5.   Drooling

  6.   Bradykinesia

  7.   Slow cycle tremor

  8.   No muscle weakness

9. No alteration in deep tendon reflexes or plantar response

10. Slow shuffling steps; loss of automatic arm swing

- Diagnostic Tests/Findings

    1. None specific to Parkinson's disease

    2. As indicated to rule out toxins

    3. As indicated to rule out differential diagnoses

- Management/Treatment

    1. Levodopa/carbidopa 25/100 or sustained release form 50/200 t.i.d.

        a. Improves all clinical features but does not halt progression

        b. Contraindicated in:

            (1) Narrow angle glaucoma

            (2) Psychotic illness

            (3) Patients taking monoamine oxidase A inhibitors

        c. Use caution with malignant melanoma or active ulcer disease

    2. Dopamine agonists—stimulate dopamine receptors in brain; may be used as monotherapy or in combination with levodopa/carbidopa

        a. Ropinirole 0.25 mg to 3 mg t.i.d.—adverse effects include orthostatic hypotension, syncope, hallucinations

        b. Pramipexole 1.5 mg to 6 mg daily—adverse effects include orthostatic hypotension, hallucinations, somnolence, nausea, vomiting

        c. Bromocriptine 1.25 mg b.i.d. titrate to symptom improvement—contraindicated in:

            (1) History of mental illnes

            (2) Recent myocardial infarction

            (3) Peripheral vascular disease

            (4) Bleeding ulcers

    3. Catechol-o-methyl transferase (COMT) inhibitors

        a. Tolcapone 100 to 200 mg t.i.d.

        b. Inhibits enzyme that breaks down levodopa

        c. Should be used with levodopa

        d. Use cautiously in patients with liver disease, particularly women

    4. Selegiline 5 mg b.i.d with breakfast and lunch with Levodopa

        a. Clinical responses not consistent

     b.   Evidence that it arrests the progression of disease requires it be considered for patients with early disease or mild forms

  5. Anticholinergics to alleviate tremor and rigidity

     a.   Benztropine mesylate 1 to 6 mg daily

     b.   Trihexyphenidyl 6 to 20 mg daily

     c.   Biperiden 2 to 12 mg daily

     d.   Poorly tolerated by elderly; side effects include:

       (1) Urinary retention

       (2) Increased intraocular pressure

       (3) Dysrhythmia

       (4) Constiption

     e.   Contraindicated in:

       (1) Narrow angle glaucoma

       (2) Prostatic hypertrophy

       (3) Obstructive gastrointestinal disease

  6. Amantadine 100 mg b.i.d.

     a.   Mode of action unclear

     b.   Improves clinical features in mild disease

     c.   Side effects include confusion, depression, restlessness, hypotension and cardiac abnormalities

  7. Physical therapy and speech therapy may be helpful

  8. Surgical thalamotomy or pallidotomy a consideration for those with severe disease and medication intolerance

Multiple Sclerosis

- Definition

  1. Pathological focal areas of demyelination with reactive gliosis scattered in white matter of brain and in optic nerve; single lesions cannot explain clinical findings

  2. Months or years may pass between initial symptom appearance and recurrence or exacerbation, but eventually progressive disability usually results

  3. Less commonly, symptoms worsen steadily from onset and disability occurs early

- Etiology/Incidence

  1. Cause unknown

  2. May be familial incidence

3. Association with HLA-DR2 antigen suggests genetic predisposition

4. Immunological basis suspected

5. Greatest incidence in young adults—onset usually < 55 years of age

6. More common in persons of Western European descent

7. Certain factors may trigger exacerbation

    a. Pregnancy and postpartum period

    b. Infection

    c. Trauma

- Signs and Symptoms

1. Weakness, numbness, tingling or unsteadiness in a limb

2. Spastic paraparesis

3. Diplopia

4. Disequilibrium

5. Urinary urgency or hesitancy

6. Vertigo

7. Sphincter disturbance

- Differential Diagnosis

1. Anxiety

2. Brain tumor

3. Spinal cord lesion

4. Neurosyphilis

5. Systemic lupus erythematosus

6. Metastatic carcinoma

- Physical Findings

1. Optic atrophy

2. Nystagmus

3. Ataxia

4. Dysarthria

5. Muscle weakness

6. Decreased vibratory sense

7. Hyperactive deep tendon reflexes

8. Positive Babinski with clonus

9. Sensory deficits in some or all limbs

- Diagnostic Tests/Findings

  1. Definitive diagnosis cannot be based on laboratory findings alone

  2. Diagnostic tests as indicated to rule out other causes of symptoms

  3. Mild lymphocytosis

  4. Cerebrospinal fluid abnormalities

     a. Slightly elevated protein

     b. Elevated IgG

     c. Discrete bands of IgG called oligoclonal bands—presence of oligoclonal bands not specific but supportive

  5. Magnetic resonance imaging (MRI) preferred to computerized axial tomography (CT) scan

     a. Demonstrates multiplicity of lesions

     b. Rule out surgically treatable lesions

     c. Visualize foramen magnum to rule out Arnold-Chiari malformation

     d. Neurophysiological assessment of electrocerebral responses to evaluate subclinical involvement of cerebral pathways

- Management/Treatment

  1. No definitive method of arresting disease process, but areas of investigation include:

     a. Immunosuppressive therapy

     b. Plasmaphoresis

     c. Beta interferon used in relapsing-remitting form of disease

     d. Cop 1 (a random polymer-stimulating myelin basic protein) may be helpful to patients with relapsing-remitting form

  2. Methylprednisolone 1 g intravenously for three days followed by prednisone 80 mg daily for one week then tapered for 2 to 3 weeks

     a. May hasten recovery from acute exacerbation

     b. Does not improve the extent of recovery

     c. Does not slow progression of disease

  3. Treatment of urinary retention

     a. Various pharmacologic options to stimulate urination

     b. Intermittent self-catheterization

     c. Indwelling foley catheter last option

4. Diazepam and carbamazepine may relieve paresthesias

5. Antidepressant medications may relieve fatigue

6. Rest/activity balance

7. Treatment of constipation

    a. High fiber diet

    b. Stool softeners/laxatives as indicated

8. Emotional support/patient teaching

    a. Sexual dysfunction may be a problem

    b. Other social/intimacy issues

        (1) Questions regarding marriage

        (2) Questions regarding having children

9. Avoidance of triggers

Questions
Select the best answer

1. The most commonly diagnosed headache is:

   a. Tension
   b. Toxic
   c. Common migraine
   d. Classic migraine

2. Which of the following causes of headache is a medical emergency?

   a. Toxic headache
   b. Classic migraine
   c. Subarachnoid hemorrhage
   d. Subdural hematoma

3. Headache can be a symptom of any variety of medical conditions, as in the case of a structural lesion, or it can be the primary manifestation of a condition as in tension headache. A systematic and thorough assessment of the headache is important in making the appropriate diagnosis. Which of the following components of headache assessment is the most important?

   a. Presence of associated symptoms
   b. Chronology of headache
   c. Presence of triggers
   d. Age of onset

4. Your patient describes a headache that is quite painful and vise-like in quality. The pain is generalized about the head, and lasts for several hours at a time. There does not appear to be an aura, and the patient does not report any symptoms suggestive of focal neurological deficits. Based upon your knowledge of headache evaluation, you know that the most likely diagnosis is:

   a. Cluster headache
   b. Common migraine
   c. Tension headache
   d. Hypertensive headache

5. Migraine and cluster headache are both extremely painful headache syndromes that may be difficult to differentiate. Based on known epidemiological patterns, who is most likely to suffer from migraines?

   a. A 45-year-old male with history of excess alcohol use
   b. A 35-year-old female with history of excess alcohol use
   c. A 19-year-old female with family history of migraine
   d. A 24-year-old male with family history of migraine

6. Excess release of serotonin is proposed as possible etiological factor in:

   a. Migraine headache

b. Seizure disorder

c. Parkinson's disease

d. Multiple sclerosis

7. Which of the following is not typically a trigger of migraine headache?

   a. Menstruation
   b. Excess sleep
   c. Changes in weather
   d. Loud noise

8. Space occupying lesions, subarachnoid hemorrhage, and cerebrovascular accident are all differential diagnoses of migraine headache. If there is any question as to the etiology of the pain, the most appropriate diagnostic intervention would be:

   a. Cerebral arteriogram
   b. Doppler ultrasound of the carotid artery
   c. Complete bloodcount
   d. Computerized axial tomography (CT)

9. When a new diagnosis of migraine is being considered a variety of baseline studies must be performed to rule out an organic cause of the pain. Which of the following would suggest an organic cause of the pain?

   a. Cortical atrophy by CT scan
   b. Elevated erythrocyte sedimentation rate
   c. WBCs $6,000 \times 10^6$/L, Hgb 14.2 g/dL, Hct 43%, Platelets 300,000/μL
   d. Na+ 140 mEq/L, K+ 3.2 mEq/L, Cl 104 mEq/L, CO_2 mEq/L, BUN 11 mg/dL, Cr 0.9 mg/dL

10. Propranolol is a pharmacologic agent used in the prophylactic management of migraine, but there are several contraindications to its use. In which of the following patients is propranolol not contraindicated?

    a. A 40-year-old man with emphysema
    b. A 39-year-old man with angina
    c. A 32-year-old woman with type 1 DM
    d. A 24-year-old man with severe depression

11. Amitriptyline is an antidepressant medication that can be useful in the prophylactic management of migraine headache. Which of the following statements is true regarding amitriptyline therapy for migraine prophylaxis?

    a. It is the only antidepressant that is useful in migraine prophylaxis
    b. Improvement is usually seen in 2-4 weeks
    c. It is contraindicated in severe depression
    d. It has less side effects than paroxetine

12. Cluster headache is among the most painful of all pain inducing conditions. Acute attacks are

difficult to manage. Which of the following therapies is known to be effective only in the case of cluster headache?

    a. Oxygen
    b. Butalbital
    c. Naproxen
    d. Verapamil

13. Many headache inducing conditions are difficult to diagnose because there are no associated physical exam findings. Ptosis, eyelid edema, conjunctival injection and ipsilateral nasal congestion are findings associated with:

    a. Classic migraine
    b. Toxic headache
    c. Narrow angle glaucoma
    d. Cluster headache

14. Tapered corticosteroids are a recommended prophylactic regimen in the treatment of:

    a. Cluster headache
    b. Tension headache
    c. Migraine headache
    d. Subdural hematoma

15. Which of the following is diagnostic criteria for transient ischemic attack?

    a. Numbness or parasthesia with motor deficits
    b. Symptoms resolve in < 24 hours
    c. Symptoms include homonymous hemianopsia
    d. Lacunar infarct on CT scan

16. Medical management of transient ischemic attack (TIA) is aimed toward preventing further attacks and subsequent cerebrovascular accident (CVA). When atrial fibrillation is discovered during the clinical examination, therapy of TIA should include:

    a. Aspirin 325 mg daily
    b. Heparin infusion at 1000 u/hr
    c. Ticlopidine 250 mg b.i.d.
    d. Verapamil 80 mg b.i.d.

17. When is ticlopidine preferred in the management of TIA?

    a. When the patient is intolerant of aspirin
    b. When cardiac emboli is suspected
    c. When heparin has been administered for 5 to 7 days
    d. When the patient is dysrhythmic

18. The most common cause of seizure disorder in the elderly population is?

    a. Congenital abnormalities

b. Renal failure

c. Neurosyphilis

d. Vascular disease

19. A seizure that consists of focal motor symptoms, autonomic symptoms, no loss of consciousness and lasts approximately one minute is most likely a:

    a. Petit mal seizure

    b. Myoclonic seizure

    c. Simple partial seizure

    d. Complex partial seizure

20. Which type of seizure is almost exclusively found in children and young adults?

    a. Myoclonic

    b. Simple partial

    c. Absence

    d. Tonic-clonic

21. Postepileptic automatism is characterized by:

    a. More tonic clonic attacks with periods of consciousness in between

    b. Headache, disorientation and nausea

    c. More tonic clonic attacks without periods of consciousness in between

    d. Abnormal behavior in the immediate postictal period

22. The most important information in seizure assessment is usually provided by

    a. An eyewitness

    b. An electroencephelogram (EEG)

    c. A CT scan

    d. Magnetic resonance imaging (MRI)

23. Initial evaluation of all patients over 10 years of age who present with seizure disorder should not include which of the following?

    a. Serum glucose

    b. Syphilis serology

    c. Renal function tests

    d. Sleep study

24. An EEG is helpful in the evaluation of seizure disorder for several reasons. Which of the following is not accomplished with an EEG?

    a. Classification of the disorder

    b. Etiology of the disorder

    c. Localization of the epileptogenic source

    d. Support of clinical diagnosis

25. The drug of choice for acute seizure management is:

    a. Phenytoin
    b. Clonazepam
    c. Lorazepam
    d. Valproic acid

26. Phenytoin is not indicated for which type of seizure?

    a. Tonic-clonic
    b. Absence
    c. Simple partial
    d. Complex partial

27. When is it appropriate to withdraw seizure medication?

    a. When the patient is pregnant
    b. When the patient has been seizure free for four years
    c. When the patient is an alcoholic
    d. When the patient has untreatable pathology

28. The most common cause of Parkinsonism is:

    a. Postencephalitic
    b. Manganese dust
    c. Exposure to toxins
    d. Idiopathic

29. Immobile face with wide palpebral fissures is a common physical finding in the patient with:

    a. Absence seizure
    b. Depression
    c. Multiple sclerosis
    d. Parkinson's disease

30. Amantadine improves clinical features of mild parkinsonism but has several side effects. Which of the following is not a side effect of amantadine?

    a. Urinary retention
    b. Restlessness
    c. Hypotension
    d. Cardiac abnormalities

31. Which of the following is true regarding the use of corticosteroids in treating multiple sclerosis?

    a. It hastens recovery from exacerbation
    b. It improves the extent of recovery
    c. It slows progression of the disease
    d. It relieves paresthesias

Answers

1. a		11. b		21. d	
2. c		12. a		22. a	
3. b		13. d		23. d	
4. c		14. a		24. b	
5. c		15. b		25. c	
6. a		16. b		26. b	
7. d		17. a		27. b	
8. d		18. d		28. d	
9. b		19. c		29. d	
10. b		20. c		30. a	
				31. a	

Bibliography

Allen, T. G. (1997). Seizure disorders: A primary care guide. *Advance for Nurse Practitioners, 5*(10), 32-34, 40, 66.

Aminoff, M. J. (2001). Nervous system. In L. M. Tierney, Jr., S. J. McPhee, & M. A. Papadakis (Eds.). *Current medical diagnosis and treatment* (40th ed., pp. 969-1027). NY: Lange Medical Books/McGraw-Hill.

Bergman, G. D., Saper, J. R., & Solomon, G. D. (1996). Chronic headache: Management strategies that make sense. *Patient Care, 30*(2), 54-66.

Brodie, M. J., & Dichter, M. A. (1996). Drug therapy: Antiepileptic drugs. *New England Journal of Medicine, 334*(3), 168-175.

Cusack, T. (1996). Multiple sclerosis: Clues to diagnosis and recommended management recertification series. *Physician Assistant, 20*(10), 24, 27-28, 37-39.

Fenstermacher, K., & Hudson, B. (1997). *Practice guidelines for family nurse practitioners.* Philadelphia: W. B. Saunders Company.

Fischer, J. H., French, J., & Leppik, I. E. (1996). Making the most of new seizure treatments. *Patient Care, 30*(1), 53-54, 56, 61-63.

Haider, A., Tuchek, J. M., & Haider, S. (1996). Seizure control: How to use the new antiepileptic drugs in older patients. *Geriatrics, 51*(9), 42-45.

Hely, M. A., & Morris, J. G. L. (1996). Controversies in the treatment of parkinson's disease. *Current Opinions in Neurology, 9*(4), 308-313.

Jones, J. M. (1996). Treating acute pain in the desperate headacher. *Journal of the American Academy of Physician Assistants, 9*(3), 26-28, 33-36, 44.

Psychosocial Disorders In Adults

Sister Maria Salerno

Depression (Major)

- Definition: A clinical syndrome consisting of physical, affective, and cognitive symptoms that range from mild to severe, commonly categorized as:

    1. Adjustment Disorder with Depressed Mood

        a. Occurring within three months of an identifiable stressor

        b. Depressed mood and impairment of function or symptoms in excess of those normally expected

        c. Symptoms ease as stressor passes

        d. Often self limiting but can lead to major depression

    2. Major Depression (MD)

        a. Five of nine symptoms are present continuously during the same two week period

            (1) Presence of depressed mood, OR

            (2) Anhedonia (loss of interest or pleasure in most all activities most of the day) with:

                (a) Increased or decreased appetite or significant weight loss or gain—more than 5% of body weight in a month

                (b) Sleep disturbance—hypersomnia or insomnia

                (c) Psychomotor agitation or retardation

                (d) Fatigue or loss of energy

                (e) Feelings of worthlessness or inappropriate guilt or low self-esteem

                (f) Decreased ability to think, concentrate or make decisions

                (g) Recurrent thoughts of death, suicidal ideation without an attempt or specific plan (American Psychiatric Association, 1994)

        b. The symptoms represent a change from previous functioning and are severe and disabling

        c. The onset is variable and may be superimposed on Dysthymia

    3. Dysthymia (chronic depression)

        a. Milder than MD

            (1) Depressed mood

            (2) At least two other symptoms

            (3) Loss of self-esteem prominent

        b. Poor coping skills

        c. Often associated with chronic drug use

    d. More chronic—symptoms present for two years or more

    e. No clear onset

4. Depressive Disorder Not Otherwise Specified (NOS)

    a. Depressed mood and 2 to 4 moderate to severe symptoms

    b. Does not meet criteria for MD or Dysthymia

    c. Includes several sub-categories

        (1) Atypical Depression—characterized by:

            (a) Hypersomnia

            (b) Hyperphagia

            (c) Lethargy

            (d) Rejection sensitivity

        (2) Seasonal Affective Disorder

            (a) Disturbance of circadian rhythm

            (b) Related to light spectrum exposure

            (c) Carbohydrate craving, lethargy, hyperphagia, and hypersomnia are characteristic

        (3) Premenstrual Dysphoric Disorder—symptoms occur year round during the late luteal phase of the cycle

        (4) Prenatal and Post-Partum Depressions

            (a) 10 to 15% accompanied by obsessive concerns about ability to care for infant or fear of doing harm to the infant

            (b) Usually occurs 2 weeks to 6 months postpartum

5. Bipolar Disorder—recurrent episodes of depression interspersed with bouts of mania

    a. Heredity a strong factor

    b. Tricyclic antidepressants (TCA) often precipitate a manic response called ''hypomania''

    c. Early onset, usually before age 30

    d. Incidence in African-Americans and Whites similar

    e. Incidence is similar in males and females

6. Organic Mood Syndrome—major depressive episode associated with a general medical condition or medications (see Table 1); examples include:

    a. Substance abuse (alcoholism is a common cause)

    b. Endocrinopathy, e.g., hypothyroidism, Cushing's disease, Addison's disease

    c. Neurological disorders—left sided stroke, Parkinsonism

    d. Pancreatic cancer

    e. Antihypertensives

- Etiology/Incidence

  1. Psychosocial and/or biochemical causes for depression have been theorized

    a. Psychosocial

        (1) Psychoanalytical

            (a) Anger turned inward

            (b) Regression to a less mature stage of functioning

        (2) Environmental

            (a) Stressful life events

            (b) Changes or inadequacies in social support

        (3) Psychodynamic

            (a) Personality development

                (i) Passive/dependent

                (ii) Obsessive/compulsive

            (b) Effects of past relationships and developmental task on coping styles, particularly use of defense mechanisms

                (i) Denial

                (ii) Suppression

                (iii) Sublimation

        (4) Cognitive

            (a) Self-reinforcing habit of unrealistic negative ideas

            (b) Recent or past style of thinking and relating

            (c) Learned "helplessness"

    b. Biochemical

        (1) Catecholamine

            (a) Poorly functioning neurotransmitter

            (b) Primarily dopamine, norepinephrine, epinephrine, and serotonin

        (2) Endocrine

            (a) Cortisol

            (b) Thyroid releasing hormone

Table 1
Some Medications and Medical Conditions Which Cause Depressive Symptoms

Anemias
Cardiovascular
    Congestive heart failure
    Hypertension
    Myocardial infarction
    Stroke
Neurological
    Brain tumors
    Dementia
    Parkinsonism
    Multiple sclerosis
    Seizure disorders
Endocrinopathies
    Addison's disease
    Cushing's syndrome
    Diabetes mellitus
    Thyroid disorders
Electrolyte imbalances
Malignancies
    Pancreatic cancer
    Lymphomas
Other
    Chronic fatigue syndrome
    Chronic obstructive pulmonary disease
    Chronic pain
    Hepatitis
    Substance abuse/stimulant withdrawal
    Rheumatoid arthritis
    Renal disease
Medications
    Anabolic steroid withdrawal
    Analgesics
    Antihypertensives (methyldopa, reserpine, clonidine)
    Antitubercular
    Benzodiazepines
    Barbiturates
    Chemotherapeutic agents
    Corticosteroids
    Levo-dopa
    Withdrawal of psychostimulants (amphetamines, cocaine)
    Analgesics

2. Incidence

    a. Depressive illness most common mental health problem seen in general practice

    b. Estimated 9 to 16 million Americans suffer from depressive illness, yet fewer than a third will receive treatment

    c. Twice as many women as men with major depression worldwide

    d. Lifetime risk for developing depressive illness

        (1) 20% for females

        (2) 10% for males

    e. Major depression can occur in any age group

      (1) Adolescents and the elderly at higher risk

      (2) Other risk factors

        (a) Family history of depressive illness, alcoholism, or major medical illness

        (b) Prior depressive episode

        (c) Being postpartum

        (d) Unanticipated or prolonged stress

    f. Major depression has a 50% to 85% recurrence rate within three to nine years

- Signs and Symptoms

  1. None specific

    a. Aggravation of any physical pathology

    b. Pains of undetermined etiology in a variety of anatomical sites

  2. Mnemonic device to recall major symptoms—IN SAD CAGES

    a. *I*nterest—loss of interest or pleasure in just about any activity

    b. *S*leep disturbances

      (1) Hypersomnia or insomnia

      (2) Early morning awakenings with painful ruminations

    c. *A*ppetite change/weight change

    d. *D*epressed mood

      (1) Tends to be most pervasive symptom

      (2) May manifest as crying spells

    e. *C*oncentration poor; indecisiveness, inability to act, procrastination

    f. *A*ctivity—agitation or retardation

    g. *G*uilt/low self-esteem

    h. *E*nergy loss/fatigue

    i. *S*uicidal ideation, thoughts of death, suicide attempts

- Differential Diagnosis

  1. Since depression may be a manifestation of many illnesses the differential diagnosis must include a thorough search for factors or organic diseases which may be responsible for symptom manifestation including:

    a. Infections, inflammation

    b. Neurological neoplasms, stroke, trauma

    c. Endocrine disorders

    d. Nutritional deficiencies

    e. Electrolyte disturbances

2. Differentiate major depression from other mental disorders, e.g., schizophrenia, dementia, adjustment disorder with depressed mood

3. Currently the trend is to address the signs and symptoms of major depression; if criteria presented previously are met the diagnosis is made regardless of co-morbidity

- Physical Findings

    1. General—may show lack of personal grooming and hygiene, inattention to dress, slouched posture, slowed speech and movements, long pauses in response to questions, tearfulness; weight may be less than or more than ideal for body size, may appear dehydrated

    2. Mental status—poor concentration, decreased memory, indecision, pessimism

- Diagnostic Tests/Findings

    1. Initial tests

        a. CBC—normal

        b. Chemical profile including liver function—normal

        c. Urinalysis and urine toxicology screen—normal

        d. Thyroid function—normal

        e. VDRL—normal

        f. B_{12} level—normal

        g. EKG—normal

        h. Chest radiograph—normal

        i. In first or second episode

            (1) Computer tomography (CT) scan or magnetic resonance image (MRI) of the brain—normal

            (2) HIV screen—normal

    2. Depression screening instruments—scores indicative of depression

        a. Beck Depression Inventory

        b. Yesavage Geriatric Depression Scale

        c. Zung Self-Rating Depression Scale

    3. Special tests (primarily used in psychiatric and research settings)

        a. Thyroid stimulating hormone (TSH) response to thyroid releasing hormone (TRH) may be decreased

    b. Dexamethasone suppression test (DST) used to distinguish between major and minor depression

    c. EEG sleep profile—may show reduction in REM sleep

    d. Platelet monoamine oxidase (MAO) activity—increased

    e. Biogenic amines (norepinephrine, serotonin)—increased levels

- Management/Treatment

  1. General considerations

    a. Assess degree of problem related to daily functioning

    b. Refer those with evidence of:

      (1) Hallucinations, delusions

      (2) Loss of contact with reality

      (3) Suicidal thoughts, wishes, tendencies (see section on suicide)

  2. Mild depression (no clear criteria but general functional status tends to be high)

    a. Structured monitoring with weekly appointments with phone contact for backup

    b. Use therapeutic communication skills to:

      (1) Encourage verbalization, clarification of feelings and fears, as well as relationship of feelings to specific events if known

      (2) Assess and discuss losses that have occurred and their meaning

      (3) Help correct cognitive errors in thinking

    c. Use crisis or social skills models to teach and promote more effective coping strategies

      (1) Help client recognize need for and identify alternative coping methods

      (2) Encourage interaction with other people

      (3) Encourage planned, regular physical activity

      (4) Teach relaxation techniques

      (5) Provide client with anticipatory guidance regarding feelings and usual course of the problem, e.g., gradual improvement and abatement of symptoms

    d. Provide consistency and caring, avoiding a judgmental or blaming attitude

    e. Reinforce positive behaviors

    f. Avoid actions or response that could be interpreted as punishment

    g. Consult with physician or psychiatrist regarding psychotherapy and use of antidepressants; both have been shown to be of help in mild depression; see Tables 2 and 3

Table 2

Antidepressants

Drug Name	Anticholinergic Effect	Sedative Effect	Orthostatic Hypotension	Cardiac Conduction	Adult dose range per day (mg)[a]
Tertiary tricyclics					
Amitriptyline	+4	+4	+4	+4	25–300
Clomipramine	+3	+2	+3	+3	25–250
Doxepine	+3	+4	+4	+2	25–300
Imipramine	+3	+2	+4	+4	25–300
Trimipramine	+3	+4	+3	+4	25–300
Secondary Tricyclics					
Amoxapine	+3	+2	+1	+2	50–600
Desipramine	+2	+2	+2	+3	25–300
Nortriptyline	+2	+3	+1	+3	25–250
Protriptyline	+2	+1	+4	+4	15–60
Tetracyclics					
Maprotiline	+2	+4	+2	+3	50–225
Mirtazapine	+3	+2	+2	+2	15–45
Others					
Alprazolam[b]	0	0	0	0	5–6
Buproprion	0	0	0	+1	100–450
Nefazodone	0	+3	+2	0/+1	200–600
Trazadone	0	+4	+4	+1	50–600
Venlafaxine	+1	0	0	+1	75–375
Selective Serotonin Reuptake Inhibitors (SSRI)					
Fluoxetine	0	0	0	0	20–80
Fluvoxamine	0	0	0	0	50–300
Sertraline	0/+1	0	0	0	50–200
Paroxetine	+1	0	0	0	20–50
Monoamine Oxidase Inhibitors (MAO)					
Phenelzine	+1	+1	+1	+3	45–90
Tranylcypromine	0	+1	+1	+2	30–60

Note: Data derived from Bhatia & Bhatia, 1997; Eisendrath, 1997; Pinkowish, 1997; Sussman & Stahl, 1997,
[a]Generally lower doses are recommended for adolescents and the elderly
[b]Only benzodiazepine approved for depression

3. Moderate to severe depression

    a. Hospitalization of those thought to:

        (1) Be a potential danger to self or others; unable to meet basic needs; suicidal ideation or behavior

        (2) Have impaired cognition or judgment

        (3) Need skilled observation for diagnosis, assessment, or monitoring of therapy

        (4) Have inadequate social supports for outpatient treatment

b. Antidepressant and/or antianxiety medications; most appropriate initial therapy for reasonably healthy individual; see Tables 2 and 3

   (1) Those with delusions, hallucinations, profound psychomotor retardation less responsive

   (2) Only 65% have complete remission with any one drug

   (3) No concrete evidence that any one is more efficacious than another

   (4) Choice based on predominant symptoms, side effects, cost, and complexity of dosing—affect compliance

   (5) Most will respond within three weeks of reaching therapeutic levels

   (6) Continue medication full 6 to 12 months after complete remission of symptoms

   (7) When drugs are discontinued taper over 6 to 8 weeks

   (8) Long term prophylaxis—full treatment dosage for those with recurrent episodes (at least three)

   (9) Some controversy regarding efficacy in Minor Depression, Dysthymia, and Adjustment Disorder

  (10) Heterocyclics (tricyclics, tetracyclics, and others)

     (a) Major advantage over newer agents is cost

     (b) Start with low dose and build to therapeutic level

     (c) Plasma levels provide crude indication of compliance with regimen

     (d) May require up to three weeks at therapeutic levels before effects are noticed

     (e) Side effects—anticholinergic, antihistaminic, antiadrenergic, and quinidine-like (except trazadone) effects

     (f) Among tricyclics, desipramine and nortriptyline are least anticholinergic, sedating, and least likely to cause postural hypotension

     (g) Among heterocyclics, trazodone lacks conduction problems and anticholinergic effects, but very sedating; also very low lethality in overdose

     (h) Dispense in small amounts; 10 day supply in many cases can be lethal

  (11) Newer agents include the serotonin reuptake inhibitors (SSRI) and the phenylaminoketones

     (a) Relatively safe for use in elderly

     (b) Do not cause postural hypotension

     (c) Little if any effect on cardiac conduction

   (d) Do not have antihistaminic effects

   (e) With the exception of paroxetine do not have anticholinergic effects

   (f) Starting dose may be effective treatment dose

   (g) SSRI all inhibit cytochrome P-450 system in the liver; must monitor for potential toxicity of other drugs such as anticonvulsants, digitalis, and coumadin

   (h) Buproprion has no effect on liver enzymes, and does not cause sexual side effects common to other antidepressants

   (i) Side effects of anxiety, insomnia, agitation with newer agents may require concomittant use of sedating antihistamine, antidepressant, or anxiolytic

   (j) Pharmacokinetic differences in the elderly can lead to toxicity or efficacy at lower than expected doses

   c. Psychotherapy

   d. Electroconvulsive therapy (ECT)

   (1) More rapid improvement than with pharmacologic agents

   (2) Indicated for severely depressed or suicidal persons for whom pharmacologic agents are contraindicated or ineffective

   (3) Barbiturates and muscle relaxants used prior to the procedure

   (4) Confusion, headache, temporary amnesia lasting one to two weeks are common side effects in about 40%; may be clinically apparent up to one month

   (5) Avoided in persons with brain tumor, recent (three months) MI, CVA, or perforated viscus repair

   e. Other options include exercise and light therapy

4. Client education

   a. Disease course, expected outcomes, and usual treatment modalities

   b. Purpose, dosage, side effects of medication

   (1) Improvement in symptoms not evident for 3 to 4 weeks

   (2) Importance of adhering to prescribed pharmacologic regimen; avoid abrupt discontinuation of medications

   (3) Caution against concomitant use of over-the-counter preparations

   (4) Interactions with food or other medications; see Table 3

5. Persons with major depression should be followed at least weekly for first 6 to 8 weeks, preferably by a mental health professional for medication adjustment and brief psychotherapeutic support

Table 3

Antidepressants and Anti-Anxiety Medications: Contraindications and Precautions

Drug Group	Contraindications	Precautions
Antidepressants		
Tricyclics	Acute M.I., hypersensitivity; concurrent administration of MAO inhibitors	In patients with urinary retention; prostatic hypertrophy; narrow angle glaucoma, convulsive disorders; cardiovascular disease; thyroid disease; pregnant patients
MAO inhibitors	Hypertension, cardiovascular disease, headaches, liver disease or advanced renal disease, concurrent use of a tricyclic; schizophrenia	Safety during pregnancy not established; avoid fermented foods, pickles, cheeses, red wine, beer, fava beans, raisins, chocolate; cold remedies, weight reduction meds, e.g., anything with tyramine
Lithium Carbonate	Significant renal disease, dietary salt restriction; cardiovascular disease; brain damage	Use caution with pregnant patients; elderly; patient who is breast feeding; persons with thyroid disease; mild renal and cardiovascular disease; epilepsy
Anti-anxiety Drugs		
Benzodiazepines	Glaucoma, hypersensitivity	Use caution if hx of allergies; psychological addiction to these drugs; hepatic or renal impairment; lower dose for elderly or breast feeding mothers
Carbamazepine	Severe renal, cardiovascular, or liver disease	Use with caution if liver, renal disease, or blood dyscrasias
SSRI[a]	Do not administer with MAO inhibitors or with tryptophan supplements	Caution in persons with history of seizures; impaired renal or hepatic function; mania or hypomania; in pregnant or nursing women; in the elderly

[a]Selective Serotinin Uptake Inhibitors

6. Persons known to be on antidepressants or receiving care for depression, who are being seen for other reasons should be routinely checked for:

   a. Suicidal feelings, plans, intentions, risks

   b. Tremor, blurred vision, dry mouth, tachycardia, postural hypotension

Suicide

- Definition

   1. The intentional taking of one's own life

   2. Usually described as:

      a. Attempted—unsuccessful conscious attempt to take one's own life

      b. Threatened—verbal or physical indication of intent for self-destruction

      c. Ideation—thoughts or behaviors indicating conscious intent for self-destruction

- Etiology/Incidence

   1. Often a manifestation or complication of depressive illness or anxiety states

   2. About 15% of depressed patients commit suicide

   3. Risk factors include:

    a. Sudden crisis or loss

    b. Destructive coping mechanisms

    c. Few or no significant others

    d. Poor social or personal resources

    e. Past suicide attempts or family history of suicide

    f. Previous psychotic problems

    g. Unstable life style

    h. Specific plan

    i. Substance abuse

4. Eight of 10 persons who state an intent to commit suicide do so; risk for depressed patients is greatest during the first month of treatment when the individual begins to feel better and has more energy

5. In the U.S. women attempt suicide more often, but men are three times as likely to succeed; in elderly, suicide among males outnumber those among women

    a. Female rates peak at age 55

    b. Male rates peak at age 75

6. Adolescents and white males over the age of 45 have a higher incidence rate; second leading cause of death in adolescent

7. In adolescents increased risk has been associated with:

    a. Extreme parental control or permissiveness

    b. Loss of communication with parents and teachers

    c. Hostility and difficulty in school or with the law

    d. Lack of social supports (peers, social, work, and school)

- Signs and Symptoms

1. Feelings of worthlessness and/or helplessness

2. Preoccupation with a dead relative or friend

3. Excessive denial, indignation, or anger in response to being questioned about suicide

4. Verbalization of a plan or rehearsal of a plan

5. Sudden mood elevation in a depressed patient often accompanied by more energy and calmer, more placid manner

6. Giving possessions away

7. Setting affairs in order

8. Making a will

9. Presence of hallucinations or delusions

10. Intuition on the part of the health professional

11. In adolescents these may be more prominent

    a. Taking excessive risks

    b. Self-destructive behaviors, e.g., drug abuse, accident proneness

    c. Negative self-concept

    d. Expression of wish to die

    e. Withdrawal from family and persons

    f. Increased interest and companionship with animal/pets

12. All depressed clients need to be asked about suicide. If client does not volunteer information, ask directly about thoughts of taking their own life. Also ask direct questions to elicit information about a plan, its lethality, and any mental or actual rehearsals of the plan. Risk is highest if planned in 24 hours; low or moderate if planned for a later time

    a. Presence of five or more risk factors constitutes high risk

    b. Mnemonic device to recall risk factors—SAD PERSONS

        (1) *S*ex

        (2) *A*ge

        (3) *D*epression

        (4) *P*revious attempt

        (5) *E*thanol abuse

        (6) *R*ational thinking diminished

        (7) *S*ocial support loss or absence

        (8) *O*rganized plan

        (9) *N*o spouse

        (10) *S*ick

- Differential Diagnosis

    1. Depression with melancholic features

    2. Depression with seasonal pattern (seasonal affective disorder)

    3. Organic disease

- Physical Findings

    1. No specific physical findings, however those of depression may be evident

        a. General appearance—unkempt, slumped or stooped posture, slow speech pattern, lack of expression or dejected look or agitation, hostility, tremulousness

      b. Mental status—disorientation, poor concentration, agitation, hallucinations or delusions

    2. Old scars or evidence of injury from past attempts or high risk behaviors

- Diagnostic Tests/Findings: There are no specific laboratory tests. See Diagnostic Tests/ Findings in section on Depression

- Management/Treatment

    1. Treatment usually includes hospitalization with psychotherapy, antidepressant medications, and/or ECT; see previous section on Management and Treatment of Depression

    2. If a client is deemed suicidal or if there is concern about the client's potential for suicide, do not leave the client alone but obtain immediate psychiatric consultation

Anxiety

- Definition

    1. An unpleasant feeling of dread, apprehension, foreboding, or tension resulting from an unexpected threat to one's feelings of self-esteem or well-being

    2. Major categories

        a. Generalized Anxiety Disorder—unrealistic or excessive anxiety and worry about life circumstance

        b. Panic Disorders—unfounded morbid dread of seemingly harmless object or situation often leads to agoraphobia

        c. Obsessive Compulsive Disorder (OCD)—repetitive thoughts (obsession) that a person is unable to control and/or urge to perform an act that cannot be resisted without great difficulty (compulsion), and which interferes with functional abilities

        d. Post-traumatic Stress Disorder (PTSD)—delayed (at least six months) anxiety after a severe trauma often perceived as a threat to physical integrity or self-concept; intrusive thoughts, flashbacks, and nightmares form the symptomatic triad

        e. Other categories include adjustment disorder with anxious mood, simple and social phobias; refer to psychiatric or major primary care text for detailed discussion

- Etiology/Incidence

    1. Various theories related to etiology include:

        a. Psychodynamic

            (1) Freudian—conflict between id and superego; ego not strong enough to resolve the conflict

            (2) Sullivanian—fear of disapproval from mother figure; conditional love

leads to fragile ego, lack of self-confidence, lack of self-esteem, fear of failure

      (3) Dollar and Miller—learned response to innate drive to avoid pain; anxiety the result of two competing drives or goals

  b. Biologic

      (1) Genetic influence with high family incidence

      (2) Autonomic nervous system response—fight or flight mechanism

      (3) Biologic abnormalities of neurotransmitter receptors in the central nervous system, particularly gamma aminobutyric acid (GABA) receptors

  c. Family dynamics

      (1) Individual with dysfunctional behavior is representative of family system problems

      (2) Carrier of problems resulting from disrupted interrelationships

2. Incidence

  a. Anxiety disorders occur in 10% to 15% of clients seen in health care settings

      (1) Only 1 in 4 diagnosed and treated

      (2) 3% of Americans will experience an anxiety disorder in their lifetime

      (3) Slight preponderance in woman

  b. Panic disorders

      (1) Occur more frequently in women than in men

      (2) Onset usually in late teens or early adulthood

      (3) More common in those who have had an early traumatic event, e.g., the death of a parent

  c. Obsessive compulsive disorder

      (1) Most often seen in adolescence and early adulthood

      (2) Males and females affected equally

      (3) More frequent in upper middle class and in persons with higher levels of intellectual functioning

- Signs and Symptoms

  1. Generalized anxiety and panic attacks

    a. A feeling of tightness in the throat

    b. Difficulty breathing; feelings of suffocation

    c. Palpitations

    d. Chest tightness or pain

    e. Tachypnea, tachycardia

    f. Gastric distress or discomfort

    g. Nausea

    h. Diarrhea

    i. Feeling of weakness in lower limbs

    j. Tingling, numbness of extremities

    k. Feeling of light-headedness

    l. Dryness of the mouth

    m. Feeling of something caught in the throat

    n. Cold sweaty hands

    o. Feelings of loss of control; irritability; impatience

    p. Motor tension—shakiness, jitteriness, trembling, restlessness

    q. Anxiety insomnia, difficulty falling asleep

    r. Symptoms of panic generally develop suddenly and have been related to mitral valve prolapse

2. OCD

    a. Recurrent, persistent thoughts, ideas or images experienced as intrusive

    b. Repetitious, purposeful, intentional behaviors which are distressing, time consuming, or interfere with functioning

3. PTSD

    a. Intrusive thoughts, flashbacks, nightmares related to the traumatic event

    b. Poor impulse control, unpredictability, and/or aggressiveness

    c. Avoidance symptoms

        (1) Avoids reminders of event

        (2) Memory difficulty

        (3) Detachment and restricted affect

    d. Hyperarousal symptoms

        (1) Hypervigilance

        (2) Insomnia

        (3) Irritability, poor concentration

- Differential Diagnosis

  1. Drug abuse, withdrawal, or intoxication

  2. Thyrotoxicosis

    3.   Hypoglycemia

    4.   Acute hypoxia

    5.   Myocardial infarction

    6.   Pheochromocytoma

    7.   Seizure disorder

    8.   Side effects of chemical agents or medications, e.g., caffeine, nicotine, antihistamines, tricyclics

- Physical Findings

    1.   Between attacks may all be within normal limits

    2.   During an attack

        a.   General appearance—looks worried, frightened, restless

        b.   Vital signs—tachycardia, increased respirations, elevated BP

        c.   Integumentary—pallor, flushed face, cold clammy hands

        d.   Gastrointestinal—possible loss of bowel or bladder control

        e.   Mental status—hypervigilence; easy distractibility; poor concentration

        f.   Motor tension—shakiness, jitteriness

- Diagnostic Tests/Findings.

    1.   Serum drug analysis—negative

    2.   Thyroid function tests—normal

    3.   Serum glucose—normal

    4.   ECG—normal

- Management/Treatment

    1.   Depends on careful workup and identified anxiety subtype

    2.   Obtain consult regarding testing for other emotional or physical disorders

    3.   Cognitive behavioral therapy more effective for generalized anxiety than for panic attacks

        a.   Assess usual coping mechanisms, life style, social supports

        b.   Establish a trusting, warm, empathetic, respectful relationship

        c.   Assist client to identify and describe emotional and physical feelings and to identify the relationship between them

        d.   Identify patient behaviors that cause anxiety in the health care provider

        e.   Use supportive confrontation as needed

        f.   Keep focus of responsibility on the client

    g. Encourage use of and teach or refer for relaxation techniques, biofeedback, and meditation

4. Anti-anxiety medications (see Tables 3 and 4)

    a. Most have behavioral profile similar to alcohol

    b. All have hypnotic properties

    c. All have varying potential for tolerance and physiologic dependence

    d. Benzodiazepines most widely used

        (1) Therapeutic doses usually do not result in physiologic dependence

        (2) May be misused to ''boost'' effects of methadone

    e. Antihistamines for those with COPD or potential for abuse of benzodiazepines

    f. Beta adrenergic blockers, e.g., propranolol more effective in reducing marked autonomic symptoms (tachycardia, palpations, breathlessness)

    g. Tricyclics and MAO inhibitors good for panic attacks but not for generalized anxiety

    h. Buspirone only anxiolytic not classified as a tranquilizer

        (1) Not linked to dependence or depressant effects

        (2) Does not impair motor skills

        (3) Does not potentiate alcohol effects

    i. Optimal duration of treatment not well established

5. Refer to psychiatric mental health professional for counseling and more specific therapy

6. Obtain consult regarding testing for other physical or emotional disorders

7. Patient education

    a. Disease course, expected outcome

        (1) Reassurance that anxiety rarely evolves into a more serious disorder

        (2) Reassurance that symptoms can be alleviated with appropriate therapy

        (3) Condition is temporary and with appropriate therapy and time, anxiety may be alleviated

        (4) Dosage, side effects, expected action of pharmacologic agents

    b. Chart attacks—date, time, situation, level of anxiety or symptoms on a scale of 0 to 10

Table 4

Anti-anxiety Medication

Generic	Average daily dose*
Benzodiazepines (Longer acting)	
Chlordiazepoxide	15–40 mg
Clorazepate dipotassium	15–60 mg
Diazepam	4–40 mg
Halazepam	60–160 mg
Benzodiazepines (Shorter acting)	
Alprazolam	0.75–1.5 mg
Lorazepam	2–6 mg
Oxazepam	30–60 mg
Nonbenzodiazepines	
Buspirone	20–30 mg
Hydroxyzine	30–300 mg
Meprobamate	400–2000 mg
Paroxetine	40 mg
For control of aggression/and mania	
Carbamazepine	100–200 mg initially Increase to 400–1500 mg until serum level is 8–12 µg/ml

*Most divided in 2 to 4 portions per day. Elderly would have lower averages and treatment resistant patients might have much higher averages than those shown.

Alcoholism

- Definition

    1. Recurrent use of alcohol to the extent it significantly interferes with the individual's physical, social, and/or emotional life

    2. Characterized by preoccupation with the drug, loss of control over its use, physical dependence, and tolerance

- Etiology/Incidence

    1. Multifactorial and poorly understood; several etiologic theories have been developed

        a. Psychological

            (1) Retarded ego, weak super ego

            (2) Fixed in lower level of psychosocial development

                (a) Dependent personality with poor impulse control

                (b) Low frustration tolerance

                (c) Low self-esteem

            (3) No evidence to support distinct personality predisposition

    b. Biologic

        (1) Physiologic changes in enzymes, genes, brain chemistry, hormones cause the disorder

        (2) May be familial, inherited or acquired

2. About 1 in 12 persons have serious problems related to alcohol use

    a. Children of alcoholics are four times as likely to develop alcoholism as children of non-alcoholics

    b. Three times as many men as women are alcoholics and they are more likely to develop the problem early in life

    c. Highest prevalence of drinking problems in 18 to 29 year olds

3. Risk factors include:

    a. Use of alcohol or other psychoactive substance

    b. Family history of alcohol abuse

    c. Being a young single male

    d. Heavy drinking—five or more drinks in one sitting or getting drunk once a week

    e. Family or social background that accepts or promotes intoxication

    f. Ready accessibility

- Signs and Symptoms

1. Definite (Level I)

    a. Blackouts

    b. Alcoholic hepatitis

    c. Withdrawal symptoms—hallucinations; fine tremors of face, tongue and hands; disorientation; seizures

    d. Memory loss, confabulation

    e. Nystagmus

    f. Prior exhibition of signs and symptoms of levels II and III

2. Probable (Level II)

    a. Previous diagnosis of:

        (1) Cirrhosis

        (2) Pancreatitis without cholelithiasis

    b. Loss of control over alcohol intake/increased alcohol tolerance

    c. Numbness of hands and feet

    d. Increased incidence of infection

    e.   Weight loss

    f.   Forgetfulness

    g.   Trauma from accidents or altercations—cigarette burns, healed fractures

    h.   Hypothermic injuries

    i.   Attempted suicide

    j.   Symptoms of associated diseases; see Table 5

3.   Possible (Level III)

    a.   Blurred or dim vision

    b.   Nocturnal diuresis

    c.   Anxiety or depression

    d.   Impotence

    e.   Symptoms of associated diseases; see Table 6

    f.   History of chronic gastritis, anemia, clotting disorders, marital discord or loss of significant relationships (job, family, friends)

- Differential Diagnosis

1.   Distinguish from a wide variety of medical and psychiatric problems that may account for signs and symptoms, e.g., depression, anxiety, endocrinopathies, viral hepatitis

2.   Determine level of alcoholism and look for concurrent abuse of other substances

    a.   Use history and physical evidence to determine stage and further testing

    b.   Use of CAGE screening test (Buck, Shaw, Cleary, Delbanco & Aronson, 1987)

        (1)   Four questions related to drinking patterns

        (2)   Scores > 2 indicate alcoholism

    c.   Use of an addiction severity tool such as the Michigan Alcohol Screening Test (MAST)

        (1)   25 item questionnaire with 90% sensitivity and 74% specificity

        (2)   Scores > 5 indicative of alcoholism

    d.   Short MAST (SMAST) (Pokorny, Miller & Kaplan, 1972)

        (1)   13 questions

        (2)   Score > 3 indicative of alcoholism

        (3)   Sensitivity 70%, specificity 74%

Table 5

Conditions Commonly Associated With Substance Abuse

1. Frequent upper respiratory infection
2. Slowly healing skin ulcers
3. Recurrent vaginal infections
4. Hepatitis
5. Sexually transmitted disease
6. Mononucleosis
7. Malnutrition
8. HIV infection
9. Pancreatitis
10. Tuberculosis

- Physical Findings

    1. Definite (Level I)

        a. General appearance—fearful, anxious, stuporous, hyperactive, or incoherent

        b. Vital signs—mild fever, tachycardia, increased or labile B.P.

        c. Integumentary—flushed face and/or palms, spider nevi, angiomas on face, numerous scars, ecchymotic areas; generalized tissue edema, and dry, dull hair

        d. HEENT—pupil constriction, nystagmus, parotid adenopathy, inflamed buccal cavity, alcoholic odor to breath, fissures at corners of mouth

        e. Cardiovascular—tachycardia; dysrhythmias; weak, irregular peripheral pulses

        f. Abdomen—gastric distention, ascites, enlarged liver, tenderness

        g. Musculoskeletal—muscle wasting, healed or new fractures

        h. Neurological—memory loss, confabulation, hallucinations, disorientation, fine motor tremors, unsteady ataxic gait

    2. Probable (Level II) and Possible (Level III)

        a. General appearance—no major abnormalities

        b. Vital signs—normal or possible tachycardia, hypertension, and cardiac dysrhythmias

        c. Integumentary—unexplained ecchymosis

        d. HEENT—parotid adenopathy, angiomas

        e. Abdomen—hepatomegaly, tenderness

        f. Neurological—hyperreflexia; unsteady walk, ataxia (Wernicke-Korsakoff Syndrome)

- Diagnostic Tests/Findings

    1. Blood alcohol/drug levels—may or may not be severely elevated depending on amount and time of consumption

        a. 300 mg/100 mL at anytime = definite diagnosis

      b.   100 mg/mL on routine exam = definite diagnosis

      c.   150 mg/mL without evidence of intoxication = alcohol tolerance

2. CBC—increased or depressed white count; microcytic, hypochromic or macrocytic, megaloblastic anemia; decreased platelets

3. Blood glucose—hyper or hypoglycemia

4. Electrolytes—hypokalemia and hypomagnesemia

5. Liver function—all may be increased

      a.   Gamma glutamyl transferase (GGT)— > 30 units/L suggests heavy drinking

      b.   Alanine aminotransferase (ALT)

      c.   Aspartate aminotransferase (AST)

      d.   Lactate dehydrogenase (LDH)

6. Total bilirubin, triglycerides, cholesterol, amylase—increased

7. Prothrombin time—prolonged

8. Urinalysis—infection, ketones

9. Nutritional—albumin and total protein decreased, folic acid low

10. Chest radiograph—enlarged heart, right lower lobe pneumonia

11. ECG—dysrhythmias, cardiac myopathies, ischemic heart disease

- Management/Treatment

1. Consult with physician regarding treatment and possible need for detoxification

2. Confront client with diagnosis ''Alcoholism''

3. Do not use nebulous statements, e.g., ''We think you might have a drinking problem'' or ''You need to cut down on your drinking''

4. Tell the client it is a disease and treatable

5. Tell the client it is not his/her fault but he/she IS responsible for accepting treatment and the goal of therapy is abstinence

6. Describe treatment options; many treatment programs will not accept pregnant women

7. Make appropriate referral for treatment and follow-up

      a.   Alcoholics Anonymous (most successful)

      b.   Behavioral approaches

      c.   Rational emotive psychotherapy

      d.   Psychodrama

8. Provide family members with information on alcoholism and encourage involvement in Al-Anon (for families of alcoholics) and/or Ala-Teen and Ala-Tots (for teenagers and young children of alcoholics)

9. General considerations

    a. Alcoholic women have a higher incidence of suicide attempts than both alcoholic men and the female population as a whole; see section on suicide

    b. Females, even with less alcohol consumption are more likely to develop liver disease than males

    c. Alcohol use by pregnant women is the leading cause of mental retardation

    d. Women's drinking and drug problems are often viewed as less serious than men's and are more frequently misdiagnosed

    e. If seeing a patient who was referred for treatment of alcoholism, reinforce participation in treatment and use of any agreed upon treatment aids

    f. Avoid compounding the problems or hindering recovery by prescribing sedatives or other depressants (cross tolerance)

Psychoactive Substance Abuse

- Definition

    1. Misuse of any substance capable of producing altered state of consciousness and/or euphoria

    2. Addiction or compulsive use includes:

        a. Psychologic craving

        b. Physiologic dependence (withdrawal symptoms with discontinuance)

        c. Tolerance (need for larger and larger doses to produce desired effect)

- Etiology/Incidence

    1. As with alcohol abuse, several theories have been developed to explain the cause of substance abuse which include:

        a. Psychologic

            (1) Failure to complete developmental tasks

            (2) Underdeveloped ego

            (3) Dependent personality

            (4) Poor impulse control

            (5) Ego breakdown with subsequent drug use as a coping mechanism

        b. Biologic hereditary/genetic factors

            (1) Neurotransmitter deficiency

            (2) Enzyme deficiency

    c.   Family dynamics

       (1)   Dysfunctional family system

       (2)   Absent parent

       (3)   Tyrannical or weak ineffective parent

       (4)   Negative role models

       (5)   Drugs used for stress relief

       (6)   Cultural perceptions of drug abuse

2.   Incidence

    a.   Drug use is the leading cause of death among teens

    b.   26% of female and 24% of males between the age of 12 to 17 years have used an illicit drug

    c.   More than 1 million women on legal psychoactive drugs

    d.   66% of psychoactive drugs are prescribed for women

    e.   Most commonly used substances alone or in combination (see Table 6)

       (1)   Depressants—benzodiazepines, barbiturates, opiates, morphine, heroin, alcohol, sedatives, hypnotics, and minor tranquilizers

          (a)   Most widely used and abused drugs

          (b)   Often prescribed for anxiety, depression, or sleep disorders

       (2)   Stimulants (amphetamines, cocaine, caffeine, tobacco)

          (a)   Most commonly abused stimulants other than caffeine and nicotine are amphetamine and cocaine

          (b)   Twice as many males as females use stimulants primarily in the 21 to 44 year age range

       (3)   Hallucinogens (lysergic acid diethylamide, L.S.D.; myristicene, nutmeg; dimethyltryptamine, DMT; psilocybin, magic mushroom; phencyclidine, PCP or angel dust; mescaline, peyote; cannabis, hashish and marijuana; and chemically related substances)

    f.   Solvents/gases

       (1)   Used to reproduce effects of depressants, stimulants, hallucinogenics

       (2)   Produce inebriation similar to volatile anesthetics.

       (3)   Examples include gasoline, paint thinners, correction fluid

- Signs and Symptoms

   1.   Depressants

     a.   Nausea/vomiting

Table 6

Commonly Abused Drugs

Generic or Trade Name	Street/Slang name
Depressants	
Codeine	School boy
Meperidine HCL (Demerol)	Demies
Hydromorphone HCL (Dilaudid)	Little D
Heroin	H; horse; junk; downtown; hard stuff; scag; white stuff
Methadone HCL	Meth; dollies
Morphine	M; Miss Emma; morph
Opium	Black stuff; blue velvet
Methaqualone (Qualude)	Ludes; 714s; Qs; soapers
Pentobarbital	Downers; yellow jackets
Amobarbital/secobarbital (comb.), Phenobarbital	Blues; red hearts; purple hearts; reds; F40s; rainbows
Benzodiazepines (Librium, Valium)	Tanks, downs
Stimulants	
Cocaine	Coke; snow; flake; toot; uptown; crack; blow
Dextoamphetamines;	Bennies; black beauties; copilots
Methamphetamines (Benzedrine)	Dexies; speed; meth; crank
Biphetamine (Desoxyn; Dexedrine)	Crystal; uppers
Hallucinogens	
Lysergic acid diethylamide	LSD; acid
Mescaline (peyote)	Buttons; cactus; mesc.
Myristicin	Nutmeg
Dimethyltryptamine	DMT, STP
Psilocybin	Magic mushroom
Phencyclidine HCL	PCP; angel dust; DOA; peace pill, hog
Marijuana	Pot; maryjane, chronic

    b. Myalgia, deep bone or muscle pain (methadone abusers)

    c. Rhinorrhea, sneezing, excessive lacrimation

    d. Headache

    e. Miosis

    f. Euphoria

    g. Apathy, dysphoria, depression

    h. Drowsiness, psychomotor retardation, slurred speech

    i. Impaired attention, memory, social judgment (disinhibition)

    j. Ataxia, tremors, lack of coordination

    k. Mood swings, aggression, combativeness; loss of impulse control

    l. Auditory hallucinations, paranoia

    m. Fever, perspiration (with withdrawal)

2. Stimulants

    a. Restlessness, irritability, anxiety, confusion, aggression

b. Tachycardia, cardiac dysrhythmia, chest pain (cocaine), increased blood pressure

c. Elation, grandiosity

d. Perspiration or chills

e. Hyper or hypothermia

f. Abdominal pain, nausea/vomiting, diarrhea, frequent urination

g. Insomnia

h. Paranoia, hallucinations (visual and tactile with cocaine)

i. Dilated pupils

3. Hallucinogenics

a. Dilated pupils, vertical and horizontal nystagmus

b. Flushed skin

c. Increased pulse and B.P.

d. Marked anxiety; panic paranoia

e. Hallucinations, visual and sensory distortions

f. Rapid, severe mood changes, hostility, aggression, violence

g. Depression, suicidal thoughts

h. Grandiosity, euphoria

i. Tremors

j. Flashbacks

k. Insensitivity to pain

4. Solvents/gases (inhaled)

a. Euphoria

b. Slurred speech

c. Hallucinations/confusion

d. Unconsciousness

e. Cardiopulmonary depression or failure

- Differential Diagnosis

1. Poly abuse is common and may present with intoxication, overdose, and/or in various stages of withdrawal

2. Rule out other disorders that may account for presenting signs and symptoms, e.g.

a. Seizure disorders

b. Hypo or hyperthyroidism, thyroid storm

     c. Hyper or hypoglycemia

     d. Schizophrenia, mania

     e. Head injury

- Physical Findings: In addition to drug specific signs, some general physical findings might include:

  1. General appearance—unkempt, poor hygiene

  2. Vital signs—temperature elevation, increased or decreased BP, tachycardia, tachypnea

  3. Integumentary—bruises, burns, needle marks, infections, cellulitis, ulcerations, abscesses

  4. HEENT—changes in pupil size, reaction to light, and extraocular movements; poor oral hygiene, puncture wounds under the tongue, pharyngitis, inflammation and or erosion of the nasal mucosa

  5. Abdomen—tenderness, organomegaly

  6. Cardiovascular—dysrhythmia

  7. Neuromuscular—incoordination; decreased pain perception (PCP); alterations and distortions in consciousness, attention, sensory perceptions

- Diagnostic Tests/Findings

  1. CBC—leukocytosis; anemia

  2. Urine and drug screens—positive for abused substance(s)

  3. If associated diseases are present other alterations will be noted, e.g., abnormal liver enzymes, thyroid function tests, or glucose levels; positive HIV test

- Management/Treatment

  1. Depressant abuse

     a. Identify drugs taken, when taken, and route of administration if possible

     b. Assess level of consciousness

     c. Evaluate for evidence of head trauma

     d. Refer to physician, emergency room, or drug detoxification unit if acute overdose or intoxication is noted

     e. In the meantime provide quiet, lighted room and do not leave patient alone

     f. Monitor vital signs

     g. In consultation with physician determine need for starting an IV

  2. Stimulant abuse

a. In cases of intoxication, overdose, or withdrawal refer to physician or emergency room

b. In the meantime provide quiet area with reduced stimuli and high staff profile; aggressive behavior is associated with amphetamine use

c. Monitor cardiac rate and rhythm; ventricular arrhythmia/cardiac arrest may occur with toxic levels of cocaine

d. Persons experiencing stimulant withdrawal may be suicidal as a result of profound CNS rebound depression; use suicide precautions until patient is transferred to emergency room or detoxification unit

e. For non-emergency cases refer to drug rehabilitation unit

3. Hallucinogenic abuse

a. Hallucinogenics do not have a withdrawal syndrome and do not require detoxification as such

b. Refer patients with psychotic symptoms to the psychiatric unit

c. Protect client and others from injury

(1) Darkened, quiet, non-threatening environment to decrease the likelihood of confusion, fear, and violent behavior

(2) Speak in a soft, non-threatening voice

(a) If LSD has been taken provide reassurance verbally and by touch and orient the individual (''talking down'')

(b) If PCP intoxication is present do not attempt ''talking down'' it will increase the patient's agitation and tendency for violent behavior

(3) Suspiciousness and paranoia, visual and auditory hallucinations, and agitation make suicide or accidental injury a likely possibility; take precautions early

(4) If frightened and hallucinating avoid the use of physical restraints, however, use of restraints with PCP users may be necessary for the safety of self and others; PCP is an anesthetic and alters thinking; persons on PCP are a danger to themselves as well as to others

4. General considerations

a. Primary role is diagnosis and referral

b. Consult with physician on medication use

(1) Period of drug free observation usually recommended

(2) Haloperidol may be given to control psychotic and assaultive behaviors

(3) Diazepam is used to reduce muscle spasm and restlessness

(4) Phenothiazine neuroleptics should be avoided in patients on PCP because of the possibility of potentiating the anticholinergic effects of PCP

(5) Vitamin C tablets (ascorbic acid) or cranberry juice may be used to acidify the urine and promote excretion of PCP

c. Many treatment programs will not accept pregnant women

d. Many treatment programs do not provide child care or other alternatives for woman and can be a significant barrier to help

e. Alcoholics Anonymous, Al-Anon will also accept other substance abusers; family members should be given information on Al-Anon and Ala-Teen even if patient refuses treatment

f. Narcotics Anonymous (substance abusers) and Nar-Anon (families of substance abusers) groups are available in some areas

Delirium (Acute Confusion)

- Definition: A transient global disorder of attention, with clouding of consciousness and cognitive impairment

- Etiology/Incidence

  1. Usually the result of systemic problems e.g. medications, hypoxia, dehydration, or electrolyte imbalance—examples include:

     a. Intoxication—alcohol, analgesics, bromides, sedatives, psychedelics

     b. Withdrawal from alcohol, sedatives, hypnotics, or corticosteroids

     c. Infections—urinary, respiratory, meningitis, encephalitis, septicemia, syphilis

     d. Endocrine disorders—diabetes, hyper or hypothyroidism, Addison's disease, Cushing's syndrome

     e. Nutritional deficiencies especially of B_1, B_6, B_{12}

     f. Medications—anticholinergics, antidepressants, digoxin, H_2 blockers

     g. May be related to sensory deprivation or overload

     h. Sleep deprivation

     i. Psychological stress

  2. Can occur in any age group but the elderly are particularly vulnerable

  3. Estimated that 40% to 80% of elderly patients hospitalized for acute physical illness exhibit delirium at time of admission or soon after

- Signs and Symptoms

  1. Cognitive impairment

     a. Inability to focus attention/short attention span

        b.   Impaired recent memory and recall

        c.   Problems in perceptual processing

        d.   Disorientation

        e.   Impaired judgement

  2. Emotional lability

  3. Impaired impulse control

  4. Anxiety/irritability

  5. Mild to moderate depression

  6. Visual and auditory hallucinations

  7. Confabulation

  8. Fluctuating mental status; worse in the evening "sundowning," more common in those with pre-existing dementia

  9. Psychomotor restlessness with insomnia

 10. Tachycardia, dilated pupils, sweating

- Differential Diagnosis

  1. Dementia

  2. Pseudodementia

  3. Amnestic syndrome

  4. Substance induced hallucinosis

  5. Schizophrenia

  6. Other psychoses

- Physical Findings: Varies according to the underlying cause

  1. General appearance—may be restless, hyper or hypovigilant; dazed expression

  2. Tachycardia, elevated blood pressure, increased temperature, tachypnea

  3. Focal neurological symptoms may be present

- Diagnostic Tests/Findings

  1. Thorough history and physical examination with mental status and neurological examination—may reveal clues to etiology

  2. Basic laboratory workup may include:

        a.   CBC with differential, chemical screen, blood gas analysis

        b.   Electrocardiogram

        c.   Chest radiograph

   d.   Urinalysis and urine toxicology screen

3.   Special tests as needed

   a.   EEG—tends to show general slowing in delirium

   b.   Computer tomography (CT) scan or magnetic resonance imaging (MRI) of the brain—expect to be normal

   c.   Blood levels for medications

- Management/Treatment

   1.   Diagnostic consult with physician

   2.   Identify suspected cause

   3.   Remove or modify etiology when possible, e.g., treat infections with antimicrobials, discontinue or simplify medication regimens

   4.   Nonpharmacologic interventions

   a.   Provide adequate nutrition, hydration, oxygenation

   b.   Institute environmental controls to control stimuli levels

   c.   Provide reassurance and institute safety measures

   d.   Institute reorientation measures; provide patient and family with sensitive reassurance

   5.   Pharmacologic intervention

   a.   Judicious use of sedation to promote rest, reduce anxiety, decrease agitation and restlessness

   b.   No ideal drug

   c.   Short acting anxiolytics without active metabolites

   (1)   Oxazepam 10 to 50 mg/day

   (2)   Lorazepam 0.5 to 2 mg/day

   (3)   Alprazolam 0.5 to 4 mg/day

   d.   For immediate calming of acute agitation—haloperidol 0.5 mg IV combined with 0.5 to 1 mg lorazepam, repeated in 30 minutes

   (1)   Repeat every hour till calming achieved

   (2)   Once delirium cycle is broken sedation may be continued particularly in evening and night hours

   6.   General considerations

   a.   Anticipate delirium when risk factors are present

   (1)   Being >80 years of age

   (2)   Having visual or hearing impairments

        (3)   Pain

        (4)   Multiple medications

        (5)   Urine elimination problems

        (6)   Fracture injury

        (7)   Multiple chronic diseases

        (8)   Pervious history of acute confusion

        (9)   Immobilized

     (10)   Low scores on mental status examinations

  b. Prevention strategies

        (1)   Avoid polypharmacy

        (2)   Monitor medication intake and monitor for side effects, interactions, toxicity

        (3)   Maintain adequate hydration and oxygenation

        (4)   Maintain adequate nutrition

        (5)   Assess for adequate pain control

        (6)   Control environmental stimuli to avoid sensory deprivation or overload

        (7)   Provide assistive devices to supplement sensory alterations, e.g., glasses, hearing aids, controlled lighting

Questions
Select the best answer.

1. Which of the following is associated with higher risk for Major Depression?

    a. Being male
    b. Having had a traumatic experience in the last six months
    c. Being middle aged
    d. Having a family history of alcoholism

2. Which is true of Major Depression?

    a. Majority of patients will have a reoccurrence
    b. It may be a normal grief reaction
    c. It is often self-limiting
    d. Strongly associated with chronic drug use

3. Dysthymic Disorder is distinguished from Major Depression by which of the following?

    a. It usually first manifests itself in old age
    b. It is rarely associated with drug use
    c. It has milder more chronic symptoms
    d. It is rarely chronic

4. Post-traumatic Stress Disorder is marked by which triad of findings?

    a. Intrusive thoughts, nightmares, flashbacks
    b. Tendency to globalize, psychomotor retardation, hypersomnia
    c. Weight loss, feelings of helplessness, irritability
    d. Indifference, decreased concentration, hyperphagia

5. Mrs. S. is a 65-year-old who comes in complaining of feeling depressed. She would like a prescription to make her feel better. Her husband died three weeks ago.

    The data you have at this point indicates:

    a. Her problem is a normal grief reaction, but will require surveillance
    b. Diagnostic tests will not be needed
    c. Pharmacologic intervention would not be warranted
    d. Major depression is a possibility

6. Your next step would be to:

    a. Refer her for psychologic evaluation
    b. Prescribe antidepressants
    c. Obtain additional information
    d. Reassure her that the problem is self-limiting

7. In a patient of this age it would be important to remember that:

    a. Somatic signs may be overlooked as normal changes
    b. Elderly may require higher doses of antidepressants for therapeutic effect
    c. Previously undiagnosed bipolar disorder is probable
    d. Tricyclics may cause ''hypomania''

8. With further exploration you determine that Mrs. S. has had intermittent episodes of anorexia, difficulty sleeping, has been feeling tired and listless. She has had to force herself to go out with her friends, although she did enjoy her grandson's birthday party a week ago. She denies any thoughts of harming herself. Routine physical and lab work are unremarkable.

   The most likely diagnosis for this patient is:

    a. Adjustment disorder with depressed mood
    b. Primary major depression
    c. Dysthymic disorder
    d. Bipolar disorder

9. Mrs. S. tells you that she can't help thinking that her husband might not have died if she had done things differently.

   Which response would be most appropriate?

    a. Telling her that these thoughts will decrease in a few weeks
    b. Encourage her to elaborate on these thoughts
    c. Tell her a psychologist or psychiatrist will best help her with her guilt
    d. Suggest an antidepressant will correct this kind of thinking

10. A 17-year-old male student comes into the student health service complaining of weight loss, fatigue, anorexia. He states that the symptoms began about a month ago after he broke up with his girl-friend. He has difficulty sleeping and says he wakes up thinking about her. He says that since she left him he just doesn't enjoy going out anymore and has been spending most of his free time in his room. His affect is flat and he shows little expression as he relates his problem. The physical examination is within normal limits.

   You suspect depression to be his problem. Your next step would be to:

    a. Prescribe an anti-anxiety medication
    b. Find out how he has coped with losses in the past
    c. Explain that this is a temporary situation and will probably clear up in another couple of weeks
    d. Ask him directly about feelings or thoughts of harming himself

11. Which factors in the available data might lead you to suspect that he might be suicidal?

    a. Weight loss, fatigue, anorexia
    b. Insomnia, loss of pleasure, social withdrawal
    c. Age, gender, emotional loss, signs of depression
    d. Intrusive thoughts, flat affect, with normal physical exam

12. Upon further questioning he admits to suicidal ideation. Knowing which of the following would be most helpful in assessing his suicide risk?

    a. Whether there have been any suicides in his family
    b. If he rooms alone or has a roommate
    c. If his family lives nearby
    d. If he has a plan for suicide in the next 24 hours

13. This patient has a roommate, but his family lives in another state. He denies substance abuse, or definite plan or time for suicide. What would be the best action at this point?

    a. Consult with a physician regarding psychotherapy and antidepressants
    b. Consult with a physician and arrange for hospitalization
    c. Give him a prescription for antidepressants and arrange to have him stay with his family for a week
    d. Give him a prescription for antidepressants, call his roommate, and have them both check with you in 24 hours

14. A 38-year-old married male comes to the clinic asking for an AIDS test. He has been awakening at night with sweating and his heart pounding. He has read in *Time* magazine that night sweats were a sign of AIDS and a few years ago he had to have a transfusion after a car accident. He would also like to have a radiograph of his throat as he feels like there's something stuck in it and wonders if it might be cancer. At times he feels like he's losing control. He denies IV drug use or high risk sexual activities. He denies marital or work problems. In fact, he just got a promotion two weeks ago and he and his wife have bought a new home.

    What other information would be most helpful to you in your diagnosis?

    a. How long has he had these symptoms
    b. Whether he has nightmares
    c. If anyone in his family has had a major mental health problem
    d. If he has a prolapsed heart valve

15. If he denies nightmares and has had the symptoms for about two weeks and the physical findings are normal, you should:

    a. Order a barium swallow
    b. Refer to a gastroenterologist
    c. Consider a post traumatic stress syndrome as the probable diagnosis
    d. Consider situational anxiety as the probable diagnosis

16. Benzodiazepines are used in anxiety disorders. They are:

    a. Contraindicated in glaucoma
    b. Not helpful for short term use in situational anxiety
    c. Usually physiologically addicting
    d. As effective as beta blockers for control of palpitations

17. The most common mental health problem seen in general practice is:

a. Anxiety
b. Depression
c. Alcoholism
d. Schizophrenia

18. Which of these symptoms is least characteristic of anxiety?

    a. Sleep disorder
    b. Decreased concentration
    c. Irritability
    d. Indifference

19. Which of the following would least likely be a cause of anxiety symptoms?

    a. Thyrotoxicosis
    b. Hyperglycemia
    c. Hormone-releasing tumor
    d. Prolapsed mitral valve

20. Tricyclics are not used for bipolar disorders because:

    a. They may precipitate mania
    b. They cause liver dysfunction
    c. They may lead to physiologic dependance
    d. They may cause a hypertensive crisis

21. Mrs. J. is a 65-year-old widow who completed a series of E.C.T. treatments a week ago with positive results. Both she and her daughter are concerned that she continues to experience a significant memory loss.

    You could be most helpful by:

    a. Reporting the problem to her psychiatrist
    b. Allow her to ventilate her feelings without any comment regarding the memory loss
    c. Explain that the loss is temporary and full memory will return
    d. Inform her that many individuals of her age begin to experience memory loss

22. Mr. P. is a 45-year-old divorced male who comes in for a physical exam required for a new job. During the interview he reveals previous hospitalization for pancreatitis and long term self-medication for gastritis. His physical exam is normal except for slight tenderness in the RUQ. A CBC reveals macrocytic, megaloblastic anemia.

    Which diagnostic test would be most helpful at this point?

    a. ECG and electrolytes
    b. Liver function, B_{12} and folic acid levels, and electrolytes
    c. Chest radiograph and ultrasound of the gallbladder
    d. Blood albumin levels and bone marrow studies

23. Ms. Z, a 35-year-old female, comes into the clinic demanding to be seen immediately. She is agitated and complaining loudly of police brutality. She states that she was unjustly jailed overnight because of a misunderstanding and that she was shackled for more than three hours causing bruises on her wrists and ankles. Upon further elaboration she states the police altered a blood test and said her blood alcohol level was 300.

    This information alone indicates:

    a. Paranoid ideation
    b. Alcoholism
    c. Need for legal services referral
    d. The patient may have a drinking problem

24. Non-compliance with medication is a concern in outpatient treatment of patients with mental health problems. Which of the following would be least helpful in promoting medication regimen compliance?

    a. Client involvement in treatment decision making
    b. Providing the client with information about expected action and side effects of the medications
    c. Arranging follow-up visits with whatever staff are available
    d. Maintaining telephone communication with the patient to monitor effects and response to medication

25. One of the most effective treatments for alcoholism is:

    a. Psychoanalysis
    b. Active participation in A.A.
    c. Aversion therapy with Antabuse
    d. Active participation in Al-Anon

26. Ms. C is brought to the emergency room from a party by her friends. She is stuporous, confused, and has pinpoint pupils.

    These signs are consistent with:

    a. PCP intoxication
    b. Heroin use
    c. LSD
    d. Amphetamine withdrawal

27. A 23-year-old male comes to the clinic to obtain treatment for a cut on his arm he received in a street fight. His face is badly bruised from a previous fight. He is unkempt and shows evidence of poor personal hygiene. He has a history of alcohol abuse. At present he is tachycardic and has an elevated blood pressure. His pupils are dilated and he is slightly diaphoretic. He complains of chest pain.

    These signs are consistent with:
    a. Acute alcohol intoxication

b. Chronic heroin use
c. Recent use of hallucinogenics
d. Recent use of cocaine

28. A young male adult is brought into the emergency room by the police. He is highly agitated and hostile and verbally abusive and threatening. He has several lacerations and bruises he sustained in a fight at a disco where he "tore the place apart."

You should:

a. Suspect police brutality
b. Suspect LSD use
c. Try to talk the patient down and keep him oriented
d. Be prepared to administer Haldol

29. Which of the following IS NOT associated with physiologic dependance?

a. Heroin
b. Phenobarbital
c. LSD
d. Amphetamines

30. Mark is an 18-year-old brought to the student health clinic complaining of chest pain and palpitations. He is highly anxious and perspiring. His roommate states he thinks he took some kind of drug.

In addition to myocardial infarction (MI) these symptoms could indicate intoxication or overdose of which of the following?

a. Heroin
b. Alcohol
c. PCP
d. Cocaine

31. Your first action in this case should be to:

a. Arrange for emergency room transfer
b. Prepare for cardiopulmonary support
c. Draw blood gasses
d. Do nothing until he is seen by a physician

32. To enhance the excretion of PCP from the body give:

a. Haloperidol
b. Ascorbic acid
c. Valium
d. A phenothiazine

33. Which pharmacologic agent is contraindicated in persons on PCP?

a. Valium
b. Phenothiazine
c. Haloperidol
d. Ascorbic acid

34. CNS rebound is seen in withdrawal of:

a. Depressants
b. Stimulants
c. Hallucinogenics
d. Alcohol

35. Aggressive behavior can be seen with abuse of which of the following?

a. Amphetamines
b. Depressants
c. Hallucinogenics
d. Any psychoactive substance

Answers

1. d	13. b	25. b
2. a	14. a	26. b
3. c	15. d	27. d
4. a	16. a	28. d
5. d	17. b	29. c
6. c	18. d	30. d
7. a	19. b	31. b
8. a	20. a	32. b
9. b	21. c	33. b
10. d	22. b	34. b
11. c	23. c	35. d
12. d	24. c	

Bibliography

American Psychiatric Association. (1994). *Diagnostic and statistical manual of mental disorders* (4th ed.). Washington, DC: Author.

Buck, B., Shaw, S., Cleary, P., Delbanco, T. L., & Aronson, M. D. (1987). Screening for alcohol abuse using the CAGE questionnaire. *American Journal of Medicine, 82,* 231–235.

Cole, S., & Raju, M. (1996). Making the diagnosis of depression in the primary care setting. *The American Journal of Medicine, 101,* (supplement 6A), 10S–17S.

Deblinger, L. (2000). Alcohol problems in the elderly. *Patient Care for The Nurse Practitioner, 3*(10), 69–87.

Eisendrath, S. J., & Lichtmacher, J. E. (2000). Psychiatric disorders. In L. M. Tierney, S. J. McPhee, & M. A. Papadakis (Eds.). *Current medical diagnosis and management* (39th ed., pp. 1019-1078). Stamford, CT: Appleton & Lange.

Foreman, M. D., & Zane, D. (1996). Nursing strategies for acute confusion in elders. *American Journal of Nursing, 96*(4), 44–52.

Gianni, A. J. (2000). An approach to drug abuse, intoxication, and withdrawal. *American Family Physician, 61*(9), 2763–2774.

Isaacs, A. (1998). Depression & your patient. *American Journal of Nursing, 8*(12), 26–32.

Longo, L. P., & Johnson, B. (2000). Addiction: Part I. Benzodiazepines-side effects, abuse risk, and alternatives. *American Family Physician, 61*(7), 2121–2128.

Longo, L. P., Parran, T., Johnson, B., & Kinsey, W. (2000). Addiction: Part II. Identification and management of the drug-seeking patient. *American Family Physician, 61*(7), 2401–2408.

Lundquist, R. S., Bernens, A., & Olsen, C. G. (1997). Comorbid disease in geriatric patients: Dementia and depression. *American Family Physician, 55,* 2687–2694.

Miller, J. L. (2000). Post-traumatic stress disorder in parimary care practice. *Journal of The American Academy of Nurse Practitioners, 12*(11), 475–485.

Pinkowish, M. D. (1997). Rational use of the newer antidepressants. *Patient Care,* March 30, 49–50, 55–57, 62, 67–77.

Primary Care Update. (2000). Acute major depression and dysthymia: A review of newer pharmacologic agents, *Consultant, 40*(11), 1938–1940.

Pokorny, A., Miller, B. A., & Kaplan, H. B. (1972). The brief MAST: A shortened version of the Michigan alcoholism screening test. *American Journal of Psychiatry, 129,* 342–345.

Simon, L., Jewell, N., & Brokel, J. (1997). Management of acute delirium in hospitalized elderly: A process improvement project. *Geriatric Nursing, 18,* 151–154.

Valente, S. M. (1996). Diagnosis and treatment of panic disorder and generalized anxiety in primary care. *The Nurse Practitioner, 21*(8), 26–47.

Dermatologic Conditions Infancy Through Adolescence

Beverly Bigler

Newborn Exanthema

Cutis Marmorata

- Definition: Transient mottling of the neonate's skin with a lacy bluish appearance
- Etiology/Incidence
    1. Physiologic response of uneven blood flow which results in constriction of small blood vessels while others dilate
    2. Often precipitated by exposure to cold
    3. More common in premature infants
    4. Persistence after neonatal period found in Down syndrome
- Signs and Symptoms: Generalized lacy, reddish-blue appearance to the skin
- Differential Diagnosis
    1. Cutis marmorata telangiectatica congenita
    2. Cyanosis
    3. Erythema toxicum neonatorum
- Physical Findings: Generalized reddish-blue reticulated pattern to most of body surface
- Diagnostic Tests/Findings: None
- Management/Treatment
    1. Keep neonate at an even warm temperature
    2. Reduce exposure to cold environment
    3. Don't overdress or keep environment overly warm

Erythema Toxicum Neonatorum

- Definition: Transient benign skin rash with lesions of varied morphology; erythematous macules; wheals, vesicles, and pustules
- Etiology/Incidence:
    1. Unknown cause
    2. Occurs in 50% to 60% of neonates
    3. More common in full-term and post-term neonates
    4. More common in neonates with birth weight > 2500 g
    5. Onset usually within first 24 to 48 hours of life, but occasionally present at birth
- Signs and Symptoms
    1. Yellow-white lesions on reddish-pink base; may be blotchy

2. Extent of rash varies from minimal to most of body surface; palms and soles are usually spared

- Differential Diagnosis

    1. Congenital candidiasis

    2. Incontinentia pigmenti

    3. Miliaria rubra

    4. Neonatal pustular melanosis

    5. Urticaria pigmentosa

    6. Bacterial infestation

- Physical Findings

    1. Lesions of varied morphology—erythematous macules 2 to 3 cm in diameter appear first, followed by wheals, vesicles, and rarely pustules

    2. Lesions usually arise from erythematous base with macular erythema fading within 2 to 3 days

    3. Occurs predominately on the trunk, however, may occur anywhere on body except soles and palms

    4. Number of lesions varies from few to many

    5. Spontaneous resolution in 5 to 7 days

- Diagnostic Tests/Findings: Wright's stained smear of pustules identifies presence of eosinophils rather than neutrophils which rules out neonatal pustular melanosis

- Management/Treatment

    1. Obtain detailed history of onset, duration, and progression

    2. Describe and monitor lesions in terms of morphology/structure, size, shape, number, color, location, distribution

    3. No treatment necessary

    4. Educate regarding characteristics of condition and expected resolution

    5. Refer for evaluation if condition does not improve

Milia

- Definition: Benign condition of small yellow-white inclusion cysts filled with cheesy keratinous material on face of newborn

- Etiology/Incidence

    1. Caused by superficial keratinous material accumulated within developing pilosebaceous follicle

    2. Occurs in 50% of newborns

- Signs and Symptoms: Numerous small yellow-white raised lesions on face of newborn

- Differential Diagnosis: Sebaceous hyperplasia

- Physical Findings

    1. Numerous firm pearly yellow-white 1 to 2 mm inclusion papular cysts on the cheeks, forehead, and nose; predominantly on face; may be found on other body surfaces

    2. Oral counterpart are yellow papular lesions on hard palate known as Epstein's pearls

    3. Condition resolves spontaneously without treatment within a few weeks as lesions exfoliate

- Diagnostic Tests/Findings: None

- Management/Treatment

    1. Describe and monitor lesions in terms of morphology/structure, size, shape, number, color, location, distribution

    2. No treatment necessary

    3. Educate regarding characteristics of condition and expected resolution

Sebaceous Hyperplasia

- Definition: Numerous small pale yellow macules or papules at the openings of pilosebaceous follicles on face of newborn

- Etiology/Incidence: Caused by sebaceous gland enlargement and overgrowth due to maternal androgenic hormonal influence

- Signs and Symptoms: Numerous small yellow-white flat and raised lesions on newborn's face

- Differential Diagnosis: Milia

- Physical Findings

    1. Numerous small yellow-white macular and/or papular lesions on cheeks, forehead, nose and upper lip of newborn

    2. Condition resolves spontaneously without treatment as lesions gradually decrease in size and finally disappear within first month of life

- Diagnostic Tests/Findings: None

- Management/Treatment

    1. Describe and monitor lesions in terms of morphology/structure, size, shape, number, color, location, distribution

    2. No treatment necessary

    3. Educate regarding characteristics of condition and expected resolution

Vascular Lesions

Salmon Patch (Nevus Simplex)

- Definition: Benign flat light red to orange vascular birthmark on head and face
- Etiology/Incidence
    1. Caused by overgrowth of blood vessels within dermis skin layer
    2. Seen in approximately 40% to 50% of newborns
    3. More common in girls
- Signs and Symptoms: Flat light red to orange lesions on face and head of newborn
- Differential Diagnosis
    1. Contact irritation or chronic rubbing
    2. Nevus flammeus
    3. Child abuse
- Physical Findings
    1. Single or multiple irregular light red to orange macular lesions on eyelids, nape of neck, glabella, and/or occiput; vary in size
    2. Lesions gradually fade and disappear spontaneously with time
        a. Eyelid lesions fade first resolving completely within 3 to 6 months
        b. Nape of neck lesions fade but may persist into adulthood
        c. Other lesions resolve completely by 7 years of age
- Diagnostic Tests/Findings: None
- Management/Treatment
    1. Describe and monitor lesions in terms of morphology/structure, size, shape, number, color, location, distribution
    2. No treatment necessary
    3. Educate regarding characteristics of condition and expected resolution

Nevus Flammeus

- Definition: Benign permanent flat dark red to purple vascular lesion predominately on head and face
- Etiology/Incidence
    1. Caused by proliferation of dilated capillaries in the dermis
    2. Lesions may be associated with other conditions
        a. Lesions covering entire half of face or bilateral; may be associated with Sturge-Weber syndrome

b. Lesions on extremities may be associated with hypertrophy of soft tissue and bone

c. Lesions on the back, especially crossing the mid-line, may be associated with defects in the spinal cord and vertebrae

3. Seen in approximately 0.4% of newborns

- Signs and Symptoms: Flat dark red or purple lesions on body surface

- Differential Diagnosis: Child abuse

- Physical Findings

1. Irregular dark red or purple macular lesions occurring on any body surface, predominately on face and head

2. Size varies from less than 1 cm to more than 20 cm

3. May initially appear pink in infancy and gradually become darker

4. Lesion never fades and may become raised in adulthood

- Diagnostic Tests/Findings: None

- Management/Treatment

1. Describe and monitor lesions in terms of morphology/structure, size, shape, number, color, location, distribution

2. Refer for MD evaluation to rule out Sturge-Weber syndrome and other associated conditions

3. No treatment necessary

4. Later in childhood

a. May be camouflaged later in childhood with water resistant cosmetics

b. Refer for MD evaluation and consideration of pulsed dye laser treatment

c. Counseling as needed for related psychological concerns

5. Educate regarding characteristics of condition

Capillary Hemangioma (Strawberry Nevus)

- Definition: Bright red or blue-red nodular lesions of varying sizes and shape with a rubbery and rough surface predominately on head and face

- Etiology/Incidence

1. Caused by proliferation of capillary endothelial cells which may be superficial or deep

2. Seen in approximately 2.5% of newborns

3. More common in girls

4. More common in light-skinned infants

- Signs and Symptoms: Red or blue-red lesions on skin surface
- Differential Diagnosis
    1. Cystic hygroma
    2. Neonatal hemangiomatosis
    3. Blue rubber bleb nevus syndrome
- Physical Findings
    1. Often is not present at birth, however, area of eventual lesion is blanched or slightly colored
    2. Size varies from less than 1 cm to over 4 cm
    3. Pattern of growth and resolution
        a. Grows quickly within 2 to 4 weeks to a red or blue-red, protuberant nodule
        b. Gradual resolution usually begins between 12 to 15 months with gray areas developing, followed by flattening from center to periphery
        c. A flat or involuted area of hyperpigmentation often remains following dissolution of the lesion
    4. Complications may occur resulting from size, location, and depth of lesion
        a. Lesions involving eye area and orbit may cause visual disturbances
        b. Lesions of head and neck may be associated with subglottic hemangiomas causing airway obstruction
        c. Lesions may cause cardiovascular disturbances through compression
    5. Complication of thrombocytopenia may occur resulting from trapped platelets within lesion
    6. Lesions resolve spontaneously and completely disappear with age
        a. 50% are cleared by 5 years of age
        b. 90% are cleared by 10 years of age
        c. Remainder clear during adolescence
- Diagnostic Tests/Findings: None
- Management/Treatment
    1. Describe and monitor lesions in terms of morphology/structure, size, shape, number, color, location, distribution
    2. Refer for MD evaluation to rule out involvement with vital organs
    3. No treatment necessary
    4. Educate regarding characteristics of condition and expected resolution

Melanocyte Cell and Pigmentation Conditions

Café au lait Spots

- Definition: Light to medium brown pigmented macular lesions of varying sizes and shapes found anywhere on the body; the color of coffee with milk from which the name is derived
- Etiology/Incidence
    1. Caused by increased pigmentation activity of melanocyte cells
    2. Overall incidence is higher in dark-skinned populations than light-skinned
    3. Lesions larger than 1.5 cm occur in 10% of light-skinned population and 20% of darker-skinned populations
    4. Lesions are usually present at birth however, may develop at any age
    5. Lesions are present throughout life, however, color intensity may fade
    6. Six or more lesions and/or lesions larger than 1.5 cm in diameter may be associated with neurofibromatosis or Albright's syndrome (Hay, Groothuis, Hayward, & Levin, 1997; Hurwitz, 1993). (see Neurological Disorders chapter.)
- Signs and Symptoms: Flat light brown lesions on skin; may be deeper in color in dark-skinned populations
- Differential Diagnosis: None
- Physical Findings
    1. Macular light to medium brown lesions on any skin surface
    2. Size varies from less than $\frac{1}{2}$ cm to 20 cm in diameter
    3. May be single or multiple
    4. Vary in shape, frequently oval
    5. Six or more lesions and/or lesions larger then 1.5 cm may be associated with neurofibromatosis or Albright's syndrome
- Diagnostic Tests/Findings: None
- Management/Treatment
    1. Describe and monitor lesions in terms of morphology/structure, size, shape, number, color, location, distribution
    2. If suspected that lesions may be associated with any other condition, refer to MD for further evaluation
    3. No treatment necessary
    4. Educate regarding characteristics of condition

Mongolian Spots

- Definition: Blue-black and gray macular lesions of irregular shape and varying sizes usually on sacrococcygeal region, buttocks, and lumbar areas but may also involve extremities, upper back and shoulders

- Etiology/Incidence

    1. Lesions consist of migrating spindle-shaped pigmented/melanocyte cells deep within dermis layer

    2. Occurs in 90% of darker skinned infants; 5% of light-skinned infants

- Signs and Symptoms: Blue-black or gray lesions of irregular shape and varying size on lower aspect of back

- Differential Diagnosis: Child abuse

- Physical Findings

    1. Blue-black or gray macular lesions of irregular shapes

    2. Vary in size from < 2 cm to > 10 cm

    3. Located on dorsal body surface, predominately on sacrococcygeal area of buttocks, and lumbar areas, but also on upper back, shoulders, and extremities

    4. Lesions not seen on palms or soles

    5. Lesions resolve spontaneously without treatment

        a. Most fade completely during childhood and adolescence

        b. Some may still be evident in adulthood

- Diagnostic Tests/Findings: None

- Management/Treatment

    1. Describe and monitor lesions in terms of morphology/structure, size, shape, number, color, location, and distribution

    2. No treatment necessary

    3. Educate regarding characteristics of condition and expected resolution

Malignant Melanoma

- Definition: Lethal form of skin cancer involving melanocyte cells; may occur on any skin surface

- Etiology/Incidence

    1. Caused by abnormal growth within melanocyte cells

    2. Severe sunburn or excessive exposure to the sun before the age of 10 years predisposes developing melanoma later in childhood or in adult life

        a. Sun damaged skin cells may be dormant for years

      b.   Melanocyte cells provide mechanism to activate malignant process

  3.   Melanoma cells spread through the lymphatic system and invade other skin surfaces and organs

      a.   90% survival rate with localized condition

      b.   20% survival with metastasis

  4.   Increasing incidence in general population

  5.   More common in males and light-skinned individuals

  6.   Increased incidence with family history (Cohen, 1999)

  7.   More lethal and faster growing than basal cell or squamous cell cancers

- Signs and Symptoms

  1.   Localized change in skin color or increase in size of existing nevus

  2.   May have itching with bleeding and tenderness

- Differential Diagnosis: Other skin cancers

- Physical Findings

  1.   Asymmetrical lesion with irregular, ragged and blurred borders

  2.   Uneven color with shades of blue, black, brown, tan, and red; all colors may exist within same lesion

  3.   More common on arms and lower legs of females and on chest of males

  4.   Single or multiple (clusters) lesions may be found in distant areas with metastasis

  5.   Bleeding and ulceration—usually late signs

- Diagnostic Tests/Findings: Skin biopsy confirms diagnosis

- Management/Treatment

  1.   Obtain detailed history of onset, duration, and progression

  2.   Refer to MD for evaluation immediately if suspected; surgical excision is indicated

  3.   Educate regarding characteristics of condition, treatment and expected prognosis

  4.   Educate regarding specific preventive measures

      a.   Protect skin from exposure to sunlight

         (1)   Cover-up clothing and hats

         (2)   Sunglasses

         (3)   Water resistant sunblocks that protect against UVB and UVA ultraviolet light with > 15 sun protection factor (SPF)

      b.   Avoid exposure to sunlight especially during 10 a.m. to 3 p.m.

      c.   Avoid sun lamps

Albinism

- Definition: Inherited congenital defect of total or partial lack of pigmentation in which affected body parts lack normal color

  1. Total form—affects entire skin, hair, and retina

  2. Partial or localized forms—confined to specific area of skin, hair (forelock of hair), or eyes (pupil or retina)

- Etiology/Incidence

  1. Metabolic process within melanocyte cells required for melanin production is impaired—melanin, giving skin its distinctive color, is not secreted

  2. Occurs in all ethnic groups

- Signs and Symptoms

  1. Milky-white skin (localized or generalized)

  2. Light sensitivity

- Differential Diagnosis

  1. Vitiligo

  2. Phenylketonuria

- Physical Findings

  1. Skin is milky-white, hair is white or yellow, iris is usually blue, pupil usually appears red and becomes darker in adulthood

  2. Skin is sensitive to light and sunburns easily

  3. Other symptoms not involving skin include decreased visual acuity, photosensitivity

- Diagnostic Tests/Findings: None

- Management/Treatment

  1. Describe skin and areas of hypopigmentation and monitor routinely for any skin changes that may occur including development of lesions

  2. Educate regarding need to protect from exposure to sunlight

     a. Cover-up clothing and hats

     b. Sunglasses

     c. Water resistant sunblocks that protect against UVB and UVA ultraviolet light with > 15 SPF

  3. Educate regarding characteristics and prognosis of condition

  4. Counsel as indicted regarding

     a. Related psychologic effects

     b. Genetic counselling related to potential inheritance factors

5. Refer to dermatologist for evaluation if skin changes occur

6. Refer to ophthalmologist for evaluation of vision and eye involvement

Vitiligo

- Definition: Acquired condition involving patches of hypopigmentation on skin surface and in mouth and genitalia
    1. Segmented form—unilateral involving two dermatones
    2. Generalized form—involves more than two dermatones, often has bilateral distribution
- Etiology/Incidence
    1. Unknown cause
        a. Affected areas of hypopigmentation have loss or destruction of melanocyte cells
        b. May be associated with autoimmune conditions—diabetes mellitus, Addison's disease, or thyroiditis
    2. Occurs in approximately 4% of all ethnic populations
    3. Onset is usually before 20 years of age
- Signs and Symptoms: Milky-white patches on skin
- Differential Diagnosis
    1. Albinism
    2. Pityriasis alba
    3. Pityriasis rosea
    4. Tinea versicolor
- Physical Findings
    1. Milky-white patches of hypopigmentation occur in unilateral or bilateral pattern on skin of normal texture
    2. Shape varies from round, oval, to irregular
    3. Size varies from less than 2 cm to well over 20 cm
    4. Varies in number from one to many
    5. Condition is often permanent without repigmentation
- Diagnostic Tests/Findings: None
- Management/Treatment
    1. Obtain detailed history of onset, duration, severity, progression, and possible precipitating factors

2. Describe skin and areas of hypopigmentation and monitor for any skin changes that may occur including development of lesions

3. Protect skin from exposure to sunlight especially during 10 am to 3 pm

   a. Use cover-up clothing, hats, and sunglasses

   b. Apply water resistant sunblocks that protect against UVB and UVA ultraviolet light with > 15 SPF

4. Refer for MD evaluation and treatment to stimulate repigmentation

   a. Topical steroid applications and controlled ultraviolet light exposure

   b. Repigmentation efforts have varying degrees of success

5. Educate regarding characteristics and expected prognoses

6. Recommend camouflage with water resistant cosmetics for adolescent

7. Counsel regarding

   a. Related psychological impact of condition

   b. Serious need for protection to reduce risk for skin cancer and sunburn

8. Refer for MD evaluation if complications develop

Pityriasis Alba

- Definition: Acquired condition of scaly hypopigmented lesions of varying sizes and shapes with indistinct borders occurring predominately on cheeks

- Etiology/Incidence

  1. Unknown cause

  2. May be associated with overdrying of skin causing inflammation and hypopigmentation

  3. Occurs most often in children ages 3 to 12 years

  4. Occurs more commonly in dark-skinned populations

- Signs and Symptoms

  1. Scaly white patches on cheeks

  2. May be pruritic

- Differential Diagnosis

  1. Pityriasis rosea

  2. Tinea corporis

  3. Vitiligo

- Physical Findings

1. Scaly hypopigmented lesions of varying sizes or shapes with non-distinct borders occurring predominately on cheeks, less commonly on other skin surfaces

2. Some lesions may be slightly erythematous

3. Number of lesions varies from one to many

4. Exposure to sunlight may exacerbate lesions, making them more pronounced

5. Repigmentation occurs as condition resolves spontaneously in 3 to 4 months

- Diagnostic Tests/Findings: KOH preparation to rule out tinea corporis

- Management/Treatment

1. Obtain detailed history of onset, duration, severity, progression of symptoms, and possible precipitating factors

2. Describe and monitor lesions in terms of morphology/structure, size, shape, number, color, location, distribution

3. Educate child and parents regarding need to protect skin from exposure to sunlight especially during 10 a.m. to 3 p.m.

    a. Use cover-up clothing, hats, and sunglasses

    b. Apply water resistant sunblocks that protect against UVB and UVA ultraviolet light with > 15 SPF

4. Use bland moisturizer to reduce overdrying

5. Educate regarding characteristics and expected prognoses

6. Recommend camouflage with water resistant cosmetics for adolescent

7. Refer for MD evaluation if condition does not improve

Papulosquamous Conditions

Pityriasis Rosea

- Definition: Acquired common mild inflammatory condition characterized by scaly, pale, salmon-pink lesions predominately on the trunk, upper arms and upper thighs

- Etiology/Incidence

1. Unknown cause

2. Possible viral association

3. Occurs more often in fall and spring months

4. Occurs especially in older children of all ethnic groups

- Signs and Symptoms

1. Scaly pink marks on skin

2. Periodic pruritus of varying degrees of severity especially at onset

3. Lack of energy and low grade fever before onset of rash

- Differential Diagnosis

    1. Pityriasis alba

    2. Seborrheic dermatitis

    3. Secondary syphilis

    4. Tinea corporis

- Physical Findings

    1. Scaly, pink to salmon lesions with progressive pattern

        a. "Herald" patch of 1 cm to 5 cm on trunk or buttocks usually occurs 5 to 10 days before generalized rash

        b. Round and oval macular to papular lesions develop over two week period on skin lines and in parallel fashion suggestive of a Christmas tree pattern

        c. Individual lesions clear in central to peripheral pattern

    2. On darker-skinned populations lesions are more predominant on neck, axillary and inguinal regions

    3. Condition is self-limiting and resolves spontaneously in 3 to 4 months

- Diagnostic Tests/Findings

    1. KOH test to rule out tinea corporis

    2. VDRL to rule out secondary syphilis, especially in sexually active individuals

- Management/Treatment

    1. Obtain detailed history of onset, duration, severity, progression of symptoms, and possible precipitating factors

    2. Describe and monitor lesions in terms of morphology/structure, size, shape, number, color, location, distribution

    3. Educate regarding characteristics of condition and prognosis

    4. Use symptomatic treatment for pruritus

        a. Topical calamine lotion on lesions

        b. Oral antipruritic agents for severe pruritus, e.g., diphenhydramine

        c. Cool bath or compresses on lesions

    5. Educate regarding medication dosage, signs of irritation, sensitivity

    6. Use controlled and limited sunlight exposure to shorten resolution time

    7. Refer for MD evaluation if condition worsens or does not resolve

Psoriasis

- Definition: Acquired chronic condition characterized by thick silver-gray-white scales
    1. Psoriasis vulgaris—large lesions occurring predominately on elbows and knees
    2. Psoriasis guttate—small lesions occurring predominately on trunk, upper arms and thighs
- Etiology/Incidence
    1. Specific cause is unknown
    2. Associated with overproduction and too rapid migration of epithelial cells to skin surface; cells migrate in 3 to 4 days in comparison to usual 28 days
        a. Psoriasis vulgaris—often associated with constant rubbing, or with trauma to the affected area known as Koebner's response
        b. Psoriasis guttate—often follows streptococcal infection
    3. Occurs in over 33% of children
    4. More common in light-skinned than dark-skinned populations
    5. More common in males
    6. Positive family history in approximately $\frac{1}{3}$ of cases suggests familial or environmental connection
- Signs and Symptoms
    1. Silvery, gray-white scaling of skin mainly on trunk or extremities, especially elbows and knees; less commonly on scalp and face
    2. Bleeding may occur if scales are picked at or removed
    3. Changes in nails—thickening with pits and ridges
- Differential Diagnosis
    1. Atopic dermatitis
    2. Candida
    3. Pityriasis rosea
    4. Seborrhea
    5. Secondary syphilis
    6. Tinea corporis
- Physical Findings
    1. Psoriasis vulgaris—large 5 to 10 cm lesions with thick silvery-white scales located on elbows and knees
    2. Psoriasis guttate—small 3 to 10 mm multiple teardrop round or oval papular lesions which become covered by a silvery-gray-white scale on trunk and proximal extremities

3. Bleeding occurs when scale is removed

4. Nail plates may be thicker and show signs of pits, ridges, splinter hemorrhages; not all nail plates are involved

- Diagnostic Tests/Findings

    1. VDRL to rule out secondary syphilis

    2. KOH to rule out fungal infections

- Management/Treatment

    1. Obtain detailed history of onset, duration, severity and progression of symptoms, and possible precipitating factors

    2. Describe and monitor lesions in terms of morphology/structure, size, shape, number, color, location, distribution

    3. Reduce hypertrophy of lesion

        a. Use controlled and limited sunlight exposure

        b. Apply topical steroids, e.g., hydocortisone, triamcinolone

        c. Apply mineral oil and moisturizers to decrease drying

    4. Educate regarding medication dosage, signs of irritation, sensitivity

    5. Educate regarding characteristics of condition and prognosis

    6. Refer for MD evaluation if condition does not improve

Dermatitis Conditions

Atopic Dermatitis

- Definition: Common skin disorder with lesions of varied morphology commonly known as eczema

    1. Acute form—occurs predominately in infants

    2. Chronic form—occurs predominately in children and adolescents

- Etiology/Incidence

    1. Specific cause is unknown

    2. May be associated with a disorder of immunity in some cases due to elevated levels of IgE

    3. Positive family history may be predisposing factor in some cases

    4. Occurs in approximately 10% to 15% of children

    5. Up to 50% of affected infants develop asthma and/or other respiratory manifestations, e.g., allergic rhinitis, hay fever and progress to chronic form

6. Up to 25% of children and adolescents continue to have symptoms throughout adulthood

- Signs and Symptoms
    1. Skin changes
        a. Infant—red, swollen skin rash with crusted areas
        b. Older children—areas of darker, thickened, leathery skin
    2. Pruritus for both, worsens with sweating
- Differential Diagnosis
    1. Contact dermatitis
    2. Psoriasis
    3. Seborrheic dermatitis
    4. Scabies
    5. Impetigo or other secondary bacterial infection
- Physical Findings
    1. Acute form in infants usually develops between ages of 2 to 6 months with 50% cases resolving by 3 years and remainder progressing to chronic form
        a. Lesions erupt on reddened and edematous skin of face, head, trunk and extensor surfaces
        b. Lesions of varied morphology, e.g., papules, vesicles, crusts, dry scales are present in various locations
    2. Chronic form develops in children and adolescents between ages 3 to 10 years; may continue into adulthood
        a. Skin is hyperpigmented, leathery, and thickened in the flexor surfaces of the neck, antecubital areas, wrists, popliteal area, ankle, fingers and toes
        b. Scratch marks on affected areas
    3. Other findings include:
        a. Circles under eyes
        b. Facial pallor
        c. Nasal crease on top of nose from frequent rubbing
        d. Dry hair
    4. Pustules may be present as sign of secondary bacterial infection
- Diagnostic Tests/Findings
    1. No specific test confirms diagnosis—serum level of IgE may support diagnosis in some cases

2. Skin scraping to rule out scabies

- Management/Treatment

    1. Obtain detailed history of onset, duration, severity/progression of symptoms, and possible precipitating factors

    2. Describe and monitor lesions in terms of morphology/structure, size, shape, number, color, location, distribution

    3. Treat secondary infections if present

        a. Oral antibiotics, e.g., erythromycin, cefaclor, cefadroxil, cephalexin, nafcillin, penicillin

        b. Topical antibiotics for localized infection—of little value with the exception of mupirocin; others may lead to sensitivity reactions

    4. Reduce and prevent pruritus with oral antipruritics, e.g., hydroxyzine, diphenhydramine

    5. Use topical steroids to reduce inflammation, immune response, and pruritus, e.g., hydrocortisone, triamcinolone

    6. Rehydrate skin if lesions are weeping and oozing

        a. Wet compresses and baths using

            (1) Aluminum acetate preparations

            (2) Oatmeal preparations

        b. Avoid skin drying agents such as harsh soaps, perfumes, lotions

        c. Apply cream emollients and lubricants, e.g., petroleum jelly

    7. Educate regarding medication dosage, signs of irritation, sensitivity

    8. Use mild soaps for general bathing and hygiene habits

    9. Eliminate exposure to all substances and agents that may dry or irritate the skin and exacerbate condition; individually determined

        a. Soaps, perfumes, hand and body lotions, makeup, household cleaning agents, bleach, chlorine, turpentine

        b. Materials and fabrics such as wool, feathers, polyesters, stuffed animals and other fabric toys

        c. Food substances such as cow's milk, eggs, nuts, citrus fruits

        d. Pets and other animals

        e. Dust and dust mites

    10. Monitor environment

        a. Maintain cool temperature to reduce sweating

        b. Increase humidity

11. Educate regarding characteristics of condition and expected prognosis

12. Refer for MD evaluation if condition does not resolve

Contact Dermatitis

- Definition: Allergic response to local contact with an allergen manifested by development of skin eruptions at site of contact

- Etiology/Incidence

    1. Caused by hypersensitivity to an allergen

        a. Initial contact—allergic response usually delayed for several days

        b. Re-exposure—allergic response usually occurs within 24 hours due to prior sensitization

    2. Numerous substances are associated with producing hypersensitivity reactions in sensitive individuals with the most common including:

        a. Perfumes, soaps, cosmetics, fabric dyes,

        b. Topical medications, e.g., neomycin

        c. Animal products—animal dander, feathers, fur, wool, leather

        d. Plastics, synthetics—latex, rubber

        e. Plants—poison sumac/ivy/oak

        f. Metals—jewelry

- Signs and Symptoms

    1. Redness and swelling at site of contact

    2. Pruritus with varying degrees of intensity

- Differential Diagnosis

    1. Bacterial infection

    2. Candida

    3. Diaper dermatitis

    4. Seborrhea dermatitis

- Physical Findings

    1. Erythema and edema with development of lesions of varying morphology—papules, vesicles, and denudation

    2. Lesions confined to area of direct contact with allergen

    3. Pruritus with varying degrees of intensity

    4. Excoriation/scratch marks and bleeding

    5. Chronic exposure may produce areas of hyperpigmentation and lichenification

- Diagnostic Tests/Findings: Skin testing to determine allergen hypersensitivities after acute stage

- Management/Treatment

    1. Obtain detailed history of onset, duration, severity, progression of symptoms, and possible precipitating factors

    2. Describe and monitor lesions in terms of morphology/structure, size, shape, number, color, location, distribution

    3. Avoid contact with allergen if sensitivity is known; if unknown, consider skin testing after acute phase to determine allergen

    4. Cool compresses of Burow's solution to affected areas

    5. Steroids to reduce inflammation, immune response, and pruritus

        a. Apply topical steroids to affected areas, e.g., hydrocortisone, triamcinolone

        b. Oral steroids for severe cases, e.g., hydrocortisone

    6. Oral antihistamines for pruritus, e.g., hydroxyzine, diphenhydramine

    7. Oral antibiotics if secondary infection present, e.g., erythromycin, dicloxicillin

    8. Educate regarding medication dosage, signs of irritation, sensitivity

    9. Educate regarding characteristics of condition and expected resolution

    10. Refer to MD for:

        a. Evaluation if condition does not show improvement in 2 days

        b. Consideration of skin testing for hypersensitivities after acute episode to identify specific allergens

Diaper (Irritant) Dermatitis

- Definition: Common disorder of genital-perineal area due to skin breakdown, characterized by erythema and other skin lesions

- Etiology/Incidence

    1. Breakdown of skin associated with:

        a. Exposure to chemical irritants in soaps, bleach, water softeners, skin lotions, diaper cleansing tissues

        b. Excessive contact with urine, feces; lax hygiene habits (primary irritant)

    2. Occurs in over 95% of all infants

    3. Peak incidence is 9 to 12 months of age

    4. Monilial rash caused by *Candida albicans*

    5. May persist until completion of toilet training

- Signs and Symptoms

1. Redness, sores in diaper area, blisters

2. Fiery red rash with monilial

3. May have general irritability and/or crying especially after elimination

- Differential Diagnosis

  1. Atopic dermatitis

  2. Allergic/contact dermatitis

  3. Psoriasis

  4. Secondary bacterial infection

  5. Child abuse

- Physical Findings

  1. Erythema with varying degrees of severity which may be generalized to entire area or localized to small area

  2. Lesions of varied morphology may develop—papules, vesicles, crusts, erosions and ulcerations

  3. Pustules may be present signaling secondary bacterial infection

  4. Monilial rash—fiery red, papular lesions within folds and on genitals; may also be pustular; may have associated oral thrush

  5. Poor genital hygiene may be present in some children

- Diagnostic Tests/Findings: No specific test confirms diagnosis

- Management/Treatment

  1. Obtain detailed history of onset, duration, severity, progression of symptoms, and possible precipitating factors

  2. Describe and monitor lesions in terms of morphology/structure, size, shape, number, color, location, distribution

  3. Treat secondary bacterial infection if present with topical antibiotics, e.g., bacitracin, mupirocin

  4. Treat present diaper dermatitis

     a. Mild erythema—emollients to affected areas with each diaper change, e.g., petroleum jelly, zinc oxide

     b. Erythema with papules—topical steriods, e.g., hydrocortisone, triamcinolone

     c. Severe erythema and edema with papules, vesicles, and ulcerations—wet dressings may be soothing, e.g., Burow's compresses; topical antibiotics may be indicated

     d. Monilial rash—topical nystatin, clotrimazole, ketoconazole; oral nystatin for thrush

e.   Avoid occlusive diapers and plastic pants

f.   Expose diaper area to air as often as possible

g.   Use appropriate preventive measures

5.   Educate regarding medication dosage, signs of irritation, sensitivity

6.   Preventive measures

a.   Expose diaper area to air several times each day

b.   Increase oral fluids to make urine less irritating

(1)   Water for infant under 12 months

(2)   Cranberry juice for older child

c.   Change diaper immediately after soiling

d.   Wash diaper area with nonirritating agents after each diaper change, e.g., mild soap and water

e.   Avoid occlusive diapers and plastic pants

f.   Diaper selection and care

(1)   Home laundry—mild soap and double rinse using 1 ounce of vinegar per gallon of water in last rinse

(2)   Disposable diapers—select alternate brand if sensitivity occurs

g.   "Diaper-wipes", may need to be avoided because of irritation or sensitivity

h.   Use lubricating ointment when diaper area skin is overly dry, e.g., petroleum jelly

7.   Refer for MD evaluation if no improvement within 2 to 3 days or if condition worsens

Seborrhea Dermatitis

- Definition: Chronic inflammatory condition usually on scalp and face

1.   Newborn and young infant—cradle cap

2.   Adolescents—dandruff

- Etiology/Incidence

1.   Associated with over production of sebum in areas abundant with sebaceous glands

2.   Increase in sebaceous gland activity may be connected with hormonal stimulation at times when hormonal influence is highest

3.   Occurs more often in spring and summer months

- Signs and Symptoms

1.   Newborns and infants—areas of redness under yellow crusts and greasy scales on scalp and face

2. Adolescents—white flakes and greasy scaling on scalp, forehead, eyebrows, and face

- Differential Diagnosis
    1. Atopic dermatitis
    2. Bacterial infection
    3. Candida
    4. Contact dermatitis
    5. Psoriasis
- Physical Findings
    1. Newborns and infants—areas of underlying erythema with yellow crusts and greasy scaling on scalp and face; in more severe cases lesions may be present on trunk and in diaper area
    2. Adolescents—white flakes and greasy scaling on scalp, forehead, eyebrows, and face; severity varies from simple dandruff to extensive, giving appearance of psoriasis; mild underlying erythema may be present
- Diagnostic Tests/Findings: No tests necessary to confirm diagnosis
- Management/Treatment
    1. Obtain detailed history of onset, duration, severity, progression of symptoms, and possible precipitating factors
    2. Describe and monitor lesions in terms of morphology/structure, size, shape, number, color, location, distribution
    3. Treat existing condition
        a. Shampoo and wash affected areas with antiseborrheic soaps and shampoos
        b. Mineral oil with brushing to loosen crusts prior to washing
        c. Topical steroid creams for extreme cases to reduce inflammation, e.g., hydrocortisone
    4. Educate regarding medication dosage, signs of irritation, sensitivity
    5. Educate regarding characteristics of condition and expected prognosis
    6. Refer for MD evaluation if condition persists without improvement

Burn Conditions

Burns

- Definition: Injury of skin from exposure to hot surfaces and agents
    1. Classified according to depth of injury to skin layers
        a. First degree/superficial burns—involve epidermis layer only

      b. Second degree/partial thickness burns—involve epidermis and part of dermis which may be superficial dermis or deep dermis

      c. Third degree/full thickness burns—involve epidermis, dermis, and dermal appendages

  2. Classified also according to extent of affected area

      a. Minor burns—less than 10% of body surface if burn is superficial, and less than 2% if burn is partial or full thickness

      b. Major burns—10% or more of body surface if burn is superficial and 2% or more if burn is partial or full thickness

      c. Major burns—hand, feet, face, eyes, ears, and perineal burns are always considered major burns, regardless of extent of body surface affected

- Etiology/Incidence

  1. Caused by exposure to hot chemicals, electrical and thermal substances and materials including electrical cords and outlets, irons, sun, flames, fireworks, hot water and foods, cigarettes, light bulbs

  2. Affected cells in epidermis, dermis, or subcutaneous skin layers are injured and no longer capable of providing protective, electrolyte storage, sensory, and other functions of normal skin cells

  3. Third leading cause of death in children and adolescents

      a. More common in toddlers and males

      b. Commonly occurs in kitchen in late afternoon during dinner preparation

      c. Approximately 10% of burns are thought to be intentional in infant, toddler, and young child

- Signs and Symptoms: According to degree, appearance, and healing time

  1. Superficial—red, swollen, and dry areas with tenderness

  2. Partial thickness and superficial burns—red, swollen, moist, and blistered areas with tenderness

  3. Partial thickness and deep burns—white, dry areas with loss of sensation

  4. Full thickness burns—white, brown, black, swollen dry areas with loss of sensation

- Differential Diagnosis

  1. Child abuse

  2. Staphylococcal scalded skin syndrome

- Physical Findings

  1. Superficial burns—erythema, mild edema, dryness, tenderness, and general discomfort of affected areas

2. Partial thickness and superficial burns—erythema, edema, moist, few vesicles/blisters may develop, sensitive to touch and air

3. Partial thickness and deep burns—white, dry, decreased sensitivity to touch, pain, temperature, and may blanch with pressure

4. Full thickness burns—white, brown, to black; swollen, dry; lack full touch, pain, temperature sensitivity

5. Physical findings associated with secondary bacterial infection may be present

- Diagnostic Tests/Findings

    1. Electrolyte studies especially if burn is extensive

    2. Culture to determine causal agent if secondary bacterial infection is present

- Management/Treatment

    1. Obtain detailed history of onset, duration, severity and symptom progression

    2. Describe and monitor burn area in terms of morphology/structure, extent of burn area, location, distribution

    3. Inpatient hospital management for all children with major burns, suspected abuse, esophageal and airway burns, and/or injuries such as fractures

    4. Outpatient management for children in stable environment with minor burns

        a. Partial thickness burn if < 10% of body surface area (BSA) or full surface burn is < 2% BSA

        b. Monitor daily healing process by documenting changes

        c. Cool compresses to affected areas

        d. Medication for pain control, e.g., acetaminophen, ibuprofen

        e. Topical antimicrobial agents to prevent infection on open blistered areas, e.g., silver sulfadiazine (except on face due to potential for hyperpigmentation), bacitracin, mupirocin

        f. Do not excise vesicles/blisters

        g. Fluids to reduce possibility of dehydration, e.g., water, juices

        h. Topical emollients if skin is dry, e.g., petroleum jelly

    5. Educate regarding need to protect skin from exposure to sunlight especially during 10 a.m. to 3 p.m.

        a. Cover-up clothing, hats, and sunglasses

        b. Water resistant sunblocks that protect against UVB and UVA ultraviolet light with > 15 SPF

    6. Educate regarding medication dosage, signs of irritation, sensitivity

    7. Educate regarding characteristics of condition and prognosis

8. Educate regarding measures to prevent further burn episodes and injuries

9. Refer for MD evaluation if condition does not show improvement

Sunburns

- Definition: Thermal burn due to excessive sunlight exposure

- Etiology/Incidence

    1. Exposed skin results in altered cell function and properties

        a. Increased blood flow

        b. Increased melanin production

    2. Fair-skinned populations are most sensitive

    3. Other factors involving sensitivity include high altitude, nearness to equator, and exposure to sun during hours of 10 a.m. and 3 p.m. when UVB waves are strongest

- Signs and Symptoms

    1. Redness, swelling, blisters, and tenderness of sun exposed areas

    2. Fatigue, chills, and headache after sun exposure

- Differential Diagnosis

    1. Child abuse

    2. Photosensitivity from medications

    3. Systemic viral exanthema

    4. Systemic drug reaction

- Physical Findings

    1. Dependent on degree of exposure and injury; develops within several minutes to several hours after exposure

        a. First degree burns—erythema and tenderness

        b. Second degree burns—increased intensity of erythema and tenderness with edema, some vesicles/blisters

        c. Third degree burns—increased intensity of erythema, tenderness, edema, and vesicles/blisters

    2. Systemic symptoms of malaise, fever, headache may be evident especially in younger child with second and third degree burns

    3. Epidermis cells scale and desquamate within 3 to 7 days after injury

    4. Exposed areas may become hyperpigmented with development of freckles and moles

- Diagnostic Tests/Findings: None used to confirm diagnosis

- Management/Treatment
    1. Obtain detailed history of onset, duration, severity, progression of symptoms and precipitating factors
    2. Describe and monitor location, color, and degree of burn, and symptoms
    3. Treat existing condition
        a. Remove from sunlight exposure
        b. Cool water or saline compresses to affected areas
        c. Do not use warm or hot showers/baths
        d. Increase oral fluids to prevent dehydration
        e. Oral pain medications, e.g., acetaminophen, ibuprofen
        f. Topical emollients for dry skin, e.g., petroleum jelly
    4. Educate regarding medication dosage, signs of irritation, sensitivity
    5. Educate regarding measures of prevention
        a. Risk factors of sun exposure
            (1) Teach early signs of skin cancer
            (2) Teach regarding individuals most vulnerable to sun exposure
        b. Use sun screens and blocks with 15 or greater SPF
            (1) Apply at least 20 minutes before exposure
            (2) Apply frequently if sustained exposure—every hour
            (3) Use waterproof agents when in water
            (4) Discontinue if sensitivity is suspected
            (5) Avoid use in infants under 6 months
        c. Use cover-up clothing and hats designed to block UVB waves
    6. Refer for MD evaluation if condition does not improve or becomes worse

Bacterial Conditions

Cellulitis

- Definition: Localized infection often precipitated by an insect bite (spider, mosquito, flea) or trauma that penetrates the protective skin barrier
- Etiology/Incidence: Caused when surface streptococci, *Haemophilus influenzae,* or *Staphylococcus aureus* bacteria invade all skin layers—epidermis, dermis, and subcutis, after a break in the skin has occurred
- Signs and Symptoms
    1. Irregular-shaped areas of skin with redness, swelling

2. Warm and tender to touch

3. Fever, chills, and malaise may be present

- Differential Diagnosis

    1. Influenza

    2. Furuncle

- Physical Findings

    1. Erythema and edema with ill-defined, irregular borders

    2. Tenderness and warmth

    3. Regional lymphadenopathy may be present

    4. Fever, chills, and malaise indicates systemic involvement

    5. Facial, periorbital, or orbital involvement is vulnerable to development of more severe conditions

- Diagnostic Tests/Findings: Blood culture to confirm causal agent

- Management/Treatment

    1. Detailed history of onset, duration, severity, progression of symptoms and precipitating factors

    2. Describe and monitor

        a. Affected skin areas in terms of morphology/structure, size, shape, color, location, distribution

        b. Systemic signs and symptoms of fever, chills, and malaise

    3. Hospitalization for severe cases and those involving face and eyes

    4. Treat with intramuscular, intravenous, and/or oral antibiotics according to severity of condition, organism, and site of involvement

        a. If streptococcus suspected—penicillins

        b. If *Haemophilus influenzae* suspected—amoxicillin

        c. If *Staphylococcus aureus* suspected—dicloxacillin

    5. Educate regarding medication dosage, signs of irritation, sensitivity

    6. Educate regarding characteristics of condition and expected prognosis

    7. Refer for MD evaluation if condition shows no improvement

Impetigo

- Definition: Localized infection of skin often precipitated by insect bites (spider, mosquito, flea) or other trauma that breaks protective skin barrier; predominately involves face and less commonly other body surfaces including perineum

- Etiology/Incidence

    1. *Staphylococcus aureus* and streptococci bacteria invade epidermis after break in skin

    2. Highly communicable with incubation period of 1 to 10 days

    3. Autoinoculable

- Signs and Symptoms

    1. Itching and tenderness may be present

    2. Areas of red swollen skin, blisters and/or moist honey-colored crusts

- Differential Diagnosis

    1. Eczema

    2. Herpes simplex

- Physical Findings

    1. Two major forms

        a. Nonbullous—underlying erythema with vesicles that erupt resulting in honey/serous colored crusts with erosion of epidermis

        b. Bullous—underlying erythema with pustules and vesicles that erupt resulting in smooth shiny appearance

    2. Regional adenopathy with tenderness

- Diagnostic Tests/Findings: Culture will confirm diagnosis and causative organism

- Management/Treatment

    1. Obtain detailed history of onset, duration, severity, progression of symptoms and precipitating factors

    2. Describe and monitor lesions in terms of morphology/structure, size, location, distribution

    3. Apply compresses of Burow's solution several times daily to aid in cleaning and removing crusts

    4. Apply topical antibiotics to areas of involvement, e.g., bacitracin, mupirocin, neosporin

    5. Prescribe oral antibiotics according to specific bacterial cause (Hay, Groothuis, Hayward & Levin, 1997; Bernstein & Shelov, 1996)

        a. For staphylococci—dicloxacillin

        b. For streptococci—penicillin or erythromycin

    6. Educate regarding medication dosage, signs of irritation, sensitivity

    7. Educate regarding characteristics of condition, treatment regime, prognosis, and good hygiene for prevention

8. Exclude from school and other public programs until treated for 48 hours due to high communicability

9. Refer for MD evaluation if condition does not improve

Staphylococcal Scalded Skin Syndrome

- Definition: Systemic bacterial infection with skin manifestations; also known as staphylococcal scarlet fever

- Etiology/Incidence

    1. Caused by effects of toxin produced by *Staphylococcus aureus* bacteria

    2. Occurs any season

    3. More common in neonates and infants than older children

    4. Incubation is variable, commonly 3 to 10 days

- Signs and Symptoms

    1. May present with abrupt onset of fever, irritability, and general malaise

    2. Bright, red, painful rash more pronounced around eyes, mouth, neck, underarms, elbow, groin, and knees

    3. Pain on pressure

    4. Blistering and/or scaling of skin

- Differential Diagnosis

    1. Streptococcal scarlet fever

    2. Burns

    3. Child abuse

    4. Drug toxicity

- Physical Findings

    1. Abrupt onset of fever and general malaise

    2. General exanthema with erythema and swelling; more pronounced in perioral, periorbital areas, flexure surfaces of neck, axilla, antecubital, groin, and popiteal areas

    3. Light pressure causes extreme pain and exfoliation of top epidermal layers

    4. After peeling, skin appears glistening and scalded

    5. Vesicles/bullae may occur in more toxic cases

- Diagnostic Tests/Findings

    1. Blood culture to confirm *Staphylococcus aureus*

    2. Culture secretions to confirm *Staphylococcus aureus*

- Management/Treatment

1. Obtain detailed history of onset, duration, severity, progression of symptoms and precipitating factors

2. Describe and monitor in terms of morphology/structure, size, shape, number, color, location, distribution

3. Hospitalization is indicated for all neonates; treat more severe cases with IV antibiotics and monitor fluid and electrolytes

4. Outpatient management may be considered with less toxic cases if environment is stable

    a. Oral antistaphylococcal antibiotics, e.g., dicloxacillin

    b. Oral antipyretics and analgesics for fever and pain control, e.g., acetaminophen, ibuprofen

    c. Increase fluids to maintain hydration and prevent dehydration, e.g., water, juices

5. Educate regarding medication dosage, signs of irritation, sensitivity

6. Educate regarding characteristics of condition, treatment, and prognosis

7. Refer for MD evaluation if condition does not improve

Bacterial Conditions Involving Pilosebaceous Unit

Acne

- Definition: Inflammatory chronic skin disorder involving the pilosebaceous follicle unit
  1. Occurs predominately on the face, neck, chest and upper back skin surfaces; less commonly in other areas
  2. Often occurs in cyclic periods of exacerbation and remission
- Etiology/Incidence
  1. Specific cause is unknown

      a. Associated with breakdown of follicle wall

      b. Cells combine with sebum and plug follicle

      c. Enzymes from *Corynebacterium acnes* mix with trapped debris causing edema and irritation

  2. Proven factors which may contribute to acne development

      a. Increased androgenic hormonal influence

      b. Positive family history

      c. Stress

  3. Unproven factors with questionable and unsubstantiated contribution

      a. Food—nuts, eggs, cheese, chocolate

    b. Poor hygiene

  4. Affects more than 70% of adolescents with varying degrees of severity

    a. Onset parallels puberty

    b. More common in females

    c. More males develop severe acne

    d. More females experience continuation of acne into adult years

- Signs and Symptoms

  1. Open and closed pimples/bumps

  2. Soreness at site of lesions

  3. Scars at site of previous lesions

- Differential Diagnosis

  1. Folliculitis

  2. Contact dermatitis

  3. Urticaria

  4. Allergic drug reaction

- Physical Findings

  1. Lesions of varying morphology

    a. Mild acne—lesions are scattered covering small areas

      (1) Open comedones/blackheads—lesions filled with dry oxidized sebum; brown in color

      (2) Closed comedones/whiteheads—lesions filled with follicle cells and sebum

    b. Moderate acne—lesions are more numerous covering large areas

      (1) All lesions of mild acne

      (2) Pustules—lesions filled with follicle cells, sebum, and white blood cells

    c. Severe acne—lesions are much more numerous covering larger areas

      (1) All lesions of mild and moderate acne

      (2) Erythema with papules and pustules

      (3) Nodules and cysts—deep dermal lesions filled with follicle debris often with communicating tracks to other cysts

  2. Increased oiliness of hair and skin

  3. Scarring especially when

    a. Lesions at any stage have been manipulated and squeezed

      b.   Cysts have erupted deep within the dermis

    4.   Signs of related psychological distress/depression may be present

- Diagnostic Tests/Findings: None; clinically determined diagnosis

- Management/Treatment

    1.   Obtain detailed history of onset, duration, severity and progression of symptoms and possible precipitating factors

    2.   Describe in terms of morphology/structure, size, shape, number, color, location, distribution

    3.   Wash and dry face and affected areas with mild non-oil base soap

    4.   Apply warm compresses

    5.   Use topical exfoliates and comedolytic preparations

        a.   Mild acne—tretinoin

        b.   Moderate acne—benzoyl peroxide

        c.   Severe acne: tretinoin and benzoyl peroxide

    6.   Use topical antibiotics for moderate to severe acne, e.g., clindamycin, erythomycin

    7.   Add oral antibiotics for persistent and unresponsive cases of moderate and severe acne

        a.   Tetracycline, erythromycin, doxycycline, minocycline

        b.   Oral clindamycin contraindicated due to adverse GI side effects

    8.   Consider using isotretinoin for unresponsive, persistent severe acne

        a.   Contraindicated in pregnancy

        b.   For sexually active females, birth control measures indicated

    9.   Educate regarding medication dosage, signs of irritation, sensitivity

    10.   Consider counseling for signs of psychological distress and depression

    11.   Educate regarding characteristics of condition, treatment regime, and expected prognosis

        a.   Condition may become worse with treatment before improvement

        b.   Treatment will improve but not cure most cases; may take months

        c.   Treatment must be consistent to be effective

    12.   Monitor progress every 2 to 4 weeks initially; less often as indicated when improvement is evident

    13.   Refer for MD evaluation if condition does not meet prognostic expectations

Folliculitis/Furuncle

- Definition: Infectious condition involving pilosebaceous follicle occurring on any skin surface where hair follicles are present but predominately on face, neck, scalp and buttocks

    1. Folliculitis—superficial involvement of upper follicle

    2. Furuncle or boil—deeper involvement of follicle and dermal appendages

- Etiology/Incidence

    1. Caused most often by *Staphylococcus aureus*; less commonly by streptococcus bacteria

    2. Also seen with some tinea infections

    3. More common in males

- Signs and Symptoms

    1. Areas of redness and swelling

    2. Nodules may be present with deep-seated furuncles

    3. Tenderness and warmth at site

- Differential Diagnosis

    1. Candida

    2. Impetigo

- Physical Findings

    1. Localized areas of erythema and edema with papular or pustular lesions on face, scalp, neck, buttocks and other areas

    2. Nodules are present with deep-seated furuncles

    3. Tenderness and warmth may be present

    4. Regional adenopathy may be present

- Diagnostic Tests/Findings: Culture confirms specific bacterial agent

- Management/Treatment

    1. Obtain detailed history of onset, duration, severity, progression of symptoms and possible precipitating factors

    2. Describe and monitor lesions in terms of morphology/structure, size, shape, number, color, location, distribution

    3. Wash with antimicrobial soap and apply warm moist compresses to affected areas

    4. Topical antibiotics, e.g., bacitracin, mupirocin, neosporin

    5. Oral antibiotics

        a. For staphylococci—use dicloxacillin

b. For streptococci infection—penicillin or cephalosporin, erythromycin for penicillin allergic patients

6. Educate regarding medication dosage, signs of irritation, sensitivity

7. Educate regarding characteristics of condition, treatment regime, prognosis, and good hygiene measures

8. Refer for MD evaluation if condition does not follow prognostic expectation

Viral Conditions

Herpes Simplex/Common Cold Sore

- Definition: Contagious infection predominately of lips and oral mucosa, commonly known as fever blisters

    1. Initial infectious state—more severe, lasts longer, and is more painful

    2. Dormant state—virus lives on ending of selected nerves, asymptomatic

    3. Secondary infectious state—activated at times of increased stress, illness, fatigue, sun exposure, menses

- Etiology/Incidence

    1. Herpes simplex virus type 1—most common cause

    2. Herpes simplex virus type 2—considered in situations of oral sex

    3. Incubation varies, commonly 2 to 12 days

- Signs and Symptoms

    1. Redness with small blisters and crusting on lips

    2. Redness and swelling with painful white ulcerated patches inside mouth

    3. Fever, generalized malaise, and sore throat may occur

    4. Mild itching, tingling, pain, and burning may precede blisters

- Differential Diagnosis

    1. Erythema multiforme

    2. Hand-foot-mouth disease

    3. Candida

    4. Localized bacterial infection

    5. Sexual abuse

- Physical Findings

    1. Lip lesions—grouped or singular vesicles on an erythematous base erupt and form crusts; usually can be found on mucocutaneous border of lips

2. Oral cavity lesions—erythema and edema of mucous membranes with singular or multiple vesicles and white ulcerations; may include tongue, palate, and gums

3. Regional adenopathy may be present

4. Halitosis may be present with oral lesions

5. Lesions are present 10 to 14 days, gradually resolving

6. Secondary infection may be present—most caused by staphylococcus bacteria

- Diagnostic Tests/Findings

    1. Tzanck smear confirms presence of multinuclear giant cells indicative of herpes

    2. Culture to confirm causal agent

- Management/Treatment

    1. Obtain detailed history of onset, duration, severity and progression of symptoms, and precipitating factors

    2. Describe and monitor lesions in terms of morphology/structure, size, shape, number, color, location, distribution

    3. Treat lip lesions

        a. Burow's compresses to alleviate discomfort

        b. Topical antiviral applications, e.g., acyclovir, for recurrent disease

    4. Treat oral lesions

        a. Avoid spicy and acid foods

        b. Cool, bland fluids especially when lesions are most painful

        c. Anesthetic mouth rinses, e.g., lidocaine (with caution), or diphenhydramine

    5. Oral antiviral medication with recurrent disease at first sign of prodrome (skin tingling), e.g., acyclovir

    6. Oral antibiotic to treat secondary bacterial infection, e.g., erythromycin, dicloxacillin, cefadroxil, cephalexin

    7. Educate regarding medication dosage, signs of irritation, sensitivity

    8. Educate regarding cause, characteristics of condition, communicability, and prognosis

    9. Educate regarding preventive measures

        a. Avoid direct exposure of others to lesions (kissing)

        b. Wash hands before and after applying topical medications or touching lesions

        c. Avoid sharing personal items—cosmetics, cups, eating utensils

    10. Refer for MD evaluation if condition does not improve

Molluscum Contagiosum

- Definition: Common infectious, self-limiting skin condition characterized by waxy firm papules which may occur on any skin surface predominately on face, axillae, abdomen, and arms

- Etiology/Incidence

  1. Caused by a poxvirus

  2. Most common in children and adolescents

  3. Common in children with HIV or AIDS

  4. Incubation is usually 2 to 8 weeks but may be up to 6 months

  5. Period of communicability uncertain

     a. May persist as long as lesions are present

     b. Spread by direct contact and through autoinoculations

- Signs and Symptoms

  1. Mild itching may be present

  2. Few or multiple small, firm, raised pinkish-white or skin colored lesions

- Differential Diagnosis

  1. Warts

  2. Closed comedones

  3. *Condylomata acuminata*

- Physical Findings

  1. Papular pink-white, or skin colored lesions of 1 to 5 mm in size usually on face, neck, axillae, abdomen, and arms

  2. Occasionally lesions grow to 1 to 2 cm

  3. Secondary bacterial infection may be present

  4. Lesions may become umbilicated (central pitting, dimpled, or depressed)

  5. Lesions are self-limiting but may be present for 2 to 3 years if left untreated

  6. May occur in genital area in sexually active and sexually abused

- Diagnostic Tests/Findings

  1. Usually not necessary

  2. Wright or Giemsa stain of papule core will show characteristic intracytoplasmic inclusions

- Management/Treatment

  1. Obtain a detailed history of onset, duration, severity and progression of symptoms, and precipitating factors

2. Describe and monitor lesions in terms of morphology/structure, size, shape, number, color, location, distribution

3. Rule out child abuse if lesions in genital area

4. Treatment options:

    a. Lesions may resolve spontaneously without treatment over time

    b. Curretage removal of lesions provides more expedient resolution; not recommended for facial lesions due to potential scarring

    c. Topical application of keratolytics; not recommended for lesions near eyes

        (1) Tretinoin cream

        (2) Cartharidin

    d. Topical antibiotics for secondary bacterial infection, e.g., erythromycin, bacitracin, mupirocin

5. Education regarding medication dosages, signs of irritation, sensitivity

6. Education regarding cause, characteristics of lesions, communicability, and prognosis

7. Education regarding preventive measures

    a. Avoid direct exposure of others to lesions

    b. Wash hands before and after application of topical medications and/or touching lesions

    c. Avoid sharing personal items—cosmetics, towels, cups, eating utensils

8. Refer for MD evaluation if condition does not resolve with selected treatment

Verruca (Warts)

- Definition: Common self-limiting skin condition characterized by firm, well-circumscribed smooth to irregular, singular or multiple papules, predominately on fingers, palms, and soles of feet; commonly known as warts

- Etiology/Incidence

1. Human papillomaviruses with more than 50 identified types

2. Virus enters skin through minor trauma

3. Occurs in 10% of children and adolescents with school-age children having the highest incidence

4. Incidence may be increased with ongoing exposure to moisture

5. Period of incubation varies widely, and estimated from 2 months to 2 years

6. Period of communicability unknown

    a. May persist as long as lesions are present

b. Spread by direct and indirect contact and through autoinoculations

- Signs and Symptoms
    1. Raised gray, brownish to skin colored, smooth to rough, singular or multiple lesions on hands
    2. Painful flat ingrown lesions on soles
    3. Bleeding may occur with trauma or picking
- Differential Diagnosis
    1. Molluscum contagiosum
    2. Calluses
- Physical Findings
    1. Common verruca—gray, brown or skin colored, rough singular or multiple papular lesions, most common on hands and fingers
    2. Flat verruca—skin colored, smooth round multiple lesions slightly elevated; most common on the face and extremities
    3. Plantar verruca—skin colored, irregular, single or multiple lesions that appear flush with sole of foot and grow inward
    4. May occur in genital area of sexually active and sexually abused
    5. Lesions are self-limiting, usually 6 to 9 months but due to reinfection through auto-inoculation; condition may persist for several years
- Diagnostic Tests/Findings: Excision and histological examination may confirm diagnosis
- Management/Treatment
    1. Obtain a detailed history of onset, duration, severity, progression of symptoms, and possible precipitating factors
    2. Describe and monitor lesions in terms of morphology/structure, size, shape, number, color, location, distribution
    3. Rule out child abuse if genital lesions are present
    4. Consider treatment options
        a. No treatment is usually necessary due to self-limiting condition
            (1) Ideal treatment has not been established
            (2) Frequently recur regardless of treatment choice
        b. Topical applications of keratolytics, e.g., cantharidin, tretinoin
        c. Applications of waterproof plastic tapes treated with keratolytics
        d. Excision of lesions except those on face due to potential scarring
    5. Topical antibiotics to treat secondary bacterial infection, e.g., erythromycin, bacitracin, mupirocin, neosporin

6. Educate regarding medication dosages, signs of irritation, sensitivity

7. Educate regarding cause, characteristics of condition, communicability, and prognosis

8. Consider congenital or acquired immunodeficiency if no resolution and/or wide-spread (Cohen, 1999)

9. Refer for MD evaluation if condition does not improve or bleeds with light trauma

Fungal Infections

Tinea Capitis (Ringworm of the Scalp)

- Definition: Superficial dermatophyte (parasitic) fungal skin infection of the scalp
- Etiology/Incidence
  1. Caused predominately by *Trichophyton tonsurans* (90%); also by *Microsporum canis, Microsporum audouinii*, and *Trichophyton mentagrophytes* (less common)
  2. Dermatophytes attach to epidermis skin layer of host's scalp and multiply within stratum corneum; do not involve lower layers of epidermis or dermis
  3. Spreads through direct and indirect contact with infected individuals, animals, caps, combs, brushes, glasses and other personal articles
  4. *Microsporum canis* may be transmitted through contact with infected dogs or cats
  5. Occurs more often in hot humid climates
  6. More common in darker skinned individuals; boys more than girls
  7. Incubation period is unknown, possibly 10 to 14 days
  8. Communicability occurs as long as lesions with dermatophytes are present
- Signs and Symptoms
  1. Itching with varying degrees of severity
  2. Slightly raised round or angular scaly areas with pink borders
  3. Some yellow honey-comb crusts
  4. Broken hairs and balding may be present
- Differential Diagnosis
  1. Impetigo
  2. Eczema
  3. Seborrhea dermatitis
  4. Psoriasis
  5. Trichotillomania
- Physical Findings

1. Several presentations may occur singularly or at the same time

   a. Diffuse scaly plaques of varying sizes with or without alopecia

   b. Pustules, papules with areas of honey-comb crusts

   c. Tender erythematous areas with broken hairs at scalp level leaving a "black-dot" appearance

2. Regional adenopathy may be present, especially occipital nodes

- Diagnostic Tests/Findings

   1. Wood's lamp will fluoresce the *Microsporum canis* only and is of limited use in confirming tinea capitis

   2. KOH scraping from the areas of scalp with alopecia, "black dots," or broken hairs will confirm hyphae and spores of dermatophytes

- Management/Treatment

   1. Obtain detailed history of onset, duration, severity and progression of symptoms, and precipitating factors

   2. Describe and monitor lesions in terms of morphology/structure, size, shape, number, color, location, and distribution

   3. Treat with oral antifungal medication

      a. Griseofulvin

      b. May require treatment up to 6 weeks before resolution

      c. Topical antifungal medications are ineffective

   4. Shampoo 2 to 3 times weekly with selenium sulfide to reduce spore count and infectivity

   5. Although condition is communicable, exclusion from school and other groups is not indicated unless treatment is refused or not followed

   6. Educate regarding medication dosage, signs of irritation, sensitivity

   7. Educate regarding characteristics of condition, treatment regime, and prognosis

   8. Educate regarding communicability and prevention

      a. Avoid sharing personal items of caps, combs, brushes, towels, pillows, glasses, razors; wash these items frequently

      b. Wash hair immediately after barbershop or salon haircut

      c. Maintain personal hygiene, wash hands before/after treatment

      d. Avoid touching or scratching affected areas

   9. Refer for MD evaluation if condition does not improve

Tinea Corporis (Ringworm of the Body)

- Definition: Superficial dermatophyte (parasitic) fungal skin infection of less-hairy surfaces of body and face; commonly known as "ring worm" due to pattern of healing centrally while spreading peripherally

- Etiology/Incidence

  1. Primary source—*Trichophyton rubrum, Trichophyton mentagrophytes,* as well as *Microsporum canis,* and *Epidermophyton floccosum*

  2. Dermatophytes attach to epidermis skin layer of host and multiply within stratum corneum; do not involve lower layers of the epidermis or dermis

  3. Spreads through direct and indirect contact with infected individuals, animals, shower stalls, benches, and other articles

  4. *Microsporum canis* may be transmitted through contact with infected dogs or cats

  5. Occurs more often in hot humid climates

  6. Incubation period is unknown, possibly 4 to 14 days

  7. Communicability occurs as long as lesions with dermatophytes are present

- Signs and Symptoms

  1. Mild itching at site of affected areas

  2. Slightly raised round or angular scaly areas with pink borders

- Differential Diagnosis

  1. Contact dermatitis

  2. Eczema

  3. Psoriasis

  4. Pityriasis rosea

- Physical Findings

  1. Typical lesions are scaly plaques of varying sizes from less than 5 mm to more that 3 cm with mild erythematous active borders

  2. Lesions spread peripherally as they heal centrally

  3. Lesions may be singular or several; numerous lesions are uncommon

- Diagnostic Tests/Findings

  1. Wood's lamp will fluoresce the *Microsporum canis*

  2. KOH scraping of lesion border—confirms hyphae and spores

  3. Dermatophyte test medium (DTM)—confirm diagnosis

- Management/Treatment

1. Obtain a detailed history of onset, duration, severity, progression of symptoms, and precipitating factors

2. Describe and monitor lesions in terms of morphology/structure, size, shape, number, color, location, and distribution

3. Treat with topical antifungal medications

   a. Clotrimazole, miconazole, econazole, terbinafine, tolnaftate, naftifine, ciclopirox, ketoconazole

   b. May require treatment up to 8 weeks before resolution

4. Treat with oral antifungal medication for extensive, recurrent, and unresponsive conditions, e.g., griseofulvin

5. Educate regarding medication dosage, signs of irritation, sensitivity

6. Educate regarding characteristics of condition, treatment regime, and prognosis

7. Educate regarding communicability and prevention

   a. Avoid sharing personal items of clothing, towels, pillows, razors and wash these items frequently

   b. Maintain personal hygiene and wash hands before and after applying treatment

   c. Avoid touching or scratching affected areas

   d. Avoid or shower after using public pools

   e. Wash clothing touching affected areas after each use

8. Refer for MD evaluation if condition does not improve

Tinea Cruris (Jock Itch)

- Definition: Superficial dermatophyte (parasitic) fungal skin infection of the groin, upper thighs, and/or inguinal folds; commonly called "jock-itch"

- Etiology/Incidence

  1. Caused by *Epidermophyton floccosum, Trichophyton rubrum,* and *Trichophyton mentagrophytes*

  2. Dermatophytes attach to epidermis skin layer of host and multiply within stratum corneum; lower layers of epidermis or dermis are not involved

  3. Occurs more often during hot humid weather with increased sweating

  4. More common in adolescents, athletes, obese children, and males

  5. Spreads through direct and indirect contact with infected individuals, including sexual contact

  6. Incubation period is unknown, possibly 4 to 14 days

  7. Communicability occurs as long as lesions with dermatophytes are present

- Signs and Symptoms

1. Pain and tenderness with varying degrees of severity
2. Itching with varying degrees of severity reported especially during healing
3. Red slightly raised scaly areas with defined borders
4. Blisters may also be present

- Differential Diagnosis
    1. Contact dermatitis
    2. Eczema
    3. Intertrigo
    4. Psoriasis
    5. Seborrheic dermatitis

- Physical Findings
    1. Erythematous scaly red to brown lesions of varying sizes with well defined raised borders
        a. Small vesicles, central clearing, and peripheral spreading may or may not be present
        b. Affected areas may be singular or multiple
        c. In chronic cases, lichenification may be present
    2. All areas of the groin may be affected including scrotum, gluteal folds, buttocks, inner aspect of thighs
    3. Painful to touch and with movement
    4. Often concurrent with tinea pedis

- Diagnostic Tests/Findings
    1. KOH scraping of lesion border—confirms hyphae and spores
    2. DTM—confirms diagnosis

- Management/Treatment
    1. Obtain a detailed history of onset, duration, severity, progression of symptoms, and precipitating factors
    2. Describe and monitor lesions in terms of morphology/structure, size shape, number, color, location, and distribution
    3. Treat with topical antifungal medications
        a. Clotrimazole, haloprogin, miconazole, terbinafine, tolnaftate, ciclopirox, econazole, ketoconazole, naftifine, oxiconazole, sulconazole
        b. May require treatment up to 4 to 6 weeks before resolution

4. Treat with oral antifungal medication for extensive, recurrent, and/ or unresponsive conditions, e.g., griseofulvin

5. Educate regarding medication dosage, signs of irritation, sensitivity

6. Educate regarding characteristics of condition, treatment regime, and prognosis

7. Educate regarding communicability and prevention

   a. Avoid sharing undergarments—pants, jock straps,

   b. Wash personal undergarments frequently

   c. Maintain good daily personal hygiene and dry well after bathing

   d. Wash hands before and after applying topical treatment

   e. Avoid touching or scratching affected areas

   f. Avoid or shower after using public pools

   g. Launder clothing touching affected areas after each use

   h. Don't wear tight clothes next to affected area including jeans and undergarments

   i. Use cotton undergarments and change daily

8. Refer for MD evaluation if condition does not improve

Tinea Pedis (Athlete's Feet, or Ringworm of the Feet)

- Definition: Superficial dermatophyte (parasitic) fungal skin infection of toes and feet
- Etiology/Incidence

  1. Caused by *Trichophyton rubrum, Trichophyton mentagrophytes,* and *Epidermophyton floccosum* fungal dermatophytes

  2. Dermatophytes attach to epidermis skin layer of host and multiply within stratum corneum; do not involve lower layers of epidermis or dermis

  3. Occurs more often during hot humid weather with increased sweating

  4. Occurs worldwide; more common in adolescents, athletes, and males

  5. Spreads through direct and indirect contact with infected individuals, public baths, swimming pools, and locker rooms

  6. Incubation period is unknown

  7. Communicability occurs as long as lesions with dermatophytes are present

- Signs and Symptoms

  1. Pruritus of affected areas

  2. Reddened, scaly and occasionally blistered areas anywhere on foot; cracks and scaling between toes

  3. Stinging or pain if cracks between toes

- Differential Diagnosis

  1. Atopic dermatitis

  2. Contact dermatitis

  3. Candida

  4. Eczema

- Physical Findings

  1. Erythematous scaly lesions of varying sizes

     a. Small vesicles, central clearing, and peripheral spreading may or may not be present

     b. Affected areas may be anywhere on foot, most commonly on lateral and planter portions

  2. Lesions on or between toes are scaly with mild erythema

     a. Interdigital fissures are present

     b. One or multiple toes may be involved, most commonly between third and fourth toes

  3. Dystrophy of toenails may be present

- Diagnostic Tests/Findings

  1. KOH scraping of lesion border confirms hyphae and spores

  2. DTM of skin scraping or nail clippings confirms diagnosis

- Management/Treatment

  1. Obtain a detailed history of onset, duration, severity, progression of symptoms, and precipitating factors

  2. Describe and monitor lesions in terms of morphology/structure, size, shape, number, color, location, and distribution

  3. Treat with topical antifungal medications

     a. Clotrimazole, haloprogin, miconazole, econazole, ciclopirox, terbinafine, tolnaftate, ketoconazole, naftifine, oxiconazole, sulconazole

     b. May require treatment up to 4 to 6 weeks before resolution

  4. Treat vesicular and fissured lesions with compresses of Burow's solution

  5. Use absorbent antifungal powder

  6. Treat with oral antifungal medication for extensive, recurrent, and unresponsive conditions, e.g., griseofulvin

  7. Educate regarding medication dosage and signs of irritation and sensitivity

  8. Educate regarding characteristics of condition, treatment regime, and prognosis

9. Educate regarding communicability and prevention
    a. Avoid sharing personal items of shoes, socks, and towels
    b. Wash personal items items frequently
    c. Maintain good daily personal hygiene and dry well after bathing
    d. Wash hands before and after applying topical treatment
    e. Avoid touching or scratching affected areas
    f. Avoid using public pools or shower after each use
    g. Launder clothing touching affected areas after each use
    h. Don't wear tight and closed shoes
    i. Use cotton socks instead of nylon or polyester
10. Refer for MD evaluation if condition does not improve

Insect Conditions

Common Insect Bites

- Definition: Wound inflicted by bite of a blood sucking arthropod
- Etiology/Incidence
    1. Caused when mosquitos, fleas, chiggers, and bedbugs feed on human blood
        a. Are attracted to host's moisture, odor, and warmth
        b. Serve as vectors for diseases such as malaria
    2. Pet dogs and cats act as hosts for some fleas that are also attracted to humans
    3. More bites occur:
        a. In warm and humid weather
        b. Around stagnant water
        c. In outside grassy and sandy areas
        d. On uncovered body areas
    4. Itching caused by sensitivity to insect's saliva
- Signs and Symptoms
    1. Itching is major symptom—may persist 5 to 7 days after exposure
    2. Pain—variable
    3. Single or multiple pink/red raised lesions on legs, abdomen, and exposed areas of upper body
- Differential Diagnosis
    1. Folliculitis

2. Insect sting

3. Spider bite

4. Scabies

- Physical Findings

    1. Single or multiple erythematous papules and wheals on lower extremities, abdomen, and exposed upper body parts

    2. Lesions from bed bug and chigger bites are smaller, more erythematous and more numerous

    3. Vesicles may develop signaling greater sensitivity

    4. Excoriation may be present with intense pruritus

    5. Pustules may develop indicating secondary bacterial infection

- Diagnostic Tests/Findings: Culture of pustules confirms causal organism of secondary infection

- Management/Treatment

    1. Obtain detailed history of bite, progression of symptoms, and precipitating factors

    2. Describe and monitor lesions in terms of morphology/structure, size, shape, number, color, location, and distribution

    3. Provide symptomatic treatment of pruritus

        a. Cool compresses

        b. Topical histamines, e.g., hydroxyzine, diphenhydramine

        c. Oral antihistamines if topical treatment is ineffective, e.g., hydroxyzine, diphenhydramine

    4. Topical steroids to reduce inflammation and immune response, e.g., hydrocortisone, triamcinolone

    5. Treat secondary bacterial infection

        a. Use topical antibiotics, e.g., bacitracin, mupirocin, neosporin

        b. Treat with oral antibiotics if extensive, recurrent, or unresponsive, e.g., erythromycin, cefadroxil, cephalexin

    6. Educate regarding characteristics of condition, treatment regime, and prognosis

    7. Educate regarding medication dosage, signs of irritation, sensitivity

    8. Educate regarding prevention

        a. Outside environmental controls—clearing areas, pesticide spraying, removing stagnant water

        b. Inside environmental controls—routine cleaning, vacuuming

        c. Bathe flea-infested pets

      d.   Wear cover-up clothing

      e.   Wear insect repellants

      f.   Avoid wearing fragrances that may attract

      g.   Avoid scratching to prevent infection

  9. Refer for MD evaluation if condition does not resolve

Spider Bites

- Definition: Wound inflicted by spider characterized by both local and systemic manifestations

- Etiology/Incidence

  1. Most spider bites are harmless, causing small localized reaction at site of bite

  2. In U.S. bites from two non-aggressive venomous spiders produce severe toxic reactions in some individuals

     a. Black widow

        (1) Mature female is shinny, black, gray or brown with an orange hour glass marking on the ventral surface

        (2) Overall size is 2.5 to 4.5 cm including legs

        (3) Male is smaller with fangs that can not penetrate human skin

        (4) Most common in Ohio, South, Southwest, and West coast

        (5) Likes dry, warm, dark areas; found in grass, wood piles, gardens, sheds, basements, closets, and trunks

        (6) Spin irregular asymmetrical web to catch flies and other prey

     b. Brown recluse

        (1) Mature spider is gray, or varying shades of red to pale brown with a violin shaped marking on cephalothorax

        (2) Overall size is 1.5 to 2.5 cm including legs

        (3) Most common in the Midwest and South

        (4) Likes trunks, carpets, old shoes, old clothes, closets, crates, shelves

  3. Most bites are in self-defense when spider feels threatened

  4. Most bites occur in warmer months

  5. Infants and small children are most vulnerable to developing serious reactions

- Signs and Symptoms

  1. Black widow

     a. Initial sensation of pinch or sting is often unnoticed

    b.   Later within 1 hour of the bite

        (1)   Dull burning or pain at site of bite

        (2)   Two red puncture marks surrounded by white area with bluish-red border

        (3)   Muscle cramps and sweating

        (4)   Muscle spasms can spread to rest of body

        (5)   In severe cases can progress to shock, coma, and death

  2. Brown recluse

    a.   Initial sensation of bite is most often unnoticed or moderately painful

    b.   Later within 2 to 7 hours

        (1)   Mild localized tingling

        (2)   Redness or blanching

    c.   After 48 to 72 hours

        (1)   Blister surrounded by blue-gray area

        (2)   Flu-like symptoms may be experienced

  3. Reactions from bites of both spiders may become more intense and last for days with more serious life-threatening signs/symptoms developing in a few cases

- Differential Diagnosis—Black widow and Brown recluse

  1. Other insect bites (both)

  2. Tetanus (black widow)

  3. Appendicitis (black widow)

  4. Diabetic ulcers (brown recluse)

  5. Stevens-Johnson syndrome (brown recluse)

- Physical Findings—specifics vary by type of spider

  1. Black widow spider bite

    a.   Symptoms begin within one hour

    b.   Dull, burning or pain at site

    c.   Two red puncture marks surrounded by a blanched area with bluish erythematous border

    d.   Muscle spasms, hypertension, tachycardia, diaphoresis

  2. Brown recluse spider bite

    a.   Initial symptoms begin within 2 to 7 hours

        (1)   Mild, localized tingling

      (2) Erythema or blanching at site

  b. Delayed symptoms after 48 to 72 hours

      (1) Hemorrhagic vesicle surrounded by bluish, gray areas of developing necrosis

      (2) Flu-like symptoms

3. Both (black widow and brown recluse)

  a. Reactions may last for days to weeks

  b. Potential to become serious and life-threatening with major renal, respiratory, cardiovascular, and neurological system involvement

- Diagnostic Tests/Findings

  1. No tests confirm specific diagnosis

  2. Dead spider specimen may help to confirm specific species

- Management/Treatment

  1. Obtain detailed history of onset, duration, severity and progression of symptoms, and precipitating factors

  2. Describe and monitor symptoms, and lesions in terms of morphology/structure, size, shape, number, color, location, and distribution

  3. If bite from black widow or brown recluse spider is suspected

    a. Apply cold compresses to site of bite

    b. Refer immediately for MD evaluation and hospitalization due to potential risk of severe reaction

  4. If bite from another less harmful spider is suspected

    a. Apply cool compresses to site of bite

    b. Use oral antihistamines to reduce severe pruritus, e.g., hydroxyzine, diphenhydramine

    c. Monitor for hypersensitivity reaction

  5. Educate regarding characteristics of condition, treatment regime, and prognosis

  6. Educate regarding medication dosage, signs of irritation, sensitivity

  7. Educate regarding prevention

    a. Outside environmental controls—clearing areas, pesticide spraying

    b. Inside environmental controls—routine cleaning, vacuuming

    c. Avoid and/or be observant around areas of natural habitat

    d. Wear protective clothing and hats

  e. Wear gloves when cleaning closets and trunks

  f. Inspect clothing and shoes prior to wearing

Insect Stings

- Definition: Wound inflicted by sting of an insect, characterized by systemic and/or local manifestations
- Etiology/Incidence
  1. Caused by bees, hornets, wasps, yellow-jackets, and fire ants
  2. Hypersensitivity to venom develops after initial exposure with more severe reactions upon subsequent exposures
     a. Mild reactions occur in 90% of children
     b. Anaphylaxis occurs in approximately 7% of general population
  3. Most stings occur in self-defense when insect feels threatened
  4. Most stings occur in warmer months
  5. Multiple stings may occur when around nests or swarms of insects
- Signs and Symptoms
  1. Usual reaction after initial exposure lasts up to 24 hours
     a. Pain with varying degrees of severity
     b. Redness and swelling at site of sting
  2. More pronounced reaction after re-exposure
     a. Nausea and abdominal pain
     b. Sneezing and coughing
     c. Itching
     d. Larger area of redness and swelling
  3. Anaphylactic reaction may occur after initial or re-exposure
     a. Early signs within minutes of exposure
        (1) Dizziness
        (2) Swelling of lips and throat
        (3) Difficulty breathing
        (4) Difficulty swallowing
     b. Later signs
        (1) Weakness and collapse
        (2) Confusion

             (3)   Coma

- Differential Diagnosis

  1. Spider bites

  2. Other insect bites

- Physical Findings

  1. Usual reaction after initial exposure may last up to 24 hours

     a. Pain with varying degrees of severity

     b. Erythema and edema surrounding central punctum at site of sting

  2. Thin white to gray stinger may project from center

  3. More pronounced reaction may last several days especially after re-exposure

     a. Nausea, abdominal pain

     b. Sneezing, coughing

     c. Pruritus

     d. Larger area of redness, swelling

  4. Anaphylactic reaction may occur after initial or re-exposure

     a. Could result in ultimate collapse and death

     b. Early signs within minutes of exposure

        (1) Dizziness

        (2) Swelling of lips and throat

        (3) Difficulty breathing

        (4) Difficulty swallowing

     c. Later signs

        (1) Weakness and collapse

        (2) Confusion

        (3) Coma

        (4) Stridor

- Diagnostic Tests/Findings: None

- Management/Treatment

  1. Obtain detailed history of onset, duration, severity, progression of symptoms

  2. Describe and monitor area in terms of size, color, and location

  3. If known sensitivity, life threatening, and/or severe reaction

     a. Administer epinephrine as indicated

      b.   Apply cool compresses

      c.   Refer immediately for MD evaluation and hospitalization

  4. If mild reaction

      a.   Remove stinger by flicking off, do not squeeze

      b.   Apply cool compresses to site of sting

      c.   Use oral antihistamines to reduce severe pruritus, e.g., hydroxyzine, diphenhydramine

      d.   Monitor for hypersensitivity reaction

  5. Provide emotional support as needed to child and family

  6. Educate regarding characteristics of condition, treatment regime, and prognosis

  7. Educate regarding medication dosage, signs of irritation, sensitivity

  8. Educate regarding prevention

      a.   Outside environmental controls—clearing areas, pesticide spraying

      b.   Inside environmental controls—routine cleaning, vacuuming

      c.   Avoid and/or be observant around areas of natural habitat

      d.   Wear protective clothing, hats and gloves

      e.   Avoid wearing bright clothing when hiking around natural habitat

      f.   Avoid wearing perfumes when around natural habitat

      g.   If known sensitivity wear medical alert tag and carry epinephrine kit

Insect Infestations

Scabies Infestation

- Definition: Highly contagious condition caused by parasitic mite infestation

- Etiology/Incidence

  1. Caused by the *Sarcoptes scabiei* (itch mite); gravid female mite burrows into stratum corneum to lay ova which hatch in 4 to 14 days

  2. Incubation period of 4 to 6 weeks with initial exposure; 1 to 5 days with re-exposure causing intense itching

  3. Worldwide distribution in all population groups regardless of hygiene

  4. Major infestations have occurred in cyclic patterns of every 15 to 30 years

  5. Spreads through direct contact with infected person or indirect contact with clothing, bed linens, and other personal items

6. Communicability is present until all mites, larva, and ova are destroyed on body surface and in surrounding environment

- Signs and Symptoms
  1. Irritability in infants
  2. Intense itching especially at night in older children and adolescents
  3. Red bumps, blisters, pustules, and small burrow marks which may be obliterated by scratch marks

- Differential Diagnosis
  1. Insect bites
  2. Impetigo
  3. Secondary bacterial infection

- Physical Findings
  1. Intense itching
  2. Fine gray to skin-colored superficial 2 to 8 mm linear curved burrows with small papule at proximal end; burrows may be obliterated by scratch and excoriation marks due to scratching
  3. Infants—typically have red-brown papular, vesicular lesions on head, neck, palms and soles
  4. Older child and adolescent—typically have red papular lesions on webs of fingers and folds of wrists, elbows, axillae, waist, buttocks, groin, umbilicus, abdomen, knees, ankles
  5. Pustules indicate secondary bacterial infection
  6. Regional adenopathy may be present

- Diagnostic Tests/Findings
  1. Skin scrapings of burrow or papule material and microscopic examination for body parts of mite, ova, or feces
  2. Culture of pustule will confirm agent of secondary infection

- Management/Treatment
  1. Obtain a detailed history of onset, duration, severity and progression of symptoms
  2. Describe and monitor lesions in terms of morphology/structure, size shape, number, color, location, and distribution
  3. Bathe and dry skin, then treat with topical medication
     a. Infants and young children—permethrin 5% (drug of choice)
     b. Older children and adolescents—permethrin 5%; lindane, crotamiton 10%, sulfur in petrolatum

4. Use topical steroids to reduce inflammation, immune response, and pruritus, e.g., hydrocortisone, triamcinolone

5. Use oral antihistamines to reduce pruritus, e.g., hydroxyzine, diphenhydramine

6. Treat secondary bacterial infection

    a. Use topical antibiotics, e.g., bacitracin, mupirocin, neosporin

    b. Use oral antibiotics if extensive, recurrence, or unresponsive, e.g., erythromycin, dicloxacillin, cefadroxil, cephalexin

7. Educate regarding medication dosage, signs of irritation, sensitivity

8. Treat household and other close contacts

9. Wash clothes, bed linens, towels, and hats with hot water and dry in hot dryer

10. Store non-washable items in plastic bags for one week; do not use

11. Educate regarding characteristics of condition, treatment regime, and prognosis

12. Educate regarding medication dosage and signs of irritation and sensitivity

13. Educate regarding communicability and prevention

    a. Avoid sharing personal items of clothes, linens, towels, and wash these items frequently

    b. Maintain good daily personal hygiene and dry well after bathing

    c. Wash hands before and after applying topical treatment

    d. Avoid touching or scratching affected areas

14. Refer for MD evaluation if condition does not improve

Pediculosis Infestation (Lice)

- Definition: Highly contagious parasitic louse infestation affecting hairy body surfaces
- Etiology/Incidence
  1. Caused by several species of lice
     a. *Pediculus capitis*—affects scalp
     b. *Pediculus humanus*—affects less hairy body surfaces
     c. *Phthirus pubis*—affects pubic, and axilla areas, eyelashes, eyebrows
  2. Worldwide distribution in all population groups regardless of hygiene practices
  3. More common in school age and adolescents due to sharing of personal items
  4. More common in Caucasians, less common in African-Americans
  5. Spreads through direct contact with infected person or indirect contact with clothing, bed linens, and other personal items

6. Incubation of 6 to 10 days from laying of eggs to hatching; hatched lice mature in 2 to 3 weeks

7. Communicability present until all lice, neophytes, and ova are destroyed on body surface and environment

- Signs and Symptoms

  1. Itching

  2. White flakes on hair

  3. Red blotches and bumps (rare)

- Differential Diagnosis

  1. Bites from other insects

  2. Bacterial infection

  3. Dandruff

  4. Hair casts

  5. Scabies

- Physical Findings

  1. Small white nits (eggs) on hair strands—$\frac{1}{4}$ inch from skin surface; difficult to remove

     a. Head lice most common on back of head, behind ears

     b. Body lice most common in seams of clothing

  2. Macular, papular lesions with mild erythema and excoriation

  3. Pustules secondary to scratching (secondary bacterial infection)

  4. Regional adenopathy may be present

- Diagnostic Tests/Findings

  1. Clinical examination of hair shaft for ova is usually sufficient to confirm diagnosis

  2. Microscopic examination of ova may confirm questionable diagnosis

- Management/Treatment

  1. Obtain detailed history of onset, duration, severity and progression of symptoms

  2. Describe and monitor lesions in terms of morphology/structure, size, shape, number, color, location, and distribution

  3. Treat infestation with topical antiparasitics to destroy louse and ova, e.g., permethrin, pyrethrins; lindane indicated for treatment failures or for those who do not tolerate permethrin or pyrethrins

  4. Educate regarding medication dosage, signs of irritation, sensitivity

  5. Remove ova/nits after topical treatment

    a. Head lice—manually with fine tooth comb

    b. Vinegar and water preparation may help soften cement

    c. Eye lashes—may coat with petroleum jelly for several days

6. Use topical antibiotics to treat secondary bacterial infection antibiotics, e.g., bacitracin, mupirocin, neosporin

7. Treat other infested family members

8. Remove infestation from surrounding environment

    a. Wash clothes, bed linens, towels, and hats with hot water and dry in hot dryer

    b. Wash personal items such as combs and brushes with pediculocide

    c. Vacuum and store nonwashable items 10 days in plastic bag

    d. Vacuum drapes, rugs, floors, and furniture (beds, chairs, sofa)

9. Educate regarding characteristics of condition and prognosis

10. Educate regarding communicability and prevention

    a. Avoid sharing personal items of towels, hats, hair brushes, combs; wash these items frequently

    b. Maintain personal hygiene, wash hands before/after treatments

    c. Avoid touching or scratching affected areas

11. Refer for MD evaluation if condition does not resolve

Miscellaneous Conditions of Hypersensitivity

Drug Reactions

- Definition: Acute condition of the skin involving an allergic hypersensitivity reaction to a drug characterized predominately by a morbilliform generalized rash

- Etiology/Incidence

1. Caused by release of histamine in reaction to immune system's response to drug allergen

2. Most common drugs

    a. Sulfates

    b. Penicillins

    c. Barbiturates

    d. Dilantin

3. Onset usually occurs within first week of exposure; may be delayed for more than 2 weeks and/or after drug has been discontinued

4. Reoccurrences are frequent with re-exposures—response varies depending on

antigen exposure

- Signs and Symptoms
    1. Intense generalized and localized itching
    2. Generalized red rash beginning on trunk and progressing to extremities
- Differential Diagnosis
    1. Scarlet fever
    2. Contact dermatitis
    3. Erythema multiforme
    4. Rubeola
    5. Urticaria
- Physical Findings
    1. Generalized and localized pruritus
    2. Generalized morbilliform erythematous rash occurring first on trunk and progressing to extremities; initially macular becoming papular and confluent
    3. Wheals are less typical, and less frequent
- Diagnostic Tests/Findings: None
- Management/Treatment
    1. Obtain detailed history of onset, duration, severity, progression of symptoms, and possible precipitating factors
    2. Describe and monitor lesions in terms of morphology/structure, size, shape, number, color, location, distribution
    3. Discontinue contact with drug/medication allergen if known sensitivity
    4. Oral steroids to reduce inflammation and immune response in severe and extensive cases, e.g., hydrocortisone
    5. Oral antihistamines for pruritus, e.g., hydroxyzine, diphenhydramine
    6. Educate regarding medication dosage, signs of irritation, sensitivity
    7. Educate regarding characteristics of condition, cause, treatment prognosis, and reoccurrence
    8. Refer to MD for evaluation if condition does not improve in 2 days or if becomes more severe at any time

Erythema Multiforme Minor

- Definition: Acute condition of the skin involving hypersensitivity reaction characterized by multi-morphology skin and mucous membrane eruptions; lasts approximately 2 to 3 weeks with spontaneous resolution

- Etiology/Incidence
    1. Hypersensitivity caused by exposure to variety of substances
        a. Infectious organisms—most common are enteroviruses, *Mycoplasma pneumoniae,* and herpes simplex especially in recurrent conditions
        b. Drugs—most common are barbiturates, sulfa, and penicillin drugs
        c. Other substances—food reactions
    2. More common in adults, however, approximately 20% of cases are in children and adolescents
    3. Recurrent episodes occur in approximately $\frac{1}{3}$ of cases
- Signs and Symptoms
    1. Itching may be present
    2. Pain especially in mouth
    3. Redness and swelling may present with blisters and/or ulcers on hands, elbows, knees, ankles, feet, eyes, lips, mouth
    4. Develop in crops over period of 1 to 2 weeks with each crop lasting 1 week
- Differential Diagnosis
    1. Allergic vasculitis
    2. Kawasaki disease
    3. Urticaria
    4. Varicella or other viral infections
- Physical Findings
    1. Pruritus and pain may be present at site of lesions, especially those in oral cavity
    2. Redness and swelling with lesions progressing from macules, to papules, blisters, and petechiae
    3. Lesions occur on bilateral exposed areas predominately—includes hands, elbows, knees, ankles, feet, eyes, lips, oral mucous membranes, tongue, oral cavity; and less commonly on chest and trunk
    4. Lesions develop in crops over period of 1 to 2 weeks with each crop lasting 1 week
    5. Target or "bull's-eye" lesions may be present which have three distinct characteristics—a necrotic or vesicular center, a pale middle macular ring and an outer erythematous peripheral ring
    6. Lasts from 2 to 3 weeks with spontaneous resolution
- Diagnostic Tests/Findings
    1. Chest radiograph to rule out *Mycoplasma pneumoniae*
    2. Tzanck test to rule out herpes simplex

- Management/Treatment

  1. Obtain detailed history of onset, duration, severity and progression of symptoms, and possible precipitating factors

  2. Describe and monitor lesions in terms of morphology/structure, size, shape, number, color, location, distribution

  3. Cool compresses for pain and pruritus

  4. Antihistamines for pruritus, e.g., hydroxyzine, diphenhydramine

  5. Oral analgesics for generalized pain, e.g., ibuprofen, acetaminophen

  6. Topical anesthetics and mouth washes for oral lesions, e.g., lidocaine

  7. Maintain hydration with cool fluids, e.g., water, nonirritating juices

  8. Determine underlying trigger and remove or treat as indicated

  9. Educate regarding medication dosages, signs of irritation, sensitivity

  10. Educate regarding characteristics of condition, cause, prognosis, and reoccurrence

  11. Refer for MD evaluation if:

      a. Condition does not improve

      b. Systemic symptoms of fever and malaise develop

Erythema Multiforme Major (Stevens-Johnson Syndrome)

- Definition: Skin condition involving hypersensitivity reaction characterized by multi-morphology mucous membrane and skin eruptions with associated systemic involvement; also known as Stevens-Johnson Syndrome

- Etiology/Incidence

  1. Hypersensitivity caused by exposure to a variety of substances

     a. Infectious organisms—most common are enteroviruses, *Mycoplasma pneumoniae,* and herpes simplex especially in recurrent conditions

     b. Drugs—most common are barbiturates, sulfa, and penicillin

     c. Other substances—food reactions

  2. More common in adults, however, approximately 20% of cases are in children and adolescents

  3. Recurrent episodes occur in approximately $\frac{1}{3}$ of the cases

  4. Can be life threatening; approximately 5% mortality of diagnosed cases

- Signs and Symptoms

  1. Fever, fatigue, sore throat, headache, nausea, vomiting, diarrhea, muscle pain, and/or joint pain

  2. Skin rash develops in 2 to 3 days after generalized symptoms

      a.   Areas of redness and swelling

      b.   Variety of skin reactions on hands, elbows, knees, ankles, feet, eyes, lips, mouth, chest and/or trunk

  3.   Itching may be present

  4.   Pain, especially in mouth

- Differential Diagnosis

  1.   Gingivostomatitis

  2.   Pemphigus

  3.   Toxic epidermal necrolysis

  4.   Urticaria

  5.   Varicella

  6.   Staphlococcal scalded syndrome

- Physical Findings

  1.   Sudden onset of prodromal state—high temperature, malaise, weakness

  2.   Multimorphology rash develops in progressive pattern

      a.   Macular erythematous with edematous areas

      b.   Progress to papules, vesicles, erosions, and petechiae

  3.   Pruritus and pain, especially lesions in oral cavity

  4.   Lesions occur on bilateral exposed areas predominately—includes hands, elbows, knees, ankles, feet, eyes, lips, oral mucous membranes, tongue; less common on chest and trunk

  5.   Target or herald lesions may be present which have three distinct characteristics— necrotic or vesicular center, pale middle macular ring, and an outer erythematous peripheral ring

  6.   Lesions develop in crops over period of 1 to 2 weeks with each crop lasting 1 week

  7.   Condition may progress to more severe stage involving the respiratory, renal, and gastrointestinal systems

- Diagnostic Tests/Findings

  1.   Chest radiograph to rule out *Mycoplasma pneumoniae*

  2.   Tzanck to rule out herpes simplex

  3.   Skin biopsy to confirm diagnosis

- Management/Treatment

  1.   Obtain detailed history of onset, duration, severity and progression of symptoms, and possible precipitating factors

2. Describe and monitor lesions in terms of morphology/structure, size, shape, number, color, location, distribution

3. Immediate MD referral for evaluation and hospitalization due to potential life threatening situation

4. Educate regarding characteristics of condition, cause, and prognosis

Urticaria

- Definition: Acute or chronic condition of the skin involving an allergic hypersensitivity reaction characterized by pale or skin colored skin lesions

- Etiology/Incidence

  1. Caused by release of histamine as reaction to immune system's response to an allergen

     a. Foods

     b. Temperature changes of heat and cold

     c. Viral infections

     d. Vibrations and scratching

     e. Emotional elation or stress

     f. Insect bites

     g. Materials and fabrics

  2. Symptoms may last for minutes or up to 24 hours after initial exposure to antigen

  3. Reccurrences are frequent with re-exposure to allergen; response is varied

- Signs and Symptoms

  1. Intense generalized and localized itching

  2. Mild redness and swelling of irregular shaped hives—may involve eyelids, lips, hands, feet, mouth, and genitalia

- Differential Diagnosis

  1. Atopic dermatitis

  2. Contact dermatitis

  3. Erythema multiforme

- Physical Findings

  1. Intense generalized and localized pruritus at site of lesions

  2. Mild erythema and swelling with irregular shaped wheals on any skin surface

     a. May have swelling of eyelids, lips, hands, feet, and genitalia

     b. May have swelling and redness of mucous membranes

3. Individual lesions range in size from under 1 cm to over 15 cm

4. Distribution pattern is generalized and scattered

5. Become more pronounced with heat

6. Will blanch with pressure

7. Excoriation due to scratching secondary to severe pruritus

- Diagnostic Tests/Findings: No tests confirm condition

- Management/Treatment

    1. Obtain detailed history of onset, duration, severity and progression of symptoms, and possible precipitating factors

    2. Describe and monitor lesions in terms of morphology/structure, size, shape, number, color, location, distribution

    3. Discontinue contact with allergen if known sensitivity

    4. Cool compresses of Burow's solution for comfort

    5. Topical steroids to reduce immune response and pruritus, e.g., hydrocortisone, triamcinolone

    6. Oral steroids for severe and extensive reactions, e.g., hydrocortisone

    7. Oral antihistamines for pruritus, e.g., hydroxyzine, diphenhydramine

    8. Educate regarding characteristics of condition

    9. Educate regarding medication dosages, signs of irritation, sensitivity

    10. Teach measures for prevention, e.g., avoid known allergens

    11. Refer to MD for evaluation:
        a. If acute episode does not improve
        b. Consideration of skin testing for hypersensitivities after acute episode resolves

Questions:
Select the best answer

1. J.D. is a postterm infant with lesions of varying morphology including wheals, vesicles, and pustules on her trunk. You suspect J.D. has:

   a. Cutis marmorata
   b. Erythema toxicum neonatorum
   c. Milia
   d. Sebaceous hyperplasia

2. In order to confirm your diagnosis of J.D., you order a Wright's stained smear. If your diagnosis is correct, what are the expected results of the smear?

   a. Presence of eosinophils
   b. Presence of neutrophils
   c. Presence of keratinous material
   d. Presence of staphylococcus bacteria

3. In addition to monitoring the skin for any changes, what is the best management for J.D.?

   a. Topical antibiotics on lesions
   b. Topical steroids on lesions
   c. A moisturizer on lesions
   d. No treatment necessary since J.D.'s condition will resolve spontaneously in 5 to 7 days

4. You examine C.C., a newborn, and observe numerous white papular lesions on the cheeks, forehead, and nose. You suspect either milia or sebaceous hyperplasia. Which physical finding helps to confirm a diagnosis of milia?

   a. Papular lesions are intermixed with pale yellow macules.
   b. Papular lesions have an erythematous circular ring at the base
   c. Papular lesions are surrounded by lacy-blue area with erythematous mottling
   d. Papular lesions, yellow in color, are observed on the hard palate

5. Newborn K.T. is three weeks premature and you observe a macular erythematous lacy appearance to her skin when you undress her. K.T. has which condition?

   a. Curtis marmorata
   b. Erythema toxicum neonatorum
   c. Salmon patch
   d. Nevus flammeus

6. In addition to monitoring the skin for any changes, what is the best management for K.T.?

   a. Keep K.T. warm
   b. Decrease the environmental temperature.
   c. Use a moisturizer on affected skin areas
   d. Do nothing as condition will resolve spontaneously in 5 to 7 days without intervention

7. Newborn W.R. has a vascular lesion that will not fade as she gets older. What is your diagnosis?

    a. Salmon patch
    b. Capillary hemangioma
    c. Café au lait
    d. Nevus flammeus

8. W.R.'s parents are concerned about her appearance and the psychological effect on their daughter as she becomes aware of her condition. In educating the parents, you tell them about several options that will be available when W.R. is older. Which of the following is not an appropriate management or treatment consideration for W.R.?

    a. Application of topical steroids to the affected area to prevent pruritus
    b. Camouflage affected areas with cosmetics
    c. Pulsed laser treatment of affected area
    d. Counseling for psychological concerns

9. Which condition is thought to be more common in darker skinned individuals?

    a. Tinea corporis
    b. Psoriasis
    c. Pityriasis alba
    d. Pityriasis rosea

10. J.R., an eight year old boy, has scaly pale salmon lesions predominately on his trunk. One lesion on the buttocks is larger than all the other lesions and measures 4 cm in diameter. What is your likely diagnosis?

    a. Psoriasis
    b. Eczema
    c. Pityriasis alba
    d. Pityriasis rosea

11. What symptom is commonly experienced in J.R.'s condition?

    a. Pruritus
    b. Pain at site of lesions
    c. Nausea
    d. Headache

12. What management would you not recommend for J.R. with his condition?

    a. Cool bath or cool compresses to lesions
    b. Topical steroids to lesions
    c. Oral antihistamine
    d. Monitored and controlled daily sunlight exposure

13. You have diagnosed D.L. with acute atopic dermatitis. Which of the following is not correct regarding the incidence of this condition?

a. D.L. is most likely an infant
b. D.L. has a greater chance of developing asthma later in childhood than the average individual
c. D.L. has a greater chance of developing malignant melanoma in adulthood than the average individual
d. D.L. has a condition associated with familial predisposition

14. Which of the following management measures or treatments would you not recommend for D.L.?

a. Topical steroids to affected areas
b. Wet compresses to affected skin areas
c. Maintain a dry warm environment
d. Eliminate all substances that dry the skin

15. In addition to having atopic dermatitis, you have diagnosed D.L. with a secondary bacterial infection at the site of several lesions. What is the best management for the infection?

a. Topical antibiotics to affected areas
b. Oral antibiotics
c. Hot compresses to affected areas
d. Monitored and controlled daily sun exposure until lesions resolve

16. Many skin conditions have lesions that may be oozing, weepy, crusting and itchy. Which of the following would you routinely recommend?

a. Dry the affected skin areas with topical preparations
b. Apply topical antibiotics to lesions to prevent secondary bacterial infection
c. Increase the room temperature to enhance drying of lesions
d. Wet dressings/compresses to soothe the skin and relieve itching

17. You see B.D. for the first time at age six weeks. B.D. has a bright red raised rubbery lesion of irregular shape and 2 cm in diameter on the occiput. What condition do you suspect B.D. has?

a. Malignant melanoma
b. Nevus flammeus
c. Capillary hemangioma
d. Burn

18. Which of the following is not characteristic of the lesion B.D. has?

a. It was not present at birth, however, B.D.'s mother noticed site was blanched
b. It will continue to gradually grow for the first 12 to 15 months of B.D.'s life
c. It will begin to gradually resolve when B.D. is between 12 to 15 months
d. It is expected to completely resolve by the time B.D. is ten years

19. You notice ten macular tan lesions of varying sizes on D.D. and refer him for a medical evaluation to rule out neurofibromatosis or Albright's syndrome. What kind of lesion does D.D. have?

   a. Malignant melanoma
   b. Café au lait spots
   c. Mongolian spots
   d. Vitiligo

20. What is characteristic of the lesion that D.D. has?

   a. More common in Caucasians than dark-skinned individuals
   b. More common in males than females
   c. Lesions are usually present at birth, however, more lesions may develop at any age
   d. Lesions usually fade spontaneously and completely resolve in adult life

21. Which condition is not more common in dark-skinned populations?

   a. Café au lait spots
   b. Mongolian spots
   c. Pityriasis alba
   d. Atopic dermatitis

22. You suspect that A.F., age nine years, has either pityriasis alba or vitiligo. Which of the following would not confirm the diagnosis of pityriasis alba?

   a. A.F.'s skin would be normal in all aspects except for areas of hypopigmentation
   b. A.F.'s skin would have one or more scaly areas of hypopigmentation
   c. A.F. complains of mild itching in areas of hypopigmentation
   d. A.F.'s lesions became more pronounced when she was exposed to sunlight

23. A.F. was diagnosed with pityriasis alba. Which of the following is proper management of A.F.'s condition?

   a. Bland moisturizers to reduce overdrying
   b. Topical steroids to the affected areas
   c. Expose affected areas to short periods of sunlight each day
   d. Burow's wet compresses to affected areas

24. Patient education is a major part of the PNP's role. What would you teach A.F. and her parent regarding the progress and prognosis of pityriasis alba?

   a. A.F. will continue to develop lesions until she completes puberty
   b. A.F.'s condition should clear completely in three to four months
   c. A.F.'s condition is permanent and affected areas will not repigment
   d. A.F.'s condition will resolve completely, however, the affected areas will become slightly reddened when exposed to sunlight

25. Malignant melanoma is a form of much dreaded skin cancer. Which of the following is not characteristic of this condition?

   a. Occurs in all ethnic groups but more commonly in light-skinned individuals
   b. Severe sunburn or excessive exposure to sunlight before the age of ten years predisposes developing melanoma later in childhood or in adult life

    c. Spreads through the lymphatic system and invades other distant skin surfaces and organs

    d. Spreads primarily by invading skin surfaces that surround the major lesion

26. Which of the following does not characterize the lesion of malignant melanoma?

    a. Irregular asymmetrical nodule with blurred borders

    b. Raised with distinct symmetrical borders

    c. Uneven coloring in which blue, black, brown, tan, and red may all be present in the same lesion

    d. Bleeding, ulceration in later stages

27. Patient education regarding prevention of malignant melanoma is essential. Which of the following is not considered best prevention education?

    a. Avoid sunlight especially during the hours of 9:00 a.m. and 1:00 p.m.

    b. Avoid sun tanning lamps

    c. Use cover-up clothing, hats, and sunglasses

    d. Use sun blocks that protect against ultraviolet exposure with > 15 SPF

28. You suspect M.N. as having chronic psoriasis. Which of the following is characteristic of her lesions if she has psoriasis vulgaris?

    a. Scaly red small areas 3 to 10 mm in diameter

    b. Round or oval in shape

    c. Large scaly silver-white areas 5 to 10 cm in diameter

    d. Located mainly on her trunk

29. M.N.'s condition of psoriasis is common in approximately 33 percent of children. Which of the following is not correct regarding the etiology or incidence of this condition?

    a. Occurs more commonly in dark-skinned ethnic individuals

    b. Associated with constant rubbing or trauma to exposed affected areas such as elbows

    c. Associated with overproduction of epithelial cells

    d. Associated with epithelial cells that migrate to the skin surface much more quickly than normal

30. What would you not advise regarding the management or treatment of M.N.'s condition?

    a. Excise lesions

    b. Apply topical steroids

    c. Apply mineral oil and moisturizers

    d. Expose to monitored short periods of sunlight

31. You have diagnosed Jale as having contact dermatitis. Which symptom is most characteristic of his condition?

    a. Headache

    b. Difficulty breathing

    c. Pruritus at site of affected areas

    d. Pain at site of affected areas

32. Which of the following is not characteristic of Jale's condition?

    a. He has hypersensitivity to a substance within his environment when direct contact is made
    b. He may experience a delayed reaction of several days with re-exposure to an allergen
    c. His dermatitis may be caused by direct contact with topical medications, soaps, cosmetics, fabrics, and plants
    d. Typical response is redness and edema at the site of contact which may progress to papules and vesicles

33. What would you not recommend as management and treatment of Jale's condition?

    a. Skin testing during the acute episode to determine if Jale has an allergy
    b. Cool compresses of Burow's solution to affected areas
    c. Topical steroids to affected areas for five days
    d. Oral antihistamines

34. You diagnose Kelli, age seven months, with diaper dermatitis. Which of the following should not be included in the differential diagnosis?

    a. Atopic dermatitis
    b. Child abuse
    c. Contact dermatitis
    d. Pityriasis alba

35. What management measure would you not prescribe to treat Kelli's condition?

    a. Oral antihistamines
    b. Emollients such as petroleum jelly to mildly affected areas
    c. Topical steroids to severely affected areas with erythema and papules
    d. Topical antibiotics to severely affected areas with ulcerations

36. What would not be an appropriate recommendation to prevent Kelli from having subsequent episodes of diaper dermatitis?

    a. Expose diaper area to air several times each day
    b. Increase oral fluids using orange juice to dilute urine
    c. Make diaper changes immediately after soiling
    d. Use a double rinse of vinegar and water for home-laundered diapers

37. Seborrhea dermatitis is common in both infants and adolescents. Which of the following is not correct of this condition?

    a. Occurs more often in the spring and summer months
    b. Is associated with an over production of sebum in areas abundant with sebaceous glands
    c. The condition in infants is known as "cradle cap" in which lesions have erythematous base with yellow crusted areas and greasy scales
    d. The condition in adolescents is known as acne with comedomes, papular, and pustular lesions

38. What is the best treatment of seborrhea in the infant?

    a. Mineral oil to loosen crusts prior to washing affected areas with an antiseborrheic shampoos
    b. Topical antibiotics
    c. Oral antibiotics in severe cases
    d. Oral steroids for severe cases

39. F.P., age three years, sustained a burn when she pulled a pan of boiling water over on her. Since burns are classified according to the depth of injury to the skin layers and the amount of area involved, how would you rate burn if 5 percent of her body surface is burned involving the epidermis and upper part of the dermis?

    a. She has a minor first and second degree burn
    b. She has a major second degree burn
    c. She has a major full thickness burn
    d. She has major first and second degree burns

40. F.P.'s burn should appear:

    a. Dry, with mild edema and erythema
    b. Dry whitish areas that blanch with pressure
    c. Dry whitish to brownish areas with edema
    d. Moist with edema, erythema and a few vesicles

41. What is the best treatment for F.P.'s burn?

    a. Warm compresses to affected areas and mild analgesic for discomfort
    b. Topical emollients to affected areas
    c. Butter to affected areas
    d. Refer for MD evaluation and hospitalization

42. Jerry has been diagnosed as having folliculitis, an inflammatory condition involving the pilosebaceous follicle. What is the most common cause of this condition?

    a. *Microsporum canis tinea*
    b. Poxvirus
    c. *Staphylococcus aureus*
    d. Streptococcus group A

43. Jerry has a condition that most commonly occurs on which body surface?

    a. Neck and scalp
    b. Upper arms
    c. Chest and abdomen
    d. Legs

44. You order a culture and the results confirm that Jerry's condition is caused by the most common organism for this condition. What treatment do you prescribe?

a. Oral penicillin
b. Dicloxacillin
c. Tinactin
d. Tretinoin

45. Sandra, age twelve years, has several vesicles and honey colored crusted lesions on her face above the right nares. She has a history of having had a scratch in the same area several days ago. What condition do you suspect?

a. Acne
b. Impetigo
c. Herpes simplex
d. Eczema

46. Judy, age fifteen years, has been diagnosed as having acne. Which of the following is not true of this condition?

a. Poor hygiene is a contributing factor
b. Associated with increased androgenic hormonal activity
c. Mild acne is more common among females
d. Severe acne is more common among males

47. Judy has a history of remission and exacerbation that has followed the pattern of menses for two years. However, the condition over the last six months has worsened to a moderate degree of severity and has been chronic and persistent. You prescribe antibiotic therapy. Which of the following antibiotics would you not consider?

a. Topical clindamycin
b. Topical erythomycin
c. Oral clindamycin
d. Oral tetracycline

48. K.C., age thirteen years, has several firm, small (2 mm) white skin-colored umbilicated papules on her neck. The lesions have been present for three months and have increased in number. What is your diagnosis?

a. Acne
b. Molluscum contagiosum
c. Warts
d. Cellulitis

49. What is the cause of K.C.'s condition?

a. *Microsporum canis* tinea
b. Poxvirus
c. *Staphylococcus aureus*
d. Streptococcus group A

50. Which treatment would you not recommend for K.C.'s condition?

    a. Curettage lesions
    b. Topical antibiotics
    c. Topical steroids
    d. Tretinoin applications

51. Paul has four superficial lesions on his anterior lower abdomen of one week duration. The lesions are 4 cm in diameter scaly irregular shaped plaques with skin colored centers and erythematous borders The affected areas are slightly pruritic. What condition do you suspect Paul has?

    a. Psoriasis
    b. Eczema
    c. Tinea corporis
    d. Pityriasis rosea

52. You performed two tests to confirm your diagnosis of Paul's condition. The KOH scraping was positive for the presence of hyphae. The Wood's lamp did not fluoresce the lesions. You are sure that Paul's condition was not caused by which organism?

    a. *Epidermophyton floccosum*
    b. *Microsporum canis*
    c. *Trichophyton tonsurans*
    d. *Trichophyton rubrum*

53. You see Paul after eight weeks of treatment with a topical antifungal preparation. The original lesions have almost resolved, however, the condition has worsened with the development of several other larger lesions on the abdomen and groin area. Which of the following would you not consider?

    a. Oral antifungal medication, griseofulvin
    b. Topical antibiotic preparation
    c. Continue with the topical antifungal applications
    d. Educate again regarding not sharing personal items

54. Dale, age 7 years, is complaining of pain and burning on his right leg where you observe two small red puncture marks surrounded by a blanched area with an erythematous border. He had been playing with his dog all morning outside in a grassy wooded area near his home and was wearing shorts. You suspect he has been bitten by which insect?

    a. Mosquito
    b. Bee
    c. Recluse spider
    d. Black widow spider

55. Which of the following is not true of insect stings from bees, wasps, and fire ants?

    a. Greater reaction of hypersensitivity occurs most often with the initial exposure than with subsequent exposures
    b. For mild reactions cool compresses to the site of injury is the usual management

c. Occurs more often during the spring and summer months

d. Most stings occur in self-defense when the nonaggressive insect feels threatened or irritated

56. You diagnose W.A. with scabies. Which of the following is not characteristic of this condition?

a. He has several erythematous papular, pustular, and crusted lesions on his face

b. He has several excoriated scratched areas around the umbilicus and waist area

c. He has several linear curved lines approximately 4 mm in length with a papule at the proximal end linear line

d. He complains of severe pruritus which is worse at night

57. Which of the following is not recommended as a management and treatment strategy for W.A.?

a. Put nonwashable items in a plastic bag and store for one week

b. Prescribe topical antifungal applications

c. Prescribe topical antiparasitics

d. Prescribe topical steroids and/or oral antihistamines for pruritus

58. Pediculosis is a highly communicable common condition in children. Which of the following is not correct of pediculosis humanus?

a. Caused by an insect that does not fly or jump

b. Gravid females lay ova in seams of clothing

c. Likes hairy areas of the body better than the non-hairy body surfaces

d. Same medication used for scabies may be used to effectively eradicate this condition

59. Hypersensitivity may occur to a variety of substances causing a variety of reactions. It is important to determine if the body's hypersensitivity reaction will cause erythema multiforme condition. Which of the following is not typical of the erythema multiforme reaction?

a. Target "bulls-eye" lesion with a necrotic center surrounded by a pale macular middle area and then by a erythematous peripheral ring

b. Itching at site of affected skin areas

c. Pain at site of affected areas, especially in the oral cavity

d. Lesions which all have the same morphology on the trunk

60. You see D.Y. in your clinic and suspect she has a form of erythema multiforme. Erythema multiforme minor must be differentiated from erythema multiforme major. Which of the following is the most important confirming evidence for making a diagnosis of erythema multiforme major?

a. Presence of deeper lesions within the dermis

b. Presence of lesions on the exposed areas of the body

c. Presence of pustules indicating a secondary infectious process

d. Occurrence of prodromal systemic symptoms of fever, malaise, sore throat, headache, nausea, and/or vomiting

61. You suspect D.Y. has erythema multiforme major. What treatment or management is most indicated?

    a. Prescribe topical antibiotics due to secondary infection
    b. Prescribe topical steroids to lesions for pruritus
    c. Refer for medical evaluation
    d. No treatment is indicated as condition will resolve spontaneously in one week

62. Urticaria is a hypersensitivity allergic reaction to a variety of substances and agents. You suspect W.P. has urticaria due to the typical morphology of lesions on her trunk and arms which are:

    a. Erythematous papules
    b. Vesicles
    c. Pustules
    d. Wheals

63. During W.P.'s acute episode of urticaria which of the following is not considered an appropriate management or treatment measure?

    a. Oral antibiotics to prevent secondary infection
    b. Oral antihistamines for pruritus
    c. Topical steroids to affected areas to reduce the immune response
    d. Cool compresses to affected areas

Answers

1. b	22. a	43. a
2. a	23. a	44. b
3. d	24. b	45. b
4. d	25. d	46. a
5. a	26. b	47. c
6. a	27. a	48. b
7. d	28. c	49. b
8. a	29. a	50. b
9. c	30. a	51. c
10. d	31. c	52. b
11. a	32. b	53. b
12. b	33. a	54. d
13. c	34. d	55. a
14. c	35. a	56. a
15. b	36. b	57. b
16. d	37. d	58. c
17. c	38. a	59. d
18. b	39. d	60. d
19. b	40. d	61. c
20. c	41. d	62. d
21. d	42. c	63. a

Bibliography

American Academy of Pediatrics. (2000). In L. K. Pickering (Ed.). *Red Book 2000: Report of the committee on infectious diseases* (25th ed.). Elk Grove Village, IL: Author.

Burns, C. E., Barber, N., Brady, M. A., & Dunn, A. M. (2000). *Pediatric primary care: A handbook for nurse practitioners.* Philadelphia: W. B. Saunders.

Cohen, B. A. (1999). *Pediatric dermatology* (2nd ed.). St. Louis: Mosby Year Book.

Goldgeier, M. H. (1996). Fungal infections: Tips from a dermatologist. *Contemporary Pediatrics, 13*(9), 21-50.

Goldman, M. P., & Hooper, B. J. (1999). *Primary dermatologic care.* St. Louis: Mosby Year Book.

Hay, W. W., Groothuis, J. R., Hayward, A. R., & Levin, M. J. (Eds.). (1997). *Current pediatric diagnosis and treatment* (13th ed.). Norwalk, CT: Appleton & Lange.

Hurwitz, S. (1993). *Clinical pediatric dermatology: A textbook of skin disorders of childhood and adolescence* (2nd ed.). Philadelphia: W. B. Saunders.

McCance, K. L., & Huether, S. E. (1994). *Pathophysiology: The biologic basis for disease in adults and children* (2nd ed.). St. Louis: Mosby.

Odom, R. B., James, W. D., & Berger, T. G. (2000). Diseases of the skin: Clinical dermatology (9th ed.). Philadelphia: W. B. Saunders.

Dermatological Disorders In Adults

Sylvia Fletcher
Susan Chaney

Acne Vulgaris

- Definition: Self limited disorders characterized by development of open comedones (black heads) and closed comedones (white heads) due to an increase in sebum release by the sebaceous gland after puberty; if further inflammation is present, pustules, cysts, and nodules on erythematous bases may be present

- Etiology/Incidence
    1. Four primary pathogenic factors
        a. *Propionibacterium acnes*
        b. Increased sebum production
        c. Abnormal follicular keratinization
        d. Chemotactic factors
    2. Factors that predispose to comedone formation
        a. Cosmetics and hair products
        b. Coal tar and insoluble oils
        c. Corticosteroids (topical and systemic), oral contraceptives
    3. Contributing host factors
        a. Heredity
        b. Environment
        c. Stress
    4. May occur as a result of polycystic ovarian disease
    5. May be worse in fall and winter seasons
    6. Seen primarily in adolescents and young adults; may persist to fifth decade
    7. More common in males than females

- Signs and Symptoms
    1. Lesions are nonpruritic, may be tender
    2. Females may notice an increase in symptoms prior to menses

- Differential Diagnosis
    1. Acne rosacea
    2. Eosinophilic folliculitis (seen in HIV patient)
    3. Drug induced folliculitis
    4. Pyogenic folliculitis

- Physical Findings
    1. Morphology

    a. Closed comedones "white heads" are papular lesions found in hair follicles due to blockage of sebum and keratinous materials

    b. Open comedones, "black heads", dilated follicular orifice with easily expressed darkened oily debris

    c. Inflamed comedones, pustules, cysts, and nodules

2. Distribution

    a. Forehead

    b. Cheek, nose, and chin

    c. Chest, upper arms, back, and buttocks

- Diagnostic Tests/Findings: Culture for causative agent rarely necessary

- Management/Treatment

1. Reduce bacterial population on skin

    a. Mild skin cleansing twice daily

    b. Benzoyl peroxide 2.5% to 10%—apply 1 to 2 times daily

    c. Topical erythromycin, clindamycin, tetracycline, minocycline or adapalene once daily for moderate papulopustular lesions

    d. For widespread distribution on chest and back

        (1) Tetracycline 250 to 500 mg, initially 1 g/day, may increase to 2 to 3 g/day (teratogenic with females)

        (2) Minocycline 50 to 100 mg twice daily

        (3) Doxycycline 50 to 100 mg twice daily

        (4) Erythromycin 250 to 500 mg, 1 g/day, if no response in 2 to 3 weeks, 2 to 3 g/day

        (5) Females—combination oral contraceptives with high estrogen component

2. Prevent development of comedone with comedolytic agent

    a. Retinoic acid cream 0.025% applied nightly

    b. Caution patient about photosensitivity

    c. Apply benzoyl peroxide in a.m. if used concurrently

3. Severe nodulocystic acne may requires aggressive treatment to decrease sebum production—13-cis-retinoic acid 0.5 to 2.0 mg/kg/day for 16 to 20 weeks

    a. Teratogenic—use with extreme caution in child bearing females

    b. Multiple systemic side effects

    c. Monitor liver function tests (LFT), CBC, triglyceride levels

4. Patient education

    a. Noticeable improvement may not be apparent for six weeks

    b. Reassure patient, advise on stress reduction

    c. Skin care including mild skin cleansing twice daily; advise patient to not squeeze or pick lesions

Alopecia

- Definition: The complete or partial loss of hair from areas where it normally is present; may be total, diffuse, patchy, or localized

- Etiology/Incidence

    1. Hair loss involving hair matrix or follicle destruction due to chemical, physical agents, or both, and by infectious or immunologically mediated inflammation; may also result from a slowing of hair growth due to metabolic diseases

    2. Cicatricial alopecia—scarring

        a. Hair cannot regrow due to follicle loss

        b. Caused by *Lichen planopilaris,* severe fungal or bacterial infections, physical trauma

        c. Other causes include severe cases of herpes zoster, chronic lupus erythematosus, or excessive ionizing radiation

        d. Permanent and irreversible

    3. Noncicatricial alopecia—nonscarring alopecia

        a. 95% of alopecia seen in primary care

        b. Most common is male or female baldness which is genetic or developmental

        c. Other causes include secondary syphilis, systemic lupus erythematosus, pituitary insufficiency, or iron deficiency anemia

- Signs and Symptoms

    1. Usually the client is symptom free, but verbalizes distress over hair loss

    2. Hair loss resulting from physical agents or infectious disease such as tinea capitis may cause pain or pruritus

- Differential Diagnosis

    1. Tinea capitis

    2. Lichen planus

    3. Folliculitis

    4. Lupus erythematosus

    5. Dermatomyositis

- Physical Findings

    1. Genetic pattern baldness of

        a. Males—frontotemporal hairline recession with various amounts of hair loss at scalp vertex

        b. Females—diffuse or vertex hair loss

    2. Traumatic alopecia findings are patchy hair loss and breakage of hairs

    3. Infectious alopecia—patches of partial hair loss

    4. Alopecia areata (immunologic)—smooth, salmon-colored patches

- Diagnostic Tests

    1. Usually a clinical diagnosis

    2. Hair pull test of 10 or 20 grouped hairs; if over 40% of shafts are removed, disease is more advanced

    3. KOH preparation—negative for fungus

    4. Wood's light—nonfluorescence rules out fungal infections

    5. Refer for scalp biopsy for uncertain cases

    6. Hair count of actual hairs lost daily; over 100 would be considered abnormal

- Management/Treatment

    1. Treatment of genetic alopecia

        a. Topical minoxidil 1 mL of 2% b.i.d.

        b. Finasteride 5 mg daily for 6 to 12 months

        c. Best results with baldness under 5 years, under age 50, and smaller diameters of alopecia

    2. Refer clients with scarring alopecia for surgical hair transplants.

    3. For premenopausal women, order serum testosterone, DHEAS, iron, TIBC, TSH, CBC to reveal other causes of hair loss

    4. Topical estrogen may be of some value for baldness in women

    5. Refer alopecia areata clients for intralesional corticosteroids

    6. Patient education

        a. About 40% of clients have moderate hair growth within one year

        b. Treatment with minoxidil must be continued indefinitely

        c. Discontinuation of treatment will result in regression to pretreatment levels of baldness within 2 to 3 months

        d. Side effects of minoxidil are minimal; some clients may experience dryness or pruritus

Bacterial Infections/Pyodermas

- Definitions:

    1. Impetigo—contagious and autoinoculable bacterial infection of skin; the two types are small vesicle and bullous

    2. Folliculitis—infection surrounding hair follicle caused by occlusion of ostium

    3. Furunculosis—deep-seated, autoinoculable infection involving entire hair follicle and adjacent subcutaneous tissue

    4. Carbuncle—several furuncles developing in adjoining hair follicles and coalescing to form deep mass with multiple drainage points

    5. Hidradenitis suppurativa—chronic suppurative disease of the apocrine gland-bearing areas of the skin

    6. Cellulitis—spreading infection of epidermis, subcutaneous tissue, and superficial lymphatic system

- Etiology/Incidence

    1. Impetigo

        a. Most frequent causative organisms—*Staphylococcus aureus* (*S. aureus*), group A beta hemolytic *Streptococcus pyogenes* (GAS)

        b. Seen primarily in children, bullous in children and young adults

        c. Predisposing factors

            (1) Humid, warm climate

            (2) Pre-existing skin disease, especially atopic

            (3) Prior antibiotic therapy

            (4) Poor hygiene, crowded living conditions,

            (5) Chronic staph carrier (nose, axilla, perineum, bowel)

    2. Folliculitis, furunculosis, carbuncle

        a. Most frequent causative organism—*S. aureus*

        b. Predisposing factors

            (1) Chronic staph carrier (nose, axilla, perineum, bowel

            (2) Diabetes

            (3) Obesity

            (4) Poor hygiene

    3. Hidradenitis suppurativa

        a. Variety of pathogens—most commonly staphylococcus, streptococcus, *E. coli*

        b. Males—anogenital involvement; females axillary involvement

    c. Predisposing factors

        (1) Obesity

        (2) Seen in all races, most severe in African-Americans

        (3) Family history of nodulocystic acne, hidradenitis suppurativa

  4. Cellulitis

    a. Most frequent causative organisms *S. aureus.* and GAS

    b. Less common—*H. influenzae*, group B streptococci (GBS), pneumococci

    c. Diabetic/immunocompromised—*E. coli, Proteus mirabilis, Acinetobacter, Enterobacter, Pseudomonas aeruginosa*

    d. Predisposing factors:

        (1) Multiple dermatoses—tinea, inflammatory, bullous, ulceration, pyodermas

        (2) Trauma

        (3) Surgical wounds

        (4) Infections

    e. Risk factors

        (1) Immunocompromised, cancer, and diabetes

        (2) Alcohol and drug abuse

- Signs and Symptoms

  1. Localized pain, redness, swelling, or heat

  2. More severe infections—malaise, fever, chills, e.g., cellulitis

- Differential Diagnosis

  1. Contact dermatitis

  2. Allergic dermatitis

  3. Fungal dermatitis

  4. Herpes dermatitis

- Physical Findings

  1. Severe infections

    a. Regional lymphadenopathy

    b. Fever

    c. Skin tracking

  2. Morphology

    a. Impetigo—small vesicle caused by sreptococcus

      (1)   Small red macules that progress to water filled vesicles

      (2)   Ruptured vesicles leave characteristic honey-colored crusted area

  b. Bullous impetigo caused by *Staphylococcus aureus*

      (1)   Large flaccid blister

      (2)   Cloudy to purulent contents

  c. Folliculitis, furuncle, carbuncle,

      (1)   Abscess—tender, fluctuant nodule

      (2)   Furuncle—firm, tender nodule with central necrotic plug

      (3)   Carbuncle—multiple abscess/furnuncles with sieve like openings draining purulent material

  d. Hidradenitis suppurativa

      (1)   Initial—inflamed nodule/abscess with serous/purulent drainage and sinus tracks; open, black comedones when active nodules are absent

      (2)   Late phase—fibrous ''bridge'' scarring and contractures

  e. Cellulitis

      (1)   Bright red plateau, sharply demarcated from surrounding skin.

      (2)   Lymphangitis (red streaking from the area of cellulitis toward proximal lymph nodes) may be present

3. Distribution

  a. Impetigo—anywhere

  b. Folliculitis, furuncle, carbuncle

      (1)   Hair bearing area—beard, axilla, occipital scalp, back of neck

      (2)   Any non-weight bearing area, buttock, upper trunk, puncture wound site

  c. Hidradenitis suppurativa

      (1)   Axilla

      (2)   Inguinal area

      (3)   Anogenital area

      (4)   Buttocks, scalp

  d. Cellulitis

      (1)   Any area where normal lymphatic drainage has been disrupted

      (2)   Recent venous and lymphatic surgical sites

      (3)   Previous cellulitis sites

      (4)   Cheek or cheek bone and lower extremities

- Diagnostic Tests/Findings

  1. Gram's stain—positive for cocci

  2. Culture and sensitivity of exudate especially on immunocompromised patient

  3. KOH—negative

  4. Wood's lamp—no fluorescence

  5. Tzanck test—negative

- Management/Treatment

  1. Impetigo

     a. Prevention

        (1) Wash with benzoyl peroxide soap

        (2) Evaluate family members; highly contagious

     b. Gently wash lesion to remove crust

     c. Small area not involving the face

        (1) Mupirocin 2% applied q.i.d. for 10 days

        (2) Effective against GAS and methicillin-resistant *S. aureus* (MRSA)

     d. GAS—small vesicular impetigo

        (1) Pen VK 500 mg q.i.d.

        (2) Erythromycin 500 mg q.i.d. for 7 to 10 days

        (3) Cephalexin 500 mg q.i.d. for 7 to 10 days

        (4) Azithromycin 500 mg on day one and 250 mg days 2 to 5

     e. *S. aureus*—bullous impetigo

        (1) Dicloxacillin 500 mg q.i.d. for 7 to 10 days

        (2) Cephalexin 500 mg q.i.d. for 7 to 10 days

     f. MRSA

        (1) Vancomycin plus rifampin plus gentamycin

        (2) Sulfamethoxazole/trimethoprim (DS) b.i.d.

        (3) Minocycline 100 mg every 12 hours

        (4) Ciprofloxacin 750 mg every 12 hours

  2. Folliculitis, furuncle, carbuncle and hidradenitis suppurativa

     a. Mild folliculitis

        (1) Benzoyl peroxide 5% b.i.d. for 10 days

        (2) Erythromycin 2% solution b.i.d. for 10 days

b. Moderate infection

   (1) Warm moist compresses to promote spontaneous drainage

   (2) Incision and drainage (I & D) usually required

   (3) Culture recurrent abscesses

   (4) Dicloxacillin 500 mg q.i.d. for 7 to 10 days

   (5) Cephalexin 500 mg q.i.d. for 7 to 10 days

   (6) MRSA (see impetigo)

c. Hidradenitis suppurativa—additional measures to reduce inflammation

   (1) Intralesional triamcinalone 3 to 5 mg/mL diluted with lidocaine

   (2) Prednisone 70 mg tapered over 14 days

3. Cellulitis

   a. Facial involvement—consult with physician for possible inpatient management

   b. I & D may be required

   c. Antibiotic should be selected based upon suspected pathogen

      (1) Penicillin VK 500 mg q.i.d. for 10 days (*S. aureus*, GAS); see impetigo for alternative drugs

      (2) Dicloxacillin 500 mg q.i.d. for 7 to 10 days (*S. aureus*); see impetigo for alternative drugs

      (3) Vancomycin plus rifampin plus gentamycin (MRSA), see impetigo for alternative drugs

   d. Rest, immobilization, elevation, moist heat, analgesia

   e. Re-evaluate in 48 hours

Dermatitis

- Definition: Group of inflammatory pruritic skin diseases that have different etiologies but share common symptoms and clinical manifestations

   1. Atopic dermatitis—acute, subacute, but usually chronic, pruritic inflammation of the epidermis and dermis; term often used synonymously with eczema, IgE dermatitis

   2. Contact dermatitis—acute or chronic inflammatory reactions to substances that come in contact with the skin

   3. Stasis dermatitis—inflammatory response to extravasated blood in dermis and subcutaneous tissue resulting from stasis

   4. Seborrheic dermatitis—chronic dermatosis characterized by redness and scaling reaction where sebaceous glands are most active

- Etiology/Incidence

  1. Atopic dermatitis

     a. Thought to have genetic basis; often seen as part of an ''atopy'' triad; dermatitis, asthma and allergic rhinitis

     b. Two-thirds of patients have personal or family history of respiratory atopy

     c. Seen in all populations and geographic locations

     d. More common in males than in females

     e. Highest incidence in childhood, usually resolves by third decade

     f. More prevalent in urban areas and developed countries

     g. Exacerbated by allergies, skin dehydration, emotional stress, hormonal changes, and infection

  2. Contact dermatitis

     a. Irritant contact dermatitis

        (1) More common than allergic contact dermatitis

        (2) Most irritants used daily in work and home environments

        (3) Accounts for high percentage of work-related skin disorders

             (a) Low-caustic irritants—soapy water, cleansers, rubbing alcohol, kerosene

             (b) High-caustic irritants—bleach, strong acids, alkalis

        (4) Higher incidence in those with compromised skin integrity

     b. Allergic contact dermatitis

        (1) Delayed (type IV) cell-mediated hypersensitivity to a substance

             (a) Substance (antigen) binds with epidermal protein

             (b) Antigen-protein complex presented to T-helper cells causing release of mediators

             (c) T-helper cell expansion occurs in regional lymph nodes producing T-effector lymphocytes

             (d) T-effector lymphocytes circulate in bloodstream and produce the epidermal response

             (e) Entire process occurs in 5 to 21 days

             (f) Re-exposure—dermatologic response in 12 to 48 hours

        (2) Most common sensitizer in U.S. is oleoresin of Rhus family of plants—poison oak, ivy, and sumac

        (3) Other common sensitizers are nickel in jewelry, fragrances, and preservatives in topical preparations

3. Stasis dermatitis

    a. Occurs as a result of chronic venous insufficiency

    b. Complicated by low grade tissue ischemia associated with stasis at capillary level

    c. History of varicosities, thrombophlebitis, or postphlebitic syndrome

    d. Often complicated by allergic contact dermatitis and chronic infection

4. Seborrheic dermatitis

    a. Etiology unknown, thought to have a genetic basis

    b. Overgrowth of naturally occurring yeast, *Pityrosporum ovale*

    c. Often begins in early adulthood, aggravated by stress

    d. Can be an early cutaneous sign of HIV infection

    e. Often severe in patients with chronic neurological diseases

    f. Seen in patients with severe acne

    g. More common in males

- Signs and Symptoms: Pruritic scaly rash
- Differential Diagnosis
  1. Scabies
  2. Tinea
  3. Atopic/eczema dermatitis
  4. Contact dermatitis
  5. Nummular dermatitis
  6. Psoriasis (seborrheic dermatitis)
  7. Cellulitis (stasis dermatitis)
- Physical Findings
  1. Common clinical findings for all types of dermatitis

         a. Initial stage—erythema, papules, microvesicles, and excoriation

         b. Chronic stage—lichenification

  2. Atopic dermatitis

         a. Papules, erythema, excoriations and lichenification

         b. Pustules represent secondary infections with staphylococci

         c. Distribution—flexural areas of neck, antecubital fossae, and popliteal fossae

         d. Other locations—face, wrist, and forearm

  3. Irritant contact dermatitis

    a. Mild irritants—erythema, chapped skin, dryness, and fissuring

    b. Severe cases—edema, serous oozing, tender, crusting, scaling

    c. Painful bullae may develop with potent irritant

    d. Distribution—hands most common, also face and eyes

4. Allergic contact dermatitis

    a. Erythema, edema, papules, vesicles, serous oozing, crusting, scaling

    b. Distribution—corresponds to exposed area

    c. Lesions outline site of irritant, often linear pattern with plant exposure

5. Stasis dermatitis

    a. Early stage—mottled pigmentation and slight erythema

    b. Evidence of varicosities, ankle edema

    c. Mild tenderness with deep palpation; pulses normal

    d. Chronic stage—subcutaneous tissue becomes thick, fibrous

    e. Distribution—lower legs

6. Seborrheic dermatitis

    a. Ill defined, greasy yellow scales overlying erythematous patches

    b. Distribution—scalp, within external ear, postauricular area, eyebrows, nasolabial folds, central chest, and at times axilla, groin, submammary folds

- Diagnostic Tests/Findings

  1. Serum IgE—levels elevated in patients with atopy

  2. KOH—negative for spores/hyphae

  3. Skins scrapings—negative for burrows

- Management/Treatment

  1. Three goals of therapy

    a. Treatment of inflamed skin

    b. Control of pruritus

    c. Control of exacerbating factors

  2. Treatment of inflamed skin

    a. Mild disease—low-potency steroid cream

      (1) Hydrocortisone 1% to 2.5% cream 2 to 4 times daily

      (2) Desonide 0.05% b.i.d. (face or areas resistant to hydrocortisone)

    b. Severe disease—medium potency steroid cream (2 to 4 weeks)

      (1) Triamcinolone acetonide 0.1% cream 2 to 4 times daily

       (2)   Fluocinolone acetonide 0.025% cream b.i.d.

   c.   Topical corticosteroid with occlusion may be helpful

       (1)   Treat area with steroid cream and cover with plastic wrap

       (2)   Leave on overnight and remove plastic wrap in morning

   d.   Lesions resistant to medium potency steroids use ultra-high potency—beta-methasone dipropionate 0.05% b.i.d., with or without occlusion

   e.   Acute flares may require short term oral glucocorticoids

       (1)   Prednisone 40 to 60 mg tapered over 14 to 21 days

       (2)   Solu-medrol dose pak

   f.   Ultraviolet light therapy and oral glucocorticoids for most severe cases

   g.   Wet to dry compresses with water or aluminum acetate (Burow's solution) to dry vesicular lesions

   h.   Bullous lesions—may be drained; do not remove top thin skin

3.   Control of pruritus

   a.   Antihistamines

       (1)   Hydroxyzine 25 mg t.i.d./q.i.d. prn

       (2)   Diphenhydramine 25 to 50 mg every 4 to 6 hours prn

       (3)   Doxepin 10 to 25 mg b.i.d./t.i.d. prn

   b.   Tepid bathes to cool and hydrate skin

   c.   Mild soaps

   d.   Emollients

   e.   Control of exacerbating factors

       (1)   Treat secondary bacterial infections, usually staphylococcus

       (2)   Maintain good hydration and integrity of skin

       (3)   Gently towel dry skin, no brisk rubbing

       (4)   Continued use of emollients to prevent skin drying

       (5)   Wear gloves to avoid contact irritants

       (6)   Identify and avoid offending irritants

       (7)   Stasis dermatitis—special measures

          (a)   Elevate legs; support stockings

          (b)   Exercise daily to help reduce venous pressure and edema

       (8)   Seborrheic dermatitis—special measures

          (a)   Daily use of shampoos containing tar, sulfur, salicylic acid, or selenium

    (b)   Ketoconazole 2% cream and shampoo (twice weekly) is an alternative to topical steroids

    (c)   Low-potency topical steroid, hydrocortisone 1%

  (9)   Educate patient on stress reduction to avoid exacerbation

  (10) Follow-up in 1 to 2 weeks

Fungal and Yeast Infections

- Definitions:

  1. Tinea (dermatophytosis)—fungal infection of skin, nails, and hair; characteristic lesions varies by site

  2. Tinea (pityriasis)versicolor—chronic, asymptomatic, scaly dermatitis

  3. Candidiasis—yeast-like fungal infection of skin and mucous membrane

- Etiology/Incidence

  1. Tinea

    a. Causative organisms—*Trichophyton, Microsporum,* and *Epidermophyton*

    b. Transmitted by fomites, animals (pets), and to a lesser extent, soil

  2. Tinea versicolor

    a. Causative organism—nondermatophyte fungus *Pityrosporum orbiculare;* normal inhabitant of skin

    b. Most common in young adults when sebum production high

  3. Candidiasis

    a. Causative organism usually *Candida albicans;* normal saprophytic inhabitant of GI tract; overgrowth often due to antibiotic use

    b. Occurs in intertriginous, moist, cutaneous areas

  4. Contributing factors

    a. Warm moist environments for fungal infections

    b. Obesity

    c. Altered immunity

      (1) HIV

      (2) Diabetes

      (3) Pregnancy

      (4) Inhaled or oral steroids

    d. Oral contraceptives

e. Antibiotic therapy

- Signs and Symptoms (depends upon area of involvement)
  1. Mild pruritus
  2. Inflamed, tender rash
  3. Thickened nails
  4. Hair loss
- Differential Diagnosis
  1. Seborrheic dermatitis
  2. Psoriasis
  3. Alopecia
  4. Atopic dermatitis
  5. Contact dermatitis
  6. Pityriasis rosea
  7. Bacterial infection
- Physical Findings
  1. Morphology
     a. Tinea (dermatophytosis)—characteristic lesion varies by site
        (1) Tinea capitis—well defined or irregular, diffuse areas of scaling and hair loss on scalp
        (2) Tinea corporis—annular appearance (ringworm), deep inflammatory nodules, or granulomas
        (3) Tinea cruris—sharply demarcated, erythematous scaly patches
        (4) Tinea pedis—erythema/edema, scaling, and occasional vesiculation; fissured toe webs
        (5) Tinea unguium—opacified thickened nails with subungal debris
        (6) Immunocompromised patient—may see abscess or granulomas
     b. Tinea (pityriasis) versicolor—oval scaly hyper or hypopigmented macules
     c. Candidiasis
        (1) Skin (intertrigo)—erythematous macerated areas with satellite pustules
        (2) Mucous membranes—white friable patches on mucous membranes
  2. Distribution
     a. Tinea
        (1) Capitis—scalp

       (2)   Corporis—non-hair-bearing skin

       (3)   Cruris—(males) groin and upper thigh sparing scrotum

       (4)   Pedis—feet, usually between 4th and 5th toes

       (5)   Unguium—nails, usually 1st and 2nd toenails

   b.   Tinea versicolor

       (1)   "Shawl like" back, chest, and shoulders

       (2)   Less common—groin, thigh, genitalia

   c.   Candidiasis

       (1)   Body folds—axillae, submammary, groin, intergluteal, webspaces of fingers and toes

       (2)   Oral and vaginal mucous membranes

- Diagnostic Test/Findings

   1.   Wood's lamp (T. versicolor)—golden fluorescence

   2.   KOH—positive for hyphae, pseudohyphae, and/or spores

   3.   Fungal culture—may be useful for inflammatory T. corporis and T. capitis

- Management/Treatment

   1.   Tinea

      a.   Scalp

         (1)   Selenium sulfide shampoo 2.5% twice weekly for two weeks

         (2)   If boggy, edematous suppurative (kerion) present—prednisone 1 to 2 mg/kg/d (25 to 50 mg) for 7 to 10 days

         (3)   Oral antifungals

            (a)   Terbinafine 250 mg daily 4 to 6 weeks, (most effective)

            (b)   Itraconazole 100 mg b.i.d. 4 to 6 weeks

            (c)   Ketoconozole 200 to 400 mg daily for 4 to 6 weeks

            (d)   Griseofulvin 500 mg daily 4 to 8 weeks

         (3)   Advise hair regrowth will be slow

      b.   Body

         (1)   Multiple topical imidazoles and triazoles applied b.i.d. until 1 to 2 weeks after clinical clearing, e.g., clotrimazole 1% cream b.i.d., miconazole 2% t.i.d. after clinical clearing

         (2)   Terbinafine 1% cream b.i.d. 1 to 2 weeks after clinical clearing

         (3)   If topical antifungals fail, use oral agents (see T. capitis)

(4) Avoid occlusive footwear for tinea pedis

c. Nails

(1) Terbinafine 250 mg daily (most effective)

(a) Fingernails—six weeks

(b) Toenails—12 weeks

(2) Poor results with topical agents; usually reserved for maintenance after successful systemic treatment

d. Follow up in two weeks to re-evaluate treatment

2. Tinea versicolor

a. Selenium sulfide lotion 2.5%—apply at bedtime, rinse in morning

b. Clotrimazole 1% cream b.i.d. for four weeks

c. Ketoconazole shampoo

(1) Cure rate 80%

(2) No shower for 12 to 18 hours following treatment

d. Oral ketoconazole 200 mg daily for one week or 400 mg single dose for resistant cases

e. Retreat if no improvement in one month

f. Recurrence common as organism is normal inhabitant of skin

3. Candidiasis

a. Nystatin cream or powder b.i.d. 2 to 4 weeks

b. Ketoconazole cream daily for 2 to 4 weeks

c. Fluconazole 150 mg orally once

d. Dry intertriginous area—wet Burow's compresses 3 to 4 times daily

e. Rule out HIV or diabetes in patients with multiple recurrences

Papulosquamous Disorders

- Definition: Group of disorders with unique scales due to abnormal keratinization process; these lesions are sharply delineated, distinguishing them from scaling lesions of eczematous diseases

  1. Psoriasis vulgaris—genetically determined, chronic, epidermal proliferate disease of unpredictable course

  2. Pityriasis rosea—self-limited mild, inflammatory skin disease lasting 3 to 8 weeks

- Etiology/Incidence

  1. Psoriasis

a. Genetic predisposition, although not totally understood

b. Affects 2% of population in U.S., Caucasians > African-Americans

c. Type 1, early onset, occurring in 2nd decade

d. Type 2, late onset, occurring in 6th to 8th decades

e. Approximately 5% of patients will develop psoriatic arthritis affecting primarily distal interphalangeal (DIP) joints

f. Abrupt onset seen with early HIV infection

g. Trigger factors

  (1) Physical trauma

  (2) Infection

  (3) Stress

  (4) Drugs—corticosteroids, lithium, antimalarial, interferon, beta-blockers

2. Pityriasis rosea

a. Etiology unknown; viral cause suspected

b. Seen primarily in the spring and fall seasons

c. Patients frequently report recent upper respiratory infection

d. 50% more common in females

- Signs and Symptoms
  1. Psoriasis

a. Frequently asymptomatic

b. Severe pruritus in body fold eruptions

c. Chronic, recurring

  2. Pityriasis rosea

a. Mild pruritus

b. Initial lesion precedes general eruption by one to two weeks

c. Self-limiting—heals without scarring in four to eight weeks

- Differential Diagnosis
  1. Psoriasis

a. Seborrheic dermatitis

b. Candidiasis

c. Intertrigo

d. Onychomycosis

e. Reiter's syndrome

2. Pityriasis rosea

    a. Secondary syphilis

    b. Tinea infections

    c. Seborrheic dermatitis

- Physical Findings

  1. Psoriasis

     a. Cutaneous lesions reveal four prominent features:

         (1) Sharply demarcated lesions with clear-cut borders

         (2) Erythematous plaque base

         (3) Overlapping silvery scales

         (4) Auspitz sign—removal of scales results in small blood droplets

     b. Fingers/nails

         (1) Stippling or pitting of nail plate

         (2) Yellow or brown-red staining of oncholytic patches with accumulation of yellow debris under nails

         (3) Swelling, redness and scaling of paronychial margins

  2. Pityriasis rosea—classic disease pattern

     a. A single lesion termed "herald patch" precedes generalized eruption by 7 to 10 days

     b. "Herald patch" is found usually on neck or lower trunk; oval, slightly erythematous, rose or fawn-colored

     c. Oval patches seen in general eruption have an unusual fine, white scale located near the border of the plaques, forming a collarette

     d. Lesions follow skin cleavage lines in a "Christmas tree" pattern

- Diagnostic Tests/Findings

  1. Psoriasis

     a. Diagnosis generally based on clinical presentation

     b. Biopsy may be necessary

     c. Rheumatoid factor

     d. Sedimentation rate

  2. Pityriasis rosea

     a. Diagnosis generally based on clinical presentation

     b. KOH—negative for spores/hyphae

    c.   Throat culture or rapid strep test—negative for scarlatina

    d.   RPR—negative for syphilis

- Management/Treatment
  1. Psoriasis—localized to palm/soles/scalp < 5% involvement
     a. Strong potency topical corticosteroid—adjunctive therapy for two to three weeks
        (1) Fluocinolone acetonide cream 0.05% b.i.d./q.i.d.
        (2) Occlusion with plastic wrap
        (3) More effective if scales removed prior to application
     b. Tar-based preparations are useful adjuncts
     c. Anthralin cream 0.1% to 1% at bedtime
     d. Calcipotriene ointment or cream twice daily
     e. Goeckerman regimen—phototherapy ultraviolet B radiation, sun (UVB) exposure 4 to 6 hours daily for 4 weeks
     f. Coal tar 15 to 25 mL in tepid bath
     g. Ingram regimen—phototherapy ultraviolet B radiation (UVB) used in combination with anthralin 0.1% to 0.5% applied daily
  2. Psoriasis—generalized (> 30% body surface affected)
     a. Referral to dermatologist
     b. May include some combination of UVB, PUVA (psoralan with UVA), etritinate, metrotrexate, cyclosporine
     c. Patient education for localized and generalized psoriasis—family issues, emotional support, stress reduction, National Psoriasis Foundation
  3. Pityriasis rosea
     a. Treatment often not necessary
     b. UVB light treatments for one week
     c. Topical corticosteroids and antihistamines for control of pruritus

Scabies

- Definition: Common highly pruritic transmissable ectoparasite infection
- Etiology/Incidence
  1. Caused by itch mite *Sarcoptes scabiei*
  2. Adult female mite burrows into skin shortly after contact; lives for 4 to 6 weeks
  3. Incubation period four weeks from initial contact; generalized hypersensitivity eruption 1 to 2 weeks later

4. Transmitted primarily by person to person or sexual contact

5. Transmission via clothing, bedding less common—mite cannot survive more than one day without host

6. May affect entire families

7. Frequently seen in institutionalized persons, such as homeless shelters, nursing homes, correctional facilities

- Signs and Symptoms

  1. Pruritus always present; most intense when individual is in bed or after a hot shower

  2. Pruritus frequently less intense in the HIV client

- Differential Diagnosis

  1. Atopic dermatitis

  2. Contact or irritant dermatitis

  3. Urticaria

  4. Pediculosis

- Physical Findings

  1. Burrows, small pruritic vesicles, or wavy dark lines a few millimeters to 1 cm in length with papule at open end

  2. May be difficult to visualize since client scratching destroys burrows

  3. Lesions are believed to be due to a hypersensitivity reaction to the excreta deposited by mite

  4. Generalized excoriations surrounding vesicles and pustules on fingers, palms, wrists, elbows, axillae, feet, nipples in females, scrotum or penis in males, buttocks

  5. Usually spares the head and neck, except in the elderly or patients with AIDS—in the client with HIV, hyperkeratotic plaques may be located on any area of the body

- Diagnostic Tests/Findings: Microscopic examination of skin scraping in oil immersion—presence of mite, eggs, or fecal pellets

- Management/Treatment

  1. Treatment of choice is 5% permethrin cream applied to all areas of the body from the neck down; left on for 8 to 14 hours, and then removed with soap and water; may be repeated in one week

  2. Alternative is 1% lindane (no longer the drug of choice)

     a. Lotion or cream applied from neck down to all areas of the body and removed with soap and water after eight hours

     b. Not recommended for pregnant or lactating women, patients with extensive dermatitis, nor infants

3. Alternative is 10% crotamiton cream applied to the body from the neck down for two consecutive nights and then removed with soap and water 48 hours after the last application

4. All household members and sexual contacts should be evaluated and treated if necessary to prevent reinfection

5. For persistent pruritus, triamcinolone 0.1% cream to affected areas b.i.d.

6. Secondary pyoderma is generally due to staphylococcus; treat with topical mupirocin or oral erythromycin

7. Patient education

   a. Launder all bedding and clothing in hot water and on hot dryer cycle

   b. Place clothing that cannot be laundered in plastic storage bags for at least four days— mites will not survive off the host longer than four days

   c. Advise client that pruritus may continue for several weeks

Skin Cancer

- Definition:

  1. Basal cell carcinoma (BCC)—slow growing locally destructive carcinoma of basal cell layer of epidermis; limited potential for metastasis

  2. Squamous cell carcinoma (SCC)—malignant, nodular, tumor arising from squamous cells in epithelium; hyperkeratotic growth

  3. Malignant melanoma (MM)—cancer that arises in melanocytes; accounts for 5% of all skin cancers; two most common types are superficial spreading melanoma (SSM) and nodular melanoma (NM)

  4. Kaposi's sarcoma (KS)—multisystem vascular neoplasm characterized by mucocutaneous and violet lesions and edema; involves nearly all body organs

- Etiology/Incidence

  1. Basal cell carcinoma

     a. Cause is multifactorial; cumulative sunlight exposure (UVB) is most significant factor

     b. Primarily affects fair-skinned persons with tendency to sunburn easily

     c. Most common form of human cancer

     d. Over 400,000 new cases in U.S. per year; mostly persons in 4th decade

     e. Additional risk factors

        (1) Extensive sun exposure as a youth

        (2) History of treatment with x-ray for facial acne

  2. Squamous cell carcinoma

    a. Causal/contributing factors

      (1) UVB light

      (2) Human papillomaviruses have also been implicated

      (3) Immunocompromised

      (4) Chemical carcinogens—topical nitrogen mustard; oral PUVA (psoralens with UVA [used to treat psoriasis]); industrial carcinogens

      (5) Increased risk of oral and lip SCC in cigarette and cigar smokers

    b. Mainly seen on sun-damaged areas of fair-skinned persons, but can appear anywhere on the body

    c. Also found in brown and black-skinned person

    d. Frequency of metastasis is by location; SCC of the cutaneous tissue has an overall metastatic rate of 3% to 4%; invasive SCC arising from chronic osteomyelitis sinus tracts, burn scars, and sites of radiation dermatitis have metastatic rates of 31%, 20%, and 18% respectively

3. Malignant melanoma

    a. All causes not known

    b. Brief, intense exposure to long-wave ultra-violet radiation contributes to development

    c. Predisposing/risk factors:

      (1) Presence of precursor lesions, e.g., Clark's dysplastic melanocytic nevus, congenital melanocytic nevus

      (2) Family history of melanoma

      (3) Fair complexion; red or blonde hair; freckles; tendency to sunburn easily

      (4) Excessive sun exposure

    d. Peak age distribution 30 to 50 years

    e. Slightly more common in men

    f. Incidence has increased 300% in 40 years

4. Kaposi's sarcoma

    a. Human herpesvirus 8 present in all forms

    b. Epidemic clusters in U.S. predominantly found in HIV infected individuals—incidence has decreased from 40% to 18% of HIV population

    c. Occurs when $CD4^+$ count < 500

    d. Non-HIV related forms are less common but do occur

      (1) African-endemic—accounts for 8% to 12% of malignancies in Zaire

      (2)   Classic (European)—occurs predominantly in elderly white males, rarely fatal

      (3)   Iatrogenic immunosuppressive drug associated—occurs infrequently in patients on immunosuppressive or cytotoxic chemotherapy, resolves when drug withdrawn

- Signs and Symptoms
  1. BCC/SCC—painless sore that will not heal
  2. Malignant melanoma—6 signs ABCDEE
     a. **A**symmetry in shape
     b. **B**order is irregular
     c. **C**olor is mottled
     d. **D**iameter is usually large > 6.0 mm
     e. **E**levation is almost always present
     f. **E**nlargement or a history of an increase in size is perhaps the most important sign
  3. Kaposi's sarcoma—small reddish-purple to brown lesions
- Differential Diagnosis
  1. BCC/SCC
     a. Seborrheic keratosis
     b. Malignant melanoma
     c. Actinic keratosis
     d. Psoriasis
     e. Nummular eczema
  2. Malignant melanoma
     a. Melanoma in situ
     b. Solar lentigo
     c. Dysplastic melanocytic nevus with marked atypia
     d. Recurring melanocyte nevus
     e. Hemangioma
     f. Pyogenic granuloma
     g. Pigmented BCC
  3. Kaposi's sarcoma
     a. Sclerosing hemangioma

b. Ecchymosis

c. Stasis dermatitis

- Physical Findings

  1. Basal cell carcinoma

     a. Most commonly found on face and head

     b. Papular, nodular, ulcerated, sclerosing pigmented lesions

     c. Pearly appearance with telangiectatic vessels is most diagnostic

     d. Lesions may have a central crust or erosion

     e. Slow growing—may reach 1 to 2 cm diameter after several years

  2. Squamous cell carcinoma

     a. In situ (Bowen's Disease)

        (1) Erythematous plaque, slightly raised, sharp borders with little infiltration

        (2) Presents most commonly on mouth and lower lip

     b. Invasive squamous cell carcinoma

        (1) Highly differentiated SCC

            (a) Keratinization within or on surface of tumor

            (b) Firm or hard upon palpation

        (2) Poorly differentiated SCC

            (a) Shows no sign of keratinization

            (b) Fleshy, granulomatous; soft on palpation

  3. Malignant melanoma

     a. SSM

        (1) Pigment variation of dark brown, black, pink, or gray; starts as flattened papule, progressing to plaques, and then nodules.

        (2) Asymmetrical to 12 mm (early), to 25 mm (late)

        (3) Isolated single lesions found primarily on sun exposed areas—back, legs, anterior chest (males)

        (4) Regional lymphadenopathy (later stages)

     b. NM

        (1) Dark blue, black uniformly elevated "blueberry-like" nodule ranging in size from 1 to 3 cm; oval or round with smooth sharply defined borders

        (2) Distribution and regional lymphadenopathy same as SSM

  4. Kaposi's sarcoma

a. Red, purple or dark color palpable plaques or nodules on cutaneous or mucosal surfaces

b. Lymph node involvement in 50% of patient's with HIV associated KS

c. May also involve the lung, gastrointestinal tract, or urogenital system

- Diagnostic Tests/Findings—total excisional biopsy with narrow margins for SSM and NM

- Management/Treatment

  1. Basal cell carcinoma

     a. Simple excision—5% to 10% recurrence

     b. Referral to oncology for therapy

        (1) Three cycles of curretage and electrodessication

        (2) Radiotherapy with 4000-5000 rads in 6 to 10 doses (cure 95%)

        (3) Mohs surgery—removal of tumor; 98% cure rate

  2. Squamous cell carcinoma

     a. Referral to oncologist for therapy

     b. Surgical excision, Mohs surgery, cryotherapy

     c. Referral for 5-fluoracil chemotherapy

  3. Malignant melanoma

     a. Refer to oncologist for therapy

        (1) Initial excision to establish histologic diagnosis

        (2) Re-excision of the area with adequate margins—margins range from 0.5 to 3.0 cm based upon depth of invasion

        (3) Elective lymph node dissection controversial

     b. Close follow up for evidence of recurrence of metastasis

  4. Kaposi's sarcoma

     a. Referral for cryotherapy, radiation or laser surgey—treatment depends upon underlying condition and location of sarcoma

     b. Supportive care, counseling for HIV progressive disease

Viral Dermatoses

- Definitions

  1. Herpes simplex I (HS-I) (''fever blister'')—recurrent cutaneous viral infection characterized by single or multiple clusters of small vesicles on an erythematous base; lesions appear on the lips, in the mouth or pharynx

2. Herpes (varicella) zoster ("shingles")—an acute CNS cutaneous viral infection characterized by vesicular eruptions and neurologic pain; involves primarily the dorsal root ganglia

3. Warts—common contagious epithelial tumors; usually benign

- Etiology/Incidence

  1. Herpes Simplex (HS-I)

     a. Caused by herpes simplex virus (HSV-I)

     b. Usually follows a minor infection, trauma, stress or sun exposure

     c. 90% of adults have serologic evidence of virus

     d. Prolonged incubation period 2 to 18 months

  2. Herpes (varicella) zoster

     a. Reactivation of varicella zoster virus (VZV) in chickenpox

     b. Proposed that VZV is dormant in dorsal root ganglia

     c. May occur at any age, but most common after age 50

     d. May precede marked immunosuppresion in patients with HIV or Hodgkin's disease

     e. Post-transplant patients on immunosuppression medication are also at risk

  3. Warts

     a. Caused by over 60 human papillomaviruses (HPV)

     b. Squamous cell carcinoma associated with HPV infections in anogenital region

     c. Common in young adults, but uncommon in the aged

- Signs and Symptoms

  1. HS-I

     a. Small vesicles appear after a short prodrome of tingling, burning, or itching

     b. Vesicles dry to a yellow crust within a few days

  2. Herpes zoster

     a. Pain along nerve root precedes eruption by 48 hours

     b. Characteristic crops of vesicles then appear

  3. Warts—generally asymptomatic

- Differential Diagnosis

  1. HS-I

     a. Contact dermatitis

  b. Pyoderma

  c. Chickenpox (VZV)

  d. Chancroid syphilis

2. Herpes zoster (local lesion and pre-eruptive pain)

  a. Contact dermatitis

  b. Herpes simplex

  c. Migraine

  d. Myocardial infarction

  e. Acute abdomen

3. Wart

  a. Squamous cell carcinoma

  b. Hypertrophic actinic keratosis

  c. Molluscum contagiosum

  d. Seborrheic keratosis

- Physical Findings

  1. Regional lymphadenopathy may be seen with herpetic diseases

  2. HS-I

    a. Small grouped vesicles on an erythematous base that progress to a crusted erosion

    b. Duration 5 to 7 days

    c. Distribution lips, mouth, pharynx

  3. Herpes zoster

    a. May present 3 to 4 days prior to pain and vesicular eruptions with prodrome of chills, fever, malaise

    b. Painful unilateral vesicular eruptions within a dermatome

    c. Duration 2 to 3 weeks

    d. Distribution—face and trunk

    e. Regional lymph glands may be tender or edematous

    f. Complication of post-herpetic neuralgia involving trigeminal region

  4. Warts

    a. Common wart (verrucae vulgaris)

      (1) Solitary flesh-colored papule with scaly irregular surface 2 to 10 mm in diameter

    (2) Appear most often on fingers, around nail plate, elbows, knees

   b. Flat wart (verruca plantaris)

    (1) Groups of smooth flat-topped, flesh-colored lesions

    (2) Distribution—face and extremities

   c. Plantar warts

    (1) Endophytic (growing inward) with thick keratin surface

    (2) Common on sole of foot

    (3) May be exquisitely painful

- Diagnostic Tests/Findings

  1. HS-I and zoster

   a. Direct immunofluorescent antibody (ELISA)—positive

   b. Tzanck smear—multinucleated cells (least sensitive)

   c. Viral culture—positive (not highly sensitive)

   d. Consider testing for HIV or Hodgkin's if recurrence of herpes

  2. Warts

   a. Acetic acid 5%—lesions turn white

   b. Biopsy—rule out squamous cell carcinoma

- Management/Treatment

  1. HS-I

   a. Immunocompetent patient

    (1) Initial episode—7 to 10 days

     (a) Acyclovir 200 mg 5 times/day

     (b) Acyclovir 800 mg t.i.d.

     (c) Valacyclovir 1000 mg t.i.d. for 7 days

     (d) Famciclovir 250 mg t.i.d.

    (2) Recurrant episodes—5 days

     (a) Acyclovir 200 mg 5 times/day

     (b) Valacyclovir 500 mg b.i.d.

     (c) Famciclovir 125 mg b.i.d.

    (3) Topical acyclovir not recommended

   b. Immunosuppressed patient

    (1) Initial episode

        (a)   Acyclovir 200 mg 5 times/day for 7 to 10 days

        (b)   Acyclovir 5 mg/kg/IV every 8 hours for severe cases

    (2)   Localized external lesion

        (a)   Topical acyclovir 5% 4 to 6 times/day

        (b)   Limit use to this group of patients due to development of resistant HS-1 viral strain

    (3)   To prevent reactivation (i.e., immediate post-transplant)—acyclovir 400 mg 3 to 5 times/day

  c.   Caution family—virus may remain on fomites for several hours

2.   Herpes zoster

  a.   Immunocompetent

    (1)   Acyclovir 800 mg five times/day for seven days started within 48 to 72 hours

    (2)   Famciclovir 500 mg t.i.d. for 7 days started within 48 to 72 hours

    (3)   Valacyclovir 1000 mg t.i.d. for 7 days started within 48 to 72 hours

    (4)   Good hydration essential

    (5)   Nerve block for analgesia may be necessary

    (6)   Acute pain—prednisone 60 mg/day for 3 weeks

    (7)   Monitor renal function in patient with renal disease

  b.   Immunosuppressed

    (1)   Consult with physician

    (2)   Antiviral therapy as with immunocompetent except of longer duration until lesions have completely crusted

  c.   Post-zoster neuralgia

    (1)   Capsaicin ointment 0.025% to 0.075%

    (2)   Chronic regional nerve blockade

    (3)   Gabapentin 300 mg t.i.d. (maximum of 3600 mg/day)

    (3)   Amitriptyline 25 to 75 mg at bedtime

  d.   Warts

    (1)   Most are unresponsive to all therapeutic modalities

    (2)   Most will resolve spontaneously in 1 to 2 years

    (3)   Multiple keratolytic agents—salicylic acid or salicylic acid and lactic acid combination

    (4)   Tretinoin—good for facial lesions

   (5) Liquid nitrogen every two weeks for several weeks

   (6) Carbon dioxide laser excision

Questions
Select the best answer.

1. Mrs. Trevino is a 35-year-old patient with patchy hair loss as a result of chronic systemic lupus erythematosus. You have determined that she has scarring or cicatrical alopecia. The most effective treatment you can offer is:

   a. Topical minoxidil
   b. Intralesional corticosteroids
   c. Topical estrogen
   d. Referral to dermatologist

2. Mr. Johnson is a 45-year-old patient with diabetes who is homeless. He presents with tender fluctulant nodules on the skin around his beard. He has been previously treated with benzoyl peroxide 5% with minimal response. You order warm moist compresses and:

   a. Dicloxacillin 500 mg q.i.d. for 10 days
   b. Trimethoprim/sulfamethoxazole every day for 5 days
   c. Acyclovir topical
   d. Clotrimazole 1% b.i.d. for 10 days

3. Mr. Johnson returns to your office with his friend. His friend presents with multiple abscesses and ''boils'' on the back of his neck that have coalesced and developed sieve-like openings draining pus. Your diagnosis is:

   a. Scabies
   b. Folliculitis
   c. Carbuncle
   d. Contact dermatitis

4. To reduce inflammation in a hidradentitis suppurativa lesion, immediately prior to incision and drainage you would:

   a. Apply cold packs to axilla
   b. Order solu-medrol dosepak
   c. Apply tretinoin topically
   d. Inject intralesional triamcinlone 3 to 5 mg/mL diluted with lidocaine

5. The most common sensitizer in the U.S. responsible for allergic contact dermatitis is:

   a. Oleoresin
   b. Tinea
   c. Rubbing alcohol
   d. Bleach

6. Mrs. Waterman is a 64-year-old with a history of varicosities and a single episode of thrombophlebitis. On inspection of both lower extremities you note mottled pigmentation, erythema, varicosities, and ankle edema. Your initial impression is:

   a. Cellulitis

    b. Stasis dermatitis

    c. Atopic dermatitis

    d. Contact dermatitis

7. The most effective antifungal agent used in the treatment of tinea capitis is:

    a. Terbinafine orally

    b. Clotrimazole 1% cream

    c. Triamcinolone 0.025% cream

    d. Nystatin cream

8. Janet is a 22-year-old white female who presents for evaluation of lesions on the palm of her right hand. The lesions consist of silvery scales on an erythematous base and are isolated by a sharply demarcated border. You remove the scales and minute drops of blood appear giving a positive Auspitz sign. Your diagnosis is:

    a. Pityriasis rosae

    b. Squamous cell carcinoma

    c. Psoriasis

    d. Eczema

9. Common mode(s) of transmission of scabies include:

    a. Moist fomites

    b. Person to person

    c. Household pets

    d. Soil

10. A 24-year-old presents to clinic with a 5 cm purple, palpable plaque on the upper right posterior chest. He admits to unprotected homosexual activity for the past 10 years. On further exam you note axillary and inguinal lymphadenopathy. You suspect this patient may have:

    a. Squamous cell carcinoma

    b. Malignant melanoma

    c. Basal cell carcinoma

    d. Kaposi's sarcoma

11. Initial laboratory evaluation(s) for this patient should include:

    a. HIV antibody screening

    b. Complete blood count

    c. GC/chlamydia cultures

    d. Liver function tests

12. The common wart, *Verrucae vulgaris,* is characterized as:

    a. Solitary flesh colored papule with scaly irregular surface

    b. Group of flat-topped flesh colored papules

    c. Thick, endophylitic papules or plaques

    d. Papular, nodular, ulcerated sclerosing pigmented lesion

13. Joan is a 15-year-old with multiple closed comedones, and a few pustules on her face and upper back. She has been on tretinoin for her face but is distressed at the progression of acne to her back. You would prescribe:

    a. 13-cis-retinoic acid (Accutane)
    b. Erythromycin 250 mg q.i.d. for 10 days
    c. Benzoyl peroxide cleansing soap
    d. Amoxil 250 mg t.i.d. for 10 days

14. Janice is an 18 year old who presents to your clinic with a scaly, pruritic rash on the dorsal aspect of her toes. This rash has occurred each winter for the past eight years. Her family history is unremarkable except for her father who has asthma. The most likely diagnosis is:

    a. Psoriasis
    b. Candidiasis
    c. Contact dermatitis
    d. Atopic dermatitis

15. Overgrowth of *Pityrosporum obiculare* in the young adult results in:

    a. Tinea corporis
    b. Tinea versicolor
    c. Tinea capitis
    d. Tinea pedis

16. A 30-year-old male presents with multiple, scattered, discrete vesicular lesions on the right leg for 5 days. There are honey-colored ''stuck-on'' crusts and erosions in some of these lesions. The culture yields *Staphylococcus aureus*. The most likely diagnosis is:

    a. Herpes simplex
    b. Herpes zoster
    c. Stasis dermatitis
    d. Impetigo

17. A 19-year-old female presents with small grouped vesicles on an erythematous base on her lower lip. The lesion is painful. She has had this before and it has always gone away in a week or so. You suspect herpes simplex 1. You would confirm your diagnosis with which of the following laboratory test?

    a. Direct immunofluorescent antibody (ELISA)
    b. KOH test
    c. Culture and sensitivity
    d. Wood's lamp

18. Mr. Smith, age 46, presents to the FNP with fever, malaise, and a painful, linear vesicular rash on just one side of his trunk. The most likely diagnosis is

    a. Tinea corporis
    b. Carbuncle

    c. Herpes simplex

    d. Herpes zoster

19. Mr. Thompson has chronic eczema. He presents with pruritic, dry, leathery patches with accentuated skin markings on his forearm. The most appropriate treatment is:

    a. Amoxicillin orally

    b. Clotrimazole 1% cream

    c. Desonide 0.05%

    d. UVB with coal tar

20. Melissa, age 22, presents to the FNP's office with a slightly pruritic red rash on her trunk and breast following the line of skin cleavage giving a "Christmas tree" configuration. She states that the rash started as a single red patch on her abdomen. Medical history is unremarkable, except for a recent upper respiratory infection. Your initial diagnosis is:

    a. Tinea versicolor

    b. Folliculitis

    c. Pityriasis rosea

    d. Seborrheic dermatitis

21. Mr. Kirk is a 45-year-old African American who presents with a sore on his lip that will not heal. Medical history includes psoriasis treated with oral PUVA. Upon inspection you note an erythematous plaque, slightly raised with sharp borders and no sign of infiltration or telangiectatic vessels. You make a referral to the dermatologist for further evaluation of what you suspect is:

    a. Basal cell carcinoma

    b. Squamous cell carcinoma

    c. Kaposi's sarcoma

    d. Psoriasis refractory to treatment

22. Mrs. Summers presents to the FNP with a complaint of red rash and large blister after wearing a new prosthetic leg for three days. This prosthesis has a new polyurethane material she did not have with her old prosthesis. She is a below the right knee amputee secondary to an accident as a child. Upon inspection you note a tender, erythematous, scaly, maculopapular rash. It is warm and edematous with a large bullous lesion on the posterior popliteal fossae. Your initial diagnosis is:

    a. Eczema

    b. Severe irritant contact dermatitis

    c. Herpes zoster

    d. Carbuncle

23. Your management of Mrs. Summers includes oral glucocorticoids steroids, UVB (sunlight exposure) and:

    a. Reducing bullae with sterile needle and syringe

    b. Leaving bullae alone and let rupture spontaneously

c. Advising continued use of new prosthesis

d. Removing top of bullae and applying high potency steroid cream

24. The following medication has no severe teratogenic properties and is safe for use in the sexually active young female with acne:

   a. Erythromycin
   b. Tretinoin
   c. Accutane
   d. Tetracycline

25. Mrs. Lopez is a 45-year-old who presents with a tender, mildly pruritic rash under both breasts and on her abdomen. She is a diabetic with poor control due to poor medication compliance and is at 160% ideal body weight (IBW). Upon inspection you note moist erythematous macerated areas with satellite pustules under both breasts. Your initial impression is:

   a. Candidiasis intertrigo
   b. Tinea corporis
   c. Herpes zoster
   d. Pityriasis rosea

26. Along with better control of Mrs. Lopez's diabetes and continued effort at weight modification, you would prescribe the following:

   a. Nystatin cream or powder
   b. Selenium sulfide lotion 2.5%
   c. Terbinifine 1% cream
   d. Hydrocortisone 1% cream

Answers

1. d	10. d	19. c
2. a	11. a	20. c
3. c	12. a	21. b
4. d	13. b	22. b
5. a	14. d	23. a
6. b	15. b	24. a
7. a	16. d	25. a
8. c	17. a	26. a
9. b	18. d	

Bibliography

Brodell, R. T., & Elewski, B. (2000). Antifungal drug interactions. *Postgraduate Medicine,* 107(1), http://www.postgradmed.com/issues/2000/01_00/brodell.htm

Colyar, M. R., & Ehrhardt, C. (1999). *Ambulatory care procedures for the nurse practitioner.* Philadelphia: F. A. Davis.

DiPiro, J. T., Talbert, R. L., Yee, G. C., Matzke, G. R., Wells, B. G., & Posey, L. M. (Eds.). (1999). *Pharmacotherapy: A pathophysiologic approach.* NY: Lange Medical Books/McGraw Hill.

Fauci, A. S., Isselbacher, K. J., Braunwald, E., Wilson, J. D., Martin, J. B., & Kasper, D. L. (Eds.). (1998). *Harrison's principles of internal medicine* (14th ed.). NY: McGraw Hill.

Fitzpatrick, T. B., Johnson, R. A., Wolff, K., Polano, M. K., & Suurmond, D. (1997). *Color atlas and synopsis of clinical dermatology common and serious diseases* (3rd ed.). NY: McGraw-Hill.

Fleischer, A. B. (1999). Atopic dermatitis. *Postgraduate Medicine,* 106(4), 49-55. http://www.postgradmed.com/issues/1999/10_01_99/fleischer.htm

Hay, W. W., Hayward, A. R., Levin, M. J., & Sondheimer, J. M. (2001). *Current pediatric diagnosis and treatment* (15th edition). NY: Lange Medical Books/McGraw-Hill.

Landow, K. (1997). Dispelling myths about acne. *Postgraduate Medicine,* 102(2), 94-114. http://www.postgradmed.com/issues/1997/08_97/landow.htm

Stobo, J. D., Hellmann, D. B., Ladenson, P. W., Petty, B. G., & Traill, T. A. (1996). *The principles and practice of medicine* (23rd ed.). Stamford, CT: Appleton & Lange.

Tierney, L. M., McPhee, S. J., Papadakis, M. A. (Eds.). (2001). *Current medical diagnosis and treatment* (40th ed.). NY: Lange Medical Books/McGraw Hill.

Uphold, C. R., & Graham, M. V. (1998). *Clinical guidelines in family practice.* Gainesville, FL: Barmarrae Books.

Wasson, J. (1997). *The common symptom guide.* NY: McGraw-Hill.

Relevant Web Sites

Dermatology Online Atlas: http://www.derma.med.uni-erlangen.de/biddb/index_e.htm

Electronic Textbook of Dermatology: http://telemedicine.org/stamfor1.htm

Genitourinary/Gynecological Disorders In Infants Through Adolescence Adolescent Pregnancy

Sandra L. Elvik
Mary A. Baroni

Urinary Tract Infection (UTI)

- Definition: A generic term referring to the presence of bacterial infection of the urinary tract including the bladder (cystitis), urethra (urethritis), or kidney (pyelonephritis)

- Etiology/Incidence

  1. Multifactorial etiology including agent virulence and host predisposing factors

     a. Agent virulence

        (1) *Escherichia coli*—pathogenic agent in 75% to 90% of all childhood UTIs

        (2) Other enteric bacteria agents—*Klebsiella, Enterobacter sp.*

        (3) *Staphylococcus saprophyticus*—common in males

        (4) Viral agents rare with exception of adenovirus

     b. Host predisposing factors

        (1) Immature kidneys associated with premature and low birth weight infants

        (2) Congenital urologic abnormalities, reflux, neurogenic bladder

        (3) Gender differences in anatomy of urinary tract predisposes females, e.g., short urethra and proximity to anus

        (4) Infrequent voiding—urinary stasis

        (5) Obstruction—constipation, pregnancy

        (6) Trauma/irritants—catheterization, bubble baths, sexual intercourse, sexual abuse, pinworms

  2. Incidence—most common pediatric urinary tract problem

     a. Newborns—1.4 to 5 per 1,000 live births

     b. Accounts for 4% to 8% of infant febrile episodes without apparent source of infection

     c. Infancy—increased incidence in males (5:1) than females in first year of life; 10 fold increased risk in uncircumcised male infants

     d. Increased incidence among females (8:1 to 10:1) after infancy and through adolescence

- Signs and Symptoms

  1. May be asymptomatic or with nonspecific symptoms especially in infancy

  2. Symptom clusters by age group (Todd, 1995)

     a. Newborns—jaundice, hypothermia, fever, vomiting, sepsis, failure to thrive

     b. Infants/preschoolers—diarrhea, vomiting, fever, failure to thrive, strong/foul-smelling urine

   c. School age/adolescents—fever, vomiting, strong/foul-smelling urine, abdominal pain, frequency, painful urination

- Differential Diagnosis

   1. Acute abdomen—appendicitis, sexually transmitted diseases, ectopic pregnancy

   2. Chemical irritation—soaps, bubble baths

   3. Vulvovaginitis

   4. Dysfunctional voiding—enuresis

   5. Sexual abuse

   6. Foreign body

   7. Pelvic inflammatory disease (PID)

- Physical Findings

   1. May be normal

   2. Infancy—weight loss, jaundice, failure to thrive

   3. Fever and irritability

   4. Blood pressure may be elevated—reflux nephropathology

   5. Abdominal examination—pain, tenderness, guarding

   6. Urethral or vaginal irritation/discharge—with vulvovaginitis due to irritation or STD

- Diagnostic Tests/Findings

   1. Urine analysis—presence of urinary leukocyte esterase, nitrate, and blood suggestive of UTI but NOT diagnostic

   2. Urine culture mandatory for accurate diagnosis—technique for specimen collection depends on age and developmental status of child, severity of condition and urgency of need for unequivocal results

      a. Random voids/bagged urine—minimal usefulness due to high potential for contamination from external genitalia

      b. Clean-catch midstream—often contaminated from external genitalia, especially in girls; more reliable from circumcised males

         (1) Appropriate for mild symptoms or follow-up

         (2) Positive with colonies $> 10^5$/mL of single organism

      c. Straight catheterization—used with infants/children who cannot void voluntarily; lower risk for nocosomial infection than indwelling catheters

         (1) Appropriate for moderate or severe symptoms

         (2) Positive with colonies $> 10^3$/mL of single or multiple organisms

      d. Suprapubic aspiration—used with infants/children unable to void voluntarily, when culture is urgently needed due to severity or equivocal results from alternative techniques

    (1)   Appropriate for moderate or severe symptoms

    (2)   Positive with colonies > 10^3/mL of single or multiple organisms

3.   Blood culture—collected in infants < 12 months with suspected sepsis

4.   Radiologic studies—for localizing infection and to rule out urinary abnormalities as part of UTI work up

    a.   Indications for imaging studies—recommendations vary but generally include:

        (1)   Symptoms of pyelonephritis regardless of age and gender

        (2)   UTI in any child < 8 years of age

        (3)   Males with first infection and females with second if above criteria are not met

    b.   Types

        (1)   Bladder and renal ultrasound—usually first step in evaluation of structural and developmental anomalies/disorders

        (2)   Voiding cystourethrogram (VCUG)—detects regurgitation (reflux) of urine into ureter; delay 4 to 6 weeks after diagnosis to exclude UTI related reflux; continue antibiotic prophylaxis until after VCUG

        (3)   Intravenous pyelogram (IVP) or nuclear renal cortical scans—detects scarring and examines renal function; usually done if VCUG is positive

- Management/Treatment

   1.   Antibiotic treatment

    a.   Parenteral antibiotics—newborns, infants, or older children with vomiting or severe symptoms

    b.   Oral antibiotic

        (1)   Generally treated for 10 day regimen

        (2)   Short-term treatment regimen (3 to 5 days) gaining greater acceptance for uncomplicated cystitis in girls

        (3)   Single dose regimen remains controversial

    c.   First-line drugs of choice

        (1)   Trimethoprim-sulfamethoxazole (TMP/SMX)—infants > 2 months of age

           (a)   TMP 6 to 10 mg/kg/day + SMX 30 to 60 mg/kg/day b.i.d.

           (b)   Recommended until sensitivities are available since most UTIs are caused by *E. coli*

        (2)   Amoxicillin—30 to 50 mg/kg/day t.i.d.

(3) Amoxicillin/clavulanate—40 mg/kg/day t.i.d.

(4) Sulfisoxazole—150 mg/kg/day q.i.d.

(5) Cephalexin—50 mg/kg/day t.i.d.

2. Follow-up urine cultures

a. Second culture at 48 to 72 hours after initiating treatment

b. Third culture one week after completion of treatment

c. Close monitoring of periodic urine cultures with recurrent infections and/or un-explained fevers

3. Prophylactic antibiotics—vesicoureteral reflux (VUR) trimethoprim-sulfamethoxa-zole, one-half daily dose usually at bedtime for 6 months to 2 years

a. Most grades I to III resolve as child grows

b. Annual VCUG to assess status of reflux

4. Education/prevention

a. Increased fluid intake

b. Frequent voiding with complete emptying of bladder

c. Good perineal hygiene with front-to-back wiping

d. Avoid bubble baths and other urethral irritants

Enuresis

- Definition: Involuntary urination after child has reached age when bladder control is usu-ally attained; may occur during daytime (diurnal) or at night, especially while sleeping (nocturnal); usually resolves by 5 to 6 years of age

1. Primary enuresis—child has never attained control

2. Secondary enuresis—recurrence of incontinence following 3 to 6 months of dryness

- Etiology/Incidence

1. Many causes suggested

a. Primary—small bladder capacity; toilet-training problems; delayed maturation of voiding inhibitory reflex; sleep problems (''deep sleeper''); lack of inhibi-tion of antidiuretic hormone (ADH); ingestion of increased amounts of fluid; inattention (too busy to void)

b. Secondary

(1) Diseases—UTI, diabetes, GU abnormalities

(2) e.g., Medications—e.g., theophylline, diuretics

(3) Family disruptions, stress

2. Primary enuresis most common form in children—75% to 80%

3. Over 12 years of age—50% have secondary enuresis

4. Familial predisposition

    a. One parent—44% increased risk

    b. Both parents—77% increased risk

- Signs and Symptoms

  1. Bed wetting or daytime "accidents"

  2. Odor of urine in clothing

  3. May have withdrawal/isolation from peers

- Differential Diagnosis

  1. UTI

  2. GU anomalies—ectopic ureter

  3. Mechanical obstruction

- Physical Findings: Genitalia

  1. Hypospadias, epispadias

  2. Labial fusion

  3. Dribbling of urine during examination

- Diagnostic Tests/Findings

  1. Urinalysis/urine culture—to rule out UTI

  2. Renal ultrasound/vesicoureterogram—with abnormal urine studies; GU anomaly on examination

- Management/Treatment

  1. Primary nocturnal

     a. Limit fluid intake after dinner

     b. Voiding before bedtime

     c. Avoid punishment/criticism

     d. Usually self-limited; spontaneous resolution of 10% per year after 5 years of age (Rosenstein & Fosarelli, 1997)

  2. Motivational therapy

     a. May be unsuccessful as exclusive treatment

     b. Verbal praise for dryness

     c. Reward system

     d. Dryness calendar

  3. Conditioning therapy—enuresis alarm

a. Triggered by urine

b. Children awakened by alarm

c. Alarm sensitizes child to sensation of full bladder

d. Restrictions

    (1) Expensive—not covered by all insurance plans

    (2) Treatment 2 to 3 months, often up to 6 months for greater success rate

    (3) May awaken other family members

    (4) Child's age, motivation, cooperation, family support important success factors

e. Bladder stretching exercises

    (1) Exercise to increase bladder capacity

    (2) Child given fluid load—child encouraged to hold urine as long as possible

f. Pharmacologic treatment

    (1) Desmopressin acetate

        (a) Synthetic analog of antidiuretic hormone vasopressin

        (b) Dose—oral tablet (0.2 mg to 0.6 mg at bedtime or nasal spray (10 μg/1 spray) in each nostril at bedtime (maximum dose of 40 μg

        (c) Rapid response—1 to 2 weeks once initiated

        (d) Increase or decrease according to response

        (e) Relapse 90% once discontinued

        (f) Side effects—headache, congestion, nasal irritation, epistaxis

    (2) Imipramine (use is becoming controversial)

        (a) Tricyclic antidepressant; unclear mechanism of action; may depress bladder contractions

        (b) Used in children over 6 years of age

        (c) Dose—0.9 to 1.5 mg/kg/day, 1 to 2 hours before bedtime;

        (d) Results seen within a few weeks

        (e) Treat 3 to 6 months, then taper

        (f) Relapse after treatment—75% to 90%

        (g) Side effects—arrhythmias, sedation, dry mouth

4. Secondary enuresis

a. Evaluation of underlying etiology—disease process, medication; modification of current treatment

b. Therapeutic intervention for individual/family stress

Cryptorchidism (Undescended Testes)

- Definition: Absence of one or both testes in scrotal sac due to failure of normal descent from abdomen during fetal development

- Etiology/Incidence

  1. Normal fetal descent of testes

     a. Hormonal mediation of normal testicular descent

        (1) Abdominal descent to inguinal ring—12 to 14 weeks gestation

        (2) Inguinal descent into scrotum—28 to 36 weeks

     b. Increased incidence among premature infants secondary to gestational development

  2. Failure of normal descent associated with hormonal imbalance, chromosomal abnormalities, structural disorders

  3. May be unilateral (usually right-sided) or bilateral

  4. Incidence

     a. Common (20% to 30%) among premature male births with birth weight < 1500 g

     b. Lower incidence (3% to 5%) among full-term male infants

     c. Incidence decreases to approximately 1% by one year due to spontaneous descent in most cases

- Signs and Symptoms

  1. May be asymptomatic

  2. Family history of undescended testes

  3. Testes may be palpable or nonpalpable

- Differential Diagnosis

  1. Rectractile testes

  2. Ectopic testes

  3. Anorchia

  4. Chromosomal disorders

- Physical Findings

  1. Palpable testes—may be retractile or ectopic

  2. Nonpalpable testes—may be abdominal or absent

3. Presence or absence of testes should always be documented

- Diagnostic Tests/Findings

  1. Unilateral—usually none

  2. Bilateral nonpalpable testes

     a. Karyotyping for chromosomal abnormalities

     b. Follicle-stimulating and luteinizing hormones may suggest anorchia

     c. Imaging studies occasionally utilized

- Management/Treatment

  1. Routine assessment at each well-child visit during first year of life; most spontaneous descents occur by 6 months

  2. Refer to urologist if undescended by one year

     a. Hormonal therapy—human chorionic gonadotropin (hCG); gonadotropin-releasing hormone (GnRH) currently used in Europe but not yet approved for use in U.S.

     b. Surgical intervention—orchiopexy

  3. Family education and support regarding potential complications

     a. Infertility—greater risk in bilateral cryptorchism

     b. Testicular malignancy—20 to 25 times increased risk

     c. Hernia

Hydrocele

- Definition: Painless scrotal swelling due to collection of peritoneal fluid within the tunica vaginalis surrounding the scrotum

  1. Noncommunicating type—tunica vaginalis is closed limiting fluid collection to scrotum; size of hydrocele is constant

  2. Communicating type—tunica vaginalis remains open allowing fluid to flow between peritoneum and hydrocele sac; often associated with hernia

- Etiology/Incidence

  1. Incomplete closure of processus vaginalis which usually isolates tunica vaginalis from peritoneum

  2. Most common cause of painless scrotal swelling; uncertain incidence

- Signs and Symptoms

  1. Swelling in scrotum—alternating or fixed

     a. Usually asymptomatic

     b. May become painful, if full or tense, secondary to coughing or straining

     c. Variable size with child's state; larger when active, decreases with rest

     d. Smaller on awakening—enlarges as day progresses

- Differential Diagnosis
    1. Cryptorchidism
    2. Retractile testes
    3. Hernia
    4. Inguinal lymphadenopathy
- Physical Findings
    1. Scrotal swelling or asymmetry—tense appearance; scrotal skin normal, nontender
    2. Fluctuance
    3. Translucent with transillumination
- Diagnostic Tests/Findings: Abdominal ultrasound to differentiate hydrocele from hernia
- Management/Treatment
    1. Noncommunicating
        a. Most resolve spontaneously without intervention
        b. Refer for evaluation:
            (1) Persists beyond one year
            (2) Significant increase in size
            (3) Causes discomfort
    2. Communicating
        a. Occasional spontaneous resolution
        b. Frequently develops into hernia requiring surgical intervention
        c. Refer for surgical evaluation if persists beyond one year

Hypospadias

- Definition: Congenital defect with urethral meatus on ventral surface of penis
- Etiology/Incidence
    1. Urethral folds along midline fail to fuse
    2. Common disorder—1 in 300 newborns; genetic predisposition
    3. Occurs more frequently in Caucasians
    4. Occurs in approximately 1:500 newborns
- Signs and Symptoms: Deflected urinary stream
- Differential Diagnosis: Ambiguous genitalia; female masculinization

- Physical Findings
  1. Location of urethral meatus
     a. Anterior—glans, corona, anterior shaft
     b. Midshaft
     c. Posterior—scrotal, penoscrotal junction, posterior shaft
  2. Inguinal hernia, undescended tests, incomplete foreskin
  3. Chordee—ventral curvature of penis due to fibrous band of tissue
- Diagnostic Tests/Findings
  1. Radiography if meatus in perineum (severe)
  2. Karyotype for chromosomal analysis
- Management/Treatment
  1. Avoid circumcision—foreskin used for repair
  2. Mild cases—primarily cosmetic surgery
  3. Increasing severity—functional, psychological and cosmetic surgery
     a. Repair early—6 to 18 months
     b. Family preparation for procedure and expected results

Phimosis and Paraphimosis

- Definition
  1. Phimosis—foreskin not fully retractable to expose glans
     a. Newborns normally have adhesions, glans to foreskin
     b. May not be fully retractable until 10 years of age or older
  2. Paraphimosis—inability to replace foreskin over glans after retraction
- Etiology/Incidence
  1. Most childhood phimosis physiologically normal
  2. Phimosis may be due to congenital narrowing/tightness
  3. Phimosis may be due to inflammation/infection under foreskin
  4. Paraphimosis may be due to forcible retraction of foreskin for "cleaning" purposes
- Signs and Symptoms
  1. May be asymptomatic
  2. Painful urination
  3. Weak urine stream
  4. Pain/tenderness with paraphimosis

5. Ballooning of foreskin when urinating; may be normal if voiding uncompromised

- Differential Diagnosis
    1. Balanitis (inflammation of glans penis)
    2. Balanoposthitis (inflammation of glans penis and prepuce)
- Physical Findings
    1. Phimosis—unretractable foreskin
    2. Paraphimosis—edema/discoloration of foreskin and glans
- Diagnostic Tests/Findings—none indicated
- Management/Treatment
    1. Maintain good hygiene
    2. Gentle stretch of foreskin during bath—advise family against forceful retraction; scarring and balanitis may occur
    3. Paraphimosis may respond to ice—reduction of swelling to reduce foreskin; may be surgical emergency
    4. Surgery—circumcision in phimosis with urinary obstruction

Meatal Stenosis

- Definition: Narrowing of distal end of urethra
- Etiology/Incidence
    1. Post-circumcision
        a. Mechanical irritation by diaper
        b. Ischemia from frenular artery damage during procedure
        c. Inflammation secondary to dermatitis
    2. Almost never seen in uncircumcised males
- Signs and Symptoms
    1. Penile pain/discomfort with urination
    2. Narrow, dorsally-diverted urine stream
- Differential Diagnosis
    1. Hypospadias
    2. Chordee
- Physical Findings
    1. Inflammation of glans
    2. Slit-like or narrowed meatus—best to observe urination; appearance alone may be misleading

- Diagnostic Tests/Findings: None
- Management/Treatment
    1. Air exposure
    2. Warm soaks/baths
    3. Frequent diaper changes
    4. Meatotomy may be necessary in some cases
    5. Prevention
        a. Care exercised at circumcision to avoid damage to frenular artery
        b. Cover glans following procedure—petrolatum gauze commonly used
        c. Observe for early sign of irritation/inflammation

Testicular Torsion

- Definition: Torsion of the spermatic cord; can result in gangrene of testes (emergency)
- Etiology/Incidence
    1. Abnormal fixation of testis to scrotum—permits testis to twist/rotate; impedes lymphatic and blood flow
    2. Occurs after trauma, physical exertion
    3. Most common between 7 to 12 years of age
- Signs and Symptoms
    1. Acute, progressive unilateral pain of scrotum
    2. Nausea, anorexia, vomiting
    3. Minimal fever, if any
    4. Lack of urinary symptoms is the norm
- Differential Diagnosis
    1. Trauma
    2. Orchitis
    3. Acute epididymitis
- Physical Findings
    1. Enlarged, highly tender testis
    2. Scrotum on involved side edematous, warm, erythematous
    3. Anxious patient, resistant to movement
    4. Lifting testis does not relieve pain (Prehn's sign)
    5. Solid mass may be visualized with transillumination

- Diagnostic Tests/Findings
  1. Complete Blood Count (CBC)—may see slight increase in white blood count
  2. Doppler ultrasound
  3. U/A—normal
- Management/Treatment: Immediate referral for surgery
  1. Emergently performed within first 6 hours—preservation of fertility great concern; prevention of atrophy and abscess
  2. Untreated torsion can lead to testicular loss

Labial Adhesions (Labial Fusion, Synechia Vulvae, Labial Agglutination)

- Defintion: Generally benign fusion of labial minora
- Etiology/Incidence
  1. Results from tissue irritation/inflammation and hypoestrogenization of labia minora
  2. Potential sources of irritation—trauma, infection, poor hygiene, sexual abuse
  3. Incidence—rarely present at birth; usually occurs after 2 months of age
     a. Estimated incidence is 10% to 20% of all girls in first year
     b. Highest incidence between 2 and 6 years of age, but may occur anytime up to menarche
- Signs and Symptoms
  1. Generally asymptomatic
  2. Parental concern regarding potential anatomic abnormality
  3. Difficulty voiding, general discomfort
  4. Enuresis—primarily diurnal
     a. Pooling of urine behind adhesion after voiding may occur depending upon degree of meatal obstruction
     b. Results in dribbling of urine throughout the day
- Differential Diagnosis
  1. Intersex anomalies
  2. Imperforate hymen
  3. Genital scarring
- Physical Findings: Thin, flat, membrane of variable length found midline extending from clitoris to posterior fourchette when labia majora are gently separated
  1. Complete fusion—entire vestibule covered; may see pinpoint opening
  2. Partial fusion—much of genital structures visible

- Diagnostic Tests: None indicated

- Management/Treatment

  1. In most cases, parental reassurance and observation for resolution without intervention

  2. Previous practice of mechanical lysis no longer recommended due to high frequency of refusion

  3. Observation for UTI symptoms

  4. Topical application of conjugated estrogen cream twice a day for 2 to 3 weeks results in separation within 8 weeks in 90% of cases

     a. Overuse may stimulate signs of precocious puberty which resolve when cream is discontinued

     b. Following separation

        (1) Maintain good hygiene

        (2) Topical applications of bland creams or petroleum jelly

  5. Inspection of vulvae on routine well-child visits to monitor baseline anatomy, hygiene, sexual development and detect problems

Vulvovaginitis

- Definition: Perineal inflammation and/or infection of the vulva (vulvitis) or vagina (vaginitis) often associated with vaginal discharge

- Etiology/Incidence

  1. Sources of vulvovaginitis may be noninfectious or infectious

  2. Noninfectious vulvovaginitis

     a. Chemical irritation—bubble bath, powder, detergents, soaps, over the counter (OTC) douches

     b. Mechanical irritation—tight clothing, nylon underwear

     c. Foreign body irritation—toilet tissue, retained tampon

     d. Trauma/sexual abuse

     e. Masturbation

  3. Infectious vulvovaginitis

     a. Nonspecific—bacterial overgrowth due to poor hygiene

     b. Specific

        (1) Bacterial—Group A beta hemolytic streptococcus, *Pneumococcus, Enterococcus, Shigella flexneri/sonnie, N. gonorrhea, Chlamydia trachomatis*

        (2) Viral—Herpes simplex virus (HSV)

(3) Parasitic—*Enterobius vermicularis* (pinworms); *Trichomonas vaginalis*

(4) Mycotic/fungal—candidiasis (common following antibiotic use)

4. Uncertain incidence; 30% to 85% are noninfectious/nonspecific inflammation with normal flora

- Signs and Symptoms

    1. Vaginal discharge

    2. Genital discomfort/itching

    3. Dysuria/burning

    4. Erythema/edema of vulva or vagina

- Differential Diagnosis

    1. Physiologic leukorrhea—thin, clear or white discharge

    2. UTI

    3. Dermatologic disorders—psoriasis, seborrheic dermatitis, atopic dermatitis

- Physical Findings

    1. May have no physical findings

    2. Discharge

        a. White to yellow—chemical, mechanical, *Chlamydia trachomatis*

        b. Pale yellow to gray green—trichomoniasis

        c. White, thick, cheesy—candidiasis (''yeast'')

        d. Thin white, frothy—bacterial vaginosis

        e. Brown, bloody, foul odor—foreign body

    3. Genital erythema

    4. Lesions

    5. Perianal soiling

    6. Examination techniques—sensitive, gentle

        a. Prepubertal female

            (1) Pelvic examination usually deferred; visual inspection only

            (2) Exploratory procedure under anesthesia may be needed for vaginal bleeding and should be referred

        b. Pubescent female

            (1) Pelvic examination—especially if sexually active

            (2) Cervix best site for culture

- Diagnostic Tests/Findings

1. Urinalysis for presence of WBC, trichomonads

2. Tape test for pinworms

3. Saline preparation for wet mount

    a. Clue cells—bacterial vaginosis

    b. Presence of WBC—may indicate bacterial vaginosis in the absence of clue cells/trichomonads

    c. Trichomonads

4. Potassium hydroxide (KOH) 10% preparation

    a. Hyphae—candidiasis

    b. "Whiff test"—positive (fishy odor of bacterial vaginosis)

- Management\Treatment (see section on sexually transmitted diseases for specific management)

    1. Foundation of treating childhood vulvovaginitis is improvement of local perineal hygiene

    2. Nonspecific vaginitis often resolves without intervention

    3. Discontinue genital irritants—bubble bath, harsh bath soap and laundry detergents

    4. Cotton or cotton-lined underwear—avoid tight fitting clothing (tights, pants, undergarments)

    5. Bacterial

        a. Penicillin 125 to 250 mg orally t.i.d., q.i.d.

        b. Erythromycin 30 to 50 mg/kg/day orally t.i.d., q.i.d.; for 10 days recommended

    6. Parasitic

        a. Mebendazole, 100 mg, orally in single dose—may repeat in 3 weeks

        b. Pyrantel pamoate 11 mg/kg/dose (maximum 1 g) in single dose—may repeat in 2 weeks

    7. Fungal

        a. Prepubertal—clotrimazole cream, 1% to external genital area

        b. Postpubertal

            (1) Terconazole 0.8% cream, 1 full applicator intravaginally at bedtime for 3 days

            (2) Miconazole 2% cream, 1 full applicator, intravaginally at bedtime for 7 days

            (3) Fluconazole 150 mg orally in single dose

    8. Foreign body

   a.   Prepubertal—attempt irrigation; warm saline via small feeding tube

   b.   Postpubertal

      (1)   Pelvic examination to locate object

      (2)   Moistened cotton-tip applicator or forceps for removal

   c.   Unsuccessful irrigation/pelvic or anxious child—refer for examination under general anesthesia

9.   Positive cultures suspicious for sexual abuse or sexual activity—see section on sexually transmitted diseases

10.   Physiologic leukorrhea

   a.   Some benefit from ''mini-pads'' in underwear to absorb moisture/prevent wetness from staining clothing

   b.   Avoid use of douches and creams

Dysmenorrhea

- Definition: Pain during menstrual cycle; usually first 1 to 2 days; cramping discomfort felt mid-to-lower abdomen

   1.   Primary dysmenorrhea—no pelvic abnormality; common in adolescents; usually develops 6 to 12 months after menarche; ovulation necessary component

   2.   Secondary dysmenorrhea—underlying pelvic pathology

      a.   Congenital anomalies (septate uterus)

      b.   Cervical stenosis or strictures

      c.   Cysts, tumors of ovary or uterus

      d.   Endometriosis

      e.   Pelvic inflammatory disease

- Etiology/Incidence (Primary Dysmenorrhea)

   1.   Increased production of uterine prostaglandins; uterine contractions, ischemia

   2.   Ovulation is required for development of primary dysmenorrhea

   3.   Most common gynecological complaint

   4.   Some degree of pain with menses in over 60% of ovulating women

      a.   Significant limitation for 10% to 15% of females

      b.   Leading cause of adolescent female school absenteeism—14%

- Signs and Symptoms

   1.   Pain usually starts with flow or several hours later or may precede flow by several hours to 2 days

2. Crampy/spasmodic pain, primarily lower abdominal area; may radiate to inner thighs, lower back

3. Systemic symptoms

    a. Nausea/vomiting/diarrhea

    b. Lightheadedness/dizziness

    c. Fatigue or general malaise

- Differential Diagnosis

  1. Reproductive system malformations

  2. Endometriosis

  3. PID

  4. Psychogenic problems

- Physical Findings: May be none; defer pelvic examination only if adolescent is not sexually active

  1. Bimanual and rectovaginal exams indicated

  2. Cervical motion tenderness with PID

- Diagnostic Tests/Findings

  1. Suspicion of PID—see section on sexually transmitted diseases

  2. Pelvic ultrasound for palpable masses or concern of GU abnormalities

- Management/Treatment

  1. Primary dysmenorrhea—mild

    a. Heat to abdomen

    b. Exercise

    c. Acetaminophen

    d. Ibuprofen—400 mg orally immediately at onset of pain, then every 4 to 6 hours for 1 to 3 days; take with food, milk, antacid to avoid GI distress

    e. Well balanced diet

    f. Acknowledgment of symptoms, pain is real

  2. Primary dysmenorrhea—moderate to severe; unresponsive to treatment for mild disorder

    a. Nonsteroidal anti-inflammatory drugs (NSAIDS)

        (1) Inhibit prostaglandin synthesis

        (2) Naproxen sodium—500 mg orally at onset, then 250 mg every 6 to 8 hours

(3) Mefenamic acid—500 mg orally at onset, then 250 mg every 6 to 8 hours

(4) Assess efficacy of NSAIDS after 3 to 4 cycles before using another medication

(5) NSAIDS contraindicated in clotting disorders, renal or peptic ulcer disease

3. Severe dysmenorrhea—unresponsive to NSAIDS alone

    a. Low-dose combination oral contraceptives (OC); effective in 90% of cases with severe pain

    b. Minimum 3 to 4 cycles for symptom improvement

    c. Continuous symptoms after 4 months

        (1) OC used in conjunction with NSAIDS

        (2) Consider gynecological referral

4. Secondary dysmenorrhea—gynecological referral

Premenstrual Syndrome

- Definition: Cluster of symptoms, both physical and behavioral, that occur in second half of menstrual cycle (last week of luteal phase); usually resolve with onset of menses

- Etiology/Incidence

    1. Numerous mechanisms postulated

        a. Vitamin B_6 deficiency

        b. Fluid retention

        c. Steroid hormone fluctuation

        d. Alteration in serotoninergic neuronal mechanisms

        e. Inappropriate prostaglandin activity

        f. Food/environmental allergies

    2. Significant complaints from 30% to 70% older adolescents

- Signs and Symptoms

    1. Onset of symptoms usually within one week of menses

        a. Breast tenderness

        b. Headache

        c. Weight gain

        d. Mood swings, lethargy, anxiety

        e. Fatigue

     f. Appetite changes

     g. Lower back pain

     h. Loss of concentration

- Differential Diagnosis

  1. Pregnancy

  2. Primary/secondary dysmenorrhea

- Physical Findings: Pelvic examination normal

- Diagnostic Tests/Findings: None indicated

- Management/Treatment

  1. Diet/nutrition

     a. Frequent small meals

     b. Increase intake—complex carbohydrates, protein, fresh fruits, vegetables, foods rich in pyridoxine (B$_6$)

     c. Vitamin/mineral supplement—Vitamin B$_6$, magnesium

     d. Limit intake—refined sugar, salt, red meat, alcohol, coffee, tea, chocolate

  2. Life style

     a. Regular exercise (especially aerobic)

     b. Stress management

     c. Avoid active and passive cigarette smoke

  3. Pharmocological management

     a. Diuretics

     b. NSAID

     c. Selective serotonin reuptake inhibitors (SSRIs), e.g., fluoxetine, sertraline, paroxetine—more useful for emotional rather than somatic symptoms; currently recommended as first line of treatment in adult females (Hofmann & Greydanus, 1997)

Genitourinary Trauma

- Definition: Injury to the genitourinary tract; refers to accidental injury (for nonaccidental trauma refer to section on sexual abuse)

- Etiology/Incidence

  1. Blunt insult generally from athletic activities, motor vehicle accidents, falls

  2. No specific incidence—commonly seen; over 50% associated with trauma to intraperitoneal organs

- Signs and Symptoms

1. Frank urethral bleeding

2. Hematuria

3. Bluish-red mass in perineal area

- Differential Diagnosis

    1. Hemorrhagic cystitis

    2. Vaginitis

    3. Sexual abuse

- Physical Findings

    1. Hematomas—urethral/scrotal/perineal

    2. Periurethral lacerations

- Diagnostic Tests/Findings: Referral necessary if extensive injury suspected

- Management/Treatment

    1. Urethral/vulvar trauma

        a. Mild bruising, superficial lacerations (symptomatic relief)—ice pack, sitz baths, analgesics

        b. Blunt or penetrating trauma—surgical intervention

    2. Testicular trauma—surgical referral

    3. Suspected renal injury—referral

    4. Penetrating injury—immediate surgical exploration

Glomerulonephritis (GN)

- Definition: Disease characterized by diffuse inflammatory changes in the glomeruli; immune-mediated response

    1. Primary acute form—poststreptococcal glomerulonephritis; most common form in children; true incidence unknown

    2. Primary chronic form

        a. Primarily seen with IgA nephropathy

        b. Other types—membranoproliferative glomerulonephritis (MPGN), mesangial proliferative glomerulonephritis

    3. Secondary forms—associated with other disorders, e.g., systemic lupus erythematosus, anaphylactoid purpura, vascular problems

- Etiology/Incidence

    1. Multifactorial etiology—not completely understood

    2. Combination of factors induce injury

a. Immune complex deposits in glomerular basement membrane

b. Coagulation factors—fibrin deposits

c. Exogenous nephrotoxins

    (1) Penicillamine, trimethadione, captopril, probenecid

    (2) Heavy metals—gold, mercury

3. Uncertain incidence

- Signs and Symptoms

  1. Acute disease

    a. Hematuria

    b. Decreased urine output

    c. Edema

    d. Dark urine—acute poststreptococcal glomerulonephritis (APSGN)

  2. Chronic disease

    a. Fatigue

    b. Failure-to-thrive

- Differential Diagnosis

  1. Benign hematuria

  2. Hereditary nephropathy

  3. Lupus erythematosus

  4. Anaphylactoid purpura

- Physical Findings

  1. May be asymptomatic or severely ill depending upon extent of renal involvement

  2. Gross hematuria

  3. Edema—facial (especially periorbital) in the morning

  4. Hypertension

  5. CVA tenderness

- Diagnostic Tests/Findings

  1. Urinalysis

    a. Casts—RBC, leukocytes and/or casts indicate glomerular inflammation

    b. Hematuria

    c. Protein—correlates with degree of hematuria

    d. pH—low

      e.   Specific gravity—increased

   2.   Titers—serum ASO, AHT, anti-Dnase B

   3.   Cultures—throat, skin; may be negative when signs of nephritis appear

   4.   Chest radiograph—assess pulmonary edema

   5.   Serum complement

      a.   Returns to normal in APSGN

      b.   Chronic elevation in MPGN

- Management/Treatment

   1.   All treatment is supportive

      a.   Hypertension/relieve edema

         (1)   Fluid restriction

         (2)   Diuretics

         (3)   Vasodilators

      b.   Antibiotic (penicillin) if throat or skin infection persists

Hydronephrosis

- Definition: Unilateral or bilateral dilation of kidney(s)
- Etiology/Incidence

   1.   Caused by anatomic block of urine flow from kidney

   2.   Obstruction in 1 per 1000 births—slight male prevalence

   3.   Ureteropelvic junction (UPJ)—most common site of blockage

- Signs and Symptoms

   1.   Nausea

   2.   Abdominal or flank pain

   3.   Decreased urine output

- Differential Diagnosis

   1.   Prune belly syndrome

   2.   UPJ obstruction

   3.   Ectopic ureterocele

   4.   Urethral/ureterovesical obstructions

- Physical Findings

   1.   Pain—abdominal/flank

   2.   Failure-to-thrive

- Diagnostic Tests/Findings
    1. May have been detected during prenatal ultrasound
    2. IVP—late emptying of renal pelvis
    3. Renal scan—impact of obstruction on total renal function
- Management/Treatment
    1. Surgery to relieve obstruction
    2. Obstruction will lead to destruction of renal parenchyma; early exploration and repair advocated
    3. Must follow-up long term to assess final renal function

Renal Tubular Acidosis (RTA)

- Definition: Defect in normal urine acidification with resulting persistent metabolic acidosis; primary RTA includes 2 types
    1. Type 1 (distal tube)—defect in distal tube secretion of hydrogen ions
    2. Type 2 (proximal tube)—defect in reabsorption of bicarbonate
- Etiology/Incidence
    1. Cellular basis of defect is unknown; distal RTA may have genetic transmission as autosomal dominant disorder
    2. Incidence of primary RTA is unknown
- Signs and Symptoms
    1. Growth failure
    2. Gastrointestinal complaints
    3. Muscle weakness
- Differential Diagnosis
    1. Diarrhea
    2. Diabetes mellitus
    3. Renal failure
    4. Lactic acidosis
- Physical Findings: Growth failure
- Diagnostic Tests/Findings
    1. Urine pH—first morning specimen; pH less than 5.5 supports diagnosis of proximal RTA; 5.8 or greater indicates distal RTA
    2. Serum electrolytes—serum bicarbonate less than 16 mEq; hyperkalemia
- Management/Treatment

1. Correction of acidosis; balance serum bicarbonate to normal level

   a. Intravenous therapy for infants with severe hyperkalemia/acidosis

   b. Oral therapy for most children

2. Alkali administration as sodium bicarbonate or sodium citrate

   a. Potassium supplement if needed

   b. Sodium bicarbonate tablets—325 mg and 650 mg

3. Mineralocorticoid deficiency corrected; diuretics reduce serum potassium

4. Carnitine supplements if needed

5. Risk of nephrocalcinosis, renal failure—continuous alkali therapy and long term clinical monitoring

6. Normal growth resumes with corrected acidosis

Sexually Transmitted Diseases

Gonorrhea

- Definition: Acute infectious process primarily involving genital tract, anorectum, throat and ophthalmic epithelium; street terms—clap, drip, strain

- Etiology/Incidence

  1. *Neisseria gonorrhoeae*—gram-negative diplococcus

  2. Reportable disease in all States; 1 million new cases/year

  3. Highest incidence among females 15 to 19 years of age

  4. Incidence among inner-city, poor adolescents as high as 14% (Hofmann & Greydanus, 1997)

  5. Associated with sexual abuse in children beyond newborn period and nonsexually active adolescents

- Signs and Symptoms

  1. Varies by site and gender; asymptomatic in 10% to 40% males and 50% to 80% females

  2. Vaginal or penile creamy discharge

  3. Perineal discomfort

  4. Menstrual irregularities

  5. Frequent, urgent, painful urination

  6. Rectal pain/itching

  7. Sore throat

  8. Fever, malaise, chills

- Differential Diagnosis

    1. *Chlamydia trachomatis* infection (may be concurrent)

    2. Genital mycoplasmas (may be concurrent)

    3. Bacterial vaginosis (may be concurrent)

    4. Trichomoniasis (may be concurrent)

    5. PID

- Physical Findings

    1. External Genitalia

        a. Erythema, edema

        b. Thick, purulent, greenish-yellow discharge (penile or vaginal)

    2. Female—pelvic examination

        a. Cervical erythema, friability, exudate

        b. Vaginal wall discharge/erythema

        c. Cervical/adnexal tenderness

    3. Male

        a. Thick, creamy penile discharge

        b. Enlarged, tender prostate

        c. Scrotal or groin pain (unilateral)

        d. Tender swelling above testis

- Diagnostic Tests/Findings

    1. Gram stain for presence of gram-negative, intracellular diplococcus

        a. Specimen sites—vagina, urethra, anus, oropharynx

        b. Oldest and least expensive method

        c. Basis of initiating treatment pending culture results

    2. Culture on selective media (Thayer-Martin) to confirm diagnosis

        a. Specimen sites—as above

        b. Most sensitive and specific test

    3. Non-culture tests (DNA probes, enzyme immunoassay); not recommended for use in pediatric patients—false positive

    4. No useful serologic test available to distinguish current from past infection

- Management/Treatment (see AAP *Red Book* for most current treatment guidelines)

    1. Uncomplicated infections

        a. Cefriaxone 125 mg IM in single dose (drug of choice)

b. Spectinomycin 50 mg/kg IM in single dose if allergic to Penicillin; maximum dose of 2 g

c. Concomitant treatment for *C. trachomatis*

(1) Erythromycin or azithromycin—if < 8 years and/or < 100 lbs

(2) Doxycycline or azithromycin if > 100 lbs and/or > 8 years of age

2. Complicated (disseminated) infections

a. Ceftriaxone 50 mg/kg/day IV or IM daily for 7 days; maximum dose of 1 g/day

b. IV administration may change to oral dose (Cefixime) for 7 days after 1 to 2 days of initial improvement

c. Concomitant treatment for *C. trachomatis* (as above)

3. Prophylaxis after sexual victimization

a. Cefixime

(1) Weight less than 100 lb 8 mg/kg (maximum 400 mg) orally in single dose

(2) Weight greater than 100 lb 400 mg orally in single dose

4. General guidelines

a. See current AAP Red Book for up-to-date treatment guidelines

b. Child protection referral for sexual abuse investigation for children beyond newborn period and nonsexually active adolescents

Chlamydia

- Definition: Most common sexually transmitted disease in U.S. with primary sites of infection being genital tract, cornea and respiratory system

- Etiology/Incidence

1. *Chlamydia trachomatis;* obligate intracellular bacteria; fifteen variants

2. Reportable disease most states

3. Incidence among sexually active females 15% to 37%; sexually active males 3%. (Hofmann & Greydanus, 1997, p. 497)

4. Congenital chlamydia—See Multisystem Disorders chapter

a. Perinatal transmission from infected mothers to infants estimated from 40% to 70%

b. Manifestation primarily as conjunctivitis or pneumonia

- Signs and Symptoms: Genital Tract Infection

1. Often asymptomatic for months to years

2. Abdominal/pelvic pain

3. Dysuria/burning

- Differential Diagnosis

  1. Gonorrhea

  2. Genital mycoplasmas

  3. Trichomoniasis

  4. Bacterial vaginosis

  5. PID

- Physical Findings: Genital Tract Infection

  1. May be normal

  2. Erythema of external genitalia

  3. Vaginal/penile discharge—yellowish, watery

  4. Tenderness on bimanual examination

- Diagnostic Tests/Findings: Judson & Ehret, 1994; Hoffmann & Greydanus, 1997

  1. Tissue culture—"gold standard" method for definitive diagnosis

     a. Culture specimen must contain epithelial cells to be accurate

     b. Only acceptable method for suspected child sexual abuse

     c. Culture processing requires 2 to 3 days; results available in 3 to 7 days depending on laboratory

  2. Alternative nonculture techniques

     a. Direct fluorescence assay (DFA)—stained direct smear of endocervical or urethra cells

        (1) Less expensive with results available within hours

        (2) Requires sufficient specimen collection

        (3) Good specificity but lower sensitivity resulting in false-positives

     b. Enzyme immunoassay (EIA)—genital secretions

        (1) Less expensive with rapid processing

        (2) Good sensitivity and specificity

     c. DNA hybridization—detects both chlamydia and gonorrhea

        (1) Results available within several days

        (2) Good sensitivity and specificity

     d. Polymerase chain reaction (PCR)—nucleic acid amplification

        (1) Good sensitivity and specificity

Genitourinary/Gynecological Disorders — 1127

(2) Not recommended for infants and young children

e. Lipase chain reaction (LCR)—for confirmation

- Management/Treatment (See AAP, *Red Book* for additional treatment guidelines)

    1. Antibiotic treatment for uncomplicated genital tract infection

        a. Adolescents—doxycycline, 100 mg b.i.d. for 7 days OR azithromycin 1 g in single dose

            (1) Doxycyline is contraindicated in pregnancy

            (2) Alternative treatment regimens—erythromycin base, 500 mg q.i.d. for 7 days

        b. Children (6 months to 12 years)—erythromycin, 50 mg/kg/day, q.i.d. for 7 days OR azithromycin 20 mg/kg in single dose

        c. Infants < 6 months—erythromycin, 50 mg/kg/day, q.i.d. for 7 days

        d. Identify, examine, test, and treat any sexual contacts

    2. Evaluate for other STDs, e.g., gonorrhea, syphilis and treat as necessary

    3. No need for retest following treatment with doxycycline, azithromycin unless symptoms persist or if possibility of reinfection

    4. Retest may be recommended at 3 or more weeks following treatment with erythromycin, sulfisoxazole or amoxicillin (AAP, 1997)

Acquired Syphilis

- Definition: A contagious systemic infectious disease characterized by three progressive clinical stages

    1. Primary stage—painless chancres

    2. Secondary stage—skin rash

    3. Tertiary stage—multisystem involvement including neurosyphilis

    4. Street terms—siff, lues, bad blood

- Etiology/Incidence

    1. Infectious agent—*Treponema pallidum,* a thin, motile spirochete

    2. Transmission—sexual contact, transplacental, direct contact with infected tissue (see Multisystem and Genetic Disorders chapter for congenital syphilis)

    3. Reportable communicable disease in all States

    4. Increased incidence during later 1980s and early 1990s

        a. Incidence has begun to decline except in large urban areas and rural south

        b. 10% to 12% of all reported cases are among adolescents between 15 and 19 years of age

- Signs and Symptoms

  1. Primary stage—one or more painless lesions usually on genitalia but may be on lips, tongue or extremities

  2. Secondary stage—fever, malaise, sore throat, skin rash, hair loss

  3. Tertiary stage—symptoms recur 15 or more years after initial infections; rarely seen among adolescents

- Differential Diagnosis

  1. Primary syphilis

     a. Genital herpes

     b. Condylomata acuminata

     c. Molluscum contagiosum

  2. Secondary syphilis

     a. Pityriasis rosea

     b. Psoriasis

     c. Drug sensitivity reactions

     d. Infectious mononucleosis

- Physical Findings

  1. Primary stage

     a. Chancre—one or more painless ulcers

     b. Most common on genitalia but seen at other sites of inoculation

  2. Secondary stage

     a. Generalized maculopapular/papulosquamous rash—classic if palms and soles included

     b. Round to oval, reddish-brown, ''copper-colored'' lesions

     c. Lymphadenopathy, arthralgia, fever, malaise

     d. Hypertrophic lesions of vulva/anus—condylomata lata

  3. Latency period follows with recurrences of secondary rash

  4. Tertiary phase

     a. 15 or more years after chancre

     b. Neurosyphilis, aortitis, gummous changes of bone, skin or viscera

- Diagnostic Tests/Findings

  1. Dark-field microscopic tests or direct fluorescent antibody tests (DFA)—presence of spirochetes from scrapings or washings of primary lesions; inexpensive, definitive diagnosis

2. Serologic tests—presumptive diagnosis

   a. Nontreponemal tests—rapid plasma reagin (RPR), venereal disease research laboratory (VDRL), automated reagin test (ART)

      (1) Measure nonspecific antigens

      (2) False-positive rate of 1% to 2%

      (3) False-negatives with recently acquired infections prior to seroconversion

      (4) Serial testing used to monitor response to treatment

   b. Treponemal tests—fluorescent treponemal antibody absorption (FTA-ABS, and microhemagglutination assay for antibody to *Treponema pallidum* (MHA-TP)

      (1) Detect specific treponemal antigens

      (2) Greater specificity than nontreponemal methods

      (3) More expensive and time-consuming

      (4) Useful to distinguish/confirm positive vs. false-positive nontreponemal results

      (5) May show false-positive results in presence of lyme disease, genital herpes, autoimmune disorders, and IV drug use

   c. High probability of infection in sexually active person with reactive nontreponemal and trepomenal tests

   d. VDRL/RPR screening in early pregnancy and at delivery for all women to prevent transplacental transmission

- Management/Treatment: See AAP *Red Book* for additional treatment guidelines

   1. Primary and secondary, latent syphilis (less than 1 year's duration)

      a. Benzathine penicillin G, 50,000 U/kg IM in single dose, not to exceed 2.4 million units (treatment of choice)

      b. Alternative regimens if allergic to penicillin

         (1) Doxycycline, 100 mg, orally, b.i.d. for 2 weeks; contraindicated in pregnancy and children < 8 years of age

         (2) Tetracycline, 500 mg, orally, q.i.d. for 2 weeks; contraindicated in pregnancy and children < 8 years of age

   2. Late latent or tertiary syphilis

      a. Benazthine penicillin G, (50,000 U/kg; not to exceed 2.4 million units), IM weekly for 3 successive weeks

      b. Alternative treatment for penicillin sensitivities

         (1) Doxycycline, 100 mg, orally b.i.d. for 4 weeks (contraindicated in pregnancy)

(2) Tetracycline, 500 mg, orally, q.i.d. for 4 weeks (contraindicated in pregnancy)

(3) Doxycycline and tetracycline not given to children < 8 years of age

3. Evaluation of patient and all recent sexual contacts for syphilis and other STDs

4. Prevention and Control

a. Patient education/discussion of sexuality, contraception and STDs as part of adolescent well-child visits

b. Counseling regarding safe sexual practices including abstinence and proper use of condoms

Genital Herpes Simplex Virus (HSV)

- Definition: Most common HSV infection among adolescents characterized by clusters of painful lesions of the genital tract, perineum, mouth, lips or pharynx

- Etiology/Incidence

1. Agent (herpes simplex viruses)—large, DNA viruses of two major types

a. Type 2 (HSV-2)—primary source of genital herpes, usually affecting skin below the waist

b. Type 1 (HSV-1)—less common source of genital herpes, usually sites include face, and skin above the waist

2. Primary transmission through sexual contact and/or direct contact with open lesions; may be transmitted by autoinoculation of HSV-1 to genital area

3. Transplacental transmission results in congenital herpes—see Multisystem and Genetic Disorders chapter

4. Genital herpes is rare in prepubertal children except in cases of child abuse

5. Estimated prevalence of 20% among sexually active adolescents

- Signs and Symptoms

1. Painful genital lesions

2. Burning with urination

3. Tender, swollen lymph nodes

4. Fever, malaise

- Differential Diagnosis

1. Chancre of early syphilis

2. Chancroid

3. Molluscum contagiosum

4. Allergic reaction

- Physical Findings
    1. Vesicular/ulcerated lesions—genital tract, perineum, mouth, lips, pharynx
    2. Genital, perianal erythema and/or edema
    3. Cervical friability, discharge
    4. Lymphadenopathy
- Diagnostic Tests/Findings
    1. Tissue culture—standard, most reliable diagnostic test
        a. Sensitivity varies by stage of disease—highest with vesicular lesions; lowest with recurrent infections and crusted lesions
        b. Results available within 1 to 3 days
    2. Newer diagnostic techniques
        a. DNA probe testing—relatively new technique with good sensitivity and specificity; results available within 1 to 3 days
        b. Direct fluorescent antibody/enzyme immunoassay—more rapid results than cultures but less sensitive results
        c. Polymerase chain reaction (PCR)—very sensitive; lower specificity resulting in false-positive results
    3. Serologic testing—may show rise in HSV antibodies; of limited value
        a. May be used to confirm initial diagnosis
        b. Often shows no rise in titers with recurrences
- Management/Treatment: See AAP *Red Book* for additional treatment guidelines
    1. Primary episode of genital infection
        a. Acyclovir, 200 mg, orally, 5 times/day for 7 to 10 days
        b. Initiation of treatment within 6 days of onset of lesions may reduce duration and severity of symptoms
    2. Recurrent episodes—alternative doses/frequency
        a. Acyclovir, 200 mg, orally, 5 times/day for 5 days
        b. Acyclovir, 400 mg, orally, 3 times/day for 5 days
        c. Acyclovir, 800 mg, orally, 2 times/day for 5 days
        d. Acyclovir less effective in treatment of recurrent vs. primary episodes
    3. Topical acyclovir no longer recommended; limited benefit
    4. Suppressive therapy—with frequent recurrences of > 6 per year
        a. Acyclovir 400 mg, orally, b.i.d. OR 200 mg, orally, 3 to 5 times/day
        b. Discontinue after one year to reassess recurrences

5. Sitz baths may provide relief

6. Education—recurrences; viral shedding; abstinence when lesions are present; use of condoms during sexual activities

Genital Warts (Condylomata Acuminata)

- Most common symptomatic viral reproductive tract infection in U.S. (Hatcher, 1998); characterized by epithelial warts/tumors of mucous membranes and skin

- Etiology/Incidence

  1. Causative agent—Human papillomavirus (HPV), a small DNA virus with more than 70 subtypes; types 6 and 11 usually cause genital warts and types 16, 18, 31, 33, 35 vaginal, anal and cervical dysplasia (Hatcher, 1998)

  2. Primary mode of transmission is sexual contact; sexual abuse must be considered when present in prepubertal child

  3. Genital HPV infection may be as high as 38% among sexually active female adolescents

- Signs and Symptoms

  1. Firm bumps in anogenital area

  2. Occasional local symptoms—burning, pain, itching, bleeding

  3. Often asymptomatic

- Differential Diagnosis

  1. Chancre of secondary syphilis

  2. Molluscum contagiosum

- Physical Findings

  1. Firm, flesh-colored anogenital lesions resembling cauliflower in configuration

  2. Range in size from few millimeters to centimeters

  3. Males—warts on shaft of penis, meatus, scrotum and perianal areas

  4. Females—warts usually seen on labia and perianal areas

- Diagnostic Tests/Findings

  1. Diagnosis usually based on clinical inspection; no culture is available

  2. Colposcopy to detect cervical lesions—application of 3% to 5% acetic acid (vinegar) causes lesion to blanch; not definitive

  3. Pelvic examination—pap smear for cytological analysis may be diagnostic

  4. Biopsy of lesion for histologic examination—may be diagnostic

  5. DNA probe—may detect asymptomatic HPV infection

- Management/Treatment

1. No definitive treatment yet available to eradicate HPV virus; palliative treatment focusing on removal of lesions, symptom relief, and close follow-up for recurrences and sequelae

2. Spontaneous resolution within 3 months in 25% cases; recurrences are common

3. External visible lesions

   a. Self-treatment with podophyllum resin solution or gel (contraindicated in pregnancy)

      (1) Topical application b.i.d. for 3 days; need not be washed off

      (2) First application should be done in office to assure proper technique

      (3) Treatment may be repeated up to 4 cycles with 4 day rest period between cycles

   b. Podophyllin, 10% to 25% in compound tincture of benzoin (contraindicated in pregnancy)

      (1) Weekly treatment up to total of 6 applications

      (2) Must be washed off in 1 to 4 hours

   c. Trichloracetic acid (TCA 80% to 90%)

      (1) Topical application followed by careful drying and application of talc or baking soda

      (2) Weekly treatments up to total of 6 applications

      (3) Causes more local discomfort than podophyllin

   d. Liquid nitrogen or cryotherapy

   e. Laser surgery, cryosurgery, excision, electrodessication—reserved for extensive, severe, and/or resistent cases

4. Gynecologic referral necessary for cervical warts

5. Monitoring of Pap smears for increased risk of cervical cancer

   a. Every 3 months during active disease; then every 3 to 6 months for 2 years

   b. Annual Pap smears for all HPV positive asymptomatic females thereafter

6. Screening serology for syphilis; evaluate for any other concommitent STDs and treat accordingly

7. Education regarding safe sexual practices

Trichomoniasis

- Definition: Common sexually transmitted infection of the genital tract

- Etiology/Incidence

   1. Causative agent—*Trichomonas vaginalis,* a flagellated protozoan

2. Transmitted primarily through sexual contact; presence in prepubertal child should alert practitioner to possible sexual abuse

3. Often associated with other STDs, e.g., gonorrhea, chlamydia

4. Unknown incidence

- Signs and Symptoms

    1. Females—asymptomatic in 25% to 50% of all cases

        a. Vaginal discharge

        b. Vulvovaginal irritation and itching

        c. Vaginal odor

        d. Difficult urination

    2. Males—usually asymptomatic

        a. Mild dysuria

        b. Itching

- Differential Diagnosis

    1. Candidiasis

    2. Chemical vaginitis

    3. Bacterial vaginosis

    4. UTI

    5. Poor hygiene

    6. Gonorrhea

- Physical Findings

    1. Vaginal discharge—frothy, light yellow to grey-green, musty odor

    2. Pelvic examination—evidence of vaginitis, cervicitis; erythema, edema and pruritus of external genitalia may be present

    3. Males generally asymptomatic

- Diagnostic Tests/Findings

    1. Wet mount of vaginal secretions or spun urine sediment—presence of motile trichomonads

    2. Motile trichomonads may also be seen on Pap smears and urine analysis

    3. Other tests—culture (trypticase yeast extract iron serum (TYI) medium); antibody tests using enzyme immunoassay; direct/indirect immunofluorescence techniques are available

        a. More sensitive techniques than wet mount

        b. Rarely needed to make diagnosis

- Management/Treatment: See AAP, *Red Book*, for additional treatment guidelines

    1. Metronidazole—treatment of choice

        a. Prepubertal—15 mg/kg/day orally t.i.d. for 7 days (maximum 2 g for 7 days) or 40 mg/kg (maximum 2 g) orally in single dose

        b. Adolescent—2 g orally in single dose

        c. Avoid alcohol during treatment

        d. Contraindicated in first trimester of pregnancy

    2. No sexual activity during treatment

    3. Partners should receive concurrent therapy

    4. Evaluate for presence of other STD—treat accordingly

Bacterial Vaginosis (BV)

- Definition: Clinical syndrome characterized by vaginal symptoms, primarily in sexually active adolescents/adults

- Etiology/Incidence

    1. Not an actual infection but classified as a sexually transmitted disease

    2. Results from replacement of normal vaginal flora (*Lactobacillus*) with high concentrations of anaerobes—*Gardnerella vaginalis, Mycoplasma hominis*

    3. Transmission may be sexual or nonsexual

    4. Incidence unknown

- Signs and Symptoms

    1. Profuse vaginal discharge with "fishy" odor

    2. May be asymptomatic

- Differential Diagnosis

    1. Foreign body

    2. Gonorrhea/chlamydia/trichomoniasis

    3. Vulvovaginitis—group A streptococci, shigella organisms

    4. Candidiasis

    5. Physiologic leukorrhea

- Physical Findings

    1. Vaginal/cervical discharge—thin, white, malodorous; adherent to vaginal wall

    2. Itching, swelling, redness of external genitalia

- Diagnostic Tests/Findings

    1. Vaginal secretions

a. pH greater than 4.5

b. KOH 10% mixed with vaginal discharge—releases amine, "fishy odor" (whiff test)

c. Saline wet mount—clue cells

2. Culture available—rarely helpful, expensive

- Management/Treatment (See AAP, *Red Book* for additional treatment guidelines)

    1. Metronidazole

        a. 500 mg, orally, b.i.d. for 7 days OR

        b. 2 g orally, single dose with 2nd dose in 48 hours

    2. Alternative Treatment

        a. Clindamycin cream 2%, one full applicator (5 g) intravaginally at bedtime for 7 days

        b. Metronidazole gel 0.75%, one full applicator (5 g), intravaginally b.i.d. for 5 days

        c. Clindamycin, 300 mg, orally, b.i.d. for 7 days

    3. Clindamycin recommended for pregnant women due to possible teratogenicity of metronidazole

    4. Education regarding possible complications

        a. Increased risk for PID

        b. Pregnancy risk for chorioamnionitis and premature delivery

Contraception

- Abstinence—most effective method

    1. Half of all adolescents select this option

    2. Should be discussed as viable option regardless of prior history

- Male Condoms—most effective barrier method

    1. Mechanism—mechanical barrier preventing semen from entering vagina; some brands provide additional protection with spermicide coating

    2. Types of male condoms—over 100 brands currently on the market

        a. Latex—recommended

        b. Polyurethane (latex-free) if latex sensitive

        c. Natural skin (lambskin)—not recommended (inadequate STD and HIV protection)

    3. Failure rates

        a. Theoretical—3%

       b.   Actual—12% primarily due to nonuse/misuse

       c.   Combined with spermicide—0.1%; comparable to oral contraceptive

   4.   Risks/precautions

       a.   Breakage rate— ~1% to 2%

       b.   Only water-based lubricants should be used—latex breaks down in contact with petroleum-based products

       c.   Latex breakdown over time and/or when exposed to heat

- Vaginal Spermicides—topical creams, jellies, foams, suppositories, and films to prevent pregnancy; used alone or in combination with condoms

   1.   Active spermicidal agent—nonoxynol-9 or octoxynol-9

   2.   Failure rates— ~6%

   3.   Risks/precautions

       a.   Few side effects—occasional reports of local burning/irritation

       b.   Timing of insertion varies by form used

       c.   Must be used with repeated intercourse

- Diaphragm—female barrier contraceptive methods

   1.   Thin latex dome with flexible ring for vaginal insertion prior to intercourse; positioned with posterior rim on posterior fornix and anterior rim behind pubic bone

   2.   Requires pelvic examination for proper fitting for appropriate size

   3.   Failure rate among adolescents—10% to 25%

   4.   Risks/precautions

       a.   Requires technical skill/comfort with body for correct placement

       b.   Must be kept in place for 6 hours post-intercourse

       c.   Spermicidal agent must be used for subsequent intercourse

       d.   Side-effects—UTI, vaginitis

- Oral Contraceptives (OC)

   1.   Mechanisms

       a.   Prevents ovulation

       b.   Increases viscosity of cervical mucus inhibiting sperm penetration

       c.   Alters endometrium to resist implantation

   2.   Estrogen-progestin combinations

       a.   Estrogens—ethinyl estradiol and mestranol

          (1)   Ethinyl estradiol—1.2 to 1.4 times stronger than mestranol

(2) Ethinyl estradiol effective at doses as low as 20 μg

(3) Usually select lowest effective estrogen dose (20 to 35 μg)

b. Basic progestins—norethindrone, norethindrone acetate, norethynodrel, ethynodiol diacetate, norgestrel

c. Newer progestins—norgestimate, desogestrel, gestodene

d. Monophasic, biphasic, or triphasic combinations—deliver constant or progressively increasing progestin during cycle

3. Failure rates—0.5% (theoretical) to 2% to 3% (actual)

4. Risks/precautions

    a. OC-drug—interactions

        (1) Drugs that may reduce OC effectiveness—antibiotics, antifungals, anticonvulsants, antacids

        (2) Drugs that enhance OC effectiveness—ascorbic acid, co-trimoxazole

    b. Major side-effects—thrombosis

    c. Minor side-effect—vaginal spotting, nausea, bloating, irritability

    d. OCs do not protect against AIDS and other STDs

    e. Absolute contraindications for OC use

        (1) History of clotting disorder

        (2) Impaired liver function

        (3) Abnormal vaginal bleeding (undiagnosed)

        (4) Pregnancy

        (5) Estrogen-dependent carcinoma

    f. Relative contraindications for OC use

        (1) Severe hypertension

        (2) Migraines

        (3) Chronic diseases, e.g., diabetes, heart disease, sickle cell etc.

        (4) Rheumatologic disorders

- Long-Acting Progestins (Injectable and Implantable to Inhibit Ovulation)

1. Depo-medroxyprogesterone acetate (injectable)

    a. Dosage and administration—150 mg/mL intramuscular injection every 3 months during first 5 days of normal period to assure non-pregnant status

    b. Failure rate—0.25%

    c. Precautions/risks

    (1) If > 3 months between injections, pregnancy test as precaution

    (2) Should not be given to postpartum, lactating adolescent mothers

    (3) Spotting, weight gain, bloating, headaches, mood changes

    (4) Risk of decreased bone density

  2. Norplant (subdermal implants)

    a. Six match-stick size tubes filled with levonorgestrel implanted in subcutaneous tissue of upper inner arm

    b. Effective for up to 5 years

    c. Failure rates—0.04% (1st year) to 1.1% (5th year)

    d. Precautions/risks

      (1) Appropriate screening, education and follow-up associated with continued effective use

      (2) Side effects similar to injectable—spotting, weight gain, headaches, and moodiness

- Postcoital or "Morning After" Contraception: Use of oral contraceptive within 72 hours of unprotected intercourse (50 µg ethinyl estradiol and 0.5 mg norgestrel)

  1. 2 tablets initially followed by additional 2 tablets 12 hours later

  2. Simplest, most common method used in U.S.

  3. Side-effects of nausea and vomiting common

  4. Failure rate—1.6%

- Contraceptive Methods Less Suitable for Adolescents

  1. Coitus interruptus—failure rate > 19%

  2. Natural family planning—high failure rate even among motivated adults

  3. Cervical cap—difficulties with proper placement; risk of cervical dysplasia

  4. Intrauterine device (IUD)—risk of PID

  5. Progestin-only mini-pill—failure rates up to 13% among mature adults

  6. Female condom—failure rates of 12% to 20% among adult users

Issues of Pregnancy and Birth for the Adolescent

- Pregnancy: Diagnosis and counseling

  1. Risk factors

    a. Early onset of sexual activity; inadequate concept of fertility and contraception

    b. Low socioeconomic level

    c. Poor academic achievement

d. Low self-image; few options for future

e. Early pregnancy in mother or sister

f. Substance abuse

g. Physical/sexual abuse

2. Incidence

a. U.S. has the highest rates of adolescent pregnancy and births among industrialized nations; estimates of one million each year

b. More than 4 out of 10 U.S. teens have at least one pregnancy before 20 years of age

c. Rates have shown a slow decline from 1991 to 1996; overall decline of 12% among 15 to 19 year olds with largest decline among African-American teens

d. Birth rate among 15 to 19-year-old females—54.7:1000 (1996)

e. Recidivism common—17% to 40% pregnant again within 1 year, 28% to 50% within 2 years

f. Only $\frac{1}{3}$ of adolescent mothers complete high school

3. Signs and Symptoms

a. First trimester

(1) Irregular menses/amenorrhea

(2) GI—nausea, vomiting

(3) Urinary frequency

(4) Breast tenderness/tingling

(5) Other—headache, vertigo, abdominal cramps

b. Second trimester

(1) Increased/darkening skin pigmentation

(2) Fetal movement—"quickening" 16 to 20 weeks

(3) Contractions—Braxton-Hicks 16 to 27 weeks

c. Third trimester—increased contractions

4. Physical Findings

a. First trimester

(1) Breast—fullness/tenderness, nipple tingling/discharge/darkening areola

(2) Abdomen—fullness/pelvic mass; uterine fundus at symphysis pubis at 12 weeks

(3) Pelvic examination

(a) Softening of uterine isthmus (Hegar sign) 6 to 8 weeks

          (b)   Bluish hue to cervix/vaginal epithelium (Chadwick sign) 6 to 8 weeks

          (c)   Cervical softening (Goodell sign) 6 to 8 weeks

          (d)   Increased leukorrhea

      (4)   Weight gain—2 pounds (1 kg)

      (5)   Fetal heart tones (FHT)—doppler 10 to 12 weeks

  b.   Second trimester

      (1)   Stretch marks ''striae'' on abdomen and breasts

      (2)   Fundus midway between symphysis pubis and umbilicus by 14 to 15 weeks, at umbilicus 20 to 22 weeks

      (3)   Fetal outline 20 weeks

      (4)   Fetal heart tones (FHT) by fetoscope at 20 weeks

      (5)   Weight gain—11 pounds (5 kg)

  c.   Third trimester

      (1)   Colostrum from breasts 28 to 40 weeks

      (2)   Fundus between umbilicus and xiphoid 28 weeks; at xiphoid 38 weeks

      (3)   Weight gain—11 pounds (5 kg)

      (4)   Bloody show—impending labor

      (5)   Ruptured membranes

  d.   Labor

      (1)   Stage 1—effacement and dilatation of cervix

      (2)   Stage 2—delivery of fetus

      (3)   Stage 3—separation and delivery of placenta

5. Differential Diagnosis

  a.   Ectopic pregnancy

  b.   Incomplete spontaneous abortion

  c.   Molar pregnancy

  d.   PID

  e.   Corpus luteum cyst (Emans, 1998)

  f.   UTI

6. Diagnostic Tests/Findings

  a.   Urine for human chorionic gonadotropin (hCG)—positive 7 to 10 days after conception

    b.   Radioimmunoassay (RIA)—serology; more specific than urine, expensive; positive 7 to 10 days after conception

    c.   Cervical cultures—gonorrhea/chlamydia screen

    d.   Wet mount—saline, KOH

    e.   Papanicolaou smears

    f.   Serology—syphilis, hepatitis B surface antigen, blood type/Rh factor, CBC with indices, rubella, human immunodeficiency virus

    g.   Urinalysis/culture (if indicated)

    h.   Pelvic ultrasound

7.   Counseling/Education

    a.   Impact on future plans, finances, family structure

    b.   Identity and age of father—anticipated involvement

    c.   Options

        (1)   Continue pregnancy and maintain custody

        (2)   Place child for adoption

        (3)   Termination of pregnancy

    d.   Prenatal care—examinations, adequate diet, vitamins (include folic acid) and iron

    e.   Avoidance of medications/drugs/alcohol

- Prenatal Diagnosis: Identify potential inherited/acquired defects

1.   Variety of causes—genetic factors (25%); environmental (15%); combination of both genetic and environmental (30%); unaccountable (30%)

2.   Incidence—3% to 5% infants in U.S.

3.   Risk factors—maternal

    a.   Disease—diabetes, thyroid, immune deficiency or compromise

    b.   Age—young, especially less than 16 years; over 35 years

    c.   Previous child with Down syndrome, anencephaly, meningomyelocele

4.   Screening tools

    a.   Family pedigree—graphic record, family medical history

    b.   Alpha-fetoprotein

        (1)   Screens for neural tube defects; Meckel syndrome

        (2)   Serum levels less accurate than amniotic fluid analysis but can be done earlier in pregnancy for initial screen

    c.   Amniocentesis—collection of amniotic fluid, 15 to 16 weeks gestation; karyo-type/chromosomal analysis; inborn errors of metabolism; confirmatory test with abnormal serum alpha-fetoprotein

    d.   Chorionic villus sampling—tissue (villus) sample from fetal placenta at 9 to 11 weeks gestation; chromosomal abnormality; usually reserved for women over 35 years

    e.   Metabolic disease, hemaglobinopathies from DNA analysis

- Genetic counseling: Communication process regarding risk/problems surrounding certain disorders

    1.   Often initiated following birth of affected child

    2.   Both parents included—family history, medical/psychological consequences for child/family; possibility of future children affected; options

    3.   Utilizes results from prenatal diagnostic tools/tests

- Pregnancy termination

    1.   Spontaneous termination—miscarriage

        a.   Miscarriage/spontaneous abortion of pregnancy prior to fetal viability

        b.   May be complete or incomplete

        c.   Occurs in 14% of all pregnancies including adolescents

        d.   Often associated with genetic abnormality in fetus

    2.   Elective termination—induced abortion

        a.   Induced or elective abortion—35% of adolescent pregnancies

        b.   Procedural options—dependent on trimester of termination

        c.   First trimester abortion options—rule out STD prior to procedure

            (1)   Manual syringe evacuation/early suction curettage—4 to 6 weeks of pregnancy

                (a)   Cannula positioned into uterus with aspiration or suction of conceptus (menstrual extraction)

                (b)   Low risk of genital injury or complications

            (2)   Suction curettage/vacuum aspiration—up to 12 to 14 weeks of pregnancy

                (a)   Cervical dilation 6+ hours prior to procedure using *Laminaria* (hydrophilic seaweed sticks)

                (b)   Cannula position into uterus with suction followed by curettage

                (c)   Considered safest first trimester method

      (3)   Mifepristone—abortifacient which induces abortion when administered in early pregnancy (49 days or less)

          (a)   Acts as antiprogesterone

          (b)   Initial dose of 600 mg followed with 400 μg of misoprostol (a prostaglandin) two days later

   d.   Second trimester

      (1)   Dilatation and evacuation curettage (D&E)—20 to 24 weeks of pregnancy

          (a)   Cervical dilation prior to procedure with osmotic dilators

          (b)   Conceptus removed via curettage, aspiration, or ring forceps under general anethesia; risk of cervical trauma

          (c)   Antibiotics recommended post-procedure

      (2)   Prostaglandin suppository technique—16 to 24 weeks of pregnancy

          (a)   Cervical dilation with osmotic dilators followed by vaginal suppositories of prostaglandin E; has largely replaced more controversial intraamniotic instillation techniques

          (b)   20 mg prostaglandin suppositories used every 3 to 4 hours induces labor and subsequent abortion within 4 to 60 hours

          (c)   Complications include significant flu-like symptoms and possible delivery of live fetus

   e.   Referral and follow-up

      (1)   Referral to obstetrician-gynecologist or family-planning clinic once decision to terminate pregnancy is made

      (2)   Continue supportive care and counseling options on follow-up

- Birthing methods: Greater risk of cesarean delivery due to immature pelvic skeletal development; cephalopelvic disproportion

- Prematurity/Low Birth Weight

   1.   Maternal risk factors—maternal age less than 16; poor prenatal care/poor nutrition

   2.   Prevention aimed at prenatal management

      a.   Good nutrition; avoid dieting—daily calories 2500 to 2700 Kcal/day

      b.   Supplements—vitamins (include folic acid), iron (anemia possible), calcium

   3.   Early/consistent prenatal care

      a.   Avoid all medications unless specifically approved by health care provider

      b.   Potential for multisystem complications—infant

(1) Respiratory—respiratory distress syndrome, bronchopulmonary dysplasia, apnea

(2) Cardiovascular—patent ductus arteriosus, bradycardia, malformations

(3) Hematologic—hyperbilirubinemia, subcutaneous hemorrhage

(4) Gastrointestinal—poor motility

(5) Metabolic/endocrine—hypocalcemia, hypoglycemia or hyperglycemia, hypothermia

(6) Central nervous system—intraventricular hemorrhage, hypotonia

(7) Renal abnormalities

(8) Infections

- Home monitoring/follow-up care

  1. Frequent contact with mother/infant—early discharge follow-up recommended within 48 hours

     a. Infant feeding patterns

     b. Adaptation of mother to sleep changes

     c. Social support—father of baby, mother's family

  2. Follow-up (well-child visits)

     a. Adolescent problems—repeated pregnancy; STD

     b. Optimal health of mother/infant

     c. Future plans—completion of high school, college/technical training, career

- Maternal substance abuse

  1. Use of substances among adolescents high—more likely to stop during and after pregnancy

  2. Drug/alcohol use

     a. Counsel at initial prenatal visit

     b. Reinforce impact of all substances on developing fetus—tobacco, alcohol, marijuana, inhalants

- Screening for potentially abusive parents

  1. Increased risk of battering by partner when pregnant

     a. Assess relationship between girl and partner

     b. Some states require mandatory reporting of victims of domestic violence

  2. Many risk factors for child abuse

     a. Parental factors

        (1) Young and/or immature parents

        (2)   Minimal education

        (3)   Financial stress

        (4)   Lack of social support

        (5)   Unplanned or unwanted pregnancy

        (6)   Unrealistic expectations of parenting

   b. Infant factors

        (1)   Prematurity

        (2)   Perception as ''different/bad''; difficult temperament

        (3)   Congenital defect/malformation

- Perinatal complications of neonate

   1. Low birth weight and prematurity—see earlier section

   2. Infant mortality—almost 6% die in first year

   3. Cognitive/social development—possible low self-esteem, less responsive/expressive, decreased ability to trust others

   4. Sudden Infant Death Syndrome (SIDS)

Questions
Select the best answer

1. Urinary tract infections (UTI) are the most common pediatric urinary tract problems seen in primary care. Which of the following statements is not true regarding UTIs?

   a. Symptoms are often nonspecific especially in infancy
   b. Urine culture is required for definitive diagnosis
   c. Trimethoprim-sulfamethoxazole is drug of choice for most children
   d. Radiologic studies are rarely indicated with first infection

2. A 3-year-old girl presents with symptoms of painful urination, frequency, and occasional incontinence over the past week. When seen in your office, she has a temperature of 101.6° F. Which of the following would be your approach in establishing a definitive diagnosis?

   a. Clean-catch midstream collection of specimen for urine analysis
   b. Clean-catch midstream collection of specimen for urine culture
   c. Straight catheterization collection of specimen for urine culture
   d. Voiding cystourethrogram (VCUG)

3. The most likely organism to cause a UTI in the pediatric population is:

   a. *Staphylococcus saprophyticus*
   b. Klebsiella
   c. Chlamydia
   d. *E. coli*

4. One of the most commonly suggested reasons for primary enuresis is:

   a. Certain medications, such as theophylline
   b. Genitourinary abnormalities
   c. Family disruptions and stress
   d. Delayed maturation of voiding inhibitory reflex

5. Suzanne, a 7-year-old, comes to you for a physical examination prior to participation in soccer. Suzanne's mother is concerned that the child "still has accidents at night." You determine that Suzanne has primary nocturnal enuresis and your first recommendation to her mother is to:

   a. Avoid use of criticism or punishment
   b. Use a sticker/star chart
   c. Treat with medication
   d. Purchase an enuresis alarm

6. The incidence of cryptorchidism at one year of age is about 1%. The best explanation for this is:

   a. Examination of the scrotum begins at this age
   b. A child can usually stand, making palpation of the testes easier
   c. Spontaneous resolution often occurs in first year
   d. Surgical repair can now be done in neonatal period

7. Communicating hydrocele is best differentiated from the noncommunicating type by the fact that:

    a. There is no association with hernia
    b. It usually resolves on its own
    c. The fluid is static in the scrotum
    d. Frequently develops into hernia

8. In counseling parents when their child is diagnosed with mild hypospadias, suggest that the following may be part of the management:

    a. Circumcision
    b. Radiography
    c. Chromosomal analysis
    d. Surgical correction at 2 years of age

9. On physical examination of a 2-year-old uncircumcised male, you note that the foreskin is retracted and discolored. There is swelling of the glans. The most likely diagnosis is:

    a. Phimosis
    b. Balanitis
    c. UTI
    d. Paraphimosis

10. Meatal stenosis, narrowing of the distal urethra, is seen following:

    a. Orchiopexy
    b. Circumcision
    c. Epididymitis
    d. Hypospadias repair

11. During a track meet, a 14-year-old male pole vaulter falls to the ground screaming in pain. He complains of intense, searing pain in his right scrotum. He vomits twice while waiting for the ambulance. He most likely has:

    a. Orchitis
    b. Hydrocele
    c. Acute epididymitis
    d. Testicular torsion

12. Treatment for this disorder is primarily:

    a. Scrotal elevation
    b. Ice
    c. Immediate surgical referral
    d. Bedrest

13. Labial adhesions are a relatively common finding among infants and young girls. Which of the following statements about this condition is true?

    a. Adhesions are usually present at birth but may be missed on examination

    b. Highest incidence is from birth to 3 years

    c. Simple lysis of adhesions is often recommended

    d. Most cases resolve without intervention

14. Which of the following statements is true regarding the use of topical application of conjugated estrogen cream with labial adhesions?

    a. It is highly successful in resolving most adhesions within 2 months

    b. It is no longer recommended because it may stimulate precocious puberty

    c. Topical applications of bland creams or petroleum jelly are equally effective

    d. Mechanical lysis is preferred treatment today

15. Sheryl, a 12-year-old, complains of a vaginal discharge for the past 8 to 9 months. She tells you her underpants are frequently wet. When she wipes after urinating, there is "white stuff" on the tissue. Sheryl denies urinary problems, genital itching or odor. She also denies sexual activity. Her menses have not yet started, but she reports she "started to develop" in her breasts at about age 10. Her vaginal discharge is most likely a result of:

    a. A fungal infection

    b. Poor hygiene

    c. Retained foreign body

    d. Physiologic leukorrhea

16. Your recommendations to Sheryl regarding management of the discharge includes which one of these?

    a. Vinegar and water douche

    b. Placing a sanitary "mini pad" in her underpants

    c. A 10 day course of penicillin or erythromycin

    d. Use of a monilial cream for 1 week

17. Which of the following is not true of dysmenorrhea?

    a. Onset is usually within the first two to three months following menarche

    b. A leading cause of school absenteeism in adolescent females

    c. Systemic symptoms include vomiting and dizziness

    d. Pain is from start of menses to about 24 to 48 hours later

18. Amy, a 16-year-old, has symptoms of premenstrual syndrome. She refuses to take NSAIDS, preferring instead more "natural" treatments. Her options include:

    a. Eating foods rich in sodium and fat

    b. Including more foods or supplements with Vitamin C

    c. Limited fluid intake, to avoid "bloating"

    d. Adequate rest, a healthy diet, and exercise

19. In cases of accidental genitourinary trauma, which of the following is not commonly seen:

    a. Extensive tears of the vaginal wall

b. Hematuria

c. Hematoma of the urethra, scrotum, lower abdomen

d. Periurethral lacerations

20. The most common form of glomerulonephritis in children is:

a. Mesangial proliferative

b. Poststreptococcal

c. Membranoproliferative

d. Mesangiostreptococcal

21. Which of the following signs/symptoms is not associated with acute forms of glomerulone-phritis:

a. Edema

b. Hematuria

c. Increased urine output

d. Dark urine

22. One of your male patients presents with weight loss, abdominal pain, and decreased urine output. On examination, you palpate a right-sided mass, noting tenderness in the abdomen and flank. Urinalysis reveals significant leukocytosis. An intravenous pyelogram is ordered, which shows marked delay of emptying from the renal pelvis. The most likely diagnosis is:

a. Glomerulonephritis

b. Pyelonephritis

c. Hydronephrosis

d. UTI

23. Which of the following is true of renal tubular acidosis—type 1?

a. Genetically transmitted as autosomal recessive disorder

b. Distal tube defect affecting secretion of hydrogen ions

c. Distal tube defect affecting bicarbonate reabsorption

d. Most children remain short in stature in spite of early treatment

24. Vulvovaginitis may be caused by all of the following except:

a. Poor hygiene

b. Herpes simplex virus

c. Pinworms

d. Condylomata acuminata

25. Meatal stenosis can be identified by all of these with the exception of:

a. Crying with urination

b. Inflammation of glans penis

c. Slit-like meatus

d. Wide urinary stream

26. Trina, age 14, comes in with complaints of headache and nausea. She admits to having a boy-friend, whom she has sex with "once in a while," and sometimes he uses a condom. She had a period last month, but it lasted 2 days instead of the usual seven. Which of the following are not usually perceived as risk factors for adolescent pregnancy?

    a. Early onset of sexual activity
    b. Familiarity with fertility knowledge
    c. Sporadic, if any, contraceptive use
    d. Low self-image

27. Trina's urine pregnancy test is positive and confirmed by serology. Which of the following physical findings is not consistent with a gestation of less than 12 weeks?

    a. Hegar sign
    b. Goodell sign
    c. Doppler auscultation of fetal heart sounds
    d. 4 to 6 pound weight gain

28. Congenital defects are present in approximately 3 to 5% of infants born in this country. Which of the following factors is the lowest contributor to defects?

    a. Genetic
    b. Unknown
    c. Environmental
    d. Combination of environmental and genetic

29. Which of the following is the earliest screening test that you would use in managing Trina's care during her first trimester of pregnancy?

    a. Amniocentesis
    b. Chorionic villus sampling
    c. Serum alpha-fetoprotein
    d. Fetal ultrasound

30. Trina expresses to you that she may want to terminate the pregnancy. She has heard that abortion is a simple procedure, without complications. Your discussion with her is based on the fact that:

    a. Adolescents only choose to terminate pregnancy 10% of the time
    b. Menstrual extraction could be done at this point
    c. The risk is high for hemorrhage and fever
    d. Cervical injury overall from induced abortion is rare

31. You know that if Trina delivers her baby, close follow-up of both is important. What is not a focus of care in the first few weeks after delivery?

    a. Social support for the family
    b. Mother's goals for education
    c. Infant's continued weight gain
    d. Adaptation of mother to sleep changes

32. While child abuse occurs across age barriers, the adolescent parent may be at greater risk for abusing their child because:

    a. The pregnancy may be unplanned or unwanted
    b. Adolescents continue substance abuse after the baby is born
    c. The infant mortality rate is low
    d. Education becomes more important than parenting

33. A thick, purulent vaginal discharge that is greenish-yellow is most likely an infection caused by:

    a. *Chlamydia trachomatis*
    b. Herpes simplex virus
    c. *Neisseria gonorrhea*
    d. Human papillomavirus

34. The primary treatment for this infection would be:

    a. Amoxicillin
    b. Ceftriaxone
    c. Ofloxacin
    d. Penicillin

35. The most common sexually transmitted disease in the United States is:

    a. Gonorrhea
    b. Human immunodeficiency virus (HIV)
    c. Chlamydia
    d. Herpes

36. Which of the following tests provide the most definitive diagnosis for suspected syphilis?

    a. VDRL
    b. ART
    c. Dark-field microscopy
    d. FTA-AB$_s$

37. Which of the following is not true regarding the use of acyclovir in the treatment of herpes simplex virus?

    a. Topical treatment not recommended
    b. Treatment is equally effective for active primary and recurrent lesions
    c. The focus of treatment is decrease in intensity symptom duration, and viral shedding
    d. Therapy is best initiated within 6 days of onset of lesions

38. Your 15-year-old female patient presents with genital lesions. Your work-up is based on the knowledge that:

    a. Human papillomavirus (HPV) is often associated with malignancy
    b. HPV manifests itself as molluscum contagiosum

   c. Most HPV infections cause genital itching and pain

   d. Syphilis serology should be included to distinguish HPV from condylomata lata

39. After your examination, you determine that your patient has condylomata acuminata. Which of the following is not commonly used to treat these lesions?

   a. Topical podophyllum resin
   b. Laser treatment for unresponsive lesions
   c. Topical acyclovir
   d. Treatment is often not needed; many lesions regress spontaneously

40. During your evaluation of Lisa, a 16-year-old female patient, she relates recent, first-time sexual intercourse with her boyfriend. Now she complains of a "frothy" substance in her underwear that "smells weird." She also has slight itching in her vaginal area. You suspect:

   a. Trichomoniasis
   b. Gonorrhea
   c. Chlamydia
   d. Herpes

41. What education needs to be included in prescribing metronidazole to treat trichomoniasis?

   a. It is safe for use during pregnancy
   b. Sexual contact may resume after 48 hours of treatment
   c. Sexual contacts do not require therapy
   d. Alcohol should not be used during treatment

42. A patient with a thin, white, malodorous vaginal discharge most likely has:

   a. Trichomoniasis
   b. Monilia
   c. Bacterial vaginosis
   d. Chlamydia

43. At which point of life is UTI more common in males?

   a. Toddler
   b. Adolescent
   c. School-age
   d. Newborn/infant

44. The organism primarily responsible for UTI is:

   a. Proteus
   b. *E. coli*
   c. Enterobacter
   d. Pseudomonas

45. Most patients with uncomplicated UTI can be treated on an outpatient basis. The first antibiotic you would consider using is:

    a. Amoxicillin

    b. Trimethoprim-sulfamethoxazole

    c. Cephalexin

    d. Amoxicillin/clavulanate

46. Cryptorchidism is more prevalent in:

    a. Term infants

    b. Premature infants

    c. Babies at 1 year of age

    d. Toddlers

47. A 3 year old boy is in the process of toilet-training. The parents come to see you because when the child urinates, all of the urine goes on the floor. You suspect hypospadias because:

    a. It is a rare disorder and would indicate a more serious problem

    b. Normally, the urine stream is directed downward

    c. The child is circumcised

    d. Fusion of the urethral folds has occurred

48. Which of the following is not used in the management of the child with phimosis?

    a. Ice packs

    b. Gentle stretching when bathing

    c. Circumcision in cases of urinary obstruction

    d. Good hygiene

49. Jeanine, an 8-year-old Hispanic girl, presents with a 2 week history of a brownish-red, very foul smelling, vaginal discharge. It is most likely caused by:

    a. Sexual abuse

    b. Accidental genital trauma

    c. Foreign body

    d. Poor hygiene

50. Which of the following is not a proposed etiologic factor in premenstrual syndrome?

    a. Imbalance of water and sodium

    b. Fluctuation in steroids

    c. Vitamin B_{12} deficiency

    d. Synthesis of prostaglandins

51. Treatment of a child with glomerulonephritis would include:

    a. Vasoconstrictors for hypotension

    b. Antibiotics for persistent infection

    c. Increased fluids to maintain hydration

    d. Avoidance of diuretics

52. Which of the following is not a frequent sign of gonorrhea infection:

  a. Diarrhea
  b. Urinary symptoms
  c. Menstrual problems
  d. Fever

53. The most significant finding in the case of chlamydia infection is:

  a. The vaginal discharge is grey and frothy
  b. Most examinations are normal
  c. The external genitalia is markedly inflamed
  d. Infection by *Chlamydia trachomatis* alone is the rule

54. One difference between the lesions of primary syphilis (chancre) and HSV genital lesions that may help in differentiating the two is:

  a. Syphilis chancre is painless while HSV lesions are painful
  b. Syphilis lesions have a flat edge while HSV lesion edges are more raised
  c. Syphilis chancres are more likely to ulcerate than HSV lesions
  d. Erythema and edema is greater with syphilis chancre than HSV lesions

55. Education of sexually active adolescents concerning use of condoms to prevent STDs would include:

  a. Only latex or natural skin condoms should be used
  b. Polyurethane condoms have inadequate STD protection
  c. Condom use is only method to prevent STDs and AIDS
  d. Only petroleum-based lubricants should be used

56. Which of the following contraceptive methods would be least suitable for adolescents?

  a. Condoms with spermicides
  b. Progestin only, mini-pill
  c. Long-acting progestins
  d. Estrogen-progestin combination

57. Which of the following is not an absolute contraindication for oral contraceptives?

  a. Clotting disorder
  b. Impaired liver function
  c. Severe hypertension
  d. Undiagnosed vaginal bleeding

Answers

1. d	20. b	39. c
2. c	21. c	40. a
3. d	22. c	41. d
4. d	23. b	42. c
5. a	24. d	43. d
6. c	25. d	44. b
7. d	26. b	45. b
8. c	27. d	46. b
9. d	28. c	47. b
10. b	29. c	48. a
11. d	30. b	49. c
12. c	31. b	50. c
13. d	32. a	51. b
14. a	33. c	52. a
15. d	34. b	53. b
16. b	35. c	54. a
17. a	36. c	55. c
18. d	37. b	56. b
19. a	38. d	57. c

Bibliography

AAP Committee on Adolescence (1996). The adolescent's right to confidential care when considering abortion. *Pediatrics, 97*(5), 746–751.

AAP Committee on Child Abuse and Neglect. (1998). Gonorrhea in pre-pubertal children. *Pediatrics, 101*(1), 134–135.

AAP Committee on Adolescence (1999). Adolescent pregnancy—Current trends and issues 1998. *Pediatrics, 103*(2), 1516–1520.

AAP Committee on Adolescence (1999). Contraception and adolescents. *Pediatrics, 104*(5), 1161–1166.

American Academy of Pediatrics. (2000). *Red Book 2000: Report of the committee on infectious diseases* (25th ed.). Elk Grove Village, IL: American Academy of Pediatrics.

Barratt, T. M., Avner, E. D., & Harmon, W. E. (1999). *Pediatric nephrology.* Baltimore: Lippincott, Williams, & Wilkens.

Behrman, R. E., Kliegman, R. M., & Jenson, H. B. (Eds.). (2000). *Nelson textbook of pediatrics* (16th ed.). Philadelphia: W. B. Saunders.

Berkowitz, C. D. (Ed.). (2000). *Pediatrics: A primary care approach (2nd ed.).* Philadelphia: W. B. Saunders.

Burns, C. E., Barber, N., Brady, M., & Dunn, A. (Eds.). (2000). *Pediatric primary care: A handbook for nurse practitioners (2nd ed.).* Philadelphia: W. B. Saunders.

Coupey, S. M. (2000). *Primary care of adolescent girls.* Philadelphia: Hanley & Belfus, Inc.

Emans, S. J., Laufer, M. R., & Goldstein, D. P. (Eds.). (1998). *Pediatric and adolescent gynecology* (4th ed.). Philadelphia: Lippincott-Raven.

Friedman, S. B., Fisher, M., Schonberg, S. K., & Alderman, E. M. (1998). *Comprehensive adolescent health care* (2nd Ed.). St. Louis: Mosby.

Gonzales, E. T. (1999). *Pediatric urology practice.* Philadelphia: Lippincott, Williams, & Wilkins.

Hatcher, R. A., Trussell, J., Stewart, F., Cates Jr. W., Stewart, G. K., Guest, F., & Kowal, D. (1998). *Contraceptive technology* (17th rev. ed.). NY: Ardent Media.

Hoekelman, R. A., Adam, H. M., Nelson, N. M., Weitzman, M. L. & Wilson, M. H. (Eds.). (2001). *Primary pediatric care* (4th ed.). St. Louis: Mosby.

Hofmann, A. D., & Greydanus, D. E. (Eds.). (1997). *Adolescent medicine.* Stamford, CT: Appleton & Lange.

Judson, F., & Ehret, J. (1994). Laboratory diagnosis of sexually transmitted infections. *Pediatric Annals, 23*(7), 361–369.

National Campaign to Prevent Teen Pregnancy. (1997). *Whatever happened to childhood? The problem of teen pregnancy in the United States.* Washington, DC: Author.

Perdad, R., Sharma, S., McTavish, J., Imber, C., & Mouriquand, P. D. (1995). Clinical presentation and pathophysiology of meatal stenosis following circumcision. *British Journal of Urology, 75,* 91–93.

Rosenstein, B. J., & Fosarelli, P. D. (1997). Genitourinary disorders. *Pediatric pearls: The handbook of practical pediatrics* (3rd ed., pp. 137–167). St. Louis: Mosby.

Starr Barber, N. (1996). Labial adhesions in childhood. *Journal of Pediatric Health Care, 10,* 26–27.

Todd, J. K. (1995). Management of urinary tract infections: Children are different. *Pediatrics in Review, 16*(5), 190–196.

Genitourinary and Gynecologic Disorders In Adults

Pamela A. Shuler
Mary D. Knudtson

Acquired Immunodeficiency Syndrome (AIDS)

- Definition: Secondary immunodeficiency syndrome resulting from Human Immunodeficiency Virus (HIV) infection and characterized by opportunistic infections, neurologic dysfunction, malignancies, systemic wasting and a variety of other disorders

- Etiology/Incidence

  1. HIV invades, multiplies within one or more types of susceptible cells; circulating $CD4^+$ lymphocytes, macrophages and monocytes are most commonly affected, destroying the host's immune system

  2. Median time from HIV infection to AIDS is 10 years

  3. Estimated 1.5 million Americans are infected with HIV, half are unaware they are infected

  4. 40,000 to 80,000 new infections diagnosed each year

  5. Most diagnoses are made in persons 20 to 49 years old; women and minorities aged 15 to 44 constitute one of the fastest growing segments of the U.S. epidemic

  6. HIV is transmitted through direct contact with bodily fluids (blood, semen, vaginal secretions) and breast milk

  7. Major routes of HIV transmission

     a. Sexual intercourse (homosexual and heterosexual)

     b. Needle sharing (IV drug users)

     c. Transfusions of contaminated blood and blood products

     d. Needle stick, open wound and mucous membrane exposure to health care workers (0.4% incidence according to the Centers for Disease Control and Prevention [CDC])

     e. Injection with previously used unsterilized needle (acupuncture, tattooing, medical injection)

     f. Pregnancy (mother to unborn fetus)

     g. Breastfeeding (mother to infant)

  8. Trends

     a. Plateau in number of newly infected homosexual males since 1991

     b. African-Americans and Hispanics are disproportionately represented

     c. One in four new HIV infections occur in people younger than 20

     d. Sexual contact leading mode of transmission for women

- Signs and Symptoms—CDC Classification

  1. Asymptomatic HIV infection (may last > 10 years)—inoculation to seroconversion 90% by three months and 98% by six months

  2. Acute HIV infection

a. Two to eight weeks after infection 30% to 40% may have acute viremia symptoms

(1) High fever, lymphadenopathy, rash, aseptic meningitis, fatigue, myalgias, arthralgias

(2) Usually mistaken for flu or mononucleosis

b. Months to years before AIDS—may have chronic fatigue, weight loss, nightsweats, persistent dermatitis, shingles, persistent diarrhea, oral candidiasis, hairy leukoplakia, chronic vaginal candidiasis, tuberculosis, cognitive changes

3. Persistent generalized lymphadenopathy (PGL)

a. Palpable lymph node enlargement (2 sites other than inguinal)

b. No concurrent illness to explain lymphadenopathy

4. HIV diseases that contribute to progression of AIDS

a. *Pneumocystis carinii* pneumonia, Kaposi's sarcoma, cytomegalovirus and/or other opportunistic infections/cancers

b. Encephalopathy

c. Wasting syndrome (involuntary weight loss greater than 10% of baseline body weight, plus either chronic diarrhea or chronic weakness and documented fever)

- Differential Diagnosis:

1. Cancer

2. Tuberculosis

3. Enterocolitis

4. Endocrine diseases

- Physical Findings: Variable, depending upon infection stage

- Diagnostic Tests/Findings

1. Informed consent with pretest counseling required prior to HIV testing

2. Post test counseling also required

3. Initial blood test for antibody detection

a. Enzyme immunoassay (EIA) (screening test)

b. Western blot or immunofluorescent antibody test—confirmatory blood tests for HIV specific antibody profile

c. Some individuals may not generate an antibody response for up to 36 months

4. Detection/quantification of HIV

a. HIV-1 p24 antigen used to diagnose infection before antibodies measurable

    b.   Qualitative polymerase chain reaction (PCR) circulating cells or plasma—can use in early disease instead of p24

    c.   Quantitative viral RNA levels—used to decide when to initiate treatment, as a prognostic indicator, and as a basis for evaluating response to treatment

    d. $CD4^+$ count used to assess magnitude of disease and to monitor effectiveness of treatment

  5. Additional recommended tests if HIV positive

    a.   HIV viral load test

    b.   Toxoplasma antibody test

    c.   Tests for hepatitis B viral markers

    d.   PPD

    e.   Chest radiograph

    f.   VDRL or RPR

- Management/Treatment
  (All STD treatment regimens throughout this chapter based on *1998 Sexually transmitted treatment guidelines*, published by CDC)
  Treatment of HIV and AIDS changing rapidly; recommendations may have changed due to new or better treatment options; consult with specialist or expert in AIDS care for latest information

  1. No cure or vaccination for HIV infection at present

  2. New treatment regimens are constantly evolving

  3. Treatment of HIV and opportunistic infections, malignancies and prophylaxis against opportunistic infections continue to evolve rapidly; basic guidelines include:

    a.   Therapy for opportunistic infections and malignancies

       (1) Conditions include *P. carinii* pneumonia, toxoplasmosis, cryptococcus, lymphoma, cytomegalovirus, esophageal candidiasis, Herpes simplex and zoster, Kaposi's sarcoma

       (2) Medications include antibiotics, antifungals and corticosteroids

    b.   Antiretroviral treatment (CDC, 1998); treatment of HIV changes very rapidly, consultation with a specialist is recommended

       (1) Initial use of combination therapy is recommended; monotherapy is no longer standard

       (2) Antiretroviral therapy is based upon disease progression risk

          (a) Option 1—in any patient with $CD4^+$ count < 500 or viral RNA levels > 5000; general consensus regarding need to initiate treatment in these patients

(b) Option 2—treat any patient with detectable plasma viral RNA > 500 regardless of CD4$^+$ count or clinical stage

(c) Option 3—treat all patients who are HIV positive even if viral RNA levels are negative and CD4$^+$ counts > 500

(d) Therapy should be initiated in all patients with symptomatic HIV, e.g., night sweats, recurrent candidiasis

(3) Medications:

    (a) Three classes of therapy—NRTs, NNRTI, PI (USPHS/IDSA, 1999)

    (b) Nucleoside reverse transcriptase inhibitors (NRT)

        (i) Zidovudine (AZT)—major adverse effects include anemia, headache, nausea, myositis

        (ii) Stavudine (d4T)—major adverse effects include peripheral neuropathy

        (iii) Didanosine (ddl)—major adverse effects include pancreatitis, diarrhea, peripheral neuropathy

        (iv) Zalcitabine (ddC)—major adverse effects include oral ulcers, peripheral neuropathy, pancreatitis

        (v) Lamivudine (3TC)—major adverse effects nausea, headache

    (c) Non-nucleoside reverse transcriptase inhibitors (NNRTI)

        (i) Nevirapine—major adverse effect is rash

        (ii) Delavirdine—major adverse effect is rash

        (iii) Efavirenz—dizziness, confusion, somnolence

    (d) Protease inhibitors (PI)

        (i) Saquinavir—major adverse effects include diarrhea, nausea, headache

        (ii) Indinavir—major adverse effects include nephrolitiasis, hyperbilirubinemia

        (iii) Ritonavir—major adverse effects include significant drug interactions, bitter after taste

        (iv) Nelfinavir—major adverse effects include diarrhea, elevated liver function tests (LFT)

        (v) Amprenavir—GI upset

    (e) Viral load monitoring—measure viral RNA every 3 to 4 months, more frequently if:

        (i) Non-compliance suspected

(ii)   CD4$^+$ count drops

(iii)   Clinical symptoms appear

(iv)   Drug adjustments are made (measure at 4 to 8 weeks then again at 3 to 4 weeks to document drug effect)

(f)   Initial therapy regimens—important to determine if patient can be compliant with regimen; complicated schedules are extremely difficult to adhere to; viral replication accelerates immediately with non-compliance

(g)   Acute retroviral syndrome—AZT + 3TC + indinavir for two years

c.   Prophylaxis of opportunistic infections

(1)   *P. carinii* pneumonia (begin when CD4$^+$ count < 200)

(a)   Trimethoprim-sulfamethoxazole (TMP/SMX) one double-strength tablet daily or three times a week

(b)   Dapsone 100 mg per day or aerosolized pentamidine 300 mg monthly if unable to tolerate TMP/ SMX

(2)   *Mycobacterium tuberculosis*

(a)   Isoniazid—10 mg/kg/day up to 300 mg plus pyridoxine 50 mg daily for one year

(b)   All patients with positive PPD reaction (5 mm of induration or greater) without positive chest radiography should receive prophylactic treatment

(3)   Toxoplasmosis—begin when CD4+ count < 100)—trimethoprim-sulfamethoxazole (TMP/SMX) one double strength tablet orally three times per week or daily

(4)   *Mycobacterium avium* complex—begin when CD4$^+$ count < 50

(a)   Clarithromycin 500 mg orally b.i.d. or

(b)   Azithromycin 500 mg orally three times a week or

(c)   Rifabutin 150 mg orally b.i.d.

d.   Recommended immunizations for HIV infected persons

(1)   Pneumococcal vaccination

(2)   Annual influenza vaccination

(3)   Three-dose schedule of hepatitis B vaccine for those who lack immunity

(4)   Tetanus-diptheria booster

(5)   Inactivated polio virus vaccine (IPV)

(6)   Measles, mumps, rubella vaccine

4.   Thorough psychosocial evaluation to include:

  a. Signs of severe psychologic distress

  b. Behavioral factors related to risk for transmitting HIV

  c. Information concerning partners who should be notified of possible HIV exposure

5. Discuss therapeutic and diagnostic plans

6. Educate regarding prevention, transmission and treatment of the disease

7. Emphasize importance of behavioral measures to protect and enhance the immune system

  a. No tobacco, street drugs, alcohol use

  b. Nutritious diet

  c. Stress management, imagery

  d. Exercise as tolerated

  e. Decrease exposure to infectious agents since HIV virus is spread when immune system is activated

8. Encourage continued ''safer sex'' practices and/or abstinence

9. Assist patient, as appropriate, in meeting physical, psychological, social, cultural, environmental and spiritual needs

10. Report AIDS cases to local health department

Gonorrhea (Uncomplicated Gonococcal Infections)

- Definition: A sexually transmitted bacterial infection that produces urethritis in men and cervicitis in women

- Etiology/Incidence

 1. Causative organism is *Neisseria gonorrhoeae*, a gram-negative diplococcus

 2. Approximately 600,000 infectious new cases reported annually

 3. Greatest incidence in the 15 to 30 year-old-age group

 4. Incubation period usually 3 to 10 days

 5. Spectrum of infection—cervicitis, urethritis, salpingitis, proctitis, P.I.D., pharyngitis, conjunctivitis, arthritis

 6. A leading cause of infertility among U.S. females

- Signs and Symptoms

 1. Female

  a. Often asymptomatic

  b. Dysuria, urinary frequency, urgency with a purulent urethral discharge

  c. Vaginal discharge

      d. Pelvic pain

      e. Abnormal menstrual bleeding

      f. Pharyngitis

      g. Septic arthritis

      h. Rash—petechial or pustular skin lesions

  2. Male

      a. One quarter are asymptomatic

      b. Dysuria (urethra most common site in male), frequency

      c. Copious penile discharge (serous/milky to yellow with blood-tinge)

      d. Testicular pain

      e. Pharyngitis

      f. Septic arthritis

      g. Rash—petechial or pustular skin lesions

      h. Proctitis—common in homosexual males

- Differential Diagnosis

  1. Nongonococcal cervicitis, vaginitis, urethritis or epididymitis

  2. Reiter's syndrome (chlamydia)

  3. Pelvic inflammatory disease (PID)

  4. Proctitis (other origin)

  5. Nongonococcal pharyngitis or arthritis

- Physical Findings

  1. Female

      a. Purulent discharge from cervix (primary site in reproductive age women)

      b. Inflammation of Bartholin's glands

      c. Evidence of PID (untreated infection)

  2. Male

      a. Evidence of urethritis, prostatitis

      b. Evidence of epididymitis (with untreated infection)

      c. Copious purulent discharge

- Diagnostic Tests/Findings

  1. Female tests

    a. Gram stain of endocervical discharge in women shows WBC with gram negative intracellular diplococci; sensitivity only 40 to 70% in women; greater than 90% in men

    b. Wet prep of purulent cervical discharge may show polymorphonuclear leukocytes (WBC) > 10/HPF

    c. Culture material from endocervix and other suspect sites on to Thayer-Martin or Transgrow media to confirm diagnosis

    d. DNA probe—sensitivity comparable to culture, two hour turn around time, only one specimen needed for chlamydia and *N. gonorrhoea*

    e. Urine-based ligase chain reaction—highly sensitive and specific in men and women

2. Male tests

    a. Gram stain of urethral discharge smear shows gram-negative diplococci and WBC

    b. Culture of urethra and other suspect sites

    c. DNA Probe

3. Test for concomitant infection from other STD including HIV, syphilis, and chlamydia

4. Test partners

- Management/Treatment

1. Treat all contacts

2. First choice—ceftriaxone 125 mg IM once, or ciprofloxacin 500 mg orally once, or cefixime 400 mg orally once, or ofloxacin 400 mg orally once, *plus* doxycycline 100 mg orally b.i.d. for 7 days, or erythromycin base or stearate 500 mg orally q.i.d. for seven days if the patient is pregnant; or azithromycin 1 g orally in a single dose (may use if pregnant and over 16 years of age); high incidence of co-existing chlamydia

3. Alternative regimens—spectinomycin 2 g IM once or ceftizoxime 500 mg IM once, or cefotaxime 500 mg IM once, or cefotetan 1 g IM once, or cefoxitin 2g IM once, with probenecid 1 g orally, enoxacin 400 mg orally once, or lomefloxacin 400 mg orally once, or norfloxacin 800 mg orally once, *plus* doxycycline as above

4. Test of cure not essential; repeat culture if symptoms persist or recur

5. Discuss therapeutic and diagnostic plans

6. Emphasize importance of complete treatment

7. Avoid sexual intercourse until patient and partner(s) cured

8. Educate regarding prevention, transmission and treatment of the disease; encourage continued use of condoms

9. Report cases to health department

10. Can cause disseminated infection, acute arthritis, hepatitis or endocarditis

Genital Chlamydial Infection

- Definition: A sexually transmitted disease that produces urethritis in men and cervicitis in women

- Etiology/Incidence

    1. Causative organism is *Chlamydia trachomatis*

    2. Approximately 4 million new cases occur annually

    3. The most common bacterial sexually transmitted disease in the U.S.

    4. A leading cause of female infertility and ectopic pregnancy in U.S.

    5. Incubation period 7 to 21 days

    6. Screening for high risk individuals recommended—sexually active adolescents and young adults, multiple partners, history of previous or current STD

- Signs and Symptoms

    1. Female

        a. Often asymptomatic

        b. Dysuria

        c. Mucopurulent vaginal discharge/spotting

        d. Lower abdominal/pelvic pain

        e. Dyspareunia

        f. Dysmenorrhea, menstrual irregularity

        g. Infertility

        h. Enlarged, tender inguinal lymph nodes

        i. Friable cervix

    2. Male

        a. Often asymptomatic

        b. Urethral discharge (any color)

        c. Dysuria

        d. Testicular pain/swelling

        e. Enlarged, tender inguinal lymph nodes

        f. Rectal pain, bleeding and diarrhea

- Differential Diagnosis

1. Gonococcal cervicitis

2. Urethritis

3. Proctitis

4. P.I.D.

5. Urinary tract infection

6. Epididymitis

7. Prostatitis from other infective agent

8. Vaginitis

- Physical Findings

   1. Female

      a. Mucopurulent urethral and/or cervical discharge

      b. Hypertropic, eroded and friable cervix (maybe)

      c. Evidence of P.I.D. (advanced infection)

   2. Male

      a. Mucopurulent urethral discharge

      b. Evidence of prostatitis

      c. Evidence of epididymitis (untreated infection)

- Diagnostic Tests/Findings

   1. Female

      a. Wet prep or gram stain shows WBC > 10/HPF

      b. Most common tests—enzyme immunoassay (EIA) and direct fluorescence assay (DFA) *or* lipase chain reaction (LCR) for confirmation

      c. Other tests include tissue culture, DNA hybridization and polymerase chain reaction (PCR)

   2. Male

      a. Gram stain or wet prep shows WBC > 10/HPF

      b. Same indirect antigen-detection tests

   3. Test for concomitant infection from other STD in patient (HIV, gonorrhea, syphilis, trichomonas)

   4. Test partners

- Management/Treatment

   1. Treat all contacts

2. First choice—doxycycline, 100 mg orally b.i.d. for 7 days or azithromycin one g orally once (may be used in pregnancy if > 16 years of age)

3. Ofloxacin 300 mg orally b.i.d. for 7 days, or erythromycin base 500 mg orally q.i.d. for 7 days, or erythromycin ethylsuccinate 800 mg orally q.i.d. for 7 days

4. During pregnancy—erythromycin base or stearate, 500 mg orally q.i.d. for 7 days or erythromycin base 250 mg orally q.i.d. for 14 days, erythromycin ethylsuccinate 800 mg orally q.i.d. for 7 days or erythromycin ethylsuccinate 400 mg orally q.i.d. for 14 days, or amoxicillin, 500 mg orally t.i.d. for 7 days or azithromycin 1 g orally once if > 16 years of age

5. No test-of-cure after treatment unless symptoms persist or re-infection suspected (wait more than three weeks after treatment to determine if test-of-cure needed)

6. Discuss therapeutic and diagnostic plans

7. Emphasize importance of complete treatment

8. Avoid sexual intercourse until patient and partner(s) complete treatment

9. Educate regarding prevention, transmission and treatment of the disease; encourage continued use of condoms

10. Report cases to health department

Syphilis

- Definition: A complex infectious disease that can affect almost any organ or tissue in the body and mimics many diseases

- Etiology/Incidence

  1. Causative organism is *Treponema pallidum*, a spirochete

  2. Transmission primarily occurs through minor skin or mucosal lesions during sexual encounters; genital and extragenital areas may be inoculated

  3. Can be transmitted via placenta (after 10th week) from mother to fetus (congenital rate—1 in 10,000 pregnancies)

  4. Incidence has declined since 1990; approximately 50,000 cases (primary and secondary types) reported in U.S. annually since 1990

  5. Risk of contraction—30 to 50% (partner-primary syphilis)

- Signs and Symptoms

  1. Primary

     a. Painless chancre

     b. Regional lymphadenopathy

  2. Secondary

     a. Skin rash—especially palmar, plantar and oral mucosa

     b. Malaise, anorexia

     c. Alopecia

     d. Arthralgias/myalgias/flu-like symptoms

     e. Other symptoms depending on affected organs

     f. Generalized lymphadenopathy

     g. Low-grade fever

     h. Condylomata lata

3. Latent

     a. May be asymptomatic

     b. Integumentary, ocular, cardiovascular, gastrointestinal, respiratory or neurological manifestations may be present

4. Neurosyphilis

     a. May occur during any stage of syphilis

     b. Optic, auditory, cranial nerve and/or meningeal symptoms are most common

- Differential Diagnosis

1. Primary

     a. Herpes genitalis

     b. Chancroid

     c. Neoplasm

     d. Lymphogranuloma venereum (LGV)

     e. Granuloma inguinale

2. Secondary

     a. Conditions associated with rash or other presenting symptoms, e.g., flu, mononucleosis, pityriasis rosea, drug eruptions

     b. Infectious hepatitis

3. Latent

     a. Neoplasms of skin, liver, lung, stomach or brain

     b. Other forms

        (1) Meningitis

        (2) Cardiovascular disorders

        (3) CNS disorders

        (4) Arthritis

        (5) Primary neurologic lesions

- Physical Findings

1. Neurological signs may be present at any stage

2. Primary

   a. Indurated ulcer (chancre) on:

      (1) Genitals

      (2) Mouth

      (3) Rectum

      (4) Nipple

   b. Regional lymphadenopathy

3. Secondary

   a. Low-grade fever

   b. Highly variable skin rash (including palms and soles)

   c. Mucous patches

   d. Evidence or manifestations of condyloma latum

   e. Generalized lymphadenopathy

   f. Evidence of meningitis, iritis, hepatitis, glomerulonephritis

4. Latent

   a. May have no clinical signs of infection

   b. Granulomatous lesions (gummas)—skin, mucous membranes, bone

   c. Leukoplakia

   d. Evidence of periostitis, osteitis or arthritis

   e. Gummatous infiltrates in larynx, trachea, pulmonary parenchyma, stomach and/or liver

   f. Diminished coronary circulation

   g. Acute myocardial infarction

   h. Cardiac insufficiency

   i. Aortic aneurysm

   j. Meningitis

   k. Hemiparesis

   l. Hemiplegia

   m. Tabes dorsalis

   n. General paresis

- Diagnostic Tests/Findings

1. Early syphilis—primary, secondary or latent syphilis of less than one year's

duration

 a. Definitive methods

  (1) Darkfield microscopy

  (2) Direct fluorescent antibody tests of lesion exudate or tissue

 b. Presumptive methods (neither test alone is sufficient for diagnosis)

  (1) Treponemal serologic tests

   (a) Fluorescent treponemal antibody absorption (FTA-ABS) test

   (b) Microhemagglutination assay for antibody to *T. pallidum* (MHA-TP)

   (c) Tests/titers should be reported as positive or negative and used to confirm nontreponemal tests

   (d) FTA-ABS or MHA-TP confirmation tests positive in 85% to 95% of primary and in 100% of secondary cases

  (2) Nontreponemal serologic tests

   (a) Veneral Disease Research Laboratory (VDRL)

   (b) Rapid Plasma Reagin (RPR)

2. Latent syphilis of more than one year's duration and cardiovascular syphilis

 a. VDRL or RPR test (+ in 75% of cases)

 b. FTA-ABS or MHA-TP confirmation test (+ in 98% cases)

 c. Lumbar puncture with tests on cerebrospinal fluid (CSF)

3. Neurosyphilis (occurs at any stage)

 a. Treponemal and nontreponemal serologic tests results dependent upon stage of disease

 b. CSF examinations as above

4. Test for concomitant infection from other STD in patient and contacts

 a. HIV

 b. Gonorrhea

 c. Chlamydia

5. Test partners

- Management/Treatment

1. Pregnant patients allergic to penicillin should be treated with penicillin after desensitization for all stages

2. Penicillin alternative treatment for all stages of syphilis except neurosyphilis

3. Early syphilis and persons exposed within last 90 days

    a.   Treat all partners

    b.   First choice—benzathine penicillin G, 2.4 million units IM once

    c.   Penicillin allergy—doxycycline 100 mg orally b.i.d. for 2 weeks or tetracycline 500 mg orally q.i.d. for 2 weeks

4.   Late latent cases and cardiovascular syphilis (normal CSF examination)

    a.   First choice—benzathine penicillin G, 2.4 million units IM weekly for 3 weeks

    b.   Penicillin allergy—doxycycline 100 mg orally b.i.d. for 4 weeks or tetracycline 500 mg orally q.i.d. for 4 weeks

5.   Neurosyphilis

    a.   First choice—18 to 24 million units aqueous crystalline penicillin G daily, administered as 3 to 4 million units IV every 4 hours for 10 to 14 days

    b.   Alternate regimen if compliance assured—2.4 million units procaine penicillin IM daily, plus probenecid 500 mg orally q.i.d., both for 10 to 14 days

6.   Post-treatment follow-up

    a.   Primary and secondary baseline RPR or VDRL at time of treatment and repeated every 3 months; titer should fall fourfold in 3 months, eightfold in 6 months and become negative within 2 years (MHA-TP and FTA-ABS will be positive for lifetime)

    b.   Latent—RPR or VDRL repeated at 6 month and 12 month intervals; titer should fall fourfold in 12 to 24 months

    c.   Neurosyphilis—CSF examination every 6 months until normal

7.   Discuss therapeutic and diagnostic plans

8.   Emphasize importance of complete treatment

9.   Avoid sexual intercourse until patient and partner(s) cured

10.   Educate regarding prevention, transmission and treatment of the disease; encourage continued use of condoms

11.   Report cases to health department

Herpes Genitalis

- Definition: A viral STD that produces recurrent, painful genital lesions and has no cure
- Etiology/Incidence

   1.   Caused by herpes simplex virus (HSV) types 1 (5% to 15%) and 2 (85 to 95%)

   2.   Initial (primary) and recurrent infections affect approximately 270,000 and 30 million persons respectively annually

   3.   Duration of initial infection—10 to 14 days; recurrent 7 to 10 days; viral shedding (without clinical symptoms) occurs during latency (interval between outbreaks)

4. Virus resides in presacral ganglia during latency

5. Can lead to neuralgia, meningitis, ascending myelitis, urethral strictures, and lymphatic suppuration

6. Infection during pregnancy can lead to spontaneous abortion or fetal morbidity/mortality; risk for transmission to neonate appears highest among women with first episode near time of delivery

7. Incubation period 2 to 21 days after exposure

- Signs and Symptoms

  1. First clinical episode

     a. Fever/chills

     b. Malaise

     c. Headache

     d. Dysuria

     e. Vaginal discharge, abnormal bleeding

     f. Dyspareunia

     g. Lymph nodes tender, enlarged, firm

     h. Pruritic/burning genital vesicles that rupture and become painful ulcers—mean duration 12 days

  2. Recurrent episodes—pruritic/burning vesicles that rupture into less painful ulcers; mean duration 4.5 days

- Differential Diagnosis

  1. Syphilis

  2. Lymphogranuloma venereum

  3. Gonorrhea

  4. Chlamydia

  5. Chancroid

  6. Vaginitis

  7. Herpes zoster

  8. Condyloma latum

  9. Erythema multiforme

  10. Neoplasm (especially cervical)

- Physical Findings

  1. Fever—first episode

  2. Single or multiple vesicles surrounded by inflammation/edema on external genitalia,

penis, scrotum, anus, vagina or cervix (75%); vesicles spontaneously rupture and form painful, erythematous ulcers, scab over and heal

3. Cervix may appear diffusely inflamed, edematous with large punched-out ulcers or a granulomatous-appearing tumor-like mass covered with gray exudate

4. Profuse, watery vaginal discharge often present and may be only sign

- Diagnostic Tests/Findings

    1. Tzanck stain—identification of multinucleated giant cells with intranuclear inclusions in a cytologic smear

    2. Identification of HSV virus(es) from tissue (vulvar, vaginal, cervical) cultures, antigen test, DNA probe or PCR assay

    3. Serologic tests for HSV types 1 and 2 antibodies are also available

    4. Test for concomitant infection of other STD in patient and contacts

        a. HIV

        b. Syphilis

        c. Condylomata acuminata

        d. Gonorrhea

        e. Chlamydia

        f. Chancroid

- Management/Treatment

    1. Symptomatic treatment—drying and antipruritic agents and topical anesthetic agents

    2. Chemotherapeutic agents—acyclovir (available in topical, oral and intravenous formulation), famciclovir, or valacyclovir

        a. Topical therapy—minimal benefit except may be useful for immunocompromised patients, use is discouraged

        b. Oral therapy

            (1) Recurrent herpes simplex infections

                (a) Famciclovir 125 mg b.i.d. for 5 days

                (b) Valacyclovir 500 mg b.i.d. for 5 days

                (c) Acyclovir 400 mg t.i.d. for 5 days or 200 mg 5 times per day for 5 days or 800 mg b.i.d. for 5 days

            (2) Uncomplicated primary herpes simplex infections

                (a) Acyclovir 200 mg 5 times per day for 7 to 10 days or 400 mg t.i.d. for 7 to 10 days

                (b) Famciclovir 250 mg t.i.d. for 7 to 10 days

                (c) Valacyclovir 1 g b.i.d. for 7 to 10 days

(3) Prophylactic or suppressive therapy (if 6 or more outbreaks per year)

    (a) Acyclovir 400 mg b.i.d. or 800 mg daily

    (b) Famciclovir 250 mg b.i.d.

    (c) Valacyclovir 250 mg b.i.d. or 500 mg daily or 1000 mg daily

c. Intravenous therapy

    (1) Used in severe disease and when complications necessitate hospitalization

    (2) Acyclovir 5 to 10 mg/kg IV every 8 hours for 5 to 7 days

d. Acyclovir is eliminated by the kidneys; hydration is particularly important

e. Safety of systemic treatment has not been established during pregnancy

3. Discuss therapeutic and diagnostic plans

4. Avoid sexual intercourse when lesions present; encourage continued use of condoms

5. Educate regarding prevention, transmission and treatment of the disease and dangers during pregnancy

6. Up to 80% may have viral shedding during asymptomatic periods

Genital Warts (Condylomata acuminata)

- Definition: Sexually transmitted warty growths appearing on any part of the genitalia

- Etiology/Incidence

  1. More than 30 types of human papillomavirus (HPV) cause genital warts; types 6, 11, 16, 18, 31, 33, 35, 39, 45, 51, 52 are predominately detected in high-grade neoplastic lesions and cervical cancer

  2. HPV increases risk of penile, vulvar and cervical cancers

  3. Greatest incidence in the 15 to 25 year old age group; correlated with multiple sex partners, early coitus and lack of contraceptive barrier methods

  4. Approximately 3 million cases diagnosed annually

  5. The most common symptomatic viral STD in the U.S.; highly contagious

- Signs and Symptoms

  1. Painless, pruritic or burning warts on external genitalia (male and female)

  2. Possibly—dyspareunia, dysuria, bleeding

- Differential Diagnosis

  1. Condyloma latum

  2. Neoplasm

  3. Granuloma inguinale

      4. Moles

      5. Molluscum contagiosum

- Physical Findings

  1. Single or multiple soft, fleshy, papillary or sessile, painless keratinized growths (may be multilobulated papules and quite large) around anus, vulvovaginal area, penis, urethra, perineum or oral cavity

  2. In women, similar lesions may appear in vagina/on cervix; vaginal discharge from co-existing infection(s) may be present; men may have lesions in urethra

  3. May have no signs since flat warts are visible only by colposcopy

- Diagnostic Tests/Findings

  1. Tissue sample (biopsy) for detection of viral DNA is available, but expense limits clinical utility

  2. Biopsies may be taken to rule out dysplasia and carcinoma

  3. Pap smear may indicate HPV infection on cervix; see section on dysplasia

  4. Test for concomitant infection of other STD

     a. HIV

     b. Gonorrhea

     c. Syphilis—RPR or VDRL to rule out Condyloma latum

     d. Chlamydia

- Management/Treatment

  1. New treatment regimens are evolving to ameliorate symptoms; no current methods are curative

     a. Small vulvar and perianal warts

        (1) Self-treatment with podofilox 0.5% solution or gel— apply with cotton tip applicator b.i.d. for 3 days followed by no treatment for 4 days; cycle can be repeated 4 times

        (2) 80% to 90% solution of trichloroacetic acid (TCA) or tincture of podophyllin weekly for 6 weeks (patient must wash off podophyllin in four hrs); protect surrounding skin with petroleum jelly

        (3) TCA is preferred since it is more effective, not absorbed and can be used during pregnancy and on penis; treatment may be slightly more painful than podophyllin; immediate application of sodium bicarbonate paste following treatment will decrease pain

        (4) Imiquimod 5% cream applied at bedtime 3 times a week for 16 weeks; wash off 6 to 10 hours after application

        (5) Surgical removal with tangential scissor or shave excision, curretage or electrosurgery

      (6)   Intralesional interferon

      (7)   Cryotherapy with liquid nitrogen

   b.   Large warts (> 2 cm), vulvar/vaginal warts

      (1) CO_2 laser

      (2)   Electrodesiccation, electrocautery, cryocautery, Leep

2. NO MORE THAN 1/3 OF LESION ENCIRCLING AN ORIFICE SHOULD BE TREATED AT SINGLE VISIT

3. Cervical warts—see section on dysplasia

4. Discuss therapeutic and diagnostic plans

5. Educate regarding prevention, transmission and treatment of the disease; encourage continued use of condoms

6. Emphasize importance of follow-up particularly if Pap abnormal

7. Discuss possible chronicity

   a.   Treatment may not be successful

   b.   High recurrence rate due to dormant and asymptomatic viral shedding

   c.   Individuals who smoke have more difficulty with recurrence

   d.   Smoking is HPV co-factor for cervical cancer

Pelvic Inflammatory Disease (PID)

- Definition: Infection of the upper genital tract, including the endometrium, oviducts, ovaries, uterine wall/serosa, broad ligaments and pelvic peritoneum

- Etiology/Incidence

1. A disease of polymicrobial infection caused by a variety of aerobic and anaerobic bacteria including *N. gonorrhoeae, Chlamydia trachomatis*, group β streptococcus, *Escherichia coli*, bacteroides bacterial vaginosis organisms, *Mycoplasma hominis* and *Ureaplasma urealyticum*

2. Clinical PID is usually a polymicrobial infection

3. More than 1 million episodes occur annually

4. Most prevalent serious infection for women 16 to 25 years of age

5. After initial infection, women more susceptible to reinfection, ectopic pregnancy and infertility

6. Oral contraceptives and barrier methods with spermicide provide significant protection

7. Depo-medroxyprogesterone acetate and Norplant cause changes in cervical mucosa which provide some protection from PID

8. Annual costs of PID and its sequelae is $4.2 billion

- Signs and Symptoms
    1. Often symptoms are mild, atypical, subtle or absent
    2. Fever/chills
    3. Nausea/vomiting
    4. Dysuria
    5. Vaginal discharge
    6. Dysmenorrhea
    7. Abnormal menstrual bleeding
    8. Lower abdominal/pelvic pain (usually < 1 week duration)
    9. Dyspareunia
    10. Infertility
- Differential Diagnosis
    1. Appendicitis
    2. Ectopic pregnancy
    3. Septic abortion
    4. Hemorrhagic or ruptured ovarian cysts or tumors
    5. Twisted ovarian cyst
    6. Degeneration of a myoma
    7. Enteritis
- Physical Findings and Diagnostic Tests/Findings (clinical criteria for diagnosing PID)
    1. Minimum criteria—empiric treatment required if all three present
        a. Lower abdominal tenderness
        b. Cervical motion tenderness
        c. Adnexal tenderness
    2. Additional criteria to increase specificity of diagnosis
        a. Laboratory documentation of cervical infection with *C. trachomatis* or *N. gonorrhoeae*
        b. Fever > 38.3° C or 101° F
        c. Abnormal cervical or vaginal discharge
        d. Elevated erythrocyte sedimentation rate and/or C-reactive protein
    3. Definitive criteria for diagnosis—warranted in select cases
        a. Histopathologic evidence of endometritis on endometrial biopsy
        b. Tubo-ovarian abscess on sonography or other radiologic tests

c. Laparoscopic abnormalities consistent with PID

- Management/Treatment

  1. Resolution of symptoms and preservation of tubal function are the primary goals in management of PID; ideally all patients are hospitalized; however, for economic and practical reasons many are treated as outpatients

  2. Hospitalization is highly recommended if:

     a. Diagnosis is uncertain and surgical emergencies cannot be excluded

     b. Tubo-ovarian abscess is suspected

     c. Patient is pregnant, an adolescent or HIV infected

     d. Severe illness, e.g., nausea and vomiting precludes outpatient treatment

     e. Patient unable to follow or tolerate outpatient regimen

     f. Patient has failed to clinically respond to outpatient treatment

     g. Clinical follow-up within 72 hours of starting antibiotic therapy cannot be arranged

  3. Outpatient treatment

     a. First choice—ofloxacin 400 mg orally b.i.d. for 14 days plus metronidazole 500 mg orally b.i.d. for 14 days

     b. Cefoxitin 2g IM plus probenecid, 1 g orally once or ceftriaxone 250 mg IM or other parenteral third-generation cephalosporins plus doxycycline 100 mg orally twice daily for 14 days

  4. Follow-up appointment in 72 hours, then tests-of-cure 4 to 6 weeks post-treatment

  5. Test and treat partners

  6. Discuss therapeutic and diagnostic plans

  7. Emphasize importance of complete treatment

  8. Avoid sexual intercourse until patient and partner(s) cured

  9. Education regarding prevention, transmission and treatment of the disease; encourage continued use of condoms

  10. Discuss fertility issues as appropriate

Vulvovaginitis

- Definition: Inflammation and infection of the vulva/vagina

- Etiology/Incidence

  1. Commonly caused by *Trichomonas vaginalis* (a motile protozoan), bacterial vaginosis (a polymicrobial bacterial vaginal infection) or *Candida albicans* (a fungi or yeast)

2. Trichomonas—transmitted through intercourse, can infect the lower urinary tract in men and women

3. Bacterial vaginosis (BV)—the most frequently diagnosed symptomatic vaginitis in the U.S.; unclear whether BV results from sexually transmitted pathogen; should be treated in pregnant women since the infection has been associated with premature rupture of membranes, preterm labor and preterm birth

4. Candida vaginitis—occurs in close to 40% to 75% of women; is not considered to be a STD; is predisposed by pregnancy, diabetes, use of broad-spectrum antibiotics or corticosteroids; heat, moisture and occlusive clothing also increase risk

5. Several types of vaginitis may co-exist

- Signs and Symptoms
    1. Trichomoniasis

        a. Malodorous yellow-green discharge with pruritus

        b. Dyspareunia

        c. Dysuria (male partners may also have dysuria)

    2. Bacterial vaginosis

        a. Malodorous, white (''fishy'') discharge

        b. Spotting

        c. 50% of patients are asymptomatic

    3. Candida vaginitis

        a. Thick discharge with pruritus

        b. Erythema of vagina and vulva

- Differential Diagnosis
    1. Chlamydia

    2. Gonorrhea

    3. Herpes genitalis

    4. Condylomata acuminata

    5. Allergy, contact dermatitis

    6. Atrophic vaginitis

- Physical Findings
    1. Trichomoniasis

        a. Diffuse vaginal erythema

        b. Intensely inflamed lesions on cervix and vaginal mucosa— ''strawberry patches''

    c. Discharge

        (1) Ranges from white/watery to green, thick and frothy

        (2) Vaginal pH—higher than 4.5

  2. Bacterial vaginosis

    a. Watery, grayish or white homogenous discharge, fishy odor

    b. Discharge slightly adherent to vaginal walls

  3. Candida vaginitis

    a. White, "cottage-cheese" discharge

    b. Marked vulvovaginal erythema/edema with intense pruritus

- Diagnostic Tests/Findings

  1. Wet prep microscopic examination of vaginal secretions viewed on low or high power

    a. Trichomoniasis—discharge mixed with saline will show motile trichomonas on microscopic examination

    b. Bacterial vaginosis—discharge mixed with saline will show clue cells on microscopic examination; amine-like odor present when discharge alkalinized with 10 to 20% potassium hydroxide (KOH) "whiff test"; vaginal pH of 4 to 5 or more

    c. Candida vaginitis—discharge mixed with 10% KOH will show branched and budding pseudohyphae on microscopic examination

  2. Test for concomitant infection from other STD

    a. HIV

    b. Syphilis

    c. Condylomata acuminata

    d. Gonorrhea

    e. Chlamydia

- Management/Treatment

  1. Trichomoniasis—recommended treatment is metronidazole 2 g orally as a single dose, alternative treatment metronidazole 500 mg b.i.d. for 7 days; treat partner

  2. Bacterial vaginosis

    a. Drugs of choice

        (1) Clindamycin cream 2%, one full applicator 5 g intravaginally at bedtime for 7 days

        (2) Metronidazole 500 mg orally b.i.d. for 7 days or

   (3) Metronidazole gel, 0.75%, one full applicator (5 g) intravaginally q.d. or b.i.d. for 5 days

  b. Alternative regimens

   (1) Clindamycin, 300 mg orally b.i.d. for 7 days (safe during pregnancy)

   (2) Metronidazole 2 g orally in a single dose

3. Candida vaginitis—many different preparations and treatment regimens exist; the following are commonly prescribed

  a. Miconazole 2% or clotrimazole 1% cream, 5 g intravaginally at bedtime for seven days

  b. Terconazole 80 mg suppository, 1 suppository intravaginally at bedtime for three days

  c. Resistant cases may need partner treatment

  d. Fluconazole 150 mg orally once

4. Discuss therapeutic and diagnostic plans

5. Avoid sexual intercourse until patient and partner(s) cured

6. Education regarding prevention, transmission and treatment of the disease; encourage continued use of condoms

7. Emphasize importance of BV treatment for pregnant patients

8. Education regarding dangers of douching and incidence of infection

9. Education regarding PID; association with bacterial vaginosis

Urinary Tract Infection (UTI, Cystitis: Acute, Uncomplicated)

- Definition: Inflammation and infection of the urinary bladder; urethra may be involved

- Etiology/Incidence

 1. Most common causative organisms—*Escherichia coli*, (women) and *Proteus species* (men)

 2. More common in women than men; urological evaluation required for men with UTI

 3. 30 to 40% of women will experience at least 1 UTI

 4. Contributing factors in women

  a. Sexual intercourse; diaphragm use

  b. Pregnancy

  c. Diabetes

  d. Catheterization

  e. Instrumentation

      f.   Retaining urine in bladder despite urge to void

   5. Contributing factors in men

      a.   Residual urine (prostatic enlargement)

      b.   Neuropathic bladder

      c.   Calculi

      d.   Prostatitis

      e.   Catheterization

      f.   Instrumentation

- Signs and Symptoms

   1. Dysuria, frequency, urgency

   2. Suprapubic discomfort

   3. Foul smelling urine

- Differential Diagnosis

   1. Vaginitis (females)

   2. Prostatitis (males)

   3. Gonorrhea

   4. Chlamydia infection

   5. Renal calculi

   6. Pyelonephritis

   7. Epididymitis

- Physical Findings

   1. Urinary meatus may be erythematous/edematous

   2. Negative costovertebral angle tenderness

   3. Negative pelvic or prostate examination

   4. May have suprapubic tenderness on palpation

- Diagnostic Tests/Findings

   1. Pyuria—> 10 WBC/HPF

   2. Complete urinalysis (clean catch) with culture and sensitivity testing

      a.   Bacteria count over 100,000 organisms per mL in fresh ''clean catch'' midstream specimen is reliable indicator of active urinary tract infection; women with acute cystitis may have more than 10^3 but less than 10^5 per mL in midstream urine cultures

      b.   Leukocyte esterase dipstick test—positive

c. Urine dipstick positive for protein, blood, nitrites suggestive of UTI

- Management/Treatment

    1. Single-dose regimens—trimethoprim/sulfamethoxazole (TMP/SMX) 2 double-strength (DS) tablets, amoxicillin 500 mg times 6 or fosfomycin 3 g

    2. Three-day regimen examples (uncomplicated lower tract infection)—TMP/SMX DS tablet b.i.d., ciprofloxacin 250 mg b.i.d., nitrofurantoin 100 mg q.i.d.; amoxicillin/clavulanate 500 mg t.i.d., amozicillin 500 mg b.i.d.; norfloxacin 400 mg b.i.d., ofloxacin 200 mg b.i.d.

    3. Seven to ten day regimen examples (usually for complicated lower tract infections)—TMP/SMX 1 DS tablet b.i.d., trimethoprim 100 mg b.i.d., norfloxacin 400 mg b.i.d., ciprofloxacin 250 to 500 mg b.i.d.

    4. Treatment during pregnancy—nitrofurantoin 100 mg b.i.d. for 7 to 10 days or amoxicillin 500 mg orally t.i.d. for 7 to 14 days; cephalosporin 500 mg q.i.d. for 7 to 14 days

    5. Consider adding phenazopyridine hydrochloride 200 mg orally t.i.d. for two days for discomfort associated with urinary tract irritation (caution patient of orange/red tinge to urine)

    6. Increase water and decrease carbonated drink intake

    7. Repeat urinalysis with culture and sensitivity after medication regimen completed if still symptomatic

    8. Discuss therapeutic and diagnostic plans

    9. Advise return appointment if symptoms increase or no improvement

    10. Emphasize importance of complete treatment and follow-up for repeat urinalysis

Acute Pyelonephritis (Upper UTI)

- Definition: An acute bacterial infection of the upper urinary tract (kidney and renal pelvis); usually results from an ascending infection

- Etiology/Incidence

    1. *Escherichia coli* (gram negative) accounts for 80% of infections; *Staphylococcus saprophyticus* and *Streptococcus faecalis* (gram positive) account for 5 to 10%

    2. If urologic abnormalities or calculi present, the following organisms may cause infection—Enterobacter, Proteus, Klebsiella, Serratia and Pseudomonas

    3. Majority of infections occur in young women; rare occurrence in men under age 50 years

    4. Most commonly occurs in patients who are pregnant or have disruptive urinary flow, neurogenic bladder dysfunction or vesicoureteral reflux

- Signs and Symptoms—usually develop rapidly over a few hours

    1. Shaking chills

2. Malaise, generalized muscle tenderness

3. Nausea, vomiting and diarrhea

4. Flank/back pain (unilateral or bilateral)

5. Abdominal pain

6. Dysuria, frequency or urgency (may be absent)

- Differential Diagnosis

  1. Cystitis

  2. Prostatitis

  3. Musculoskeletal back pain

  4. Appendicitis

  5. Diverticulitis

  6. Pelvic inflammatory disease

  7. Ectopic pregnancy

- Physical Findings

  1. Fever, tachycardia

  2. Costovertebral angle pain (unilateral or bilateral) upon percussion

  3. Peritoneal signs are usually absent

  4. Patient may appear very ill

- Diagnostic Tests/Findings

  1. Microscopic urinalysis

     a. 5 to 10 WBC/HPF

     b. Occasional erythrocytes

     c. White cell casts may be present

     d. Mild proteinuria

  2. Urine culture—> 100,000 bacteria per mL of urine; sensitivity testing should be done

  3. Gram stain of uncentrifuged urine—one bacterium per oil-immersion correlates with 100,000 bacteria per mL of urine or more

  4. Complete blood count (CBC)—leukocytosis with left shift

  5. Elevated ESR

  6. BUN and creatinine are usually normal

  7. Electrolytes may be abnormal if dehydrated

- Management/Treatment

1. MD referral or consult may be required

2. Inpatient therapy

   a. Patients who are pregnant, have underlying illness, have decreased renal reserve, very toxic (high fever, hypotensive, etc) or unable to tolerate oral therapy should be hospitalized for parenteral antibiotics

   b. IV antimicrobial therapy is based upon culture and sensitivity report

   c. IV hydration is also required

3. Outpatient therapy—if compliant/reliable and have immediate access to health care services if condition worsens

   a. Antibiotics may include trimethoprim-sulfamethoxazole (if gram stain indicates gram negative organism), norfloxacin, ciprofloxacin, or amoxicillin/clavulanate for 14 days

   b. Resistance to ampicillin is 30%, therefore should not be used as sole therapy

   c. Follow-up within 24 hours

   d. Hydration measures

4. Repeat urine culture two weeks after completed course of antibiotics

5. Discuss therapeutic and diagnostic plans

6. Emphasize importance of complete treatment and follow-up appointments

7. Instructions regarding no sexual intercourse until treatment completed

8. Education regarding emergency signs and symptoms if managed as outpatient

9. Second episode of acute pyelonephritis requires urologic consultation or work-up

Acute Bacterial Prostatitis

- Definition: Inflammation/infection of the prostate gland

- Etiology/Incidence

   1. *Escherichia coli* or other gram-negative bacteria are common causative agents

   2. Occasionally acute urinary retention develops, requiring urgent hospitalization; suprapubic drainage may be necessary; URINARY CATHETERIZATION SHOULD BE AVOIDED

   3. Absence of zinc in prostatic fluid can predispose patient to infection

   4. Young adult men may be more prone to nonbacterial prostatitis or prostatosis

      a. WBC are present in expressed prostatic secretions, but no organisms are cultured

      b. Causative agents include mycoplasma, ureaplasma, gonorrhea and chlamydia

- Signs and Symptoms

1. Fever/chills, malaise, myalgias

2. Low back pain

3. Dysuria, urgency, nocturia, frequency

4. Perineal pain increased with defecation

- Differential Diagnosis

   1. Acute/chronic bacterial cystitis (urinary retention)

   2. Chronic prostatitis

   3. Nonbacterial prostatitis

   4. Prostatodynia

   5. Prostatic or seminal vesicle abscesses

   6. Benign prostatic hypertrophy

   7. Prostatic cancer

   8. Epididymitis

   9. Acute diverticulitis

- Physical Findings

   1. Fever

   2. Prostate—edematous, firm or "boggy," warm and tender; AVOID VIGOROUS MASSAGE, CAN LEAD TO BACTEREMIA

- Diagnostic Tests/Findings

   1. Urine cultures—positive

   2. Prostatic secretions—expressed prostatic secretions (EPS), WBC > 20 cells/HPF is abnormal

   3. Diagnosis is best made by performing simultaneous quantitative bacterial cultures of urethral urine, bladder urine, and EPS, the three glass test

   4. Patient often treated based only on physical findings and urine culture

- Management/Treatment

   1. Patients who appear septic and/or have urinary retention should be hospitalized

   2. Outpatient treatment

      a. First choice if age > 35 years is trimethoprim/sulfamethoxazole double-strength tablet b.i.d. for 2 to 4 weeks; if age < 35 years doxycycline 100 mg orally b.i.d. for 10 days

      b. Alternative choices are carbenicillin 2 tablets orally q.i.d. for 2 to 4 weeks or ciprofloxacin 250 to 500 mg orally b.i.d. for 2 to 4 weeks

   3. Bed rest

4. Sitz bath t.i.d. for 30 minutes

5. Follow-up appointment 48 to 72 hours

6. Discuss therapeutic and diagnostic plans

7. Avoid sexual intercourse until acute phase resolved; encourage continued use of condoms if multiple partners

8. Education regarding signs/symptoms of urinary retention and epididymitis

9. Emphasize importance of follow-up appointments

Chronic Bacterial Prostatitis

- Definition: Chronic inflammation/infection of prostate gland
- Etiology/Incidence
  1. Causative organisms are *Escherichia coli*; enterobacter organisms, *Proteus species*, *Chlamydia trachomatis*
  2. Often associated with urethritis or infection of lower urinary tract
  3. One of the most common causes of recurrent urinary tract infection in men
- Signs and Symptoms
  1. Symptoms similar to, but milder than acute bacterial prostatitis
  2. Hallmark of disease is relapsing UTI due to same pathogen found in prostatic secretions
  3. Urinary frequency, dysuria, decreased flow, hesitancy, dribbling
  4. Vague lower abdominal pain
  5. Lumbar and perineal pain
  6. Fever and urethral discharge uncommon
  7. May experience swelling and severe tenderness of scrotum
- Differential Diagnosis: Same as acute bacterial prostatitis
- Physical Findings
  1. May involve scrotal contents, producing intense local discomfort, swelling, erythema, and severe tenderness to palpation
  2. Prostate may be tender, irregularly indurated, or boggy
- Diagnostic Tests/Findings: Diagnosis made by examination of EPS and quantitative bacterial cultures
  1. EPS—abnormal if greater than 10 WBC/HPF
  2. More than 1 or 2 lipid-laden macrophages/HPF—abnormal
  3. EPS culture—positive

- Management/Treatment

    1. Often difficult to treat

    2. Usual antibiotics—trimethoprim/sulfamethoxazole, carbenicillin, ciprofloxacin, norfloxacin for 4 to 12 weeks

    3. Sitz baths, prostatic massage, intercourse, masturbation

    4. Avoid over-the-counter decongestants if urinary outlet symptoms

Epididymitis

- Definition: An acute intrascrotal infection

- Etiology/Incidence

    1. Caused by infection from bladder urine, the prostate, or an ascending urethral infection

    2. Common affliction of men 35 years and younger; chlamydia usual causative organism for this population (*Neisseria gonorrhoeae* far less common)

    3. Infection in men > 35 years usually arises from bladder bacteriuria secondary to coliform organisms or following instrumentation, catheterization or surgery (prostatectomy)

    4. "Sterile" epididymitis associated with vigorous physical activity is caused by vasal reflux of sterile urine which leads to a chemical inflammation of the epididymis

    5. Epididymitis in boys may indicate underlying congenital anatomic abnormalities (i.e., ectopic ureter, posterior urethral valve)

    6. Condition is usually unilateral

    7. Epididymitis may be complicated by development of testicular necrosis, testicular atrophy or infertility

- Signs and Symptoms

    1. Painful, scrotal swelling (pain may radiate up the spermatic cord into the lower abdomen)

    2. Sensation of scrotal heaviness

    3. Symptoms of prostatitis or UTI may be present

    4. Systemic symptoms may develop—fever, chills and malaise

- Differential Diagnosis

    1. Mumps

    2. Testicular torsion

    3. Testicular abscess

    4. Tumor of testicle with or without hemorrhage

    5. Hydrocele

6. Trauma

7. Infarction

- Physical Findings

    1. Enlarged, tender indurated epididymis

    2. Urethral discharge may be present

    3. Massaging prostate may exacerbate epididymitis

- Diagnostic Tests/Findings

    1. Men

        a. STD testing (chlamydia, gonorrhea and syphilis)

        b. Culture and gram-stained smear of uncentrifuged urine

        c. Scrotal ultrasonography if condition initially severe or if fever continues while on antibiotics (rule out abscess)

        d. CBC—may show increased white blood cell count with left shift

    2. Boys—require more extensive work-up; refer for consult

        a. Intravenous urography

        b. Cystourethroscopy

        c. Voiding cystourethrography

        d. Scrotal ultrasonography (with or without Doppler imaging)

        e. Radionuclide scanning

        f. Surgical exploration may be required

- Management/Treatment

    1. MD referral or consult required if:

        a. Patient is a child

        b. Systemic symptoms of infection (leukocytosis, fever) present in adults; patient should be hospitalized for parenteral antibiotics

        c. Possible torsion of testes

    2. Outpatient therapy

        a. Antibiotic therapy based on patient's age and symptoms

            (1) Adult < 35 years of age—first choice is ceftriaxone 250 mg IM in a single dose plus doxycycline 100 mg orally b.i.d.; alternative choice for men 17 years of age or older is ofloxacin 200 to 400 mg orally b.i.d. for 10 days

(2) Adult > 35 years of age—trimethoprim/sulfamethoxazole one double-strength tablet orally b.i.d. or ciprofloxacin 250 mg orally b.i.d. for 10 days; treat for 4 weeks if underlying prostatitis present

  b. Scrotal elevation, support and bed rest

  c. Analgesics—nonsteroidal anti-inflammatory agents

  d. Ice (early), heat (late)

  e. Spermatic cord block with lidocaine may be used

3. Follow-up within 48 hours if symptoms persist or worsen

4. If STD present or suspected, instruct patient to refer sex partners for evaluation and treatment

5. Discuss therapeutic and diagnostic plans

6. Emphasize importance of complete treatment

7. Avoid sexual intercourse until course of antibiotics completed

8. Inform patient that swelling and discomfort may persist for weeks or months after eradication of infecting organism; epididymis may remain enlarged or indurated indefinitely

9. Educate regarding prevention, transmission and treatment of sexually transmitted disease (if causative agent); encourage continued use of condoms

10. Encourage patient to discuss concerns and/or fears

Benign Prostatic Hyperplasia (BPH)

- Definition: Progressive, benign hyperplasia of prostate gland tissue

- Etiology/Incidence

  1. Cause is uncertain

  2. Approximately 50% of men have BPH by age 60; incidence increases to 90% by age 85

  3. The most common cause of bladder outlet obstruction in males > 50 years

  4. Symptoms are attributed to mechanical obstruction of the urethra by the enlarged prostate gland

- Signs and Symptoms

  1. Frequency, urgency, urge incontinence

  2. Nocturia, dysuria

  3. Weak urinary stream, dribbling, hesitancy

  4. Sensation of full bladder immediately after voiding

  5. Retention

- Differential Diagnosis
    1. Urethral stricture
    2. Prostate or bladder cancer
    3. Neurogenic bladder
    4. Bladder calculus
    5. Acute or chronic prostatitis
    6. Bladder neck contracture
    7. Medications that affect micturition
- Physical Findings
    1. Abdomen—may have distended bladder secondary to retention
    2. Prostate (patient should void prior to examination)
        a. Nontender with asymmetrical or symmetrical enlargement; gross enlargement atypical
        b. Consistency is smooth and rubbery (consistency of a pencil eraser)
        c. Distinct nodules (spheroids) may be present—differentiation between BPH nodules and cancerous ones is based on induration or firmness of gland; may require biopsy
- Diagnostic Tests/Findings
    1. Urinalysis—NO hematuria or urinary tract infection
    2. Urinary flow rate—voided volume and peak urinary flow rate (uroflowmetry) tests prostatic obstruction
    3. Abdominal ultrasound—rules out associated upper tract pathology
    4. Serum creatinine and BUN—normal
    5. Prostate-specific antigen (PSA) levels should be normal
- Management/Treatment
    1. Observation
    2. Urology consult required for pharmacologic, mechanical, or surgical treatments
    3. Pharmacologic—drugs selected that reduce bulk and/or tone of gland
        a. Terazosin—1 mg orally at bedtime, increase up to 10 mg at bedtime
        b. Prazosin—1 mg orally b.i.d. to t.i.d.; increase up to 6 to 15 mg per day
        c. Doxazosin—1 mg orally every day up to 16 mg if required
        d. Finasteride—5 mg orally daily
        e. Tamsulosin—0.4 mg orally daily

4. Mechanical—balloon dilation of prostatic urethra

5. Surgery—indications

    a. Acute urinary retention (urgent urology referral)

    b. Gross hematuria

    c. Epididymitis (especially if recurrent)

    d. Recurrent urinary tract infections

    e. Renal failure from obstruction

    f. Intolerable chronic symptoms

6. Discuss therapeutic and diagnostic plans

7. Educate regarding signs/symptoms of urinary retention, renal failure and epididymitis

8. Emphasize importance of follow-up appointments

9. Avoid caffeine and alcohol to decrease bladder irritation

10. Avoid decongestants, antihistamines, tricyclic antidepressants, anticholinergics

Prostate Cancer

- Definition: A malignant neoplasm of the prostate gland

- Etiology/Incidence

  1. Etiology is unknown; environmental factors may be involved; adenocarcinoma is most common type

  2. Most common malignancy in American men and second most common cause of cancer deaths in men over 65

  3. The relative survival rates have improved over the past 30 years (due to increased awareness and early detection, rather than improved therapy)

  4. May be associated with high-fat diet

  5. Risk factors—family history, age, African-American

- Signs and Symptoms

  1. Many patients are asymptomatic

  2. Symptoms may mimic BPH with frequency, dribbling, nocturia, hesitancy

  3. Occasionally bone pain from metastases (advanced stage)

  4. Occasionally symptoms of uremia due to urethral obstructions (advanced stage)

- Differential Diagnosis

  1. BPH, urethral stricture

  2. Bladder cancer

    3.   Neurogenic bladder

    4.   Bladder calculus

    5.   Acute/chronic prostatitis

    6.   Bladder neck contracture

    7.   Medications that affect micturition

- Physical Findings

    1.   May present with lymphadenopathy, signs of uremia, or urinary retention with distended bladder

    2.   More common physical findings are confined to prostate—on rectal examination prostate feels harder than normal and normal boundaries of gland may be obscured; nodules may be present

    3.   Prostate may have asymmetric enlargement

- Diagnostic Tests/Findings (performed by consultant M.D.)

    1.   Transperineal or transrectal needle biopsy of prostate—diagnostic accuracy rate > 90%

    2.   PSA levels between 4 to 10 ng/mL may indicate BPH, levels > 10 ng/mL are suggestive of carcinoma; false negatives occur

    3.   Transrectal ultrasound can aid in identification of solid nodules and is used to guide biopsy

    4.   Other tests such as bone scans may be conducted

- Management/Treatment

    1.   Consult/referral required

    2.   Treatment predicated largely on stage of tumor; accurate staging is therefore essential

    3.   Methods of treatment include surgery, radiation, hormonal therapy

    4.   Assistance as appropriate in meeting physical, psychological, social, cultural, environmental and spiritual needs

    5.   Emphasize importance of follow-up appointments

Fibrocystic Breast Changes

- Definition: Benign breast condition characterized by increased growth of fibrous tissue, proliferation of the ductal epithelial lining and/or formation of cysts

- Etiology/Incidence

    1.   Cause is unknown, estrogen dependency is suspected; condition occurs clinically in 50% and histologically in 90% of women

    2.   Three types of fibrocystic changes have been identified

    a. Nonproliferative lesions—most common type; no increased risk of breast cancer

    b. Proliferative lesions without atypia—minimal increased risk of breast cancer

    c. Cellular atypia—five-fold increased risk of breast cancer

3. May be related to dietary intake of methylxanthines, e.g. coffee, chocolate (inconclusive)

- Signs and Symptoms (more pronounced premenstrually)

1. Cyclic breast tenderness, engorgement, increased density, increased nodularity, enlargement of cystic lump(s)

2. Nipple discharge may be present

3. Symptoms of discomfort decrease after menopause

- Differential Diagnosis

1. Fibroadenosis

2. Fat necrosis

3. Fibroadenoma

4. Carcinoma (especially in women > 40 years)

5. Breast cysts

- Physical Findings

1. Skin and contour usually normal

2. Mass or thickened area present

    a. Location—upper outer quadrant or any area

    b. Size—varies

    c. Shape—round, oval or nodular

    d. Mobility—mobile

    e. Consistency—soft to firm (depends on tension of fluid within cysts)

    f. Number—solitary or multiple (may give impression of "beads on a string")

    g. Nipple—clear/serous discharge may be present (rare)

- Diagnostic Tests/Findings

1. Fine needle aspiration (FNA)—fluid should return if cyst

2. Excisional biopsy (most definitive test)—no cancer cells

3. Mammography—negative (for women > 35 years)

4. Ultrasound—distinguishes cyst vs. solid mass

- Management/Treatment
    1. Warm compresses applied t.i.d.; supportive brassiere
    2. Low-salt diet; diuretics may also be given premenstrually
    3. Elimination of dietary methylxanthines (coffee, tea, colas, chocolate) (inconclusive) and tobacco use
    4. Vitamin E—400 to 600 international units orally daily
    5. Vitamin B_6—50 to 100 mg daily
    6. Evening primrose oil 1000 mg/day (Pizzomo & Murray, 1999)
    7. Hormonal and anti-hormonal therapy are controversial; the following agents may be used in severe cases
        a. Oral contraceptives—low estrogen with relatively high progesterone
        b. Danazol
        c. Bromocriptine
        d. Tamoxifen
    8. Surgical excision is controversial
    9. Discussion of diagnostic and therapeutic plans
    10. Reassurance of low risk for malignancy
    11. Instruction and demonstration of breast self-examination
    12. Encouragement to report any new mass that does not resolve following menstruation
    13. At follow-up, assess for progression of condition and/or concurrent malignancy

Breast Cancer

- Definition: A malignant neoplasm of the breast
- Etiology/Incidence
    1. Most common cancer in women; second leading cause of death from cancer in women
    2. Frequency increases steadily after age 35
    3. 12% of women will develop breast cancer in the U.S.
    4. Whites have higher incidence than nonwhites in U.S.
    5. Approximately 182,000 new cases occur annually
    6. Risk factors include:
        a. Increasing age
        b. Postmenopausal long-term estrogen therapy—conflicting data

    c.   Nulliparity

    d.   Late first pregnancy (over age 30)

    e.   Early menarche and late menopause after age 55

    f.   Cellular atypia

    g.   Previous endometrial cancer

    h.   Alcohol intake

    i.   High fat diet (polyunsaturated)

    j.   Obesity

7. Patients with higher risk:

    a.   Positive family history (premenopausal more significant)

    b.   Family history suggestive of an inherited predisposition to breast cancer

    c.   Confirmation of an inherited mutation (BRCA, or $BRCA_2$) on a breast cancer susceptibility gene

    d.   Prior personal history of breast cancer

    e.   Fibrocystic changes associated with cellular atypia

- Signs and Symptoms

  1. Often asymptomatic

  2. Single, firm, nontender, painless mass is usual presenting sign

  3. Later manifestations

         a.   Skin erythema, dimpling, ulceration

         b.   Breast pain

         c.   Nipple retraction, eczema, or ulceration

         d.   Nipple discharge

- Differential Diagnosis

  1. Fibrocystic breast changes

  2. Fibroadenoma

  3. Intraductal papilloma

  4. Lipoma

  5. Fat necrosis

  6. Mastitis

  7. Dermatitis (Paget's disease)

- Physical Findings

1. Most common manifestation is single, firm, nontender, ill-defined lump in breast; associated findings may include:

    a. Diffuse nodularity

    b. Skin dimpling

    c. Nipple retraction, discharge (usually bloody)

    d. Lymphadenopathy

    e. Ulcerated/fungating mass (rare)

    f. Palpable supraclavicular and/or axillary lymph nodes

2. Inflammatory cancer—skin erythema/edema, pain

3. Paget's disease

    a. Associated with about 5% of mammary carcinomas

    b. Nipple erosion, crusting, bloody discharge

    c. Eczema-like change in skin

- Diagnostic Tests/Findings

    1. Mammography—mass or calcifications indicated; may be negative since 10% of palpable masses are missed on mammogram

    2. Ultrasound—distinguishes cyst vs. solid mass

    3. FNA cytology—fluid vs solid mass, 10% false-negative

    4. Large-needle (core needle) biopsy—histological examination reveals cancer cells (problems with sampling occur)

    5. Excisional biopsy—most reliable diagnostic test where staging of the tumor is done

    6. Determination of hormone receptor tumor cells

    7. Various tests may be conducted if metastasis is suspected including bone and organ scans

- Management/Treatment

    1. Referral to an oncology team is required

    2. Dependent upon tumor stage, presence of hormone receptors and patient's symptoms/preferences

    3. May include surgery, chemotherapy, radiation therapy and/or hormonal therapy

    4. Discussion of diagnostic and therapeutic plans

    5. Encouragement to express concerns and fears

    6. Education and demonstration of breast self-examination to patient and family members, especially daughters

    7. Encouragement to report new mass or changes

8. Assistance, as appropriate, in meeting physical, psychological, sexual, social, cultural, environmental and spiritual needs

9. Emphasis on importance of maintaining follow-up with specialists and primary care providers

Dysfunctional Uterine Bleeding (DUB)

- Definition: Excessive, abnormal uterine bleeding, that occurs at irregular intervals, with no demonstrable organic cause

- Etiology/Incidence

    1. Usually results from irregular sloughing of endometrium during anovulatory cycles (90% of cases); but occasionally occurs with poor quality ovulatory cycles

    2. Most frequently due to abnormalities of endocrine function

    3. Estrogen withdrawal or estrogen breakthrough bleeding

    4. Progesterone breakthrough bleeding—continuous low-dose contraceptives

    5. Heaviest bleeding due to high sustained levels of estrogen and seen with:

        a. Polycystic ovarian disease

        b. Obesity

        c. Immaturity of the hypothalamic-pituitary-ovarian axis (postmenarchal teenagers)

        d. Late ovulations (perimenopausal women)

        e. Unopposed estrogen replacement therapy

    6. Not related to oral contraceptive use

- Signs and Symptoms

    1. A carefully obtained history and character of bleeding pattern is critical to assist in ruling-out other conditions

    2. Bleeding is usually characterized by one or more of the following

        a. Persistent or intermittent uterine bleeding

        b. Episodes of extremely heavy bleeding

        c. Oligomenorrhea

    3. DUB bleeding patterns

        a. Intermenstrual bleeding—variable amounts of bleeding that occur between regular menstrual periods

        b. Menometrorrhagia—prolonged, frequent, excessive uterine bleeding that occurs at irregular intervals

        c. Menorrhagia (hypermenorrhea)—prolonged (> 7 days) and excessive (> 80 mL) uterine bleeding occurring at regular intervals

     d.   Metrorrhagia—uterine bleeding between normal cycle

     e.   Polymenorrhea—frequent, irregular bleeding < 18 day intervals

     f.   Oligomenorrhea—infrequent, irregular uterine bleeding that occurs at intervals > 40 days

- Differential Diagnosis

    1. *Inappropriate* to assume that abnormal uterine bleeding is endocrine in origin; other conditions must be ruled-out according to reproductive age

    2. Adolescents

        a.   Vaginal trauma secondary to athletics or early sexual exposure

        b.   Hypothalamic-pituitary dysfunction secondary to exercise

        c.   Pregnancy

        d.   Genital infection

        e.   Oral contraceptive use/misuse

        f.   Blood dyscrasias

    3. Women in reproductive years

        a.   Previously noted causes

        b.   Endocrine-related anovulatory abnormal uterine bleeding, common with exercise

        c.   Organic pathology

            (1)   Uterine fibroids

            (2)   Endometrial polyps

            (3)   Chronic systemic illness, e.g., liver cirrhosis, renal failure

        d.   Neoplasia

        e.   Secondary to stress

        f.   Excessive weight change

    4. Perimenopausal women

        a.   Previously listed causes

        b.   Follicular dysfunction (predominant cause)

    5. Postmenopausal women

        a.   Previously noted causes

        b.   Hormone replacement therapy

        c.   Cancer

- Physical Findings

1. A thorough general and pelvic examination should be performed to assist in ruling out conditions included in the differential diagnosis; source of bleeding must be determined

2. For DUB, the examination may be essentially negative, or an adnexal mass may indicate polycystic ovaries or other pathology

- Diagnostic Tests/Findings

    1. Of secondary importance and usually only substantiates a diagnosis already determined by history and physical examination findings

    2. Three most important initial tests

        a. Pregnancy test (quantitative Beta hCG)

        b. Prolactin determination (hyperprolactinemia may initially present as ovulatory dysfunction or anovulation and abnormal uterine bleeding)—may be elevated after breast examination

        c. Thyroid stimulating hormone (TSH)

    3. Additional initial tests should include:

        a. Follicle stimulating hormone (FSH) and luteinizing hormone (LH)

        b. Complete blood count, blood smear, platelet count

        c. Cervical Pap smear

        d. STD screening tests

    4. Additional tests may be done to rule out other conditions as indicated by the history and physical examination, such as:

        a. Coagulation profile

        b. Serum iron studies if anemic

        c. Pelvic ultrasound

    5. Tests more important in older women

        a. Endometrial biopsy

        b. D & C

- Management/Treatment

    1. Should be considered according to amount of blood loss and with an age-related perspective

    2. Medical consult may be required

    3. Arrest of heavy acute or prolonged bleeding may require intravenous conjugated estrogens followed by combined oral contraceptives or medroxyprogesterone acetate to prevent recurrence

    4. Induction of ovulation is reserved for those desiring pregnancy (use of clomiphene citrate)

5. Iron supplementation if indicated

6. Patient should maintain a basal body temperature chart and record symptoms during cycles

7. Instruction regarding basal body temperature monitoring

8. Discussion of therapeutic and diagnostic plans

9. Review of emergency instructions for acute, heavy bleeding

10. Review of nutritional requirements and encourage intake of iron-rich foods

11. Encouragement of expression of concerns and fears

12. Emphasis on importance of maintaining follow-up

Endometriosis

- Definition: Presence of endometrial glands and stroma outside the endometrial cavity and uterine musculature

- Etiology/Incidence

    1. Etiology is unknown, theories include:

        a. Familial tendency, seven fold increase if first degree female relative

        b. Retrograde menstruation

        c. Metaplastic transformation of epithelium to endometrial tissue at extrapelvic sites

        d. Spread of endometrial tissue through lymphatic and vascular channels

    2. Estimated to affect 5 to 20% of all women of reproductive age

    3. Median age at diagnosis 29 years

- Signs and Symptoms

    1. Presence and severity of symptoms correlate poorly with degree of disease

    2. Pain (most common complaint)

        a. Cyclic pelvic pain due to blood and menstrual debris in surrounding tissues

        b. Constant pain with secondary dysmenorrhea

        c. Pelvic heaviness

        d. Chronic pelvic pain

    3. Dysmenorrhea, primary or secondary

    4. Dyspareunia from fixed uterine retroversion

    5. Infertility

    6. Menstrual irregularities, especially premenstrual spotting

- Differential Diagnosis

1. Chronic pelvic inflammatory disease

2. Pelvic adhesions

3. Ovarian cyst or tumors

- Physical Findings

    1. Uterosacral ligament nodularity and/or tenderness

    2. Fixed uterine retroversion

    3. Adnexal enlargement and/or tenderness

    4. Endometrioma

    5. Tenderness in vaginal cul de sac or cervical motion tenderness

- Diagnostic Tests

    1. Visualization of disease by laparoscope gold standard "powder burn lesions"

    2. Ultrasound—detection of endometrioma (cannot be used as specific test of endometriosis)

    3. Cancer antigen-125 (CA-125)—chemical marker and noninvasive test; of limited value in following course of disease and response to treatment (Mishell, Stenchever, Droëgemueller and Herbst, 1997)

- Management/Treatment (since condition is chronic and recurrent, long-term integrative care is required)

    1. Medication:

        a. Combined low-estrogen monophasic oral contraceptive pills taken continuously to produce amenorrhea

        b. Non-steroidal anti-inflammatory medications for pain relief

        c. Medroxyprogesterone acetate (MPA)—30 mg orally daily causes atrophy of endometrial tissue

        d. Depot MPA—100 to 400 mg intramuscularly monthly causes atrophy of endometrial tissue

        e. Danazol—200 to 400 mg orally twice a day creates anovulation and amenorrhea

        f. GnRH agonists—leuprolide acetate 1 mg subcutaneously daily or 3.75 mg (depot) intramuscularly monthly or nafarelin acetate 200 μg intranasally twice a day creates anovulation and amenorrhea

    2. Surgery:

        a. Ablation of endometrial implants laser or electrocautery

        b. Hysterectomy with salpingo-oopherectomy is curative 90%

3. Optimal treatment depends on goal, pain relief or fertility

4. Complications—infertility

Dysplasia—Abnormal Papanicolaou (Pap) Smear Management

- Definition: Squamous intraepithelial lesions (SIL) refers to precancerous cellular development of the cervix (includes mild, moderate and severe dysplasia) and carcinoma in situ (CIS) of the cervix

- Etiology/Incidence

  1. Etiology is most likely related to a sexually transmitted factor; the human papillomavirus (HPV) is suspected to be an initiator of malignant transformation

  2. Suspected HPV co-factors include cigarette smoking and folate deficiency

  3. Major risk factors for cervical cancer

     a. Sexual intercourse prior to age 18

     b. More than three sexual partners in a lifetime

     c. Intercourse with a male who has had multiple sexual partners

     d. Smoking or history of smoking

     e. Presence or history of HPV (types 16, 18, 31, 33, 35, 39, 45, 51 and 52) more commonly associated with high-grade lesions—see section on Genital Warts or Condylomata acuminata

     f. Intercourse with man who has HPV

  4. SIL may persist, spontaneously regress or advance to invasive disease

  5. Globally, carcinoma of the cervix is the most common female malignancy; in the U.S. it ranks as the third most common gynecologic malignancy (behind endometrial and ovarian cancer)

- Cervical Cancer Screening

  1. The Papanicolaou (Pap) smear has reduced disease-related mortality in the U.S. by 50% in the past 40 years

  2. Screening has also increased detection of preinvasive cervical neoplasms including dysplasia and carcinoma in situ (CIS)

  3. 30% of Pap smears may have false-negative results

  4. Risk of invasive cervical cancer significantly increases when screening exceeds 3 year intervals

  5. Recommended screening criteria (U.S. Preventive Task Force)

     a. Initiate at age 18 or at the age of first intercourse

     b. Between the ages of 18 and 65, Pap smears should be repeated every one to three years depending upon patient's risk factors for cervical cancer

c. After age 65

    (1) Routine screening may be discontinued if findings are normal on two consecutive Pap smears

    (2) If abnormal Pap smear, annual screening should occur until two consecutive Pap smears are normal

- Pap smear interpretation: The Bethesda Classification System is most commonly used

  1. Statement on specimen adequacy

    a. Satisfactory for interpretation

    b. Less than optimal

    c. Unsatisfactory

  2. General categorization

    a. Within normal limits

    b. Other

      (1) Infection

      (2) Reactive or reparative changes

      (3) Squamous cell abnormalities

        (a) Atypical—undetermined significance

        (b) Low grade squamous intraepithelial lesion (LSIL)— associated with HPV and/or mild dysplasia (cervical intraepithelial neoplasia 1 (CIN 1)

        (c) High grade squamous intraepithelial lesion (HSIL)—moderate dysplasia (CIN 2), severe dysplasia (CIN 3) or carcinoma in situ (CIS)

        (d) Squamous cell carcinoma

      (4) Glandular cell abnormalities

        (a) Presence of endometrial cells—menstruating or postmenopausal women

        (b) Atypical—undetermined significance (endometrial or endocervical)

        (c) Adenocarcinoma

      (5) Nonepithelial malignant neoplasm

      (6) Hormonal evaluation (vaginal smears only, i.e., hysterectomy)

- Management of Pap smear results

  1. Within normal limits—repeat annually or as indicated according to cervical cancer risk factors and age

2. Infection

   a. Treat based on agent causing inflammation

   b. Repeat Pap smear in one year

3. Reactive or reparative changes

   a. Treat if infectious agent present

   b. May be related to contraceptive mechanical devices (IUD), atrophic changes, chemotherapy and/or radiotherapy etc.

   c. Repeat Pap in 4 to 6 months

4. Atypical squamous cells of undetermined significance (ASCUS)

   a. 10% to 40% risk of SIL and 5% to 10% of these are HSIL

   b. Repeat Pap smear every 4 to 6 months, three times

   c. Colposcopy and cervical biopsies with ECC if HSIL develops or HIV positive

   d. If peri- or postmenopausal, treat with vaginal estrogen cream prior to repeat Pap or colposcopy (even if patient is on HRT)

5. Low and high grade SIL

   a. Colposcopy and cervical biopsies with ECC

   b. Low-grade lesions may be monitored with Pap smears every 6 months for two years if ECC is negative

   c. Common treatments include cryotherapy, large loop excision of transformation zone (LLETZ), laser vaporization

   d. Referral to M.D. specialist if carcinoma in situ present

6. Squamous cell carcinoma, adenocarcinoma and other epithelial or nonepithelial malignant neoplasm—refer to M.D. specialist

7. Hormonal evaluation—treat atrophic changes if present (see Pregnancy, Contraception, Menopause chapter)

8. Discuss therapeutic and diagnostic plans along with common complications of treatment

9. Emphasize importance of regular screening

10. Review patient's individual risk factors as appropriate

11. Educate regarding recommended management and treatment as appropriate

12. Encourage patient to discuss concerns and/or fears

Amenorrhea

- Definition

   1. Primary amenorrhea—absence of normal spontaneous menstrual period by age 16

2. Secondary amenorrhea—cessation of menses after a variable period of normal function, usually 3 to 6 consecutive cycles

- Etiology—potential underlying conditions
  1. Primary amenorrhea
     a. Hypergonadotropic hypogonadism
     b. Turner's syndrome (gonadal dysgenesis)
     c. Severe malnutrition
     d. Pituitary tumors
     e. Head trauma
     f. Encephalitis
     g. Uterine malformations, congenital absence of uterus
     h. Imperforate hymen, cervical stenosis
     i. Androgen insensitivity
     j. Polycystic ovaries
  2. Secondary amenorrhea
     a. Pregnancy (most common cause)
     b. Oral contraceptives
     c. Menopause
     d. Emotional stress
     e. Malnutrition
     f. Excessive exercise
     g. Lactation
     h. Hyperprolactinemia (pituitary tumor)
     i. Anorexia/obesity
     j. Drug use
     k. Polycystic ovaries, anovulation
     l. Hypothalamic suppression
     m. Hyper and hypothyroidism
     n. Addison's disease
     o. Cervical stenosis

- Signs and Symptoms
  1. Primary amenorrhea
     a. Absence of menarche

    b.   Failure to develop pubic hair and other secondary sex characteristics may or may not occur

    c.   Abnormal growth and development may be present

    d.   Normal breast development may or may not occur

    e.   Patient symptoms are dependent upon the etiology of the amenorrheic condition

  2. Secondary amenorrhea

    a.   Absence of menses at expected time intervals

    b.   Previous regular menses

- Differential Diagnosis

  1. First, rule out pregnancy

  2. All the potential underlying conditions listed under etiology should be considered in the differential diagnosis

  3. A thorough and complete history/physical examination, with supplemental diagnostic/laboratory testing will assist in ruling out unrelated etiologies

- Physical Findings

  1. A thorough general and pelvic examination should be performed, partially directed by the history

  2. Findings will be related to the underlying etiology

  3. The examination may be essentially negative if the amenorrhea is secondary to such conditions as oral contraceptive use or unreported emotional stress

- Diagnostic Tests/Findings

  1. Primary amenorrhea—refer to endocrinologist if suspected

  2. Secondary amenorrhea

    a.   Pregnancy test (quantitative Beta hCG)—initial test

    b.   Prolactin (if negative pregnancy test), FSH, LH

      (1) Elevated prolactin—rule out micro and macroadenomas with CT scan of sella turcica

      (2) MD consult may be required if prolactin, FSH or LH elevated

    c.   Progestin challenge test

    d.   TSH

      (1) Elevated TSH—hypothyroid

      (2) Normal TSH—rule out pituitary adenoma

    e.   Cervical Pap smear

  f. STD screening tests

  g. Urinalysis

 3. Additional tests may be done to rule out other conditions as indicated by the history and physical examination

- Management/Treatment

 1. Dependent upon underlying etiology

 2. Medical consult is often required

 3. Discuss therapeutic and diagnostic plans

 4. Encourage expression of concerns and fears

 5. Emphasize importance of maintaining follow-up

Dysmenorrhea

- Definition: Crampy pain that occurs prior to or during menses, often with a constellation of other symptoms

 1. Primary—usually begins in women under 20 years; related to menses with no other organic cause

 2. Secondary—usually occurs after age 20 in women with pelvic pathology or IUD use

- Etiology/Incidence

 1. Primary—probably the result of excessive uterine prostaglandin production; usually appears shortly after onset of ovulatory cycles; affects approximately 50% or more of all menstruating females

 2. Secondary—usually occurs in the presence of organic disease, e.g., endometriosis, pelvic adhesions, adenomyosis, cervical stenosis, uterine fibroids, chronic pelvic infection or with the use of an IUD

- Signs and Symptoms

 1. Primary

  a. Pain usually crampy in nature, may radiate to back, thighs and lower abdomen

  b. May also have other symptoms, e.g., nausea, vomiting, diarrhea, headache, fatigue

  c. Usually begins at onset of menstruation or several hours before; duration is usually 48 to 72 hours

 2. Secondary

  a. Signs and symptoms associated with organic disease listed under Etiology/Incidence

  b. Pain occurs at any point in cycle

c. Associated symptoms may include dyspareunia, infertility and abnormal bleeding

- Differential Diagnosis

    1. Differentiation between primary and secondary dysmenorrhea

    2. Rule out secondary pathologic conditions as noted under Etiology/Incidence

- Physical Findings

    1. Primary—usually no significant physical findings; uterine corpus may be tender during menstruation; no pelvic masses or uterine fixation

    2. Secondary—findings associated with organic disease

- Diagnostic Tests/Findings

    1. Primary—usually none, but if diagnosis unclear, CBC, erythrocyte sedimentation rate and genital culture for pathogens

    2. Secondary—tests related to suspected organic pathology; may include pelvic ultrasound, hysterosalpingogram, laparoscopy, hysteroscopy or dilatation and curretage

- Management/Treatment

    1. Primary

        a. Prostaglandin synthetase inhibitors (PGSI), e.g., naproxen, indomethacin, mefenamic acid, ibuprofen

        b. Oral contraceptives for sexually active individuals

        c. Moderate exercise on a regular basis

        d. Diet high in whole grains, beans, vegetables, fruit

        e. Elimination of or decreased salt, sugar, caffeine

    2. Secondary—treatment related to organic pathology

Premenstrual Syndrome (PMS)

- Definition: A group of somatic and affective symptoms occurring during the luteal phase of the menstrual cycle, decreasing shortly after onset of menstruation

- Etiology/Incidence

    1. Exact cause unknown

    2. Postulated etiologic factors include insufficient progesterone, fluid retention, nutritional problems, glucose metabolism disorders, vitamin deficiencies, ovarian infections, altered serotonin, endorphin levels; elevated prolactin levels

    3. Peak prevalence in the thirties with a decline noted in the forties

    4. Incidence ranges from 5% to 95%; generally agreed about 40% of women are significantly affected at one time or another; only 2% to 3% of women of childbearing age suffer severe symptoms

5. Most women experience some physical and emotional changes before onset of menstrual flow

- Signs and Symptoms
    1. Bloated feeling, feeling of weight increase
    2. Breast pain or tenderness
    3. Skin disorders
    4. Hot flushes
    5. Headache
    6. Pelvic pain
    7. Change in bowel habits
    8. Irritability, aggression, tension, anxiety, depression, crying, lethargy
    9. Insomnia, fatigue
    10. Change in appetite, thirst
    11. Change in libido
    12. Loss of concentration
    13. Poor coordination, clumsiness, accidents
- Differential Diagnosis
    1. Depression
    2. Anxiety disorders
    3. Marital discord
    4. Substance abuse
    5. Thyroid disease
    6. Impaired glucose tolerance or diabetes
    7. Early menopause
- Physical Findings
    1. Because etiology is still unknown, diagnosis is made by history
    2. Complete history and physical examination should be conducted to rule out any medical problems that could be influencing symptomatology
- Diagnostic Tests/Findings
    1. Thyroid profile
    2. Fasting blood sugar
    3. FSH, LH (if early menopause suspected)
- Management/Treatment

1. Exercise 3 to 4 times per week, especially during luteal phase

2. Appropriate diet with reasonable amounts of protein (from fish and poultry rather than red meats), vegetables, and fruit

3. Elimination of tobacco, alcohol, caffeine

4. Pyridoxine, multiple vitamins

5. Diuretics, if fluid retention predominates

6. Progesterone is controversial; in several studies no more effective than placebo

7. Prostaglandin inhibitors, e.g., mefenamic acid, naproxen sodium

8. Oral contraceptives

9. Danazol

10. Bromocriptine

11. PMS support group referral

12. Fluoxetine hydrochloride or alprazolam for severe cases

Questions
Select the best answer

1. Which of the following statements regarding AIDS is incorrect?

    a. Most diagnoses are made in persons 20 to 49 years old
    b. Over 1.5 million Americans are infected with HIV
    c. HIV is transmitted through casual kissing
    d. The EIA is a screening test

2. During the acute phase of HIV infection (first 2 to 8 weeks) which of the following symptoms may be present?

    a. Rash
    b. Shingles
    c. Persistant dermatitis
    d. Pulmonary symptoms

3. Which of the following is not considered in a HIV treatment program?

    a. Zidovudine (AZT)
    b. Didanosine (ddI)
    c. Nutritious diet and stress management
    d. Acyclovir

4. Which of the following may not develop with AIDS?

    a. Kaposi's sarcoma
    b. Cytomegalovirus
    c. Wasting syndrome
    d. Prostatic hypertrophy

5. Which of the following is a diagnostic test for gonorrhea?

    a. Western blot assay
    b. VDRL
    c. Wet prep with WBC
    d. Culture of endocervix on Thayer-Martin media

6. Which of the following is not a correct statement regarding *Neisseria gonorrhoeae?*

    a. One of the leading causes of infertility among U.S. females
    b. The majority of male patients are asymptomatic
    c. P.I.D. is a possible complication
    d. Incubation period is usually 3 to 10 days

7. Which of the following is not recommended for the treatment of gonorrhea?

    a. Ceftriaxone
    b. Ciprofloxacin

    c. Acyclovir
    d. Ofloxacin

8. The most common serious gonococcal complication that occurs in women is:

    a. PID
    b. Cervicitis
    c. Arthritis
    d. Conjunctivitis

9. The most common sexually transmitted disease in the U.S. is:

    a. Gonorrhea
    b. Syphilis
    c. Chlamydia
    d. Herpes

10. The causative organism of chlamydia is:

    a. *Chlamydia coli*
    b. *Chlamydia megalovirus*
    c. *Chlamydia trachomatis*
    d. *Chlamydia hominos*

11. A 20-year-old female presents to your clinic with dysuria, dyspareunia, mucopurulent discharge. She reports that her boyfriend was recently treated for nongonococcal urethritis, what STD has she most probably been exposed to?

    a. Gonorrhea
    b. HPV
    c. Chlamydia
    d. Trichomonas

12. Which of the following is a diagnostic test for chlamydia?

    a. Culture of endocervical smear on Thayer-Martin
    b. Tissue culture
    c. RPR
    d. VDRL

13. Which of the following does not apply to syphilis?

    a. It cannot be transmitted via the placenta
    b. Incidence has steadily declined since 1990
    c. Risk of contraction through sexual intercourse approaches 50%
    d. It can affect any organ or tissue in the body

14. Which of the following is not a characteristic of secondary syphilis?

    a. Skin rash

b. Arthralgias

c. Chancre

d. Malaise

15. The treatment of choice for a 32-year-old male with early syphilis who is allergic to penicillin is:

    a. Ciprofloxacin
    b. Doxycycline
    c. Erythromycin
    d. Amoxicillin/clavulanate

16. A 38-year-old female presents to your clinic with meningeal symptoms; what stage of syphilis must you rule-out?

    a. Primary
    b. Secondary
    c. Latent
    d. Any stage

17. One of the definitive methods of diagnosis of early syphilis is:

    a. FTA-ABS
    b. Darkfield microscopy
    c. VDRL
    d. MHA-TP

18. A 24-year-old female seen in your clinic has been diagnosed with urethral strictures. What STD is probably included in her past history?

    a. Chlamydia
    b. Herpes genitalis
    c. Syphilis
    d. HPV

19. Which of the following statements regarding herpes genitalis is not true?

    a. Causative agent is a virus
    b. Genital lesions are painless
    c. Infection during pregnancy can lead to spontaneous abortion
    d. Treatment focuses on relieving symptoms

20. The most common symptomatic STD in the U.S. is:

    a. Gonorrhea
    b. Chlamydia
    c. Genital warts (HPV)
    d. Herpes genitalis

21. Which of the following statements regarding genital warts is incorrect?

a. More than 30 types of HPV cause genital warts
b. Increased risk of developing cervical, penile and vulvar cancer
c. Lesions on the vulva, cervix and penis are treated with TCA
d. RPR aids in diagnosing cervical lesions

22. All of the following conditions are included in the differential diagnosis for PID except:

    a. Enteritis
    b. Appendicitis
    c. Degeneration of a myoma
    d. Cholecystitis

23. After an initial case of PID, a woman is more susceptible to experience:

    a. Multiple births
    b. Dysmenorrhea
    c. Twisted ovarian cysts
    d. Infertility

24. Which of the following is not found in P.I.D.?

    a. Direct abdominal tenderness
    b. Cervical motion tenderness
    c. Vulvovaginal tenderness
    d. Adnexal tenderness

25. A 22-year-old female seen in your clinic has the following signs and symptoms—malodorous, greenish discharge, perineal itching, red macular cervical lesions, and a vaginal pH of 5.0 to 7.0. What type of vulvovaginitis does she probably have?

    a. Candidiasis
    b. Gardnerella
    c. Bacterial vaginosis
    d. Trichomoniasis

26. Which of the following is not related to bacterial vaginosis?

    a. Multiple bacterial causative agents
    b. ''Curdy'' white discharge
    c. Positive ''whiff test''
    d. Metronidazole is a treatment of choice

27. A classic description of the discharge associated with candida vaginitis is:

    a. ''Cottage-cheese''
    b. ''Fishy'' odor
    c. Green, frothy
    d. Nonpruritic

28. One of the most common causative organisms of UTI in women is:

a. Klebsiella

b. Beta-hemolytic streptococci

c. Chlamydia

d. *E. coli*

29. Which of the following statements regarding UTI is not relevant?

    a. 30 to 40% of women will experience at least 1 UTI in life-time
    b. Men with UTI should be referred to a urologist
    c. Condom use by sex partner is a contributing factor in women
    d. Prostatitis is a contributing factor in men

30. Which of the following is not a characteristic sign or symptom associated with a UTI:

    a. Fever
    b. Pyuria
    c. Urgency
    d. Negative CVA tenderness

31. Which of the following activities is contraindicated in a patient with suspected acute bacterial prostatitis?

    a. Ejaculation
    b. Urinary catheterization
    c. Prostate examination
    d. Masturbation

32. The drug of choice for a 40-year-old, monogamous male with prostatitis is:

    a. Ciprofloxacin
    b. Doxycycline
    c. TMP/SMX
    d. Carbenicillin

33. Which of the following statements regarding BPH is incorrect?

    a. 90% of men by 85 years of age have BPH
    b. BPH often leads to bladder outlet obstruction
    c. Drugs to reduce bulk of gland may be prescribed
    d. Upon palpation, the prostate surface is roughened

34. The most common type of prostate cancer is:

    a. Adenocarcinoma
    b. Squamous cell
    c. Lymphoma
    d. Sarcoma

35. What is the most common physical finding associated with prostate cancer?

    a. Boggy prostate
    b. Tender prostate
    c. Enlarged, smooth prostate
    d. Hard, nodular prostate

36. Which of the following statements regarding prostate cancer is incorrect?

    a. The largest cancer mortality rate in men over 65 years of age
    b. Relative survival rates have improved over the past 30 years
    c. Prostate-specific antigen is used as a laboratory marker
    d. Bladder calculus is considered in the differential diagnosis

37. The type of fibrocystic breast change that has been associated with malignancy is:

    a. Proliferative changes without atypia
    b. Nonproliferative changes
    c. Cellular atypia
    d. Dysplasia

38. What diagnostic test is most definitive in diagnosing fibrocystic changes?

    a. Mammography
    b. Fine needle aspiration
    c. Excisional biopsy
    d. Ultrasound

39. A 30-year-old woman is diagnosed with fibrocystic breast changes in your office. All of the following components may be included in the treatment plan except:

    a. Yearly mammograms starting now
    b. Low-salt diet
    c. Limited consumption of caffeine
    d. Oral contraceptives

40. The most common cancer in women is:

    a. Cervical
    b. Breast
    c. Ovarian
    d. Endometrial

41. Which of the following is not considered a risk factor for breast cancer?

    a. Nulliparity
    b. Alcohol intake
    c. Positive family history
    d. Late menarche and early menopause

42. Which description is most characteristic of breast cancer?

   a. Single, firm, non-tender, ill-defined breast lump
   b. Multiple, firm, non-tender, ill-defined breast lumps
   c. Single, firm, tender, circumscribed breast lump
   d. Single, rubbery, non-tender, circumscribed breast lump

43. Which of the following does not apply to breast cancer?

   a. 10% of palpable masses are missed on mammography
   b. Core needle biopsy is the most reliable diagnostic test
   c. Paget's disease affects the nipple
   d. Inflammatory breast cancer may be painful

44. Dysfunctional uterine bleeding is most often (90%) associated with:

   a. Polycystic ovaries
   b. Ovulatory cycles
   c. Anovulatory cycles
   d. Late ovulation

45. Menorrhagia refers to:

   a. Uterine bleeding that occurs at regular intervals < 21 days apart
   b. Prolonged and excessive uterine bleeding occurring at regular intervals
   c. Infrequent uterine bleeding that occurs at intervals > 40 days apart
   d. Uterine bleeding that occurs at irregular but frequent intervals

46. Which of the following is least likely to be included in the differential diagnosis of dysfunctional uterine bleeding for a perimenopausal women?

   a. Neoplasia
   b. Blood dyscrasias
   c. Pregnancy
   d. Vaginal trauma

47. Which one of the following characteristics is not associated with primary amenorrhea?

   a. Irregular menses
   b. Absence of menarche
   c. Lack of pubic hair
   d. Abnormal growth and development

48. The most common cause of secondary amenorrhea is:

   a. Oral contraceptives
   b. Polycystic ovaries
   c. Pregnancy
   d. Anovulation

49. What is the first test that should be ordered in a woman who presents with secondary amenorrhea?

a. Thyroid profile
b. Prolactin
c. Pregnancy test
d. Progestin challenge

50. Which of the following does not apply to abnormal Pap smears?

a. Cancer of the cervix is the third most common gynecologic cancer in the U.S.
b. 10% of Pap smears may have false negative results
c. Colposcopy and cervical biopsies with ECC are warranted if LSIL or HSIL present
d. Smoking is a risk factor for cervical cancer

51. Medical treatment options for endometriosis include:

a. DES
b. Triphasic oral contraceptives
c. Methyltestosterone
d. Medroxyprogesterone acetate

52. Endometriosis:

a. Is the development and deposition of endometrial tissue in the myometrium
b. Is not a significant factor in infertility
c. Is common in postmenopausal women
d. Is a common cause of pelvic pain

Answers

1. c	18. b	35. d
2. a	19. b	36. a
3. d	20. c	37. c
4. d	21. d	38. c
5. d	22. d	39. a
6. b	23. d	40. b
7. c	24. c	41. d
8. a	25. d	42. a
9. c	26. b	43. b
10. c	27. a	44. c
11. c	28. d	45. b
12. b	29. c	46. d
13. a	30. a	47. a
14. c	31. b	48. c
15. b	32. c	49. c
16. d	33. d	50. b
17. b	34. a	51. d
		52. d

Bibliography

Buttaro, T. M., Trybulski, J. A., Bailey, P. P., & Sandberg-Cook, J. (Eds.). (1999). *Primary care: A collaborative practice*. St. Louis: Mosby Year Book.

Centers for Disease Control and Prevention. (1998). ''1998 Sexually transmitted diseases treatment guidelines'' *Morbidity and Mortality Weekly Report*. January 23, (47) RRI

Copeland, L. J. (Ed.). (2000). *Textbook of gynecology*. Philadelphia: W. B. Saunders.

Cunningham, F. G., MacDonald, P. C., Gant, N. F., Leveno, K. J., & Gilstrap, L. C. (1997). *Williams obstetrics* (20th ed.). Norwalk, CT: Appleton & Lange.

DiPiro, J. T., Talbert, R. L., Yee, G. C., Matzke, G. R., Wells, B. G., & Posey, L. M. (1999). *Pharmacology: A pathophysiologic approach*. NY: Lange Medical Books/McGraw-Hill.

Fanning, M. M. (1997). *HIV infection: A clinical approach* (2nd ed.). Philadelphia: W. B. Saunders.

Gompel, C., & Silverberg, S. G. (Eds.). (1994). *Pathology in gynecology and obstetrics* (4th ed.). Philadelphia: J. B. Lippincott.

Harris, J. R., Lippman, M. E., Morrow, M., & Osborne, L. K. (Eds.). (2000). *Diseases of the breast*. Philadelphia: Lippincott Williams & Wilkens.

Hatcher, R. A., Trussell, J., Stewart, F., Cates Jr. W., Stewart, G. K., Guest, F., & Kowall, D. (1998). *Contraceptive technology* (17th rev. ed.). NY: Ardent Media.

Holmes, K. K., Sparling, P. F., Mardh, P. A., Leman, S. M., Stamm, W. E., Piot, P., & Wasserhert, J. N. (1999). *Sexually transmitted diseases* (3rd ed.). NY: Lange Medical Books/ McGraw Hill.

Mishell, D. R., Stenchever, M. A., Droëgemueller, W., & Herbst, A. L. (1997). *Comprehensive gynecology* (3rd ed.). St. Louis: Mosby Year Book.

Pizzomo, J., & Murray, M. (1999). *Textbook of natural medicine* (2nd ed.). NY: Churchill Livingstone.

Sanfilippo, J. S., Muram, D., Dewhurst, J., & Lee, P. A. (Eds.). (1998). *Pediatric and adolescent gynecology*. Philadelphia: W. B. Saunders.

Scott, J. R., Philip, J. D., Hammond, C. B., & Spellacy, W. N. (Eds.). (1999). *Danforth's obstetrics and gynecology*. Philadelphia: Lippincott Williams & Wilkins.

Tierney, L. M., McPhee, S. J., & Papadakis, M. A. (Eds.). (2000). *Current medical diagnosis and treatment* (39th ed.). NY: Lange Medical Books/McGraw-Hill.

USPHS/IDSA (1999). Guidelines for the prevention of opportunistic infections in persons infected with human immunodeficiency virus. U.S. Public Health Service (USPHS) and Infectious Diseases Society of America (IDSA). *MMWR Morb Mortal Wkly Rep—1999 Aug 20; 48 (RR-10): 1–59, 61–6*.

Walsh, P. C., Retik, A. B., Vaughn, E. D., & Wein, A. J. (Eds.). (1998). *Campbell's urology* (7th ed.). Philadelphia: W. B. Saunders.

Pregnancy, Contraception and Menopause

Susan B. Moskosky

Pregnancy

- Definition: The condition of having a developing embryo or fetus within the female body (usually within the uterus)

- Incidence

  1. Birth rate, or number of births per 1,000 total population, in the U.S. for the year ending 1996 was 14.8—same rate as 1995

  2. Birth rate for teenagers during 1996 was 54.7 per 1,000 women aged 15 to 19 years, down 4 percent compared with 1995; teenage birth rate has declined by 12 percent since 1991

  3. Fertility rate, or number of births per 1,000 women of childbearing age (15 to 44 years), for the year ending 1996 was 65.7

  4. Pregnancy rate, or number of pregnancies per 1,000 women of childbearing age (15 to 44 years), for the year ending 1992 was 109.9

- Preconception Care Improves Pregnancy Outcome

  1. Goal is to maximize health of mother and infant

  2. Includes history-taking, physical examination and laboratory/diagnostic testing

  3. Preconception counseling

     a. Menstrual record—record first day of last normal menstrual period (LNMP)

     b. Exercise and nutrition

        (1) 0.4 mg of folic acid per day recommended to reduce risk of neural tube defects

        (2) Encourage attainment of ideal weight prior to conception

        (3) Begin exercise program to improve cardiovascular status, assist with weight loss, and lessen potential for hypertension and diabetes in pregnancy

        (4) Avoid teratogens—environmental and medications

        (5) Identify genetic risks

        (6) Affirm readiness for parenthood

        (7) Appropriate vaccinations/immunizations (e.g., rubella, tetanus, hepatitis)

- Early Diagnosis of Pregnancy is Essential

  1. Begin prenatal care; physical examination; laboratory tests; risk assessment; discontinue use of tobacco, alcohol, street drugs and/or teratogenic medications; provide educational materials

  2. If pregnancy is unintended, make timely decision regarding pregnancy options (e.g., continuation, termination, adoption)

- Signs and Symptoms of Pregnancy

1. Presumptive—subjective; frequently reported with pregnancy, but not conclusive for pregnancy

    a. Nausea with or without vomiting

    b. Urinary frequency

    c. Fatigue

    d. Perception of fetal movement by mother (quickening); with pregnancy, usually occurs 16 to 20 weeks

    e. Amenorrhea

    f. Breast changes

    g. Vaginal mucosa discoloration (Chadwick's sign)

    h. Increased skin pigmentation and abdominal striae

2. Probable—more objective; often noted on physical examination or with laboratory testing

    a. Enlargement of abdomen and uterus

    b. Uterine changes in size, shape, consistency; softening of lower uterine segment at 6 to 8 weeks gestation (Hegar's sign)

    c. Softening of cervix at 6 to 8 weeks gestation (Goodell's sign)

    d. Braxton-Hicks contractions—often present by 4th month

    e. Ballottement

    f. Outlining of fetus by examiner

    g. Pregnancy tests—endocrine tests that detect human chorionic gonadotropin (hCG) in maternal blood or urine

3. Positive—noted with absolute confirmation of pregnancy

    a. Detection of fetal heartbeat—auscultation with fetoscope at 17 to 20 weeks gestation; auscultation with doppler by 10 to 12 weeks gestation

    b. Perception of fetal movement by examiner

    c. Visualization of fetus by ultrasonography

- Differential Diagnosis

    1. Myomas, hematometra, adenomyosis

    2. Ovarian tumor or extrauterine mass

    3. Amenorrhea/irregular menses of other origin

    4. Urinary tract infection

    5. Gastrointestinal problem

    6. Gestational trophoblastic disease

- Physiologic Changes (Maternal)

  1. Cardiovascular/Respiratory

     a. Blood volume increased by 30% to 50% at term

     b. Increased cardiac output

     c. Heart displaced by uterus upward and to left

     d. Pulse rate increased by 10 to 15 beats per minute

     e. Dependent edema of feet and hands by third trimester—assess for vena caval syndrome and/or aorta caval compression

     f. Exaggerated heart sounds; functional systolic murmurs common

     g. Physiologic anemia common due to unequal expansion of red cell volume (30%) and plasma volume (50%)

     h. Increased respiratory tidal volume

     i. Dyspnea common during early pregnancy related to hormonal changes; also common later in pregnancy due to progressive elevation of diaphragm

  2. Gastrointestinal

     a. Decreased smooth muscle tone and decreased motility due to progesterone resulting in:

        (1) Decreased intestinal peristalsis may lead to constipation

        (2) Gastric reflux and heartburn

     b. Abdominal distention secondary to increased uterine size and flatus

     c. Hypertrophy and bleeding of gums possibly due to estrogen

  3. Musculoskeletal

     a. Progesterone-induced relaxation of pelvic structures and joints (may cause discomfort)

     b. Center of gravity shifts causing lordosis and posture changes; lower back pain common; waddling gait develops

     c. Diastasis recti possible (separation of rectus abdominis muscles)

  4. Integumentary

     a. Cutaneous vascular changes—spider angiomas, palmar erythema

     b. Increased pigmentation of face (chloasma), areolae, abdomen (linea nigra), and genitalia

     c. Striae gravidarum

     d. Increased sebaceous and sweat gland activity

  5. Endocrine

a. Diffuse thyroid gland enlargement

b. Insulin needs increase due to action of human placental lactogen (hPL)

6. Breasts

a. Early tenderness and tingling

b. Increase in size and nodularity; striae may develop

c. Veins prominent

d. Nipples erectile; arealoe darken

e. Montgomery follicles hypertrophy

f. Colostrum after first few months

7. Genitalia/reproductive

a. External genitalia

(1) Increased pigmentation

(2) Pelvic congestion; swelling of labia majora near term

(3) Vulvar varicosities possible

b. Vagina

(1) Increased vascularity causing bluish/purple color (Chadwick's sign)

(2) Rugations of vaginal mucosa prominent

(3) Increased secretions (leukorrhea)

c. Cervix

(1) Pronounced softening and cyanosis (early)

(2) Proliferation of endocervical glands (cervical ''erosion'')

(3) Mucus plug blocks endocervical canal

d. Musculature—broad ligament softening

e. Uterus

(1) Increases in size and weight

(2) Softening of lower uterine segment (Hegar's sign)

(3) Blood supply increased

f. Ovaries

(1) Corpus luteum—continues for first 10 to 12 weeks of pregnancy; produces progesterone until placenta develops

(2) Ovarian function ceases during pregnancy

g. Urinary

      (1) Dilation of ureters and kidneys (especially on right), decreased bladder tone—increased risk for urinary stasis and infection

      (2) Urinary frequency common early and late in pregnancy

      (3) Incontinence common, particularly with multiparity

- Prenatal Care

    1. Initial visit

        a. Laboratory confirmation of pregnancy—urine and serum tests available, all test for hCG

           (1) Agglutination inhibition test—urine test, reliable 14 to 21 days post-conception

           (2) Enzyme-linked immunosorbent assay (ELISA); immunometric test (urine or serum) reliable 7 to 10 days post-conception

           (3) Beta subunit radioimmunoassay (RIA)—serum test, reliable 7 days post-conception

        b. Expected date of birth (EDB)—Nagele's rule subtract 3 months from LNMP and add 7 days

        c. History—emphasize factors that may affect maternal or fetal outcome

           (1) Menstrual history—extremely important for estimating gestational age

           (2) Contraceptive history

           (3) Maternal history—attention to acute or chronic health problems

           (4) Family history—multiple gestation, congenital anomalies, inherited diseases, maternal family history of diabetes or hypertension

           (5) Medication history

           (6) Substance use—tobacco, alcohol or other drugs

           (7) Exposure to environmental or occupational toxins or hazards

           (8) History of domestic violence

           (9) Reproductive/obstetric history

               (a) Each previous pregnancy including outcome— e.g., **T**erm birth, **P**reterm birth, **A**bortion (spontaneous or induced) and number of **L**iving children (T-P-A-L)

               (b) Complications during previous pregnancy/delivery/postpartum— e.g., gestational diabetes, pregnancy induced hypertension (PIH), preterm labor (PTL) and/or preterm birth, postpartum hemorrhage, postpartum depression

               (c) Previous pregnancy loss including gestational age and related factors

(d) Method of delivery for previous pregnancies—vaginal or cesarean

d. Physical examination

(1) Vital signs and complete head-to-toe examination—attention to ruling out pre-existing medical conditions

(2) Assess uterine size to confirm pregnancy and determine gestational age—most accurately assessed by bimanual examination up to 14 weeks

(a) 8 weeks—approximately 9 cm

(b) 10 weeks—approximately 10 cm

(c) 12 weeks—uterine fundus at symphysis pubis

(d) 16 weeks—fundus midway between symphysis pubis and umbilicus

(e) 20 weeks—fundus at umbilicus

(f) 20 weeks to term—abdominal measurement of fundal height

(i) Measure from top of symphysis pubis to top of uterine fundus

(ii) Between 18 and 32 weeks gestation, good correlation between gestational age in weeks and measurement of fundal height in centimeters

(3) Evaluate pelvic dimensions (pelvimetry)

(4) Obtain Pap smear and cervical cultures

(5) Auscultation of fetal heart by doppler (usually audible by 10 to 12 weeks with doppler) or fetoscope (usually audible by 17 to 20 weeks)

e. Laboratory testing (routine)

(1) ABO blood group/Rh factor determination

(2) Complete blood cell count (CBC) with indices

(3) Antibody screen and titer

(4) Rubella titer—titer of > 1:10 indicates immunity

(5) Syphilis screening—Venereal Disease Research Laboratories test (VDRL), rapid plasma reagin (RPR)

(6) Hepatitis B surface antigen screening

(7) Urinalysis; urine culture if indicated

(8) Chlamydia/gonorrhea screening

(9) Offer human immunodeficiency virus (HIV) antibody testing

(10) Other tests indicated by individual risk status or general patient population, e.g., postprandial 50 g glucose screen, sickle cell screen, tuberculin testing

f. Risk assessment

    (1) Referral for genetic counseling if indicated

        (a) Maternal age of 35 or older by delivery

        (b) Family history of genetic anomaly—e.g., Down syndrome, other chromosomal abnormality, hemophilia, muscular dystrophy, cystic fibrosis

        (c) History of three or more spontaneous abortions

        (d) Previous unexplained pregnancy loss

        (e) Parents possible carriers of sickle cell, thalassemia, or Tay-Sachs disease

    (2) PTL risk assessment

        (a) Medical/obstetrical factors—multiple gestation, diethylstilbestrol (DES) exposure, hydramnios, uterine anomaly, cervical effacement or dilatation at 32 weeks gestation, previous history of PTL and/ or preterm delivery, history of cone biopsy, uterine irritability, febrile illness, history of pyelonephritis

        (b) Behavioral factors—smoking, substance use/abuse, malnutrition

g. Education

    (1) Nutrition

        (a) Dietary assessment

        (b) Ideal weight gain during pregnancy is 25 to 35 pounds for woman of normal weight; obese (> 120% of ideal body weight) 15 to 25 pounds; underweight (< 90% of ideal body weight) 28 to 40 pounds

            (i) First trimester—2 to 5 pounds

            (ii) Second and third trimesters—0.8 to 1 pound per week

        (c) Discourage weight loss during pregnancy

        (d) Nutritional requirements

            (i) Calories—1800 to 2400 kilocalories per day (increase by 300 over normal consumption)

            (ii) Protein—75 to 100 grams per day

            (iii) Calcium—1200 mg per day

            (iv) Iron—30 to 60 mg supplement per day

(v) Folic acid—0.4 mg per day

(vi) Other vitamin and mineral needs can usually be met from a balanced diet; encourage fiber and fluids

(2) Encourage good hygiene; douching not recommended

(3) Exercise

(a) Regular exercise recommended throughout pregnancy

(b) May continue with pre-pregnancy exercise routine, but should not begin new strenuous exercise program

(c) Walking and swimming are ideal during pregnancy

(d) Avoid excessive fatigue and excessive overheating

(4) Sexual activity

(a) Coitus not contraindicated during normal pregnancy

(b) Changes in position may be required as pregnancy progresses

(c) Sexual intercourse contraindicated during pregnancy with undiagnosed vaginal bleeding, rupture of membranes, preterm labor, threatened abortion

(5) Warning signs—patient should contact provider promptly

(a) Signs of ectopic pregnancy or threatened abortion

(i) Abdominal pain

(ii) Vaginal bleeding

(iii) Passage of tissue

(iv) Syncope

(b) Hyperemesis—severe nausea and vomiting; unable to retain food or fluids

(c) Signs of pyelonephritis

(i) Fever above 100.6° F

(ii) Dysuria, flank pain

(d) Signs of PIH

(i) Severe headache, dizziness

(ii) Scotomata, blurring of vision

(iii) Swelling of face; severe dependent edema that does not respond to rest/elevation

(iv) Epigastric pain

(e) Signs of PTL

(i) Loss of fluid from vagina

(ii) Lower back pain or lower abdominal cramping

(iii) Frequent, palpable uterine contractions with or without pain

(iv) Heaviness or pressure

(v) Increased vaginal discharge, especially if blood-tinged, mucoid or watery

(f) Decreased or absent fetal movement

(6) Signs and symptoms of labor

  (a) True labor

    (i) Contractions—timed from beginning of one contraction to beginning of the next

      a) Occur at regular intervals which gradually shorten

      b) Initially felt in back, then radiate to lower abdomen

      c) Duration and strength of contractions increase

      d) Intensity of contractions increase with walking

      e) Sedation does not stop contractions

    (ii) Bloody "show"—pink or blood-tinged mucous discharge from cervix may indicate loss of mucus plug

    (iii) Cervix dilates and effaces

    (iv) Presenting part has descended into pelvis

  (b) False labor

    (i) Contractions irregular in timing, duration and intensity

    (ii) Discomfort is felt mainly in abdomen

    (iii) Intensity of contractions not affected by walking

    (iv) No changes in cervix; no bloody show, dilatation or effacement

    (v) Fetal head remains free in pelvis

    (vi) Sedation will stop contractions

  (c) Rupture of membranes

    (i) Occurs spontaneously at onset of labor in 50%

    (ii) Premature rupture of membranes associated with increased risk for:

      a) PTL if occurs prior to 37 weeks gestation

       b) Ascending intrauterine infection if not delivered within 24 hours

       c) Prolapse of umbilical cord

2. Interval visits

   a. For low risk, routine monthly visits up to 28 weeks, every 2 to 3 weeks until 36 weeks, then weekly until delivery

   b. Components of routine visits

     (1) Measurement of maternal weight and blood pressure

     (2) Screen urine for protein and glucose; ketones and nitrites if indicated

     (3) Obtain interval history, evaluate client complaints and risk-related symptoms, answer questions and provide anticipatory guidance

     (4) Assess fetal heart tones by fetoscope or doppler (normal rate is 120 to 160 beats per minute)

     (5) Evaluate fetal growth

       (a) Determine fundal height

       (b) Leopold's maneuvers—abdominal palpation performed using four maneuvers to determine fetal presentation and position (used later in pregnancy—beginning approximately 26 weeks)

     (6) Specific needs or screening tests as indicated by gestational age or patient history

       (a) First trimester (LNMP through 13th week)

         (i) Chorionic villus sampling (CVS)—refer when indicated for genetic reasons; optimal time 9 to 11 weeks

         (ii) 1 hour postprandial 50 g glucose screen (initial visit or first trimester) for women with risk factors for gestational diabetes mellitus (GDM)—prior history of GDM; first degree relative with diabetes; prior delivery of macrosomic infant; previous unexplained stillbirth or spontaneous abortions; obesity; glucosuria; advanced maternal age (≥ 35)

         (iii) Assess physical and psychological impact of pregnancy, including support system

         (iv) Discuss warning signs and early complications

       (b) Second trimester (14th through 27th week)

         (i) Maternal serum alpha-fetoprotein (MSAFP) and Multiple Marker Screening—screen at 15 to 19 weeks (16 to 18 weeks optimal)

a) Elevated levels of MSAFP associated with fetal congenital abnormalities— open neural tube defects, congenital nephrosis, abdominal wall defects; also elevated with multiple gestation

b) Low levels of MSAFP associated with Down Syndrome (Trisomy 21)

(ii) Amniocentesis—performed at 15 to 18 weeks if indicated

a) Genetic screening—mother of ≥ 35, history of previous child with chromosomal, congenital or metabolic abnormality

b) Rh sensitization—spectrophotometric examination of amniotic fluid predictive of severity of hemolytic disease

c) Fetal lung maturity—lecithin/sphingomyelin ration (L/S) ration ≥ 2:1 indicates lung maturity

(iii) 1 hour postprandial 50 g glucose screen— screen all women between 24 to 28 weeks

a) If 1 hr glucose screen is 140 to 199 mg/dL, order 3 hour 100 g glucose tolerance test (3 hr OGTT); if 2 or more values are abnormal, diagnosis of GDM is made

b) If 1 hr glucose screen is > 200 mg/ dL, order fasting blood sugar (FBS); if FBS is > 130 mg/dL, omit OGTT and refer for treatment

(iv) Assess for fetal movements (quickening)— usually between 16 to 20 weeks

(v) Evaluate for signs of PTL

(c) Third trimester (28th week to term—usually 40 weeks)

(i) Repeat VDRL and hemoglobin (Hgb)

(ii) Re-evaluate antibody screen titer

(iii) Rh (D) immune globulin (RhoGAM) to unsensitized Rh-negative mother—28 weeks

(iv) Discuss importance of monitoring fetal movement as indicator of fetal well being

(v) Review signs and symptoms of labor

(vi) Perform cervical assessment for position, consistency, length and dilation

(vii) Assess fetal lie and presentation (36 to 40 weeks)

3. Tests for assessment of fetal well-being

    a. Ultrasound (ultrasonography)

        (1) Definition: High-frequency sound waves reflected from tissues of varying densities and converted into images

            (a) Level 1 (Basic Ultrasound)—establishes gestational age, location and grade of placenta; determines fetal presentation, number of fetuses, stage of fetal growth, cardiac activity; assesses amniotic fluid volume; detects gross fetal anomalies and maternal pelvic masses

            (b) Level II (Targeted Ultrasound)—confirms information obtained in Level I and surveys fetal anatomy for malformations

        (2) Indications—determination of gestational age; assess fetal growth pattern; size/date discrepancy; suspected ectopic pregnancy; determine fetal presentation/lie; suspected hydramnios/oligohydramnios; suspected fetal anomaly or fetal demise; determine placental location, integrity, maturity; identify number of fetuses; aid in diagnostic procedures, e.g., amniocentesis, CVS

    b. Nonstress test (NST)

        (1) Definition: Diagnostic test that monitors fetal heart rate acceleration in response to fetal movement (noninvasive); both NST and contraction stress test (CST) were developed to assess any indication of uteroplacental insufficiency and to predict ability of fetus to endure stress of labor

        (2) Procedure—fetal heart rate (FHR), fetal movement and uterine contractions are assessed (using external monitoring) over a 20 minute period; may be extended to 40 minutes if no FHR accelerations occur

        (3) Interpretation

            (a) Reactive NST—appropriate heart rate accelerations; fetal well-being assured for one week (repeat weekly)

            (b) Nonreactive NST—absence of appropriate heart rate accelerations over a 40 minute period; consider additional testing, e.g., contraction stress test (CST) or biophysical profile

    c. Contraction stress test (CST)

        (1) Definition: Diagnostic test performed to evaluate fetal response to uterine contractions; mimics labor

        (2) Procedure—baseline tracing obtained prior to stimulating uterine contractions; if fewer than 3 contractions occur in 10 minutes, contractions stimulated by intravenous oxytocin infusion or nipple stimulation

        (3) Interpretation

(a) Positive CST—late decelerations following 50% or more of contractions; delivery recommended or further tests (test has 30% false-positive rate)

(b) Negative CST—no late or variable decelerations; subsequent testing based on fetal and maternal conditions and institutional protocol

(c) Equivocal CST—late decelerations in fewer than 50% of contractions, or significant variable decelerations; repeat in 24 hours or do biophysical profile

(4) Contraindications—premature rupture of membranes, history of PTL during current pregnancy, incompetent cervix or cerclage, previous vertical uterine incision, third trimester bleeding, polyhydramnios, placenta previa, multiple pregnancy

d. Biophysical profile (BPP)

(1) Definition: Use of real-time ultrasound combined with NST to assess four parameters of fetal well-being which include fetal tone, breathing, body movements and amniotic fluid volume

(2) Indications—high-risk pregnancy, e.g., post-date pregnancy, decreased fetal movement, maternal disease, suspected oligohydramnios, intrauterine growth retardation

(3) Interpretation—each of five components is scored as 2 (normal) or 0 (abnormal), with total possible score of 10

(a) 8 to 10—normal

(b) 6—equivocal (repeat according to agency protocol)

(c) ≤ 4—abnormal (consider delivery)

- Common Complaints in Pregnancy

   1. Nausea and vomiting

      a. Etiology—high levels of hCG in first trimester, changes in carbohydrate metabolism, delayed gastric emptying

      b. Management

         (1) Rule out hyperemesis gravidarum, pyelonephritis

         (2) Small, frequent high carbohydrate meals; avoid high-fat or spicy meals; avoid empty or overdistended stomach

   2. Backache

      a. Etiology—softening and relaxation of pelvic structures and joints; increased lordosis of spine caused by shift in center of gravity

      b. Management

(1) Rule out pyelonephritis, labor, musculoskeletal disease

(2) Teach pelvic tilt exercise; use proper body mechanics; avoid excessive twisting, bending and stretching

3. Varicosities

    a. Etiology—pressure of enlarged uterus causing impaired venous circulation and increased venous pressure in lower extremities; relaxation of vein walls and valves; hereditary factors; weight gain

    b. Management

        (1) Rule out thrombophlebitis

        (2) Support pantyhose; frequent leg elevation; avoid standing for long periods, crossing legs, and knee high hose

4. Hemorrhoids

    a. Etiology—pressure of enlarging uterus; constipation; predisposition to varicosities

    b. Management

        (1) Rule out abscessed or thrombosed hemorrhoids

        (2) Topical anesthetics; prevent or treat constipation by increasing fluids and roughage in diet; warm or cool sitz baths; ice packs or cold compresses

5. Constipation

    a. Etiology—decreased intestinal motility caused by progesterone and compression of bowel by enlarging uterus; oral iron supplements

    b. Management—increase high-fiber foods and fluids; regular exercise; bulk-forming, nonnutritive laxative

6. Heartburn

    a. Etiology—decreased gastrointestinal peristalsis and relaxation of cardiac sphincter; reflux of gastric contents into lower esophagus; upward displacement and compression of the stomach by uterus

    b. Management

        (1) Rule out cardiac, gallbladder, epigastric or pancreatic disease, PIH

        (2) Small frequent meals; avoid fatty foods; fluids between but not with meals; do not lie down after eating for at least one hour; low sodium antacids

7. Pica and food cravings

    a. Etiology—unknown

    b. Management—evaluate diet to determine adequacy; explain need to maintain healthy diet; problems may occur if craved substance is substituting for nutritious food or is harmful to mother or fetus

8. Ptyalism (increased salivation)

   a. Etiology—unknown

   b. Management—reassurance of resolution following pregnancy; good oral hygiene; avoid excessive starch intake; adequate fluid intake

9. Fatigue—most common in first and third trimesters

   a. Etiology

      (1) Early pregnancy—increased oxygen consumption, increased progesterone level, fetal demands

      (2) Late pregnancy—sleep deprivation from physical discomforts

   b. Management

      (1) Rule out iron deficiency anemia, depression

      (2) Reassurance; encourage adequate sleep and rest periods

10. Headache

    a. Etiology—increased circulatory volume; vasodilation caused by high progesterone levels; vascular congestion; stress; fatigue; hypoglycemia

    b. Management

       (1) Rule out PIH, migraine headache, sinus infection

       (2) Teach symptoms of PIH; encourage adequate rest; stress reduction; massage; moist hot or cold compresses; avoid intake of foods that trigger headaches; acetaminophen

11. Vaginal discharge (leukorrhea)

    a. Etiology—estrogen-induced increase in vascularity and hypertrophy of cervical glands and vaginal cells

    b. Management

       (1) Rule out ruptured membranes, vaginitis, cervicitis, sexually transmitted disease (STD)

       (2) Reassurance; cotton underwear and loose clothing; avoid douching or tampon use; keep vulva clean and dry

12. Urinary frequency

    a. Etiology—enlargement of uterus compresses bladder; hyperplasia and hyperemia of pelvic organs and increased kidney output

    b. Management

       (1) Rule out urinary tract infection (UTI)

      (2) Void frequently; maintain adequate fluid intake; discontinue fluids 2 to 3 hours prior to bedtime; avoid caffeine

13. Leg cramps

    a. Etiology—pressure of uterus on pelvic nerves and blood vessels; imbalance in phosphorus/calcium ratio caused by inadequate or excessive calcium intake (postulated)

    b. Management

        (1) Rule out thromboembolic disease, varicosities

        (2) Avoid stretching legs, pointing toes, and lying on back; dorsiflexion of foot to relieve cramp in calf; diet evaluation to correct excessive or inadequate intake of calcium

14. Round ligament pain

    a. Etiology—growth of uterus causes round ligaments to stretch

    b. Management

        (1) Rule out PTL, ectopic pregnancy, ruptured ovarian cyst, appendicitis

        (2) Reassurance of resolution following pregnancy; avoid sudden, twisting movements; heating pad; avoid excessive exercise, standing or walking

15. Dyspnea (breathlessness)

    a. Etiology—increased sensitivity to lower levels of CO_2 (progesterone effect) in early pregnancy; later in pregnancy caused by displacement of diaphragm by enlarging uterus

    b. Management

        (1) Rule out upper respiratory infection, pulmonary or cardiac problem

        (2) Sleep with head elevated; reassure improvement will occur when fetus drops into pelvis; avoid exercise if a precipitating factor

16. Edema

    a. Etiology—increased capillary permeability (hormonal); pressure of uterus impedes venous return; increased fluid in intracellular spaces

    b. Management

        (1) Assess for PIH

        (2) Instruct about symptoms of PIH; rest in left lateral recumbent position for 1 to 2 hours during day and at night; elevate legs several times during day; avoid constrictive clothing; avoid long periods of sitting or standing

- Pregnancy Complications

  1. Bleeding disorders

a. Spontaneous abortion (SAB)

   (1) Definition: Naturally occurring termination of pregnancy before 20 weeks gestation

   (2) Etiology—chromosomal abnormalities of fetus; maternal disease, infection, or endocrine imbalance; blighted ovum; faulty implantation; immune factors; advanced maternal age

   (3) Signs and symptoms/physical examination findings

      (a) Threatened abortion—occurs in 1 of 4 pregnancies

         (i) Vaginal bleeding with or without cramping; may be accompanied by low backache

         (ii) No cervical changes; cervix closed

      (b) Inevitable

         (i) Vaginal bleeding with contractions; possible gush of fluid from vagina

         (ii) Cervical dilatation and rupture of membranes

      (c) Missed abortion—prolonged retention of fetus after fetal death

         (i) Loss of symptoms of pregnancy; may have brownish vaginal discharge

         (ii) Gradual decrease in uterine size; cervix closed and firm

      (d) Incomplete abortion—incomplete expulsion of products of conception (POC), usually placenta retained

         (i) Bleeding (may be profuse); cramping

         (ii) May observe tissue in cervical canal

      (e) Complete abortion—complete expulsion of all POC

         (i) Bleeding; cramping

         (ii) No retained POC; cervix dilated

   (4) Differential diagnosis

      (a) Vaginal infection

      (b) Cervical polyp

      (c) Ectopic pregnancy

      (d) Molar pregnancy

      (e) Incompetent cervix

   (5) Diagnostic tests/findings

      (a) Ultrasound for evidence of fetal heart action and uterine size

        (b)   Serial hCG levels

        (c)   Pelvic exam to evaluate cervical dilation, uterine size and bleeding

   (6)   Management/treatment

        (a)   Bedrest; pelvic rest; hydration; counsel regarding signs of infection and when to report symptoms

        (b)   May require hospitalization, dilatation and curettage (D & C), transfusion, IV fluids

b.   Ectopic pregnancy

   (1)   Definition: Implantation of fertilized ovum outside the uterine cavity (usually in fallopian tube)

   (2)   Etiology—any condition that prevents or slows passage of fertilized ovum into uterus—e.g., tubal damage from previous pelvic infection, tubal surgery, previous ectopic; progestin-only contraceptive use

   (3)   Signs and symptoms/physical findings

        (a)   Before rupture—early pregnancy symptoms; amenorrhea followed by spotting/bleeding; lower abdominal pain, usually unilateral; uterus normal to slightly enlarged

        (b)   After rupture—sharp, unilateral abdominal pain, may radiate to shoulder; syncope/fainting/shock; spotting/bleeding; adnexal tenderness, possible fullness; cervical motion tenderness; bulging of posterior cul-de-sac

   (4)   Differential diagnosis

        (a)   Acute appendicitis

        (b)   Pelvic inflammatory disease (PID)

        (c)   Ruptured corpus luteum cyst

        (d)   SAB

   (5)   Diagnostic tests/findings

        (a)   Ultrasound—no evidence of intrauterine pregnancy

        (b)   CBC—may indicate anemia, slight leukocytosis

        (c)   Serum Beta hCG—positive, but hCG level lower than expected for gestational age

        (d)   Serial Beta hCG levels—level rises slowly or plateaus; with intrauterine pregnancy, doubles every 2 days

   (6)   Management/treatment—hospitalization; surgery for repair or removal of damaged tube; fluid replacement; transfusion if needed; RhoGAM administration for Rh-negative woman

   c. Placenta previa

     (1) Definition: Abnormal implantation of placenta in lower uterine segment

     (2) Etiology—unknown; may be associated with multiparity, multiple gestation, previous cesarean, previous uterine surgery

     (3) Signs and symptoms/physical findings

       (a) Painless bleeding after 20 weeks gestation; usually in third trimester

       (b) Uterus nontender; usually no evidence of fetal distress

     (4) Differential diagnosis

       (a) Abruptio placentae

       (b) Cervical lesion or cervicitis

       (c) Nonvaginal bleeding (rectal or urinary)

     (5) Diagnostic tests/findings

       (a) Ultrasound—indicates low-lying placenta

       (b) *No* pelvic exam

     (6) Management/treatment

       (a) Gestation is less than 36 weeks—expectant management; hospitalization and bedrest; fetal surveillance; monitor mother for increased bleeding

       (b) Gestation 36 weeks or more—anticipate delivery; may need amniocentesis to assess fetal lung maturity

   d. Abruptio placentae

     (1) Definition: Partial or complete detachment of normally implanted placenta anytime prior to delivery

     (2) Etiology—unknown; contributing factors include PIH, cocaine use, decreased blood flow to placenta, advanced maternal age, multiparity, trauma, underlying vascular problems

     (3) Signs and symptoms/physical findings

       (a) Vaginal bleeding of varying amount with severe, unremitting abdominal pain

       (b) Uterine tenderness, increased uterine tone, contractions, signs of fetal distress, signs of shock

     (4) Differential diagnosis

       (a) Placenta previa

       (b) Appendicitis

(c) Ovarian cyst

(d) Hematoma of rectus muscle

(5) Diagnostic tests/findings—ultrasound for placental location

(6) Management/treatment

(a) Immediate transport for emergency care

(b) Immediate delivery if massive bleeding or fetal distress

(c) Expectant management in emergency facility if fetus immature, no evidence of fetal distress or maternal hypovolemia or anemia

2. Pregnancy induced hypertension (PIH)

a. Definition

(1) Hypertension (HTN)—blood pressure of at least 140/90 mm Hg, or systolic rise > 30 mm Hg or diastolic rise ≥ 15 mm Hg above baseline on at least 2 occasions, 6 hours or more apart

(2) Preeclampsia—HTN with proteinuria and/or generalized edema after 20 weeks gestation; may occur earlier with gestational trophoblastic disease

(3) HELLP Syndrome—variant of severe preeclampsia including **H**emolysis, **E**levated **L**iver enzymes, and **L**ow **P**latelets

(4) Eclampsia—when convulsions, not caused by neurological disease, occur in woman with clinical criteria for preeclampsia

b. Etiology

(1) Unknown

(2) Predisposing factors—primigravidas; maternal age < 20 or > 35; maternal family or personal history of preeclampsia; preexisting hypertensive, vascular, autoimmune or renal disease; multiple gestation; gestational trophoblastic disease

c. Signs and symptoms/physical findings

(1) Preeclampsia—HTN, sudden weight gain; generalized edema; frontal or occipital headaches; visual disturbances, e.g., scotomata, blurred vision; hyper-reflexia; oliguria; decreased fetal movement; fetal size small for dates; proteinuria

(2) HELLP Syndrome—preeclampsia signs and symptoms; fatigue; nausea with or without vomiting; jaundice; right upper quadrant tenderness; epigastric pain; enlarged, firm liver

(3) Eclampsia—seizure; drowsiness following seizure; cyanosis and tachypnea; oliguria; decreased or absent FHT

d. Differential diagnosis

(1) Brain tumor

(2) Renal failure

(3) Chronic HTN

e. Diagnostic tests/findings

(1) Preeclampsia

(a) Proteinuria—up to ≥ 5 g/24 hour urine collection with severe pre-eclampsia

(b) CBC—hemoconcentration

(c) AST, serum creatinine, uric acid—elevated

(d) Ultrasound—may indicate intrauterine growth retardation

(e) Coagulation studies—decreased clotting factors, platelets and increased fibrin

(2) HELLP Syndrome—above plus

(a) Extremely low platelets (< 50,000) and decreased clotting factors

(b) Severe hemoconcentration (elevated hematocrit)

(c) Serum glucose—may be significantly decreased

(d) Elevated liver enzymes

f. Management/treatment—delivery is only cure

(1) Antepartum

(a) Bedrest in left lateral recumbent position—indicated with mild to moderate preeclampsia

(b) Adequate nutrition and hydration

(c) Careful monitoring of mother and fetus—NST, CST, BPP, fetal movement counts

(d) Hospitalization if condition worsens to decrease possibility of convulsions and increase chance for fetal survival

(2) Intrapartum

(a) Prevent convulsions and deliver

(b) Medications used to control or prevent seizure activity

(i) Magnesium sulfate

a) Prevents convulsions without central nervous system depression

b) Monitor for signs of toxicity—nausea, thirst, depression of reflexes, flushing

(ii) Hydralazine—antihypertensive usually reserved for cases when diastolic BP is 110 mm Hg or higher

(iii) Diazepam—reserved for most severe cases to arrest seizures

Early Pregnancy Termination

- Mifepristone

  1. Description: Abortifacient which induces abortion when administered in early pregnancy

  2. Mechanism of action

     a. Approved for termination of early pregnancy (49 days or less)

     b. Acts as antiprogesterone; high affinity for progesterone receptors

     c. Progesterone support in early pregnancy essential; blocking this support results in expulsion of conceptus

  3. Effectiveness: Followed by misoprostol is approximately 92% to 95% effective with pregnancy durations of 7 weeks or less

  4. Advantages

     a. Usefulness extends beyond the 72 hour time-frame required for the Yuzpe method

     b. Medication guide given to all patients describing drug schedule, contraindications and side effects

  5. Disadvantages

     a. Only available through physicians who have met certain criteria, e.g., can accurately determine duration of a patient's pregnancy, can detect an ectopic pregnancy, be able to provide surgical intervention in cases of incomplete abortion or severe bleeding

     b. Cramping, bleeding common side effects; heavy bleeding in approximately one of 100 women

     c. May also cause nausea/vomiting, diarrhea, headache, dizziness, fatigue, back pain

  6. Precautions

     a. Contraindicated in women with confirmed or suspected ectopic pregnancy, IUD in place, chronic adrenal failure, long-term corticosteroid use, allergy to mifepristone, misoprostol or other prostaglandins, hemorrhagic disorders or current anticoagulant therapy

     b. Action may be enhanced by ketoconazole, itraconazole, erythromycin, grapefruit juice (Mifepristone, 2001)

     c. Action may be inhibited by rifampin, dexamethasone, St. John's wort, phenytoin, phenobarbital, carbamazepine (Mifepristone, 2001)

  7. Guidelines for use

a. Duration of pregnancy (49 days or less; initial dose of 600 mg, two days later 400 μg of misoprostol (a prostaglandin)

b. Follow-up visit fourteen days after mifepristone to determine if pregnancy has been terminated

Contraception

- Oral Contraceptives

    1. Combined oral contraceptives (OC)

        a. Description

            (1) Pills containing both an estrogen and a progestin

                (a) Estrogenic compounds currently used in U.S.— ethinyl estradiol (EE) and mestranol

                (b) Currently available progestins

                    (i) First generation progestins—norethindrone; norethindrone acetate; ethynodiol diacetate; norgestrel; levonorgestrel

                    (ii) New generation progestins—desogestrel; norgestimate; gestodene

            (2) Types of OC

                (a) Monophasic—constant dose of estrogen and progestin delivered throughout the cycle

                (b) Multiphasic—dosage of estrogen and progestin are varied during the cycle

        b. Mechanism of action—suppression of ovulation through combined actions of estrogen and progestin

            (1) Estrogenic effects

                (a) Ovulation inhibited, partially by suppression of follicle stimulating hormone (FSH) and luteinizing hormone (LH)

                (b) Uterine secretions altered, inhibiting implantation

                (c) Acceleration of ovum transport

                (d) May cause degeneration of corpus luteum (luteolysis)

            (2) Progestin effects

                (a) Suppression of LH inhibits ovulation

                (b) Cervical mucus thickens, inhibiting sperm transport and sperm penetration of ovum

                (c) Ovum transport may be slowed

                (d) Alteration of endometrium hampers implantation

c. Effectiveness: First year failure rate

    (1) Perfect use—0.1%

    (2) Typical use—5%

d. Noncontraceptive benefits and advantages

    (1) Menstrual cycle effects

        (a) Regulation of menstrual cycle

        (b) Decreased menstrual cramps and pain

        (c) Decreased duration and amount of menstrual flow

    (2) Affords some protection against:

        (a) PID

        (b) Ovarian and endometrial cancer

        (c) Benign breast disease

        (d) Ectopic pregnancy

        (e) Functional ovarian cysts

        (f) Premenstrual symptoms

        (g) Iron deficiency anemia

    (3) Improvement of some medical conditions

        (a) Symptoms of estrogen deficiency—e.g., osteoporosis

        (b) Endometriosis

        (c) Acne

e. Disadvantages

    (1) No protection against STD and HIV/AIDS

    (2) Must be taken every day

    (3) Potential side effects

        (a) Unwanted menstrual cycle changes—may include missed periods, scanty periods, spotting, breakthrough bleeding

        (b) Potential side effects caused by hormonal properties of OC—estrogenic, progestogenic and androgenic

            (i) Estrogenic effects—breast tenderness and possible increase in breast size; nausea; cyclic weight gain caused by fluid retention; cervical ectopia or erosion; growth of leiomyomata; spider angiomas; thromboembolism; pulmonary emboli; cerebrovascular accidents; hepatocellular adenomas and cancer

         (ii) Progestogenic effects—breast tenderness; headaches; hypertension; myocardial infarction

         (iii) Androgenic effects—appetite increase and weight gain; depression, fatigue and tiredness; decreased libido; acne and oily skin; increased breast size due to alveolar tissue; increased LDL and decreased HDL cholesterol levels; diabetogenic effects including decreased carbohydrate tolerance; pruritus

    (4) Chlamydial cervicitis more common in women on OC

    (5) Potential but rare serious complications

      (a) Thrombophlebitis

      (b) Pulmonary emboli

      (c) Cardiovascular disease (CVD)

f. Precautions

    (1) Should not be provided to women who are pregnant or in whom pregnancy is strongly suspected

    (2) Should not be provided to women with current or previous diagnosis of:

      (a) Thrombophlebitis or thromboembolic disorder

      (b) Cerebrovascular accident

      (c) Coronary artery or ischemic heart disease

      (d) Known or strongly suspected breast cancer

      (e) Known or strongly suspected estrogen-dependent neoplasia

      (f) Benign hepatic adenoma or liver cancer

      (g) Markedly impaired liver function (currently)

      (h) Older than 35 and heavy smoker ($\geq$ 20 cigarettes per day)

    (3) Exercise caution in prescribing and monitor closely for development of adverse effects

      (a) Older than 35 and light smoker (< 20 cigarettes per day)

      (b) Migraine headaches that start after initiation of OC (without focal neurological symptoms)

      (c) Hypertension with resting diastolic BP of $\geq$ 90 mm Hg or resting systolic BP of $\geq$ 140 mm Hg on 3 separate visits, or diastolic BP of $\geq$ 110 mm Hg on single visit

      (d) Diabetes mellitus

      (e) Impending major surgery requiring immobilization in next four weeks

      (f)   Undiagnosed abnormal vaginal bleeding

      (g)   Sickle cell disease or sickle C disease

      (h)   Lactation

      (i)   Gestational diabetes

      (j)   Active gallbladder disease

      (k)   Congenital hyperbilirubinemia

      (l)   Over age 50

      (m)   Completion of term pregnancy within past 21 days

      (n)   Current or past cardiac or renal disease

      (o)   Conditions likely to make it difficult for woman to take OC correctly and consistently

      (p)   Family history of dyslipidemia

      (q)   Family history of death of parent or sibling prior to age 50 due to myocardial infarction

  g. Prescribing guidelines

    (1) Most women started on OC containing ≤ 35 mcg estrogen (low-dose)

    (2) Efficacy of low-dose OC may be lowered when used concurrently with medications that affect liver metabolism

      (a)   Anticonvulsants—phenobarbital, phenytoin, carbamazepine, primidone, ethosuximide

      (b)   Antibiotics—particularly ampicillin and tetracycline

      (c)   Rifampin

      (d)   Griseofulvin

    (3) OC may potentiate the effects of the following:

      (a)   Antidepressants—amitriptyline, desipramine, imipramine

      (b)   Benzodiazepines

      (c)   Beta-blockers—nadolol, propanolol, metoprolol, atenolol

      (d)   Theophylline

2. Progestin-only pills (minipills)

  a. Description—oral contraceptive containing fixed dose of a progestin only

  b. Mechanism of action

        (1) Inhibition of ovulation—although does not consistently inhibit ovulation; regular, cyclic bleeding pattern indicates ovulation is not being suppressed

        (2) Cervical mucus thickens and decreases in amount inhibiting sperm penetration

        (3) Creation of thin, atrophic endometrium

        (4) Premature luteolysis

  c. Effectiveness: First year failure rate

        (1) Perfect use—0.5%

        (2) Typical use—5%

  d. Noncontraceptive benefits and advantages

        (1) No estrogen-related side effects or complications

        (2) No adverse effects on lactation

        (3) Scanty or no menses; decreased anemia; decreased dysmenorrhea

        (4) Decreased risk of developing endometrial cancer, ovarian cancer, and PID

        (5) Immediately reversible upon discontinuation

  e. Disadvantages

        (1) No protection against STD and HIV/AIDS

        (2) Menstrual cycle disturbances—irregular bleeding

        (3) Generally less effective than combined OC—must be taken consistently at the same time every day

        (4) Functional ovarian cysts occur more often

        (5) If pregnancy occurs, greater likelihood of ectopic

  f. Precautions—exercise caution in prescribing and monitor closely for development of adverse effects

        (1) Unexplained abnormal vaginal bleeding

        (2) Liver conditions such as severe decompensated cirrhosis; adenoma or cancer; active viral hepatitis

        (3) Breast cancer—effect of progestin not completely understood

        (4) Use of rifampin and most antiseizure medications (phenytoin, carbamazepine, phenobarbital) which induce hepatic enzymes

  g. Managing side effects

        (1) Allow time for adjustment to pills

        (2) Determine if pills are taken correctly

(3) Determine whether any symptoms are indicative of health problems

(4) Determine if hormonal component may be responsible

- Implants and Injectables
  1. Norplant
     a. Description
        (1) Long-acting progestin-only contraceptive
        (2) Levonorgestrel administered through six slender, flexible silicone capsules that are 2.4 × 34 mm each
        (3) Silicone capsules are implanted under the skin of the upper, inner arm
        (4) Effective for five years
     b. Mechanism of action
        (1) Ovulation inhibited
        (2) Cervical mucus changes—thickens and decreases in amount making sperm penetration more difficult
        (3) Creation of thin, atrophic endometrium
        (4) Premature luteolysis
     c. Effectiveness: First year failure rate
        (1) Perfect use—0.05%
        (2) Typical use—0.05%
     d. Noncontraceptive benefits and advantages
        (1) No estrogen-related side effects or complications
        (2) Noncontraceptive benefits—scanty or no menses; decreased anemia; decreased dysmenorrhea; suppression of ovulation-related pain; decreased risk of endometrial cancer, ovarian cancer and PID
        (3) Immediately reversible
        (4) Extremely effective, long-term contraception
        (5) Not related to intercourse
        (6) Low risk of ectopic as compared with women not using a contraceptive method
        (7) Safe for women over 35 years of age
     e. Disadvantages
        (1) No protection against STD and HIV/AIDS
        (2) High initial cost

    (3)   Irregular bleeding patterns—most common reason for removal in first two years; if heavy, anemia may occur

    (4)   If pregnancy occurs, must consider ectopic

    (5)   Effectiveness significantly lowered with anticonvulsants and rifampin

    (6)   Implants may be visible or may cause scarring

    (7)   Side effects may include—bloating, weight gain, acne, hair loss, breast tenderness, local inflammation or infection at insertion site, depression

    (8)   Ovarian cysts—usually regress spontaneously

    (9)   Removal may be difficult—especially if insertion was too deep

  f.   Precautions

    (1)   Do not provide to women with following diagnoses

       (a)   Known or suspected pregnancy

       (b)   Unexplained abnormal vaginal bleeding

       (c)   Active thrombophlebitis or pulmonary emboli

       (d)   On antiseizure medications (except valproic acid) or rifampin

       (e)   Known or suspected current or past breast cancer

       (f)   Active liver disease

       (g)   Hypercholesterolemia

    (2)   Exercise caution in prescribing and monitor closely for development of adverse effects

       (a)   Intolerant of irregular bleeding

       (b)   Migraine or other headaches

       (c)   Heart lesions that predispose to subacute bacterial endocarditis

       (d)   History of heart attack, stroke, chest pain due to heart disease, thrombophlebitis, pulmonary embolism or blood clots in the eye, diabetes which predisposes to cardiovascular disease

       (e)   History of allergic reaction with use of pills containing levonorgestrel

       (f)   History of acne that worsened on combined OC

2. Depo-Provera (DMPA)

  a.   Description

    (1)   Injectable progestin (depo-medroxyprogesterone acetate)

    (2)   150 mg of DMPA administered by deep intramuscular injection every 12 weeks

b. Mechanism of action

  (1) Inhibits ovulation by suppressing FSH and LH levels and eliminating LH surge

  (2) Development of shallow, atrophic endometrium

  (3) Thickens cervical mucus that decreases sperm penetration

c. Effectiveness: First year failure rate

  (1) Perfect use—0.3%

  (2) Typical use—0.3%

d. Noncontraceptive benefits and advantages

  (1) Long-acting, highly effective, reversible contraceptive

  (2) No estrogen-related side effects or complications

  (3) No interference with intercourse

  (4) Noncontraceptive benefits—scanty or no menses; decreased anemia; decreased dysmenorrhea; suppression of ovulation-associated pain; decreased risk of developing endometrial cancer, ovarian cancer, and PID

  (5) Low risk of ectopic as compared with women not using any contraceptive method

  (6) Decreases frequency of seizures

  (7) No drug interactions

  (8) No adverse effects on lactation

e. Disadvantages

  (1) No protection against STD and HIV/AIDS

  (2) Menstrual cycle changes—during first year of use, more spotting and breakthrough bleeding; the longer DMPA is used, the greater likelihood of amenorrhea

  (3) Weight gain, depression, breast tenderness

  (4) Return visits every 12 weeks for repeat injections

  (5) No immediate discontinuation—side effects, including menstrual irregularities may continue for 6 to 8 months following discontinuation of method

  (6) Lipid changes—decrease in HDL cholesterol levels

  (7) Decrease in bone density; reversible when DMPA stopped

  (8) Allergic reactions—anaphylactic reactions are rare, but may occur immediately following Depo-Provera injections

f. Precautions

(1) Should not be provided to women with following:

    (a) Known or suspected pregnancy

    (b) Unexplained vaginal bleeding past three months

    (c) Breast cancer—current or past

(2) Exercise caution in prescribing and monitor closely for development of adverse effects

    (a) Pregnancy planned in fairly near future

    (b) Concern over weight gain

    (c) Severe, acute liver disease, liver tumors, or gallbladder disease

    (d) Diabetes with nephropathy, retinopathy, and neuropathy

g. Prescribing guidelines

  (1) Administer

    (a) During first five days after onset of menses

    (b) Within first seven days postpartum if not breastfeeding

    (c) At six weeks postpartum if breastfeeding

  (2) Do not massage injection site—may lower effectiveness

3. Lunelle

a. Description

  (1) Injectable progestin (25 mg medroxprogesterone acetate) and estrogen (5 mg estradiol cypionate)

  (2) 0.5 mL aqueous suspension administered by deep muscular injection every 28 to 33 days (not to exceed 33 days)

b. Mechanism of action

  (1) Inhibits ovulation by suppressing secretion of gonadotropins (FSH and LH), which prevents follicular matruation and ovulation

  (2) Possible thickening and reduction in volume of cervical mucus, which decreases sperm penetration

  (3) Possible thinning of endometrium, which may reduce likelihood of implantation

c. Effectiveness—precise rate not yet available, but likely in range from 0.1 to 1%

d. Noncontraceptive benefits and advantages—not yet available, but likely same as combined OC

e. Disadvantages

  (1) No protection against STD and HIV/AIDS

    (2)   Injection must be administered monthly

    (3)   Potential side effects—same as combined OC, plus

        (a)   Alteration of menstrual bleeding pattern—may include frequent bleeding, irregular bleeding, prolonged bleeding, infrequent bleeding, and amenorrhea

        (b)   Weight gain

        (c)   Possible anaphylaxis or anaphylactoid reaction to injection—rare

f.   Precautions—same as combined OC

g.   Prescribing guidelines

    (1)   Administer

        (a)   First injection

            (i)   Within 5 days after onset of normal menses

            (ii)   Within 5 days of a complete first trimester abortion

            (iii)   No earlier than 4 weeks postpartum if not breastfeeding

            (iv)   No earlier than 6 weeks postpartum if breastfeeding

            (v)   If switching from OC, should be administered within 7 days after last active pill

        (b)   Second and subsequent injections

            (i)   Monthly (28 to 30 days) after previous injection, not to exceed 33 days

            (ii)   If client has not adhered to prescribed schedule, pregnancy should be ruled out, and client should not receive another injection until pregnancy is ruled out

    (2)   Drug interactions—same as combined OC, plus

        (a)   Possible decreased effectiveness of aminoglutethamide

        (b)   Efficacy of Lunelle may be lowered when used concurrently with

            (i)   Rifampin

            (ii)   Anticonvulsants—phenobarbital, phenytoin, and carbamazepine

            (iii)   Antibiotics—particularly ampicillin, tetracycline, and griseofulvin

            (iv)   Herbal products—containing St. John's Wort (hypericum perforatum)

        (c)   May increase plasma concentration of—cyclosporine, prednisolone, and theophylline

- Intrauterine Device (IUD)
    1. Description
        a. Plastic contraceptive device inserted into uterus
        b. Two types currently available in U.S.
            (1) Progesterone T (Progestasert System)
                (a) Must be removed and replaced every year
                (b) Releases 65 mcg of progesterone per day
            (2) Copper T 380A (Paragard)—most widely used in U.S.
                (a) T-shaped polyethylene device with copper wound around vertical stem
                (b) Approved for 10 years use
            (3) Levonorgestrel-IUD (LNg IUD)—not currently approved in U.S., but approval is expected
                (a) Releases 20 mcg levonorgestrel per day into uterus
                (b) Effective for five years
    2. Mechanism of action
        a. Exact mechanism not completely understood
        b. Immobilizes sperm
        c. Interferes with migration of sperm from vagina to fallopian tubes
        d. Speeds transport of ovum through the fallopian tubes
        e. Local effects on endometrium
    3. Effectiveness: First year failure rate
        a. Copper T 380A
            (1) Perfect use—0.6%
            (2) Typical use—0.8%
        b. Progesterone T
            (1) Perfect use—1.5%
            (2) Typical use—2.0%
        c. LNg 20
            (1) Perfect use—0.1%
            (2) Typical use—0.1%
    4. Noncontraceptive benefits and advantages
        a. Less expensive per year and easier to use than some other methods

    b. Copper IUD can be used by women who have contraindications to hormonal methods

    c. IUDs that release progesterone decrease menstrual blood loss and dysmenorrhea

5. Disadvantages

    a. No protection against STD and HIV/AIDS

    b. Increased risk of PID—greatest risk at time of insertion

    c. May have increased dysmenorrhea and minor increase in blood loss

    d. Spontaneous expulsion may occur—2% to 10% expelled within first year

    e. Pregnancy complications possible if pregnancy occurs with IUD in situ—if IUD left in place, 50% will end in spontaneous abortion; if IUD removed early in pregnancy, 25% will spontaneously abort

    f. Possible risks at time of insertion include—vasovagal reaction, uterine perforation, cramping and pain

    g. Potential side effects and complications

        (1) Spotting, bleeding, and hemorrhage—abnormal bleeding common in first 3 months; after first 3 months, may be a sign of infection or pregnancy

        (2) Anemia—remove IUD if Hgb < 9 g

        (3) Cramping and pain—except at time of insertion, may be sign of pregnancy, infection or expulsion

        (4) Expulsion—symptoms may include unusual vaginal discharge, cramping or pain, intermenstrual spotting, postcoital spotting, dyspareunia, absence or lengthening of IUD string, presence of hard plastic of IUD at cervical os or in vagina

        (5) Pregnancy—5% will be ectopic; higher risk of ectopic with Progesterone T

        (6) Uterine perforation, embedding and cervical perforation—most common sites are uterine fundus, body of the uterus, and cervical wall

        (7) PID—remove IUD and treat

6. Precautions

    a. Should not be provided to women with following:

        (1) Active, recent or recurrent pelvic infection—PID, postpartum endometritis, infection following abortion

        (2) Known or suspected pregnancy

        (3) Severely distorted uterine cavity caused by anatomical abnormalities of the uterus

    b. Exercise caution in prescribing, counsel thoroughly, and monitor closely for development of adverse effects

      (1) Risk factors for PID—purulent cervicitis; recent positive gonorrhea or chlamydia test; recurrent history of chlamydia or gonorrhea

      (2) High risk for STD—multiple partners or partner with multiple partners

      (3) Impaired response to infection—diabetes, steroid treatment, HIV disease

      (4) Risk factors for HIV infection and/or HIV disease

      (5) Undiagnosed, irregular, heavy or abnormal vaginal bleeding; known or suspected cervical or uterine cancer, including unresolved abnormal Pap smear

      (6) Previous problems with IUD use

      (7) History of vasovagal reactions or fainting

      (8) Lack of access to emergency medical care if complications occur

      (9) Valvular heart disease such as aortic stenosis; increased susceptibility to subacute bacterial endocarditis

     (10) Anatomical abnormalities that do not distort uterus—leiomyomata, endometrial polyps, cervical stenosis, bicornuate uterus, small uterus

     (11) Women who have never had a child tend not to tolerate the IUD as well as women who have carried to term

7. Prescribing guidelines

  a. Review IUD instructions with patient

    (1) Check strings

    (2) Be aware of infection signs or symptoms

    (3) Carefully monitor menstrual periods

  b. Teach patient IUD warning signs—PAINS

    (1) **P**eriod late (pregnancy), abnormal spotting or bleeding

    (2) **A**bdominal pain, pain with intercourse

    (3) **I**nfection exposure (any STD), abnormal discharge

    (4) **N**ot feeling well, fever, chills

    (5) **S**tring missing, shorter or longer

- Condoms

1. Male condom

  a. Description

    (1) Sheath-like covering for the penis

      (2)   Three types—Latex (rubber); polyurethane (plastic); lambskin (from intestinal membrane)

  b. Mechanism of action

      (1)   Acts as a mechanical barrier, preventing sperm from entering vagina

      (2)   Placed on erect penis before any contact with vagina

  c. Effectiveness: First year failure rate

      (1)   Perfect use—3%

      (2)   Typical use—14%

  d. Noncontraceptive benefits and advantages

      (1)   Accessible and inexpensive—over 100 brands available, some with spermicide

      (2)   Can effectively reduce transmission of STD and HIV/AIDS (latex and polyurethane)

      (3)   Male involvement needed

      (4)   May help maintain erection and prevent premature ejaculation

      (5)   May prevent sperm allergy

  e. Disadvantages—interruption of foreplay; interference with erection; male involvement essential; reduced sensitivity; decreased pleasure; embarrassment; possibility of breakage; allergy to latex

  f. Precautions

      (1)   ''Skin'' condoms do not prevent STD and HIV transmission

      (2)   Petroleum-based lubricants and some vaginal medications break down latex

2. Female condom

  a. Description—polyurethane sheath with flexible rings at each end

  b. Mechanism of action—physical barrier that lines the vagina and partially covers the perineum

  c. Effectiveness: First year failure rate

      (1)   Perfect use—5%

      (2)   Typical use—21%

  d. Noncontraceptive benefits and advantages

      (1)   Polyurethane stronger than latex, may not tear as easily as male condom

      (2)   Theoretical protection against STD and HIV exposure— has been tested in laboratory

      (3)   Does not require prescription

       (4)   May be inserted up to eight hours prior to intercourse

    e. Disadvantages

       (1)   May be difficult for some women to insert

       (2)   May affect sexual sensation, cause irritation or discomfort

       (3)   May be used only once—expensive

       (4)   May become displaced

    f. Precautions

       (1)   Some may be allergic to polyurethane

       (2)   May be difficult to use with some anatomic abnormalities

- Diaphragm

1. Description

    a. Dome-shaped, latex rubber cup with flexible ring that is inserted into the vagina prior to intercourse, with anterior rim positioned behind the pubic bone and posterior rim in the posterior fornix; spermicidal jelly is placed within the dome and around rim prior to insertion

    b. Available in a variety of rim types (flat, coil, and arcing) and sizes (50 to 100 mm)

2. Mechanism of action—barrier plus spermicide

3. Effectiveness: First year failure rate

    a. Perfect use—6%

    b. Typical use—20%

4. Noncontraceptive benefits and advantages

    a. No systemic side effects

    b. Some protection against STD, including gonorrhea and chlamydia; irritation related to spermicide may increase susceptibility to HIV transmission

    c. Protection against cervical neoplasia

5. Disadvantages

    a. Requires fitting by clinician and instruction in use

    b. Slight increased risk for toxic shock syndrome

    c. Increases risk for vaginal and urinary tract infections

6. Precautions—conditions that may preclude satisfactory use

    a. Allergy to spermicide, rubber, latex, or polyurethane

    b. Abnormalities in vaginal anatomy that interfere with satisfactory fit or stable placement of diaphragm

    c.   Inability to learn correct insertion technique

    d.   History of toxic shock syndrome

    e.   Repeated urinary tract infections that persist despite refitting

    f.   Lack of trained personnel to fit or provide instruction

    g.   Full-term delivery within the past six weeks, recent spontaneous or induced abortion, vaginal bleeding

7.   Prescribing guidelines

    a.   Review instructions for use

       (1)   Must be left in place six hours after last intercourse, with maximum time of 24 hours in vagina

       (2)   Avoid oil-based lubricants and medications

    b.   Teach warning signs for toxic shock syndrome—requires immediate treatment

- Cervical Cap (Prentif Cavity Rim Cervical Cap)

   1.   Description—deep, soft rubber cup with a firm round rim; covers the cervix and fits with suction around the base of the cervix; available in 4 sizes (22, 25, 28, 31 mm); small amount of spermicide placed in cap prior to insertion

   2.   Mechanism of action—barrier plus spermicide

   3.   Effectiveness: First year failure rate

    a.   Perfect use—parous women 20%; nulliparous women 9%

    b.   Typical use—parous women 40%; nulliparous women 20%

   4.   Advantages—continuous protection for up to 48 hours; STD and HIV protection has not been studied

   5.   Disadvantages

    a.   Requires trained clinician to fit

    b.   May be difficult for some women to insert or remove

    c.   May cause odor, especially with prolonged use

    d.   Slightly increased risk for toxic shock syndrome

   6.   Precautions—conditions that may preclude satisfactory use

    a.   Allergy to latex, rubber, polyurethane or spermicide

    b.   Anatomical abnormalities that interfere with satisfactory fit

    c.   Inability to learn insertion or removal technique

    d.   History of toxic shock syndrome; vaginal bleeding

    e.   Lack of trained personnel to fit and provide instruction

    f.   Full-term vaginal delivery within past six weeks, recent spontaneous or induced abortion, vaginal bleeding

    g.   Known or suspected cervical or uterine cancer, abnormal Pap smear, vaginal, cervical, or urinary tract infections

- Spermicides

    1.   Description—consists of two components

        a.   Inert base or carrier—foam, jelly, cream, suppository, film

        b.   Spermicidal chemical that kills sperm—Nonoxynol-9 or Octoxynol-9

    2.   Mechanism of action—spermicides are surfactants that destroy sperm cell membrane; immobilize and kill sperm

    3.   Effectiveness: First year failure rate

        a.   Perfect use—6%

        b.   Typical use—26%

    4.   Noncontraceptive benefits and advantages

        a.   Relatively inexpensive; available without prescription or clinic visit

        b.   May provide some protection against bacterial STD although protection greatest when used in conjunction with barrier method

        c.   Can be used as back-up with other methods

    5.   Disadvantages

        a.   Possible allergic reaction to spermicide or base

        b.   Increased colonization of *Candida albicans*

        c.   Increased colonization of vagina with anaerobic bacteria and uropathogens (bacterial vaginosis)

        d.   Nonoxynol-9—ineffective against HIV transmission and may increase transmission

    6.   Precautions—spermicide not the best choice in following circumstances

        a.   Client at high risk for HIV

        b.   Inability to learn correct insertion technique

        c.   Allergy or sensitivity to spermicide or base ingredients

        d.   Abnormal vaginal anatomy that interferes with appropriate placement or retention of spermicide

    7.   Guidelines for use

        a.   Jellies, creams, foams—inserted into vagina prior to each act of intercourse; protection is immediate and remains effective for no more than one hour when used alone; jelly and cream when used with diaphragm remain effective for 6 to 8 hours

    b. Film and suppositories—inserted into vagina before each act of intercourse; contraceptive protection begins 10 to 15 minutes after insertion and lasts no more than one hour

- Emergency Contraception

    1. Description

        a. Postcoital contraception used after an act of unprotected intercourse

        b. Methods used include OC (Yuzpe method), progestin-only minipills or insertion of copper-releasing IUD within 5 days

    2. Mechanism of action (Yuzpe method—emergency contraceptive pills)

        a. Are not effective if woman is already pregnant

        b. Act by delaying or inhibiting ovulation, and/or altering tubal transport of sperm and/or ova (inhibiting fertilization), and/or altering the endometrium (altering implantation)

    3. Effectiveness—depends on when unprotected intercourse occurs in cycle; effectiveness ranges from 55.3% to 94.2% (average effectiveness 74.0%)

    4. Advantages

        a. Only option available after unprotected intercourse has occurred

        b. Simple, easy to use

        c. Side effects are of short duration

    5. Disadvantages

        a. Nausea and vomiting are common side effects (nausea in 50% to 70%)

        b. May alter timing of next menstrual period—need to evaluate for pregnancy if no menstrual period within three weeks

    6. Precautions—not appropriate for woman who has serious problems that would contraindicate OC

    7. Guidelines for use

        a. Four regimens are currently approved by FDA—all require two doses, 12 hours apart, of an estrogen (ethinyl estradiol) and progestin (norgestrel or levonorgestrel)

        b. Must be initiated within 72 hours after unprotected intercourse

- Fertility Awareness Methods

    1. Description

   a. A variety of methods that help couples prevent or plan pregnancies by identifying fertile days of the menstrual cycle; natural family planning methods are based on fertility awareness

   b. Methods include calendar rhythm method, basal body temperature (BBT) method, cervical mucus charting (ovulation or Billings method), and sympto-thermal method

2. Mechanism of action—calculation of fertile period based on four assumptions

   a. Sperm remain viable for two to seven days (average three days)

   b. Ovum remains fertile for 24 hours

   c. Ovulation occurs on day 14 ($\pm$ 2 days) before onset of next menses

   d. Span of fertility may be from seven days before ovulation to three days after

3. Effectiveness: First year failure rate

   a. Perfect use—calendar 9%; ovulation method 3%; sympto-thermal 2%; BBT 1%

   b. Typical use—25% for all

4. Advantages

   a. No serious side effects

   b. Increases users' knowledge of reproductive physiology—can be used to plan conception, detect pregnancy, and prevent pregnancy

   c. Low cost

   d. No interruption of normal body functions

   e. Acceptable to most religious groups

   f. Encourages communication between partners

5. Disadvantages

   a. No protection against STD or HIV

   b. Lack of cooperative male partner is an obstacle

   c. Women must abstain (or use another method) when libido is at peak

   d. Requires copious record keeping

   e. Periodic abstinence may be problem for some couples

   f. Unreliable during lactation and perimenopausal period

6. Precautions

   a. Certain conditions may make fertility awareness more difficult to use—irregular menstrual cycles; irregular temperature charts; recent discontinuation of hormonal methods; recent menarche; approaching menopause; unable to keep careful records

    b. Not recommended postpartum prior to resumption of normal menses

7. Specific methods

    a. Calendar charting—fertile days are predicted based on records of past menstrual cycles

        (1) Earliest day of fertility is calculated by subtracting 18 days from length of shortest cycle

        (2) Latest day of fertility is calculated by subtracting 11 days from length of longest cycle

    b. Basal body temperature (BBT) charting—BBT is lowest body temperature of healthy person taken upon awakening

        (1) Record BBT for 3 to 4 consecutive months to determine time of ovulation

        (2) Drop in BBT sometimes precedes ovulation by 12 to 24 hours followed by sustained rise in BBT for several days

        (3) Progesterone increases BBT by 0.4 to 0.8° F

        (4) To avoid pregnancy, abstain until temperature elevation is sustained for three consecutive days

    c. Cervical mucus method (Ovulation, Billings)

        (1) Mucus just before and at ovulation—clear, thin, watery, elastic, abundant

        (2) Mucus following ovulation—thick, cloudy, whitish, tacky, scant

        (3) To prevent pregnancy, avoid intercourse or use another method until day four after peak (ovulatory) mucus

    d. Sympto-thermal method

        (1) Combines various charting techniques—mucus, cervix, BBT

        (2) To prevent pregnancy, abstain or use another method until four days after peak mucus and three days after temperature rise

- Voluntary Sterilization

1. Female sterilization

    a. Description—a surgical procedure in which the fallopian tubes are occluded to prevent the sperm and egg from uniting

    b. Mechanism of action

        (1) Surgical interruption of fallopian tubes

        (2) Methods for tubal interruption include—surgical ligation, excision, electrocoagulation, mechanical devices

    c. Effectiveness—first year failure rate 0.5% with perfect and typical use

    d. Advantages

        (1) Safe operative procedure; no long-term side effects

        (2) Permanent and highly effective

    e. Disadvantages and precautions

        (1) Risks of surgery—anesthesia, infection, hemorrhage

        (2) Post-operative pain and discomfort

        (3) Expensive at time it is performed

        (4) No protection against STD and HIV

        (5) Considered permanent—reversibility difficult and expensive; success cannot be guaranteed

        (6) If pregnancy occurs, high probability of ectopic

2. Male sterilization—vasectomy

    a. Description—male surgical procedure in which the vas deferens are blocked, preventing passage of sperm

    b. Mechanism of action—surgical interruption of sperm

    c. Effectiveness: First year failure rate

        (1) Perfect use:—0.1%

        (2) Typical use:—0.15%

    d. Advantages

        (1) Extremely safe and effective

        (2) Permanent

        (3) Non-scalpel technique carries lower complication rate; simple procedure; very quickly performed

    e. Disadvantages

        (1) Expensive in short term

        (2) Reversal is difficult, expensive, and results cannot be guaranteed

        (3) No protection against STD and HIV

        (4) Post-operative side effects—bruising, swelling, hematoma, infection at operative site

        (5) Vasectomy is not effective until sperm are ejaculated from reproductive system—usually 15 ejaculations

        (6) One-half to two-thirds of men will develop sperm antibodies following vasectomy—no evidence that it causes pathology

    f. Precautions—should not be provided to men with following diagnoses

(1) Local skin infection

(2) Varicocele, large hydrocele, inguinal hernia, scar tissue from previous surgery

(3) Special precautions with clotting disorders, diabetes and recent coronary artery disease

g. Counseling guidelines

(1) **B**enefits—permanent and highly effective

(2) **R**isks of surgery—small chance of future pregnancy

(3) **A**lternatives—other reversible contraceptive methods

(4) **I**nquiries—encourage and answer questions

(5) **D**ecision to change—without loss of medical or financial benefits

(6) **E**xplanation—of entire procedure and possible side effects

(7) **D**ocumentation—of method and timing of surgery, any complications

Menopause

- Definition: Ovarian failure marked by cessation of menses for 12 months or by a serum FSH level of over 40 mIU per mL on two occasions one week apart, outside of normal FSH surge; climacteric refers to transitional period of up to 15 years leading up to the last menstrual period marked by waning ovarian function; term "perimenopause" may be used interchangeably

- Etiology/Incidence

  1. Results from changes in the ovary, with gradual atresia of ovarian follicles leading to decline in ovarian production of estrogen and progesterone; fewer available follicles to produce estradiol (most potent estrogen)

  2. Estrogen deficiency increases woman's risk for cardiovascular disease and osteoporosis; also responsible for majority of symptoms associated with menopause

  3. Cessation of menses usually occurs between 45 and 55 years—average age in U.S. is 50; ovarian failure prior to age 30 is premature; between 31 and 40 is considered early; after age 40 considered normal

- Signs and Symptoms of Menopause

  1. Menstrual changes—irregular menses with wide variations in cycle length and anovulatory cycles

  2. Hot flashes/hot flushes experienced during day or night

  3. Hormonal changes

     a. Immediately preceding menopause

        (1) Lower estradiol levels

        (2) Increased FSH levels

         (3)   LH levels somewhat increased

    b. Following menopause

         (1)   Primary estrogen is estrone—derived from conversion of androstenedione to estrone in extraglandular sites

         (2)   FSH elevated 10 to 20 fold (> 40 mIU/mL)

         (3)   LH elevated three fold

4. Physical changes due to aging and estrogen loss

    a. Vulva—atrophy; pruritus; pubic hair thinning; labia majora decrease in size and labia minora almost nonexistent

    b. Vagina—decreased lubrication leading to dyspareunia; vaginitis; dryness; loss of rugae; becomes shorter and narrower; vaginal pH more alkaline (6.5 to 7.5)

    c. Pelvic floor—muscular tissue loss causing uterine prolapse, cystocele and rectocele

    d. Bladder/urethra—atrophy; frequency and urgency; stress incontinence

    e. Uterus—decreases in size and weight

    f. Breasts—decrease with gradual atrophy of glandular tissue; nipples smaller and flatter

    g. Skin—dryness; decreased sebaceous and sweat gland activity; less elasticity; hyperpigmentation/hypopigmentation; atrophy and thinning of epidermal and dermal skin layers; decrease in scalp, pubic and axillary hair

    h. Cardiovascular—changes in lipids (gradual increase in LDL and decrease in HDL) favor formation of atherosclerosis; coronary artery disease; gradual increase in total cholesterol and triglycerides

    i. Lungs—lung expansion decreases; thorax more rigid and tissues less elastic

    j. Musculoskeletal—muscle tone related to exercise; if sedentary, tone and strength diminish; atrophy if muscles not used

         (1)   Osteoporosis

            (a)   Definition—imbalance between bone formation and bone resorption; associated with skeletal fractures

               (i)   Type I—on average, occurs 15 to 20 years after menopause; trabecular bone loss; common fracture sites include vertebrae and distal radius

               (ii)   Type II—occurs in men and women in 7th decade; common fracture site is hip

            (b)   Risk factors—sedentary lifestyle, smoking, small-boned, Caucasian or Asian, low dietary intake of calcium throughout reproductive years, family history of osteoporosis

      (c)   Management—estrogen replacement therapy to treat and prevent progression; adequate calcium intake to maintain calcium balance; weight-bearing exercise 30 minutes 3 times per week; eliminate smoking

          (i)   Selective Estrogen Receptor Modules (SERMS) (raloxifene)—suppresses bone resorption; approved for prevention and treatment; estrogen agonist (bone and heart); estrogen antagonist (breast and uterus); seems to mimic estrogen's effect on bones and heart, but not negative effects; shown to reduce risk of breast cancer; lowers total cholesterol and LDL, but little effect on HDL

         (ii)   Bisphosphonates (alendronate, risedronate)—inhibits osteoclast mediated bone resorption; approved for prevention and treatment

        (iii)   Salmon calcitonin—inhibits osteoclastic resorption; approved for treatment; analgesic effect in some patients

   k.   Neuroendocrine

      (1)   Vasomotor instability (hot flashes and night sweats)

      (2)   Sleep disturbances; insomnia

      (3)   Many sources suggest decreased estrogen levels may contribute to an increased risk of Alzheimer's disease

      (4)   Anxiety, depression, irritability

      (5)   Libido changes

      (6)   Impaired concentration and memory

- Diagnostic Tests/Findings

   1.   Pregnancy test (if suspected)—negative

   2.   Pap smear—low estrogen effect with predominantly parabasal cells

   3.   Serum FSH—level > 40 mIU/mL is diagnostic of menopause

- Management/Treatment (see Osteoporosis in Musculoskeletal Disorders in Adults chapter)

   1.   Discuss diet, exercise, stress management, calcium supplementation, hormone replacement therapy (HRT), estrogen replacement therapy (ERT), SERMS, bisphosphonates and salmon calcitonin

   2.   Minimum daily calcium requirements—supplementation reduces bone loss and decreases fractures

      a.   Women not on estrogen, 50 to 64 years of age 1500 mg

      b.   Women on estrogen, 50 to 64 years of age 1000 mg

      c.   All women over age 65 1500 mg

  3.   Hormone replacement therapy (HRT)

      a.   Indications

          (1)   Relief of menopausal symptoms related to estrogen deficiency—hot flashes, urinary symptoms, vaginal dryness

          (2)   Prevention and treatment of osteoporosis

          (3)   Protection against cardiovascular disease

      b.   Select methods of regimen options

          (1)   Along with estrogen, progestin is indicated to decrease risk of endometrial hyperplasia or cancer if patient has a uterus

          (2)   Sequential regimen—0.625 mg conjugated estrogen or 1.0 mg micronized estradiol daily or from day 1 to 25 each month; medroxyprogesterone acetate (Provera) 10 mg per day added for first 14 days of month or for last 10 days of estrogen administration

          (3)   Continuous regimen—0.625 mg conjugated estrogen, or 0.625 estrone sulfate, or 1.0 mg micronized estradiol daily with daily progestin administration of 2.5 or 5mg medroxyprogesterone acetate or 0.35 mg norethindrone

          (4)   Transdermal estradiol (skin patch)—0.05 to 0.1 mg estradiol; changed once or twice a week; add medroxyprogesterone acetate 10 mg for 12 days per month or 2.5 mg per day continuously for those women with intact uterus

          (5)   Transdermal estradiol/norethindrone acetate—continuous combined therapy; applied twice weekly

          (6) .   Topical estrogens—may be used for atrophic vaginitis and dyspareunia while on oral or transdermal therapy

      c.   Contraindications to HRT

          (1)   Known or suspected breast cancer

          (2)   Known or suspected estrogen-dependent neoplasia

          (3)   Undiagnosed abnormal vaginal bleeding

          (4)   Past or present history of deep vein thrombosis

          (5)   Thrombophlebitis

          (6)   Liver dysfunction or disease

          (7)   Known or suspected pregnancy

          (8)   Active clotting disorders

      d.   Guidelines for HRT provision

    (1)   If not contraindicated, decision for HRT should rest primarily with the woman

    (2)   Before initiating HRT—should have negative clinical breast examination and mammogram; endometrial biopsy indicated with abnormal vaginal bleeding

    (3)   For patients with abnormal vaginal bleeding beyond three to six months of initiating HRT, endometrial biopsy indicated

- General Guidelines

    1.   Pharmacological and nonpharmacological options should be thoroughly discussed with patient

    2.   Educate patient on nonpharmacological symptom relief strategies; e.g., nutritional options, exercise, stress management

    3.   If HRT/ERT is prescribed, thoroughly discuss side effects

    4.   Review/teach self breast examination

    5.   Annual mammogram

    6.   Annual breast examination by health professional

Note: This chapter was written by Susan Moskosky in her private capacity. No official support or endorsement by the Department of Health and Human Services or any component thereof is intended or should be inferred.

Note: Appreciation is extended to Marjorie A. Maddox, Ed.D., C.R.N.P. RN, CS, associate professor, Mary Jane Miskovsky, MSN, C.R.N.P., CNS and Virginia Clark, MSN, RN adjunct faculty, University of Scranton, Department of Nursing, Scranton, Pennsylvania for their contributions and review of this chapter.

Questions
Select the best answer

1. Which of the following is a positive sign of pregnancy?

   a. Goodell's sign
   b. Urinary frequency/urgency
   c. Braxton-Hicks contractions
   d. Fetal movement felt by examiner

2. Which of the following statements is correct regarding maternal physiologic changes in pregnancy?

   a. Pulse rate decreases
   b. Insulin requirements decrease
   c. Increased sweat gland activity
   d. Increased intestinal peristalsis

3. Examination of the breasts in pregnancy may normally show:

   a. Increased nodularity
   b. Linea nigra
   c. Retractions in skin
   d. Loss of nipple pigmentation

4. Examination of a woman in the 30th week of pregnancy would normally reveal:

   a. Cervical dilation of 2 cm
   b. Complaint of nausea and vomiting
   c. Fundal height of 29 cm
   d. Increased platelet count

5. Examination of a woman in her 14th week of pregnancy would normally reveal:

   a. Fundal height of 14 cm
   b. Fetal heart tones audible with fetoscope
   c. Milk expressed from breasts
   d. Cyanosis of the cervix

6. Which of the following is considered to be a common complaint of pregnancy?

   a. Facial edema
   b. Varicosities
   c. Scotomata
   d. Dysuria

7. Which of the following complications is most likely to occur in the first trimester?

   a. Pregnancy induced hypertension
   b. Bleeding

    c. Placenta previa

    d. Gestational diabetes

8. Recommended weight gain in pregnancy for a woman of normal weight for height is:

    a. Less than 20 pounds

    b. 20 pounds

    c. 25 pounds

    d. Over 30 pounds

9. How is the EDB determined using Nagele's rule?

    a. Subtract 3 months from LNMP and add 7 days

    b. Subtract 7 days and add 9 months from the start of the LNMP

    c. Add 9 months from start of the LNMP

    d. Subtract 7 from last day of LNMP and count back 3 months

10. During pregnancy, sexual relations are contraindicated when:

    a. Increased whitish vaginal discharge is present

    b. 36 weeks gestation has been reached

    c. Rupture of membranes is suspected

    d. Weight gain is inadequate

11. Which of the following statements is true regarding diagnostic testing during pregnancy?

    a. Chorionic villus sampling is performed between weeks 14 and 24 when indicated for genetic reasons

    b. Alpha-fetoprotein in maternal blood is assessed between weeks 16 and 18

    c. Gestational diabetes screening is performed between weeks 15 and 18

    d. Amniocentesis between weeks 22 and 26 when indicated for advanced maternal age

12. Which of the following should be avoided during pregnancy?

    a. Intercourse during the third trimester

    b. Swimming

    c. Daily caloric increase of 300 kcal

    d. Douching

13. True labor is characterized by:

    a. Contractions initially felt in back and radiate to lower abdomen

    b. Decrease of intensity of contractions with walking

    c. Discomfort of contractions felt mainly in abdomen

    d. Contractions relieved with sedation

14. A predisposing factor for preterm labor is:

    a. Hypothyroidism

    b. Gestational diabetes

   c. Pyelonephritis
   d. Oligohydramnios

15. Which of the following is a risk factor for the development of gestational diabetes?

   a. Multiple gestation
   b. Prior macrosomic infant
   c. Oligohydramnios in prior pregnancy
   d. Maternal age under 19

16. A woman with a ruptured ectopic pregnancy is likely to have which of the following?

   a. Urinary frequency and urgency
   b. Hypertension
   c. Referred shoulder pain
   d. Fever with nausea and/or vomiting

17. Which of the following increase a woman's chances of having an ectopic pregnancy?

   a. Use of combined oral contraceptives
   b. Uterine myoma
   c. Endometriosis
   d. Previous ectopic pregnancy

18. Inevitable abortion refers to:

   a. Death of embryo or fetus without expulsion
   b. Gross rupture of membranes in the presence of cervical dilatation
   c. Expulsion of products of conception without medical intervention
   d. Presence of bleeding and uterine cramping without cervical dilation

19. Which of the following is a sign of increasingly severe preeclampsia?

   a. Hemoconcentration with decreased platelets
   b. Increased urinary output
   c. Patellar hyporeflexia
   d. Elevated serum glucose

20. Presentation with placenta previa is differentiated from abruptio placentae by:

   a. Abruptio placentae occurs earlier in gestation
   b. Amount of bleeding is more with placenta previa
   c. Severe abdominal pain with abruptio placentae
   d. PIH usually accompanies placenta previa

21. Typical failure rates for combined oral contraceptives approach:

   a. 0.5%
   b. 0.1%
   c. 1%

d. 5%

22. Estrogen in combined oral contraceptives has which of the following effects?

    a. Decrease in HDL and increase in LDL
    b. Thickening of cervical mucus, inhibiting sperm transport
    c. Suppression of FSH and LH
    d. Ovum transport slowed

23. Noncontraceptive benefits of oral contraceptives include which of the following?

    a. Protection against ovarian and endometrial cancer
    b. Protection against breast cancer
    c. Increased libido
    d. Protection against cervical neoplasia

24. The efficacy of combined oral contraceptives may be lowered when used concurrently with which of the following?

    a. Antihypertensives
    b. Antiseizure medications
    c. Beta-blockers
    d. Antidepressants

25. Which of the following side effects is more characteristic of the minipill than the combined oral contraceptive?

    a. Nausea
    b. Increased breast size
    c. Cervical ectopia
    d. Irregular bleeding that persists after 3 months

26. A disadvantage of the minipill is:

    a. Incidence of functional ovarian cysts is increased
    b. Adversely affects lactation
    c. Delayed return to fertility after discontinuation
    d. Increased risk of PID

27. The Norplant system is effective for:

    a. 1 year
    b. 3 years
    c. 5 years
    d. 10 years

28. Which of the following statements about Norplant is true?

    a. Effectiveness not altered by medications
    b. Menstrual irregularities most common reason for removal

c. Menstrual irregularities may continue for 6 to 8 months after removal

d. Risk of decreasing bone density

29. A patient considering use of Depo-Provera should be counseled regarding:

a. Failure rate of 3%
b. Potential menstrual cycle changes
c. Intensification of ovulatory pain
d. Risk of developing hypertension

30. Which of the following is true with regard to administering Depo-Provera?

a. Should be initiated within five days after onset of normal menses
b. Injection site should be massaged to enhance absorption
c. Should be initiated at six weeks postpartum if not breastfeeding
d. Should not be used if breastfeeding

31. To be effective, emergency contraception must be initiated within:

a. 24 hours
b. 48 hours
c. 72 hours
d. 96 hours

32. A woman who had a ParaGard IUD inserted eight weeks ago is complaining of mild pelvic cramping and lengthening of the string. What is the most likely cause?

a. Cervicitis
b. Pregnancy
c. Uterine perforation
d. IUD expulsion

33. A woman with a ParaGard IUD is six weeks pregnant and wishes to continue the pregnancy. She should be told that:

a. The IUD should be removed today and there is a risk of spontaneous abortion
b. The IUD should be left in place to reduce the risk of spontaneous abortion
c. There is an increased risk of fetal congenital anomalies from the copper in the IUD
d. There is no increased risk of spontaneous abortion whether the IUD is left in or removed

34. Calculation of the fertile period rests on which of the following assumptions?

a. Sperm remain viable for 24 hours
b. Ovum survive an average of three days
c. Ovulation occurs on day 14 ($\pm$ 2) before onset of next menses
d. Progesterone decreases basal body temperature 0.4-0.8° F

35. Which of the following would not be considered a complication associated with IUD use?

a. Infection

    b. Ectopic pregnancy

    c. Dysmenorrhea

    d. Ovarian cyst development

36. When counseling a patient who has a ParaGard IUD, emphasis should be placed on which of the following?

    a. Need to change IUD every five years

    b. Risk factors and signs of infection

    c. Risk of developing anemia

    d. Pain control for dysmenorrhea

37. Which of the following statements about the diaphragm is true?

    a. Has a 25% failure rate

    b. Association with increased incidence of urinary tract infections

    c. More effective than cervical cap when used by parous women

    d. There are no contraindications for use other than latex allergy

38. What is the contraceptive ingredient in most vaginal spermicides?

    a. Sodium laurel sulfate

    b. Benzalkonium chloride

    c. Nonoxynol-9

    d. Surfactant

39. Which of the following statements about vaginal spermicides is incorrect?

    a. First year failure rates range from 6% to 26%

    b. Nonoxynol-9 provides some protection against HIV

    c. Spermicidal foam remains effective for up to one hour following insertion

    d. Spermicides work by destroying sperm cell membranes

40. Which of the following statements about condoms is true?

    a. Petroleum based lubricants may deteriorate latex

    b. Skin condoms are equal to latex condoms in STD and HIV protection

    c. Condom use may exacerbate premature ejaculation

    d. Spermicide may weaken the latex in condoms

41. First year failure rates for male condom use range from:

    a. 1%-5%

    b. 3%-14%

    c. 5%-10%

    d. 2%-15%

42. Which of the following is correct when calculating fertile days for a woman using calendar rhythm for contraception?

    a. Subtract 15 days from the longest cycle, and 12 days from the shortest cycle
    b. Subtract 15 days from the shortest cycle, and 12 days from the longest cycle
    c. Subtract 11 days from the longest cycle, and 18 days from the shortest cycle
    d. Subtract 11 days from the longest cycle, and add 7 days to the shortest cycle

43. A disadvantage of female sterilization is:

    a. It is less effective than Norplant
    b. Long-term side effects
    c. High incidence of ectopic pregnancy
    d. Partner's consent is required

44. When compared to female sterilization procedures, male procedures:

    a. Are more likely to result in complications
    b. Have slightly lower failure rates
    c. Are more expensive
    d. Are more common

45. Which of the following is not a potential complication associated with a vasectomy?

    a. Hematoma
    b. Development of sperm antibodies
    c. Prostatitis
    d. Pregnancy

46. Which of the following is an indication for hormone replacement therapy?

    a. Irregular vaginal bleeding
    b. Bone pain
    c. Uterine prolapse
    d. Vasomotor instability

47. The average age a woman in the U.S. experiences menopause is:

    a. 40 years
    b. 45 years
    c. 50 years
    d. 55 years

48. With regard to menopause, which of the following statements is true?

    a. FSH and LH levels decrease
    b. Depo-Provera frequently used to treat symptoms
    c. Estradiol levels increase
    d. Estrone becomes primary type of estrogen in body

49. Which of the following is characteristic of estrogen deficiency?

    a. Atrophy of vaginal epithelium

b. Increased sweat gland activity
c. Thickening of skin epidermal and dermal layers
d. Increased libido

50. Which of the following is a contraindication for hormone replacement therapy?

a. Diabetes
b. Hypertension
c. Rheumatoid arthritis
d. Liver disease

51. Which of the following may not be helpful in preventing or treating osteoporosis?

a. Hormone replacement therapy
b. Weight bearing exercise
c. Vitamin E
d. Calcium

Answers

1. d	18. b	35. d
2. c	19. a	36. b
3. a	20. c	37. b
4. c	21. d	38. c
5. d	22. c	39. b
6. b	23. a	40. a
7. b	24. b	41. b
8. c	25. d	42. c
9. a	26. a	43. a
10. c	27. c	44. b
11. b	28. b	45. c
12. d	29. b	46. d
13. a	30. a	47. c
14. c	31. c	48. d
15. b	32. d	49. a
16. c	33. a	50. d
17. d	34. c	51. c

Bibliography

Centers for Disease Control and Prevention (CDC), National Center for Health Statistics (NCHS) (1995). Trends in pregnancies and pregnancy rates: Estimates for the United States, 1980-92. *Monthly vital statistics report,* 43 (11-S). Hyattsville, MD: U.S. Department of Health & Human Services, Publication No. 95-1120.

CDC, NCHS (1997). Births and deaths: United States, 1996. *Monthly vital statistics report,* 46(1-S2). Hyattsville, MD: U.S. Department of Health & Human Services, Publication No. 97-1120.

CDC, National Center for HIV, STD and TB Prevention (NCHSTP) (2000). August 4, 2000. *Dear colleague letter: Nonoxynol-9 trial-implications.* (http://www.cdc.gov/hiv/pubs/mmwr/mmwrllaugoo.htm)

Cunningham, F. G., MacDonald, P. D., Gant, N. F., Leveno, K. J., Gilstrap, L. C., Hankins, G. D. V., & Clark, S. L. (1997). *Williams obstetrics* (20th ed.). Stanford, CT: Appleton & Lange.

Food and Drug Administration (1997). Prescription drug products: Certain combined oral contraceptives for use as postcoital emergency contraception; Notice. *Federal register, 62* (37). U.S. Department of Health & Human Services.

Hatcher, R. A., Trussell, J., Stewart, F., Cates Jr. W., Stewart, G. K., Guest, F., & Kowal, D. (1998). *Contraceptive technology* (17th ed.). New York: Ardent Media.

Heinemann, D. F. (2000). Osteoporosis: An overview of the national osteoporosis foundation clinical practice guide. *Geriatrics 55*(5), 31-36.

HHS News. (September 28, 2000). U.S. Department of Health and Human Services. *FDA approves mifepristone for the termination of early pregnancy.* http://www.fda.gov/cder/drug/infopage/mifepristone

Jacobs institute of women's health expert panel on menopause counseling (Second printing, June, 2000). *Guidelines for Counseling Women on the Management of Menopause.*

Kupecz, D. (2000). Risedronate: A new bisphosphonate for treatment of osteoporosis. *The Nurse Practitioner 25*(3), 1068.

Mifepristone (2001). *Nurse practitioners' prescribing reference,* Spring, 2001. NY: Prescribing Reference, Inc

Moore, K. L. (1998). *The developing human: Clinically oriented embryology* (6th ed.). Philadelphia: W. B. Saunders.

Olds, S. B., London, M. L., & Ladewig, P. W. (1996). *Maternal-newborn nursing: A family-centered approach* (5th ed.). Menlo Park, CA: Addison-Wesley.

Olshansky, E. (2000). *Integrated women's health: Holistic approaches for comprehensive care.* Gaithersburg, MD: Aspen Publication.

Peters, S. (1999). The politics of prevention: Issues of emergency contraception. *ADVANCE for Nurse Practitioners 7*(11), 60-62.

Rawlins, S., Burkman, R. T., & Schwarz, B. E. (2000). The power of the pill: Making evidence-based decisions. *The American Journal of Nurse Practitioners*, 4(1), 25-40.

Schmitt, M. (2000). Osteoporosis: Focus on fractures. *Patient Care for the Nurse Practitioner 3* (2), 61-71.

Speroff, L., Glass, R., & Kase, N. (1994). *Clinical gynecologic endocrinology and infertility* (5th ed.). Baltimore, MD: Williams & Wilkins.

Turner, S. L. (1999). Somewhere in between: An overview of perimenopause. *ADVANCE for Nurse Practitioners 7*(11), 63-66.

Villa, M. L. & Chen, Z. (2000). Osteoporosis: Understanding ethnic differences. *Annals of Long-Term Care 8,* 52-55.

Advanced Practice, Role Development, Current Trends and Health Policy

Leanne C. Busby
Mary A. Baroni

Introduction

Advanced practice registered nurses (APRN) must remain informed regarding role development, current issues and trends related to their practice as well as changes in health care policy, as each has an impact on the evolving practice environment. Although current information is presented, the reader is encouraged to contact local and State regulatory bodies for variations in practice requirements.

Advanced Practice Nursing

- Definition of Advanced Practice Registered Nursing (APRN)

    1. National Council of State Boards of Nursing (NCSBN)—"practice based on the knowledge and skills acquired in a basic nursing education, through licensure as a registered nurse, and in graduate education and experience, including advanced nursing theory, physical and psychosocial assessment, and treatment of illness" (NCSBN, 1992, p. 6)

    2. American Nurses Association (ANA)—"professional nurses who have successfully completed a graduate program of study in a nursing specialty or related field that provides specialized knowledge and skills that form the foundation for expanded practice roles in health care" (ANA, 1996)

    3. National Association of Pediatric Nurse Practitioners, (formerly known as the National Association of Pediatric Nurse Associates and Practitioners) (NAPNAP)—a PNP is an advanced practice registered nurse who provides patient care to children and young adults. To function in this role, the PNP must have completed a formal educational program specializing in pediatric health care and have met the State Board of Registered Nursing regulations that govern their practice (2000)

        a. 1992 Position statement on entry into practice endorsed the master's level for PNP preparation

        b. Curricular content includes growth and development, pathophysiology, physical, developmental, family and cultural assessments, laboratory skills, and the diagnosis and management of common childhood illnesses and behavioral problems

Role Development

- First PNP program established in 1964 through collaborative efforts of Loretta C. Ford, EdD, RN and Henry K. Silver, MD at the University of Colorado

    1. PNP role development provided a model for other emerging nurse practitioner (NP) specialties

    2. Original support of PNP role as "physician extender" to improve access concerns due to shortage of primary care providers

    3. Most early PNP education occurred within certificate and/or continuing education programs; e.g., Colorado program included 4 months didactic study followed by 18 months clinical practicum training

4. Early research focused on quality of care, cost-effectiveness, productivity, clinical decision-making skills and role satisfaction of the PNP

5. National Association of Pediatric Nurse Practitioners (NAPNAP) organized in 1973 to establish PNP practice guidelines

6. Early resistance to NP role as too much of a ''medical model'' from mainstream graduate nursing education, that focused on ''nursing model'' of Clinical Nurse Specialist (CNS) role development

7. During 1980 to 1989 more physicians resulted in less need for nurse practitioner (NP)

8. During 1990 to 1998 increased emphasis on primary care resulted in decreased need for specialty care; NP seen as viable, cost effective member of healthcare delivery team

- Majority of NP programs currently at the Master's degree level within mainstream nursing education

    1. By 1989, 85% federally funded NP programs were graduate level

    2. Distinction between NP and CNS roles in practice have blurred

    3. Blended NP/CNS programs focusing on Advanced Practice Nursing (APN) are emerging within graduate nursing education

    4. Advantages/disadvantages of blended NP/CNS role remains controversial

    5. Most current programs require 2 years of full-time or 3 to 4 years of part-time graduate study

- Curriculum Guidelines and Content

    1. Association of Faculties of Pediatric Nurse Practitioner and Associate Programs (AFPNP/AP)—first published terminal competencies (1981) later updated in 1996

    2. National Association of Nurse Practitioner Faculties (NONPF)—published curriculum guidelines and standards for NP education (1990) later updated in 1995

    3. Core graduate nursing content includes: Nursing theory, organizational/leadership theory, ethical/legal issues, multicultural care, economics, community based care, managed care, and health care delivery systems

    4. Advanced practice core content includes: Advanced health assessment, pharmacology, physiology, advanced pathophysiology or other related sciences depending on the APRN specialty; clinical decision making process, advanced nursing interventions/therapeutics, health promotion/disease prevention, community based practice, role differentiation, and interpersonal and family theory

    5. APRN specialty content includes information that is unique to type of APRN role, information that is unique to health care needs of respective specialty population, information that supports standards and competencies established by professional spe-

cialty organizations, clinical decision making applied to specialty practice, and faculty supervised clinical practice experience (NONPF, 1997)

- Conceptual Models For Advanced Practice Nursing
    1. Benner's model of expert practice (1985)
    2. Calkin's model of advanced nursing practice (1984)
    3. Shuler's model of NP practice (1993; 1998)
        a. Holistic patient needs
        b. NP/Patient interaction
        c. Self-care
        d. Health prevention
        e. Health promotion
        f. Wellness

Advanced Practice Trends and Issues

- Components of Advanced Practice Registered Nursing Role
    1. Coordinator of care
    2. Patient advocate
    3. Accountable for patient outcomes and cost effectiveness
    4. Direct care giver
    5. Educator
    6. Administrator
    7. Researcher
    8. Consultant
    9. Case manager
    10. Change agent
- Standards and Scope of Practice
    1. Standards of practice
        a. Described by ANA (1996) as authoritative statements by which to measure quality of practice, service or education
        b. Establishes minimum levels of acceptable performance
        c. Provides consumer with means to measure quality of care received (Hawkins & Thibodeau, 1999)
        d. Both generic and specific specialty standards exist

e. Specialty groups have also developed standards, including: National Association of Pediatric Nurse Practitioners (NAPNAP), Association for Women's Health, Obstetric, and Neonatal Nurses (AWHONN)—formerly NAACOG

f. PNP relevant standards of practice

(1) American Nurses Association (ANA) Maternal-Child Health (MCH) Standards—first published in 1983

(2) NAPNAP Standards—first published in 1987

(3) AWHONN Standards

g. Can be used to provide legal expectations of practice but were not designed to define standards of practice for clinical or legal purposes

2. Scope of practice

a. Based on what is legally allowable in each State under its Nurse Practice Act

b. Provides guidelines vs. specific mandates for nursing practice

c. Is not mandated

d. Varies widely from State to State (Hawkins & Tibodeau, 1999) and over time

e. Often based on legal requirements within State and national standards

f. NAPNAP first published Scope of Practice for PNPs in 1983 with updated statements published in 1990 and 2000

g. Fluid and evolving (Hanson, 1996)

3. Nurse practice acts

a. Authorizes Boards of Nursing in each State to establish statutory authority for licensure of registered nurse (RN)

b. Authority includes use of title, authorization for scope of practice, and disciplinary grounds (Bosna, 1997)

c. Evolves from statutory law which, after interpretation, becomes regulatory language

4. Clinical practice guidelines or protocols

a. Definition: "Systematically developed statements to assist practitioner and patient about appropriate care for specific clinical outcomes" (IOM, 1990)

b. Need/requirements for guidelines/protocol development

(1) Standards for PNP practice include the collaborative development of appropriate pediatric protocols (NAPNAP, 1987)

(2) Variable requirements depending on individual State nurse practice act and standards of practice

(3) Protocol requirements may be met with recognized reference books and published clinical guidelines

    c. Examples of pediatric related practice guidelines for preventive care

       (1) Bright futures (MCHB)

       (2) Guidelines for Adolescent Preventive Services (AMA)

       (3) Guide to Clinical Preventive Services

    d. Examples of pediatric related practice guidelines for illness management

       (1) Asthma (NIH, AAP)

       (2) Hearing Screening (NIH, AAP)

       (3) HIV—Agency for Healthcare Research and Quality (AHRQ), formerly Agency for Health Care Policy and Research (AHCPR)

       (4) Otitis media with effusion (AHRQ)

       (5) Pain (AHRQ)

       (6) Sickle Cell disease (AHRQ)

- Regulation Of Advanced Nursing Practice

  1. Credentialing—regulatory mechanism(s) to insure accountability for competent practice

    a. Mandates accountability/responsibility for competent practice

    b. Validation of required education, licensure, and certification

    c. Necessary to assure public of safe health-care provided by qualified individuals

    d. Necessary to assure compliance with federal and State laws related to nursing practice

    e. Acknowledges APRN advanced scope of practice

    f. Should provide appropriate avenues for public or individual practice complaints

    g. Allows profession to be accountable to public and its members by enforcing professional standards for practice (Hickey, Ouimette, & Venegoni, 2000)

    h. Tension between certification bodies, State Boards of Nursing, and nursing education accrediting organizations regarding role and responsibility for credentialing intensified in the 1990s with the proliferation of NP programs

    i. National task force on quality nurse practitioner education convened in 1995 with broad-based representation

       (1) National Organization of Nurse Practitioner Faculties (NONPF)

       (2) American Academy of Nurse Practitioners (AANP)

       (3) American Association of Colleges of Nursing (AACN)

       (4) American Nurses Credentialing Center (ANCC)

      (5)   National Association of Neonatal Nurses (NANN)

      (6)   The National Association of Nurse Practitioners in Women's Health (NPWH) (formerly the National Association of Nurse Practitioners in Reproductive Health)

      (7)   National Association of Pediatric Nurse Practitioners (NAPNAP)

      (8)   National Certification Board for Pediatric Nurse Practitioners and Nurses (NCBPNPN)

      (9)   National Certification Corporation (NCC)

      (10)   National League for Nursing (NLN)

      (11)   National League for Nursing Accrediting Commission (NLNAC)

  j. Credentialing as an APRN currently remains within the domain of nongovernmental professional agencies

  k. Credentialing currently available through certification agencies

      (1)   National Certification Board for Pediatric Nurse Practitioners and Nurses (NCBPNPN)
           800 South Frederick Avenue, Suite 104
           Gaithersburg, MD 20877-4250
           (301-330-2921) (1-888-641-2767)

         (a)   PNP

         (b)   Pediatric acute care NP—in developmental stages

      (2)   American Nurses Credentialing Center (ANCC)
           600 Maryland Avenue, SW Suite 100 West,
           Washington DC 20024-2572
           (1-800-284-2378)

         (a)   Adult Nurse Practitioners

         (b)   Family Nurse Practitioners

         (c)   Several types of other nurse practitioner specialties

      (3)   American Academy of Nurse Practitioners (AANP)
           Certification Administration
           P.O. Box 12926
           Austin, TX 78711
           (512-442-4262)

         (a)   Family Nurse Practitioners

         (b)   Adult Nurse Practitioners

2. Certification

  a. Definition—process by which nongovernmental agency or association confirms that an individual licensed professional has met certain predetermined standards as specified by that profession for specialty practice

    b. Purpose—to assure the public that an individual has mastered a body of knowledge and acquired skills in a particular specialty

    c. May be required for State licensure and reimbursement

    d. Required for APRN practice in some states (Hickey, Ouimette, & Venegoni, 2000)

3. Prescriptive authority

    a. Some level of prescriptive authority for NP and Certified Nurse-Midwives (CNM) since mid-1970s

    b. As of 1998, all states have approved and/or implemented some degree of prescriptive authority; Illinois legislation passed with statutory authority pending

    c. Required pharmacology education within graduate program and continuing education to maintain authority—specific requirements vary by State

    d. Scope of prescriptive authority varies by State; full scope includes ability to obtain federal DEA registration number

4. Clinical privileges

    a. Possibility of hospital staff membership opened to nonphysician providers by Joint Commission on Accreditation of Health Care Organizations (JCAHO) in 1983

    b. Current issue for APRN practice

- Practice Issues

1. Collaborative practice

    a. Definition: ANA's *Nursing: A Social Policy Statement* (1995) describes collaboration as ''true partnership'' in which all players have and value power, recognize and accept separate and combined areas of responsibility and activity, and share common goals

    b. Purpose—to enhance quality of care and improve patient outcomes through on-going continuity and coordination of care (Hickey, Ouimette, & Venegoni, 2000)

    c. Interdisciplinary teams—examples of collaborative practice

2. Case management

    a. Definition—''A collaborative process which assesses, plans, implements, coordinates, monitors, and evaluates options and services to meet an individual's health needs through communication and available resources to promote quality cost-effective outcomes.'' (Case Management Society of America, 1994)

    b. Purpose—to mobilize, monitor and control resources that patient uses over course of an illness while maintaining a balance between quality and cost (Hickey, Ouimette, & Venegoni, 2000)

    c. Components of role

      (1)   Planning care for cost effectiveness and optimal outcomes

      (2)   Procuring and coordinating care

      (3)   Monitoring and evaluating outcomes

      (4)   Performing physical assessments

      (5)   Selecting laboratory and other tests

      (6)   Prescribing medications (Hawkins & Thibodeau, 1999; Synder, 1999)

      (7)   Requires that provider have strong communication skills and clinical expertise

      (8)   Provides care along continuum, decreases fragmentation of services, enhances patient and family quality of life, and contains costs

  d. Key features associated with case management models:

      (1)   Standardized appropriate use of resources aimed at identified outcomes within appropriate time frames

      (2)   Promotes collaborative practice among disciplines

      (3)   Promotes coordinated continuity of care over course of illness

      (4)   Promotes job satisfaction for providers

      (5)   Promotes patient and provider satisfaction with care delivery while minimizing cost to institution (Hickey, Ouimette, Venegoni, 2000)

  e. Populations appropriate for case management

      (1)   Those for whom course of treatment is costly and unpredictable

      (2)   Those who experience frequent or chronic readmissions to hospital

      (3)   Those involved with multiple providers or multiple disciplines (Hickey, Ouimette, & Venegoni, 2000)

3. Quality improvement (QI)

  a. Definition—"The organized creation of beneficial change...the attainment of unprecedented levels of performance." (Juran, 1989 p. 28)

  b. Alternative terms—Total Quality Management (TQM); Continuous Quality Improvement (CQI); differs from Quality Assurance (QA) in being continuous rather than episodic process

  c. Systematic, organized structures, processes, and expected outcomes focus on defining excellence and assuring accountability for quality of care

  d. Provides framework for ongoing evaluation of practice through identification of norms, criteria, and standards that measure program effectiveness and minimize liablity

  e. QI mechanisms and strategies

      (1)   Peer review

       (a) Recognize and reward nursing practice

       (b) Leads to higher standards practice

       (c) Discourages practice beyond scope of legal authority

       (d) Improves quality of care (Cherry & Jacob, 1999)

       (e) Provides for accountability and responsibility

  (2) Other methods of evaluation

       (a) Audit—retrospective measurement of quality

       (b) Interviews and questionnaires

       (c) Patient satisfaction surveys or interviews

4. Risk management

  a. Systems and activities designed to recognize and intervene to decrease risk of injury to patients and subsequent claims against healthcare providers; based on assumption that many injuries to patients are preventable

  b. Evaluates sources of legal liability in practice such as:

    (1) Patients

    (2) Procedures

    (3) Quality of record keeping

  c. Areas of liability risk

    (1) Practitioner-client relationship

    (2) Communication and informed consent

    (3) Clinical expertise

    (4) Self-evaluation by professionals of need to stay current

    (5) Documentation

    (6) Consultation and referral

    (7) Policies, procedures, and protocols

    (8) Supervision of others

  d. Includes educational activities that decrease risk in identified areas

5. Malpractice

  a. Professional misconduct, unreasonable lack of skill; infidelity in professional or fiduciary duties; illegal, immoral conduct resulting in patient harm

  b. Alleged professional failure to render services with degree of care, diligence and precaution that another member of same profession in similar circumstances would render to prevent patient injury

  c. Malpractice insurance

(1) Does not protect APRN from charges of practicing medicine without a license if APRN is practicing outside legal scope of practice for that State

(2) National Practitioner Data Bank collects information on adverse actions against health care practitioners, including nurses

(3) Types of coverage

    (a) Occurrence coverage—covers malpractice event which occurred during policy period, regardless of date of discovery or when claim filed

    (b) Claims made coverage—covers only claims filed during policy coverage period, regardless of when event occurred; optional tail coverage contract extends the coverage of a claims made policy into the future to cover all claims filed after the basic claims made coverage period

6. Negligence—failure of individual to do what a reasonable person would do that results in injury to another

7. Reimbursement

Whether working independently, sharing a joint practice with a physician, or practicing within a hospital, or managed care system, APRNs must be reimbursed appropriately. Standards that determine private pay insurance mechanisms are often modeled after federal policies such as Medicaid and Medicare. However, even when the federal government establishes mandates that encourage direct payment of nonphysician healthcare providers, barriers to reimbursement are often encountered in State level rules and regulations
(Hamric, 2000)

  a. Medicaid

    (1) Authorized in 1965 as Title XIX of Social Security Act

    (2) Federal/State matching program with federal oversight

    (3) Financed through federal and State taxes, with between 50% and 83% of total Medicaid costs covered by federal government

    (4) Does not cover all people below federal poverty level, but State Medicaid programs are required by federal government to cover certain categories such as:

      (a) Recipients of Aid to Families with Dependent Children (AFDC)—States set own eligibility requirements for AFDC

      (b) People over 65, blind, or totally disabled who are eligible for cash assistance under federal Supplemental Security Income (SSI) program

        (c)   Pregnant women (for pregnancy-related services only) and children under six with family incomes up to 133% of federal poverty level

        (d)   Children born after September 1983 in families whose income is at or below federal poverty level

   (5)   States can choose to cover "medically needy"

   (6)   Coverage required for certain services

        (a)   Hospital and physician services

        (b)   Laboratory and radiographic services

        (c)   Nursing home and home health care services

        (d)   Prenatal and preventive services

        (e)   Medically necessary transportation

   (7)   States can add services to list and can place certain limitations on federally mandated services

   (8)   Although Medicaid recipients cannot be billed for services, States can impose nominal copayments or deductibles for certain services (Bodenheimer, 1998)

b. Medicare

   (1)   Federally mandated program established in 1965, provides health insurance for aged and disabled individuals

   (2)   Eligibility covers hospital service, physician services, and other medical services

   (3)   Income level does not impact eligibility

   (4)   Medicare Part A

        (a)   Those 65 years of age and older who are eligible for Social Security are automatically enrolled, whether or not they are retired—persons are eligible for Social Security when they (or their spouses) have paid into Social Security system through employment for 40 quarters or more

        (b)   Those who have paid into system for less than 40 quarters can enroll in Medicare Part A by paying monthly premium

        (c)   Those who are under age 65 and are totally and permanently disabled may enroll in Medicare Part A after receiving Social Security disability benefits for 24 months

        (d)   Those with chronic renal disease requiring dialysis or transplant may also be eligible for Part A without a two year waiting period

        (e)   Services covered include some hospitalization costs; some skilled nursing facility costs, although custodial care is not covered; home health care—100% for skilled care; 80% of approved amount for medical equipment; and hospice care—100% for most services

(f) Payment for hospitalization is based on projected costs of caring for patient with given problem—each Medicare patient admitted to a hospital is classified according to a diagnosis-related group (DRG); the hospital is then paid a predetermined amount for each patient admitted with the given DRG, if hospital costs are above payment rate, the hospital must absorb loss; if costs are below payment rate, hospital allowed to keep a percentage of excess

(g) APRN not paid directly for services delivered in a hospital

(5) Medicare Part B—Supplementary Medical Insurance (SMI)

(a) Monthly premium is charged

(b) Some-low income people are eligible to have monthly premium paid by Medicaid

(c) Financed by general federal revenues and by Part B monthly premiums

(d) Covers all medically necessary services—80% of an approved amount after annual deductible; includes physician services, physical, occupational, and speech therapy; medical equipment and diagnostic tests, and some preventative care such as Pap tests, mammograms, hepatitis B, pneumococcal and influenza vaccines can be included in medical expenses

c. APRN—Medicaid/Medicare coverage

(1) Omnibus Budget Reconciliation Act (OBRA) 1989—mandated Medicaid reimbursement for certified pediatric and family nurse practitioners began July 1, 1990; providers required to practice within the scope of State law and do not have to be under supervision or associated with a physician or other provider

(a) Level of payment determined by States—reimbursement rates range from 70% to 100% of fee-for-service physician Medicaid rate (Pearson, 1999)

(b) Pediatric and family nurse practitioners may bill Medicaid directly after attaining provider number from State Medicaid agency

(c) States can elect to pass laws allowing them to extend Medicaid payment to other types of NP not identified in federal statutes

(2) Legislation (1997) has expanded direct Medicare reimbursement for APRN in all geographic locations

(a)   APRN reimbursement at 85% of physician fee schedule when billing independently using APRN billing number; direct physician supervision not required

(b)   When APRN is employed by physician, the physician practice may receive 100% of customary physician charge, according to "Incident to" rules (Buppert, 1998)

(c)   APRN must be RN currently licensed to practice in the State in which services are rendered; must meet requirements for NP practice in State in which services are rendered; must be currently certified as a primary care NP; must have successfully completed a formal advanced practice educational program of at least one academic year that includes at least four months of classroom instruction and awards a degree, diploma, or certificate OR, have successfully completed a formal advanced practice educational program and have been performing in that expanded role for at least 12 months during the 18-month period immediately preceding February 8, 1978, the effective date for the provision of services of NP as reflected in the conditions for certification for rural health clinics

(d)   NP covered services are limited to services an NP is legally authorized to perform under the State law in which the NP practices and must meet training, educational and experience requirements prescribed by the Secretary of Health and Human Services

(3)   NP services covered under Part B if service would be considered physician's services if furnished by MD or Doctor of Osteopathy (DO); if NP is legally authorized to perform services in the state in which they are performed; if services are performed in collaboration with MD/DO (collaboration specified as a process whereby NP works with physician to deliver health care within scope of NP expertise with medical direction and appropriate supervision as provided for in jointly developed guidelines or other mechanisms defined by federal regulations and law of the state in which services are performed); and services are otherwise precluded from coverage because of one of the statutory exclusions

(4)   "Incident to" refers to services provided as an integral, yet incidental, part of the physician's personal, professional services in the course of diagnosis or treatment of injury or illness—these services must occur under direct personal supervision of a physician, and the APRN must be an employee of the physician group; services must occur during the course of treatment where the physician performs an initial service and subsequent services in a manner that reflects the physician's active participation and management of the course of treatment—direct personal supervision does not mean that the physician must be in the same room as the APRN, however, the physician must be present in the office suite

and available for assistance and direction while the APRN provides patient care (Buppert, 1998)

(5) When APRN performs "incident to" service in physician's office, billing must be submitted to Medicare by employing physician, under the physician's name, provider number and CPT code—payment is made at full physician rate and is paid to physician or physician practice

(6) When APRN provides service in skilled nursing facility, or nursing facility located in urban area as defined by law, Medicare payment can be obtained—medicare reimbursement is also available for APRN services in skilled nursing facilities (SNF) in nonrural areas on a reasonable charge basis; this amount may not exceed physician fee schedule amount for service and payment is made to the APRN's employer

d. Other third party payors

(1) Private insurer reimbursement is contract specific per State insurance commission

(2) Civilian Health and Medical Program of the United States (CHAMPUS)

(a) Federal health plan for military personnel, including surviving dependents, families, and retirees

(b) APRN reimbursement for services

(3) Federal Employees Health Benefit Program (FEHBP)

(a) One of largest employer sponsored group health insurance programs

(b) APRN recognized as designated health care provider

e. Methods of payment for advanced practice nurses

(1) Fee-for-service model

(a) Unit of payment by visit or procedure

(b) Can occur with utilization review in which case payor has right to authorize or deny payment of expensive medical interventions such as hospital admission, extra hospital days, and surgery

(2) Episodic model

(a) One sum is paid for all services delivered during a given illness

(b) DRG fee payment

(3) Capitation model, PPO, and HMO are covered in section on Managed Care in this chapter

- Professional Organizations
  1. Purpose and benefits
     a. Establish practice standards
     b. Collective voice to promote nursing and quality of care
     c. Monitor and influence policy and legislative initiatives
     d. Position papers on practice issues
     e. Disseminate information
  2. Examples
     a. American Nurses Association (ANA)
     b. National Association of Pediatric Nurse Practitioners (NAPNAP)
     c. National Conference of Gerontological Nurse Practitioners
     d. National Organization of Nurse Practitioner Faculties (NONPF)
     e. American Academy of Nurse Practitioners (AANP)
     f. American College of Nurse Practitioners (ACNP)
     g. Nurse Practitioner Associates for Continuing Education (NPACE)
     h. National Association of School Nurses
     i. Association for Women's Health, Obstetrics, and Neonatal Nurses (AWHONN)
     j. The National Association of Nurse Practitioners in Women's Health (NPWH) (formerly the National Association of Nurse Practitioners in Reproductive Health [NANPRH])
- Research in Advanced Practice: "Practice-based research is essential to the development of advanced practice nursing for the future." (NONPF, 1995, p. 84)
  1. Major trend is outcome studies
  2. Sources of federal funding
     a. Agency for Healthcare Research and Quality (AHRQ)
        (1) Formerly the Agency for Health Care Policy and Research (AHCPR)
        (2) *http://www.ahcpr.gov/*
     b. National Institutes of Health (NIH)
        (1) Includes the National Institute for Nursing Research (NINR)
        (2) *http://www.nih.gov/*
     c. Maternal and Child Health Bureau (MCHB)
        (1) Functions within Health Resources and Services Administration (HRSA)

(2) *http://www.mchb.hrsa.gov/*

3. Sources of research findings

   a. Conferences

   b. Scholarly publications

   c. Distribution of summaries of research studies (Hawkins & Thibodeau, 1996)

4. Use of research in practice setting

   a. Develop research-based clinical pathways

   b. Track clinical outcomes and variances

   c. Demonstrate quality and cost effectiveness of care

   d. Give structure to demonstration projects

   e. Persuade lawmakers of NP value and contributions in today's health care system

   f. Improve quality and patient outcomes

5. Benefit of research for patients

   a. Provides thorough understanding of patient situation

   b. Provides more accurate assessment of situations

   c. Increases effectiveness of interventions

   d. Increases provider sensitivity to patient situations

   e. Assists providers to more accurately determine need for and effectiveness of interventions (Hickey, Ouimette, & Venegoni, 2000)

6. Barriers to research utilization

   a. Time and cost of conducting research studies

   b. Resistance to change in work setting

   c. Lack of rewards for using research findings

   d. Lack of understanding or uncertainty regarding research outcomes (Hickey, Ouimette, & Venegoni, 2000)

7. Strategies to overcome barriers to research utilization

   a. Creation of organizational culture that values and uses research

   b. Creation of environment where questions are encouraged, critical thinking is appreciated, and nursing care is evaluated

   c. Support for research through time allocation and financial commitment (Hickey, Ouimette & Venegoni, 2000)

Health Policy

- Policy Influences

  1. Healthy People 2000

     a. Published in 1990 by U.S. Department of Health and Human Services; mid-course review of progress published in 1995; subsequent review of progress published in Decemeber 1999

     b. Purpose—committed nation to obtain three broad goals

        (1) Increase span of healthy life for all Americans

        (2) Reduce health disparities among Americans

        (3) Achieve access to preventive services for all Americans (DHHS, 1990)

     c. Contained 300 specific objectives based on 22 priority areas leading to socially and economically productive lives

     d. Objectives focused on equal access, acceptability, availability, continuity, cost and quality of care

     e. Objectives organized within broad categories of health promotion, health protection, and preventive services

     f. Identified priority of systematic collection, analysis, interpretation, dissemination, and use of data to understand national health status and plan effective prevention programs

     g. Individuals, communities and organizations were responsible for determining how they would achieve the goals by the year 2000 (Hickey, Ouimette & Venegoni, 1996)

     h. Progress (1998–1999), towards meeting Healthy People 2000 goals

        (1) Fifteen percent of objectives met in areas of nutrition, maternal and child health, heart disease and mental health

           (a) There were 17 maternal\infant health objectives; progress made on 8 of the 17 including

              (i) Perinatal/infant mortality—although U.S. ranks 25th among industrialized countries for infant mortality

              (ii) Screening for fetal abnormalities and genetic disorders

           (b) No progress on four or movement away on five of the target goals for problems including fetal alcohol syndrome and low birth weight

        (2) Fourty-four percent of objectives, including those related to childhood immunizations, breast feeding, regular dental visits, mammography screening and consumption of fruits and vegetables per day are proceeding on track (DHHS, 1999)

2. Healthy People 2010

   a. Released in 2000 by U.S. Department of Health and Human Services

   b. Builds on initiatives set in Healthy People 2000

   c. Purpose—designed to achieve two broad-based goals

      (1) Increase quality and years of healthy life

      (2) Eliminate health disparities

   d. Contains 467 objectives with twenty-eight focus areas

   e. Objectives focus on partnering for health improvements; eliminating health disparities; increasing quality and years of healthy living; and harnessing technology for health

   f. Objectives categorized into the following focus areas

      (1) Physical activity and fitness

      (2) Nutrition

      (3) Tobacco use

      (4) Educational\community-based programs

      (5) Environmental health

      (6) Food Safety

      (7) Injury\violence prevention

      (8) Occupational safety and health

      (9) Oral health

      (10) Access to quality health services

      (11) Family planning

      (12) Maternal, infant and child health—fetal, infant, child and adolescent deaths; maternal deaths and illnesses; prenatal care; obstetrical care; risk factors; developmental disabilities and neural tube defects; prenatal substance exposure; breastfeeding, newborn screening and service systems for children with special health care needs

      (13) Medical products safety

      (14) Public health infrastructures

      (15) Health communication

      (16) Prevention and health promotion

      (17) Disability and secondary conditions

      (18) Heart disease and stroke

      (19) Kidney disease

(20) Mental health and mental disorders

(21) Respiratory diseases

(22) Sexually transmitted diseases

(23) Substance abuse

g. Ten ''leading health indicators'' (LHI)—physical activity; overweight and obesity; tobacco use; substance abuse; responsible sexual behavior; mental health; injury and violence; environmental quality; immunizations; access to health care

h. Written for States and communities to tailor health objectives to their specific needs (DHHS, 1999)

(http://www.health.gov/healthypeople/)

3. Prevention guidelines

a. ''Put Prevention Into Practice''—campaign established by U.S. Public Health Service to enhance delivery of preventive care in primary care practice

b. *Clinicians Handbook of Preventive Services: Put Prevention Into Practice,* (1998)—provides practical and comprehensive reference on preventive services to primary care providers including:

(1) Health screening schedules for early disease detection and immunization

(2) Disease prophylaxis issues

(3) Risk factor counselling techniques

(4) Educational resources on preventive care (Hickey, Ouimette & Venegoni, 2000)

http://www.ahcpr.gov/clinic/ppiphand.htm

c. *Guide to Clinical Preventive Services* (U.S. Preventive Services Task Force, 1996) presents national clinical preventive services guidelines for practice and educational settings

(1) Age and gender specific

(2) Suggests targeted examinations, immunizations and health counseling that should be part of periodic health visits

4. Nursing's Agenda for Health Care Reform (ANA, 1991)

a. Supports creation of a health care system that assures access, quality, and services at affordable costs

b. Supports ongoing primary care

c. Calls for basic core of essential health services to be available to all, and for restructured health care system focusing on consumers and their health and health care delivery in familiar, convenient sites

d. Proposes shift from focus on illness and cure to orientation on wellness and caring

e. Supports provisions for long-term care and insurance reforms to assure improved access to coverage

f. Calls for establishment of public/private sector review of resource allocations, cost reduction plans, and fair and consistent reimbursement for all providers

- Utilization of Health Policy

1. Shifting trend toward primary care and early preventive measures; supports need for APRN

2. Four major factors influencing health care delivery services

a. Payors—individual health care consumers, businesses that pay for health insurance for employees, and government through public programs and entitlement programs such as Medicare and Medicaid

b. Insurers—take money from payors, assume risks, and pay providers

c. Providers—includes hospitals, physicians, nurses, APRN, physician assistants, pharmacies, home health agencies, and long term care facilities

d. Suppliers—pharmaceutical and medical supply industries

3. Legislative strategies and political involvement

a. Professional organizations monitor policy issues and keep membership informed—e.g., NAPNAP legislative newsletter

b. Local networks of APRN develop practice guidelines and advocate for policies to enhance practice

- Types of Health Care Delivery Systems

1. Primary health care

a. Definition: ''Primary care is the provision of integrated, accessible health care services by clinicians who are accountable for addressing a large majority of personal health care needs, developing a sustained partnership with patients, and practicing in the context of family and community (Institute of Medicine, Committee on Future of Primary Care, 1994)''

b. Activities and/or functions define boundaries of primary care, such as curing or alleviating common illnesses and disabilities

c. Entry point to a system that includes access to secondary and tertiary care

d. Attributes include care that is accessible, comprehensive, coordinated, continuous, and accountable

e. Strategy for organizing health care system as a whole; gives priority and allocates resources to community-based rather than hospital-based care

f. Categories of primary care providers (PCP) and nature of care

      (1)   Medical specialties—family medicine, general internal medicine, general pediatrics, obstetrics and gynecology as specified in the Clinton administration's Health
Security Act

      (2)   Other experts have included NP and physician assistants (PA) as primary care providers (PCP)

  g. Many definitions stress self-responsibility for health (Hickey, Ouimette, & Venegoni, 2000)

2. Managed care

  a. Definition: "An integrated network that combines financing and delivery of health care services to covered individuals." (Mahn & Spross, 1996, pg. 446)

      (1)   Network connects consumers, sponsors, providers, and third party payors

      (2)   Initial managed care organization was Kaiser Health Plan (California) established in 1930s (Bodenheimer, 1998)

  b. Objectives

      (1)   Manage use and price of health care delivery system

      (2)   Control type, level and frequency of treatment

      (3)   Restrict level of reimbursement for services

  c. Type of health insurance plan designed to control costs while assuring quality care

  d. Obligation to manage is shared among providers, consumers and payers

      (1)   Providers no longer dictate price of care delivery; must assume more financial risk for population assigned to them for care

      (2)   Consumers have fewer choices of coverage, providers and greater financial responsibility

      (3)   Payors manage health care dollars through benefit design, selective contracting, and shifting financial risk to providers (Hickey, Ouimette, & Venegoni, 2000)

  e. Types of managed care plans

      (1)   Health Maintenance Organizations (HMO)

         (a)   Most common type

         (b)   By 1994, enrollment at 52 million (20.3% of population)

         (c)   Offer pre-established benefit package—including preventive, inpatient and outpatient care

         (d)   HMO contracts with providers to provide care to enrollees

(e) Providers at financial risk resulting in incentive to provide high quality, cost effective care

(f) Enrollees select a primary care provider (PCP) who manages total care by authorizing specialty visits, hospitalization, and other services

(g) PCP may be MD, APRN or PA providers; serving as "gatekeepers"

(2) Preferred Provider Organizations (PPO)

(a) Compromised managed care option that is alternative between indemnity and HMO insurance

(b) Uses financial incentives to influence consumer and provider behaviors

(c) Refers to variety of arrangements between insurers, providers, and third-party payers rather than standard plan

(d) Often owned by large insurance companies such as Prudential, Travelers and Aetna

(e) Available primarily to employed commercial population

(3) Point of Service Plans (POS)

(a) Consumers decide whether to use a provider network, or seek care outside the network

(b) If variation of HMO plan, PCP coordinates care for enrollees; if variation of PPO plan, enrollees may choose lower cost options outside of provider network

(c) Most rapidly growing type of managed care

(4) Integrated delivery systems

(a) Vertical integration of services across levels of care into seamless system with improved access for enrollees

(b) Capitated payment—financial risk shifts from payor to provider; unit of value is cost per member per month (PMPM); providers receive age and sex adjusted budget to cover services to maintain wellness of specific target population

(c) Emphasis on provision of appropriate but not unlimited care with financial benefit of keeping population healthy through systematic preventive services

f. Reimbursement under managed care

(1) Providers accept financial risk for care provided to specific population of enrollees

(2) Capitated payment

          (a)   Provider receives payment in advance

          (b)   Payment level reflects expected utilization by enrolled population for which provider is responsible

     (3)   Provider must control volume and cost

     (4)   Efficiency usually rewarded through bonus payments for operating within budget and meeting goals for quality and efficiency

g.   Monitoring, evaluation and accreditation in managed care

     (1)   Health plan employer data and information set (HEDIS)—provides quality measures and compares with benchmark standards and goals

     (2)   National committee for quality assurance (NCQA)

          (a)   Major accreditation body for managed care organizations

          (b)   Standards in six critical areas are evaluated—quality management, utilization management, credentialing, preventive health services, medical records, members rights/responsibilities

     (3)   NCQA reported reviews of 30% of the 554 HMOs in the U.S. as of 1995; 31% received full accreditation; 56% received one year or provisional accreditation; 12% were denied accreditation (Mischler & Quinn, 1995)

h.   Challenges and opportunities of managed care for APRN

     (1)   Need for balance between quality of care and costs inherent in diagnosis/management per client visit

          (a)   Educational programs must incorporate managed care content into curriculum

          (b)   APRN must combine strong clinical and financial skills to determine cost of providing care to target population

          (c)   Success in managed care environment requires systems-thinking skill to complement primary care skills; blended NP/CNS models may provide this necessary linkage with added focus on case management, utilitization/resource management, quality improvement, and client education/advocacy within systems of care

     (2)   APRN strategies for success within evolving managed care environment

          (a)   Determine strategies to increase efficiency without sacrificing quality of client-provider interactions; e.g., group well-child visits

          (b)   Lobby for APN inclusion on provider panels

          (c)   Maintain partnerships with APRN educational programs for collaborative study and documentation of APRN effectiveness

Questions
Select the best answer

1. If the two broad-based goals of Healthy People 2010 are met, the nation will:

   a. Increase quality of healthy, years of healthy life span and eliminate health disparities
   b. Increase healthy life span, increase access and improve economics related to health for all Americans
   c. Increase healthy life span, reduce health disparities, and improve economics related to the health of all Americans
   d. Reduce health disparities, increase access to health care services and make life more socially acceptable for all Americans

2. Which of the following objectives from Healthy People 2000 has not made progress towards achieving its targeted goal?

   a. Low birth weight
   b. Infant mortality
   c. Fetal mortality
   d. Screening for genetic disorders

3. Preventive health guidelines include references to:

   a. Immunizations, health screening, disease prophylaxis, education and infection control
   b. Immunizations, counseling, health screening, disease prophylaxis and education
   c. Health screening, disease prophylaxis, counseling and CPR
   d. Health screening, disease prophylaxis, education, immunizations and CPR

4. Nursing's Agenda for Health Care Reform:

   a. Is supportive of equal access, cost effective, high quality care
   b. Is a mandate to all nurses in the U.S.
   c. Is a summary of nursing research related to health care reform
   d. Is a report of the status of nursing in the 1990s

5. The nurse practitioner role was initially established to:

   a. Improve access to care and partially solve physician shortage
   b. Reduce the nursing shortage and improve access to care
   c. Improve working conditions of nurses while improving access to care
   d. Improve nursing's image through expansion of the role

6. Early nursing research focused on:

   a. The response of policy makers to the nursing shortage
   b. The effectiveness of the NP as a primary care giver
   c. An effort to demonstate quality and cost effectiveness of NP
   d. The role of the NP as a physician extender

7. Which of the following is not a major factor influencing health care delivery services?

    a. Provider

    b. Payors

    c. Insurers

    d. Agencies

8. All definitions of primary health care include:

    a. The concept of universal access and accountability

    b. The concept of universal access and AIDS prevention

    c. The concept of universal access and a focus on self-responsibility for health

    d. The concept of universal access and a focus on reimbursement for services rendered

9. Standards of practice are:

    a. Authoritative statements used to measure quality

    b. Used to measure outcome but are not authoritative

    c. Designed for legal purposes

    d. Not designed for legal purposes and cannot be used to measure quality

10. Quality improvement activities include:

    a. Patient satisfaction surveys only

    b. Peer review, patient satisfaction surveys, chart audits

    c. Defining four practice domains

    d. Systems to decrease risk of injury to patients

11. Most risk management programs are based on the assumption that:

    a. Many injuries to patients are preventable

    b. Most legal liability is a result of poor documentation

    c. Most injuries to patients are not preventable

    d. Malpractice insurance is generally unnecessary

12. If an APRN practices beyond his/her scope:

    a. Malpractice insurance will protect him/her from a charge of practicing medicine without a license

    b. Malpractice insurance will not protect him/her from a charge of practicing medicine without a license

    c. He or she is legally accountable to the certifying body

    d. The collaborating physician is legally accountable to the certifying body

13. Standards of practice may be used to:

    a. Establish minimal levels of performance

    b. Establish reimbursement schemes for APRN

    c. Mandate nursing practice across the nation

    d. Mandate nursing practice in certain States

14. Scope of practice:

   a. Is identical across the States
   b. Is determined by the federal government
   c. Is mandated by the federal government
   d. Varies from State to State

15. Medicaid provides health insurance coverage to:

   a. Certain categories of people whose personal income falls below the federal poverty level
   b. Anyone whose personal income falls below the federal poverty level
   c. Newborns, pregnant women and those over 65 whose personal income falls below the federal poverty level
   d. Those who are elderly

16. Medicaid reimbursement is available to an APRN:

   a. Practicing in federally designated areas
   b. At a rate that is between 70% and 100% of the physician rate
   c. Only if the APRN is in collaborative practice with a physician
   d. Practicing in nursing homes only

17. Medicare reimbursement for services:

   a. Is not dependent on the patient's income level
   b. Depends on the patient's income level
   c. Is not available to APRN under any circumstances
   d. Is only available to APRN who is in collaborative practice with a physician

18. Medicare Part A covers:

   a. Hospital, skilled nursing facility, and hospice care
   b. All medically necessary services
   c. Skilled nursing facility care only
   d. Hospice care only

19. Medicare Part B covers:

   a. All medically necessary services
   b. Inpatient hospital care
   c. Outpatient physician services only
   d. Skilled nursing facility and hospice care

20. To receive Medicare reimbursement, APRN must:

   a. Be nationally certified and maintain prescriptive privileges
   b. Maintain a current license in the State in which they are practicing
   c. Practice in a designated medically underserved area
   d. Practice with a physician

21. The term ''incident to'' refers to:

    a. The occasions when an APRN practices independently but occasionally consults with a physician
    b. The notion that the physician must be present in the office suite and immediately available to provide assistance in order for the APRN to bill for services rendered
    c. The notion that a physician must examine the patient along with the APRN if Medicare is to be billed for services rendered
    d. Medicaid only and is not pertinent to Medicare billing

22. ''Incident to'' billing is specific to:

    a. Medicare
    b. Medicaid
    c. Medicare and Medicaid
    d. Private insurance companies

23. The Civilian Health and Medical Program of the United States (CHAMPUS):

    a. Is a federal health plan which covers health care for military personnel and their families and recognizes APRN as reimbursable provider
    b. Is a federal health plan which covers health care for military personnel and recognizes APRN as reimbursable provider
    c. Is a federal health plan which covers health care for military personnel and their families but does not recognize APRN as reimbursable provider
    d. Only covers hospital expenses of military personnel and their families

24. The knowledge base of the APRN is based on:

    a. Medical content
    b. Theoretical content only
    c. Scientific content and theory
    d. Theory and research

25. The role of the APRN has traditionally focused on:

    a. The delivery of primary health care to all people
    b. The delivery of acute health care to all people
    c. Chronic care
    d. The medical model

26. The nurse practitioner role began:

    a. With the establishment of a pediatric nurse practitioner program in an effort to expand the role of the registered nurse in order to meet the needs of the children of the nation
    b. As a result of the new entitlement programs, Medicare and Medicaid
    c. When it was evident that the medical schools across the U.S. could not prepare enough family practitioners to meet the nation's need
    d. As an experimental program at Duke University Medical Center

27. Legal authority for APRN practice is granted by:

    a. Federal law
    b. Regulations from the Department of Health and Human Services
    c. State law and regulations
    d. The Board of Medicine in most States

28. Direct reimbursement to APRN has resulted in:

    a. Increased access to cost-effective, quality primary care
    b. Increased malpractice claims against APRN
    c. Decreased consumer choice of health care providers
    d. Proliferation of APRN in independent practice

29. Malpractice insurance:

    a. Protects an APRN from charges of practicing medicine without a license when they are practicing outside the legal scope of practice
    b. Does not protect an APRN from charges of practicing medicine without a license when they are practicing outside the legal scope of practice
    c. Does not pay for legal defense if the APRN is practicing beyond the legal scope of practice
    d. Is important, but should not be purchased if the facility in which the APRN is employed carries good coverage

30. Collaborative practice:

    a. Limits autonomy and not reasonable in current managed care environment
    b. Will enhance quality of care and improve patient outcomes
    c. Will limit consumer choice of providers
    d. Excludes the concept of interdisciplinary teams

31. Case management:

    a. Balances quality and cost of patient care
    b. Has not been found to be cost effective
    c. Decreases the autonomy of the APRN
    d. Is rarely used today

32. The major trend in health policy research today is:

    a. Outcome studies
    b. Primary care studies
    c. Studies that compare practice strategies of MD and NP
    d. Studies that compare patient satisfaction with care delivered by MD versus NP

33. Current prescriptive authority for APRN:

    a. Varies among the States
    b. Is fairly consistent among the States

    c. Provides DEA numbers for APRN

    d. Allows APRN to move freely from State to State

34. Managed care is a term that describes:

    a. An established system of health care delivery that is mandated by the federal government

    b. A network of providers who contract to provide services for a specific group of enrollees

    c. A system that does not recognize APRN as a primary provider

    d. A network of hospitals and nursing homes that provide care to chronically ill people

35. Certification is:

    a. A procedure through which the government appraises and grants certification to the APRN

    b. Granted by the individual States

    c. Governed by each State's Board of Nursing

    d. A process in which a non-governmental agency or group verifies that an APRN has met certain predetermined standards for specialty practice

36. Licensure:

    a. Is a federal process that is used to standardize health care facilities

    b. Is granted by a State government agency and grants permission to engage in the practice of a given profession

    c. Cannot be used to prohibit anyone from practicing a given profession

    d. Is a federal process that is used to standardize educational programs

37. Reimbursement under managed care:

    a. Requires that the provider accept the financial risk for the care provided to a specific population of enrolled patients

    b. Requires that the managed care organization accept the financial risk for the care provided to a specific population of enrolled patients

    c. Does not reward efficient care delivery

    d. Is not available to APRN

38. An integrated delivery system:

    a. Is one that delivers high quality care but is often not cost effective

    b. Delivers a vertical integration of services with capitated payment

    c. Does not include rationing of resources

    d. Does not include a capitated payment scheme

Answers

1. a	14. d	27. c
2. a	15. a	28. a
3. b	16. b	29. b
4. a	17. a	30. b
5. a	18. a	31. a
6. c	19. a	32. a
7. d	20. b	33. a
8. a	21. b	34. b
9. a	22. a	35. d
10. b	23. a	36. b
11. a	24. c	37. a
12. b	25. a	38. b
13. a	26. a	

Bibliography

American Association of Colleges of Nursing. (1996). *The essentials of master's education for advanced practice nursing.* Washington DC: AACN

Association of Faculties of Pediatric Nurse Practitioner and Associate Programs. (1996). Philosophy, conceptual model, terminal competencies for the education of pediatric nurse practitioners. Cherry Hill, NJ: NAPNAP.

Bodenheimer, T. S. (1998). *Understanding health policy: A clinical approach.* NY: McGraw-Hill.

Bosna, J. (1997). Using nurse practitioner certification for state nursing regulation: An update. *The Nurse Practitioner: The American Journal of Primary Health Care, 22*(6), 213–216.

Buppert, C. (1998). Reimbursement for nurse practitioner services. *The Nurse Practitioner: The American Journal of Primary Health Care, 23*(1), 67–81.

Case Management Society of America. (1994). CMSA proposes standards of practice. *The Case Manager 5* (1) 59-70.

Cherry, B., & Jacob, S. R. (1999). *Contemporary nursing: Issues, trends and management.* St. Louis: Mosby.

Hamric, A. B., Spross, J. A., & Hanson, C. M. (2000). *Advanced practice nursing: An integrative approach* (2nd ed.). Philadelphia: W. B. Saunders.

Hardy Havens, D. M., Ronan, J. P., & Hannan, C. (1996). Maintaining the nurse practitioner identity in a world of managed care. *Journal of Pediatric Health Care, 10,* 86–88.

Hawkins, J. W., & Thibodeau, J. A. (1999). *The advanced practice nurse: Current issues* (5th ed.). NY: Tiresias Press.

Hickey, J. V., Ouimette, R. M., & Venegoni, S. L. (2000). *Advanced practice nursing: Changing roles and clinical applications* (2nd ed.). Philadelphia: J. B. Lippincott, Williams & Wilkins.

IOM. (1990). *Clinical practice guidelines: Directions for a new program.* Washington, DC: National Academy Press.

Juran, M. (1989). *Juran on leadership for quality: An executive handbook.* NY: The Free Press.

Mezey, M. D., & McGivern, D. O. (1998). *Nurses, nurse practitioners: Evolution to advanced practice* (3rd ed.). Philadelphia: W. B. Saunders.

Mischler, N., & Quinn, N. (1995). Research report: National committee for quality assurance (NCQA) accreditation. Milliman & Robertson.

NAPNAP. (1987). *Standards of practice for PNP/As. Cherry Hill, NJ: Author.*

NAPNAP. (1989). Risk management for pediatric nurse practitioners. Cherry Hill, NJ: Author.

NAPNAP. (2000). *Scope of practice.* Cherry Hill, NJ: Author.

National Council of State Boards of Nursing. (1992). *Position paper on the licensure of advanced practice nursing.* Chicago: Author.

National Organization of Nurse Practitioner Faculties Curriculum Guidelines Task Force.

(1995). *Advanced nursing practice: Curriculum guidelines and program standards for nurse practitioner education.* Washington, DC: NONPF

National Organization of Nurse Practitioner Faculties. (1997). *Criteria for evaluation of nurse practitioner programs: A report of the national task force on quality nurse practitioner education.* Washington, DC.

Pearson, L. (2000). Annual legislative update: How each state stands on legislative issues affecting advanced nursing practice. *Nurse Practitioner: The American Journal of Primary Care, 26*(1), 7, 11–19, 22–29, 32–39, 48–55.

Shuler, P. A., & Davis, J. E. (1993). The Shuler nurse practitioner model: A theoretical framework for nurse practitioner clinicians, educators, and researchers, Part I. *Journal of the American Academy of Nurse Practitioners, 5*(1), 11–18.

Shuler, P. A., & Davis, J. E. (1993) . The Shuler nurse practitioner model: Clinical application, Part 2. *Journal of the American Academy of Nurse Practitioners, 5*(2), 73–88.

Shuler, P. A., & Huebscher, R. (1998). Clarifying nurse practitioner's unique contributions: Application of the Shuler nurse practitioner practice model. *Journal of the American Academy of Nurse Practitioners, 10*(11), 491–499.

Snyder, M., & Mirr, M. P. (1999). *Advanced practice nursing: A guide to professional development* (2nd ed.). NY: Springer Publishing.

U.S. Department of Health and Human Services. (1990). *Healthy people 2000: National health promotion and disease prevention objectives* (DHHS Publication No. PHS 91-50213). Washington, DC: Agency for Health Care Policy and Research.

U.S. Department of Health and Human Services. (1998). *Clinicians handbook of preventative services: Put prevention into practice* (2nd ed.). Washington, DC: U.S. Government Printing Office.

U.S. Department of Health and Human Services. (1999). *Healthy people 2000 program review 1998–1999.* Washington, DC: U.S. Government Printing Office.

U.S. Department of Health and Human Services. (1999). *Healthy people 2010 fact sheet: Healthy people in healthy communities.* Washington, DC: U.S. Government Printing Office.

Pediatric Index
Infancy Through Adolescence

Adult Index

The First in Certification Review

A Full Service Nursing Education Provider

Don't forget we also offer these other programs!

Live Certification Review & Update Courses

(A wonderful compliment to our review books)

Home Study Programs

(Can not attend the live course? Our home study is just like being there, great to listen to on a long commute)

Continuing Education Programs

(Need to keep your certification current or just enjoy keeping up to date with the latest information, then these programs are for you)

Health Leadership Associates is an approved Continuing Education Provider.
Our continuing education offerings have been approved for contact hours by the Maryland Nurses' Association which is accredited by the American Nurses Credentialing Center's Commission on Accreditation.

For more information or to order these programs visit our web site at www.healthleadership.com or cal 800-435-4775.

Health Leadership Associates, Inc.
P.O. Box 59153
Potomac, MD 20859